Pediatric Dermatopathology and Dermatology

Pediatric Dermatopathology and Dermatology

Editor-in-chief

Alejandro A. Gru, MD

Associate Professor of Pathology and Dermatology
Dermatopathology Fellowship Program Director
Dermatopathology and Hematopathology Sections
University of Virginia Health Science Center
Charlottesville, Virginia

Associate Editors

Mark R. Wick, MD
Professor of Pathology
Associate Director, Surgical Pathology
University of Virginia Health Science Center
Charlottesville, Virginia

Adnan Mir, MD, PhD
Assistant Professor
Department of Dermatology
University of Texas Southwestern Medical Center
Dallas, Texas

Barrett J. Zlotoff, MD
Associate Professor
Director, Pediatric Dermatology
Residency Program Director for Dermatology
University of Virginia Health Science Center
Charlottesville, Virginia

Louis P. Dehner, MD
Professor
Department of Pathology and Immunology
Washington University in St. Louis
Attending Pathologist
Department of Pediatric and Anatomic Pathology
Barnes-Jewish and St. Louis Children's Hospitals
St. Louis, Missouri

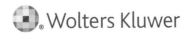

Philadelphia • Baltimore • New York • London
Buenos Aires • Hong Kong • Sydney • Tokyo

Senior Acquisitions Editor: Ryan Shaw
Development Editor: Carole Wonsiewicz
Editorial Coordinator: Emily Buccieri
Strategic Marketing Manager: Julie Sikora
Production Project Manager: Marian Bellus
Design Coordinator: Holly McLaughlin
Manufacturing Coordinator: Beth Welsh
Prepress Vendor: S4Carlisle Publishing Services

9 8 7 6 5 4 3 2 1

Printed in China

Library of Congress Cataloging-in-Publication Data

Names: Gru, Alejandro Ariel, editor. | Wick, Mark R., 1952- editor. | Mir, Adnan, editor. | Zlotoff, Barrett (Barrett J.), editor. | Dehner, Louis P., 1940- editor.
Title: Pediatric dermatopathology and dermatology / editor-in-chief, Alejandro A. Gru; associate editors, Mark R. Wick, Adnan Mir, Barrett Zlotoff, Louis P. Dehner.
Description: Philadelphia: Wolters Kluwer Health, [2019] | Includes bibliographical references and index.
Identifiers: LCCN 2018039411 | ISBN 9781496387851 (hardback)
Subjects: | MESH: Skin Diseases—pathology | Child
Classification: LCC RJ511 | NLM WS 260 | DDC 618.92/5—dc23 LC record available at https://lccn.loc.gov/2018039411

shop.lww.com

To the love of my life, Lorena, and my five beautiful children, Sofia, Camila, Santiago, Valentin, and Nicolas.

"Here is my secret. It is very simple: It is only with the heart that one can see rightly; what is essential is invisible to the eye."
The Little Prince. Antoine de Saint Exupéry.
Alejandro A. Gru

I am grateful to my wife, Jane, and my children, Robert, Morgan, and Kellyn, for giving me their support in the completion of this project.
Mark R. Wick

For my parents, whose love and sacrifices carry us to great heights.
Adnan Mir

To my wife, Ellie, who is my greatest love and support.
Thank you for everything.
Barrett J. Zlotoff

To Becky, Helen, and my children and grandchildren.
Louis P. Dehner

Contents

Contributors

Maria Eugenia Abad, MD
Staff member
Dermatology
Hospital Aleman
Buenos Aires, Argentina

Lihi Atzmony, MD
Postdoctoral Fellow
Department of Dermatology
Yale University
New Haven, Connecticut

Nima Mesbah Ardakani, MD, FRCPA
Clinical Senior Lecturer
Faculty of Health and Medical Science,
    School of Biomedical Science
The University of Western Australia
Consultant Pathologist
Department of Anatomical Pathology
PathWest Laboratory Medicine
Nedlands, Australia

Mary Barrett, MD
Dermatopathology Fellow
Department of Dermatology
Boston University
Boston, Massachusetts

Francisco G. Bravo, MD
Associate Professor
Department of Medicine
Attending Physician
Department of Pathology
Cayetano Heredia University
Lima, Peru

Michael A. Cardis, MD
Dermatopathology Fellow
Department of Dermatology
University of Pittsburgh Medical Center
Pittsburgh, Pennsylvania

Keith A. Choate, MD, PhD
Professor
Departments of Dermatology, Genetics, and Pathology
Yale University
New Haven, Connecticut

Jarish Cohen, MD
Department of Dermatology
University of California in San Francisco (UCSF)
San Francisco, California

Edward W. Cowen, MD, MHSc
Acting Chief
Department of Dermatology
National Institute of Arthritis and Musculoskeletal
    and Skin Diseases
National Institutes of Health
Bethesda, Maryland

Jonathan J. Davick, MD
Department of Pathology
University of Virginia
Charlottesville, Virginia

Jennifer A. Day, MD
Department of Dermatology
University of Texas Southwestern
Parkland Health & Hospital System
Dallas, Texas

Louis P. Dehner, MD
Professor
Department of Pathology and Immunology
Washington University in St. Louis
Attending Pathologist
Department of Pediatric and Anatomic Pathology
Barnes-Jewish and St. Louis Children's Hospitals
St. Louis, Missouri

Esteban Fernandez Faith, MD
Assistant Professor
Department of Pediatrics and Internal Medicine
Division of Dermatology
The Ohio State University College of Medicine
Pediatrics Dermatologist
Department of Pediatrics
Division of Pediatric Dermatology
Nationwide Children's Hospital
Columbus, Ohio

Richard H. Flowers, MD
Assistant Professor
Department of Dermatology
University of Virginia
Charlottesville, Virginia

Laura E. K. Gifford, MD, FAAD
Assistant Professor
Dermatology and Pediatrics
Eastern Virginia Medical School
Pediatric Dermatology Attending Physician
Dermatology
Children's Hospital of The King's Daughters
Norfolk, Virginia

Lynne J. Goldberg, MD
Jag Bhawan Professor of Dermatology and Pathology
Department of Dermatology
Boston University School of Medicine
Boston, Massachusetts

Anna L. Grossberg, MD
Assistant Professor
Departments of Dermatology and Pediatrics
Johns Hopkins University School of Medicine
Baltimore, Maryland

Alejandro A. Gru, MD
Associate Professor
Department of Pathology and Dermatology
University of Virginia, School of Medicine
Charlottesville, Virginia

Kristen P. Hook, MD
Associate Professor of Dermatology
Pediatric Dermatology Section
Department of Dermatology
University of Minnesota
Minneapolis, Minnesota

Emma F. Johnson, MD
Dermatopathology Fellow
Department of Dermatology
Mayo Clinic
Rochester, Minnesota

Benjamin H. Kaffenberger, MD
Associate Professor
Department of Dermatology
Ohio State University and Wexner Medical Center
Columbus, Ohio

Jessica Kaffenberger, MD
Associate Professor
Division of Dermatology
Ohio State University
Gahanna, Ohio

A. Yasmine Kirkorian, MD
Assistant Professor
Department of Dermatology and Pediatrics
George Washington University
School of Medicine
Attending Physician
Department of Dermatology
Children's National Health System
Washington, DC

Ellen Koch, MD
Assistant Professor
Department of Dermatology
University of Pittsburgh Medical Center
Pittsburgh, Pennsylvania

Margarita Larralde, MD
Chief
Department of Dermatology
Hospital Alemán
Buenos Aires, Argentina

Nima Mesbah Ardakani, MD, FRCPA
Clinical Senior Lecturer
Faculty of Health and Medical Science, School of
    Biomedical Science
The University of Western Australia
Consultant Pathologist
Department of Anatomical Pathology
PathWest Laboratory Medicine
Nedlands, Australia

Chyi-Chia Richard Lee, MD
Assistant Research Physician
Dermatopathology
Laboratory of Pathology
National Cancer Institute
Bethesda, Maryland

Grace L. Lee, MD
Assistant Professor of Dermatology
Texas Children's Hospital
Baylor College of Medicine
Houston, Texas

Jonathan J. Lee, MD
Department of Dermatology
University of Pittsburgh Medical Center
Pittsburgh, Pennsylvania

Paula C. Luna, MD
Staff
Department of Dermatology
Hospital Alemán
Buenos Aires, Argentina

Sheilagh M. Maguiness, MD
Assistant Professor
Department of Dermatology and Pediatrics
University of Minnesota Hospital
Minneapolis, Minnesota

Daniel D. Miller, MD
Assistant Professor of Dermatology
Dermatopathology Section
Department of Dermatology
University of New Mexico
Albuquerque, New Mexico

Adnan Mir, MD, PhD
Assistant Professor
Department of Dermatology
University of Texas Southwestern Medical Center
Dallas, Texas

Paradi Mirmirani, MD
Assistant Chief
Department of Dermatology
Kaiser Foundation Hospital
Vallejo, California

J. Olufemi Ogunbiyi, MBBS, FWACP (Lab Med)
Professor
Department of Pathology
College of Medicine
University of Ibadan
Ibadan, Oyo State

Charlene W. Oldfield, MD
Department of Dermatology
Eastern Virginia Medical School
Norfolk, Virginia

Emily J. Osier, MD
Dermatology Resident
Dermatology and Pediatrics
Eastern Virginia Medical School
Division of Dermatology
Children's Specialty Group of Children's Hospital
  of the King's Daughters
Norfolk, Virginia

Vikash S. Oza, MD
Assistant Professor of Dermatology and Pediatrics
Director of Pediatric Dermatology
The Ronald O. Perelman Department of Dermatology
New York University School of Medicine
New York, New York

Shivani S. Patel, MD
Department of Dermatology
Johns Hopkins University
Baltimore, Maryland

James W. Patterson, MD
Professor Emeritus of Pathology
Department of Pathology
University of Virginia Health System
Charlottesville, Virginia

Ifeoma U. Perkins, MD
Dermatopathology fellow
Dermatopathology and Oral Path Services
University of California San Francisco
San Francisco, California

Lori D. Prok, MD
Associate Professor
Dermatology and Pathology
University of Colorado
Pediatric Dermatologist and Dermatopathologist
Dermatology and Dermatopathology
Children's Hospital Colorado
Aurora, Colorado

Barbara Reichert, MD
Pediatric Dermatology Fellow
Division of Pediatric Dermatology
Nationwide Children's Hospital
Columbus, Ohio

Andrea Lorena Salavaggione, MD
Attending Pathologist
Department of Pathology
Universidad de Buenos Aires
Buenos Aires, Argentina

Julia Scarisbrick, MD
Consultant Dermatologist
University Hospital Birmingham
Birmingham, United Kingdom

Kevin Y. Shi, PhD
Department of Dermatology
University of Texas Southwestern Medical Center
Dallas, Texas

Aimee C. Smidt, MD
Associate Professor and Chair
Dermatology and Pediatrics
University of New Mexico School of Medicine
Albuquerque, New Mexico

Titilola Sode
Ines Wu Soukoulis, MD
Attending Physician
Charlottesville Dermatology
Charlottesville, Virginia

Thomas Stringer, MD, MS
Department of Medicine
The Mount Sinai Hospital
New York, New York

Travis Vandergriff, MD
Assistant Professor of Dermatology and Pathology
Director of Dermatopathology
UT Southwestern Medical Center
Dallas, Texas

Matthew D. Vesely, MD, PhD
Instructor
Department of Dermatology
Yale University
New Haven, Connecticut

Scott Walter, MD
Department of Dermatology
Boston University School of Medicine
Boston, Massachusetts

Mark R. Wick, MD
Professor of Pathology
Associate Director, Surgical Pathology
University of Virginia Health Science Center
Charlottesville, Virginia

Judith V. Williams, MD
Associate Professor
Pediatrics and Dermatology
Eastern Virginia Medical School
Director of Dermatology
Children's Speciality Group
Norfolk, Virginia

Benjamin Wood, MD
Clinical Associate Professor
Faculty of Health and Medical Sciences
The University of Western Australia
Consultant Pathologist
Dermatopathology
PathWest Laboratory Medicine
Nedlands, Australia

Barrett J. Zlotoff, MD
Associate Professor
Program Director
Director of Pediatric Dermatology
Department of Dermatology
University of Virginia
Charlottesville, Virginia

Preface

All books need an idea(s), an author(s), a publisher, and a certain amount of paper because even in this day and age, most books are still a stack of papers between a front and a back cover. The progenitor of this volume was a survey of the small world that we live in and the recognition that a void existed in the niche of dermatopathology of those disorders that present in the first two decades of life. These disorders occurring in pediatric patients can carry lifelong consequences in terms of management, life-ending implications, or simply a dermoid cyst in the brow line.

This project brought three of us together (AAG, MRW, LPD) who have shared a great deal of our professional and personal lives with each other. That started for two of us (MRW, LPD) at the University of Minnesota, then moved down river to Washington University in St. Louis where Alejandro joined our team. Two of us (MRW, AAG) continued the journey at the University of Virginia, where the idea of this collaboration began. Our team was then developed further by two amazing pediatric dermatologists (BZ, AM).

Once we decided that a reference on pediatric dermatopathology was the right topic, our next decision was where to find potential collaborators. In the world of dermatopathologists, there are few who self-identify as "pediatric" dermatopathologists. However, there are certified pediatric dermatopathologists who are not only interested in the topic but are also bona fide experts. A decision was made to invite several of them to join us and to provide their clinical perspective and context thus teaching the pathology collaborators some insights beyond the microscopic image.

This endeavor has resulted in a comprehensive 850 page volume because of the interaction between the clinicians and pathologists—which has its metaphorical utilitarian aspects. We often speak about that ideal interaction which we hope this volume conveys. We believe that our audience of general dermatologists who see children in their practice, pediatric dermatologists, general pathologists, pediatric pathologists and dermatopathologists will find this work as a worthy addition to their reference library.

Louis P. Dehner
Mark R. Wick
Adnan Mir
Barrett J. Zlotoff
Alejandro A. Gru

Introduction to the Field of Pediatric Dermatopathology

Barrett J. Zlotoff / Alejandro A. Gru

It is true that Pediatric Dermatology has existed since the dawn of medicine. Hippocrates described multiple pediatric dermatologic conditions in his *Corpus Hippocraticum*. But it was not until 1827 that the first book exclusively devoted to pediatric dermatology, *Cutaneous Diseases Incidental to Childhood*, by Walter Dendy was published in London.[1,2] The global establishment of Pediatric Dermatology as a recognized subspecialty did not gain momentum until the first international symposium on and founding of the International Society of Pediatric Dermatology in 1972. Before 1983, the dermatologic literature was made up of only 15% articles related specifically to children, and the pediatric literature had only 4% of articles devoted to skin disease. Since the launch of the journal *Pediatric Dermatology* in 1982, and particularly after the recognition of the subspecialty by the Accreditation Council for Graduate Medical Education in 2000, research in and the description of dermatologic disease specific to the pediatric population has blossomed.[2,3]

If the field of Pediatric Dermatology can be said to be in its infancy, Pediatric Dermatopathology may still be in the gestation process.[4] We are delighted to include Dr Louis P. Dehner, a pioneer and developer of this discipline, as one of the senior editors and contributor to our book. "Pepper" has been one of the most influential surgical pathologists of the last century. Authoring more than 450 publications, he is the premier modern pediatric pathologist. Perhaps less recognized is his role as creator of the art of pediatric dermatopathology.

Dehner has written at least 50 major publications describing, discovering, and orienting the discipline in the fields of fibrohistiocytic disorders of childhood, vascular tumors, and histiocytosis, among others. He gave birth to the theory that, although there are many similarities between adult and pediatric surgical pathology, "children get different diseases." Dehner has been one of the primary investigators who helped separate histiocytosis into two main categories in accordance with the cell which they morphologically and immunophenotypically resemble: the mature macrophage and the dendritic cells. Originally classified as histiocytosis X, nonhistiocytosis X, and malignant histiocytosis, significant reordering and reclassifications have emerged.[5,6] The largest, most eloquent and comprehensive article documenting the natural history, clinical presentation, and histopathologic findings of juvenile xanthogranulomas, the most common histiocytic disorder in children, was written by Dehner in 2003 and published in the *American Journal of Surgical Pathology*.[7] An article crucial to understanding reactive and neoplastic fibrous tumors in children was published by Dehner and Askin in Cancer in 1976.[8] Dehner also was one of the first to publish a large series of adnexal neoplasms in patients aged 20 or younger.[9] His mindful analysis and correlations between the clinicopathologic and biologic aspects of specific entities certainly qualify him as a pioneer in the field of pediatric dermatopathology.

WHY ARE CHILDREN DIFFERENT?

Skin diseases occur in both pediatric and adult individuals, but we know that skin conditions in children differ from adults.[10,11] In fact, certain conditions are limited to the pediatric age group, and some neoplasms, such as lipoblastoma, occur only in children. Many present in the context of inflammatory dermatoses and genodermatoses that clinicians, and particularly pathologists, may not be entirely familiar with. Careful histopathologic studies of many entities are limited to small series or case reports, making histologic recognition challenging. Dermatopathologists in community practice, without a significant volume of cases from pediatric hospitals, may never get to witness some conditions. We have heard many colleagues describe pediatric dermatopathology as a "no-man's land."

Most cases in adult dermatopathology practice are derived from benign tumors (particularly keratoses and epidermal tumors), malignant tumors, drug-induced hypersensitivity reactions, melanocytic proliferations, infectious processes, papulosquamous disorders (eg, psoriasis), connective tissue disorders, vasculitis, bullous dermatoses, and folliculitis. This pattern does not reflect the pediatric practice, with the exception of melanocytic lesions, which are probably some of the most common biopsies seen in the routine histopathologic examination. In contrast, in the pediatric setting, Henoch-Schonlein purpura, pityriasis lichenoides, pityriasis rubra pilaris, atopic dermatitis, erythema multiforme, granuloma annulare, and pigmented purpuras are frequent inflammatory conditions that are biopsied.

The rate of skin biopsies has been reported to be from 1.7% to 3.7% in an outpatient pediatric dermatology practice.[12] However, the rates can be as high as 17.5% to 35% in a consultation practice.[13-15] Those numbers are extraordinarily lower in comparison with those of adult practitioners. Children do not get biopsied as frequently, and this limits the understanding of the histopathologic findings in pediatric skin disorders. Dysplastic nevi are an example of the differences of histologic interpretation in the pediatric population versus adults. Biopsies of melanocytic lesions in children are typically performed because of a change in the lesion or an abnormal appearance. It is easy then to assume that the frequency of histologically diagnosed dysplastic nevi in children would be higher than in adults. But the opposite is true: there is an extremely low rate of diagnosis of dysplastic moles in the pediatric age. There is more tolerance to the degree of architectural distortion and cytologic atypia of melanocytic lesions in children when compared with adults. In fact, when we review cases with fellows and residents or other rotating physicians in evaluating a melanocytic lesion, the first question that derives is: "How old and where are we?" Frequently, we tell our fellows that a very atypical lesion that would be diagnosed as severely atypical or malignant in an adult could be entirely benign in children. But we are also careful not to miss the possibility of a malignant lesion in a child. The difficulty in making this determination is reflected in the original description of Spitz nevi by Sophie Spitz at Memorial Sloan-Kettering Cancer Center, which was titled "Malignant melanomas of childhood."[16-18]

Similarly, some papulovesicular eruptions such as pityriasis lichenoides can be encountered in both young adults and children. However, the differential diagnosis of this condition in children is different from that considered in adults and may include arthropod reactions, Gianotti-Crosti syndrome, other viral exanthems, varicella infection, and erythema multiforme. It is the case for many inflammatory dermatoses that the differential can shift greatly depending on the age of the patient.

WHEN TO DO A BIOPSY IN A CHILD?

There is often a certain amount of anxiety surrounding the skin biopsy of a pediatric patient. This is true for all parties involved: the patient, parents, the one performing the biopsy, and the pathologist. So, how do we know when to perform a cutaneous biopsy in children and how can we make the experience as valuable as possible for all parties involved?

The most common reason to do a skin biopsy from a clinician's perspective is when diagnoses or prognostic information cannot be provided on the basis of physical exam findings or laboratory testing alone. Maximum value of the cutaneous biopsy derives from the process of clinicopathologic correlation. The clinical information provided to the pathologist guides how they think about the specimen in front of them, what special stains, immunohistochemistry, or molecular biology investigations are pursued, and how to frame the final interpretation and diagnostic report. On the basis of information provided by the pathologist, the clinician is able to narrow differential diagnosis, guide further workup, and give the patient and/or family the most precise prognostic information.

In an ideal world, the practitioner would be able to see the patient, perform the biopsy, review the case, and make a clinicopathologic correlation. But in reality, this does not often happen. There are significant workforce issues for both dermatopathologists and pediatric dermatologists, and the number of practitioners with subspecialty training is low. The specialized knowledge required to evaluate dermatologic conditions in the pediatric population and analyze histopathologic specimens of pediatric skin biopsies has become increasingly extensive. Currently, many skin biopsies on children are performed by general dermatologists and primary care providers, and the histopathologic specimens are evaluated by pathologists without specific dermatopathology training or by dermatopathologists without training in pediatric skin disease.[4] This book is an attempt to bridge this gap and provide clinicians from all sides with a common language and context for clinicopathologic correlation and case discussion.

Avoiding unnecessary biopsies in children is of primary concern because of the trauma to children and parents, the difficulties with local anesthesia (particularly in small children), and the risk of scarring. This must be weighed by the provider undertaking the biopsy, who is faced with the possibility of a descriptive report that is just "not very specific."

One study evaluating results of the biopsies performed in pediatric dermatology clinics reported that the rate of providing a satisfactory definitive diagnosis was 61%, and the correct diagnosis was given to the pathologist in the differential in only 56.3% of cases.[4] One study evaluating 100 consecutive skin biopsies of inflammatory dermatoses demonstrated that the rates of accurate diagnosis improved significantly with an accurate clinical description and differential diagnosis (53% vs. 78%).[19] Another study comparing biopsy results performed by clinical dermatologists versus nondermatologists found that inflammatory skin conditions were correctly diagnosed in 71% of cases by dermatologists but in only 34% of cases by nondermatologists.[20] Such studies emphasize that the histopathologic evaluation requires "sufficient" and "accurate" clinical information. The same holds true for both adults and children.[20]

In pediatric dermatology, an experienced team of dermatologists and pathologists significantly increases the success of clinicopathologic correlation and definitive diagnosis. Today, with widespread access to digital photography, pictures can be obtained from parents or clinical providers and shared to facilitate consultation. This can be helpful, particularly if the lesion's clinical appearance has changed significantly over time.

Factors that could pose problems in the interpretation of skin biopsies include the following: sampling bias, the size of the biopsy, optimal time for obtaining the biopsy (age of the lesion), tissue quality from the histology laboratory, and fixation time. If the biopsy is taken from the edge of a lesion, particularly in tumors, the findings might not be entirely representative of the extent of the lesion. One recent illustrative scenario occurred during review of a biopsy of a "solitary lesion" for which only the periphery was sampled. It showed mostly scarring and inflammation. The possibility of an inflammatory form of morphea was considered. To my surprise, a subsequent biopsy revealed a clear-cut histiocytosis. The size of many biopsies in children is small, which can significantly challenge us when interpreting disorders of pigmentary alteration and identifying *normal* versus *lesional* skin. The age of the lesion is also important—for example, vasculitis significantly changes appearance within 24 to 48 hours and beyond from the time of its development. Tissue quality, fixation, and other laboratory-related problems can also affect the interpretation, particularly when analyzing the degree of atypia in melanocytic neoplasms.

This book written in collaboration with dermatopathologists and pediatric dermatologists serves as a handy chairside reference to provide clinical context for the pathologist reviewing a slide and pathologic context for the dermatologist interpreting histologic reports from pathology

colleagues. Our hope is that this information will advance and facilitate conversation and collaboration among all of us with special interest in the cutaneous pathology of the pediatric patient. It is an essential step forward, yet there is still much more to be learned.

REFERENCES

1. Sgantzos M, Tsoucalas G, Karamanou M, Giatsiou S, Tsoukalas I, Androutsos G. Hippocrates on pediatric dermatology. *Pediatr Dermatol.* 2015;32(5):600-603.
2. Irvine A, Hoeger P, Yan AC. Ebook Central Academic Complete, Wiley Online Library UBCM All Obooks. In: Irvine A, Hoeger P, Yan AC, eds. *Harper's Textbook of Pediatric Dermatology.* 3rd ed. Chichester, England: Wiley-Blackwell; 2011. Also available at http://RE5QY4SB7X.search.serialssolutions.com/?V=1.0&L=RE5QY4SB7X&S=JCs&C=TC0000506269&T=marc. Accessed August 1, 2018.
3. Prindaville B, Antaya RJ, Siegfried EC. Pediatric dermatology: past, present, and future. *Pediatr Dermatol.* 2015;32(1):1-12.
4. Afsar FS, Diniz G, Aktas S. Pediatric dermatopathology: an overview. *Arch Argent Pediatr.* 2017;115(4):377-381.
5. Arceci RJ. The histiocytoses: the fall of the Tower of Babel. *Eur J Cancer.* 1999;35(5):747-767; discussion 767-749.
6. Jaffe RA, Pileri SA, Facchetti F, Jones DM, Jaffe ES. *Histiocytic and Dendritic Cell Neoplasms, Introduction.* 4th ed. Lyon, France: International Agency for Research on Cancer; 2008.
7. Dehner LP. Juvenile xanthogranulomas in the first two decades of life: a clinicopathologic study of 174 cases with cutaneous and extracutaneous manifestations. *Am J Surg Pathol.* 2003;27(5):579-593.
8. Dehner LP, Askin FB. Tumors of fibrous tissue origin in childhood. A clinicopathologic study of cutaneous and soft tissue neoplasms in 66 children. *Cancer.* 1976;38(2):888-900.
9. Marrogi AJ, Wick MR, Dehner LP. Benign cutaneous adnexal tumors in childhood and young adults, excluding pilomatrixoma: review of 28 cases and literature. *J Cutan Pathol.* 1991;18(1):20-27.
10. Sardana K, Mahajan S, Sarkar R, et al. The spectrum of skin disease among Indian children. *Pediatr Dermatol.* 2009;26(1):6-13.
11. Tamer E, Ilhan MN, Polat M, Lenk N, Alli N. Prevalence of skin diseases among pediatric patients in Turkey. *J Dermatol.* 2008;35(7):413-418.
12. Wenk C, Itin PH. Epidemiology of pediatric dermatology and allergology in the region of Aargau, Switzerland. *Pediatr Dermatol.* 2003;20(6):482-487.
13. McMahon P, Goddard D, Frieden IJ. Pediatric dermatology inpatient consultations: a retrospective study of 427 cases. *J Am Acad Dermatol.* 2013;68(6):926-931.
14. McMahon PJ, Yan AC. Inpatient consultative pediatric dermatology: an emerging need in an era of increasing inpatient acuity and complexity. *Pediatr Dermatol.* 2013;30(4):508-509.
15. Srinivas SM, Hiremagalore R, Venkataramaiah LD, Premalatha R. Pediatric dermatology inpatient consultations: a retrospective study. *Indian J Pediatr.* 2015;82(6):541-544.
16. Allen AC, Spitz S. Histogenesis and clinicopathologic correlation of nevi and malignant melanomas; current status. *AMA Arch Derm Syphilol.* 1954;69(2):150-171.
17. Spitz S. Melanomas of childhood. *Am J Pathol.* 1948;24(3):591-609.
18. Spitz S. Melanomas of childhood. 1948. *CA Cancer J Clin.* 1991;41(1):40-51.
19. Rajaratnam R, Smith AG, Biswas A, Stephens M. The value of skin biopsy in inflammatory dermatoses. *Am J Dermatopathol.* 2009;31(4):350-353.
20. Sellheyer K, Bergfeld WF. A retrospective biopsy study of the clinical diagnostic accuracy of common skin diseases by different specialties compared with dermatology. *J Am Acad Dermatol.* 2005;52(5):823-830.

Disorders in the Newborn

Margarita Larralde / Paula C. Luna / Maria Eugenia Abad / Andrea Lorena Salavaggione

SCLEREMA NEONATORUM

Definition and Epidemiology

Sclerema neonatorum (SN) is a severe form of panniculitis characterized by diffuse hardening of the skin and subcutaneous tissues.[1,2] SN is an extremely rare disorder mostly seen in critically ill preterm newborns in the setting of a wide variety of comorbidities like sepsis, congenital heart disease, pneumonitis, enteritis, hypothermia, hypocalcemia, and developmental anomalies.[1-5]

Etiology

Premature newborns have a higher ratio of saturated (stearic and palmitic acids) to unsaturated (oleic acid) fatty acids in their adipose tissue when compared with term healthy neonates. High concentration of saturated fat is associated with a high melting point and a low solidification point, a tendency to harden, and fat crystallization with temperature fall.[2,4,5]

Clinical Presentation

SN usually occurs in the first week of life but can develop immediately after birth or as late as several weeks of life. It is characterized by a hardening and thickening of the skin that begins on the thighs, buttocks, and trunk (Figure 2-1). The process rapidly progresses with diffuse woody induration of large body areas, resulting in difficulties with respiration, feeding, and movements. Fat-free areas like palms, soles, and genitalia are not affected. The prognosis is poor.[1-3,5]

Histologic Findings

SN is characterized by a lobular lymphohistiocytic panniculitis[1] (Figure 2-2). The epidermis and dermis are normal-appearing. The adipose tissue undergoes partial degeneration and formation of needle-like crystals with a radial arrangement toward the adipocytes. There is no significant necrosis or marked inflammation in the majority of cases. Some can have a thickening of the fibrous septa. Occasional multinucleated giant cells are present.[1-6]

Differential Diagnosis

Subcutaneous fat necrosis of the newborn (SCFN) shows a more pronounced inflammatory infiltrate. Admixed eosinophils are frequently seen. The crystals are seen in the adipocytes and macrophages. Case reports showing overlapping features of both SN and SCFN have been reported.[7-10]

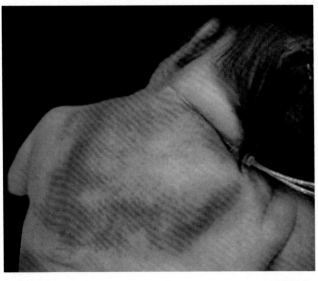

FIGURE 2-1. Sclerema neonatorum.

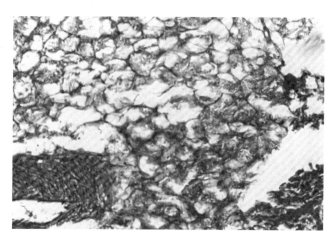

FIGURE 2-2. **Sclerema neonatorum.** The adipose tissue undergoes partial degeneration and formation of needle-like crystals with a radial arrangement toward the adipocytes. Courtesy of Dr. JW Patterson. University of Virginia.

The other main differential diagnosis is scleredema. This occurs more frequently in preterm infants, usually during the first week of life, and is characterized by generalized firm, pitting edema, which is more common in lower extremities and manifests with an increase in the volume of the affected part. It is often preceded by cold injury, vomiting, diarrhea, or other acute infections. Body temperature is usually abnormal and the infant is apathetic. Histologically, there is a lobular panniculitis with the absence of vasculitis. There is a rich infiltrate of lymphocytes and histiocytes, and marked dermal edema. The edema can also extend to the adipose tissue and sometimes skeletal muscle.[11]

CAPSULE SUMMARY

SCLEREMA NEONATORUM

SN is a severe form of panniculitis characterized by a diffuse hardening of the skin and subcutaneous tissues. SN usually occurs in the first week of life but can develop immediately after birth or as late as several weeks of life. SN is characterized by a lobular lymphohistiocytic panniculitis. The adipose tissue undergoes partial degeneration and formation of needle-like crystals.

SUBCUTANEOUS FAT NECROSIS OF THE NEWBORN

Definition and Epidemiology

Subcutaneous fat necrosis of the newborn (SCFN) is a rare, transient, and self-limiting lobular panniculitis. SCFN usually affects term and postterm babies in the first week of life, with few cases developing as late as 6 weeks of age.[12,13] Maternal risk factors to develop SCFN include preeclampsia, gestational diabetes, smoking or exposure to passive smoking, calcium channel blockers intake, and cocaine abuse. Neonatal risk factors include hypothermia, perinatal asphyxia, meconium aspiration, umbilical cord prolapse, obstetric trauma, and Rh incompatibility.[7,8,14] SCFN was reported in 1% to 3% of newborns who underwent whole-body cooling for birth asphyxia.[15-17]

Etiology

Perinatal asphyxia induces blood shunt from skin to the brain and heart, leading to impaired tissue perfusion and local hypoxia. Neonatal fat tissue has a relatively high concentration of saturated fatty acids with a high melting point that predispose to solidify and crystallize under cold injury, resulting in adipocyte necrosis and subsequent formation of granulomatous inflammation.[4,14,18,19]

Clinical Presentation

SCFN is characterized by multiple indurated, erythematous, or violaceous painful nodules and plaques located on the cheeks, back, shoulders, extremities, and buttocks (Figure 2-2A-C). The anterior trunk is typically spared. Some lesions may become calcified or fluctuant with drainage of liquefied fat. Lesions resolve spontaneously within a few weeks, leaving in some cases atrophy, fibrosis, scarring, or necrosis. Although SCFN is a benign condition with an excellent prognosis, complications such as transitory hypoglycemia, hypertriglyceridemia, thrombocytopenia, and hypercalcemia have been reported.[7-9,18]

Histologic Findings

Biopsies of SCFN are characterized by a lobular panniculitis with a diffuse and brisk inflammatory infiltrate within the fat lobules (Figure 2-4). Necrosis of the adipocytes results in crystal formation and small granulomata surrounding the inflammatory cells.[5,14-18,20,21,135-139] The crystals are needle-shaped and are present within the adipocytes and histiocytes. Abnormal eosinophilic granules can be present.[22,140] Older lesions can show dystrophic calcification. Some cases can show a very rich acute neutrophilic inflammatory infiltrate and can mimic an infectious process. In the latter, neutrophilic represented more than 75% of the cells in the infiltrate.[23,141]

Differential Diagnosis

The main differential diagnosis is with SN. Subcutaneous fat necrosis of the newborn shows a more pronounced inflammatory infiltrate. Admixed eosinophils are frequently seen.

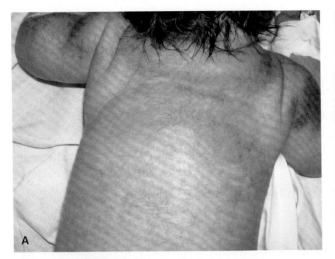

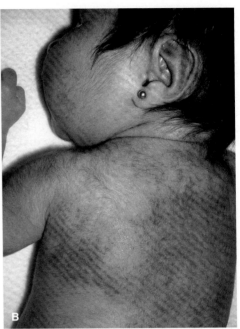

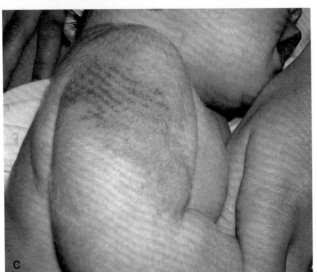

FIGURE 2-3. Subcutaneous fat necrosis. A, Extensive erythematous plaque over the back of a term newborn. B, Erythemo-edematous plaque over the back and shoulder. C, Well-circumscribed plaque over the shoulder.

CAPSULE SUMMARY

SUBCUTANEOUS FAT NECROSIS

This is a rare, transient, and self-limiting lobular panniculitis. SCFN usually affects term and postterm babies in the first week of life, with a few cases developing as late as 6 weeks of age. It is characterized by multiple indurated, erythematous, or violaceous painful nodules and plaques located on the cheeks, back, shoulders, extremities, and buttocks. Biopsies of SCFN are characterized by a lobular panniculitis with a diffuse and brisk inflammatory infiltrate within the fat lobules. Necrosis of the adipocytes results in crystal formation and small granulomata surrounding the inflammatory cells.

Milia and Miliaria

MILIA

Definition and Epidemiology

Milia is a common condition of the newborn that may be due to several causes can be found alone or associated with other diseases. These lesions affect up to 83% of newborns. Milia is a common condition of the newborn that may be due to several causes, can be found alone or associated with other diseases, and affects up to 83% of babies.

Etiology

Milia is divided into primary milia (when occurs spontaneously) or secondary milia (when develops after healing of a previous skin condition). Lesions usually appear and

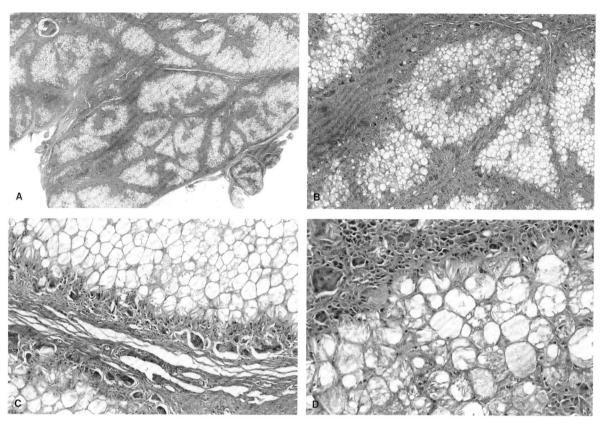

FIGURE 2-4. **Subcutaneous fat necrosis of a newborn.** Biopsy shows a lobular panniculitis (A). Necrosis of the adipocytes results in crystal formation and small granulomata surrounding the inflammatory cells (B and C). The crystals are needle-shaped and are present within the adipocytes and histiocytes (D). Digital slides courtesy of Path Presenter.com.

disappear spontaneously during the first month of life. In some cases, milia may be more persistent.[20]

Clinical Presentation

The clinical lesions of milia include pearly, superficial, firm papules that mainly affect the nose, cheeks, chin, and forehead (Figure 2-5A and B).[21,22] Lesions can vary from a single cyst to hundreds, and also vary in size, with larger lesions usually affecting foreskin, areolae, scrotum, and labia majora.[23] When milia are numerous and persistent, different types of genodermatoses should be considered (Figure 2-6).[20,24] A large congenital, milia-like, papule in the midline anterior neck (Figure 2-7) has been recently reported by Walsh et al[25] as "MANIC (Midline Anterior Neck Inclusion Cyst);"

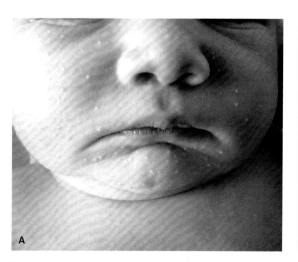

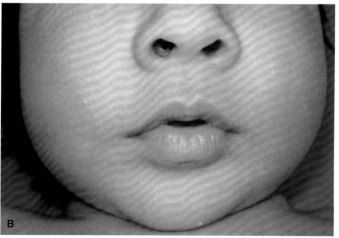

FIGURE 2-5. **Milia.** A, Multiple pinpoint white papules over the face and one isolated lesion on the chest. B, Scattered white papules over the face.

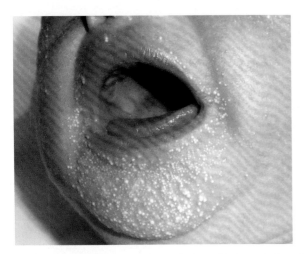

FIGURE 2-6. Profuse congenital facial milia in a baby with Basan syndrome.

it is postulated to be a forme fruste of a midline developmental defect. The histology is indistinguishable from large milia.

Histologic Findings

It is thought that primary milia arise from the pilosebaceous units and the secondary forms from the sweat ducts. These two subtypes can be distinguished on the basis of the histopathologic findings. Primary milia resemble small follicular cysts derived from the follicle infundibulum (Figure 2-8). The cysts are lined by atrophic squamous epithelium that contain a granular cell layer and show loose keratin contents. Secondary milia are also cystically dilated spaces, but are lined by ductal epithelium (eccrine). Serial sectioning can easily demonstrate the connection of the cysts to the sweat duct in most cases.[24,26-28,142]

Differential Diagnosis

Differential diagnostic considerations will include vellus hair cysts. Those can also be multiple, and only rarely present in

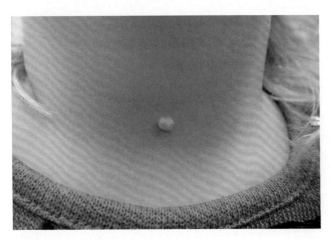

FIGURE 2-7. Midline anterior neck inclusion cyst.

the newborns or shortly thereafter.[29,143] The vellus hair cysts show a similar lining epithelium, but contain vellus hairs admixed with the loose keratinous debris. Apocrine hidrocystomas can also be multiple and be present in a congenital fashion.[30,144] The difference is that the lining shows plumped columnar epithelioid cells with apocrine decapitation.

CAPSULE SUMMARY

MILIA

Milia is a common condition seen in the newborn population that may be due to several causes. It can occur in isolation, or be associated with other conditions. These lesions may affect up to 83% of newborns. Primary milia resemble small follicular cysts derived from the follicle infundibulum. Secondary milia are also cystically dilated spaces, but are lined by ductal epithelium (eccrine).

MILIARIA

Definition and Epidemiology

Miliaria is a term used to describe the obstruction of the eccrine ducts that may occur at different levels of the apparatus. Although it may appear at any age, it is particularly frequent in neonates, affecting around 1% to 15% of newborns, especially in warm climates.

Etiology

Miliaria is caused by the extravasation of sweat into the skin because of obstruction and rupture of the eccrine duct. It can be classified into miliaria crystallina or sudamina (with the obstruction located at the stratum corneum) and miliaria rubra, which is caused by a deeper type of obstruction (intraepidermal) with secondary local inflammation. Miliaria profunda is extremely rare in neonates and is the deepest type of miliaria.[26,27]

Clinical Presentation

In miliaria crystallina, lesions are fragile, pinpoint, clear, superficial vesicles over a noninflammatory skin, affecting mainly the forehead and upper trunk appearing during the first week of life.[27] Miliaria rubra lesions are erythematous nonfollicular papules, pustules, and vesicles. It usually affects the face, neck, and trunk during the second week of life (Figure 2-9).

Miliaria profunda shows a great amount of inflammation, and lesions are deeply situated in the dermis and are intensely red.

Histologic Findings

Miliaria is characterized by a disruption of the sweat ducts at various levels throughout the outflow tract with extravasation of the secretions (Figure 2-10). The specific

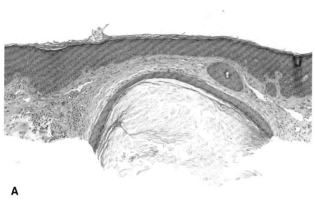
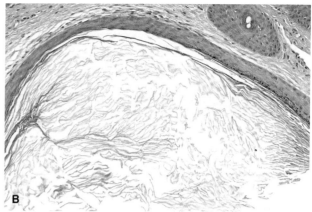

A

B

FIGURE 2-8. Milia: The cysts are lined by atrophic squamous epithelium that contain a granular cell layer and show loose keratin contents (A and B). Digital slides courtesy of Path Presenter.com.

site of disruption is associated with a diversity of clinical and histologic findings.[31-33,145-147] *Miliaria crystallina* is associated with the occlusion at the closest proximity to the surface epidermis. In this form, the secretion is present at the level of the acrosyringia within the stratum corneum. The result is the presence of acrosyringial spongiosis and intracorneal fluid collection. Inflammation is typically minimal or absent. When present, neutrophils are the predominant type of inflammatory cell. In *Miliaria rubra*, the secretion occurs in the intraepidermal portion of the eccrine duct. Spongiosis is more prominent, but dermal inflammation is also present. *Miliaria profunda* is the deepest form of this entity, occurring within the dermis. A lymphocytic infiltrate can be present. In rare occasions, large areas of miliaria profunda present as dermal plaques, and the histopathology includes a granulomatous reaction to the extravasated secretions.[34,148]

Differential Diagnosis

The spongiosis of miliaria is different from other spongiotic reactions, because it is typically more pronounced at the level of acrosyringium. However, when severe, it can be more diffuse and potentially mimic eczematous reactions. Erythema toxicum neonatorum (see below) can sometimes resemble miliaria clinically. Histologically, the former has intracorneal or intraepidermal pustules. Eosinophilic folliculitis can also resemble miliaria clinically, but it is associated with a follicular-based inflammatory infiltrate, with eosinophils extending into the hair follicle epithelium.

CAPSULE SUMMARY

MILIARIA

Miliaria is a term used to describe the obstruction of the eccrine ducts that may occur at different levels. Miliaria is characterized by a disruption of the sweat ducts at various levels throughout the outflow tract with extravasation of secretions. The specific site of disruption is associated with a diversity of clinical and histologic findings.

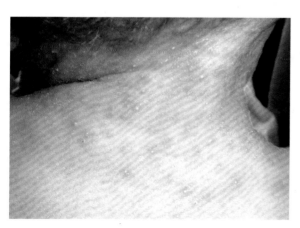

FIGURE 2-9. Miliaria pustulosa over the back navel of a 3-month-old.

ERYTHEMA TOXICUM NEONATORUM

Definition and Epidemiology

Erythema toxicum neonatorum (ETN) is a common, benign, and transient condition of healthy neonates. ETN is very frequent in full-term neonates, an incidence varying from 3.7% to 72%.[29-32] There is no gender or racial predilection. Higher incidence rates are seen in term healthy neonates born after a normal pregnancy with a birth weight of over 2500 g.[32] It is rarely seen in preterm infants with low birth weight.[26]

Etiology

The etiopathogenesis of ETN is still unclear. The identification of proinflammatory mediators aquaporin-1,

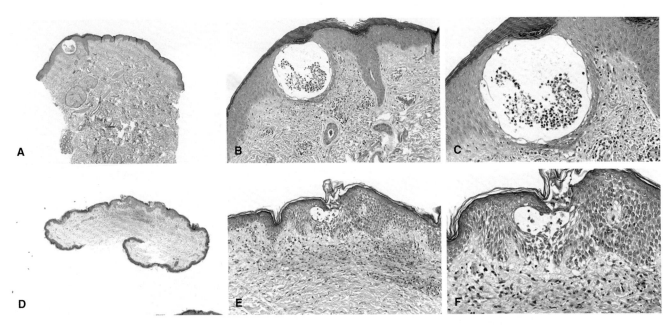

FIGURE 2-10. *Miliaria crystallina* is associated with occlusion at the closest proximity to the surface epidermis. In this form, the secretion is present at the level of the acrosyringia within the stratum corneum. Neutrophils are seen in the vesicle (A to C). In *Miliaria rubra*, the secretion occurs in the intraepidermal portion of the eccrine duct. Spongiosis is more prominent, and dermal inflammation is also present. (D to F). Digital slides courtesy of Path Presenter.com.

aquaporin-3, eotaxin, interleukin-1, interleukin-8, and psoriasin and nitric oxide synthases 1, 2, and 3 in the ETN infiltrate supports the current theory that ETN is an immunologic cutaneous response to microbial skin and hair follicles colonization from the first day of life.[29,32,33]

Clinical Presentation

Skin lesions of ETN most commonly present at 24 to 72 hours of life, but can occur since birth to 2 weeks of age, resolving in 5 to 7 days without sequelae. The occurrence may occasionally be delayed for a few days in premature neonates.[26,31] It is characterized clinically by asymptomatic erythematous macules and wheals (Figure 2-11), ranging from a few millimeters to several centimeters in diameter, centered by a papule or pustule (Figure 2-12). Lesions typically occur on the face, trunk, proximal limbs, and buttocks, whereas palms, soles, and genitalia are usually spared.[26,31,34] Lesions can vary from few to several in number, and new ones may appear during the first few days of life as the eruption waxes and wanes; recurrences may occur in up to 11% of neonates.[26,31]

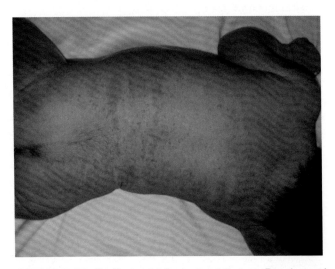

FIGURE 2-11. Erythema toxicum neonatorum. Papules and erythema over the back of a newborn.

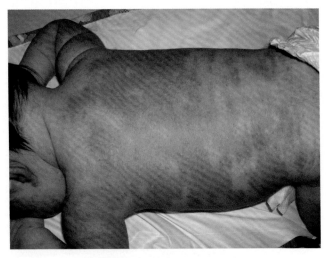

FIGURE 2-12. Erythema toxicum neonatorum. Erythema and overlying papules over the back of a boy.

Histologic Findings

Biopsies of ETN show subcorneal or intraepidermal pustules of eosinophils, and a marked inflammatory infiltrate within the pilosebaceous unit, usually just deep to the dermal-epidermal junction. Inflammation in the dermis can also be present (Figure 2-13A to D). Scattered dermal eosinophils are seen. Some have suggested that ETN and transient neonatal pustular melanosis are closely related entities.[35,36,149,150]

CAPSULE SUMMARY

ERYTHEMA TOXICUM NEONATORUM

ETN is a common, early occurring eruption in full-term neonates characterized by asymptomatic erythematous macules and wheals, ranging from a few millimeters to several centimeters in diameter, centered by a papule or pustule. Biopsies of ETN show subcorneal or intraepidermal pustules of eosinophils, and a marked inflammatory infiltrate within the pilosebaceous unit.

EOSINOPHILIC PUSTULAR FOLLICULITIS

Definition and Epidemiology

Eosinophilic pustular folliculitis (EPF) is an uncommon condition first described in adults mainly associated with HIV infection. Its pediatric variant, EPF of infancy, was first described by Lucky et al.[35] It consists of intensely pruritic crusted papules affecting mainly the scalp. The infantile variant is typically not associated with HIV, but with different hypereosinophilic states. Few cases have been reported occurring since birth or in the first few days of life. It is more frequent in males than in females.

Etiology

The exact etiology of this condition remains unknown. Given its histologic similarities to ETN, it has been suggested that this entity might represent a severe and persistent type of ETN.[36] A relation to hypereosinophilic states, as well as its manifestation in patients with hyper Immunoglobulin E (IgE) syndrome, has also been suggested in a few number of patients.

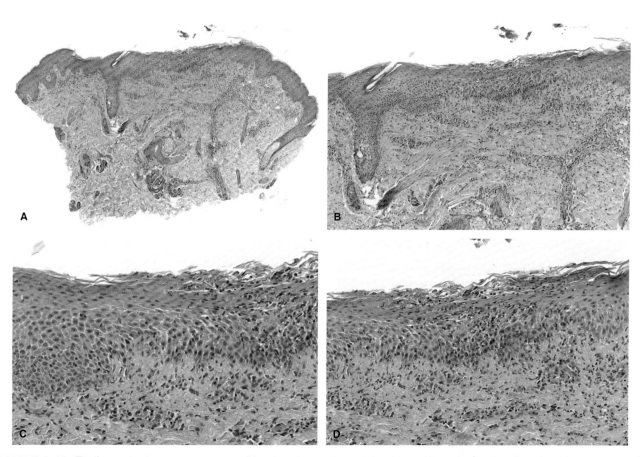

FIGURE 2-13. Erythema toxicum neonatorum. Biopsies show subcorneal or intraepidermal pustules of eosinophils and a marked inflammatory infiltrate within the pilosebaceous unit, usually just deep to the dermal-epidermal junction (A-D). Digital slides courtesy of Path Presenter.com.

Clinical Presentation

It is characterized by the presence of 1 to 3 mm pustules and crusts on the scalp and face (Figures 2-14 and 2-15), but also on the trunk and extremities.[35-41] Lesions typically appear in crops, with a waxing and waning course lasting from days to weeks; most severe cases might last several years, always healing without scarring.[39] Most cases resolve completely by age 3. Pruritus or irritability is a very common feature, in more than 77 percent of patients. Peripheral eosinophilia is present in many patients. Because this eruption has been described in patients who later developed a hyper IgE syndrome, a close follow-up of these neonates is recommended.[(41-46)]

Histologic Findings

It is important to obtain an entire papule or pustule with associated follicle during a biopsy to ensure an adequate sample for histologic examination and diagnosis. Because eosinophilic folliculitis is a folliculocentric finding, one may need to do serial sections to catch the inflamed hair follicle (Figure 2-16). An examination of unexcoriated, fresh papulopustules shows an acute and chronic infiltrate of eosinophils and lymphocytes focused at the level of the follicular isthmus that may rarely progress to complete follicle destruction. One sees eosinophils along with scattered mononuclear cells and neutrophils in the pilar outer root sheath and sebaceous glands and ducts. Perifollicular and perivascular eosinophilic invasion can be observed. In some cases, eosinophilic flame figures are present.[37-40]

Differential Diagnosis

EPF must be distinguished from other infectious and non-infectious pustular disorders in childhood: ETN, transient pustular melanosis, scabies, miliaria pustulosa, infections, acropustulosis of infancy, arthropod bites, and Langerhans

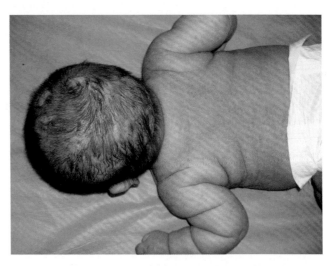

FIGURE 2-15. Widespread crusts and erosions over the scalp and erythematous papules over the back of a patient with eosinophilic pustular folliculitis who later developed a hyper immunoglobulin E syndrome.

cell histiocytosis. ETN and TNPM (Transient Neonatal Pustular Melanosis) are not typically folliculocentric processes. Scabies can be easily distinguished by the presence of scabies mites. Miliaria pustulosa is associated with an acrosyringial pattern of spongiosis with subsequent superinfection. Acropustulosis of infancy is also similar to ETN in terms of lack of folliculocentrism and is more acral in distribution. Langerhans cell histiocytosis is often folliculocentric and can show a large number of eosinophils. The main feature of Langerhans cell histiocytosis is the presence of an atypical population of Langerhans cells (demonstrated by S100, CD1a, and Langerin immunostains) that is epidermotropic, a feature that is missing in EPF.

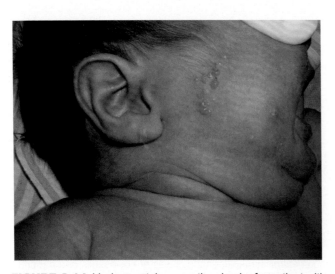

FIGURE 2-14. Vesico pustules over the cheek of a patient with eosinophilic pustular folliculitis.

CAPSULE SUMMARY

EOSINOPHILIC PUSTULAR FOLLICULITIS

ETN consists of intensely pruritic crusted papules affecting mainly the scalp. The infantile variant is typically not associated with HIV, but with different hypereosinophilic states. It is characterized by the presence of 1 to 3 mm pustules and crusts on the scalp and face. Biopsies show a folliculitis with a predominance of eosinophils.

TRANSIENT NEONATAL PUSTULAR MELANOSIS

Definition and Epidemiology

Transient neonatal pustular melanosis (TNPM) is a very infrequent, benign, self-healing condition that mainly affects full-term neonates.[47,48] It is thought to affect around 0.6% of Caucasians, with a higher incidence in African American newborns (4.4%).

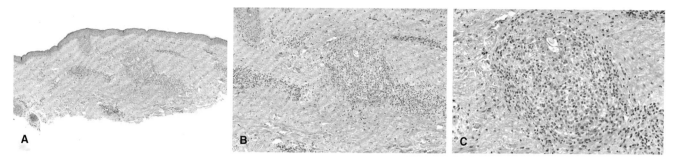

FIGURE 2-16. Eosinophilic pustular folliculitis with numerous eosinophils infiltrating into the hair follicle epithelium (A-C). Digital slides courtesy of Path Presenter.com.

Etiology

The etiology of this condition is still unknown, but some authors have suggested it might be an early manifestation of ETN because of its clinical and histologic overlap.

Clinical Presentation

Three different types of lesions can be identified—pustules that easily break and leave a fine white collarette of scale, and a hyperpigmented macule. Lesions appear usually over a normal skin and can be found in clusters or scattered around different parts of the body, including genitals, scalp (Figure 2-17A to C), palms, and soles.[49] The most important differential diagnoses include ETN, bacterial, viral, and mycotic infections, miliaria, and eosinophilic pustulosis. Under some circumstances, a clear-cut differentiation between TNPM and ETN might be really impossible.

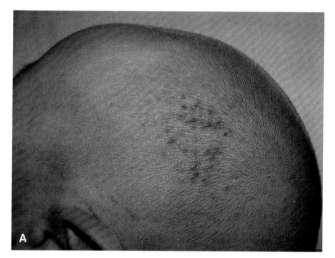

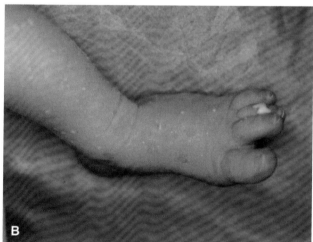

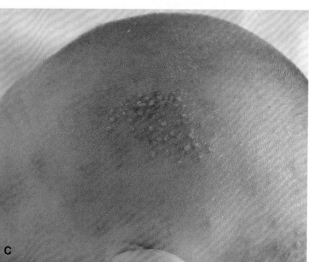

FIGURE 2-17. A, Transient neonatal pustular dermatosis—a crop of congenital pustules over the scalp of a term newborn. B, Evolution of lesions showing hyperpigmentation and scale 2 days later. C, The three coexistent states of transient neonatal pustular dermatosis: pustules, scaling, and hyperpigmentation.

Histologic Findings

Biopsies of TNPM reveal neutrophilic microabscesses within the stratum corneum and in the upper portions of the epidermis. The presence of melanin in the dermis is a result of postinflammatory hyperpigmentation. There is usually minimal inflammation in the dermis.[35,41,42]

Differential Diagnosis

Differential diagnostic considerations include pustular psoriasis. The latter is very uncommon in neonates, and can be easily distinguished on the basis of the presence of other clinical findings. ETN is characterized by eosinophils in the pustules, as opposed to TNPM, where the main inflammatory cell is neutrophils in the pustules. Some authors consider that TNPM represent a precursor lesion to what rapidly evolves into ETN.[35,41,50,51]

CAPSULE SUMMARY

TRANSIENT NEONATAL PUSTULAR MELANOSIS

TNPM is a very infrequent, benign, self-healing condition that mainly affects full-term neonates. Three different types of lesions can be identified—pustules that easily break and leave a fine white collarette, and a hyperpigmented macule. Biopsies of TNPM reveal neutrophilic microabscesses within the stratum corneum and in the upper portions of the epidermis.

ACROPUSTULOSIS OF INFANCY

Definition and Epidemiology

Acropustulosis of infancy, also known as infantile acropustulosis (IA), is a benign cutaneous disease that affects infants in their first years of life and is characterized by recurrent crops of very pruriginous papules with an acral distribution. Two variants have been described, one occurring spontaneously and another developing after scabies. It is a very infrequent disease. The spontaneous variant affects boys more frequently than girls, and although it may affect any race, it is more common in infants of African origin and among international adoptees.[52,53]

Etiology

The etiology of IA remains unknown. Theories include a reaction pattern in predisposed individuals to infection or infestation.[54] A history of scabies preceding the diagnosis of IA is common, although the relationship between the two remains unclear, as often the diagnosis of scabies is made clinically.[55,56] It is clear though, that some infants, after eradication of documented scabies infection, may have a condition with clinical manifestations, course, and histologic features identical to those of IA.

Clinical Presentation

Lesions are 1 to 2 mm papules, vesicles or flat vesicopustules together with crusts on palms, soles, dorsal hands and feet, and lateral aspects of fingers and toes are typically involved (Figure 2-18). Occasional scattered lesions on the ankles, wrists, proximal limbs, and trunk may be seen. Postinflammatory hyperpigmentation can be observed. Lesions appear in crops every 2 to 4 weeks. With time, intervals between outbreaks become longer and the intensity and length of each episode are shorter, with complete resolution at about 3 years of age.[56] Rare cases associated with eosinophilic folliculitis have been reported, suggesting they might be both part of a same hypereosinophilic spectrum.[57,58]

Histologic Findings

In IA, the epidermis shows spongiosis with microvesiculation. Neutrophilic microabscesses are seen within the vesicles (Figure 2-19). Parakeratosis is more typical of chronic lesions. The vesicles can sometimes have scattered eosinophils.[43,47,48,59]

Differential Diagnosis

Candidiasis and impetigo can both be easily distinguished with the use of special stains (Gomori Methenamine-Silver Nitrate or Periodic acid–Schiff (PAS), and Gram stains, respectively). Pustular psoriasis can be challenging to separate from IA. The presence of vascular ectasia within the dermal papillae may favor a diagnosis of psoriasis. In cases where eosinophils are present within the infiltrate, a diagnosis of ETN can also be considered. However, ETN can be separated clinically because the rash is mostly located on the scalp. Incontinentia pigmenti can also share some histologic findings. The presence of dyskeratotic cells is in favor of a diagnosis of incontinentia pigmenti.

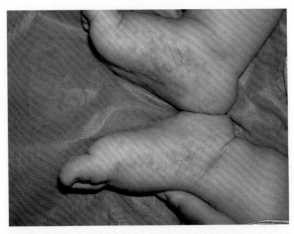

FIGURE 2-18. Acropustulosis of infancy: pustules, erythematous papules, and crusts on the lateral aspect of both feet.

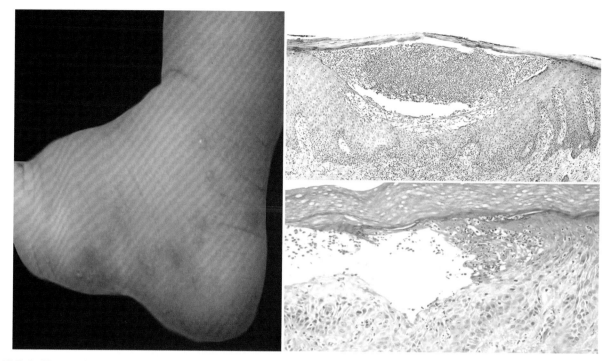

FIGURE 2-19. In infantile acropustulosis, the epidermis shows spongiosis with microvesiculation. Neutrophilic microabscesses are seen within the vesicles.

CONGENITAL EROSIVE AND VESICULAR DERMATOSIS

Definition and Epidemiology

Congenital erosive and vesicular dermatosis with reticulated supple scarring (CEVD) is an extremely rare congenital disorder first described by Cohen in 1985.[60] CEVD occurs in preterm (median 29 weeks) or small-for-gestational age newborns. Almost half of the cases are associated with chorioamnionitis, discolored amniotic fluid, and/or premature rupture of membranes.[61,62]

Etiology

CEVD is a sporadic condition of unknown etiology that is thought to be related to an intrauterine event, such as infections, trauma, amniotic adhesions, or developmental defects. Although some cases seem to be related to herpes simplex virus, the exact role in the pathogenesis of CEVD remains unclear.[63-66]

Clinical Presentation

At birth, neonates present with erythema, vesicles, erosions, ulcerations, and crusts, affecting almost 75% of the body surface area with spare of palms and soles. Lesions heal within the first months of life leaving characteristic soft, reticulated hypopigmented scars (Figure 2-20).[60,61,66] Recurrence of erosions and vesicles after the neonatal period has been described in almost 30% of the cases.[61,64] Heat intolerance observed in some cases is related to paucity of eccrine glands in scars and compensatory hyperhidrosis and hyperthermia in the remaining normal skin.[61,63] Associated features include nail dystrophy, such as hypoplasia, dysplasia, or anonychia (39%), cicatricial alopecia (39%), ophthalmologic involvement (36%), neurodevelopmental abnormalities (30%), and oral mucosal involvement (29%).[61,63,67]

Histologic Findings

The histopathologic findings of CEVD depend on the stage of the disease. In early inflammatory lesions, there is epidermal necrosis, subepidermal vesiculation, and an eroded epidermis with a predominantly neutrophilic or mixed (including eosinophils, histiocytes, lymphocytes, and neutrophils) dermal infiltrate. Histopathologic examination of biopsy specimens from

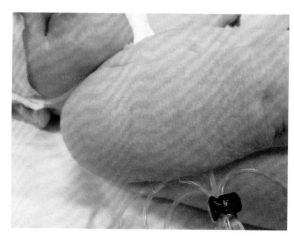

FIGURE 2-20. Congenital erosive and vesicular dermatosis: reticulated, depressed scars over the shoulder of an extremely preterm newborn.

late lesions shows scar formation with a decrease in hair follicles and absent eccrine glands, or the dermis can appear normal. Vasculitis, thrombosis, and evidence of herpes simplex virus or other infections are not observed. Electron microscopy does not show consistent abnormalities and results of direct immunofluorescence studies are negative or nonspecific.[49,52,54,55]

Differential Diagnosis

Differential diagnosis of congenital erosive vesicular dermatosis that should be considered in the neonatal period include congenital herpes simplex infection, staphylococcal scalded skin syndrome, epidermolysis bullosa, incontinentia pigmenti, focal dermal hypoplasia, and autoimmune bullous disorders. History, characteristic scarring, and histopathologic/immunofluorescence findings can help to exclude those diagnostic possibilities.

CAPSULE SUMMARY

CONGENITAL EROSIVE AND VESICULAR DERMATOSIS

At birth neonates present with erythema, vesicles, erosions, ulcerations, and crusts, affecting almost 75% of the body surface area with spare of palms and soles. Lesions heal within the first months of life leaving a characteristic soft, reticulated hypopigmented scars. In early inflammatory lesions there is epidermal necrosis, subepidermal vesiculation, and an eroded epidermis with a predominantly neutrophilic or mixed (including eosinophils, histiocytes, lymphocytes, and neutrophils) dermal infiltrate. Histopathologic examination of biopsy specimens from late lesions shows scar formation with a decrease in hair follicles and absent eccrine glands.

SEBORRHEIC DERMATITIS

Definition and Epidemiology

Infantile seborrheic dermatitis (ISD) is a self-limited inflammatory disorder occurring most often on areas with a high density of sebaceous glands. ISD usually appears in newborns by the third to fourth weeks of life, has a peak of prevalence at 3 months of age, and progressively decreases until complete recovery by the end of the first year of life in most patients.[68-70]

Etiology

The etiology of ISD is still not fully understood. The role of maternal androgens acquired transplacentally is controversial, given though sebum excretion may be normal in some patients with SD.[69] Some studies have demonstrated a link between ISD and skin commensal *Malassezia*, a lipid-dependent yeast. The efficacy of topical antifungals like selenium sulfide or ketoconazole suggests the pathogenic role of *Malassezia* on the development of ISD. *Malassezia* spp. genome encodes different enzymes which can initiate inflammation: hydrolases that produce fatty acids, and lipases and phospholipases that release free fatty acids from the sebum lipids.[71,72]

Clinical Presentation

ISD is an asymptomatic eruption that occurs most commonly on the scalp. Other affected sites include the forehead, eyebrows, eyelids, cheeks, nasolabial folds, retroauricular area, and intertriginous regions like neck, axillae, and diaper area. Scalp lesions can present as mild whitish scaly overlying erythematous skin or as thick patches of greasy yellowish hyperkeratosis ("cradle cap") (Figure 2-21A and B). Cutaneous lesions of ISD occur as erythematous scaly papules and macules that coalesce and develop

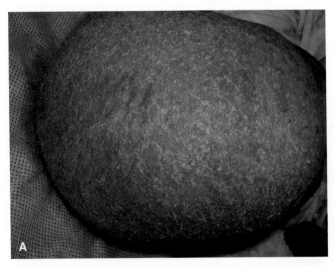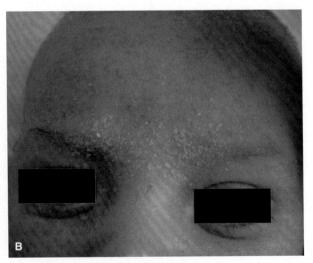

FIGURE 2-21. A, Seborrheic dermatitis with severe crusted lesions over the scalp. B, Crusts over the glabella and eyebrows in seborrheic dermatitis.

slightly elevated plaques. Intertriginous lesions, including those located on diaper area, are characterized by confluent lesions with a moist non-scaly, erythematous "slick and shiny" appearance. In rare occasions ISD can present as erythroderma.[34,68,69]

Histologic Findings

Biopsies of ISD are characterized by the presence of parakeratosis at the periphery of the opening of the hair follicles in the epidermis ("shouldering" parakeratosis) (Figure 2-22). Small clusters of neutrophils can also be present (in the epidermis or the follicles). The epidermis also show psoriasiform changes with regular elongation of the rete ridges. Hypogranulosis is present in most cases. Epidermal spongiosis is also seen, a feature that is typically more accentuated within the follicular epithelium. Superficial vascular ectasis and mild edema in the dermis can be noted. Within the dermis, there is an inflammatory infiltrate composed of lymphocytes, histiocytes, and scattered neutrophils. Colonization with *Pityrosporum* yeast forms is also typical.[56] Distinguishing seborrheic dermatitis from psoriasis can sometimes be very challenging: features of in favor of ISD include the perifollicular nature of the inflammation, the more prominent spongiosis, and partial (not diffuse) loss of the granular cell layer.

CAPSULE SUMMARY

INFANTILE SEBORRHEIC DERMATITIS

ISD is a self-limited inflammatory disorder occurring most often on areas with a high density of sebaceous glands. ISD is an asymptomatic eruption that occurs most commonly on the scalp. Other affected sites include the forehead, eyebrows, eyelids, cheeks, nasolabial folds, retroauricular area, and intertriginous regions like neck, axillae, and diaper area. Biopsies of ISD are characterized by the presence of parakeratosis at the periphery of the opening of the hair follicles in the epidermis ("shouldering" parakeratosis).

Congenital Infections in the Newborn

Although most skin lesions in newborn are benign or transient, they may also be the presenting symptom of a usually mild, but in some cases serious infection. We will focus on those congenital infections in which the skin biopsy is a useful tool for the diagnosis.

BLUEBERRY MUFFIN BABY

Definition and Epidemiology

The blueberry muffin (BBM) cutaneous lesions are a rare cutaneous transient eruption attributable to extramedullary dermal hematopoiesis secondary to congenital infections and hematologic dyscrasias.[73,74]

Etiology

During normal intrauterine development, extramedullary hematopoiesis occurs until the fifth month of pregnancy in different organs, including the dermis. The presence of BBM skin lesions at birth represents postnatal expression of this normal fetal extramedullary hematopoiesis. Among congenital TORCH (Toxoplasmosis, Other (syphilis, varicella-zoster, parvovirus B19), Rubella, Cytomegalovirus (CMV), and Herpes) infections, the most common cause is cytomegalovirus, followed by rubella and toxoplasmosis.[74-76]

Clinical Presentation

The BBM eruption is characterized by congenital generalized non-blanching, red-violaceous macules and firm papules, 0.5 to 1 cm in diameter. Resolution of the skin lesions usually occurs within the first 6 weeks of life (Figure 2-23A and B).[73,75]

Histologic Findings

Histopathologically, there are clusters of normoblastic erythropoiesis with nucleated red blood cell precursors in the dermis (Figure 2-24). Myeloid and megakaryocytic elements as well as dermal fibrosis are not typically present. CD61, Factor VIIIra, and CD31 can be used to demonstrate

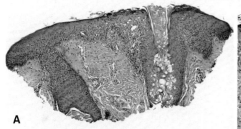
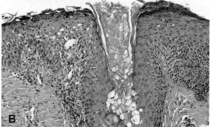
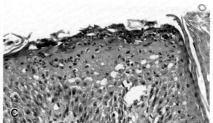

FIGURE 2-22. A to C, Biopsies of infantile seborrheic dermatitis are characterized by the presence of parakeratosis at the periphery of the opening of the hair follicles in the epidermis ("shouldering" parakeratosis). Small clusters of neutrophils can also be present (in the epidermis or the follicles). Digital slides courtesy of Path Presenter.com.

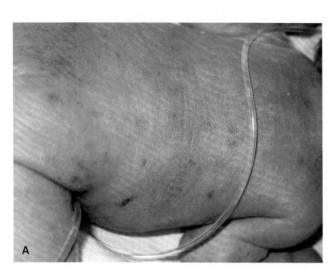
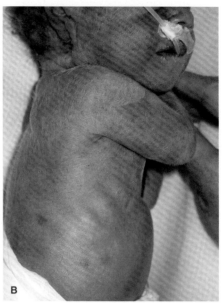

FIGURE 2-23. A and B, Blueberry muffin baby. A, Multiple erythematous lesions over the back. B, Multiple erythematous lesions over the abdomen.

the megakaryocytes, glycophorin A or hemoglobin for erythroid precursors, and CD34, CD117, and TdT for blasts. Megakaryocytes can be small and hypolobulated and might be missed without CD61 staining.

Differential Diagnosis

The differential diagnosis of blueberry muffin appearance includes congenital leukemia cutis, Langerhans cells histiocytosis, congenital vascular malformations such as multifocal hemangiomas, multifocal lymphangioendotheliomatosis, glomangiomas, and blue rubber bleb nevus syndrome.

CAPSULE SUMMARY

THE BLUEBERRY MUFFIN

BBM cutaneous lesions are a rare cutaneous transient eruption attributable to extramedullary dermal hematopoiesis secondary to congenital infections and hematologic dyscrasias. Histopathologically, there are clusters of normoblastic erythropoiesis with nucleated red blood cell precursors in the dermis. Myeloid and megakaryocytic elements as well as dermal fibrosis are not typically present.

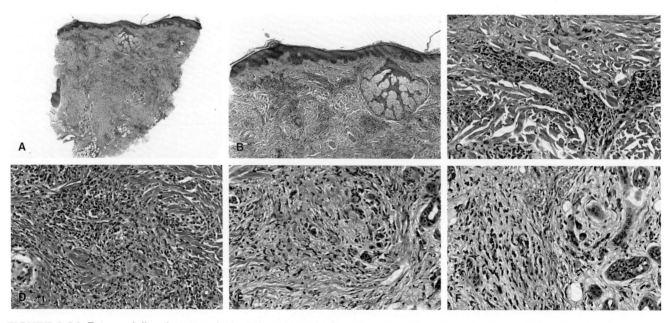

FIGURE 2-24. **Extramedullary hematopoiesis.** A dermal-based infiltrate is present (A and B). Immature myeloid and erythroid precursors are present in the dermis (C and D). Scattered megakaryocytes are also identified (E and F). Digital slides courtesy of Path Presenter.com.

NEONATAL HERPES SIMPLEX VIRUS

Definition and Epidemiology

Neonatal herpes simplex virus (HSV) infection is a serious and potentially life-threatening condition. Neonatal HSV infection occurs in about 1 case in 3200 deliveries in the United States. Considering the high prevalence of HSV infections in the general population, it occurs with less frequency than expected.[77-79]

Etiology

HSV type 1 and 2 are DNA viruses that belong to the Herpesviridae family, establish latency after primary infection, and can cause recurrent disease or asymptomatic shedding. The risk of transmission among women who acquire genital HSV during pregnancy close to the delivery period is 25% to 60%; in contrast, viral shedding secondary to a recurrent genital lesion is associated with 1% to 2% risk of transmission.[80-82]

Mother-to-child transmission of HSV can occur in three different scenarios:

- Intrautero (congenital) (5%) occurs with both primary and recurrent genital infection; clinical manifestations are present at birth.[80,82]
- Perinatally (neonatal) (85%) when there is symptomatic or asymptomatic shedding of virus from the genital tract around the time of delivery
- Postpartum (neonatal) (10%) through direct contact by a caregiver, usually from an orolabial or cutaneous infection

Clinical Presentation

Clinical manifestations of congenital HSV infection present as a triad: (1) Cutaneous: vesicles, pustules, erosions, scarring, aplasia cutis; (2) Neurologic: microcephaly, calcifications, hydranencephaly; (3) Ophthalmologic: chorioretinitis, microphthalmia, optic atrophy.[77,78,82]

Neonatal HSV acquired perinatally or postpartum cause the same clinical disease, which is divided into three categories: (1) Skin, eye, and/or mouth (mucocutaneous) disease (45%); (2) central nervous system (CNS) disease (35%); and (3) disseminated disease (20%).[82-85] Cutaneous findings of neonatal HSV infection appear within the second week of life. Skin and mucosal lesions present as 2 to 4 mm grouped clear vesicles on an erythematous base, which evolve onto pustules, crusts, or erosions (Figure 2-25A to D).[26,79,82,86]

Histologic Findings

HSV infection begins as an intraepidermal process, proceeding to the formation of subepidermal blisters. Infected keratinocytes in the epidermis and hair follicles undergo "ballooning" degeneration and acantholysis, and they may form multinucleated cells. Nuclei often have margination and homogenization of chromatin. At least some contain eosinophilic viral inclusions, surrounded by clear halos. As the lesions age, the keratinocytes become intensely eosinophilic and the cited nuclear changes tend to disappear. Dermal inflammation is variable in quantity and constituency; it may include a mixture of mononuclear cells and neutrophils, and, in rare cases, lymphoid cells in the infiltrate are numerous and cytologically atypical. Vasculitic changes are also very frequent in the biopsies. The presence of inflammation of the sebaceous glands attached to the hair follicles can also point toward the diagnosis of HSV infection. Immunostains for HSV-1 or HSV-2 are positive in active skin lesions.[57,60,61]

CAPSULE SUMMARY

NEONATAL HERPES SIMPLEX VIRUS

HSV infection is a serious and potentially life-threatening condition. Clinical manifestations of congenital HSV infection present as a triad: (1) Cutaneous: vesicles, pustules, erosions, scarring, aplasia cutis; (2) Neurologic: microcephaly, calcifications, hydranencephaly; (3) Ophthalmologic: chorioretinitis, microphthalmia, optic atrophy. The histopathology is similar to other herpetic infections occurring later in life.

CANDIDIASIS

Definition and Epidemiology

Depending of the route of infection and the age of the patient, cutaneous candidiasis in neonates can be divided into two clinical forms: congenital cutaneous candidiasis (CCC) and neonatal candidiasis (NC).[26,86] CCC is an uncommon disease acquired through ascending *Candida albicans* from maternal vulvovaginal area into the uterus. Risk factors for CCC include vaginal maternal candidiasis and the presence of a foreign body (intrauterine device or cervical cerclage sutures). NC is acquired during passage through an infected birth canal or by close contact at the nursery.[87,88]

Etiology

Both clinical forms are produced by *Candida albicans*, a commensal microorganism commonly found in skin and mucosal membranes, isolated from vaginal flora in 20% to 35% of pregnant women.[87,88]

Clinical Presentation

CCC skin eruption is present at birth in 81% of the patients, whereas in the remaining cases it develops within the first 6 days of life.[88] The rash begins as 2 to 4 mm erythematous macules and papules that quickly evolve into pustules, on

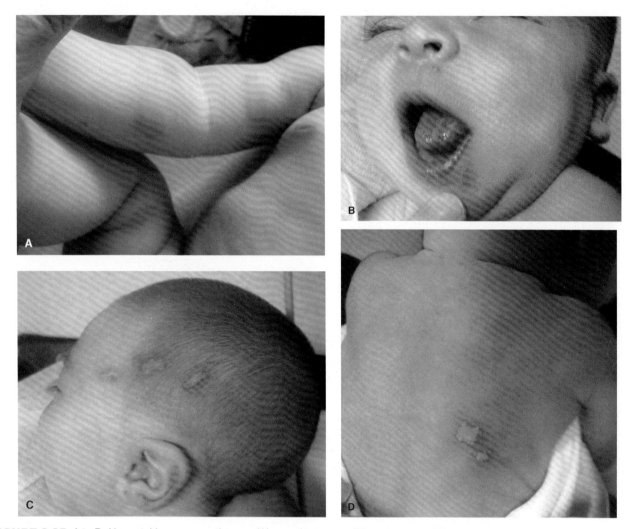

FIGURE 2-25. A to D, Neonatal herpes over the arm (A) over the tongue (B) on the scalp (C) and back (D).

a 5 to 10 mm erythematous base, diffusely scattered on the trunk, extensor surfaces of the limbs, and intertriginous areas (Figure 2-26A to D). Oral cavity and diaper area are generally spared. Characteristic pustules may be present on palms and soles. Nails can be affected with onychia and paronychia. The eruption is followed by crusting and a pronounced desquamation within 1 to 2 weeks. In full-term infants, the clinical course is benign with complete recovery.[26,87,88] Premature infants with a gestational age of <27 weeks and weighing <1000 g at birth are at greatest risk for systemic disease. Cutaneous involvement is characterized by diffuse erythematous–eroded macules and denuded areas resembling a burn.[87,88]

Lesions of NC occur after the first week of life, and include thrush, diaper dermatitis, and involvement of intertriginous areas like neck, perineum, suprapubic area, and inguinal folds. Skin lesions are characterized by erythematous scaly macules and plaques with satellite pustules and papules.[26,87]

Histologic Findings

Histopathologically, *Candida* dermatitis may have an acute-vesicular or subacute spongiotic appearance, or it may become psoriasiform if chronic. In acute infections, the tissue reaction is purulent, with possible folliculitis. The fungi may be missed in hematoxylin and eosin-stained sections, but they are readily identified in PAS or silver impregnation stains (Figure 2-27).

Candida are identified histologically by observing blastospores (yeast forms) in association with pseudohyphae. The blastospores are sharply defined, round or oval structures, 3 to 4 μm in diameter; they may contain one or more vacuoles. Rarely, candidiasis may produce a granulomatous response, with pseudoepitheliomatous epidermal hyperplasia.

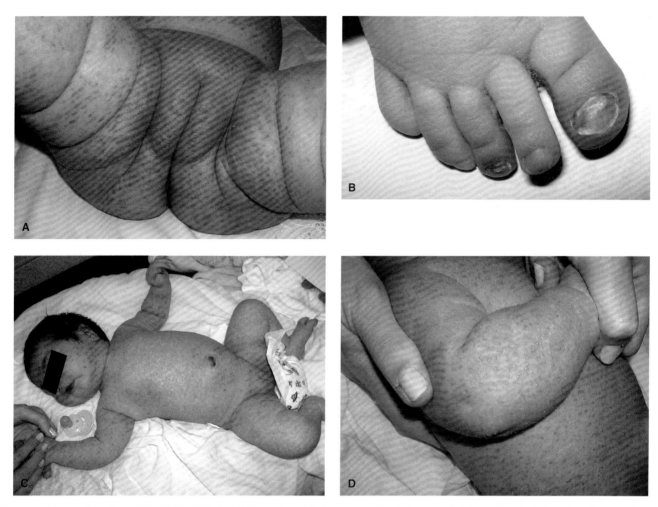

FIGURE 2-26. A to D, Diaper candidiasis (A), Onychomycosis over the hallux (B) generalized candidiasis (C), and a closeup view of the lesions on the arm (D).

CAPSULE SUMMARY

CANDIDIASIS

Depending of the route of infection and the age of the patient, cutaneous candidiasis in neonates can be divided into two clinical forms: CCC and NC. CCC skin eruption is present at birth in 81% of the patients, whereas in the remaining cases, it develops within the first 6 days of life. The rash begins as 2 to 4 mm erythematous macules and papules that quickly evolve into pustules, diffusely scattered on the trunk, extensor surfaces of the limbs, and intertriginous areas. The oral cavity and diaper area are generally spared. Lesions of NC occur after the first week of life, including thrush, diaper dermatitis, and intertriginous eruptions in areas such as the neck, perineum, suprapubic area, and inguinal folds.

NEONATAL LUPUS ERYTHEMATOSUS

Definition and epidemiology

Neonatal lupus (NL) represents a model of passive autoimmune disease in which maternal antibodies are transmitted through the placenta. It is characterized by the presence of dermatologic, cardiac, hematologic, hepatic, and/or neurologic manifestations. NL is an extremely infrequent disease with an estimated incidence of around 1 in 12 500 to 20 000 live births that affects 1% to 2% of children born to mothers with SSA/Ro, SSB/La, and less frequently, U1RNP antibodies.[89-91]

Etiology

NL is a passive autoimmune disease in which maternal antibodies are transmitted through the placenta. As the antibodies clear from the blood of the newborns, most manifestations disappear and resolve completely, except for

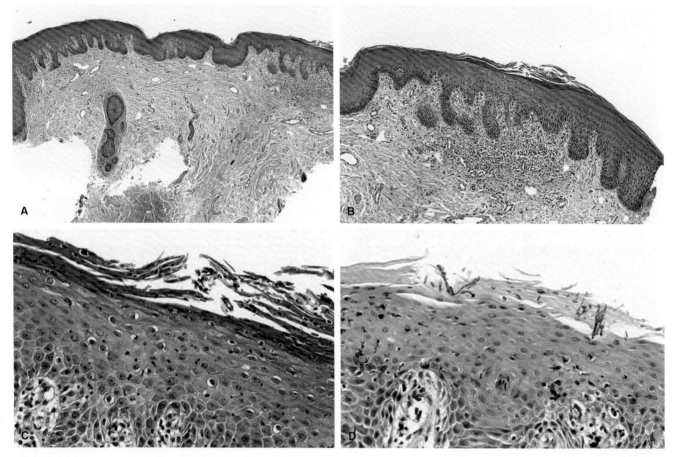

FIGURE 2-27. A to D, Candidiasis. Psoriasiform changes and spongiosis (A and B). Neutrophilic pustules are present in the stratum corneum (C). Periodic acid–Schiff stain shows pseudohyphae (D). Digital slides courtesy of Path Presenter.com.

cardiac involvement that might be life-threatening and persist throughout life.

Clinical Presentation

Affected organs include skin, heart, blood, liver, brain, and bones. Most of the literature reports a similar incidence of around 50% both for skin and heart involvement and a 15% for all the other symptoms put together. One single patient may show one to several affected organs. Skin lesions are very wide in spectrum, with several types of different morphologies and severities.[92] The most typical lesions are erythematous, arcuate, polycyclic, or annular macules, patches, and papules with slight central atrophy, with or without a fine scale, appearing mainly on the scalp and periorbital area, with a tendency to be confluent around the eyes, giving the baby an "owl eyes" or "eye mask" appearance (Figure 2-28A to D).[93] Although lesions might be present since birth, they tend to develop at around 6 weeks of life.[89] Other types of lesions such as urticaria-like lesions, atrophy, bullae, telangiectasia,[94] purpura, erythema multiforme–like lesions, widespread erosions,[95] cutis marmorata

telangiectasia congenital-like lesions,[96,97] and lesions mimicking an extensive capillary malformation[98] have all been described in patients with NL. Oral ulcers might also be present. Most of the lesions tend to completely resolve paralleling the descent of maternal antibodies around 6 to 9 months, although in some cases, residual hypo or hyperpigmentation, atrophic scars, or telangiectasias may remain.[99]

The heart is the most important target organ in NL. It might manifest as a congenital heart block (mainly complete atrioventricular block, but also other conduction alterations).[100] Most children with complete atrioventricular block will require permanent heart pacing before adulthood, with 60% paced during neonatal period.[101]

In contrast to those who have SS-A or SS-B antibodies, cardiac involvement has not been reported in the small percentage of patients who demonstrate U1RNP antibodies.[102]

The liver is affected in approximately 15% of patients with NL, usually presenting as asymptomatic elevated hepatic enzymes or hepatomegaly, transient hepatitis, hyperbilirubinemia, or even rare cases of liver failure.[103] Hematologic symptoms appear in 10% of the patients and may

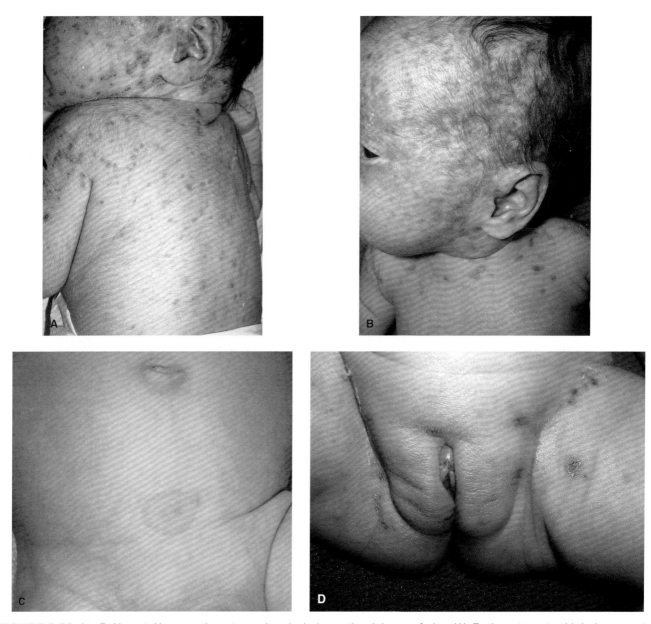

FIGURE 2-28. A to D, Neonatal lupus erythematosus. Annular lesion on the abdomen of a boy (A). Erythematous atrophic lesions over the head and upper trunk (B), Erythematous atrophic lesions over the extending to nonexposed areas (C). Erosions over the diaper area (D).

manifest as thrombocytopenia, hemolytic or aplastic anemia, and neutropenia.[92,103] CNS has also shown to be rarely affected in NL. Hydrocephalus, macrocephaly, and different degrees of neuropsychiatric dysfunction have all been previously described in patients with NL. Chondrodysplasia punctata (punctuate calcification of cartilage) has also been described in NL patients with U1RNP antibodies.[104]

Histologic Findings

The biopsy findings resemble those seen in cases of subacute lupus erythematosus in adults (Figure 2-29). There is

an interface dermatitis with vacuolar changes of the basal keratinocytes. A superficial and deep, perivascular and periadnexal lymphocytic inflammatory infiltrate is present. Epidermal atrophy and dermal pigment incontinence can also be present in some cases.[62-64,67,68,105] More recently, cases of NL showing a rich dermal neutrophilic inflammatory infiltrate have been described.[67,69,106,107] On rare occasions, the neutrophils can be admixed with large histiocytoid cells expressing CD68, CD33, and myeloperoxidase. Some cases have shown vascular telangiectasia, which can have a resemblance to the findings seen in cutis marmorata telangiectatica congenital.[71,97]

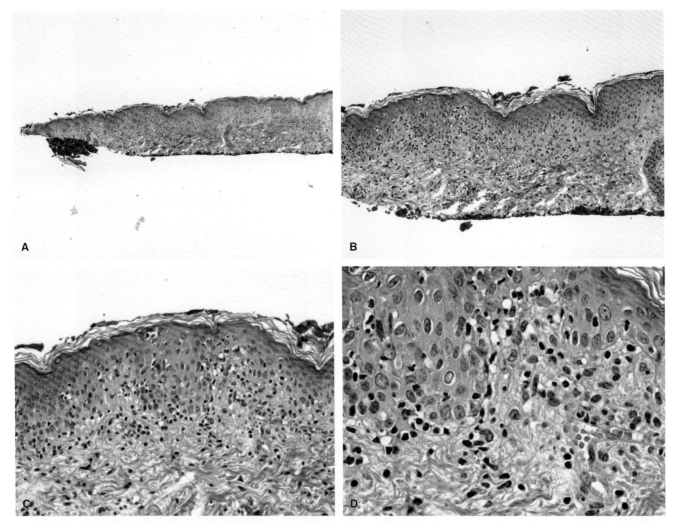

FIGURE 2-29. A to D, Neonatal lupus. The findings are equivalent to those seen in SCLE (Subacute cutaneous lupus eryday thematosus). Interface changes with mild epidermal atrophy is noted (A and B). The interface changes include vacuolar alteration of basal keratinocytes and dyskeratotic cells (C and D).

CAPSULE SUMMARY

NEONATAL LUPUS

NL represents a model of passive autoimmune disease in which maternal antibodies are transmitted through the placenta. It is characterized by the presence of dermatologic, cardiac, hematologic, hepatic, and/or neurologic manifestations. The most typical lesions are erythematous, arcuate, polycyclic, or annular macules, patches, and papules with slight central atrophy, with or without a fine scale, appearing mainly on the scalp and periorbital area, with a tendency to be confluent around the eyes, giving the baby an "owl eyes" or "eye mask" appearance. The biopsy findings resemble those seen in cases of subacute lupus erythematosus in adults.

LANGERHANS CELL HISTIOCYTOSIS

Definition and Epidemiology

Langerhans cell histiocytosis (LCH) is a rare disease characterized by a proliferation of CD1a and S100 histiocytes that may infiltrate different organs.[108] LCH might affect any age group (including adults) but is by far more frequent in neonates and infants. It affects around 9:1 000 000 infants of less than 1 year of age, with around 9% of those appearing during the newborn period (both congenital or postnatal).[109]

Etiology

Pathophysiology is not completely elucidated. Two main hypotheses have been suggested, and it is a matter of debate whether it is a reactive process or a true neoplasm. Evidence suggests a role for immune dysfunction in the pathogenesis of LCH, through the creation of a permissive immunosurveillance system.[110-113] However, in 2010, it was discovered that in a large proportion of LCH cases (greater than half of cases), there is a gain of function somatic mutation in lesional cells involving *BRAF (V600E)*, resulting in uncontrolled activation of the MAPK pathway (RAS/RAF/MEK/ERK).[72]

Clinical Presentation

Depending on the number of involved organs it can be divided into unifocal (only one organ) or multifocal (more than one organ), and depending on the number of lesions, it can be divided into single lesion to multiple lesions.[114] During the neonatal period, both unifocal solitary and multiple lesions can be present.[115] Single lesions are highly polymorphic: Crusted or flesh-colored papules, nodules, ulcers, erosions, and hemorrhagic macules have all been described (Figure 2-30A to F).

Lesions can be congenital or appear shortly after birth.[116] Most patients with this type of LCH will show no extracutaneous findings, with lesions resolving spontaneously in a few weeks. Still, patients should be granted a long-term follow-up, given rare cases of cutaneous relapse and extracutaneous manifestations, with a lethal outcome having been reported.[108,117,118]

Histologic Findings

Diagnosis of LCH can be tentatively made on the basis of characteristic morphologic findings of proliferating histiocytic cells in the proper pattern and background. Neoplastic Langerhans cells are medium to large in size, exhibit abundant eosinophilic cytoplasm, and "coffee bean"-shaped grooved nuclei. Involvement of skin shows an upper epidermal lesion that tends to infiltrate the epidermis-creating abscesses. Confirmation of diagnosis is achieved by demonstrating Langerhans granules (Birbeck granules) on electron microscopy or more easily by the characteristic positivity of Langerhans cells for the typical markers CD1a, S-100, and Langerin.[73-76,112,113]

Differential Diagnosis

LCH is often discernible on the basis of its characteristic cytology and unique immunohistochemical pattern. Nonneoplastic, reactive Langerhans cell hyperplasia secondary to an exogenous inflammatory insult such as an eczematous dermatitis, bug bites, or scabies should be considered. Non-LCH disorders such as juvenile xanthogranuloma and Erdheim-Chester disease may mimic LCH at various time points.

CAPSULE SUMMARY

LANGERHANS CELL HISTIOCYTOSIS

LCH is a rare disease characterized by a proliferation of CD1a and S100 histiocytes that may infiltrate different organs. Depending on the number of involved organs it can be divided into unifocal (only one organ)

or multifocal (more than one organ) and depending on the number of lesions it can be divided into single lesion or multiple lesions. Diagnosis of LCH can be tentatively made on the basis of the characteristic morphologic findings of proliferating histiocytic cells in the proper pattern and background. Neoplastic Langerhans cells are medium to large in size, exhibit abundant eosinophilic cytoplasm, and "coffee bean"-shaped grooved nuclei.

INCONTINENTIA PIGMENTI

Definition and Epidemiology

Incontinentia pigmenti (IP) is a rare X-linked disorder that mainly affects female patients. It is caused by a mutation in the *IKBKG* gene (formerly known as NEMO).[119] IP occurs in approximately 1:40 000 to 1:50 000 births, affecting mainly female patients. As all X-linked dominant disorders, IP is usually lethal in male fetuses. Some rare cases of IP affecting male patients have been reported because of hypomorphic alleles, postzygotic mosaicism, or an additional X chromosome (Klinefelter syndrome).[120,121]

Etiology

IKBKG is involved in the activation of nuclear factor κB, which protects cells against apoptosis and is located in the Xq28. Eighty percent of patients with IP show a deletion at exons 4 through 10.[119,122]

Clinical Presentation

It affects structures of neuroectodermal origin, with cutaneous manifestations being present in around 100% of patients. Other organs such as the brain and eyes might also be affected less frequently, but when they do, a more severe disease may result.

Cutaneous manifestations are characterized by different types of lesions that follow the Blaschko lines. Four different types of lesions characterizing the different stages can be recognized:

Stage 1 (vesiculopustular stage) where inflammation is present in a linear pattern along the lines of Blaschko. Erythematous papules, vesicles, and/or pustules can be present since birth or appear shortly after, tending to disappear before 4 months of age (Figures 2-31, 2-32 and 2-33).[119] Reactivation of this first stage later in life has been reported, mainly in association with infectious or febrile illnesses.[123,124]

Stage 2 (verrucous stage) is characterized by warty papules or plaques along the lines of Blaschko, that may or may not coincide with the lesions of the previous stage, and might even overlap with stage I lesions in different areas of the body. It usually appears around 2 to 6 weeks of life and can be quite persistent (Figures 2-34, 2-35 and 2-36).

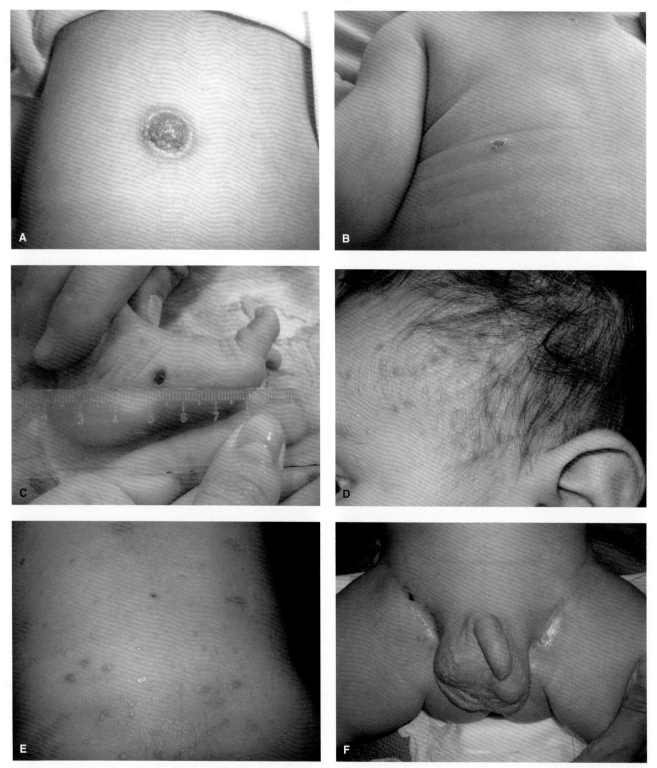

FIGURE 2-30. A to F, Langerhans cell histiocytosis. A, Deep, round, well-demarcated, congenital ulcer over the back of a newborn. B, Subtle single-crusted papule over the back of a newborn. C, Crusted single nodule over the inner aspect of the left foot of a newborn. D, Multiple flesh-colored papules and crusts over the scalp and forehead of a patient with CLCH (cutaneous langerhans cell histiocytosis). E, Multiple flesh-colored, umbilicated lichenoid papules over the back of a patient. F, Erythematous papules and erosions over the inguinal folds of a male patient.

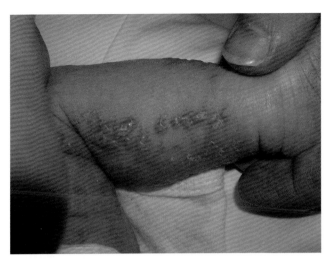

FIGURE 2-31. Vesicles following Blaschko lines over the leg of a female newborn.

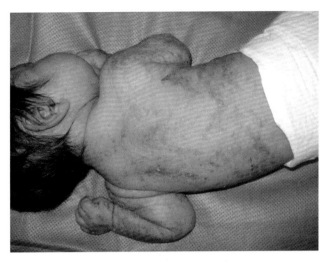

FIGURE 2-33. Crust, erosions, and erythema following lines of Blaschko over the back of a female newborn.

Stage 3 (hyperpigmented stage) is characterized by the development of linear or whorled, hyperpigmented lesions following Blaschko lines mainly affecting the trunk. Lesions appear in early infancy and may persist until adulthood.

Stage 4 (atrophic/hypopigmented stage) develops during adolescence, persisting through adult life, and is characterized by hypopigmented atrophic lines, mainly along the lower extremities.

These lesions might be the only clue in a mother of an affected child.[119,123,125] The scalp can also be affected, showing a characteristic whorled scarring alopecia of the vertex (Figure 2-37). Dental anomalies may develop with time in approximately 80% of patients with IP.[119]

CNS can be affected in around 20% of patients, and it usually correlates with the cutaneous manifestations. Patients with more severe and widespread skin lesions have a higher likelihood of having neurologic involvement. Central nervous system disease may manifest as seizures, developmental delay, paresis, and ataxia, among others. The symptoms are due to microvascular infarcts.[123]

Ocular involvement can also be present in less than 30% of patients, and it has the same characteristics as those of neurologic involvement. It is more frequent in patients with a more severe cutaneous disease. Both retinal and

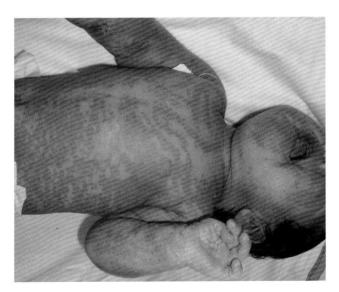

FIGURE 2-32. Widespread erythematosus lesions following lines of Blaschko over the trunk of a female newborn.

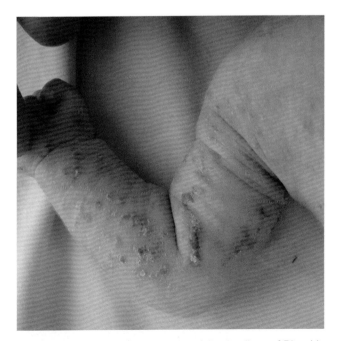

FIGURE 2-34. Erythema and crusts following lines of Blaschko over the arm of a female newborn.

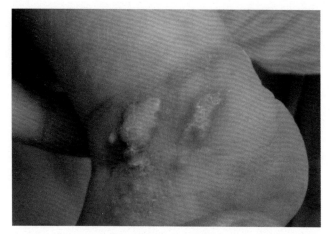

FIGURE 2-35. Linear verrucous lesions over the ankle of a 2-month-old female patient.

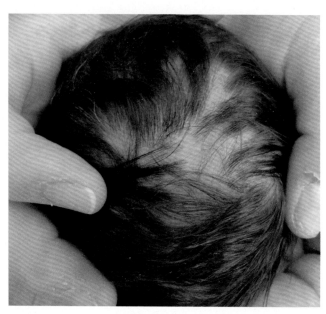

FIGURE 2-37. Whirled crusts and alopecia over the scalp of a newborn.

nonretinal manifestations might develop. Amaurosis, retinal detachment, strabismus, cataracts, optic atrophy, and microphthalmia have all been described.[119,122,123,126]

Histologic Findings

The histopathologic findings vary according to the stage of the clinical lesion. The earliest stage I lesions (vesicular stage) are characterized by eosinophilic spongiosis. The epidermis is spongiotic, often with the presence of intraepidermal vesicles containing eosinophils. Focal necrosis is seen, and there are scattered dyskeratotic keratinocytes, both in the epidermis and in hair follicle epithelium. The dermis shows a perivascular inflammatory infiltrate containing abundant eosinophils (Figure 2-38). The stage II lesions (verrucous stage) show epidermal acanthosis with hyperkeratosis on the surface (Figure 2-39 A-C). Dyskeratotic keratinocytes are numerous within the epidermis, and a "whorled" configuration of these cells have been reported. The epidermal and dermal eosinophilia is no longer a prominent feature of

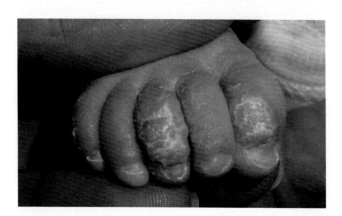

FIGURE 2-36. Warty linear lesions over the dorsum of the toes.

the biopsies at this stage (however, eosinophils can still be encountered at this stage). The stage III lesions have the features of postinflammatory hyperpigmentation (Figure 2-39 D-F). There is a loss of epidermal pigment with abundant dermal melanophages. Focal hydropic changes of the basal keratinocytes are noted, in addition to scattered dyskeratotic cells. The lesions from stage IV show epidermal atrophy and variable reduction in the number of melanocytes.[77,78,80,81,127]

Differential Diagnosis

Differential diagnostic considerations include erythema toxicum, varicella, bullous impetigo, and diffuse cutaneous mastocytosis. Erythema toxicum can be particularly challenging, as the number of intraepidermal eosinophils is prominent in both conditions. Helpful clues to separate both apart are (1) the linear pattern following the lines of Blaschko in IP and (2) the presence of dyskeratotic keratinocytes in this entity. Bullous impetigo can easily be separated on the basis of a predominance of neutrophils in it and eosinophils in IP. The presence of bacterial colonies using a Gram stain and cultures can also be helpful. Infections such as HSV and varicella-zoster virus can be excluded on the basis of the viral cytopathic changes and/or positive viral cultures of polymerase chain reaction swabs. Diffuse cutaneous mastocytosis lacks the epidermal changes seen in IP and shows a mast cell infiltrate in the dermis. The older the lesions of IP, the easier the diagnosis can be made, particularly given the distinctive verrucous changes and the prominence of dyskeratotic cells.

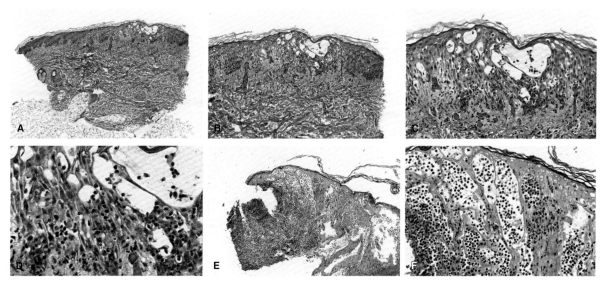

FIGURE 2-38. **Incontinentia pigmenti—histopathologic findings.** Stage I marked spongiosis with intraepidermal vesiculation (A and B). Eosinophilic spongiosis is noted (C and D). Large intraepidermal eosinophilic vesicles can be also seen (E and F). Digital slides courtesy of Path Presenter.com.

CAPSULE SUMMARY

INCONTINENTIA PIGMENTI

IP is a rare X-linked disorder that mainly affects female patients. It is caused by a mutation in the *IKBKG* gene (formerly known as NEMO). Cutaneous manifestations are characterized by different types of lesions that follow the Blaschko lines. The histopathologic findings vary according to the stage of the clinical lesion. The earliest stage I lesions (vesicular stage) are characterized by eosinophilic spongiosis. The stage II lesions (verrucous stage) show epidermal acanthosis with hyperkeratosis on the surface.

CUTANEOUS MASTOCYTOSIS

Definition and Epidemiology

Mastocytosis is a heterogeneous group of disorders, characterized by an abnormal proliferation and infiltration of mastocytes into different organs, mainly the skin. Extracutaneous involvement includes bone marrow, liver, spleen, lymph nodes, and gastrointestinal tract. Mastocytosis is divided into two different forms: cutaneous mastocytosis (CM), which is mostly seen in children, and systemic mastocytosis.[128,129]

Mastocytosis is a rare disease, with an estimated prevalence of 9 cases per 100 000 population. The true incidence of CM in children is unknown; in Spain, the annual incidence of CM has been estimated to be 0.2 cases per 100 000

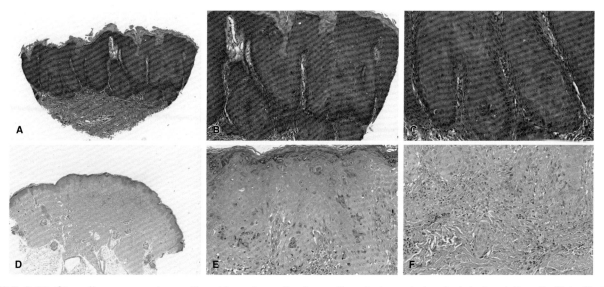

FIGURE 2-39. Stage II verrucous stage with epidermal acanthosis, papillomatosis, and abundant dyskeratotic cells (A to C). Stage III lesions show postinflammatory hyperpigmentation. In the current case, numerous dyskeratotic cells also seen (D to F). Digital slides courtesy of Path Presenter.com.

population.[128] Mastocytosis has a male preponderance, with a male-to-female ratio of 1.5:1.[130,131] The onset of CM occurs in 85% to 90% of the cases in the first year of life.[128-130] Although mastocytosis is considered a sporadic disease, identical twins and triplets have been reported; familial involvement is described in 2% to 4% of the cases.[128-130]

Etiology

Mastocytosis is a clonal disease produced by a somatic-activating mutation in the *KIT* protooncogene, which encodes KIT (CD117), a transmembrane receptor, with tyrosine kinase activity expressed in mast cells. Almost 90% of patients with adulthood-onset mastocytosis carry the *KITD816V* mutation in exon 17, whereas only 35% to 45% of pediatric patients express the former mutation, and 44% present other *KIT*-activating mutation affecting exon 8, 9, or 11.[128,132] Interaction between stem cell factor, which is released by stromal cells, and its ligand-KIT receptor, has a key role in differentiation, growth, proliferation, and survival of mast cells.[128,133]

Clinical Presentation

Currently, CM is divided into three different forms: (1) maculopapular CM (urticaria pigmentosa), (2) diffuse CM, and (3) mastocytoma. Almost 20% of mastocytosis are congenital.[131] Overall, more than 40% to 60% of mastocytomas and nearly 20% of maculopapular CM are present at birth.[130,134] Maculopapular CM is the most common clinical form of CM, characterized by erythematous or brown papules and macules of varying sizes, and in some cases, plaques and nodules, located mainly on the trunk. Mastocytoma typically presents as a single or scarce, yellowish to brownish plaques or nodules, most often located on the limbs and sparing palms and soles. A positive Darier's sign is associated with CM, and it is characterized by urtication and redding upon friction or mechanical irritation secondary to mast cell mediators' release. Most cases of both maculopapular CM and mastocytoma resolve around puberty (Figures 2-40 to 2-42).[131,132]

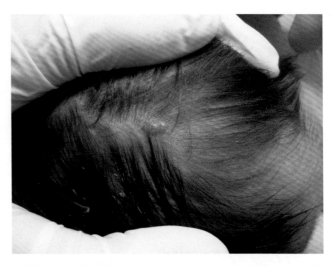

FIGURE 2-41. Urticaria pigmentosa: bullous lesion over the scalp of a newborn with bullous mastocytosis.

Histologic Findings

Cutaneous mastocytoses show a dense, nodular aggregate of mature mast cells in the dermis, with occasional extension into the deeper levels of the dermis and subcutaneous tissues (Figure 2-43). The mast cells of mastocytoses are ovoid or polygonal in shape with abundant cytoplasm and contain round to oval nuclei with inconspicuous nucleoli. The cytoplasm is filled with eosinophilic to amphophilic cytoplasmic granules that contain histamine and other bioactive chemicals.

The abnormal mast cells express CD33, CD5, CD68, CD117, tryptase, and chymase. Mast cells also express CD45 (common leukocyte antigen). Histochemical stains such as Toluidine blue, Giemsa, and chloroacetate esterase (the Leder stain) may also be used to highlight mast cells.

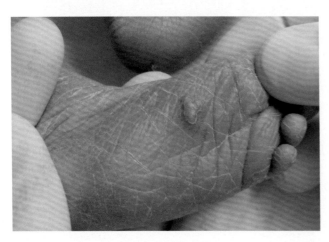

FIGURE 2-40. Urticaria pigmentosa: Vesicopustule on the sole of a newborn with bullous mastocytosis.

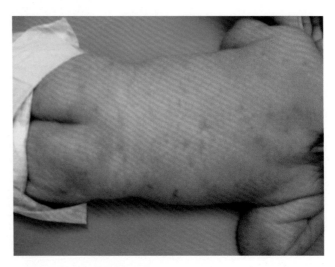

FIGURE 2-42. Widespread brown macules over the dorsum of a newborn with urticaria pigmentosa.

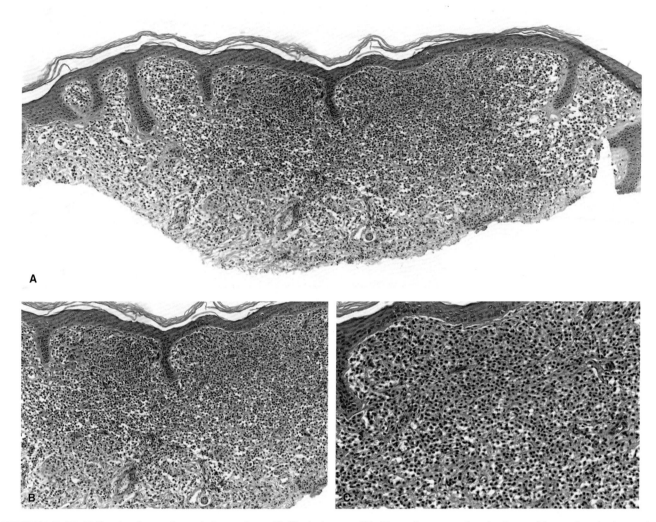

FIGURE 2-43. Urticaria pigmentosa. A dense dermal infiltrate is seen (A). The cells are medium in size and have abundant granular cytoplasm (B). Atypical mast cells typically clustered around vessels (C).

CD117 is the most sensitive marker for mast cells but is not entirely specific. Conversely, chymase is highly specific for mast cells, but less sensitive. Childhood mastocytoses very rarely express aberrant immunohistochemical markers such as CD25 and CD2, with very few cases reported in the literature. Aberrant antigen expression in solitary mastocytomas specifically is not well characterized. However, as a whole, the limited cutaneous mastocytoses (including solitary mastocytomas) express aberrant CD25 much less often than the cutaneous lesions of systemic mastocytosis.

Differential Diagnosis

The differential diagnosis includes systemic mastocytosis and other forms of CM (urticaria pigmentosa, isolated cutaneous mastocytoma, and diffuse CM). Cutaneous tumors with cell types that resemble mast cells may also be considered in the differentia. Those include LCH, non-Langerhans cell proliferations, and melanocytic lesions. The differential diagnosis will be discussed further in Chapter 26.

CAPSULE SUMMARY

CUTANEOUS MASTOCYTOSIS

Mastocytosis is a heterogeneous group of disorders, characterized by an abnormal proliferation and infiltration of mastocytes into different organs, mainly the skin. Mastocytosis is divided into two different forms: CM, which is mostly seen in children, and systemic mastocytosis. Mastocytosis is a clonal disease produced by a somatic-activating mutation in the KIT protooncogene which encodes KIT. Currently, CM is divided into three different forms: (1) maculopapular CM (urticaria pigmentosa), (2) diffuse CM, and (3) mastocytoma. Almost 20% of mastocytosis are congenital. Cutaneous mastocytoses show a dense, nodular aggregate of mature mast cells in the dermis, with occasional extension into the deeper levels of the dermis and subcutaneous tissues. The abnormal mast cells express CD33, CD5, CD68, CD117, tryptase, and chymase.

REFERENCES

1. Shrestha S, Chaudhary N, Koirala S, et al. Sclerema neonatorum treated successfully with parenteral steroids: an experience from a resource poor country. *Case Rep Pediatr.* 2017;2017:1-4.

2. Zeb A, Darmstadt GL. Sclerema neonatorum: a review of nomenclature, clinical presentation, histological features, differential diagnoses and management. *J Perinatol.* 2008;28:453-460.

3. Spohn GP, Pietras TA, Stone MS. Delayed-onset sclerema neonatorum in a critically ill premature infant. *Pediatr Dermatol.* 2016;33:e168-e169.

4. Torrelo A, Hernández A. Panniculitis in children. *Dermatol Clin.* 2008;26:491-500.

5. Polcari IC, Stein SL. Panniculitis in childhood. *Dermatol Ther.* 2010;23(4):356-367.

6. Dasgupta A, Ghosh RN, Pal RK, Mukherjee N. *Sclerema neonatorum-histopathologic study. Indian J Pathol Microbiol.* 1993;36(1):45-47.

7. Larralde M, Abad ME, Corbella C, et al. Subcutaneous fat necrosis of the newborn, report of five cases. *Dermatol Argent.* 2009;15:200-204.

8. Gomes M, Porro A, Enokihara M, et al. Subcutaneous fat necrosis of the newborn: clinical manifestations in two cases. *An Bras Dermatol.* 2013;88:154-157.

9. Horsfield GI, Yardley HJ. Sclerema neonatorum. *J Invest Dermatol.* 1965;44:326-332.

10. Joncas J. Sclerema neonatorum: report of an unusual case. *Can Med Assoc J.* 1959;80(5):365-368.

11. Heilbron B, Saxe N. Scleredema in an infant. *Arch Dermatol.* 1986;122(12):1417-1419.

12. Savić DM, Stojanović ND, Stanković VD, et al. Subcutaneous fat necrosis in newborns. *Med Glas (Zenica).* 2012;9(2):429-431.

13. Repiso-Jiménez JB, Márquez J, Sotillo I, García-Bravo B, Camacho F. Subcutaneous fat necrosis of the newborn. *J Eur Acad Dermatol Venereol.* 1999;12(3):254-257.

14. Tran JT, Sheth AP. Complications of subcutaneous fat necrosis of the newborn: a case report and review of the literature. *Pediatr Dermatol.* 2003;20:257-261.

15. Grass B, Weibel L, Hagmann C, et al. Subcutaneous fat necrosis in neonates with hypoxic ischaemic encephalopathy registered in the Swiss National Asphyxia and Cooling Register. *BMC Pediatr.* 2015;15:73.

16. Strohm B, Hobson A, Brocklehurst P, et al. Subcutaneous fat necrosis after moderate therapeutic hypothermia in neonates. *Pediatrics.* 2011;128:e450-e452.

17. Oza V, Treat J, Cook N, et al. Subcutaneous fat necrosis as a complication of whole-body cooling for birth asphyxia. *Arch Dermatol.* 2010;146:882-885.

18. Rubin G, Spagnut G, Morandi F, et al. Subcutaneous fat necrosis of the newborn. *Clin case reports.* 2015;3:1017-1020.

19. Requena L. Normal subcutaneous fat, necrosis of adipocytes and classification of the panniculitides. *Semin Cutan Med Surg.* 2007;26(2):66-70.

20. Berk DR, Bayliss SJ. Milia: a review and classification. *J Am Acad Dermatol.* 2008;59:1050-1063.

21. Monteagudo B, Labandeira J, Cabanillas M, et al. Prevalence of milia and palatal and gingival cysts in Spanish newborns. *Pediatr Dermatol.* 2012;29:301-305.

22. Gupta P, Faridi M, Batra M. Physiological skin manifestations in twins: association with maternal and neonatal factors. *Pediatr Dermatol.* 2011;28:387-392.

23. Lucky A. Transient benign cutaneous lesions in the newborn. In: Eichenfield LF, Frieden IJ, Esterly N, ed. *Neonatal Dermatology.* 2nd ed. Philadelphia, PA: Saunders Elsevier; 2008:85-97.

24. Luna PC, Larralde M. Profuse congenital familial milia with absent dermatoglyphics (Basan's syndrome): description of a new family. *Pediatr Dermatol.* 2012;29:527-529.

25. Walsh R, Cordoro KM, North J, Frieden IJ. Midline anterior neck inclusion cyst: a novel superficial congenital developmental anomaly of the neck. *Pediatr Dermatol.* 2018;35(1):55-58.

26. De Araujo T, Schachner L. Benign vesicopustular eruptions in the neonate. *An Bras Dermatol.* 2006;81:359-366.

27. Arun Babu T, Sharmila V. Congenital miliaria crystallina in a term neonate born to a mother with chorioamnionitis. *Pediatr Dermatol.* 2012;29:306-307.

28. Honda Y, Egawa K, Baba Y, Ono T. Sweat duct milia—immunohistological analysis of structure and three-dimensional reconstruction. *Arch Dermatol Res.* 1996;288(3):133-139.

29. Monteagudo B, Labandeira J, Cabanillas M, et al. Prospective study of erythema toxicum neonatorum: epidemiology and predisposing factors. *Pediatr Dermatol.* 2012;29:166-168.

30. Hulsmann AR, Oranje AP. Educational paper: neonatal skin lesions. *Eur J Pediatr.* 2014;173:557-566.

31. Morgan AJ, Steen CJ, Schwartz RA, et al. Erythema toxicum neonatorum revisited. *Cutis.* 2009;83:13-16.

32. Reginatto FP, Muller FM, Peruzzo J, et al. Epidemiology and predisposing factors for erythema toxicum neonatorum and transient neonatal pustular: a multicenter study. *Pediatr Dermatol.* 2017;34:422-426.

33. Marchini G, Nelson A, Edner J, et al. Erythema toxicum neonatorum is an innate immune response to commensal microbes penetrated into the skin of the newborn infant. *Pediatr Res.* 2005;58:613-616.

34. Connor NR, McLaughlin MR, Ham P. Newborn skin: Part I. Common rashes. *Am Fam Physician.* 2008;77:47-52.

35. Lucky A, Esterly N, Heskel N, et al. Eosinophilic pustular folliculitis in infancy. *Pediatr Dermatol.* 1984;1:202-206.

36. Duarte A, Kramer J, Yusk J, et al. Eosinophilic pustular folliculitis in infancy and childhood. *Am J Dis Child.* 1993;147:197-200.

37. Colton A, Schachner L, Kowalczyk A. Eosinophilic pustular folliculitis. *J Am Acad Dermatol.* 1986;14:469-474.

38. Giard F, Marcoux D, McCuaig C, et al. Eosinophilic pustular folliculitis (Ofuji disease) in childhood: a review of 4 cases. *Pediatr Dermatol.* 1991;8:189-193.

39. Taieb A, Bassan-Andrieu L, Maleville J. Eosinophilic pustulosis of the scalp in childhood. *J Am Acad Dermatol.* 1992;27:55-60.

40. Darmstadt GL, Tunnessen WJ, Swerer R. Eosinophilic pustular folliculitis. *Pediatrics.* 1992;89:1095-1098.

41. Larralde M, Morales S, Santos Muñoz A, et al. Eosinophilic pustular folliculitis in infancy: report of two new cases. *Pediatr Dermatol.* 1999;16:118-120.

42. Kamei R, Honig P. Neonatal Job's syndrome featuring a vesicular eruption. *Pediatr Dermatol.* 1998;5:75-82.

43. Blum R, Geller G, Fish L. Recurrent severe staphylococcal infections, eczematoid rash, extreme elevations of IgE, eosinophilia, and divergent chemotactic responses in two generations. *J Pediatr.* 1997;90:607-609.

44. Ellis E, Scheinfeld N. Eosinophilic pustular folliculitis: a comprehensive review of treatment options. *Am J Clin Dermatol.* 2004;5(3):189-197.

45. Hernández-Martín Á, Nuño-González A, Colmenero I, Torrelo A. Eosinophilic pustular folliculitis of infancy: a series of 15 cases and review of the literature. *J Am Acad Dermatol.* 2013;68(1):150-155.

46. Nervi SJ, Schwartz RA, Dmochowski M. Eosinophilic pustular folliculitis: a 40 year retrospect. *J Am Acad Dermatol.* 2006;55(2):285-289.

47. Tarang G, Anupam V. Incidence of vesicobullous and erosive disorders of neonates. *J Dermatol Case Rep.* 2011;12:58-63.

48. Agusti-Mejias A, Messeguer F, Febrer I, et al. Transient neonatal pustular melanosis. *Actas Dermosifiliogr.* 2013;104:84-85.

49. Chia P, Leung C, Hsu Y, et al. An infant with transient neonatal pustular melanosis presenting as pustules. *Pediatr Neonatol.* 2010;51:356-358.

50. Barr RJ, Globerman LM, Werber FA. Transient neonatal pustular melanosis. *Int J Dermatol.* 1979;18(8):636-638.

51. Ramamurthy RS, Reveri M, Esterly NB, Fretzin DF, Pildes RS. Transient neonatal pustular melanosis. *J Pediatr.* 1976;88(5):831-835.

52. Good L, Good T, High W. Infantile acropustulosis in internationally adopted children. *J Am Acad Dermatol.* 2011;65:763-771.

53. Kahn G, Rywlin AM. Acropustulosis of infancy. *Arch Dermatol.* 1979;115(7):831-833.

54. Dromy R, Raz A, Metzker A. Infantile acropustulosis. *Pediatr Dermatol.* 1991;8:284-287.

55. Nguyen J, Strobel M, Arnaud J, et al. Infantile acropustolosis: unusual manifestation of scabies in the infant? *Ann Pediatr.* 1991;38:479-483.

56. Mancini A, Frieden I, Paller A. Infantile acropustulosis revisited: history of scabies and response to topical corticosteroids. *Pediatr Dermatol*. 1998;15:337-341.

57. Lucky A, McGuire J. Infantile acropustulosis with eosinophilic pustules. *J Pediatr*. 1982;100:428-429.

58. Truong AL, Esterly NB. Atypical acropustulosis in infancy. *Int J Dermatol*. 1997;36(9):688-691.

59. Dorton DW, Kaufmann M. Palmoplantar pustules in an infant. Acropustulosis of infancy. *Arch Dermatol*. 1996;132(11):1365-1366, 1368-1369.

60. Cohen B, Esterly N, Nelson PF. Congenital erosive and vesicular dermatosis healing with reticulated supple scarring. *Arch Dermatol*. 1985;121:361-367.

61. Tlougan BE, Paller AS, Schaffer JV, et al. Congenital erosive and vesicular dermatosis with reticulated supple scarring: unifying clinical features. *J Am Acad Dermatol*. 2013;69:909-915.

62. Polat A, Barbarot S, Bellanger A, et al. Congenital erosive and vesicular dermatosis healing with reticulated scarring. *J Pediatr*. 2016;176:212-212.e1.

63. Mashiah J, Wallach D, Leclerc-Mercier S, et al. Congenital erosive and vesicular dermatosis: A new case and review of the literature. *Pediatr Dermatol*. 2012;29:756-758.

64. Wong V, Fischer G. Congenital erosive and vesicular dermatosis with reticulated supple scarring. *Australas J Dermatol*. 2017;58:e236-e239.

65. Plantin P, Delaire P, Guillois B, Guillet G. Congenital erosive dermatosis with reticulated supple scarring: first neonatal report. *Arch Dermatol*. 1990;126(4):544-546.

66. Srinivas SM, Mukherjee SS, Hiremagalore R. Congenital erosive and vesicular dermatosis healing with reticulated supple scarring: report of four cases. *Indian J Dermatol Venereol Leprol*. 2018;84(1):73-75.

67. Cohen RS, Wong RJ, Stevenson DK. Understanding neonatal jaundice: a perspective on causation. *Pediatr Neonatol*. 2010;51:143-148.

68. Gupta A, Bluhm R. Seborrheic dermatitis. *J Eur Acad Dermatol Venereol*. 2004;18:13-26.

69. Elish D, Silverberg NB. Infantile seborrheic dermatitis. *Cutis*. 2006;77:297-300.

70. Pagliarello C, Fabrizi G, Cortelazzi C, Boccaletti V, Feliciani C, Di Nuzzo S, et al. Psoriasis and seborrheic dermatitis in infancy and childhood. *G Ital Dermatol Venereol*. 2014;149(6):683-691.

71. Prohic A, Jovovic Sadikovic T, Krupalija-Fazlic M, et al. Malassezia species in healthy skin and in dermatological conditions. *Int J Dermatol*. 2016;55:494-504.

72. Lee YW, Lee SY, Lee Y, et al. Evaluation of expression of lipases and phospholipases of Malassezia restricta in patients with seborrheic dermatitis. *Ann Dermatol*. 2013;25:310-314.

73. De Carolis MP, Salvi S, Bersani I, et al. Fetal hypoxia secondary to severe maternal anemia as a causative link between blueberry muffin baby and erythroblastosis: a case report. *J Med Case Rep*. 2016;10:1-5.

74. Darby JB, Valentine G, Hillier K, et al. A 3-week-old with an isolated "Blueberry Muffin" rash. *Pediatrics*. 2017;140(1). doi:10.1542/peds.2016-2598.

75. Mehta V, Balachandran C, Lonikar V. Blueberry muffin baby: a pictorial differential diagnosis. *Dermatol Online J*. 2008;14:8.

76. Karmegaraj B, Vijayakumar S, Ramanathan R, et al. Extramedullary haematopoiesis resembling a blueberry muffin, in a neonate. *BMJ Case Rep*. 2015. doi:10.1136/bcr-2014-208473.

77. James SH, Kimberlin DW. Neonatal herpes simplex virus infection: epidemiology and treatment. *Clin Perinatol*. 2015;42:47-59.

78. Marquez L, Levy M, Munoz F, et al. A report of three cases and review of intrauterine herpes simplex virus infection. *Pediatr Infect Dis J*. 2011;30:153-157.

79. Crowson AN, Saab J, Magro CM. Folliculocentric herpes: a clinicopathological study of 28 patients. *Am J Dermatopathol*. 2017;39(2):89-94.

80. Wang A, Wohrley J, Rosebush J. Herpes simplex virus in the neonate. *Pediatr Ann*. 2017;46:e42-e46.

81. Corey L, Wald A. Maternal and neonatal HSV infections. *N Engl J Med*. 2009;361:1376-1385.

82. James SH, Kimberlin DW. Neonatal herpes simplex virus infection. *Infect Dis Clin North Am*. 2015;29:391-400.

83. Castillo SA, Pham AK, Dinulos JG. Cutaneous manifestations of systemic viral diseases in neonates: An update. *Curr Opin Pediatr*. 2017;29:240-248.

84. Dhar S, Dhar S. Disseminated neonatal herpes simplex: a rare entity. *Pediatr Dermatol*. 2000;17(4):330-332.

85. Jang KA, Kim SH, Choi JH, Sung KJ, Moon KC, Koh JK. Viral folliculitis on the face. *Br J Dermatol*. 2000;142(3):555-559.

86. Conlon JD, Drolet BA. Skin lesions in the neonate. *Pediatr Clin North Am*. 2004;51:863-888.

87. Tieu KD, Satter EK, Zaleski L, et al. Congenital cutaneous candidiasis in two full-term infants. *Pediatr Dermatol*. 2012;2:507-510.

88. Darmstadt GL, Dinulos JG, Miller Z. Congenital cutaneous candidiasis: clinical presentation, pathogenesis, and management guidelines. *Pediatrics*. 2000;105:438-444.

89. Wisuthsarewong W, Soongswang J, Chantorn R. Neonatal lupus erythematosus: clinical character, investigation and outcome. *Pediatr Dermatol*. 2011;28:115-121.

90. Hetem MB, Takada MH, Llorach Velludo MA, Foss NT. Neonatal lupus erythematosus. *Int J Dermatol*. 1996;35(1):42-44.

91. Lee LA. Neonatal lupus erythematosus. *J Invest Dermatol*. 1993;100(1):9S-13S.

92. Silverman E, Jaeggi E. Non-cardiac manifestations of neonatal lupus erythematosus. *Scand J Immunol*. 2010;72:223-225.

93. Lee L. The clinical spectrum of neonatal lupus. *Arch Dermatol Res*. 2009;301:107-110.

94. Guinovart R, Vicente A, Rovira C, et al. Facial telangiectasia: an unusual manifestation of neonatal lupus erythematosus. *Lupus*. 2012;21:552-555.

95. Lynn Cheng C, Galbraith S, Holland K. Congenital lupus erythematosus presenting at birth with widespread erosions, pancytopenia, and subsequent hepatobiliary disease. *Pediatr Dermatol*. 2010;27:109-111.

96. Heughan C, Kanigsberg N. Cutis marmorata telangiectatica congenita and neonatal lupus. *Pediatr Dermatol*. 2007;24:320-321.

97. Trevisan F, Cunha PR, Pinto CAL, et al. Cutaneous neonatal lupus with cutis marmorata telangiectatica congenita-like lesions. *An Bras Dermatol*. 2013;88:428-431.

98. Vílchez-Márquez F, Martín-Fuentes A, Conejero R, et al. Neonatal lupus erythematosus mimicking extensive capillary malformation. *Pediatr Dermatol*. 2013;30:495-497.

99. Monari P, Gualdi G, Fantini F, et al. Cutaneous neonatal lupus erythematosus in four siblings. *Br J Dermatol*. 2008;158:626-628.

100. Hornberger L, Al Rajaa N. Spectrum of cardiac involvement in neonatal lupus. *Scand J Immunol*. 2010;72:189-197.

101. Buyon J, Clancy R, Friedman D. Cardiac manifestations of neonatal lupus erythematosus: guidelines to management, integrating clues from the bench and bedside. *Nat Clin Pr Rheumatol*. 2009;5:139-148.

102. Dugan EM, Tunnessen WW, Honig PJ, Watson RM. U1RNP antibody-positive neonatal lupus. *Arch Dermatol*. 1992;128:1490-1494.

103. Kim K, Yoon T. A case of neonatal lupus erythematosus showing transient anemia and hepatitis. *Ann Dermatol*. 2009;21:315-318.

104. Kozlowski K, Basel D, Beighton P. Chondrodysplasia punctata in siblings and maternal lupus erythematosus. *Clin Genet*. 2004;66:545-549.

105. Peñate Y, Guillermo N, Rodríguez J, et al. Histopathologic characteristics of neonatal cutaneous lupus erythematosus: description of five cases and literature review. *J Cutan Pathol*. 2009;36(6):660-667.

106. Satter EK, High WA. Non-bullous neutrophilic dermatosis within neonatal lupus erythematosus. *J Cutan Pathol*. 2007;34(12):958-960.

107. Lee SH, Roh MR. Targetoid lesions and neutrophilic dermatosis: an initial clinical and histological presentation of neonatal lupus erythematosus. *Int J Dermatol*. 2014;53(6):764-766.

108. Paller A, Mancini A. Histiocytoses and malignant skin diseases. In: Paller A, Mancini A, eds. *Hurwitz Clinical Pediatric Dermatology*. 3rd ed. New York, NY: Elsevier Saunders; 2006:245-263.

109. Satter E, High W. Langerhans cell histiocytosis: a review of the current recommendations of the Histiocyte Society. *Pediatr Dermatol.* 2008;25:291-295.

110. Badalian-Very G, Vergilio J, Degar B, et al. Recent advances in the understanding of Langerhans cell histiocytosis. *Br J Haematol.* 2012;156:163-172.

111. Lieberman PH, Jones CR, Steinman RM, et al. Langerhans cell (eosinophilic) granulomatosis. A clinicopathologic study encompassing 50 years. *Am J Surg Pathol.* 1996;20(5):519-552.

112. Pileri SA, Grogan TM, Harris NL, et al. Tumours of histiocytes and accessory dendritic cells: an immunohistochemical approach to classification from the International Lymphoma Study Group based on 61 cases. *Histopathology.* 2002;41(1):1-29.

113. Picarsic J, Jaffe R. Nosology and pathology of Langerhans cell histiocytosis. *Hematol Oncol Clin North Am.* 2015;29(5):799-823.

114. Zunino-Goutorbe C, Eschard C, Durlach A, et al. Congenital solitary histiocytoma: a variant of Hashimoto-Pritzker histiocytosis. A retrospective study of 8 cases. *Dermatology.* 2008;216:118-124.

115. Zwerdling T, Konia T, Silverstein M. Congenital, single system, single site, Langerhans cell histiocytosis: a new case, observations from the literature, and management considerations. *Pediatr Dermatol.* 2009;26:121-126.

116. Papadopoulou M, Panagopoulou P, Papadopoulou A, et al. The multiple faces of Langerhans cell histiocytosis in childhood: a gentle reminder. *Mol Clin Oncol.* 2018;8:489-449.

117. Zinn DJ, Grimes AB, Lin H, Eckstein O, Allen CE, McClain KL, et al. Hydroxyurea: a new old therapy for Langerhans cell histiocytosis. *Blood.* 2016;128(20):2462-2465.

118. Risdall RJ, Dehner LP, Duray P, Kobrinsky N, Robison L, Nesbit ME Jr. Histiocytosis X (Langerhans' cell histiocytosis). Prognostic role of histopathology. *Arch Pathol Lab Med.* 1983;107(2):59-63.

119. Berlin A, Paller A, Chan L. Incontinentia pigmenti: a review and update on the molecular basis of pathophysiology. *J Am Acad Dermatol.* 2002;47:169-187.

120. Pacheco T, Levy M, Collyer J, et al. Incontinentia pigmenti in male patients. *J Am Acad Dermatol.* 2006;55:251-255.

121. Ehrenreich M, Tarlow MM, Godlewska-Janusz E, Schwartz RA. Incontinentia pigmenti (Bloch-Sulzberger syndrome): a systemic disorder. *Cutis.* 2007;79(5):355-362.

122. Hadj-Rabia S, Rimella A, Smahi A, et al. Clinical and histologic features of incontinentia pigmenti in adults with nuclear factor-κB essential modulator gene mutations. *J Am Acad Dermatol.* 2011;64(3):508-515.

123. Poziomczyk C, Recuero J, Bringhenti L, et al. Incontinentia pigmenti. *An Bras Dermatol.* 2014;89:26-36.

124. Dupati A, Egbers R, Helfrich Y. A case of incontinentia pigmenti reactivation after 12-month immunizations. *JAAD Case Rep.* 2015;27:351-352.

125. Hadj-Rabia S, Froidevaux D, Bodak N, et al. Clinical study of 40 cases of incontinentia pigmenti. *Arch Dermatol.* 2003;139:1163-1170.

126. Poziomczyk CS, Bonamigo RR, Santa Maria FD, Zen PR, Kiszewski AE. Clinical study of 20 patients with incontinentia pigmenti. *Int J Dermatol.* 2016;55(2):e87-e93.

127. Fraitag S, Rimella A, de Prost Y, Brousse N, Hadj-Rabia S, Bodemer C. Skin biopsy is helpful for the diagnosis of incontinentia pigmenti at late stage (IV): a series of 26 cutaneous biopsies. *J Cutan Pathol.* 2009;36(9):966-971.

128. Azaña JM, Torrelo A, Matito A. Update on mastocytosis (Part 1): pathophysiology, clinical features, and diagnosis. *Actas Dermosifiliogr.* 2016;107:5-14.

129. Castells M, Metcalfe DD, Escribano L. Diagnosis and treatment of cutaneous mastocytosis in children: Practical recommendations. *Am J Clin Dermatol.* 2011;12:259-270.

130. Ben-Amitai D, Metzker A, Cohen HA. Pediatric cutaneous mastocytosis: a review of 180 patients. *Isr Med Assoc J.* 2005;7:320-322.

131. Méni C, Bruneau J, Georgin-Lavialle S, et al. Paediatric mastocytosis: a systematic review of 1747 cases. *Br J Dermatol.* 2015;172:642-651.

132. Hartmann K, Escribano L, Grattan C, et al. Cutaneous manifestations in patients with mastocytosis: Consensus report of the European Competence Network on Mastocytosis; the American Academy of Allergy, Asthma & Immunology; and the European Academy of Allergology and Clinical Immunology. *J Allergy Clin Immunol.* 2016;137:35-45.

133. Lange M, Ługowska-Umer H, Niedoszytko M, et al. Diagnosis of mastocytosis in children and adults in daily clinical practice. *Acta Derm Venereol.* 2016;96:292-297.

134. Azaña JM, Torrelo A, Matito A. Update on mastocytosis (Part 2): categories, prognosis, and treatment. *Actas Dermosifiliogr.* 2016;107:15-22.

135. Tsuji T. Subcutaneous fat necrosis of the newborn: Light and electron microscopic studies. *Br J Dermatol.* 1976;95(4):407-416.

136. Tajirian A, Ross R, Zeikus P, Robinson-Bostom L. Subcutaneous fat necrosis of the newborn with eosinophilic granules. *J Cutan Pathol.* 2007;34(7):588-590.

137. Pasyk K. Subcutaneous fat necrosis of newborn infants (light and electron microscopic studies) [in Polish]. *Folia Med Cracov.* 1978;20(3):327-344.

138. Montes LF. Subcutaneous fat necrosis of the newborn with eosinophilic granules. *J Cutan Pathol.* 2008;35(7):699; author reply 700.

139. Friedman SJ, Winkelmann RK. Subcutaneous fat necrosis of the newborn: light, ultrastructural and histochemical microscopic studies. *J Cutan Pathol.* 1989;16(2):99-105.

140. Farinelli P, Gattoni M, Delrosso G, et al. Eosinophilic granules in subcutaneous fat necrosis of the newborn: what do they mean? *J Cutan Pathol.* 2008;35(11):1073-1074.

141. Ricardo-Gonzalez RR, Lin JR, Mathes EF, McCalmont TH, Pincus LB. Neutrophil-rich subcutaneous fat necrosis of the newborn: a potential mimic of infection. *J Am Acad Dermatol.* 2016;75(1):177-185 e17.

142. Epstein W, Kligman AM. The pathogenesis of milia and benign tumors of the skin. *J Invest Dermatol.* 1956;26(1):1-11.

143. Somer M, Peippo M, Aalto-Korte K, Ritvanen A, Niemi KM. Cardio-facio-cutaneous syndrome: three additional cases and review of the literature. *Am J Med Genet.* 1992;44(5):691-695.

144. Housholder AL, Plotner AN, Sheth AP. Multiple axillary papules in an infant. Diagnosis: Multiple congenital apocrine hidrocystomas. *Pediatr Dermatol.* 2013;30(4):491-492.

145. Engur D, Turkmen MK, Savk E. Widespread miliaria crystallina in a newborn with hypernatremic dehydration. *Pediatr Dermatol.* 2013;30(6):e234-e235.

146. Holzle E, Kligman AM. The pathogenesis of miliaria rubra. Role of the resident microflora. *Br J Dermatol.* 1978;99(2):117-137.

147. Straka BF, Cooper PH, Greer KE. Congenital miliaria crystallina. *Cutis.* 1991;47(2):103-106.

148. Doshi BR, Mahajan S, Kharkar V, Khopkar US. Granulomatous variant of giant central centrifugal miliaria profunda. *Pediatr Dermatol.* 2013;30(4):e48-e51.

149. Ferrándiz C, Coroleu W, Ribera M, Lorenzo JC, Natal A. Sterile transient neonatal pustulosis is a precocious form of erythema toxicum neonatorum. *Dermatology.* 1992;185(1):18-22.

150. Marchini G, Ulfgren AK, Loré K, Ståbi B, Berggren V, Lonne-Rahm S. Erythema toxicum neonatorum: an immunohistochemical analysis. *Pediatr Dermatol.* 2001;18(3):177-187.

3

Spongiotic, Psoriasiform, and Lichenoid Dermatoses

Laura E. K. Gifford / Emily J. Osier / Charlene W. Oldfield / Judith V. Williams / Alejandro A. Gru

ATOPIC DERMATITIS

Definition and Epidemiology

Atopic dermatitis is a chronic, relapsing inflammatory skin condition defined by pruritus.[1] The most widely used diagnostic criteria specify that a patient must have pruritus with an eczematous dermatitis of typical morphology and distribution, with a chronic and relapsing course. Additional diagnostic features include xerosis and additional signs of atopy such as asthma, allergic rhinitis, and food allergies.[2]

Atopic dermatitis affects between 10% and 27% of all children.[3,4] Initial presentation is in the first year of life in approximately 60% of patients,[3] with the vast majority, approximately 90%, presenting prior to 5 years of age.[1] Although many of these patients will outgrow their atopic dermatitis by adulthood, it persists in up to 30% into adulthood. A small percentage of affected adults initially develop atopic dermatitis during adulthood.[1] Persistent atopic dermatitis has been associated with comorbid atopic conditions and with a family history of atopy.[4]

Etiology

The etiology of atopic dermatitis is complex and is mediated by a combination of genetic and environmental factors. An estimated 70% of patients have a family history of atopy (atopic dermatitis, asthma, allergic rhinitis).[1] A recent genome-wide association study identified 136 genetic variants associated with atopic disease, including genes involved in epidermal barrier formation, immune dysregulation, and inflammation.[5,6] The Th2 cytokines, IL-4, IL-5 IL-13, IL-31, and CCL18, are often implicated, whereas some variants are associated with Th 1 cytokines IL-17, IL-22, and IL-23.[7]

Among the most well-characterized genetic risk factors for atopic dermatitis is *filaggrin* mutation. Loss-of-function mutations in this gene are seen in 10% to 50% of patients with atopic dermatitis.[5] Affected patients have decreased epidermal production of the profilaggrin protein, an important contributor to the hydration and barrier functions of the epidermis. Other proteins and lipids contributing to the hydration and barrier of the epidermis include loricrin, involucrin, ceramides, and cholesterols.[5] The resultant defective epidermal barrier increases water loss, allergen sensitization, and bacterial colonization with *Staphylococcus aureus*.[8] All of these factors, in combination with immune system variations, result in the development of atopic dermatitis.[8]

Up to 80% of patients with atopic dermatitis are colonized with *S. aureus*, compared with only 10% of nonatopic children.[9] The production of exotoxins by *S. aureus* influences the adaptive immune system, specifically increasing IL-22 and IL-31.[5] Increased IL-4, IL-13, and IL-22 levels potentiate colonization with *S. aureus*.[5] A decrease in the antimicrobial peptides, cathelicidin, and human beta-defensin-3, part of the innate immune system, further contributes to increased rates of *S. aureus* colonization.[10]

Clinical Presentation

The diagnosis of atopic dermatitis is based, in part, on a typical distribution. For newborns and infants, this includes the face, neck, and extensor extremities, and in older children and adults, the antecubital and popliteal fossae are commonly involved. The groin and axillae are typically spared.[2] Morphologically, the acute phase can present with vesicles and weeping plaques. Over time, the plaques become more lichenified and scaly (Figure 3-1).[1] Pruritus often leads to excoriations, erosions, and crusting. Variants include a papular variant resembling a lichenoid eruption and a follicular variant.[11] Associated clinical findings include cheilitis, nipple dermatitis, keratosis pilaris, hyperlinear palms, ichthyosis, follicular accentuation, facial pallor, and white dermatographism.[2] Asthma, allergic rhinosinusitis, and/or food allergies affect 70% to 80% of patients with atopic dermatitis.[12] This "atopic march" starts with atopic dermatitis, because the impaired epidermal barrier allows exposure and sensitization to both airborne and foodborne allergens.[12]

Histologic Findings

In the acute phase, the changes are usually subtle. Focal areas of parakeratosis overlie an epidermis with a mild degree of spongiosis. Scattered intraepidermal collections of Langerhans cells can be present. Within the dermis, there is a superficial and perivascular lymphocytic inflammatory infiltrate with variable numbers of scattered eosinophils (Figure 3-2). Follicular spongiosis can sometimes be seen,

a finding that has been encountered more frequently in dark-skinned individuals.[13-15]

In the chronic phase, the findings are typically nonspecific and correspond to those of a "chronic spongiotic dermatitis." There is epidermal hyperplasia with psoriasiform changes and larger areas of hyperkeratosis with parakeratosis (Figure 3-3). Lichen simplex chronicus (LSC)-like changes can be seen, with thick orthokeratotic hyperkeratosis, a thickened granular cell layer, and sometimes a zone of stratum lucidum at the base of the cornified layer. Dermal eosinophils can sometimes be seen, and a slight increased number of mast cells are found.

Differential Diagnosis

The histologic differential diagnosis for the spongiotic pattern is broad and requires adequate clinicopathologic correlation. Id reaction, allergic contact dermatitis (ACD), spongiotic drug eruptions, and nummular dermatitis may present with identical histologic features and should be included as histologic possibilities. Seborrheic dermatitis (SD) is also frequently encountered in children and can also be a mimicker. The location of the lesions, the presence of plasma cells, and perifollicular parakeratosis can be used to separate those apart.[13-15] Other conditions featuring spongiosis include pityriasis rosea and dermatophyte

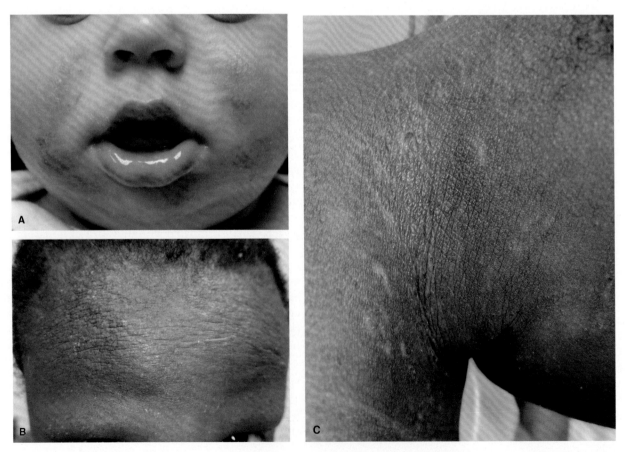

FIGURE 3-1. Infantile atopic dermatitis. A, Scaly, erythematous, eroded plaques on the cheeks. B and C, Chronic lichenified, and hyperpigmented plaques on the forehead and neck. Note loss of eyebrows due to chronic rubbing.

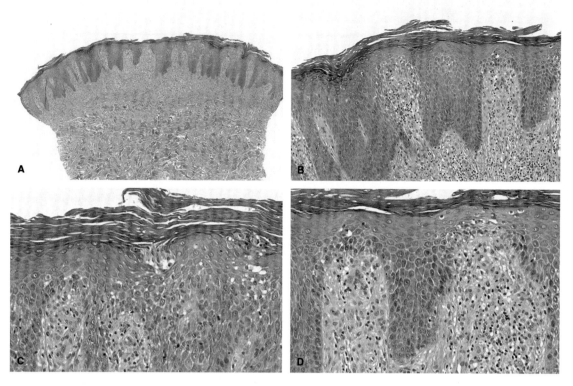

FIGURE 3-2. **Subacute spongiotic dermatitis.** A and B, Epidermal acanthosis and spongiosis. C, Clusters of Langerhans cells are noted. D, Lymphocyte exocytosis is present Digital slides courtesy of Path Presenter.com.

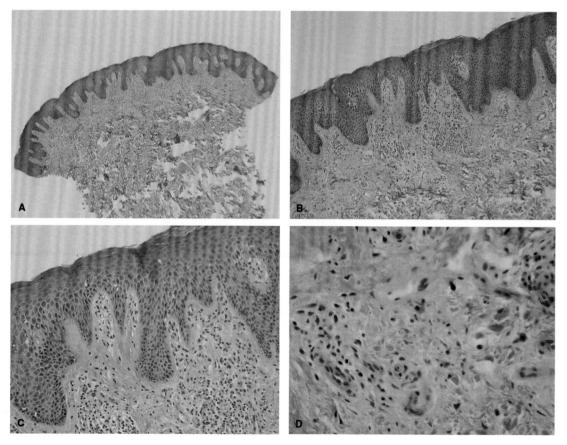

FIGURE 3-3. **Chronic spongiotic dermatitis (CSD).** A and B, In contrast to the acute phase, CSD shows more acanthosis and confluent parakeratosis on the surface. C, A mild degree of spongiosis is noted. D, Dermal pigment incontinence is present.

infection. Pityriasis rosea (PR) features mild spongiosis and mounds of parakeratosis, and dermatophyte infection may feature clusters of intraepidermal or intracorneal neutrophils. Routine performance of periodic acid–Schiff (PAS) or Grocott-Gomori's methenamine silver (GMS) staining in all biopsies of spongiotic dermatitis is common practice in some dermatopathology laboratories.

CAPSULE SUMMARY

ATOPIC DERMATITIS

Atopic dermatitis is a very common chronic, relapsing inflammatory skin condition characterized by pruritus, eczematous dermatitis, and a typical distribution. Affected children often outgrow atopic dermatitis, but there is a large percentage of patients in whom it persists in, or develops during, adulthood. The histologic findings are those of a spongiotic dermatitis, and clinical correlation is required to differentiate these findings from other primary spongiotic disorders such as Id reactions, ACD, and nummular dermatitis.

IRRITANT CONTACT DERMATITIS

Definition and Epidemiology

Irritant contact dermatitis (ICD) is an eczematous response to substances that are inherently irritating to the skin.[16] It does not require sensitization and may occur in anyone.[16]

ICD is very common. Although adults are often affected by occupational exposures, infants are at higher risk because of a weaker epidermal barrier.[17] Children under 3 years old have a lower threshold for irritation than adults, reacting more quickly and more intensely to irritants.[18]

Etiology

ICD is an "outside-in" dermatitis resulting from cytotoxic effects of irritants on the skin.[19] Contributing factors include the biology of the underlying skin, the location on the body, the strength of the irritant substance, and the duration of exposure. The homeostasis of the stratum corneum affects permeability and susceptibility to irritants.[20] Regional risk factors affecting this homeostasis include occlusion, maceration, and perspiration. Environmental factors, such as cold and humidity, both disrupt the homeostasis of the stratum corneum and may act as primary physical irritants.[20,21]

The irritant itself contributes to the speed and severity of the dermatitis; strong irritants act quickly, whereas weak irritants can require cumulative exposures.[19] Common irritants in children are soaps, bleach, detergent, disinfectants, solvent, acids, alkalis, bubble baths, foods, saliva, urine, feces, and metal salts.[16,19] Generally, alkalis are more caustic than acids.[20]

Clinical Presentation

Because of universal susceptibility for ICD, the presentation is highly variable and eruptions can be polymorphous.[16] Clinical findings include erythema, scale, edema, vesicles, erosions, fissuring, ulceration, folliculitis, and even bulla.[19,20] Areas are often sharply demarcated.[19] The most common sites of involvement are exposed areas, such as the hands and face, which are open to irritant exposure. The exception in children is the diaper area.[20,22,23]

The perioral region is frequently involved in infants and toddlers because of saliva and foods. Teething, pacifier use, and sucking on fingers are common predisposing factors.[16] Common culprit foods include citrus, carrots, shrimp, spinach/kale, corn, radish, mustard, garlic, onion, and pineapple.[16,19] Saliva exposure through lip licking is a common culprit in older children and adults.

Diaper or napkin dermatitis is most commonly caused by an ICD to urine and feces.[23] Basic excrement alters the normally acidic local pH, resulting in irritation, which is compounded by fecal proteases, lipases, and bacteria. Diaper dermatitis is typically found on the convex surfaces and perianally.[23] The gluteal cleft and inguinal creases are typically spared, although the perianal area can erode with prolonged contact with irritants.[23] The occlusive nature of the diaper/napkin amplifies the irritant effect.[22]

Different common irritants tend to cause ICD in different body locations. The dorsal hands, for example, are a hot spot for handwashing and hand-sanitizer ICD. In contrast, less than 4% of foot dermatitis is attributable to ICD, whereas nearly half of cases are caused by immunologically mediated ACD.[24] Shin guards, as worn in soccer and hockey, can cause both ICD related to trapped moisture and friction and ACD related to the materials from which the guard is made.[25,26] Infants with involvement of the bilateral elbows, upper posterior thighs, lower lateral legs, and a band-like distribution on the occipital scalp may develop ICD caused by sweat trapping related to shiny nylon-like car seat material in warmer months, with negative patch testing for relevant allergens.[27] Plaques on the posterior thighs and lower buttocks have been reported as pediatric positional sitting dermatitis, an ICD secondary to sitting cross-legged.[28] Pustular ICD on the eyelids has been reported in an 8-year-old because of dexpanthenol, a known irritant in cosmetics.[29]

Many unique irritants have been reported in children. Epidemics of fiberglass dermatitis have been reported in classrooms related to desks and airborne irritation.[30] The methylphenidate patch commonly used for attention deficit hyperactivity disorder is a relatively common cause of ICD, which can be controlled by rotating patch sites (Figure 3-4).[31] Black henna, a common cause of ACD to paraphenylene diamine, has also been reported to cause ICD, with secondary postinflammatory hypopigmentation in a 10-year-old.[32] Other reported causes include topical lidocaine/prilocaine (EMLA), green walnut (*Juglans regia*) shell and husk, and rove beetle (*Paederus*) toxin.[33-36]

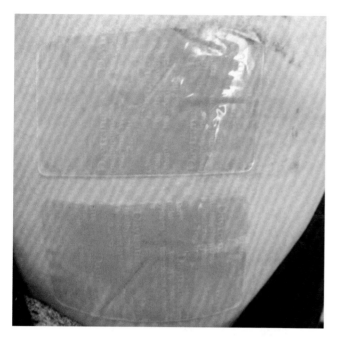

FIGURE 3-4. Irritant contact dermatitis to methylphenidate patches.

Histologic Findings

The pathologic findings depend on the potency of the irritant and the extent of exposure. Strong irritants can cause confluent epidermal necrosis with "ghost" nuclei caused by the loss of nuclear basophilia, either within the superficial epidermis or its full thickness. Epidermal spongiosis is a common finding. Dermal eosinophils may be present (Figure 3-5).[37,38]

Differential Diagnosis

In general, the differential diagnosis for ICD overlaps with that of spongiotic dermatitis, as discussed previously for atopic dermatitis. The presence of epidermal necrosis should prompt a consideration of interface dermatitis as well. However, in IDC, the injury results from external factors, and so vacuolar degeneration of the basal keratinocytes is absent. Single necrotic keratinocytes at the junction may also reflect wound healing from trauma induced externally.

CAPSULE SUMMARY

IRRITANT CONTACT DERMATITIS

ICD is a very common result of exposure to compounds that are inherently irritating and cytotoxic to the skin. Although adults are often affected by occupational exposures, infants are at high risk because of a weaker epidermal barrier. Presentations include erythema, scale, edema, vesicles, erosions, fissure, ulceration, folliculitis, and even bulla. The histologic changes are those of a spongiotic dermatitis with the presence of necrotic keratinocytes that result from the external damage.

ALLERGIC CONTACT DERMATITIS

Definition and Epidemiology

ACD is an immunologically mediated eczematous dermatitis that results from contact sensitization with a low-molecular-weight chemical or metal ion and subsequent reexposure leading to a type IV delayed hypersensitivity reaction.[39,40] Approximately 20% of people experience contact

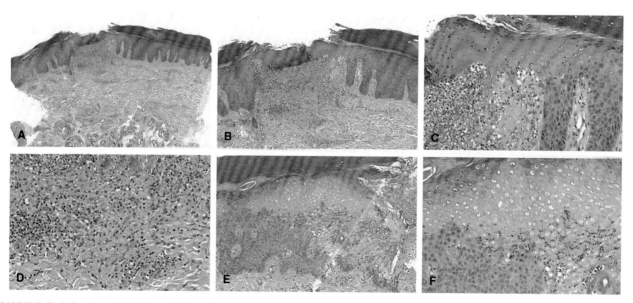

FIGURE 3-5. Irritant contact dermatitis. A-C, A localized area of epidermal necrosis is noted. D, A mixed dermal inflammation containing neutrophils is present. E and F, The areas of contact between the irritant and the epidermis show necrotic and "ghost" cells. Digital slides courtesy of Path Presenter.com.

sensitization to cutaneous or mucosal exposures, with up to 18% going on to develop ACD.[39-42] Up to 42% of children with atopic dermatitis also have ACD.[43]

Etiology

ACD is a type IV delayed hypersensitivity reaction occurring on the mucosa or skin.[39,42,43] Asymptomatic contact sensitization occurs 10 to 15 days after initial exposure to an allergen, with subsequent exposure eliciting a reaction after 72 to 96 hours.[39,40]

Contact sensitizers are polar, low-molecular-weight substances.[39-41] After penetration of the epidermal barrier, sensitizers bind with endogenous proteins, creating a complex that activates the innate immune system.[39,41] Pattern recognition receptors including Toll-like receptors 2 and 4 are activated, resulting in the activation of dendritic cells.[39,41] Mast cells, neutrophils, and natural killer cells support the sensitization response.[41] Activated dendritic cells migrate through the lymphatics to activate both regulatory and effector T cells in lymph nodes. The balance between these subsets determines susceptibility to future allergic response versus the development of tolerance. Susceptible individuals are characterized by a Th2 skewed response and subsequent inflammation.[39,44]

Although mild atopic dermatitis may be a risk factor for developing ACD, particularly to nickel,[45] some studies suggest that patients with moderate to severe atopic dermatitis may have decreased rates of ACD related to alterations in the Th1/Th2 balance.[43] The most frequent contact allergens for children, after *Toxicodendron* species (poison ivy, oak, and sumac),[46] are nickel, fragrance, Balsam of Peru, bacitracin, formaldehyde, cocamidopropyl betaine, propylene glycol, wool alcohol, lanolin, and bronopol.[43]

Clinical Presentation

Morphologically, ACD may appear similar to atopic dermatitis. Patients develop pink to erythematous, pruritic, scaly eczematous papules and plaques. Vesicles may be present acutely, whereas lichenification and fissures may be seen with chronic exposures.[45,47] The diagnosis should be suspected when the eruption shows linearity, sharp cutoffs, odd/geometric shapes, or other atypical distributions of eczematous dermatitis indicating that something external interacted with the skin.[45,47] For example, several cases of ACD to para-phenylenediamine, a dye added to make "black" henna temporary tattoos, have been reported, with the pattern of dermatitis appearing in the shape of the tattoo (Figure 3-6).[48] Another classic example presents with linear arrays of bullae on the lower legs, after brushing by poison ivy during a hike, caused by exposure to the potent contact allergen urushiol. Other typical patterns of ACD include nickel allergy on the abdomen where belts and buckles come in contact with the skin (Figure 3-7),[45] diaper wipe dermatitis to methylchloroisothiazolinone or

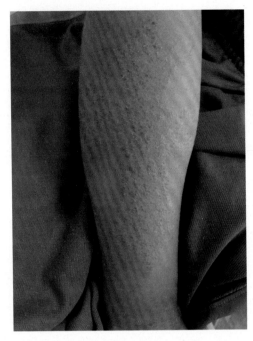

FIGURE 3-6. Allergic contact dermatitis caused by paraphenylene diamine in a black henna tattoo.

methylisothiazolinone, presenting with recalcitrant diaper dermatitis,[49] and shin guard dermatitis to adhesives and rubbers.[25] Without an obvious external exposure pattern, the diagnosis of ACD can be challenging to differentiate from atopic dermatitis, because many patients are affected with both.[47] Additionally, children are more likely to have a scattered and generalized pattern of dermatitis.[43,45,50]

Systemic contact dermatitis is a generalized, diffuse presentation of dermatitis after a noncutaneous exposure to an allergen.[51,52] The exposure is typically by ingestion but can be by parenteral exposure. Balsam of Peru is a tree resin

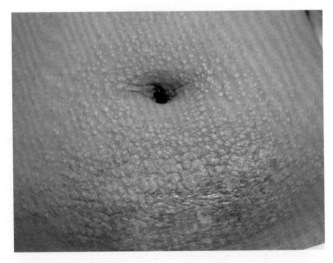

FIGURE 3-7. Allergic contact dermatitis to nickel on the lower abdomen, from the contact with the metal snap on the inside of pants, or a belt buckle. There is secondary lichen simplex chronicus change.

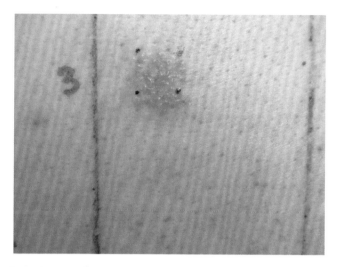

FIGURE 3-8. Positive patch test: bacitracin.

used in fragrances with significant cross-reactivity with tomato, cinnamon, clove, and orange peel. Ingestion of these foods has been implicated in several cases of systemic contact dermatitis.[51,52] Nickel in the diet, in the form of chocolate, oats, legumes, canned foods, and other items, can lead to systemic contact dermatitis as well and often improves with a nickel-free diet.[53]

The diagnosis of ACD is made by patch testing. This process involves applying known contact allergens to the skin for 48 hours under occlusion and evaluating for a localized, inflammatory response such as induration or vesiculation at 48 and 96 hours (Figure 3-8).[54] Correlation of patch testing results with clinical findings is important to determine the relevance of positives, because testing may reveal prior sensitization to substances with which patients do not regularly come into contact.

Histologic Findings

The main pathologic change in ACD is spongiotic dermatitis with frequent epidermal Langerhans cells microabscesses, typically accompanied by a superficial perivascular lymphocytic inflammatory infiltrate with eosinophils. In very florid cases, spongiosis can lead to intraepidermal vesiculation as seen in dyshidrotic eczema (seen on volar skin) and severe acute ACD (as frequently seen in exposure to poison ivy). The dermal eosinophils can also extend into the surface epidermis (eosinophilic spongiosis) (Figure 3-9). The inflammation does not extend to the deeper portions of the biopsy. Scattered dermal neutrophils can also be present, in addition to superficially papillary dermal edema. Chronic photoallergic contact dermatitis, in which contactants

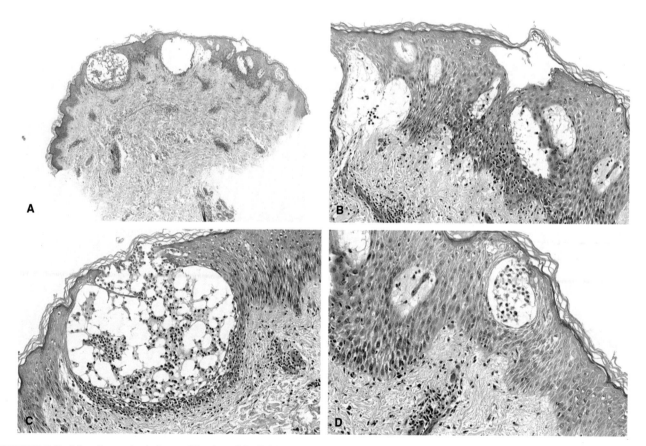

FIGURE 3-9. **Allergic contact dermatitis.** A and B, Epidermal acanthosis and spongiosis with intraepidermal vesicle formation. C, The vesicles contain neutrophils and some eosinophils. D, Collections of Langerhans cells are seen. Digital slides courtesy of Path Presenter.com.

become allergenic only after exposure to sunlight, can show deep perivascular inflammation. Variants of ACD include urticarial (eg, latex), systemic, pustular (eg, cement), purpuric (eg, textile dyes), granulomatous (eg, gold), lymphomatoid (eg, nickel), and chronic dermatitis with prominent postinflammatory hypopigmentation (leukodermic forms).[38,55,56]

Differential Diagnosis

The histologic differential diagnosis is identical to that of atopic dermatitis, as described earlier, and includes atopic dermatitis, Id reaction, nummular dermatitis, and other causes of spongiotic dermatitis.

CAPSULE SUMMARY

ALLERGIC CONTACT DERMATITIS

ACD is an eczematous dermatitis resulting from a type IV delayed hypersensitivity reaction to a substance to which an individual has been previously sensitized. It may appear clinically similar to atopic dermatitis, presenting with pink to erythematous, pruritic, scaly papules and plaques overlying an erythematous base. Vesicles may be present acutely, whereas lichenification and fissures may be seen in chronic exposures. The pathologic findings include epidermal spongiosis and dermal eosinophils accompanying superficial dermal perivascular lymphocytic inflammation.

SEBORRHEIC DERMATITIS

Definition and Epidemiology

Seborrheic dermatitis (SD) is an eczematous dermatitis that is typically seen in infancy and may reappear starting in adolescence.[16] Onset of infantile SD most commonly occurs during the 3rd and 4th weeks of life (with a range of 2-10 weeks of age) and peaks in incidence around 3 months of age.[57] Resolution can sometimes be seen as quickly as 3 to 4 weeks after onset, but findings may persist until 8 to 12 months of age. In adolescence, onset is typically seen around puberty.[16]

Etiology

Although sebaceous gland involvement has been implicated in its development given its distribution in sebaceous gland–rich locations, the exact etiology of SD is unclear and varies with age of onset. *Pityrosporum ovale (Malassezia ovalis)* is a contributor to SD of adolescence and adulthood, but its role in infantile disease has been debated.[58-60] The strong association between infantile SD and the later development of atopic dermatitis[61] has led many to consider them on a clinical spectrum.[62]

Clinical Presentation

Infantile SD begins as thin dry scaling of the scalp, commonly referred to as "cradle cap" (Figure 3-10). Although isolated scalp involvement is most commonly seen, the diaper area may be affected, with the development of well-marginated, salmon-colored plaques with thick, yellow-brown, greasy crust, and may be complicated by bacterial and candidal infections.[16] Involvement may progress to a more typical "seborrheic" distribution including the forehead, ears, eyebrows, nose, occiput, and intertriginous and flexural areas. Pruritus, if present, is usually mild.[16] Adolescent SD is similar in presentation to adult disease and is characterized by fine, dry scalp desquamation, commonly referred to as dandruff (Figure 3-11). Inflammation of varying degrees commonly affects the skin in a seborrheic distribution.[16] Unlike infantile disease, the eyes can also be affected, where blepharitis presents with erythema and scaling of the lid margins, and tends to be more chronic and recurrent in nature.[16]

Histologic Findings

SD shows characteristically a spongiotic or psoriasiform and spongiotic pattern in the epidermis. The classic feature associated with SD is the presence of parakeratosis in the outflow tracts of the hair follicles (also called "shouldering" parakeratosis). Small clusters of neutrophils in the epidermis can be seen, often within the stratum corneum. The epidermis shows psoriasiform elongation of the rete pegs and focal hypogranulosis in most cases. Mild intraepidermal spongiosis is noted (Figure 3-12). The latter is more typically seen in the areas around the hair follicles. Papillary dermal edema and superficial vascular dilatation can

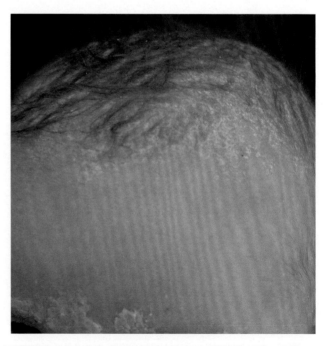

FIGURE 3-10. Infantile seborrheic dermatitis ("cradle cap").

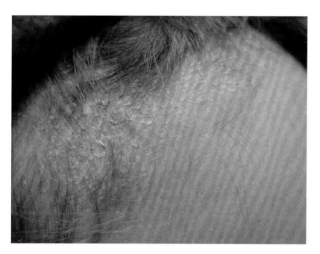

FIGURE 3-11. Childhood seborrheic dermatitis, scalp.

CAPSULE SUMMARY

SEBORRHEIC DERMATITIS

SD is an eczematous dermatitis that, within the pediatric population, is typically seen in infancy and adolescence. Although typically isolated to the scalp in infants (cradle cap), it may appear on other typical seborrheic locations such as the face, chest, and intertriginous areas, as well as the diaper area. Histologically, it is characterized by a spongiotic or psoriasiform and spongiotic pattern in the epidermis. The classic feature associated with SD is the presence of parakeratosis in the outflow tracts of the hair follicles (also called "shouldering" parakeratosis).

also be noted. Within the dermis, there is a superficial to mid-dermal, perivascular but more typically perifollicular chronic inflammatory infiltrate composed of lymphocytes, histiocytes, and scattered neutrophils. Plasma cells can also be seen. Colonization by *Pityrosporum* yeast forms is present within the follicular keratin and stratum corneum.[63]

Differential Diagnosis

The main differential diagnosis is between SD and psoriasis. Psoriasis shares the epidermal changes seen in SD. However, broader areas of parakeratosis and hypogranulosis are features more typical in the setting of psoriasis. SD also has a larger amount of intraepidermal spongiosis. Other forms of spongiotic dermatoses (previously described) should also be included in the differential diagnosis.

PITYRIASIS ALBA

Definition and Epidemiology

Pityriasis alba (PA) is a mild eczematous eruption that typically results in residual postinflammatory

hypopigmentation.[16] Its overall incidence in the pediatric population ranges from 1.9% to 5.2%, but is more frequently seen in children with darker skin types. Age of onset is typically between 3 and 16 years.[64]

Etiology

The exact etiology of PA is unclear. It has been postulated that PA is a minor form of atopic dermatitis[20,65,66] and is associated with overexposure to light,[67,68] personal hygiene practices such as long and frequent bathing and mechanical exfoliation,[68,69] microbiologic factors such as *Malassezia furfur, S. aureus,* and *Propionibacterium acnes*[64] colonization, and even low serum copper levels.[70]

Clinical Presentation

Clinically, PA is considered to be a chronic condition with multiple stages typically involving the upper body, most notably the face. Initially, erythematous changes with uplifted edges may be seen, which, upon resolution, leave hypopigmentation and fine scale (Figure 3-13). Lesions can be associated with pruritus and range in size from 0.5 to 5

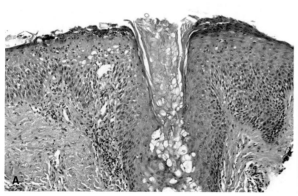
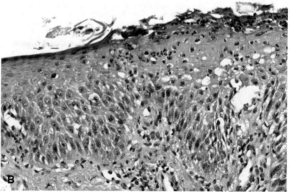

FIGURE 3-12. **Seborrheic dermatitis.** A, Acanthosis and spongiosis with "shouldering" parakeratosis around the hair follicles. B, Clusters of intracorneal and intraepidermal neutrophils are seen. Digital slides courtesy of Path Presenter.com.

cm that may resolve spontaneously or persist for months to years, and can recur.[64,69,71]

Three clinical variants of PA have been described—classic (CPA), extensive (EPA), and pigmenting (PPA). CPA is the most common form, presenting with well-defined hypopigmented patches of the lips, chin, and cheeks with scaling borders in primary school–aged children.[64] Of the three variants, CPA has the shortest course and is most responsive to treatment.[72] EPA is similar in presentation, but the individual lesions tend to be symmetric and larger (>2.0 cm) and involve the neck, trunk, shoulders, and extensor surfaces of upper extremities in teenagers and young adults, particularly females.[73,74] PPA is the least common variant and is notable among non-Caucasian individuals of the Republic of South Africa and the Middle East.[75,76] In fact, there are no documented cases within the Caucasian population. It presents with approximately 1.5 cm bluish patches with a surrounding hypopigmented halo typically involving the forehead and cheeks of females during childhood and adolescence.[64,75,77,78] PPA has been associated with mycotic infections and can coexist with CPA.[75]

Histologic Findings

The pathologic findings are relatively nonspecific. There is a mild degree of epidermal spongiosis with hyperkeratosis and areas of parakeratosis. Follicular plugging can be sometimes present. Atrophic sebaceous glands have been reported in some patients. Within the dermis, there is a superficial and perivascular lymphocytic infiltrate with focal exocytosis into the epidermis. The more characteristic finding is the presence of decreased melanin pigment in the epidermis, with normal numbers of melanocytes.

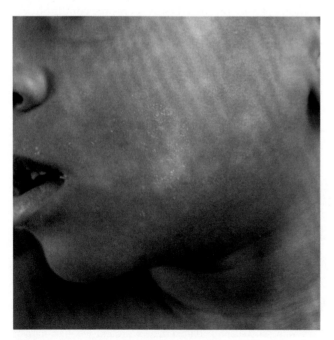

FIGURE 3-13. **Pityriasis alba.** Hypopigmented patches with fine overlying scale and minimal erythema.

Residual melanocytes within the affected areas demonstrate a decreased number of melanosomes on ultrastructural studies.[73,79-81]

Differential Diagnosis

The main clinical differential diagnoses are vitiligo and tinea versicolor. Histologically, the presence of superficial scale is a useful clue to distinguish PA from vitiligo (which is usually nonscaling). In addition, vitiligo shows absence of melanocytes within the hypopigmented patches (as opposed to the more preserved number of cells in PA). Pityriasis versicolor can be easily distinguished from PA on the basis of the presence of fungal organisms in the stratum corneum with the use of PAS or GMS stains.

CAPSULE SUMMARY

PITYRIASIS ALBA

PA is a mild eruption, often associated with residual postinflammatory hypopigmentation, most typically involving the upper body, most notably the face, and presenting as variably dyspigmented patches with fine scale. The pathologic findings are relatively nonspecific and include a mild degree of epidermal spongiosis with hyperkeratosis and areas of parakeratosis. The more characteristic finding is the presence of decreased melanin pigment in the epidermis with a relative sparing of the number of intraepidermal melanocytes.

JOB SYNDROME

Definition and Epidemiology

Job syndrome, or autosomal dominant hyperimmunoglobulinemia E syndrome (AD-HIES), is a rare primary immunodeficiency disorder characterized by elevated immunoglobulin E (IgE) (>2000 IU/mL), eczematous eruptions, and abscesses and sinopulmonary infections.[16] Onset of cutaneous symptoms can be seen as early as the neonatal period or infancy, with recurrent infections beginning as early as 3 months of age.[16]

Etiology

Job syndrome is associated with mutations in *STAT3*, which is integral to multiple cytokines' signal transduction, particularly Th17 and CD4. These mutations result in a failure of Th17 and CD4 differentiation, leading to increased susceptibility to various infections such as *S. aureus*,[82-85] mucosal candidiasis,[86-89] and lung and cutaneous infections.[89,90] Nonimmunologic abnormalities such as supernumerary teeth, delayed tooth eruption, and craniosynostosis are thought to be a consequence of impaired IL-11 signaling secondary to missense mutations in Arg296Trp, resulting in an impaired stimulation of STAT3.[91]

Clinical Presentation

Clinically, Job syndrome can have a wide phenotypic presentation because of the pleiotrophic effects of STAT3. Immunologic abnormalities can present within the first few weeks of life and even at birth. Typically, this is seen as an eczematous or pustular eruption of the face and scalp,[92,93] which can progress to an eczematoid dermatitis (Figure 3-14). *S. aureus* is implicated as a driving force behind the eruption.[94,95] Recurrent sinopulmonary infections are commonly seen, with the majority of patients experiencing at least one episode of pneumonia and more than 50% experiencing three or more episodes. Causative organisms can include *S. aureus, Streptococcus pneumoniae,* and less frequently, *Haemophilus* species.[96-98] Subsequent aberrant healing, in the form of pneumatoceles and bronchiectasis, is seen in up to 75% of patients.[95] Causative agents are similar to those associated with cystic fibrosis, making treatment difficult and resulting in significant morbidity and mortality.[95,99] Fungal infections, specifically chronic oral candidiasis, are seen in up to 80% of patients.[95] Lastly, "cold abscesses," or boils and furuncles lacking in erythema and warmth, are an almost universal feature of Job syndrome.[100] Patients with Job syndrome also have a higher incidence of malignancy, specifically non-Hodgkin lymphoma.[101-103]

Nonimmunologic features, including craniofacial, musculoskeletal, dental, and vascular abnormalities, can also be seen. Characteristic facies present in late childhood and early adolescence, including increased interalar distance, prominent forehead and chin, coarse skin, and facial asymmetry.[96,104] Musculoskeletal abnormalities include scoliosis, joint hyperextensibility, early development of degenerative joint disease, and minimal trauma fractures.[96,98] Oral and dental abnormalities, such as retention of primary teeth (often three or more), are seen in approximately 70% of patients,[95] and almost all patients demonstrate a high-arched palate with central ridging and fissuring of the palate and buccal mucosa.[105] Vascular abnormalities have been more recently identified and can include aneurysms of middle-sized arteries, lacunar infarcts, and hypertension in the absence of atherosclerosis.[95]

Histologic Findings

The pathologic findings in Job syndrome are those of a spongiotic dermatitis with dermal and/or intraepidermal eosinophils. There is hyperkeratosis with areas of parakeratosis and a small serum crust. There is epidermal acanthosis and spongiosis. A superficial and perivascular lymphocytic infiltrate is present, which sometimes extends to the epidermis (exocytosis). In some cases, an eosinophilic pustular folliculitis (resembling the eosinophilic folliculitis in newborns) can be seen. At the time of birth, many patients show a pustular eruption that is more pronounced in the face and contains abundant eosinophils on the biopsy. However, such changes resolve rapidly, and the more classic spongiotic pattern develops.[92,106]

Differential Diagnosis

As with other forms of spongiotic dermatitis, the differential diagnosis overlaps with that of eczema, contact dermatitis, atopic dermatitis, and others (previously discussed). Eosinophilic folliculitis can also be considered in the differential diagnosis, particularly in those acute presentations after birth.

CAPSULE SUMMARY

JOB SYNDROME, OR AUTOSOMAL DOMINANT HYPERIMMUNOGLOBULINEMIA E SYNDROME

AD-HIES is a rare primary immunodeficiency disorder characterized by elevated IgE (>2000 IU/mL), recurrent eczematous eruptions, abscesses, and sinopulmonary infections. Immunologic abnormalities can present within the first few weeks of life and even at birth. Typically, this is seen as an eczematous or pustular eruption of the face and scalp, which can progress to an eczematoid dermatitis. The pathologic findings in Job syndrome are those of a spongiotic dermatitis with dermal and/or intraepidermal eosinophils.

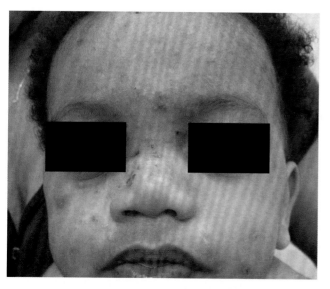

FIGURE 3-14. Job syndrome. Pustules and thin eczematous papules and plaques on the face. Courtesy of Barrett Zlotoff, MD.

JUVENILE PLANTAR DERMATOSIS

Definition and Epidemiology

Juvenile plantar dermatosis (JPD) is a very common scaling and fissuring dermatitis of infancy and childhood, localized to the distal aspects of the plantar surfaces.[16,107] It is seen more commonly among atopic children[16,107,108] and can be associated with hyperhidrosis.[16] Onset is generally between 3 and 14 years old.[107]

Etiology

The etiology of JPD is not fully understood, but is thought to represent frictional irritant dermatitis secondary to repeated maceration and subsequent drying, which results in impairment of the epidermis.[16,107]

Clinical Presentation

Clinically, JPD appears as symmetric, shiny erythematous plantar skin and toes, particularly of the great toes (Figure 3-15). There is notable sparing of the arches and interdigital web spaces. Scaling and fissuring can be seen, and if chronic, can become lichenified.[16,107] There are reports of similar cutaneous changes of the fingertips in 5% of patients with palmar hyperhidrosis.[16] JPD can persist for several years if left untreated, and flaring can be precipitated by heat, sweating, or friction secondary to socks and/or occlusive footwear.[16,107]

Histologic Findings

The pathologic findings are those of a subacute or chronic spongiotic dermatitis. Some patients can also have a spongiotic and psoriasiform pattern. A distinctive feature of JPD is the presence of perieccrine lymphocytic inflammation (Figure 3-16). The inflammation of the acrosyringium or the eccrine sweat duct at its epidermal starting edge tends to be present in the most typical clinical picture of JPD.[109,110]

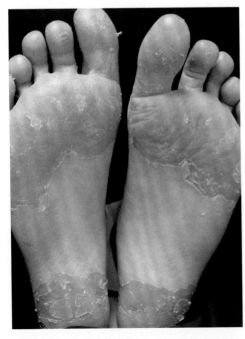

FIGURE 3-15. Juvenile plantar dermatosis. Erythema and desquamative scale over the plantar surfaces of the feet.

Differential Diagnosis

The differential diagnosis includes other entities with spongiotic tissue reactions. The presence of perieccrine inflammation can also be seen in lichen striatus. However, the blaschkoid distribution of the clinical lesions and the presence of interface changes in lichen striatus can easily distinguish those conditions.

CAPSULE SUMMARY

JUVENILE PLANTAR DERMATOSIS

JPD is a very common scaling and fissuring dermatitis of infancy and childhood, localized to the distal aspects of the plantar surfaces of the feet. Clinically, JPD will manifest as symmetric, shiny erythematous plantar skin and toes, particularly of the great toes. There is notable sparing of the arches and interdigital web spaces. The pathologic findings are those of a subacute or chronic spongiotic dermatitis. A distinctive feature of JPD is the presence of perieccrine inflammation.

LICHEN SIMPLEX CHRONICUS

Definition and Epidemiology

Lichen simplex chronicus (LSC) (also known as atopic or circumscribed neurodermatitis) is a chronic, pruritic dermatosis localized to the areas of habitual rubbing, scratching, and, less commonly, picking.[16,111]

The incidence of LSC increases with age, and patients are most likely to be adolescents or adults.[16,112] Pediatric LSC may have a slight male predominance.[111] When present in children, LSC is usually caused by underlying pruritic skin disease, such as atopic dermatitis, or by a tendency toward repetitive behaviors.[20,113] Anxiety disorders, such as obsessive–compulsive disorders and autism spectrum disorders, have characteristic repetitive behaviors that are potentially self-injurious; these behaviors often arise out of psychological distress and predispose patients to LSC.[20,113,114]

Etiology

LSC represents reactive epidermal hypertrophy in response to repetitive focal skin trauma or manipulation.[20]

Clinical Presentation

Early LSC has erythematous, slightly edematous, scaling plaques with accentuated skin markings.[16] Over time, these evolve into well-demarcated, dry, thickened plaques with a leathery appearance (Figure 3-17).[16,20,111] They can be hyperpigmented or hypopigmented over time, even developing a white hue in moist areas.[16,20,111] Excoriation may be noted.[111] LSC can arise de novo in normal skin or in areas of primary pruritic dermatoses, such as atopic dermatitis, SD, psoriasis,

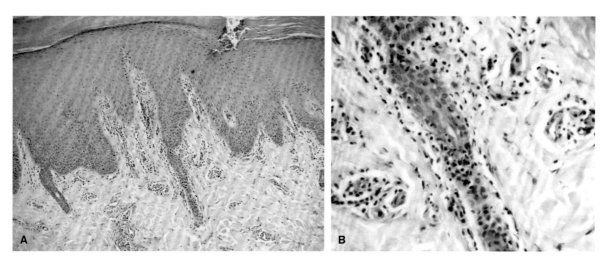

FIGURE 3-16. **Juvenile plantar dermatosis.** A, Hyperkeratosis with parakeratosis, acanthosis, mononuclear dermal infiltrate inflammatory in the superficial dermis. B, Exocytosis of lymphocytes at the point of entry of the eccrine duct into epidermis topography. With permission from Zagne V, Fernandes NC, Cuzzi T. Histopathological aspects of juvenile plantar dermatosis. *Am J Dermatopathol.* 2014;36(4):359-361.

or lichen planus (LP). LSC is usually located in areas that are easily reached and can be inconspicuously scratched: the neck, wrist, ankles, hands, forearms, and pretibial shins.[16,20] When involving the anogenital region, LSC is usually symmetric and favors the labia majora, scrotum, or perianal area.[111] The diagnosis is made clinically on the basis of lichenified plaques with severe pruritus and a history of scratching/rubbing.[16,111]

Histologic Findings

LSC and prurigo nodularis ("picker's nodules") are considered as two ends of the spectrum of clinical lesions that range from a plaque (LSC) to a nodule (PN). Pathologically, there is

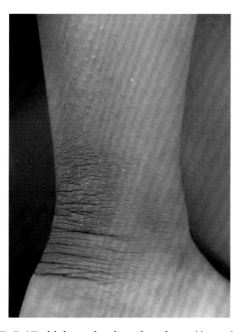

FIGURE 3-17. **Lichen simplex chronicus.** Hyperpigmented, lichenified plaque at the site of chronic rubbing.

compact hyperkeratosis, often without significant parakeratosis (Figure 3-18). The epidermis is acanthotic, with irregular or regular elongation of the rete pegs in a psoriasiform pattern. A mild degree of epidermal spongiosis can be noted. The granular cell layer is thickened, and there is usually a zone of stratum lucidum between the epidermis and the stratum corneum. In cases of continuous exogenous trauma, scattered apoptotic keratinocytes can be present. There is superficial papillary dermal fibrosis with vertically oriented collagen bundles extending from the superficial vascular plexus to the epidermis. A mild superficial perivascular lymphohistiocytic inflammatory infiltrate is seen, with or without dermal eosinophils. Neural hypertrophy has been described in LSC. LSC typically has a flat epidermal surface. Its counterpart PN shows a gradient of crescendo/decrescendo acanthosis. Epidermal excoriation can also be seen.[115-119]

Differential Diagnosis

The differential diagnosis includes psoriasis, tinea infection, LP, epidermal nevus, and verruca vulgaris. LSC and psoriasis can share the epidermal acanthosis and regular elongation of the rete. However, as opposed to LSC, the granular cell layer is markedly diminished in psoriasis. In addition, clusters of neutrophils in the epidermis and stratum corneum are seen in psoriasis, but not in LSC. LP can share the hyperkeratosis and thickening of the granular cell layer seen in LSC, but the epidermis shows more irregular acanthosis ("sawtooth" pattern). In addition, the band-like infiltration of lymphocytes obscuring the dermal–epidermal junction and interface changes are not seen in LSC. Verruca vulgaris may also be considered. Warts have viral cytopathic changes, columns of parakeratosis, and intracorneal hemorrhage. Epidermal nevi can also look similar to LSC, but lack the dermal fibrosi of LSC. Tinea can easily be excluded using special stains (which are often advocated to be performed in all cases of LSC).

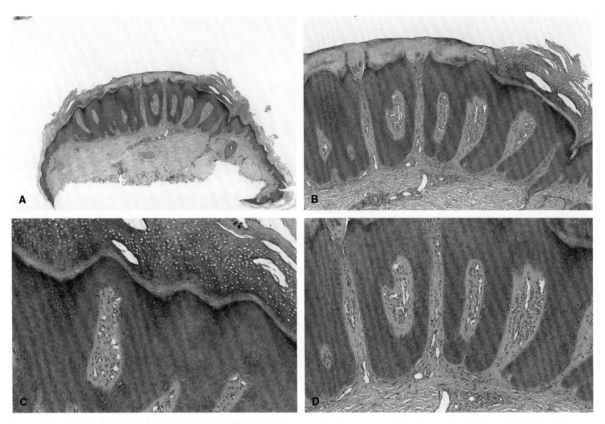

FIGURE 3-18. **Lichen simplex chronicus (LSC).** Epidermal acanthosis with a psoriasiform pattern (A and B). The arrows highlight the stratum lucidum typical of LSC. Hypergranulosis and superficial fibrosis with vertical streaks of collagen are seen (C and D). Digital slides courtesy of Path Presenter.com.

CAPSULE SUMMARY

LICHEN SIMPLEX CHRONICUS

LSC (also known as atopic or circumscribed neurodermatitis) is a chronic, pruritic dermatosis localized to the areas of habitual rubbing, scratching, and picking. It typically presents with erythematous, slightly edematous, scaling plaques with accentuated skin markings. Pathologically, LSC shows psoriasiform acanthosis, hypergranulosis, a stratum lucidum, and superficial dermal fibroplasia with vertical orientation to the epidermis.

POLYMORPHOUS LIGHT ERUPTION

Definition and Epidemiology

Polymorphous light eruption (PMLE) is the most common idiopathic photosensitive disorder. It is characterized by recurrent cutaneous reactions following exposure to natural or artificial ultraviolet (UV) radiation. Sensitivity occurs commonly to the UVA and/or UVB spectrum,[120] but occasionally to visible light as well.[121] These reactions, usually seen in spring or early summer, develop minutes to hours after exposure and can last for 1 to 2 weeks afterward.

PMLE has a slight female predominance and is more common in the 2nd to 3rd decades of life. It has a higher incidence in populations living at higher latitudes and elevations. Juvenile spring eruption, a subset of PMLE, is seen in children between 5 and 12 years of age and occurs more often in boys than in girls.

Etiology

The etiology of PMLE has not been fully elucidated. Proposed mechanisms include a delayed-type hypersensitivity reaction to endogenous cutaneous photo-induced antigens and abnormal UV-induced immunosuppression.[122] Photohardening studies suggest that decreased levels of regulatory T cells, mast cells, and epidermal Langerhans cells may play a role in the pathogenesis of PMLE.[123]

Clinical Presentation

PMLE, as the name implies, may present with a variety of findings, from erythematous nonscarring papules or vesicles to urticarial or erythema multiforme (EM)-like papules or plaques on exposed surfaces (Figure 3-19). Pruritus is also variable, ranging from none to severe. In children, it often appears as an eczematous eruption with small papules on the face, progressing to other sun-exposed areas. Individuals with darker skin types may present with a lichen nitidus–like eruption.[124] Juvenile spring eruption, considered a subset of PMLE, consists of edematous papules and vesicles, mainly on the helices of the ears but occasionally on the dorsal surfaces of the hands

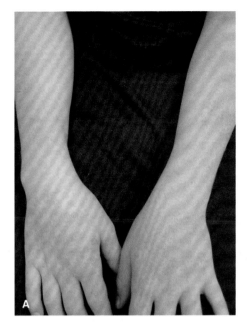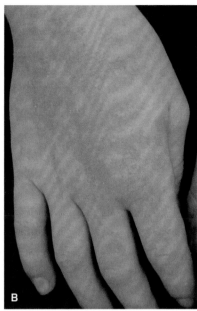

FIGURE 3-19. **Polymorphous light eruption.** Coalescing, thin, erythematous plaques on the dorsal forearms and hands (A and B).

or elbows (Figure 3-20).[125] It can occur 8 to 24 hours after UV exposure and is often pruritic. Like PMLE, the lesions resolve without scarring, usually within 2 weeks.

Histologic Findings

PMLE is pathologically characterized by a superficial and deep, relatively dense, predominantly chronic lymphocytic inflammatory infiltrate largely devoid of eosinophils and plasma cells (Figure 3-21). Depending on the type of clinical lesion, other histopathologic findings can be noted. Urticarial lesions and blisters are accompanied by marked superficial dermal edema. Eczematous or papulovesicular

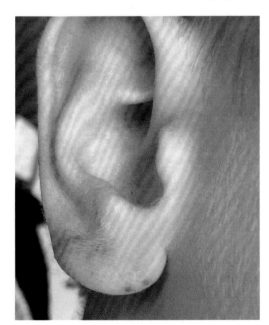

FIGURE 3-20. **Juvenile spring eruption.** Erythema and erythematous papules on the helices and lobule of a young child.

lesions show epidermal spongiosis. Purpuric lesions frequently have extravasated red blood cells. In children, the histologic findings of juvenile spring eruption are considered by some to be on the spectrum of PMLE.[126-130]

Differential Diagnosis

Actinic prurigo (AP) may present with psoriasiform epidermal changes, in addition to a deeper and denser inflammatory infiltrate when compared with PMLE. The inflammation can have eosinophils and reactive lymphoid follicles. Photoallergic contact dermatitis should be considered in the differential diagnosis if spongiosis and eosinophils are present. Acute radiation dermatitis and phototoxic dermatitis show scattered single necrotic keratinocytes in the mid-epidermis (sunburn cells) and junctional vacuolar alteration (interface changes). Lupus erythematosus can also enter the differential diagnosis and can be differentiated by the presence of superficial and deep, perivascular, and periadnexal inflammation with increased dermal mucin.

CAPSULE SUMMARY

POLYMORPHOUS LIGHT ERUPTION

PMLE is the most common idiopathic photosensitive disorder. It is characterized by recurrent cutaneous reactions following exposure to natural or artificial UV radiation. In children, it often appears as an eczematous eruption with small papules on the face, progressing to other sun-exposed areas. Individuals with darker skin types may present with a lichen nitidus–like eruption. PMLE is pathologically characterized by a superficial and deep, relatively dense, and predominantly chronic, lymphocytic inflammatory infiltrate.

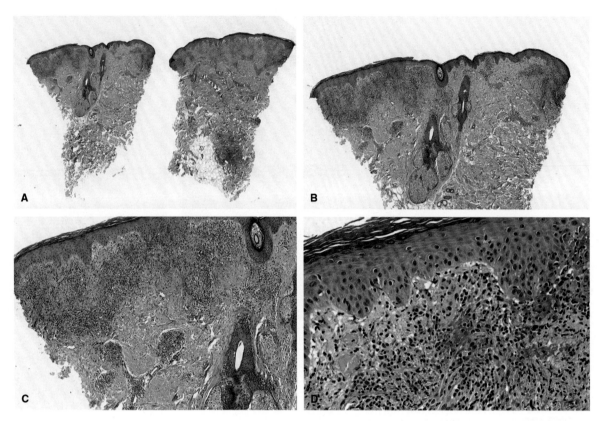

FIGURE 3-21. **Polymorphous light eruption.** A and B, There is a superficial and deep, mostly perivascular inflammatory infiltrate. C, A mild degree of acanthosis is noted, but there is significant dermal edema. D, Mild spongiosis, edema, and mixed inflammation. Digital slides courtesy of Path Presenter.com.

ACTINIC PRURIGO

Definition and Epidemiology

AP also known as *hydroa aestivale* and *Hutchinson summer prurigo*, is a chronic photodermatosis that is less common than PMLE. It usually begins in childhood and can last for many years.[131] Although patients with AP appear to have a higher percentage of first-degree relatives with PMLE,[132] it appears to be a distinct photosensitive disorder. Both UVB and UVA have been implicated, but reactivity to UVB appears to be more common.[133]

AP occurs mainly in Native Americans and Mestizo Indians from North, Central, and South America, although it can be seen in other parts of the world. Human leukocyte antigen (HLA) DRB1*0407 is found in 60% to 70% of patients with AP, but in only 4% to 8% of unaffected individuals.[134] HLA DRB1*0401 has been shown in up to 20% of affected individuals. Although both AP and PMLE can occur in the same individual, no HLA associations have been found with the latter. AP is more common in females.

Etiology

The pathogenesis of AP has yet to be determined, but an immunologic mechanism seems likely, given known HLA associations. AP lesional skin shows proliferative responses to autologous skin antigens in vitro.[135] Response to thalidomide in AP patients correlates with a decrease in TNF-α production

and an increase in IFN-γ-positive CD3[+] peripheral blood mononuclear cells.[136] A recent study suggests the role of a type IV hypersensitivity–like reaction, indicated by the presence of IgE, eosinophils, and mast cells in tissue from AP patients.[137]

Clinical Presentation

AP lesions present on sun-exposed areas but may involve covered areas as well, especially the buttocks. The lesions appear as erythematous and often crusted papules, nodules, and lichenified plaques, which can heal with pitting or linear scars, perhaps exacerbated by scratching because of intense pruritus (Figure 3-22). Ocular or lip involvement can be seen in 30% to 50% of affected patients. Cheilitis usually involves mainly the lower lip and may be the sole manifestation of the disease.[138] Ocular findings include conjunctivitis, photophobia, and exudate.[139]

Histologic Findings

The pathologic findings of AP are variable and relatively nonspecific. There is hyperkeratosis with ortho- or parakeratosis. The epidermis shows regular acanthosis, focal or multifocal spongiosis, and thickening of the basal membrane. There is a dense perivascular lymphocytic infiltrate in the superficial to mid-dermis, with papillary dermal edema. Eosinophils, melanophages, and extravasated erythrocytes can be seen (Figure 3-23).

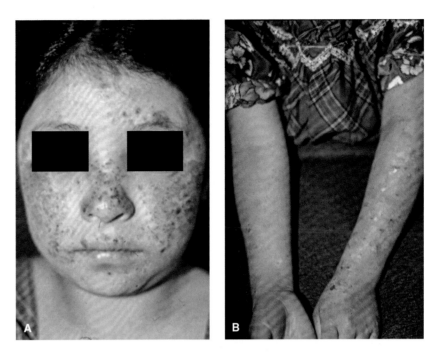

FIGURE 3-22. Actinic prurigo. Crusted and eroded erythematous papules and plaques on sun-exposed areas of the face and arms (A and B).

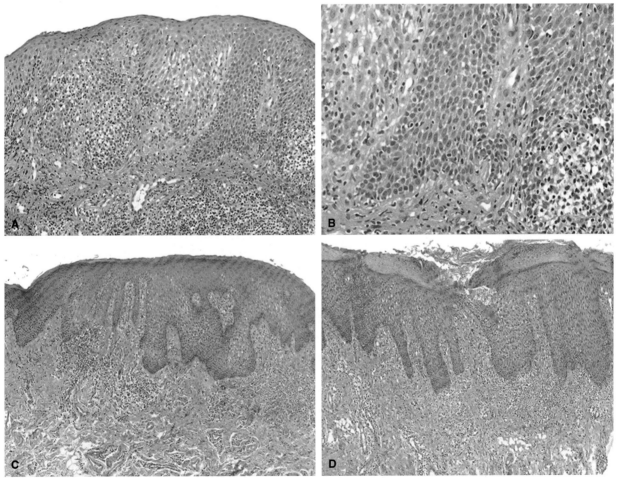

FIGURE 3-23. Actinic prurigo (AP). A, Acute phase of AP cheilitis. This biopsy of an acute lesion shows marked epidermal hyperplasia and spongiosis. B, Higher magnification shows the characteristic eosinophilic spongiosis seen in acute lesions. C, This biopsy shows epidermal hyperplasia with a lichenoid lymphocytic infiltrate. D, This case shows epidermal erosion with spongiosis, acanthosis, and hyperplasia. Lymphocytic exocytosis is also a characteristic feature of this phase of the disease. With permission from Plaza JA, Toussaint S, Prieto VG, et al. Actinic prurigo cheilitis: a clinicopathologic review of 75 cases. *Am J Dermatopathol.* 2016;38(6):418-422.

The pathologic findings on the biopsies of cheilitis vary depending on where the biopsy is taken from and at what phase of the disease the lesion has been biopsied. The biopsies from the lower vermillion show more typical changes that appear to be more specific for this condition. In the acute phase, there is acanthosis, spongiosis, and eosinophilia, along with dermal edema, congested vessels, and a lymphocytic infiltrate. Chronic lesions show an ulcerated epithelium with a dense lymphohistiocytic infiltrate and the presence of well-formed lymphoid follicles. The lymphoid follicles have been interpreted as a relatively specific finding for the diagnosis of AP cheilitis and have been termed "follicular cheilitis." The follicles can show germinal center formation and coalesce into irregular shapes but maintain a discernible polarized mantle and marginal zone (Figure 3-24).

The affected conjunctivae show epithelial hyperplasia alternating with atrophy, vacuolization of the basal layer, and dilated capillaries in the dermis. Similar to mucosal lip biopsies, lymphoid follicles can be seen.[138,140,141]

Differential Diagnosis

The most important pathologic differential diagnosis is with cutaneous lymphoid hyperplasia (CLH) and low-grade B-cell lymphomas. Follicular cheilitis and CLH have similar histologic changes. As opposed to AP, CLH typically presents as a solitary lesion on the face, with a predilection for females and Caucasian patients. The lips are not typically involved by CLH. Low-grade B-cell lymphomas include cutaneous marginal zone lymphomas and primary cutaneous follicle center lymphomas. The latter is not typically a disease of children and shows poorly formed follicles that lack germinal centers. BCL-2 can be coexpressed in 25% of the neoplastic cells. Cutaneous marginal zone lymphomas are the more common lymphomas in children, also occurring as solitary lesions in the trunk and extremities. The follicles tend to be atrophic and not reactive as in AP. Demonstration of clonality (by polymerase chain reaction [PCR] or in situ hybridization) can also help in distinguishing an

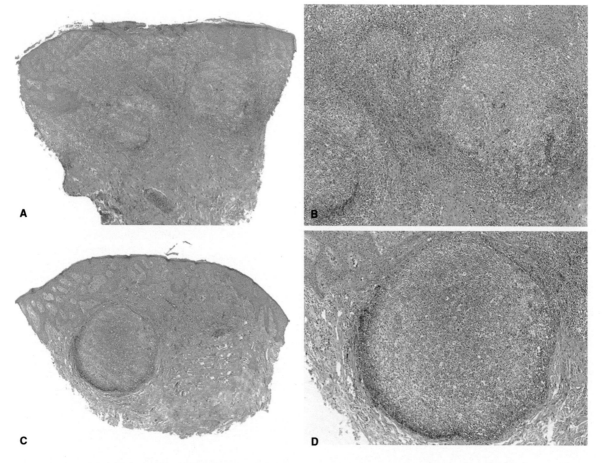

FIGURE 3-24. Actinic prurigo (AP). A, Chronic phase of AP cheilitis. This biopsy shows well-formed lymphoid follicles in superficial and mid-dermis (follicular cheilitis). B, Higher magnification shows the characteristic germinal centers with preservation of the light and dark zones. Note the increased number of interfollicular infiltrate. C, This biopsy shows epidermal hyperplasia with lymphoid follicle formation in dermis (follicular cheilitis). D, Higher magnification shows characteristic reactive germinal centers with darkly stained areas full of proliferating centroblasts and lighter zones in which centrocytes predominated. With permission from Plaza JA, Toussaint S, Prieto VG, et al. Actinic prurigo cheilitis: a clinicopathologic review of 75 cases. *Am J Dermatopathol.* 2016;38(6):418-422.

inflammatory (polyclonal) from a neoplastic (clonal) condition. Atypical marginal zone hyperplasias can also be included in the differential because they sometimes occur in children. They are characterized by clonal lambdarestriction by immunohistochemistry or in situ hybridization studies and lack a clonal population of cells by PCR analysis of the *IGH* gene.

CAPSULE SUMMARY

ACTINIC PRURIGO

AP, also known as *hydroa aestivale* and *Hutchinson summer prurigo*, is a chronic photodermatosis that usually begins in childhood and can last for many years. Clinically, it presents on sun-exposed areas but may involve covered areas as well, especially the buttocks. Lesions appear as erythematous and often crusted papules, nodules, and lichenified plaques, which heal with pitting or linear scars. Ocular or lip involvement can be seen in 30% to 50% of affected patients. The presence of follicular cheilitis, lymphoid follicles in affected areas of the lip, appears to be a distinctive histologic finding of this condition.

PHOTOTOXIC REACTIONS

Definition and Epidemiology

Phototoxic reactions occur when light activates a drug or chemical agent (Table 3-1). UVA (340–400 nm) is most often the cause, with rare cases attributable to UVB or visible light. When activated, these agents or their metabolites are converted into products that can cause direct injury to keratinocytes, resulting in an inflammatory response in the skin that is noted minutes to hours after exposure. Phototoxicity is the main mechanism of systemic drug photosensitivity.[142,143] Topical psoralens (from medications or furocoumarin-containing plants) also produce a phototoxic reaction. Prior sensitization to the agent is not required because the reaction is not immune mediated.

Phototoxic reactions are relatively common, but their prevalence is difficult to determine because many cases may not be recognized or reported as such. At several photodermatology centers, phototoxicity was the diagnosis in 5% to 16% of patients.[144,145] Not all patients exposed to the same drug exhibit a phototoxic response, and there is variability in the severity and extent of involvement.[146] Emerging drugs with phototoxic potential include voriconazole and BRAF inhibitors. A recent review of pediatric patients treated with voriconazole at a children's hospital over a 10-year period showed the incidence of phototoxicity to be 20%, increasing to 47% in patients treated for 6 months or longer.[147]

TABLE 3-1.	Phototoxic medications
Antibiotics	
Quinolones	
Doxycycline and tetracycline	
Sulfonamides	
Antifungals	
Griseofulvin	
Itraconazole	
Voriconazole	
BRAF inhibitors	
Vemurafenib	
Calcium channel blockers	
Diuretics	
Furosemide	
Thiazides	
Hypoglycemics	
Sulfonylureas	
Nonsteroidal anti-inflammatory agents	
Naproxen	
Photodynamic therapy agents	
Foscan	
Photofrin	
Psoralens	
Psychoactive drugs	
Phenothiazines	
Retinoids	
Acitretin	
Isotretinoin	
Topical tar	

Etiology

When phototoxic compounds absorb photons from radiation, a variety of reactive oxygen-intermediate compounds are formed, such as free oxygen radicals, superoxide anions, and hydrogen peroxide, which then activate proinflammatory pathways. The result is direct injury to cell membranes and cytoplasmic structures, or even nuclear DNA (as is the case with psoralens), which can lead to cell death.

Clinical Presentation

The most common presentation of a phototoxic reaction is sunburn-like erythema in exposed areas within minutes to several hours after light exposure. There may be associated stinging or burning. Edema, vesicles, or blistering may occur, followed by healing with desquamation and occasionally hyperpigmentation.

Phytophotodermatitis is the most common phototoxic reaction in children and is caused by furocoumarin-containing fruits and plants (Table 3-2).[16] When there is

TABLE 3-2.	Drugs implicated in drug-induced hypersensitivity syndrome

Aromatic anticonvulsants
    Phenytoin
    Phenobarbital
    Carbamazepine
    Lamotrigine when used with valproic acid

Antibiotics
    Sulfonamides
    Minocycline

Antiretrovirals
    Abacavir

Allopurinol

Dapsone

Gold salts

Infliximab

Protease inhibitors
    Boceprevir
    Telaprevir

Targeted oncologics
    Sorafenib
    Vismodegib
    Vemurafenib

Pseudoporphyria is another phototoxic reaction that can be seen in up to 11% of children who are taking non-steroidal anti-inflammatory agents, especially naproxen sodium for arthritis.[149-151] These patients present with lesions that clinically resemble porphyria cutanea tarda with fragile skin, tense bullae, and erythema with erosions that crust, often healing with milia and scarring. Involvement is usually seen a few months after starting the drug, and occurs in sun-exposed areas that are subject to mild trauma, especially the backs of the hands. Unlike true porphyria, there are no porphyrin abnormalities in the urine, stool, serum, or red blood cells. Similar reactions have been noted with other medications, including antibiotics and antifungals such as tetracyclines, ciprofloxacin, voriconazole, systemic retinoids, diuretics, metformin, dapsone, imatinib, and cyclosporine.[150]

Histologic Findings

Pathologically, phototoxic reactions show a mild degree of epidermal spongiosis with scattered apoptotic keratinocytes ("sunburn" cells), which are often present at all levels of the epidermis. There is a lymphohistiocytic infiltrate with a superficial dermal perivascular distribution and associated exocytosis (Figure 3-26). Eosinophils are not frequently seen.[152-154]

Differential Diagnosis

The differential diagnosis includes graft-versus-host disease (GVHD), EM, and other interface dermatitides (lupus, dermatomyositis, etc.). PMLE may also be considered. GVHD may have overlapping histopathologic changes, but can be easily differentiated on the basis of the clinical history and presentation. Lupus erythematosus shows interface changes

contact with skin followed by exposure to sunlight, erythema, and sometimes vesicles or blisters, occurs, often in a streaky pattern that reflects the areas of contact with the agent (Figure 3-25). Hyperpigmentation eventually appears in the involved areas. Phytophotodermatitis can be mistaken for ACD, cellulitis, and even child abuse.[148]

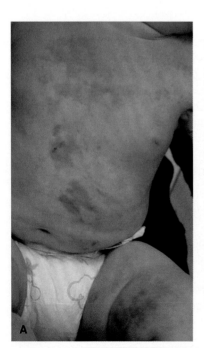 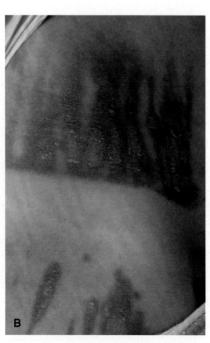

FIGURE 4-25. Phytophotodermatitis in an infant (A) and caused by lemon juice in an older child (B). Note the bizarre, streak pattern of erythema and hyperpigmentation, indicating an external contactant.

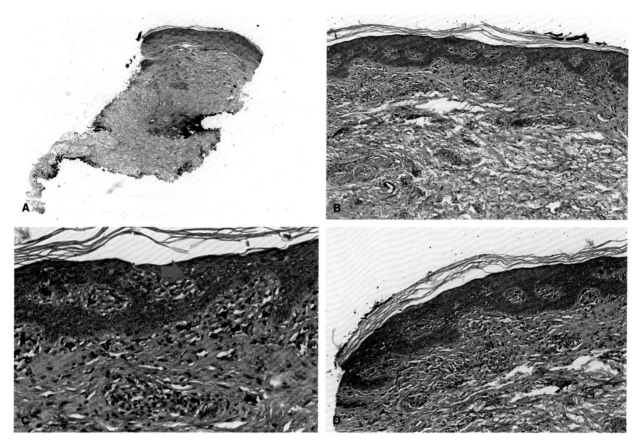

FIGURE 3-26. **Photodermatitis.** A and B, Mostly superficial and perivascular inflammation with epidermal acanthosis. C, "Sunburn" cells are shown by an arrow head. D, Spongiosis and exocytosis of lymphocytes are noted. Digital slides courtesy of Path Presenter.com.

and a superficial and deep, perivascular, and periadnexal infiltrate with increased dermal mucin. Dermatomyositis shares similar histologic findings, including the presence of interstitial dermal mucin, but typically shows epidermal atrophy. PMLE lacks apoptotic keratinocytes and often has deep perivascular inflammation and dermal edema that are not frequent in phototoxic reactions. Photoallergic dermatitis classically shows abundant dermal eosinophils and more prominent spongiosis.

CAPSULE SUMMARY

PHOTOTOXIC REACTIONS

These occur when light activates a drug or chemical agent after systemic or topical exposure. The most common presentation of a phototoxic reaction is sunburn-like erythema in exposed areas within minutes to several hours after light exposure and may be associated with stinging or burning. Edema, vesicles, or blistering may occur, followed by healing with desquamation and occasionally hyperpigmentation. Pathologically, phototoxic reactions show a mild degree of epidermal spongiosis with scattered apoptotic keratinocytes ("sunburn" cells).

DRUG-INDUCED HYPERSENSITIVITY SYNDROME

Definition and Epidemiology

Drug-induced hypersensitivity syndrome (DIHS) has been known by many names since it was described almost 70 years ago in patients taking certain anticonvulsants. Initially described as phenytoin hypersensitivity syndrome, the most familiar name is Drug Reaction with Eosinophilia and Systemic Symptoms (DRESS). Aromatic anticonvulsants still predominate as the precipitating drugs, as do sulfonamides, but multiple other medications have been implicated (Table 3-2). DIHS consists of a spectrum of clinical and laboratory features that include fever, exanthem, lymphadenopathy, facial edema, eosinophilia, and internal organ involvement. DIHS is distinguished from other drug reactions and syndromes by its longer latency until onset of findings and the relative lack of mucous membrane involvement.

In children, the frequency of DIHS has been reported to be 27.6%[155] with a mean age of about 9 years.[156] It occurs almost equally in males and females. In some ethnic groups, specific HLA allele types have been linked to a predisposition to severe drug hypersensitivity reactions, including

DIHS, with exposure to phenobarbital, carbamezepine, allopurinol, dapsone, and abacavir.[157-159]

Etiology

Although the exact mechanism has not yet been elucidated, the etiology of DIHS appears to be a manifestation of immune responses to one or more pathogenic events involving defects in drug metabolism, eosinophil production, and viral reactivation. Patients with genetic polymorphisms in genes encoding drug-metabolizing enzymes in the cytochrome P450 system accumulate toxic arene oxide and hydroxylamine metabolites, which then evoke a complex hypersensitivity response by the immune system.[147,160,161] The presence of large numbers of eosinophils as part of the immune response in DIHS can cause direct tissue damage upon release of cytotoxic granule proteins.[158,162]

Reactivation of human herpesviruses HHV-6, HHV-7, Epstein–Barr virus (EBV), and cytomegalovirus (CMV) has been found in patients with many cutaneous adverse drug reactions,[163] but it appears that reactivation of HHV-6 is found almost exclusively in patients with DIHS.[164] The massive expansion of regulatory T cells that occurs in the acute stages of DIHS may have the effect of inducing viral reactivation.[165] In children with drug hypersensitivity syndrome, patients who showed HHV-6 positivity had a more severe disease course than those children who were HHV-6 negative.[166]

Clinical Presentation

The clinical features of DIHS are similar in children and adults and usually begin on average 6 weeks after beginning the culprit medication, with a range of 2 to 8 weeks. It often starts with features similar to those of a viral prodrome with malaise, pharyngitis, and fever. Lymphadenopathy as well as arthralgia may be noted. A morbilliform rash will follow in 75% of patients accompanied by edema of the face, especially the periorbital area (Figure 3-27). The rash can be follicular based and becomes pruritic as it advances down the trunk and extremities. The development of vesicles, tense bullae, and targetoid-like lesions can occur and may suggest Stevens–Johnson syndrome (SJS), but mucous membrane involvement is not a hallmark of DIHS and is usually found only when there is progression to diffuse erythroderma.[156,160,167]

Laboratory evaluation is key to making the diagnosis of DIHS in children as it is in adults. The incidence of organ system involvement is similar regardless of age, with the most common finding being peripheral eosinophilia ($>2.0 \times 10^9$ eosinophils/L) in 50% to 80% and atypical lymphocytosis in 72% of patients. The liver is the most commonly affected visceral organ, with involvement in 50% to 90% of cases. Although rare, progression to fulminant hepatitis with liver necrosis may occur and carries a mortality of 10%. The kidney is affected in 11% to 16% of patients, especially when allopurinol is the inciting agent. Pulmonary involvement is more likely with abacavir exposure and may include interstitial pneumonitis, pleuritis, and rarely acute respiratory distress syndrome.[160,167] Myocarditis, meningitis, and encephalitis have been reported, but are rare.

Involvement of the skin and other organs can last for weeks to months. Autoimmune disorders, including thyroiditis, type 1 diabetes mellitus, and pancreatitis, can occur 2 to 3 months after resolution of DIHS.[167,168] It has been

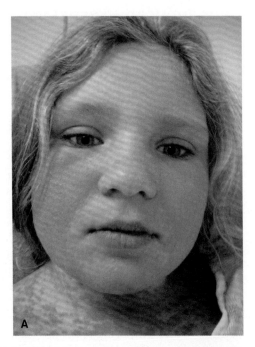
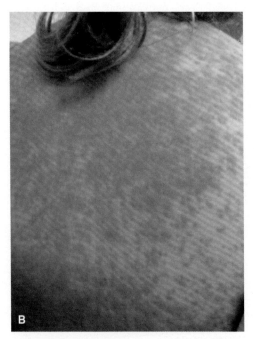

FIGURE 3-27. Drug-induced hypersensitivity syndrome/drug reaction with eosinophilia. Coalescing erythematous, edematous papules and plaques (A and B). Note the marked facial swelling.

postulated that a gradual loss of regulatory T-cell function may increase the risk of developing subsequent autoimmune disease.[165] Patients should be monitored for these disorders beginning several months after resolution of DIHS.

Histologic Findings

The pathologic findings seen in DRESS are relatively nonspecific and do not differ significantly from other medication-induced hypersensitivity reactions (for a detailed explanation of histologic findings in association with specific medications, see Chapter 8). In general, biopsies taken from DRESS show a superficial and deep, perivascular lymphocytic inflammatory infiltrate with abundant dermal eosinophils. Epidermal spongiosis can be present, and scattered apoptotic keratinocytes are seen in a minority of cases (Figure 3-28). In some circumstances, the number of dermal eosinophils can be quite low, despite the presence of peripheral blood eosinophilia. The diagnosis of DRESS is strictly based on specific clinical criteria, because the pathologic findings are relatively nonspecific. The group of drug-induced hypersensitivity reactions in association with anticonvulsants (eg, phenytoin, carbamazepine, etc.) can potentially mimic a T-cell lymphoma.[169-173]

Differential Diagnosis

Drug reactions may present with nearly every histologic inflammatory reaction pattern in the skin. In disorders characterized by superficial perivascular inflammation such as spongiotic, interface, or psoriasiform patterns, the presence of deep inflammation and eosinophils is often invoked as evidence to include the differential diagnosis of a drug reaction.

CAPSULE SUMMARY

DRUG-INDUCED HYPERSENSITIVITY SYNDROME

DIHS to medications (also known as DRESS) is a spectrum of clinical and laboratory features that includes fever, exanthem, lymphadenopathy, facial edema, eosinophilia, and internal organ involvement. Following viral prodrome-like fever and malaise, a morbilliform eruption occurs in 75% of patients accompanied by edema of the face, especially the periorbital area. The pathologic findings seen in DIHS are relatively nonspecific and do not differ significantly from other medication-induced hypersensitivity reactions.

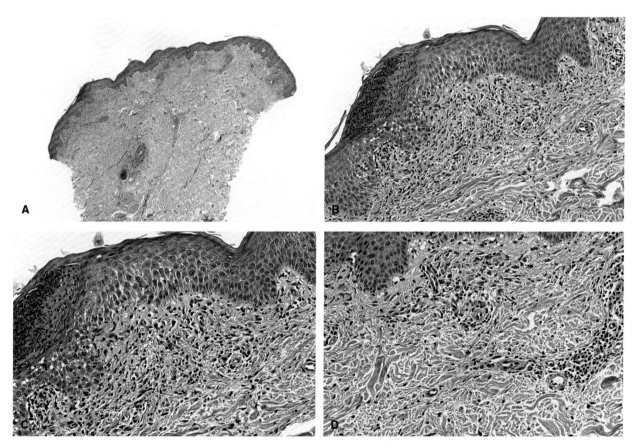

FIGURE 3-28. Drug-induced hypersensitivity syndrome/drug reaction with eosinophilia. A and B, There is epidermal acanthosis and spongiosis with lymphocyte exocytosis and a serum crust. C and D, A perivascular and interstitial superficial infiltrate rich in eosinophils is present. Digital slides courtesy of Path Presenter.com.

PITYRIASIS ROSEA

Definition and Epidemiology

PR is a common, self-limited inflammatory dermatosis that is usually seen in children.[174] It has a classic distribution and morphology, and evidence suggests a viral etiology. It occurs most commonly between the ages of 10 and 35, with 50% of cases in patients under 20 years of age.[16,174] Although less than 10% of cases occur in children under 10 years, it has been reported in those as young as 3 months of age.[16] It affects males and females equally.[174]

Etiology

A viral etiology has long been suspected because of case clustering and limited relapses (<3% of cases), which suggest immunity to an infectious process.[175-177] There is growing evidence to suggest a causal role for HHV-6 and HHV-7 infection and reactivation.[178-181]

Clinical Presentation

Classically, PR begins with a herald patch on the trunk: an asymptomatic, pink erythematous scaling patch with slight central depression.[174,182,183] The herald patch, seen in 17% to 76% of cases, can grow to several centimeters in size and precedes the rest of the eruption by at least 2 days. The secondary eruption appears 2 to 84 days after the herald patch with crops of thin-to-nonsubstantive, faint salmon-pink, scaling, oval-to-oblong plaques oriented along Langer lines of skin cleavage (Figure 3-29).[174,180,183] These give the characteristic "Christmas tree" appearance. Each lesion can have a "peripheral collarette scaling pattern."[183] PR resolves in an average of 6 to 8 weeks, but can last up to 5 months.[174,180]

Some children (5%-69%) present with a prodrome: sore throat, headache, anorexia, nausea, malaise, fever, or upper respiratory infection symptoms.[16,176,180] The eruption may be slightly pruritic.[174] There are several noted variants of PR, and an atypical presentation is not uncommon.[176] Inverse PR is characterized by predominant facial and extremity over truncal involvement.[174] African-American children with PR are more likely to have facial and scalp involvement (30%), an inverse presentation, papules (33%), and postinflammatory pigment alteration (77%).[184] Papular and vesicular PR are variants that are more common in children.[180] Vesicular PR can have intense pruritus and is diffuse. Other rarer variants include EM like, purpuric/hemorrhagic with oral hemorrhagic ulcers, urticarial, and unilateral PR.[174,176,180]

Histologic Findings

There is epidermal spongiosis with occasional mounds of parakeratosis. Prominent lymphocyte exocytosis is typical (Figure 3-30). Within the dermis, there is a perivascular lymphocytic infiltrate with associated extravasation of red blood cells. Scattered single or multiple apoptotic keratinocytes can be seen, particularly in biopsies taken from the "herald patch," but frank interface dermatitis is uncommon. Atypical presentations of PR may show a slightly more intense dermal inflammatory infiltrate with papillary dermal edema, more exocytosis, and extensive basal vacuolar alteration. Dyskeratotic cells are also seen. A vesicular form of PR, characterized by foci of more extensive spongiosis, is rare, but occurs with a higher frequency in the pediatric age group, particularly in those with darker skin color.[184-187]

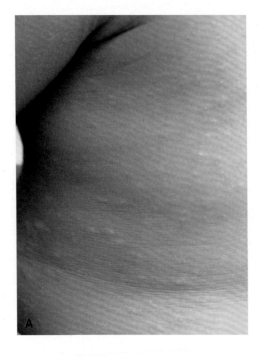
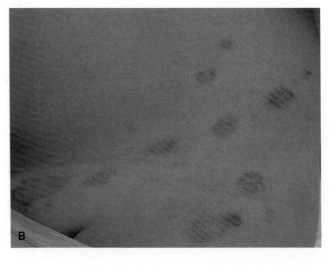

FIGURE 3-29. **Pityriasis rosea.** Discrete scaly, faintly erythematous papules and plaques on the trunk (A) and in an inverse pattern involving the groin (B).

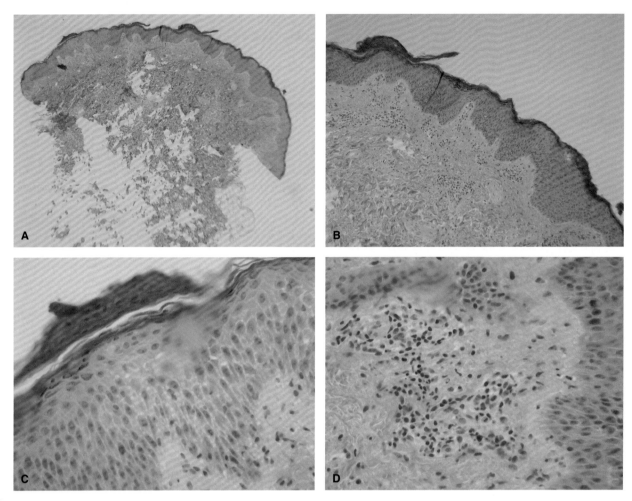

FIGURE 3-30. Pityriasis rosea. A and B, Epidermal acanthosis and spongiosis with mounds of parakeratosis. C, A closer view to the parakeratotic mounds and areas of spongiosis is shown. D, A perivascular lymphocytic infiltrate with extravasated erythrocytes is shown.

Differential Diagnosis

PR is typically diagnosed on the basis of clinical findings alone without the need for a biopsy. Classic examples of PR cannot always be differentiated reliably on a histologic basis from other forms of spongiotic dermatoses. If the epidermal changes are focal, the findings in PR might be indistinguishable from the superficial variant of erythema annulare centrifugum (EAC). Because the biopsies taken from EAC may sometimes exhibit multiple foci of parakeratosis with spongiosis, including intraepidermal vesiculation, clinicopathologic correlation is necessary to differentiate the two entities. Lymphocyte exocytosis, scattered apoptotic keratinocytes, and extravasated red blood cells are also features present in pityriasis lichenoides and morbilliform viral exanthems. Pityriasis lichenoides show more prominent interface changes than PR. In *pityriasis lichenoides et varioliformis acuta* (PLEVA), areas of epidermal necrosis are seen, features never encountered in PR. Morbilliform viral exanthems show a sparse lymphocytic infiltrate with or without extravasated red blood cells, mild vacuolar changes, minimal spongiosis with lymphocyte exocytosis, and no parakeratotic mounds.

CAPSULE SUMMARY

PITYRIASIS ROSEA

This is a common, self-limited inflammatory dermatosis that is usually seen in children. Classically, it begins with a herald patch on the trunk: an asymptomatic, pink-erythematous scaling patch with slight central depression, followed by appearance 2 to 84 days later of crops of thin, faint salmon-pink scaling, oval-to-oblong plaques oriented along Langer lines of skin cleavage. Histologically, there is epidermal spongiosis, with occasional mounds of parakeratosis. Prominent lymphocyte exocytosis is typical. Within the dermis, there is a perivascular lymphocytic infiltrate with associated extravasation of red blood cells.

PSORIASIS

Definition and Epidemiology

Psoriasis is a common, chronic, immune-mediated inflammatory dermatosis.[188-190] It has a relapsing and remitting course and may affect the skin, nails, and joints. Approximately 2% to 3% of the global population has psoriasis, and one-third of those cases begin in childhood.[189,191] The age- and sex-adjusted annual incidence of pediatric psoriasis is 40.8/100 000, which has more than doubled since 1970.[191,192] Although psoriasis is not thought to have a gender predominance, some studies show a female predilection in children.[189] The mean age at onset is 8–11 years old.[192]

Etiology

The risk for psoriasis is a complicated interplay between genetic and environmental factors. About 30% of children have a first-degree family member with psoriasis, and in children with onset before 16 years, this can be up to 71%.[188,189,193] Many genes have been associated with psoriasis, including the following: *PSOR1, CARD14/PSOR2, IL 12-B9, IL-13, IL-23R, HLABw6, PSORS6, STAT2/IL-23A, TNFAIP3,* and *TNIP1*.[16,188] *CARD14* mutations have specifically been associated with familial psoriasis vulgaris and familial generalized pustular psoriasis.[194] Many cases of pustular psoriasis have IL-36 receptor antagonist mutations.[189]

The innate and adaptive immune systems mediate psoriatic inflammation, but Th1 and Th17 cells predominate.[16,195] Proinflammatory cytokines (TNF-α, IFN-γ, IL-1β, and IL-6) activate dendritic cells to express IL-12 and IL-23. These subsequently trigger the dominant Th1 and Th17 cell responses. Th1 and Th17 cytokines (TNF-α, IFN-γ, IL-17, IL-22, IL-23) then stimulate keratinocytes and perpetuate the inflammation and immune activation of psoriasis.[16] A recent study examining the T-cell and cytokine milieu in pediatric psoriatic plaques revealed the increased prevalence of IL-22-secreting T cells more so than IL-17-secreting T cells, which contrasts with adult psoriasis.[195] Additionally, disease severity has been shown to correlate with increased levels of circulating Th-17 and T regulatory cells.[196]

Clinical Presentation

Although pediatric psoriasis can present with all of the same variations as adults, the morphology, distribution, and symptoms of pediatric psoriasis can vary.[189] Children are affected by significant psychosocial impact and adverse effects on the quality of life.[189] Additionally, pediatric psoriasis is more likely to be preceded by stress, trauma, and pharyngitis, and it exhibits the koebnerization phenomenon (development of psoriasis at sites of trauma such as scratching).[190,193] The most common form of pediatric psoriasis is chronic plaque type (73.7%), with salmon-pink, sharply demarcated, silver-white scaling, flat-topped papules and plaques (Figure 3-31).[192] They are usually symmetrically distributed on the extremities or scalp at presentation (46.8%-57.3%).[189,192,193] Plaques in childhood tend to be smaller and thinner than in adults.[189] Although the scalp (46.8%-57.3%) and extremities are the most common sites of presentation, flexural surfaces are involved more frequently in children than in adults, with potential for maceration.[189,192,193] Facial involvement, particularly periorbital, is seen more frequently in children, even in the absence of other areas of involvement.[16,189]

At 44%, guttate psoriasis is the second most common presentation in children. It presents with smaller, droplet-like papules and plaques and has a more acute onset than plaque

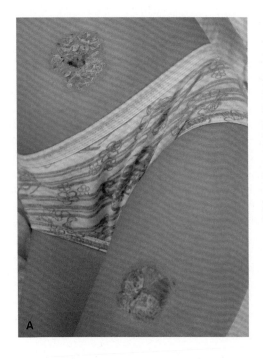

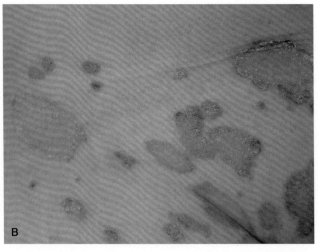

FIGURE 3-31. **Psoriasis.** A, Classic plaque type with erythematous plaques with thick overlying scale. B, Plaques in an inverse distribution, centered around a body fold.

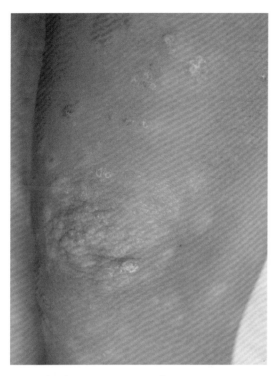

FIGURE 3-32. **Guttate psoriasis.** Small erythematous papules with overlying scale.

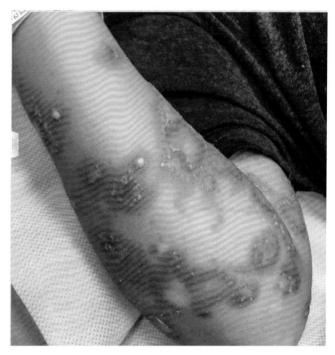

FIGURE 3-33. **Pustular psoriasis.** Erythematous plaques with pustules at the margins and central desquamation.

psoriasis (Figure 3-32). It is an often-triggered β-hemolytic *Streptococcal* infection of the pharynx or perineum.[16,189] If guttate psoriasis progresses to chronic plaque type (40%), it can herald a more severe disease course.[16,189,190] Young children and infants may present with recalcitrant diaper dermatitis that has sharp demarcation, maceration, and involvement of the inguinal folds.[189] Nail changes are seen in 40% of children and are more common in boys—these changes include pitting, oil spots, onycholysis, subungual hyperkeratosis, onychodystrophy, and splinter hemorrhage.[189,190] Nail changes may not correlate with arthritis.[190]

Pustular psoriasis is composed of superficial sterile pustules, is quite rare (1%-5.4% of childhood psoriasis), and usually presents before 5 years of age (Figure 3-33).[189] Although pustular psoriasis is more common in adult patients, the von Zumbusch (febrile, arthralgias) and annular variants are more common in children.[189] Other infrequently encountered forms of pediatric psoriasis include the following: erythrodermic (1.4%), inverse (affecting intertriginous sites), palmoplantar, isolated facial, Blaschkolinear, glossitis, and congenital.

As a systemic inflammatory condition, it is not surprising that psoriasis is associated with arthritis in 1% to 10% of cases. Psoriatic arthritis comprises 7% of juvenile idiopathic arthritides.[16,188,189] Findings of metabolic syndrome, including obesity, hyperlipidemia, and diabetes, are also seen in concert with psoriasis.[189]

Histologic Findings

Classic plaque psoriasis shows confluent hyperparakeratosis on the surface. The epidermis shows regular elongation of the rete pegs with hypogranulosis and a mild degree of spongiosis (Figure 3-34). Clusters of neutrophils in the stratum corneum (Munro microabscesses) and in the superficial portions of the epidermis (spongiform pustules of Kogoj) are seen. An increased number of mitotic figures in the basal portions of the epidermis is noted, a feature that translates into the accelerated transit of cells in the epidermis. Thinning of the suprapapillary plates with marked dilatation of the postcapillary venules is present. A modest superficial and perivascular lymphohistiocytic infiltrate is noted. Eosinophils are uncommon. Biopsies taken from the scalp typically show a marked sebaceous gland atrophy.[63,197-200]

Biopsies from *pustular psoriasis* show large neutrophilic abscesses within the stratum corneum and epidermis. A pattern of "spongiform" pustulation is typical of pustular psoriasis. Features of classic plaque psoriasis may or may not be present. The dermal inflammatory infiltrate can often include neutrophils (Figure 3-35). Vascular telangiectasis is also typical of pustular psoriasis. *Guttate psoriasis* shows only focal parakeratosis and lacks the clusters/collections of neutrophils in the stratum corneum or the epidermis. The acanthosis is only minimal, and there is no significant elongation of the rete. The vascular ectasia is the most

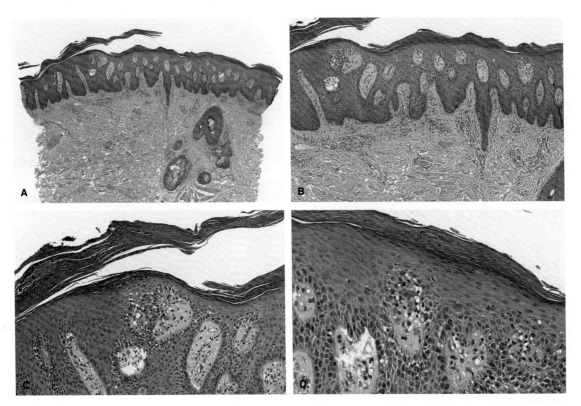

FIGURE 3-34. Psoriasis vulgaris. A and B, The classic features of psoriasis include epidermal acanthosis with regular elongation of the rete, and hypogranulosis. C, A mild degree of spongiosis, intraepidermal and intracorneal collections of neutrophils, and the hypogranular cell layer are shown. D, Superficial vascular telangiectasia is noted. Digital slides courtesy of Path Presenter.com.

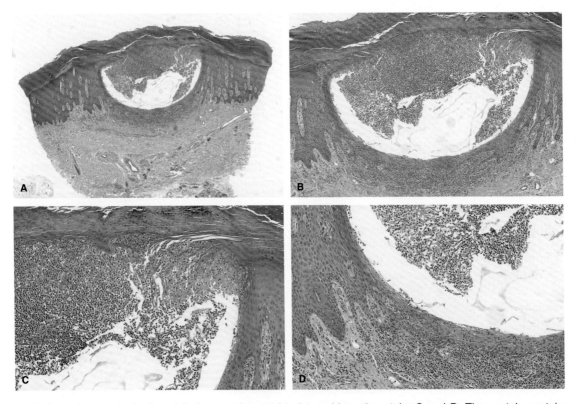

FIGURE 3-35. Pustular psoriasis. A and B, Large subcorneal to intraepidermal pustule. C and D, The pustule contains abundant neutrophils, and the surrounding epidermis is spongiotic. Digital slides courtesy of Path Presenter.com.

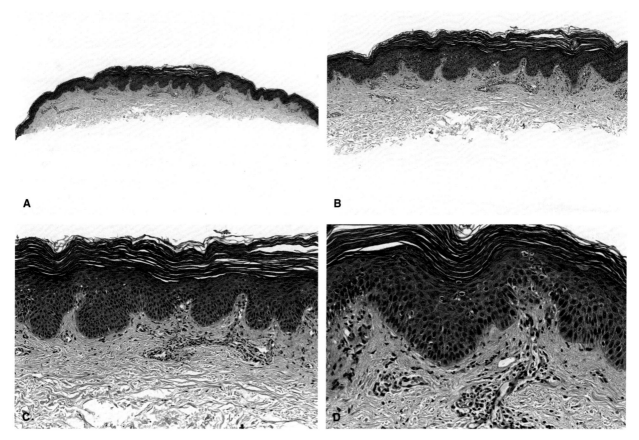

A

B

C

D

FIGURE 3-36. **Guttate psoriasis.** The findings are very mild. There is mild acanthosis and hyperkeratosis with hypogranulosis (A and B). Mild telangiectasis is noted (C and D). Digital slides courtesy of Path Presenter.com.

significant finding and is usually the clue to the diagnosis (Figure 3-36).[200,201]

Differential Diagnosis

Psoriasis can typically be diagnosed on the basis of the clinical features alone, without the need for a biopsy. Biopsies are more likely to be done when the clinical findings are unusual, or there is no significant response to therapy. The differential diagnosis varies with the type of lesion being biopsied. For classic plaques, dermatophyte infection, chronic spongiotic dermatitis, psoriasiform drug reactions, pityriasis rubra pilaris, and mycosis fungoides (MF) can enter the differential diagnosis. In chronic spongiotic dermatitis, the elongation of the rete tends to be more irregular, the granular cell layer is preserved or thickened, and the spongiosis is more prominent. If lesions of psoriasis are traumatized (as by scratching or rubbing), the distinction between psoriasis and chronic spongiotic dermatosis can be impossible. A dermatophyte infection often shows collections of neutrophils superficially, but lacks the other changes seen in psoriasis. Regardless, it is recommended to perform GMS or PAS staining on "all" biopsies that are done for a new diagnosis of psoriasis. Psoriasiform drug reactions typically show a much larger proportion of eosinophils. A recent study has shown that

up to 1 to 2 eosinophils can be encountered in a biopsy of psoriasis, but a larger number suggests a different etiology. Psoriasiform drug eruptions tend to be much less frequent in children than in adults. Pityriasis rubra pilaris (PRP) can also show a psoriasiform pattern of acanthosis. However, pityriasis rubra pilaris shows much less regular elongation of the rete, alternating areas of parakeratosis and orthokeratosis, lacks the collections of neutrophils, has a retained granular cell layer, and can have follicular plugging. MF in children typically presents as hypopigmented patches and plaques in sun-protected areas. The psoriasiform changes tend to be more irregular, and there is significant cytologic atypia of the lymphocytes. Characteristically, the atypical lymphocytes extend to the epidermis and show tagging along the dermal–epidermal junction. Perinuclear halos and cerebriform nuclear contours in addition to hyperchromasia are noted. MF in children characteristically has a CD8-positive phenotype with aberrant loss of T-cell markers (classically CD7).

Biopsies taken from pustular psoriasis can closely resemble the changes seen in acute generalized exanthematous pustulosis (AGEP). The presence of eosinophils favors AGEP. Subcorneal pustular dermatosis and IgA pemphigus can also share features similar to those of pustular psoriasis. Acantholysis is typical of IgA pemphigus, but is not a feature of psoriasis. Additionally, a positive direct immunofluorescence study can help confirm the diagnosis. Impetigo can also show pustules, but can easily be excluded with the identification of bacterial organisms in the pustules. The differential diagnosis of guttate psoriasis includes PR and small-plaque parapsoriasis (digitate dermatosis). PR shows more prominent spongiosis, lymphocyte exocytosis, mounds of parakeratosis, and extravasated erythrocytes. Small-plaque parapsoriasis shows less prominent epidermal changes and more conspicuous lymphocyte exocytosis.

CAPSULE SUMMARY

PSORIASIS

Psoriasis is a common, chronic, immune-mediated inflammatory dermatosis that often begins in childhood. The most common form of pediatric psoriasis is chronic plaque type, with salmon-pink, sharply demarcated, silver-white scaling, flat-topped plaques. Guttate psoriasis is the second most common form, presenting with small, droplet-like papules and plaques. Histologically, plaque psoriasis shows confluent hyperparakeratosis, regular elongation of the rete pegs with hypogranulosis, and a mild degree of spongiosis. Clusters of neutrophils in the stratum corneum and in the superficial portions of the epidermis are seen.

PITYRIASIS RUBRA PILARIS

Definition and Epidemiology

Pityriasis rubra pilaris (PRP) is a rare, often chronic, inflammatory dermatosis, now classified into six classic types on the basis of onset, distribution, and course (Table 3-3).[16] PRP is quite rare, found in 1 in 5000[202] individuals, and affects males and females equally.[203,204] There are rare familial cases; 0% to 6.5% of patients have a family history of PRP.

Etiology

The etiology and pathogenesis remain largely unknown, with the exception of type V PRP. Proposed causes include autoimmune processes, an abnormal immune response to antigenic triggers (such as infectious superantigens), and possible physical triggers.[20,205,206] Juvenile acute PRP (JAPRP), a subtype of type III, is proposed to be an exanthem in response to an infectious superantigen.[206] Additionally, case clustering (seven cases over 4 months) of type IV PRP supports an infectious trigger in genetically predisposed individuals.[207] Type V, atypical pediatric PRP, has been shown in multiple studies to be caused by activation of CARD14, a

TABLE 3-3.   Pityriasis rubra pilaris classifications[16,20,203,204,208-210,213,214]

Type I	Classic adult	>50% of cases[203]
Type II	Atypical adult	5%,[203] chronic, ichthyosiform
Type III	Classic juvenile	10% of cases Resembles I Clears in 3 y Presents: infancy to late teens[204,213]
Type IV	Circumscribed juvenile	Most common (25%) juvenile form Usually focal—favors knees, elbows, palms, soles. Also can involve the buttocks, bony prominences, trunk, scalp, face Usually presents before <12 y old[204]
Type V	Atypical juvenile	Similar to type II 5% of cases Chronic Ichthyosiform scale Sclerodermoid fingers Less erythema Familial (AD >AR) or sporadic CARD14 activation
Type VI	HIV associated	PRP-like eruption, lichen spinulosus, nodulocystic acne, hidradenitis suppurativa

Abbreviation: AD, autosomal dominant; AR, autosomal recessive; PRP, pityriasis rubra pilaris.

known activator of NFKB. Familial cases of type V PRP, usually autosomal dominant, are secondary to activating mutations in CARD14.[208-210] CARD14, also known as PSORS2, mutations are also seen in familial psoriasis.[16,208,209]

Clinical Presentation

Classic findings include follicular, keratotic papules, a cephalocaudal rash, keratoderma, and classic salmon color.[202] The most characteristic lesion is a small (1 mm), folliculocentric, salmon (orange-pink) papule with central keratotic plug.[203] These favor the knees, elbows, dorsal feet and hands, but spare the dorsal fingers in contrast to what is commonly seen in adults.[16,203] These papules can coalesce into symmetric, sharply demarcated patches and coarsely textured ("nutmeg grater like") diffuse psoriasiform plaques with classic islands of spared normal skin (Figure 3-37).[16,211,212] Thickened plaques are commonly found on the elbows, knees, ankles, and over the achilles.[16] The palmoplantar keratoderma is orange-red, sharply demarcated, and often extends to the dorsal aspect of the hands and feet (Figure 3-38). Edema is often seen, as is desquamation.[16,20,202,203,213] The classically described yellow keratodermic sandal on the feet and heels has subsequently been noted to be rare.[16,20,202,203,213] The original "cephalic rash" begins on the head, spreading to the neck and upper trunk in a cape-like distribution with geographic borders in 40% of children.[16,203,204] While mucosal surfaces are usually spared, ectropion is possible in more extensive cases.[16,203,204] Nail changes are seen in 11% to 33% with thickening, onycholysis, transverse striations, subungual debris, and yellow-brown discoloration, but no nail pits.[204,213] Koebnerization, photosensitivity, pruritus, or burning are not common.[16,205,204,213] Differential diagnosis includes psoriasis, disorders of cornification (keratodermas), and PRP-like dermatomyositis.[16]

Five classic types were described by Griffiths, with the addition recently of a sixth related to HIV.[214] Types I and II are seen in adulthood; types III, IV, and V are seen in childhood.[202] As many children do not perfectly fit into a type, subsequent classifications have been proposed but are not as commonly used.[211] Type IV, circumscribed juvenile PRP, is generally considered the most common pediatric form, although some studies suggest that the classic juvenile type (type III) is more common. Classic keratoderma is found in 47% to 84% of pediatric patients.[16,202-204,213]

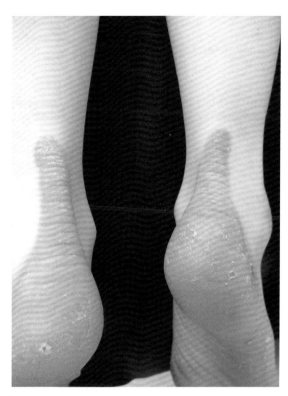

FIGURE 3-38. **Pityriasis rubra pilaris.** Orange/erythematous keratoderma on plantar surfaces of the feet and extending over the Achille's tendons.

Type III, classic juvenile PRP, can be erythrodermic and extensive.[20,204] A unique subtype of type III is JAPRP, which has scarlatiniform erythema following infection that evolves into classic PRP lesions over 1 to 2 weeks.[206] It resolves with desquamation in 2 to 3 months without recurrence.[206] Dermoscopy is an added diagnostic tool in type IV PRP, showing hyperkeratotic papules and plaques, with erythema around a central hair.[215] Type V can be hereditary or sporadic and is caused by CARD14 activation.[208-210] Hereditary cases tend to be of early onset, even congenital, and are more persistent.[16,208,209,216]

Disease course is highly variable, from self-resolution in months[204,206] to chronic and relapsing.[213] Interestingly, prognosis is not dependent upon onset or severity of disease, but is generally better in children than in adults, with self-resolution in months to years.[203,214] Pediatric PRP can have periods of remission and exacerbation, which is not typical of adult PRP.[16,203,214] There is one report of recurrence in adulthood after 15 years of quiescence, transitioning from types III to I.[205]

Histologic Findings

Biopsies of PRP show a distinctive pattern of alternating parakeratosis and orthokeratosis. Such alternation can

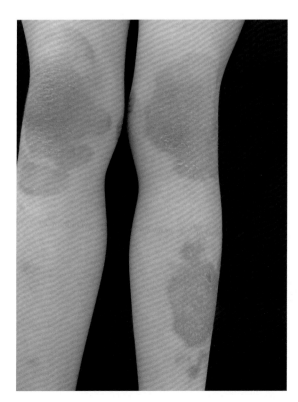

FIGURE 3-37. Pityriasis rubra pilaris. Rough-appearing, well-demarcated erythematous plaques over the knees and legs.

occur in both horizontal and vertical planes, giving rise to the "checkerboard" appearance. The areas of parakeratosis are typically seen around or within the hair ostia. Follicular plugging is also typical of PRP. The granular cell layer can be normal, increased, or decreased. The epidermis is acanthotic, with regular elongation of the rete in a psoriasiform pattern. Focal acantholysis can be seen in up to 70% of cases. The dermis has a very sparse lymphohistiocytic inflammatory response. Slight dilatation of the superficial dermal papillary vessels and hypertrophy of the piloerector muscles can also be encountered in some cases (Figure 3-39). Spongiosis is typically very mild.[201]

Differential Diagnosis

Compared with psoriasis, the epidermal hyperplasia seen in PRP tends to be more irregular (there is more variable elongation of the rete pegs). In PRP, the granular cell layer is typically preserved, and neutrophils in the stratum corneum or epidermis are not seen. Follicular plugging is also not typical of psoriasis. The focal acantholytic changes present in a minority of cases of PRP are also absent in psoriasis. If regressing chronic dermatitis is sampled, the differential diagnosis between psoriasis and PRP might be impossible to establish.

MF can also enter the differential diagnosis (please review previous differential diagnosis between MF and psoriasis).

CAPSULE SUMMARY

PITYRIASIS RUBRA PILARIS

This is a rare, often chronic, inflammatory dermatosis, classified into six classic types on the basis of onset, distribution, and course. Classic findings include follicular, keratotic papules, a cephalocaudal rash, a keratoderma, and classic salmon color, often conferring a "nutmeg grater–like" texture. Islands of spared normal skin are a classic finding. Biopsies of PRP show a distinctive pattern of alternating parakeratosis and orthokeratosis giving rise to a "checkerboard" appearance. Follicular plugging is also typical.

KERATOSIS LICHENOIDES CHRONICA

Definition and Epidemiology

Keratosis lichenoides chronica (KLC) is a very rare, inflammatory, keratotic dermatosis that is chronic and

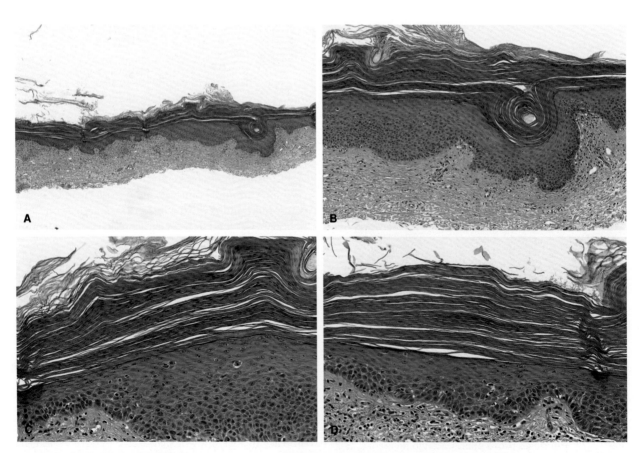

FIGURE 3-39. Pityriasis rubra pilaris. A and B, Vague psoriasiform acanthosis and follicular plugging is noted. C and D, Alternating hyperorthokeratosis and parakeratosis are noted. Digital slides courtesy of Path Presenter.com.

recalcitrant.[217-219] There have been fewer than 100 reported cases of KLC in the literature, with around 20 reported cases in children.[219-221] Pediatric KLC usually presents in infancy and before 3 years of age.[218,220]

Etiology

The etiology of this rare condition is unknown. The only case clusters are in Mexico and New Mexico, suggesting a potential genetic predisposition or ethnic predilection.[220,222]

Clinical Presentation

Classic clinical findings include keratotic, lichenoid, follicularly based papules that coalesce into strikingly linear and reticulated plaques favoring proximal and extensor surfaces (Figure 3-40). Reticulated hyperpigmented patches remain after treatment. SD-like facial plaques also result in hyperpigmentation. The disease course is chronic, progressive, and notably recalcitrant.[219]

Madarosis, keratoconjunctivitis, other ophthalmologic changes, oral aphthae, and mucous membrane keratoses can also be seen.[222] Alopecia of the scalp, eyebrows, and eyelashes is reported.[16] There is one pediatric report of pseudoepitheliomatous hyperplasia within a plaque of KLC.[221]

Histologic Findings

The findings of KLC appear to be similar in adults and children. There is an interface reaction pattern with vacuolar changes of the basal keratinocytes and frequent dyskeratotic cells, with overlying hyperkeratosis and areas of

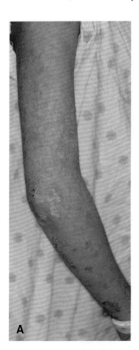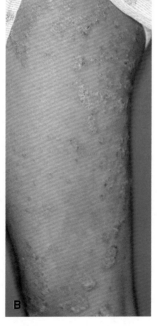

FIGURE 3-40. Keratosis lichenoides chronica. Scaly, erythematous plaques on the arm (A) and leg (B). Courtesy of Aimee Smidt, MD.

parakeratosis. A lichenoid lymphocytic infiltrate is present. Neutrophils can be present in the stratum corneum. Similar to lupus erythematosus, a deep perivascular and periadnexal lymphocytic infiltrate can be seen (Figure 3-41). As opposed to lupus, there is no significant increase in dermal mucin.[218,223,224]

CAPSULE SUMMARY

KERATOSIS LICHENOIDES CHRONICA

KLC is a very rare, inflammatory, keratotic dermatosis that is chronic and recalcitrant. Classic findings include keratotic, lichenoid follicularly based papules that coalesce into strikingly linear and reticulated plaques favoring proximal and extensor surfaces. Biopsies of KLC show an interface reaction pattern with vacuolar changes of the basal keratinocytes and frequent dyskeratotic cells. A lichenoid lymphocytic infiltrate is present. Hyperkeratosis and areas of parakeratosis are seen.

LICHEN PLANUS

Definition and Epidemiology

Lichen planus (LP) is a pruritic, inflammatory dermatosis of the skin, nails, and mucous membranes that usually affects adults, but may also be seen in children.[225] It is classically described as purple, polygonal, pruritic papules and plaques.

Only 2% to 11% of LP cases are pediatric.[225,226] Although there is no definitive racial predilection, reports from the United States show an African-American predisposition, whereas reports from the United Kingdom show mainly children from the Indian subcontinent, and most case series are from the Indian subcontinent and Africa.[225-229] Males and females are affected equally.[226] Mean age of onset in children is 7 to 11.8 years.[227]

Etiology

The etiology of LP is unknown.[16] There are reports of at least 18 cases of pediatric LP occurring after hepatitis B vaccinations, but hepatitis B itself has not been associated with LP.[226,230] Unlike adults, hepatitis C has not been associated with LP in children. There are reports of personal and family histories of autoimmune disease in affected patients (up to 17%).[227] Only 1% to 4% of childhood LP is familial.[228]

Clinical Presentation

Classic LP is the most common presentation in adults and children,[225] presenting on the limbs (lower legs, flexor wrists, and ankles), low back, scalp, or genitals as violaceous flat-topped scaling polygonal papules often coalescing into plaques (Figure 3-42).[16,225,226] Some have white-gray puncta and lacey lines known as Wickham striae.[16,226] Darker skin

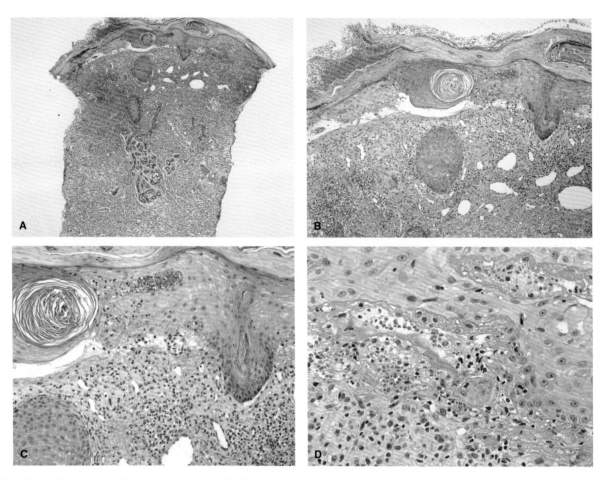

FIGURE 3-41. Keratosis lichenoides chronica (KLC). In KLC, there is a lichenoid dermatosis with deep extension of the inflammation (A). Broad areas of parakeratosis are seen (B). The interface changes noted include vacuolar alteration of the basal keratinocytes and scattered apoptotic cells (C and D).

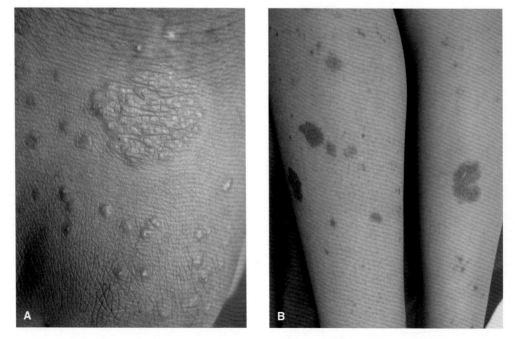

FIGURE 3-42. Lichen planus. A, Flat-topped, hyperlinear, erythematous to violaceous papules and plaques. B, More darkly pigmented skin often presents with hyperpigmented, less erythematous plaques.

tones can have a more slate-gray color.[226] Pruritus occurs in 90% of affected patients.[228]

Mucosal, oral, and genital lesions are much less frequently seen in children than in adults (6%-40% vs. 75%).[16,225,229] The most common oral location is the buccal mucosa.[231] Children may develop mucosal lesions similar to those in adults (hyperkeratotic, reticular with Wickham striae, papules, plaque-like, atrophic/erythematous, and erosive/ulcerative), but tend to fare better than their adult counterparts.[231]

Nail changes are not as commonly seen in children, found in 2.6% to 13.9% of childhood LP.[228] Classic nail changes include nail plate thinning, longitudinal ridging and fissuring, pterygium, and distal splitting.[232] Twenty-nail dystrophy (trachyonychia) and idiopathic nail atrophy are unusual presentations of nail LP. Idiopathic nail atrophy is the rapid, painless destruction of all nails over 6 to 12 months.[232]

Although classic LP is the most common presentation in children, eruptive, hypertrophic, and linear LP are not unusual.[228,229,233] The stripes and segments of linear LP follow Blaschko lines and are more than would be expected from koebnerization.[233] The variants of lichen planopilaris (LPP), actinic LP, and LP pigmentosus, can also be seen.[228,229] In contrast, bullous LP, LP pemphigoides, annular LP, atrophic LP, hemorrhagic/purpuric LP, erosive/ulcerative LP, and lupus-LP overlap are all quite rare in children.[16,225,226,228]

Overall, pediatric LP has a good prognosis; most cases resolve in fewer than 6 months, although some may take years.[16,225,228] Many cases, particularly in darker skin types, can have postinflammatory hyperpigmentation that may be slow to resolve.[225]

Histologic Findings

The pathologic findings of LP are identical in adults and children. Fully developed lesions of LP show an interface and lichenoid reaction pattern with an infiltrate of lymphocytes and histiocytes that obscures the dermal–epidermal junction. The epidermis shows irregular acanthosis with wedge-shaped areas of hypergranulosis. The acanthotic pattern has a sawtoothed pattern. Hyperorthokeratosis on the surface is present. Squamatization of the basal layer is noted, a feature that refers to the flattening of the basilar keratinocytes in the upper epidermis as they enter the granular cell layer just prior to terminal differentiation into the stratum corneum. This phenomenon is best represented in areas where the rete ridges exhibit the jagged or sawtooth shape, and the overlying hypergranulosis provides optimal contrast. Vacuolar degeneration of the basal keratinocytes, in addition to numerous apoptotic and dyskeratotic keratinocytes, is noted (Figure 3-43). When the vacuolar degeneration is very prominent, focal

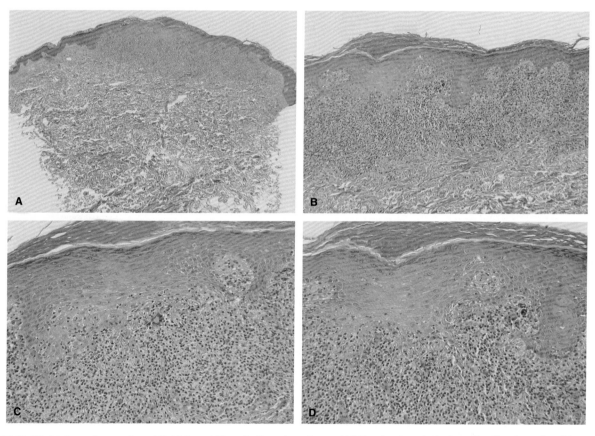

FIGURE 3-43. **Lichen planus.** A and B, Lichenoid band of lymphocytes and histiocytes is noted, obscuring the dermal–epidermal junction. C and D, Interface changes are present, Civatte bodies and pigmented melanophages.

subepidermal clefts are formed, known as Max-Joseph spaces. In some cases, this may present with clinically apparent bullae (bullous LP). The apoptotic keratinocytes exhibit homogeneous eosinophilic cytoplasm and pyknotic basophilic nuclei. The apoptotic cells can be seen in the base of the epidermis, or at all epidermal levels, and within the dermis. In the context of LP, the anucleate remnants of the apoptotic keratinocytes are known as Civatte bodies (colloid bodies, cytoid bodies) when seen in the papillary dermis. Older lesions of LP, particularly in patients of darker skin types, show postinflammatory hyperpigmentation (dermal melanophages). The inflammatory infiltrate in the dermis (within the lichenoid band) consists of lymphocytes and histiocytes with few, if any, eosinophils and plasma cells.[234-239]

In *hypertrophic LP*, there is pronounced acanthosis, vague papillomatosis, and dermal fibrosis secondary to chronic rubbing. Eosinophils are frequently seen (Figure 3-44). *Atrophic LP* shows atrophy of the epidermis with attenuation of the rete pegs (Figure 3-45). *Oral LP* demonstrates similar changes to the skin, but often with parakeratosis, rounded rete ridges as opposed to pointed, and the presence of plasma cells within the inflammatory infiltrate.

Lichen planus actinicus has similar histologic findings to LP and occurs in a photodistributed pattern. This variant is more common in individuals of darker skin, and melanophages are typically found. *Lichen planus pemphigoides* shows a histologic overlap between LP and bullous pemphigoid, including the presence of linear deposition of IgG and C3 along the dermal–epidermal junction by direct immunofluorescence. The latter has been rarely reported in children.

Differential Diagnosis

The histologic differential diagnosis of LP is broad. Lupus erythematosus shows more frequent atrophy of the epidermis and an inflammatory infiltrate that is both superficial and deep into the reticular dermis. Plasma cells are common in LE, in addition to increased dermal mucin. The latter can be demonstrated with the use of special strains (Alcian blue, colloidal iron). LE also shows thickening of the basement membrane zone (demonstrated with PAS stain). Lichen striatus can also enter the differential diagnosis. Similar to that of LE, the inflammation also extends deeper in the dermis, but with a particular perieccrine accentuation. Lichen striatus also lacks the

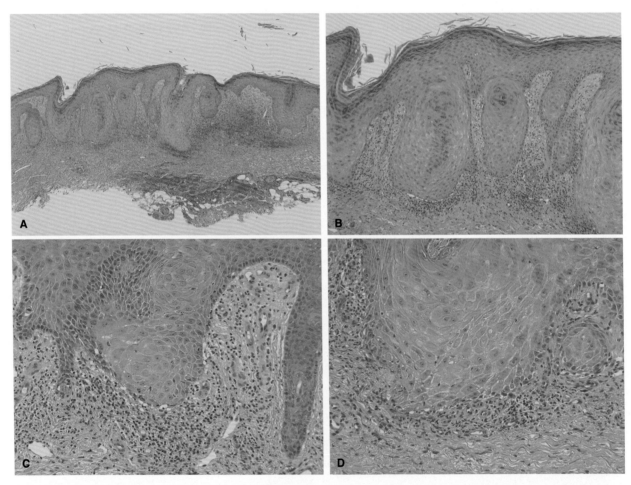

FIGURE 3-44. Hypertrophic lichen planus. A and B, Marked acanthosis and hyperkeratosis with epidermal pseudoepitheliomatous changes. C and D, The lichenoid inflammation is less intense. Interface changes are seen.

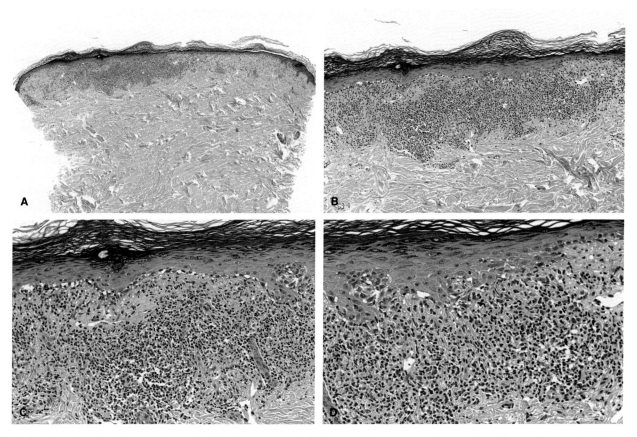

FIGURE 3-45. Atrophic lichen planus (ALP). The changes of ALP are similar to those of conventional lichen planus, with the exception of significant thinning of the surface epidermis (A-D). Digital slides courtesy of Path Presenter.com.

dense lichenoid band present at the dermal–epidermal junction of LP. Pityriasis lichenoides also shows interface changes on the surface epidermis and is relatively common in children. However, both acute (PLEVA) and chronic (PLC) forms have a lymphocytic vasculitis with extravasated red blood cells and lack the irregular acanthosis seen in LP. Lichenoid drug reactions are another potential mimicker of LP. The presence of abundant eosinophils and a history of exposure to a medication can be helpful clues to establish the latter diagnosis.

CAPSULE SUMMARY

LICHEN PLANUS

LP is a pruritic, inflammatory dermatosis of the skin, nails, and mucous membranes, classically described as purple, polygonal, pruritic, papules, and plaques. Children have similar presentation to adults, but tend to have a better prognosis. Histologically, classic LP shows an interface lichenoid reaction pattern with an infiltrate of lymphocytes and histiocytes that obscures the dermal-epidermal junction. The epidermis shows irregular acanthosis with wedge-shaped areas of hypergranulosis. The bases of the rete have a saw-toothed pattern.

LICHEN NITIDUS

Definition and Epidemiology

Lichen nitidus is a fairly rare, benign inflammatory dermatosis with characteristic small, flat-topped, uniform thin papules with central dells. It is most commonly seen in children of preschool and school ages.[16] There is no known gender or ethnic predilection. The actinic variant of lichen nitidus, however, is more common in darker complexions and in tropical locations.[240]

Etiology

The specific etiology is unknown. However, many propose an association with LP because they can be seen in the same patient and have similar early histologic findings.[241] Lichen nitidus has also been seen in families and in association with Niemann–Pick disease, Russell–Silver syndrome, and Trisomy 21.[16,242,243]

Clinical Presentation

Lichen nitidus presents with classic minute, flat-topped, shiny, skin-colored thin papules, often with a central dell. Individual lesions are round to polygonal and monomorphic.

They range from pinpoint to 2 mm in size[16,244] and most commonly present as localized clusters on the trunk, genitalia, flexor upper extremities, and dorsal hands (Figure 3-46).[20] Lichen nitidus uncommonly can be generalized, and older children have been reported to have palmar involvement.[244,245] Lichen nitidus does exhibit koebnerization. Rare mucosal findings include small, gray, flat papules on the buccal mucosa.[16] Although nail involvement is more common in adults, it can be seen in addition to cutaneous lichen nitidus or as the presenting feature in children.[20,246] Nail changes include pits, rippling, trachyonychia, distal splitting, and longitudinal ridges. Resolution is usually spontaneous over the course of months to years without residua, although postinflammatory pigmentary alteration has been reported.[245] Uniquely, lichen nitidus actinicus tends to recur seasonally every summer and is more likely to have a photo distribution.[240]

Histologic Findings

The pathologic findings in lichen nitidus include the presence of localized areas of lichenoid and interface changes that are restricted to a width of 3 to 5 rete ridges with a "ball and claw" pattern. The epidermis shows focal parakeratosis overlying the areas of thinning. At the edges of the atrophic epidermis, there is classic elongation of the rete ridges with an inward turn. Within the papillary dermis, a lichenoid lymphohistiocytic infiltrate is present, contained by the elongated rete. Vacuolar degeneration of basal keratinocytes and scattered apoptotic keratinocytes are seen (Figure 3-47). Extension around adnexal appendages has been rarely described. Many cases of lichen nitidus show focal areas of granulomatous inflammation within the lymphohistiocytic foci. Eosinophils and plasma cells are only rarely present. The inflammation is restricted to the region of the flattened epidermis. The dermis outside this area is devoid of inflammation. Some cases can show perforating features.[247-249]

Differential Diagnosis

Differential diagnostic considerations include LP and granulomatous dermatoses (including infectious processes). As opposed to LP, lichen nitidus shows only small and focal areas of lichenoid/interface changes. Additionally, the epidermis tends to be acanthotic in LP, but is thinned in lichen nitidus. The localized character of a granulomatous reaction can also suggest the possibility of a ruptured folliculitis.

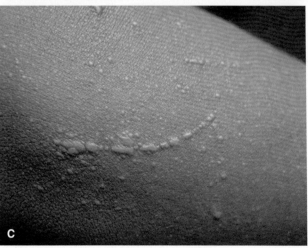

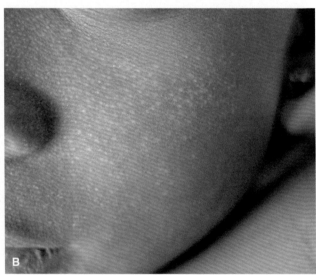

FIGURE 3-46. Lichen nitidus. A, Tiny, flat-topped, skin-colored papules. B, Lesions on the face of a young child. C, A linear arrangement of papules indicating development of lesions after scratching, known as koebnerization.

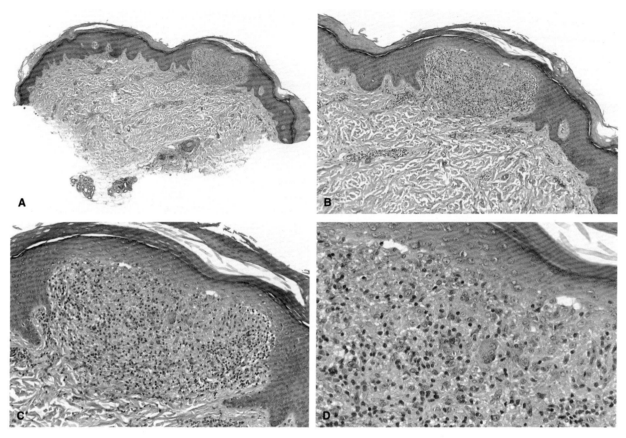

FIGURE 3-47. Lichen nitidus. Localized lichenoid and interface dermatitis, limited to two to three rete ridges (A and B). The epidermis is thinned within this area and, in addition to the interface changes, granulomas are present (C and D). Digital slides courtesy of Path Presenter.com.

CAPSULE SUMMARY

LICHEN NITIDUS

LN is a fairly rare, benign inflammatory dermatosis with characteristic small, flat-topped, uniform thin papules that range in size from pinpoint to 2 mm. It commonly presents as localized clusters of papules on the trunk, genitalia, flexor upper extremities, and dorsal hands. The pathologic findings in lichen nitidus include the presence of localized areas of lichenoid and interface changes that are restricted to 3 to 5 rete ridges with a "ball and claw" pattern.

LICHEN STRIATUS

Definition and Epidemiology

Lichen striatus is a Blaschkolinear, self-limited, inflammatory dermatosis seen primarily in children.[16] It shows a 3:1 female predominance.[250] The average age of onset is 4 years (range 4 months-15 years).[20,250,251]

Etiology

Although the specific etiology has not been elucidated, numerous hypotheses point to an underlying genetic mosaicism (possibly related to retrotransposons) combined with a potential trigger.[20,252] Reported associations or potential triggers include a viral illness, vaccines (measles, mumps, and rubella [MMR] and hepatitis B), and trauma.[16,252] Additionally, 50% to 60% of patients are atopic, suggesting that an aberrant immune status is a predisposing factor.[250,253] Further in support of a genetic predisposition are reports of cases clustering in families, including in a mother and son and siblings.[252,254]

Clinical Presentation

Lichen striatus presents with classic flat-topped scaling papules that converge into curvilinear bands along the lines of Blaschko (Figure 3-48).[16] Papules can be erythematous, hypopigmented, or skin colored. Lichen striatus favors the extremities (lower greater than upper), but can also involve the face (15% of cases) trunk, neck, and buttocks.[251,253] Typically, one line of Blaschko is involved, but up to 6% of children may have multiple.[255] Lesions usually arise over days to weeks, spreading both proximally and distally. Lichen

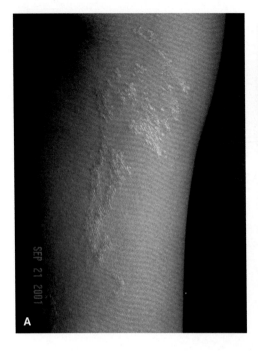
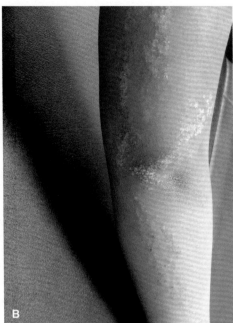

FIGURE 3-48. **Lichen striatus.** Faintly erythematous scaly plaques in a Blaschkolinear distribution (A and B).

striatus takes months to years to resolve; the average duration is 6 to 7 months with reports of up to 3.5 years duration.[16,256] It usually resolves without long-term residua, but many cases have postinflammatory hypopigmentation.[251] Nail changes can be seen if the nail matrix lies in the affected line of Blaschko; these changes include onycholysis, splitting, pitting, longitudinal ridging and fissuring, shredding, leukonychia, nailbed hyperkeratosis, and nail plate loss.[251,257] Lichen striatus is usually asymptomatic, but pruritus can occur in up to one-third of cases.[250]

Histologic Findings

Biopsies of lichen striatus show an interface pattern. There is a mild lichenoid band of lymphocytes and histiocytes with vacuolization of the basal cell layer which leads to keratinocyte apoptosis. In earlier lesions, the lichenoid inflammation is denser, and with time, this inflammation becomes less prominent. Mild acanthosis with elongation of the rete ridges is seen. Focal areas of spongiosis can also be seen, particularly within the lower portions of the epidermis. Parakeratosis can also be present. The dermis contains a superficial and deep, perivascular, perifollicular, and particularly perieccrine, lymphocytic infiltrate (Figure 3-49). Eosinophils and plasma cells are not typically found.[251,258-262]

Differential Diagnosis

The main clinical differential diagnosis includes other inflammatory skin disorders with a blaschkoid distribution. LP, particularly the linear forms, can be particularly challenging to separate from lichen striatus. As opposed to LP, the inflammation is deeper in lichen striatus, and has a perieccrine location. The parakeratosis of lichen striatus is also not typical of LP.

Although lupus erythematosus can be histologically similar to lichen striatus, they can be easily differentiated on a clinical basis. In addition, the basement membrane thickening, dermal mucin, and clusters of CD123+ plasmacytoid dendritic cells can also be useful in pointing toward a diagnosis of lupus. Another important consideration includes a diagnosis of Blaschkitis, which many consider to be a variant of lichen striatus. In contrast to LS, the lesions heal much more rapidly, which is the main clinical distinction. Blaschkitis runs its course over 2 to 6 weeks and is characterized by a high recurrence rate. The biopsies show more prominent spongiosis.[73]

CAPSULE SUMMARY

LICHEN STRIATUS

This is a Blaschkolinear, self-limited, inflammatory dermatosis usually affecting children. It presents with classic flat-topped scaling papules that converge into curvilinear bands along the lines of Blaschko. Biopsies show an interface pattern with mild lichenoid inflammation with lymphocytes and histiocytes, vacuolization of the basal cell layer, and keratinocyte apoptosis. In earlier lesions, the lichenoid inflammation is denser, and with time, the lichenoid inflammation becomes less prominent. Deep perieccrine lymphocytic inflammation is characteristic.

GRAFT-VERSUS-HOST DISEASE

Definition and Epidemiology

Graft-versus-host disease (GVHD) is a known complication of hematopoietic stem cell transplantation (HSCT) in

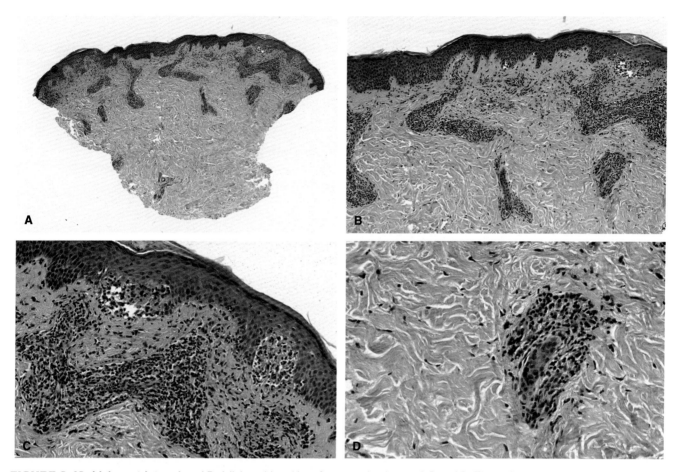

FIGURE 3-49. Lichen striatus. A and B, A lichenoid and interface reaction is noted. B and D, The main characteristic of lichen striatus is the presence of a perieccrine lymphocytic infiltrate. C, The interface changes include vacuolar degeneration of the basal keratinocytes and apoptotic cells. Digital slides courtesy of Path Presenter.com.

which the donor immune system recognizes host tissues as foreign.[16,263,264] It can affect any organ system and is classically seen after a HSCT in patients whose immune systems have been suppressed by radiation and chemotherapy. GVHD can also occur in immunodeficient children after receiving blood products or at birth and after multisolid organ transplant due to donor T-cell chimerism.[16,265] GVHD can be acute or chronic or have hybrid features, known as overlap syndrome.[266]

GVHD is the most common nonrelapse-related complication affecting long-term survivors of HSCT for malignant disease.[267,268] Children, generally, are at a lower risk of developing GVHD than adults (20%-50% vs. 60%-70%, respectively).[263,268] Moderate to severe GVHD can be seen in 10% to 50% of HLA-identical donors.[16] Chronic GVHD is seen in as few as 6% of matched sibling cord blood and as much as 65% of matched unrelated peripheral blood stem cell transplant recipients.[264,268] Having acute GVHD increases the risk of chronic GVHD. A variety of stem cell transplant factors related to the donor and recipient affect the risk of developing GVHD (see Table 3-4).

Etiology

Acute GVHD has three phases: conditioning, activation, and effector. During the conditioning phase, preparatory chemotherapy and radiation result in host tissue damage, usually in the gastrointestinal tract. Subsequently, antigen-presenting cells from the donor and the recipient activate donor-derived Th1 cells. Finally, the activated donor T cells effect cytotoxicity against host cells through a variety of pathways: fas-fas ligand, perforin-granzyme B, and TNF-α.[263]

Although the mechanism of acute GVHD has been well described, the mechanism of chronic GVHD is poorly understood and may involve a combination of alloreactivity and autoimmunity.[264] Key players in chronic GVHD include alloreactive donor T cells, B cells, antibodies to minor histocompatibility alloantigens (such as the H-Y antigen in male recipients of female donors), autoantibodies (such as antinuclear antibodies [ANA], anti-ds-DNA, anticardiolipin, antimitochondrial, antismooth muscle, platelet, and antineutrophil antibodies), and inflammatory cytokines (MCP-1, IL-6, TGF-β, IFN-γ).[268] Antiplatelet-derived growth factor antibodies, involved in the fibrosis of scleroderma, are seen in sclerotic GVHD.[268]

TABLE 3-4. Risk factors for graft-versus-host disease[16,263,267,268]

Increased Risk	Reduced Risk
Male recipient of female donor cells,[16,267] especially if the female is parous	Cord blood stem cells[263,268]
Peripheral blood stem cell[268]	Greater HLA matching (allele matching instead of group matching)[263,268]
Older age—donor or recipient	Relative/sibling donor[268]
Mismatched donor	Youth—donor or recipient[268]
Unrelated donor	
Total body radiation, pretreatment malignancy[268]	
Acute GVHD → for chronic GVHD	

Abbreviations: GVHD, graft-versus-host disease; HLA, human leukocyte antigen.

Clinical Presentation

The skin is the most commonly affected organ in all GVHD, with involvement in 75% of cases; other frequently involved organs are the mouth, liver, and eyes.[264]

Acute GVHD classically starts less than 100 days after transplant but is frequently seen in the first 2 to 4 weeks.[16] Skin findings in mild to moderate acute GVHD are very nonspecific and include erythematous macules and papules that are often morbilliform (Figure 3-50). They favor the ears, as well as the face, neck, palms, and soles.[16] In moderate to severe acute GVHD, the presentation ranges from a generalized morbilliform eruption to confluent exfoliative erythroderma. Lesions can be bullous, and severe disease may mimic toxic epidermal necrolysis (TEN).[16,263,265]

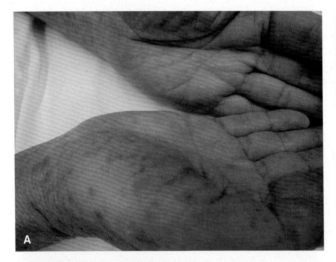

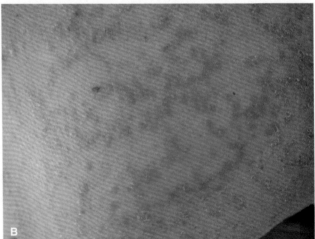

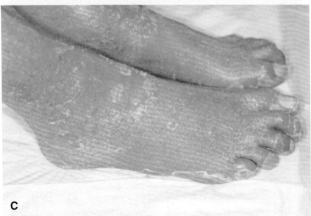

FIGURE 3-50. **Graft-versus-host disease.** A, Erythematous papules on the palms. B, Lichenoid papules on the trunk. C, Erythrodermic pattern on the feet. Courtesy of Barrett Zlotoff, MD.

Desquamation is common.[16] Other cutaneous presentations of acute GVHD include acquired ichthyosis, pustular acral erythema, columnar epidermal necrosis, and general desquamation.[265] A unique form of acute GVHD with isolated mild skin involvement can be seen after an autologous transplant; it self-resolves in 1 to 3 weeks.[16] Liver and gastrointestinal involvement are also frequently seen, with crampy abdominal pain, nausea, vomiting, diarrhea, and hepatitis.[263,264] Many other organ systems can be involved (see Table 3-5). Staging is based on the number and extent of organ involvement, with a focus on skin findings, bilirubin, and diarrhea.[263,264]

Children present very similarly to adults with chronic GVHD. Although acute GVHD increases the risk of chronic GVHD, many people develop only chronic disease. Chronic GVHD is no longer defined by time (ie, more than 100 days after transplant), but by the clinical presentation and pathology.[16,268] Most cases present an average of 6 months after transplant, but all cases are noted before 3 years post transplant.[16,268] It is graded as mild, moderate, or severe on the basis of the number of sites, functional impairment/disability, and lung involvement.[268] Similar to the autoimmune conditions that chronic GVHD often mimics, it can affect any organ.[16] Diagnosis is made on the basis of the presence of one or more diagnostic manifestations or at least one distinctive manifestation with diagnosis confirmed by biopsy, laboratory studies, or radiology (see Table 3-5).[266] Diagnostic cutaneous findings are poikiloderma, LP-like lesions, morphea-like sclerosis, lichen sclerosis–like lesions, and deep sclerosis/fasciitis.[264,266] LP-like lesions can be linear in either blaschkoid or dermatomal distribution.[16] Other skin changes include depigmentation, dyspigmentation, ichthyosis, new keratosis pilaris, and nail dystrophy (50% of patients).[264,266]

Sclerotic chronic GVHD is the most severe and recalcitrant form.[268] It is rare, but potentially deadly, with the onset

TABLE 3-5.	Clinical findings and organ involvement in acute and chronic graft-versus-host disease[16,263,267,268]		
Organ	**Acute**	**Chronic Diagnostic**	**Chronic Distinctive/Other**
Skin	Morbilliform eruption Blisters Desquamation Ear involvement Exfoliative dermatitis TEN-like Acquired ichthyosis Pustular acral erythema Columnar epidermal necrosis Pruritus	LP-like LS-like Morphea-like Poikilodermatous Sclerotic	Depigmentation Dyspigmentation Ichthyosis Keratosis pilaris Sweat alteration
Skin appendages			Dystrophy Ridging, splitting, brittle Pterygium Loss (symmetric/most) Onycholysis Alopecia scarring Alopecia, nonscarring Hair thinning or graying Scalp scaling
Oral	Mucositis Gingivitis Erythema Pain	LP-like Hyperkeratotic plaques Restricted oral opening	Xerostomia Atrophy Ulcers Mucoceles Pseudomembranes
Genital		LP-like Vaginal scarring/stenosis	Erosion Fissure Ulcer
Ocular		New dry eye Cicatricial conjunctivitis Keratoconjunctivitis sicca Keratopathy, punctate	Photophobia Periorbital pigmentation Blepharitis

(continued)

TABLE 3-5.	Clinical findings and organ involvement in acute and chronic graft-versus-host disease[16,263,267,268] (continued)		
Organ	**Acute**	**Chronic Diagnostic**	**Chronic Distinctive/Other**
GI/liver	Nausea Abdominal pain, crampy Watery/bloody diarrhea Hepatomegaly Transaminitis/hepatitis Hyperbilirubinemia	Esophageal stenosis Esophageal stricture Esophageal web	Pancreative insufficiency
Lung	BOOP	Bronchiolitis obliterans	
Blood			Thrombocytopenia Eosinophilia Lymphopenia Anemia Hyper-/hypogammaglobulinemia Autoantibodies
Musculoskeletal		Fasciitis Joint stiffness Joint contractures	(poly)Myositis Muscle cramps Arthritis/arthralgias
Other	Fever Anorexia Weight loss/failure to thrive		Effusions/ascites Neuropathy, peripheral Nephrotic syndrome Myasthenia gravis Cardiac abnormalities (conduction, myopathy, coronary artery fibrosis)

Abbreviations: BOOP, bronchiolitis obliterans organizing pneumonia; GI, gastrointestinal; LP, lichen planus; LS, Lichen sclerosus; TEN, toxic epidermal necrolysis.

of widespread ulceration portending a poor prognosis.[269] It favors the trunk and proximal limbs and can present with classic dyspigmentation referred to as a "leopard-skin eruption."[269] Alopecia and contractures are also seen in sclerotic GVHD.[269] Hepatic dysfunction is common.[269]

Histologic Findings

GVHD is an interface tissue reaction pattern. A gradient system has been developed to evaluate and assess the severity of the disease. Grade I lesions typically show minimal epidermal change: there is mild vacuolar degeneration of the basal keratinocytes and slight spongiosis. Grade II shows more prominent interface changes, with the presence of apoptotic keratinocytes along the basal layer (Figure 3-51). Lymphocyte exocytosis can also be seen. There may be a mild band of lymphocytes and histiocytes. Eosinophils can be sometimes present. The interface changes can also be present in the hair follicle epithelium and eccrine ducts. Grade III lesions show more extensive apoptosis with confluence, which results in separation of the epidermis from the dermis and early vesicle formation (Figure 3-52). Finally, the more advanced stages of acute GVHD, grade IV, have areas of full-thickness epidermal necrosis and subepidermal

vesicle formation. Many examples of GVHD show epidermal atypia or dysplasia (actinic keratosis–like changes), a pattern that has been associated with the use of chemotherapy agents, and sometimes referred to as "epidermal dysmaturation." The term "satellite cell necrosis" applies to the presence of apoptotic keratinocytes surrounded by lymphocytes in the epidermis, and is not specific for a diagnosis of GVHD. Rare examples of psoriasiform GVHD have been documented, including in children.[270-276]

Chronic GVHD shows two main reaction patterns: lichenoid (LP-like) pattern and a form that resembles scleroderma. Acute changes of GVHD can be seen in biopsies of chronic GVHD. The lichenoid form of chronic GVHD resembles or is identical to LP: there is irregular epidermal acanthosis with hyperkeratosis and wedge-shaped hypergranulosis. A lichenoid band of lymphocytes and histiocytes obscures the dermal–epidermal junction. Apoptotic keratinocytes and vacuolar alteration of basal keratinocytes are also present. Many cases show numerous dermal melanophages.

The sclerodermoid pattern has features that are indistinguishable from scleroderma or morphea (Figure 3-53).[277] Slight vacuolar changes of individual keratinocytes and melanophages are seen in this form of GVHD. There is diffuse dermal fibrosis with a decreased number of adnexal

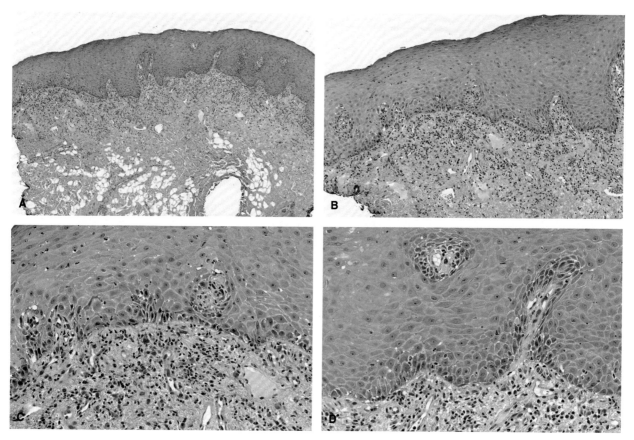

FIGURE 3-51. Graft-versus-host disease, grade II. Epidermal acanthosis (A and B). Epidermal dysmaturation is noted. In addition, the interface changes include vacuolar alteration of the basal keratinocytes and apoptotic cells (C and D). Digital slides courtesy of Path Presenter.com.

structures. The fibrosis increases the thickness of the dermis. There is a superficial and deep, perivascular, and interstitial chronic inflammatory infiltrate of lymphocytes, histiocytes, and plasma cells. The fibrosis can also extend superficially into the adipose tissue.

Differential Diagnosis

The two main differential diagnostic considerations are a viral exanthem and a drug eruption. A viral infection usually lacks keratinocyte apoptosis and shows more frequent spongiosis. A drug hypersensitivity reaction can be virtually impossible to distinguish from GVHD. Indeed, dermal eosinophils can be present in both conditions. However, abundant eosinophils and the presence of apoptotic cells in the acrosyringium have been shown to favor a diagnosis of a drug reaction.

The eruption of lymphocyte recovery is described as a generalized exanthem occurring 17 to 21 days after chemotherapy initiation. It has been debated whether this represents a distinct condition or a mild form of GVHD. The findings of this entity are identical to those present in grade I or II GVHD. A mild superficial and perivascular lymphocytic infiltrate is noted in the absence of a significant number of dermal eosinophils.

CAPSULE SUMMARY

GRAFT-VERSUS-HOST DISEASE

GVHD is a known complication of HSCT in which the donor immune system recognizes host tissues as foreign. Acute GVHD presents clinically with a range of findings from generalized morbilliform eruption to confluent exfoliative erythroderma, bullae, and a TEN-like presentation. Chronic GVHD presents with LP-like findings, sclerodermoid change, or deep involvement. Histologically, acute GVHD shows an interface reaction pattern and is graded by severity. Chronic GVHD has two forms: a LP-like reaction and a sclerodermoid.

ERYTHEMA MULTIFORME

Definition and Epidemiology

Erythema multiforme (EM) is a self-limited hypersensitivity reaction that is immune mediated and characterized by the sudden onset of classic targetoid lesions. It can be distinguished as major and minor, with severe involvement of mucosa and systemic symptoms in the former.[278] Although

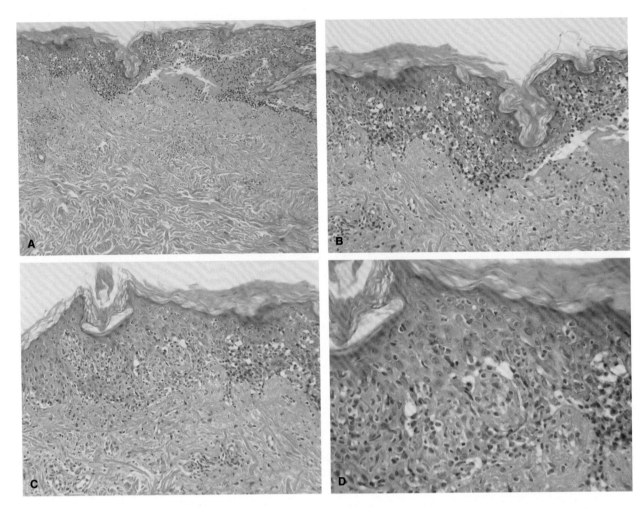

FIGURE 3-52. **Graft-versus-host disease (GVHD), grade III.** A and B, More severe lesions of GVHD show more prominent apoptosis and dyskeratosis. B, A subepidermal blister is seen. C and D, Full-thickness apoptosis and dyskeratosis are evident.

initially considered on a spectrum with SJS and TEN, it is now widely considered a unique entity that does not progress to this syndrome or TEN.[16,278] EM is most commonly seen in young adults between 20 and 40 years old.[279] Approximately 20% of cases are in children.[278] EM is even rarer in neonates, with only three biopsy-proven cases reported.[280]

Etiology

As a hypersensitivity reaction, EM requires a trigger that is usually herpes simplex virus (HSV) infection. HSV infection, usually herpes labialis, is seen in 63% of cases and 71% of recurrent cases.[16,278,281] Because herpes is such a common precipitant, the term HSV-associated EM (HAEM) was coined. In one study of pediatric EM, HSV DNA was detected in 80% of cutaneous lesions by PCR, even in the absence of a clinical history of HSV infection.[282] Other infections associated with EM include HSV2, CMV,[283] varicella zoster virus,[283] EBV,[284] orf, histoplasmosis, group A strep,[283] and mycoplasma.[283] Drugs (such as penicillin) and vaccines (diphtheria-pertussis-tetanus, hepatitis B, BCG, smallpox) are other reported causes, particularly in infants.[279,280,283]

The specific mechanism of EM is unclear, but autoreactive T cells have been implicated in studies of HAEM,[285] and some neonatal cases suggest that circulating immune complexes play a role.

Clinical Presentation

EM is usually recognized clinically with the abrupt onset of classic "target" or "iris" lesions. They appear symmetrically in groups on the palms and soles, dorsal hands and feet, and extensor arms and legs covering less than 2% of the body surface area.[16] The targets have three concentric regions: a dusky center, a pale edematous zone, and a peripheral thin erythematous ring (Figure 3-54). Atypical lesions are common and are either poorly defined or have only two zones. Additional findings can include vesicles, bulla, petechiae, and evidence of koebnerization.[16] Lesions typically progress over 72 hours to 7 days. They usually remain fixed for a week and heal over 2 to 3 additional weeks without sequelae.[16,278] These episodes can recur sporadically every year.[281] Mucosal involvement is not uncommon and is seen in 25% to 50% of children; it is typically isolated to the mouth or lips and spares the gingiva.[16,286] Lip

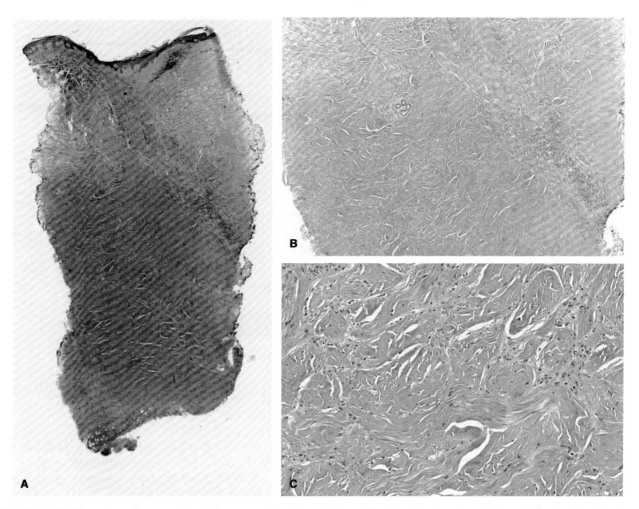

FIGURE 3-53. Chronic graft-versus-host disease, sclerodermoid form. The chronic sclerodermoid form is identical to scleroderma and morphea. There is marked dermal fibrosis with a marked loss of adnexal structures. A perivascular and interstitial chronic inflammatory infiltrate is also present (A-C). Digital slides courtesy of Path Presenter.com.

involvement can be quite extensive. Systemic symptoms such as fever and malaise are rare and mild if present.[16]

Histologic Findings and Differential Diagnosis

Because of the similarity to SJS, these topics are discussed in the following section.

CAPSULE SUMMARY

ERYTHEMA MULTIFORME

EM is an immune-mediated, self-limited hypersensitivity reaction. The sudden onset of classic targetoid lesions that appear symmetrically in groups on the palms and soles, dorsal hands and feet, and extensor arms and legs covering less than 2% of the affected body surface is characteristic. Approximately 20% of cases occur in children. Histologically, EM is characterized by vacuolar interface dermatitis with necrotic keratinocytes and prominent superficial dermal lymphocytic inflammation.

STEVENS–JOHNSON SYNDROME, TOXIC EPIDERMAL NECROLYSIS, AND MYCOPLASMA-INDUCED RASH AND MUCOSITIS

Definition and Epidemiology

Stevens–Johnson syndrome (SJS) and toxic epidermal necrolysis (TEN) constitute the spectrum of a life-threatening, mucocutaneous hypersensitivity reaction leading to extensive necrosis of the epidermis and the epithelium. It is most commonly triggered by medications but can also be caused by infectious agents. The spectrum is defined by the degree of epidermal detachment: less than 10% body surface area is seen in SJS, 10% to 30% in SJS–TEN overlap, and greater than 30% in TEN.[287] A subtype of mucosal-predominant SJS caused by *Mycoplasma pneumoniae* has been renamed mycoplasma-induced rash and mucositis (MIRM).[288]

SJS, SJS–TEN, and TEN are all exceedingly rare and are more common in adults than in children. The average age of onset in SJS is 28 years.[289] The average age of the SJS/

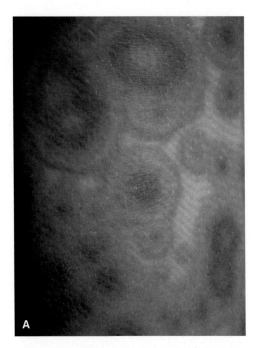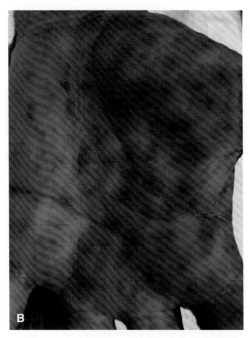

FIGURE 3-54. **Erythema multiforme.** A, Targetoid erythematous macules. B, Palmar involvement is characteristic.

TEN spectrum in children is 9 to 10 years.[290,291] Cases in neonates and infants are quite rare, but have been reported.[292] The incidence per million children per year is 5.3 cases for SJS, 0.8 for SJS–TEN, and 0.4 for TEN.[290] When comparing pediatric cases to adult cases, generally mortality is lower, recurrence risk is higher (reported 18%), and half of the children have cutaneous and ocular sequelae.[291] In mixed patient populations, reports of TEN mortality range from 9.5% to 40%, with an average of 25% to 30%.[293-295] Mortality in children is 0% for SJS, 2% to 4% with SJS–TEN overlap, and 16% for TEN.[290,291] Of note, HIV infection significantly increases the risk of SJS.[16,296]

Etiology

SJS and TEN are commonly triggered by medications, although infectious agents have also been reported. Over 200 medications have been reported to cause SJS and TEN.[297] The most common classes are antiepileptics and antimicrobials.[298] Analyses of highest-risk medications identified aromatic anticonvulsants (carbamazepine, lamotrigine, valproate, phenobarbital, phenytoin), sulfonamides, β-lactams, allopurinol, oxicam nonsteroidal anti-inflammatory drugs (NSAIDs), nevirapine, and sulfasalazine (Table 3-6).[294,297-300] Commonly used acetaminophen may also be a trigger.[294] Recent reports suggest that trimethoprim may be responsible for some cases of SJS and TEN, even in the absence of sulfamethoxazole.[301] Generally speaking, the longer the half-life of a medication, the more likely it is to trigger SJS than similar medications of the same class.[299]

Over 80% of TEN cases are triggered by medications. Identifying and discontinuing the culprit medication is essential, a process that may be aided by use of the ALDEN algorithm[302] and lymphocyte transformation tests.[296] Recently identified serum biomarkers including miR-18a-5p and HMGB1 (high-mobility group protein B1) can be used to distinguish SJS/TEN from other drug hypersensitivity reactions.[295,303] Host risk factors for developing drug-induced SJS/TEN include HIV, altered drug metabolism, and specific HLA types with specific medications (see Table 3-7).[16,296,299,300]

TABLE 3-6.	Highest risk medications for Stevens–Johnson syndrome and toxic epidermal necrolysis[299]
Common Drugs (Highest Risk)	
Allopurinol	
Carbamazepine	
Cotrimoxazole + other sulfa antibiotics	
Lamotrigine	
Nevirapine	
Oxicam NSAIDs	
Phenobarbital	
Phenytoin	
Sulfasalazine	

Abbreviation: NSAIDs, nonsteroidal anti-inflammatory drugs.

TABLE 3-7.	HLA types at high risk for Stevens–Johnson syndrome and toxic epidermal necrolysis[16,299,300]
Carbamazepine	**HLA-b*15:02-Han, Asian** **HLA-A*3101- European**
Phenytoin	HLA-b*15:02- Asian
Allopurinol	HLA-b*5801
Sulfamethoxazole	HLA-B*38
Lamotrigine	HLA-B*38
Oxicam NSAID	HLA-B*73

Abbreviation: HLA, human leukocyte antigen; NSAID, nonsteroidal anti-inflammatory drug.

Other triggers of SJS and TEN include infections, malignancy,[304] lupus,[20,294] vaccines (MMR),[300] and contrast,[300] with many cases being idiopathic.[304] An infectious etiology is much more likely to be found in children than in adults,[16,305] particularly with *M. pneumoniae* or *Chlamydia pneumoniae*.[288,306] These cases tend to be mucosal predominant. Other identified infectious triggers are dengue and CMV.[300]

The characteristic epidermal necrosis results from disordered apoptosis. Apoptosis caused by granulysin, perforin, and granzyme from cytotoxic CD8$^+$ T cells and NK cells leads to the characteristic keratinocyte death.[297,300,304] Fas-Fas ligand interactions and TNF-α have also been implicated.[300] T-cell activation is usually due to a drug-immune system interaction and potentially is a prohapten process.[300]

Clinical Presentation

SJS and TEN usually present 7 to 21 days after drug exposure and always within 8 weeks.[16] Average onset in pediatric cohorts is 9 days,[297] whereas it is 15 days in adult cohorts.[289] Onset is within 2 to 3 days of exposure and may represent a cross-reaction or reexposure.[16,297] Onset of cutaneous eruption is preceded by a prodrome that may consist of fever, malaise, anorexia, headache, cough, pharyngitis, rhinorrhea, conjunctivitis, vomiting, diarrhea, chest pain, arthralgias, and myalgias for 1 to 14 days.[16,293,299,300] This is followed by erythematous to purpuric macules, a morbilliform eruption, or atypical targetoid macules that are notably painful.[299,300] They begin on the face and upper trunk and can be symmetric, widespread, and commonly palmoplantar.[299] As the macules become confluent, gray or bullous changes emerge and subsequent denuding or sloughing results in widespread erosions (Figure 3-55).[299] Nikolsky sign, easy detachment of the epidermis with lateral pressure, is present, although it is nonspecific.[16] Epidermal detachment can continue for up to a week.[299,300] Reepithelialization may begin within days and lasts for 1 to 3 weeks.[299,300]

Mucosal involvement of at least two sites is required for a definitive diagnosis of SJS or TEN and may include the lips, tongue, buccal mucosa, eyes, nose, genitalia, and rectum (Figure 3-56).[300] Although mucosal changes may be more pronounced in SJS than in TEN,[16] 87% to 100% of TEN cases have mucosal inflammation or ulceration.[300] Findings include bulla, erosions, ulcerations, gray-white membranes, and hemorrhagic crusts.[300] Mucosal changes are painful, leading to difficulty in eating, hydrating, urinating, and defecating.[300] Mucosal sites can develop strictures over the long term, but the mouth is the least likely to do so.[300] The mouth is the most commonly affected mucosal site, followed by eyes

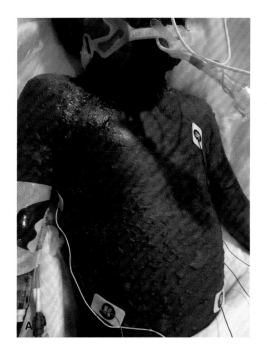
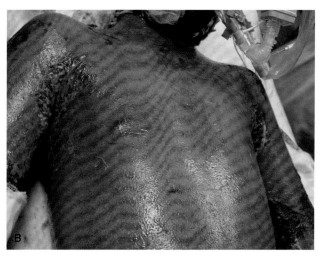

FIGURE 3-55. Toxic epidermal necrolysis. A, Extensive erosions, bullae, and dusky necrosis of the skin. **B,** Nearly total desquamation of the skin at a later stage.

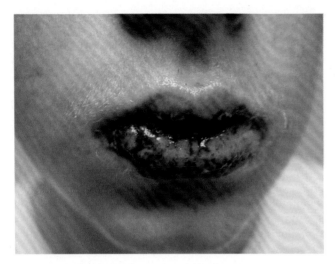

FIGURE 3-56. **Stevens–Johnson syndrome.** Crusted erosions on the lips.

and genitalia. Ocular changes include purulent conjunctivitis, photophobia, corneal ulcerations, keratitis, uveitis, and panophthalmitis[16,289] with a high risk of sequelae, making ophthalmologists crucial in management.

SJS and TEN rapidly become multisystem conditions with potential respiratory, renal, gastrointestinal, hepatic, cardiac, and hemodynamic dysfunction (see Table 3-8).[16,293] Septicemia is a frequent cause of morbidity and mortality. Children are better able to maintain hemodynamic function than adults, but airway compromise from edema remains an important risk.[293]

The Score of Toxic Epidermal Necrolysis scale is a validated composite score to predict prognosis and mortality in adults with SJS/TEN and has been shown to accurately predict prognosis in pediatric cases as well, although there are modified proposed pediatric scales.[307] Predictors of mortality are renal failure, malignancy, septicemia, bacterial infection, epilepsy, and increasing percentage of body surface involvement (>30%).[290]

Long-term sequelae are seen in at least half of cases (Table 3-8), and most commonly affect the skin and eyes. Dyspigmentation and scarring are the most common cutaneous sequelae.[16,295,298] Respiratory sequelae such as chronic cough, sinusitis, or functional airway obstruction can be seen in 19% of cases.

As previously mentioned, MIRM has been reclassified from EM major and SJS on the basis of morphology, prognosis, and treatment.[288] Although classically reported with *Mycoplasma*, *C. pneumoniae* has been shown to cause the same phenotype of disease.[306] Patients affected by MIRM are younger (average age of all affected patients is 12-14 years) and more commonly male.[278,289] Cutaneous findings are sparse to absent in 81% of cases.[288] Mucosal findings dominate the clinical picture (94% have oral involvement, 82% have eye involvement, and 63% have genital findings) (Figure 3-57).[288] The cornerstone of treatment for MIRM is appropriate antibiotics, often azithromycin or doxycycline, although steroids and intravenous immunoglobulin have been used.[288] Prognosis is good, with only 3% mortality, although there is an 8% risk of recurrence.[288] On the basis of the etiology, it is not surprising that cases can cluster,[308] and patients often have a coinciding pneumonia.[309]

Histologic Findings

The histologic findings of EM, SJS, and TEN are similar and will be described together (in addition to the differential diagnostic considerations). Each entity is characterized by an interface reaction pattern: the epidermis is often normal in

TABLE 3-8.	Multisystem findings of Stevens–Johnson syndrome/toxic epidermal necrolysis and sequelae[16,295,298,300]	
System	**Acute Involvement**	**Sequelae**
Skin (dermatologic sequelae in 42%)	Painful Dusky erythematous to purpuric macules Morbilliform eruption Atypical targetoid macules Bulla Erosion Ulceration Sloughing + Nikolsky sign	Scar Dyspigmentation Onycholysis Onychodystrophy Loss of nails Pruritus Alopecia, hair thinning Eruptive nevi
Oral	Bulla Erosions Ulcerations Gray-white membranes Hemorrhagic crusts Painful po intake	Discomfort Xerostomia Reduced saliva Increased saliva acidity Periodontal disease Gingivitis Scar/synechia Severe oral fibrosis

TABLE 3-8.	Multisystem findings of Stevens–Johnson syndrome/toxic epidermal necrolysis and sequelae[16,295,298,300] (continued)	
System	**Acute Involvement**	**Sequelae**
Ophthalmologic sequelae 27%	Purulent conjunctivitis Photophobia Corneal ulcerations Keratitis Uveitis Panophthalmitis	Reduced visual acuity or blindness, trichiasis, symblepharon, conjunctival scarring, keratoconjunctivitis sicca=dry eyes, corneal ulceration, neovascularization, subconjunctival fibrosis
Genital	Dysuria Pain with defecation Penile and scrotal erosions/ulcerations Vulvar/vaginal erosions/ulcerations	Dyspareunia Adhesions Introital stenosis Vaginal synechia Phimosis—2%
GI	Hepatitis Transaminitis Abdominal pain Diarrhea Hepatosplenomegaly	Esophageal stricture Sclerosing cholangitis
Respiratory (25% of TEN)	Airway compromise ARDS Bronchiolitis obliterans Subcutaneous emphysema Hypoxemia, dyspnea, bronchial mucosal sloughing Interstitial infiltrates on CXR Pneumonitis	Chronic bronchitis Bronchiectasis Bronchiolitis obliterans BOOP Obstruction Nasal septal synechiae
Renal	Acute renal failure Microalbuminuria Hypoalbuminemia Hyponatremia Hypernatremia Renal tube enzymes in urine Proteinuria Microscopic hematuria Nephritis	
Hematopoietic	Anemia Leukopenia, leukocytosis Eosinophilia Elevated ESR Lymphadenopathy	
Constitutional/infectious	Fevers Malaise Anorexia Pharyngitis Dehydration Septicemia	Growth delay
Other	Myocarditis Arthritis Encephalopathy	Hearing loss

Abbreviations: ARDS, Acute respiratory distress syndrome; BOOP, bronchiolitis obliterans organizing pneumonia; CXR, chest x-ray; ESR, erythrocyte sedimentation rate; GI, gastrointestinal; po, orally; TEN, toxic epidermal necrolysis.

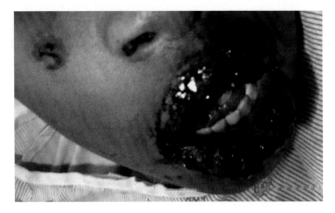

FIGURE 3-57. Mycoplasma-induced rash and mucositis. Crusted erosions on the lips, identical to that seen in Stevens–Johnson syndrome.

thickness and shows varying degrees of vacuolar degeneration of the basal keratinocytes, in addition to necrotic and apoptotic keratinocytes, frequently at all the levels of the epidermis. Lymphocyte exocytosis can be seen. The stratum corneum is orthokeratotic, with parakeratosis in biopsies taken from mucosal sites (Figure 3-58). In TEN, full-thickness epidermal necrosis is noted, often resulting in a subepidermal noninflammatory blister (Figure 3-59). Interestingly, cases of TEN typically lack significant inflammation as

opposed to EM. Scattered eosinophils can be seen in the dermis, particularly when triggered by medications. There is some evidence that keratinocyte necrosis within the acrosyringium favors a drug-induced EM possibly because of the toxic levels of the medication within these structures.[310-313] The histologic overlap between EM and lupus erythematosus has been referred to as Rowell syndrome.[314]

Differential Diagnosis

The histologic differential diagnosis of EM/SJS/TEN includes lupus erythematosus, dermatomyositis, GVHD, pityriasis lichenoides, and fixed drug reactions (particularly the more generalized forms). GVHD can usually be excluded on the basis of the clinical history (bone marrow transplant). However, the findings seen in GVHD and EM may be identical, and a histologic separation is not always possible. Lupus erythematosus can be differentiated on the basis of the basement membrane zone thickening, deep inflammation, the presence of plasma cells, and an increased amount of dermal mucin. Eosinophils are also absent in lupus, unless medication induced. Dermatomyositis, similarly to lupus, has increased dermal mucin. Pityriasis lichenoides, particularly PLEVA, can show areas of epidermal necrosis. However, PLEVA has abundant dermal inflammation. In addition, the presence of a lymphocytic vasculitis is not seen in EM/

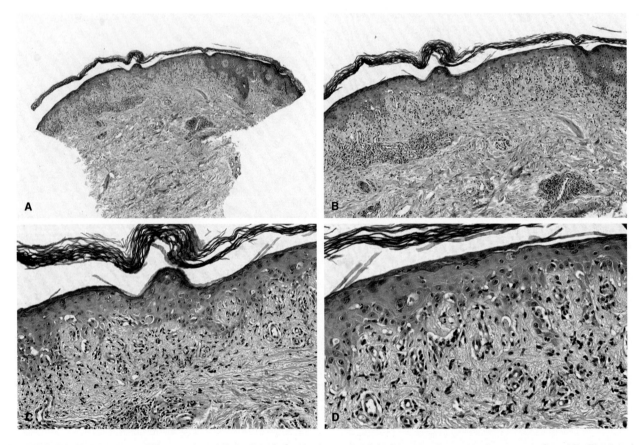

FIGURE 3-58. Erythema multiforme. A and B, An interface reaction patter interface reaction patter is present. C and D, The interface reaction shows numerous dyskeratotic and apoptotic cells along the epidermal layer. Digital slides courtesy of Path Presenter.com.

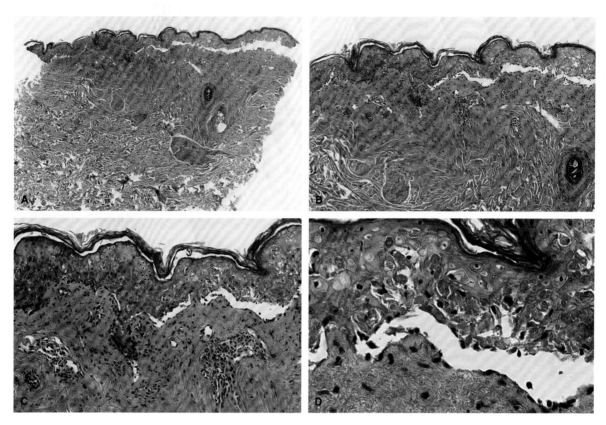

FIGURE 3-59. **Toxic epidermal necrolysis.** A and B, Areas of transepidermal necrosis and subepidermal blister formation are seen. C and D, Numerous dyskeratotic cells are seen. Digital slides courtesy of Path Presenter.com.

SJS/TEN. Fixed drug eruptions (FDEs) can be particularly challenging to distinguish from EM. FDE tends to have a greater degree of spongiosis, and the inflammatory infiltrate often includes neutrophils and eosinophils. After repeated episodes, FDE leaves abundant dermal melanophages in the papillary dermis. Infectious processes can also be considered in the differential diagnosis, particularly varicella/zoster and HSV. The viral cytopathic changes, PCR studies, and immunohistochemistry can easily exclude those conditions.

CAPSULE SUMMARY

STEVENS–JOHNSON SYNDROME AND TOXIC EPIDERMAL NECROLYSIS

SJS and TEN constitute the spectrum of a life-threatening, mucocutaneous hypersensitivity reaction leading to extensive necrosis of the epidermis and the epithelium. It is most commonly triggered by medications but can also be caused by infectious agents. Following a prodrome, there is eruption of painful erythematous to purpuric macules, a morbilliform eruption, or atypical targetoid macules. Histologically, interface dermatitis is seen with varying degrees of vacuolar degeneration of the basal keratinocytes, necrotic and apoptotic keratinocytes, and transepidermal necrosis in SJS and TEN.

ERYTHEMA DYSCHROMICUM PERSTANS

Definition and Epidemiology

Erythema dyschromicum perstans (EDP), also known as "ashy dermatosis," is an acquired dermatosis of slate-gray hyperpigmentation.[315,316] It is slowly progressive and asymptomatic- and is considered by some to be a variant of LP or LP pigmentosus.[20]

EDP usually presents before the 4th decade. It has been reported in patients as young as 2 years old, but is most common in young adults.[20,317] Only 8% of patients with EDP are less than 12 years old.[318] Although some authors suggest a slight female predominance, most report no gender predilection.[315] EDP favors darker skin tones, such as Fitzpatrick types III and IV, and it is most common in Hispanics.[16,20,315] Interestingly, one report of 14 cases suggests that children with EDP may be more likely to be Caucasian (12 cases) than Hispanic (2 cases).[315] Other reported ethnicities of affected children include African, Indian, and Asian.[316,318]

Etiology

The specific etiology of EDP is still unknown. Although there are reported triggers in adult patients (sicknesses, infections, and medications), there have been no identified potential triggers in pediatric cases.[315,318]

Clinical Presentation

EDP begins as ash-gray to gray-blue macules that spread centrifugally and symmetrically, often on the trunk.[20,318] Individual lesions range from millimeters to centimeters and can be oval, round, or polycyclic (Figures 3-60 and 3-61).[16,315] Early EDP may have an elevated, erythematous 1 to 2 mm rim.[315] The neck, trunk, and upper arms are commonly involved; the scalp, palms, soles, and mucosa are spared.[16,20,315] Some authors report lesions arranged along Blaschko lines.[20] Although adults tend to have chronic disease, 50% to 70% of prepubertal children clear spontaneously in an average of 2.5 years.[315,318]

Histologic Findings

Depending on the age of the lesion, the findings in EDP can be quite variable. The acute phase shows an interface dermatitis. The chronic phase has postinflammatory hyperpigmentation changes (Figure 3-62). In the chronic phase, a diagnosis of EDP can be very difficult to establish without an adequate clinicopathologic correlate. Early lesions show vacuolar degeneration of the basal keratinocytes and scattered apoptotic keratinocytes. Mild spongiosis can be sometimes seen. A lymphoid population is present along the dermal–epidermal junction or within the dermis with either a lichenoid or perivascular pattern. Eosinophils are not typically seen. The older lesions show less spongiosis and interface changes, a lower number of lymphocytes, and abundant dermal melanophages. Epidermal atrophy can also be seen. Other features identified in chronic lesions include papillary dermal fibrosis and telangiectasis.[319-321]

Differential Diagnosis

The histologic differential diagnosis of EDP includes other interface dermatoses. Many believe that EDP represents a form of LP. It is virtually impossible to distinguish a lesion of atrophic LP from EDP. As opposed to more conventional

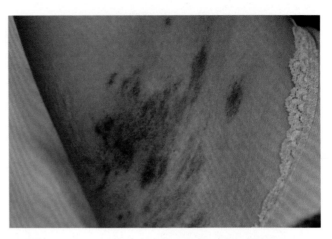

FIGURE 3-61. Lichen planus pigmentosus. Thin hyperpigmented plaques in the axilla. This entity is considered by some to be on a spectrum with erythema dyschromicum perstans. Courtesy of Barrett Zlotoff, MD.

cases of LP, EDP lacks the hyperkeratosis, irregular acanthosis, and dense lichenoid infiltrate of LP. EDP can be differentiated from lupus erythematosus by the lack of significant hyperkeratosis, follicular plugging, deep inflammation, and interstitial mucin deposition. FDE tends to have more spongiosis, neutrophils, and eosinophils when compared with EDP. EM has an acute clinical presentation, as opposed to the chronic presentation of EDP, but may have very similar histologic features. Pityriasis lichenoides shows a denser inflammatory infiltrate and evidence of lymphocytic vasculitis.

CAPSULE SUMMARY

ERYTHEMA DYSCHROMICUM PERSTANS

EDP, ashy dermatosis is an acquired dermatosis of ash-gray to gray-blue macules that spread centrifugally and symmetrically, often on the trunk. A total of 8% of affected patients are 12 years old or younger. Pathologic findings depend on the age of the lesion and can be quite variable. The acute phase shows an interface dermatitis, whereas the chronic phase may show only changes of postinflammatory hyperpigmentation.

LUPUS

Definition and Epidemiology

Lupus is an autoimmune condition related to immune complex deposition. It can involve any organ system, resulting in a diversity of disease phenotypes. The skin is frequently affected. The Systemic Lupus International Collaborating Clinics Diagnostic Criteria for systemic lupus erythematosus (SLE) are the most commonly used and have a 94% sensitivity and 92% specificity (see Table 3-9).[322] There are four types of cutaneous lupus erythematosus (CLE): acute (ACLE),

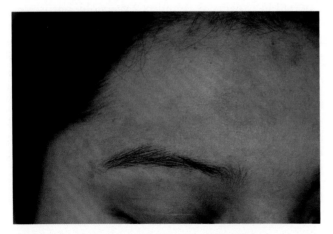

FIGURE 3-60. Erythema dyschromicum perstans. Slate-gray hyperpigmentation on the forehead. Courtesy of Barrett Zlotoff, MD.

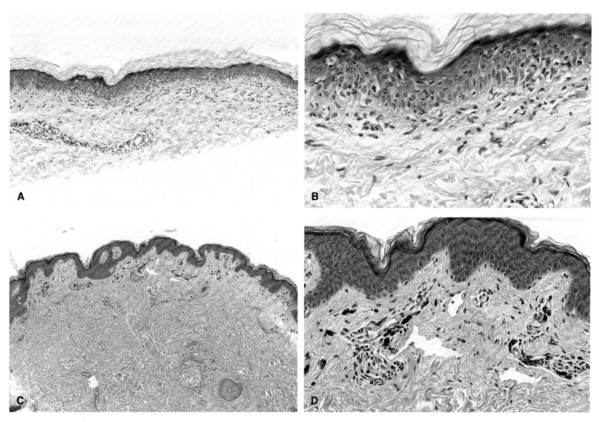

FIGURE 3-62. Erythema dyschromicum perstans. Acute phase (A and B), with evidence of basal layer vacuolar degeneration, exocytosis of lymphocytes, and a few lightly pigmented dermal melanophages. Chronic phase (C and D), with a normal epidermis and heavily pigmented dermal melanophages. These changes are indistinguishable from other causes of postinflammatory pigmentary alteration. Digital slides courtesy of Path Presenter.com.

subacute (SCLE), intermittent, and chronic (CCLE). For more information on neonatal lupus, lupus panniculitis, and chilblains lupus, see the chapters on newborn disease (Chapter 2), panniculitis (Chapter 5), and perniosis (Chapter 6).

The incidence of CLE in the general population mirrors the incidence of SLE (4/100 000).[323] Approximately one in five cases of lupus presents before 20 years of age.[16] Most (60%) pediatric SLE cases start between 11 and 15 years old,[16,324] whereas 35% of pediatric SLE occurs between 5 and 10 years old, and only 5% of SLE starts before age 5.[16,324]

Subacute CLE represents 10% to 15% of CLE in children.[16] Discoid lupus erythematosus (DLE) is the most common form of chronic cutaneous lupus, but is rare in children, with less than 3% of cases occurring prior to 10 years old.[322] There is a female predominance, which may become more pronounced as the age of onset increases.[325] Non-Caucasian children, especially African-American and Hispanic children, are at an increased risk of systemic lupus. These cases are more likely to be severe and complicated by nephritis or central nervous system involvement.[326]

TABLE 3-9.	Systemic Lupus International Collaborating Clinics diagnostic criteria[16,322]
Clinical Criteria	**Comments**
1. Acute cutaneous lupus	Malar/butterfly Bullous lupus Photosensitive lupus rash[a] Maculopapular lupus rash TEN variant SCLE lesions (polycyclic)

(continued)

TABLE 3-9.	Systemic Lupus International Collaborating Clinics diagnostic criteria[16,322] *(continued)*
Clinical Criteria	**Comments**
2. Chronic cutaneous lupus	DLE (localized or generalized) Lupus panniculitis (profundus) Tumid lupus Chilblains lupus Hypertrophic/verrucous lupus LP/LE Mucosal lupus
3. Oral ulcers	Palate, buccal, tongue, nasal[a]
4. Nonscarring alopecia	Diffuse thinning[a] Fragility/broken hairs[a]
5. Synovitis	Synovitis in ≥2 joints (swelling, effusions) Tenderness in ≥2 joints + 30 min morning stiffness
6. Serositis	Pleural cavity: pleurisy >1 d, effusions, rub Pericardium: pericardial pain >1 d, effusion, rub, pericarditis[a] by EKG
7. Renal	Urine protein/urine Cr: 500 mg protein/d RBC casts Biopsy-proven lupus nephritis[b]
8. Neurologic	Seizures Psychosis Mononeuritis multiplex[a] Myelitis Neuropathy[a]: peripheral or cranial Acute confusional state[a]
9. Hemolytic anemia	
10. Leukopenia	Leukopenia <4000/mm^{3a} Lymphopenia <1000/mm^{3a}
11. Thrombocytopenia	<100 000/mm^{3a}
Immunologic Criteria	**Comments**
1. +ANA[b]	
2. Anti-ds DNA Ab+[b]	
3. Anti-Sm Ab+	
4. Antiphospholipid Ab+	Lupus anticoagulant False-positive RPR Medium or high anticardiolipin Anti-β2 glycoprotein I
5. Low complement	C3 C4 CH50
6. Direct Coombs test[a]	
Nondiagnostic systemic findings	Livedo reticularis and racemosa Raynaud phenomenon, rare (n) Pernio Urticarial vasculitis/LCV Bullous SLE Papulonodular (dermal) mucinosis Alopecia (DLE, fragility/receding hairline of short broken hairs ("lupus hair"), telogen effluvium) Mucosa: mucositis, gingivitis, hemorrhage, erosion, ulceration, redness, silvery-whitening Periungual telangiectasia (c), periungual erythema (c) palmar erythema(c), periungual gangrene (n)

[a]absence of other causes.

[b]Four criteria, at least one in each category—OR—nephritis + ANA or dsDNA.

Abbreviations: ANA, antinuclear antibodies; DLE, discoid lupus erythematosus; dsDNA, double-stranded deoxyribonucleic acid; EKG, electrocardiography; LE, lupus erythematosus; LCV, leukocytoclastic vasculitis; LP, lichen planus; RBC, red blood cells; RPR, rapid plasma reagin; SCLE, subacute lupus erythematosus; SLE, systemic lupus erythematosus; TEN, toxic epidermal necrolysis.

Etiology

Lupus is a complex condition triggered by autoimmune and autoinflammatory activation and immune complex deposition.[16,327] Both genetic predisposition and environmental triggers play a role.[16] A genetic component is supported by familial cases as well as the identification of pathogenic mutations in autosomal recessive juvenile-onset SLE (*PRKCD*) and autosomal recessive hypocomplementemic urticarial vasculitis (*DNASE1L3*).[16] Furthermore, genetic deficiency of C1q is the strongest risk factor for SLE.[16] HLA-DR3 type has shown an increased risk for SCLE.[328] Known environmental triggers include UV radiation, various medications, pesticides, metals, tobacco, and infections.[16]

Clinical Presentation

There are both specific and nonspecific cutaneous findings in lupus patients. Of the specific types of cutaneous lupus, acute is the most common in children, followed by subacute and chronic.[325] Atypical presentations and rare CLE variants, such as chilblains, may be more common in children.[325]

Acute Cutaneous Lupus Erythematosus

ACLE is seen in patients with SLE; 80% of pediatric SLE patients have cutaneous involvement, which is often a presenting symptom.[16] ACLE classically presents as erythematous slightly scaling plaques of the malar cheeks confluent with the bridge of the nose, known as the butterfly or malar rash (Figure 3-63). Although common, seen in 60% to

74% of patients with SLE, the malar rash is not specific for SLE.[16,324] Other potential findings in acute CLE include markedly erythematous papules in a photodistributed pattern on the lower neck, upper chest, and hands. Digital involvement spares the knuckles.[16]

Subacute Cutaneous Lupus Erythematosus

SCLE presents with erythematous, scaling annular, polycyclic, or figurate plaques in photoexposed areas, commonly in the upper trunk and extensor extremities (Figure 3-64).[328,329] There is often central telangiectasia.[328] Although nonscarring, it does commonly result in postinflammatory pigment alteration.[328,329] SCLE patients are usually (70%-90%) positive for anti-SS-A(Ro) antibodies, and they can also have anti-SS-b (La) antibodies. Sixty percent to 80% are ANA positive.[328,329]

Given the rarity of SCLE in childhood, ascertaining the actual risk of SLE in these patients is difficult.[327,328] Reassuringly, a summary in 2015 of all 11 reported cases of pediatric SCLE showed a benign course with none meeting criteria for SLE,[328] although 2 of the 11 children did have C2 deficiency, a known risk factor for SLE.[328] Nonbullous histiocytoid neutrophilic dermatitis is a rare Sweet's-like presentation of SCLE with blanching violaceous papules and plaques or well-defined erythematous, edematous curvilinear crusted plaques.[330]

Intermittent Cutaneous Lupus Erythematosus

Intermittent CLE comprises tumid lupus, which presents on the face or other sun-exposed areas with fixed erythematous to violaceous urticarial plaques.[16]

Chronic Cutaneous Lupus Erythematosus

CCLE includes DLE, lupus panniculitis, lupus profundus, and chilblains lupus (lupus pernio). DLE presents with well-demarcated, raised, or indurated, telangiectatic,

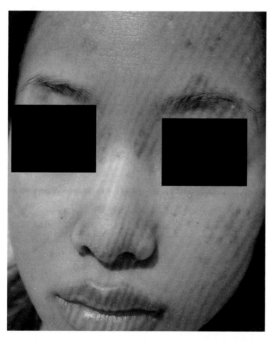

FIGURE 3-63. Systemic lupus erythematosus. Acute cutaneous lupus erythematosus on the face, with thin erythematous plaques in a photodistributed pattern on the face.

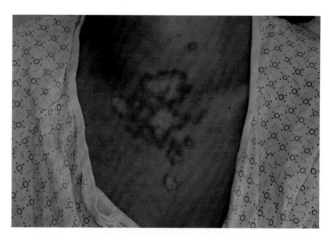

FIGURE 3-64. Subacute cutaneous lupus erythematosus. Annular erythematous plaques on the upper chest. Courtesy of Barrett Zlotoff, MD.

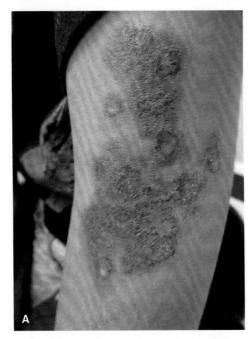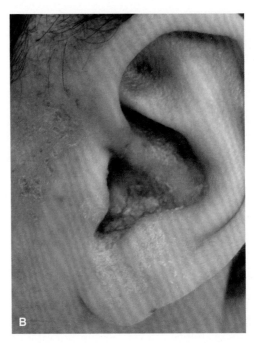

FIGURE 3-65. **Discoid lupus erythematosus.** Scaly erythematous plaques with mottled pigmentation on the arm (A), face, and conchal bowl (B).

violaceous scaling plaques (Figures 3-65 and 3-66).[16] Alopecia is noted within lesions.[20,331] Scaling is often adherent, and marked follicular plugging (carpet-tack-like) is common. Over time, plaques develop atrophy, scar, telangiectasia, and central hypopigmentation or mottled pigmentation.[331,332] About half of the cases are photosensitive.[322] The ears, particularly the conchal bowls, are classic locations.[16] DLE is "localized" if it is above the neck only and "generalized" when plaques are noted below the neck. It may present in a Blaschkolinear distribution.[331,333] Lupus profundus occurs when DLE overlies lesions of lupus panniculitis, and like DLE, this can be Blaschkolinear.[331,334]

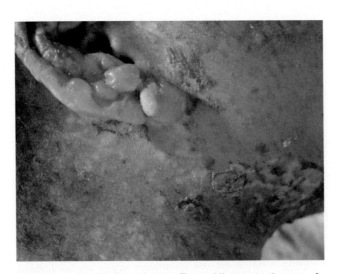

FIGURE 3-66. **Bullous lupus.** Tense blisters on the ear of a patient with lupus on a background of discoid lupus.

As with SCLE, the rarity of DLE in childhood makes ascertaining the exact risk of SLE difficult.[332,335] However, several smaller studies suggest that pediatric DLE has a faster rate and higher risk of conversion to SLE than adult DLE (23.5%-30% vs. 0%-28%).[16,322,332,335] Generalized DLE, when compared with localized DLE, has an increased risk of SLE.[322] However, the SLE in these pediatric DLE cases tends to follow a benign course, with almost 90% meeting the mucocutaneous criteria with no end-organ damage.[335,336]

Nonspecific

There are many nonspecific clinical dermatologic findings in lupus (see Table 3-9). Many are vascular phenomena such as livedo reticularis, Raynaud phenomenon, pernio, and vasculitis (Figure 3-67). Periungual telangiectasia, erythema, and gangrene can be noted.[322,324] Although alopecia is a prominent finding of DLE lesions, patients with lupus can also have telogen effluvium and hair fragility.[16,322] A variety of mucosal changes in addition to ulcers can be seen.[16,322]

Drug Induced

Many drugs have been reported to induce all types of cutaneous lupus.[16] The most commonly encountered triggers in pediatric patients include minocycline and TNF-α inhibitors for ACLE/SLE, terbinafine, griseofulvin, NSAIDs for SCLE, and TNF-α inhibitors for CCLE.[16]

Histologic Findings

Discoid lupus erythematosus shows the classic pathologic findings of LE. There is hyperorthokeratosis with lymphohistiocytic infiltrate. Scattered plasma cells can be seen. Eosinophils are not typically present. Increased interstitial dermal mucin can be shown with the use of special stains (colloidal iron, alcian blue). Clusters of plasmacytoid dendritic cells can be demonstrated by immunohistochemical staining with CD123 at the dermal–epidermal junction and within the dermis. The same changes of DLE can be encountered in biopsies taken from scarring alopecia in patients with LE.[337-339]

In *subacute LE (SCLE)*, *neonatal LE*, and early DLE, dermal lymphocytes may be sparse enough that a vacuolar rather than a lichenoid pattern and a more superficial, rather than a superficial and deep, pattern of inflammation is observed (Figure 3-69). In SCLE, the epidermis can have a more atrophic pattern. Other features that can be present in both SCLE and DLE are fibrin thrombi, or lymphocytic leukocytoclastic debris (nuclear dust) within and around vessels (small vessel vasculitis) or in the subepidermal or subcutaneous areas.

Systemic LE (SLE) shows similar changes to those seen in DLE. However and paradoxically, those changes seem to be less intense. *Tumid lupus erythematosus* or *lupus tumidus* is a less frequent variant of LE that lacks significant epidermal changes. Within the dermis, there is a very intense superficial and deep, perivascular, and periadnexal lymphocytic infiltrate with scattered plasma cells. Marked increased dermal mucin is present, which is greater in proportion to other forms of LE (Figure 3-70). Tumid lupus, reticular erythematous mucinosis, and Jessner lymphocytic infiltrate share identical histologic findings (and might represent the same clinicopathologic entity).[340-342]

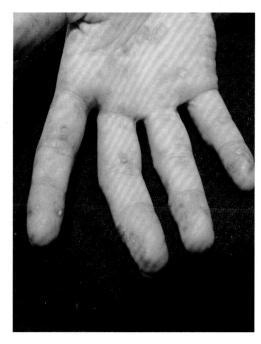

FIGURE 3-67. **Chilblain lupus (lupus pernio).** Erythematous papules and erosions on the fingertips, extending onto the hand.

follicular plugging and normal to mildly acanthotic epidermis. The interface changes include vacuolar degeneration of (Figure 3-68) keratinocytes, dyskeratotic cells, and apoptotic keratinocytes. Older lesions show thickening of the basement membrane zone, which can be demonstrated with a PAS stain. Within the dermis, there is a superficial and deep, perivascular, perifollicular, and perieccrine

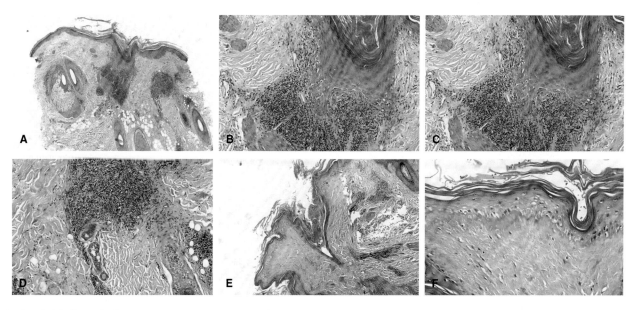

FIGURE 3-68. **Discoid lupus erythematosus.** A, Interface dermatitis with superficial and deep, perivascular, and periadnexal inflammation. B and C, Closer view of the interface changes. Perieccrine lymphocytic infiltrate (D). Follicular plugging (E) and thickening of the basement membrane zone (F). Digital slides courtesy of Path Presenter.com.

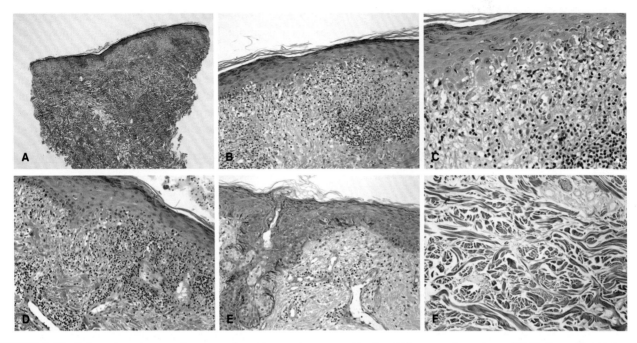

FIGURE 3-69. **Subacute cutaneous lupus erythematosus.** As opposed to discoid lupus erythematosus (DLE), the epidermis is more atrophic and the inflammation more superficial (A and B). Interface changes are noted, but less intense than DLE (C and D). Periodic acid–Schiff shows only focal thickening of the basement membrane area, and colloidal iron shows increased dermal mucin (E and F).

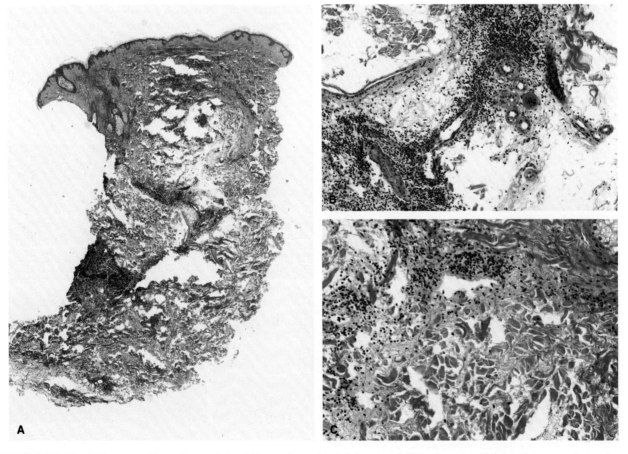

FIGURE 3-70. **Tumid lupus erythematosus.** In tumid lupus, the epidermis is normal. There is a superficial and deep, perivascular, and periadnexal infiltrate with a prominent increased amount of dermal mucin (A-C).

Bullous LE is characterized by a subepidermal blister. The underlying dermis shows a dense neutrophilic infiltrate with marked leukocytoclasis. Within the dermis, there is also a superficial and deep, perivascular, and periadnexal inflammatory infiltrate with dermal mucin, features more typical of conventional LE (Figure 3-71). Linear or mixed linear and granular deposits of IgG are present along the basement membrane zone. IgM and/or IgA can also be present.[343-345]

Lupus profundus or *lupus panniculitis* is discussed in detail in the panniculitis chapter (Chapter 5). *Neonatal lupus erythematosus (NLE)* resembles SCLE in histology. There is an interface pattern with vacuolar degeneration of the basal keratinocytes and scattered dyskeratotic cells. Epidermal atrophy can be present. There is a superficial to mid-dermal perivascular and periadnexal lymphohistiocytic infiltrate. More recently, several cases of NLE have shown a dermal infiltrate rich in neutrophils. On rare occasions, the neutrophils can be accompanied by large histiocytic cells that express CD68, CD33, and myeloperoxidase. Such changes are reminiscent to those seen in Sweet syndrome and the histiocytic variant of this disorder.[346-351]

Direct immunofluorescence is an ancillary tool that can be of significant benefit in establishing the diagnosis of LE. There is a granular staining pattern with antibodies directed against IgG, IgA, IgM, and C3 along the basement membrane zone and is most frequently seen in the biopsies of DLE and SLE. The sensitivity is much lower in cases of SCLE, tumid lupus, and lupus profundus.

Differential Diagnosis

An adequate clinicopathologic correlation is capital to separating the different forms of LE. Likewise, other connective tissue disorders, like dermatomyositis and mixed connective tissue disease, should be distinguished from LE on a clinical basis. LP can resemble LE both clinically and pathologically, including its propensity to cause a scarring alopecia (LPP). Compared with LP, LE exhibits a denser and deeper dermal inflammatory infiltrate, increased dermal mucin, basement membrane thickening, and a lack of dense lichenoid inflammation.

PMLE may sometimes resemble LE clinically and can be differentiated histologically by marked papillary dermal edema. Most cases of PMLE do not exhibit interface or other epidermal changes. Cases of tumid lupus should be distinguished from Lyme disease, CLH, arthropod bite reactions, and cutaneous marginal zone lymphoma. Lyme disease can share the superficial and deep perivascular, and periappendigeal inflammation. However, the mucin is not a common finding. In addition, the history of exposure to a tick bite and positive serologic findings can help in the differential diagnosis. Both CLH and arthropod bite reactions share the dense inflammatory infiltrate in the dermis. However, both typically have abundant eosinophils. Germinal center formation can also be present, a feature that is not typical of tumid lupus (although it can be seen in lupus profundus). Cutaneous marginal zone lymphoma can be distinguished on the basis of the presence of atrophic follicles and clonal populations of B cells or plasma cells. Frequent IgG4-positive plasma cells are present.

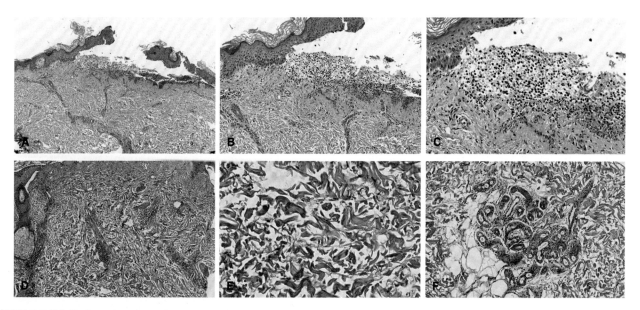

FIGURE 3-71. Bullous lupus erythematosus (BLE). A-C, In BLE, there is a subepidermal blister containing abundant neutrophils. Other parts of the biopsy show more classic lupus changes: deep inflammation (D), mucin deposition (E), and perieccrine inflammation (F). Digital slides courtesy of Path Presenter.com.

CAPSULE SUMMARY

LUPUS

Lupus is an autoimmune condition related to immune complex deposition and can involve any organ system, with the skin being frequently affected. There are four types of CLE: acute, subacute, intermittent, and chronic. Clinical findings range from erythematous slightly scaling plaques of the malar cheeks in the acute form to scaling annular plaques in the subacute form and hyperkeratotic plaques in the chronic form (discoid lupus). Interface dermatitis is seen in the vast majority of cases, with DLE showing follicular plugging, a superficial and deep, perivascular, and periadnexal lymphocytic infiltrate, and increased dermal mucin. SCLE shows less epidermal change, and sparser, more superficial inflammation. Direct immunofluorescence studies can be beneficial in establishing the diagnosis.

FIXED DRUG ERUPTION

Definition and Epidemiology

Fixed drug eruption (FDE) is a sharply demarcated, localized dermatosis that recurs with exposure to an inciting agent. It can occur at any location, but classically flares in the exact same place when reexposed to the offending compound. Acutely, it ranges from violaceous to a dusky erythema, but often results in chronic hyperpigmenation.[16,352]

FDE comprises 22% of common adverse drug reactions in children,[353] which makes it the 2nd or 3rd most common drug reaction.[352,354] Although there may be a male predominance, many studies show no gender preference.[355]

Etiology

FDE is a type IV hypersensitivity reaction. CD8[+] intraepidermal memory T cells are found at the site of eruption and, upon activation by the drug, release IFN-γ to cause direct cytolysis via Fas-Fas ligand interaction or perforin.[356] Numerous drugs have been reported to cause FDE, with the most common causes changing over time with physician prescribing habits and drug availability.[357] For example, reactions to phenolphthalein have reduced after its removal from over-the-counter laxative preparations.[16] The most common culprit is currently sulfamethoxazole–trimethoprim.[353-355] Tetracycline-induced reactions tend to involve the genitals.[259] Phenytoin has been reported to cause a more generalized FDE.[352] Ciprofloxacin is an increasingly common etiology in India.[352] Other common culprits include the following: terbinafine, omeprazole, fluconazole, diltiazem, mefenamic acid, enalapril, lansoprazole, fluoxetine, naproxen, amlodipine, amoxicillin, carbamazepine, lamotrigine,

paracetamol, ibuprofen, aspirin, sulfasalazine, and tetracyclines.[357]

Clinical Presentation

FDE present as round to oval, well-demarcated, violaceous to duskily erythematous, edematous plaques (Figure 3-72).[16,358] They recur in the same location with reexposure to the causal drug, usually within 30 minutes to 8 hours, but can take as long as 2 months.[352] Over months to years, they transition to gray-brown hyperpigmentation (Figure 3-73).[352,354] Lesions range from 2 to 10 cm in size.[352] With reexposure to

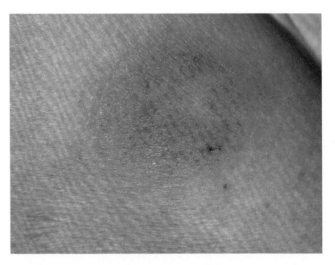

FIGURE 3-72. Fixed drug eruption, acute. An erythematous, edematous, round plaque. Courtesy of Howard Pride, MD.

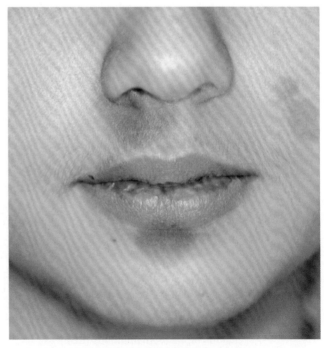

FIGURE 3-73. Fixed drug eruption, late. Round, hyperpigmented patches. Courtesy of Barrett Zlotoff, MD.

a medication, they may increase in both size and number.[16] Most cases have two to five lesions, but in rare cases, over 100 lesions can be seen.[355] Lesions can be bullous or have associated crust and scale.[16,352] Associated findings can include oral erosions, fever, and lymphadenopathy.[353] Common locations include the face, lips, hands, arms, legs, trunk, feet, and genitals (20.2%). Genital lesions are more common in males, tend to be pruritic, can become bullous, and are most commonly found on the glans (47%).[358]

Histologic Findings

The pathologic findings are similar to those seen in EM, but feature more prominent inflammation. There is a lichenoid band of lymphocytes, histiocytes, and scattered eosinophils. Areas of spongiosis and lymphocyte exocytosis into the epidermis are present. Vacuolar changes of the basal keratinocytes and apoptotic cells along the basal cell layer of the epidermis are present (Figure 3-74). The injury to the basal cell layer can result in the formation of a blister (bullous FDE). In addition to eosinophils, dermal neutrophils can be present, often extending into the epidermis. Chronic lesions show resolution of the lichenoid inflammation, leaving vacuolar changes of the basal keratinocytes and abundant pigmented melanophages.[359,260]

Differential Diagnosis

Interface dermatoses (EM, LP, lupus erythematosus) are the differential diagnostic considerations of FDE. EM lacks spongiosis and neutrophils and tends to have less inflammation. Lupus tends to have deep periadnexal inflammation, an increased amount of mucin, plasmacytoid dendritic cell clusters, and thickening of the basement membrane zone. LP can be distinguished from FDE by the presence of irregular acanthosis. They both share the abundance of pigmented melanophages.

CAPSULE SUMMARY

FIXED DRUG ERUPTION

FDE is a sharply demarcated, localized dermatosis that recurs with exposure to an inciting agent. It is a relatively common form of drug eruption in children and presents as round to oval, well-demarcated, violaceous to duskily erythematous, edematous plaques. Pathologically, there is a lichenoid band of lymphocytes, histiocytes, and scattered eosinophils. Areas of spongiosis and lymphocyte exocytosis into the epidermis are present. Vacuolar changes of the basal keratinocytes and apoptotic cells along the basal cell layer of the epidermis are present.

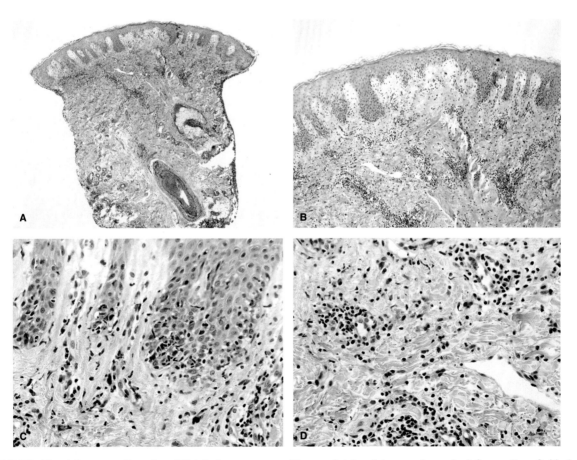

FIGURE 3-74. Fixed drug eruption. A and B, Interface process with superficial and deep perivascular inflammation. C, Marked vacuolar alteration is noted. D, The dermal inflammation includes eosinophils and neutrophils.

JUVENILE IDIOPATHIC ARTHRITIS/STILL DISEASE

Definition and Epidemiology

Juvenile idiopathic arthritis (JIA) comprises seven arthritides including systemic onset, polyarticular-rheumatoid factor positive, polyarticular-rheumatoid factor negative, psoriatic, oligoarticular, enthesitis-related, and others.[16,20] By definition, they must present with at least 6 weeks of symptoms before 16 years of age. Cutaneous findings may be present in three of the six forms (see Table 3-10).[20,361] As psoriasis and rheumatoid nodules are covered elsewhere, we will focus on systemic-onset JIA (soJIA), also known as Still disease. SoJIA consists of arthritis, a daily fever for at least 2 weeks, and one of the following: an evanescent nonpruritic eruption, generalized lymphadenopathy, serositis, or hepatosplenomegaly.[16,361,362]

JIA is the most common rheumatic condition in the pediatric population.[20] soJIA comprises 20% of JIA.[362] It affects males and females equally.

Etiology

soJIA is an autoinflammatory condition, caused by activation of the innate immune system.[363] Driving cytokines include IL-1, IL-6, and IL-18. Unlike autoimmune conditions, the effector cells are neutrophils and monocytes/macrophages.[363] The transient rash is thought to reflect fleeting vasodilatation related to vascular endothelium activation.[364]

Clinical Presentation

The evanescent eruption of soJIA satisfies a diagnostic criteria and is found in 25% to 50% of patients.[16] It is intermittent and usually not pruritic.[365] The nonsubstantive to thin erythematous papules range from 2 to 6 mm and favor the limbs and trunk (Figure 3-75).[16,365] They can coalesce into plaques up to 9 cm in diameter. The erythema varies from salmon-pink to bright red. Lesions can be linear, secondary to koebnerization, or have irregular to serpiginous to annular borders.[16,365] If pruritus is present, linear dermatographism can be seen.[365] Characteristically, the evanescent eruption coincides with late afternoon daily high fevers.[16,365]

Rheumatoid nodules are most commonly seen in patients with rheumatoid factor + polyarthritis, but rarely are found in soJIA. An eruption of rheumatoid nodules can be seen while on methotrexate; as of 2009, there were six reported cases in patients between 1 and 16 years old.[362] "Persistent pruritic papules and plaques" are seen in a subset of Still's patients, but are more common in adults.[366] Other rare cutaneous findings include telangiectasias of the cuticles and interstitial granulomatous dermatitis.[16,367]

Histologic Findings

The pathologic findings in Still disease typically consists of two consistent findings: a characteristic pattern of dyskeratosis present mainly in the superficial layers of the epidermis (upper stratum spinosum, stratum granulosum, and corneal layer) without accompanying basilar dyskeratosis; and a sparse superficial dermal infiltrate often containing neutrophils but without vasculitis (Figure 3-76). The amount of dermal inflammation is variable and can be minimal or absent. Most cases also have hyperortho- or parakeratosis. Some cases can have vacuolar alteration of the basal keratinocytes. Other reported findings include dermal mucin deposition, subcorneal or intracorneal pustules, acanthosis, and spongiosis. This histopathologic pattern is somewhat reminiscent of the verrucous phase of incontinentia pigmenti.[366-370]

CAPSULE SUMMARY

JUVENILE IDIOPATHIC ARTHRITIS/STILL DISEASE

JIA is a group of arthritides that present with at least 6 weeks of symptoms before 16 years of age. It is the most common rheumatic condition in the pediatric population. soJIA presents with nonsubstantive to thin erythematous papules that range from 2 to 6 mm favoring the limbs and trunk. The pathologic findings in Still disease typically consists of two findings: a characteristic pattern of dyskeratosis present mainly in the superficial layers of the epidermis without accompanying basilar dyskeratosis and a sparse superficial dermal infiltrate often containing neutrophils but without vasculitis.

TABLE 3-10.	Types of juvenile idiopathic arthritis and associated cutaneous findings[20,361]	
Systemic-onset JIA	**Polyarticular Rheumatoid Factor +**	**Psoriatic Arthritis**
Evanescent eruption	Rheumatoid nodules	Skin and nail psoriasis
Persistent pruritic papules and plaques		
Periorbital erythema and edema		
Rheumatoid nodules, rare		

Abbreviation: JIA, juvenile idiopathic arthritis

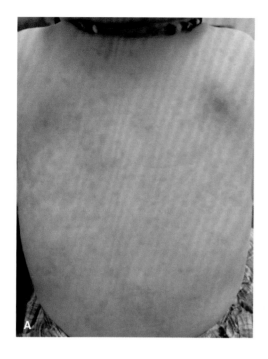
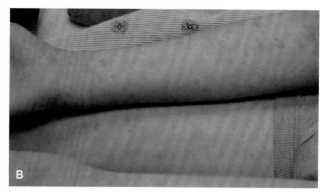

FIGURE 3-75. Systemic-onset juvenile idiopathic arthritis. Urticarial papules and plaques on the trunk (A) and extremities (B)

JUVENILE DERMATOMYOSITIS

Definition and Epidemiology

Juvenile dermatomyositis is an idiopathic inflammatory myopathy with distinct cutaneous manifestations.[371,372] Patients develop proximal muscle weakness with cutaneous findings that can include Gottron papules, heliotrope rash, and periungal telangiectasias. The clinical diagnosis is supported by the presence of autoantibodies and signs of inflammation.[372-374]

Juvenile dermatomyosis is a rare idiopathic inflammatory myopathy, with only 1 to 3 cases per million children in the United States in a given year.[372] There is a slight female over male predominance of approximately 2:1.[375,376] The median age of onset for juvenile dermatomyositis is approximately 6 years old.[375,376]

Etiology

The etiology of juvenile dermatomyositis is undetermined. It is possibly caused by a complex interplay of the immune system and environmental exposures.[374] Early in disease development, immune-mediated damage to small blood vessels affects the skin and striated muscles.[374] Several autoantibodies have been identified, including ANA, which are present in approximately 55% to 68% of patients.[374,376] Compared with adults with dermatomyositis, children are less likely to have myositis-specific antibodies.[373] When present, antibodies to Mi-2, Jo-1, MDA-5, and TIFI-γ have been reported.[374,377] Antibodies to Mi-2, found in 2% to 13% of patients, are associated with a lower risk of interstitial pneumonia and better response to therapy.[374] Juvenile cases have an increased expression of Th17 cell

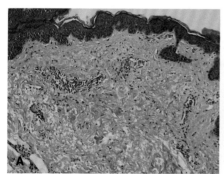
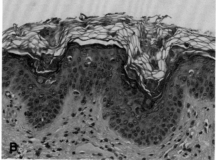
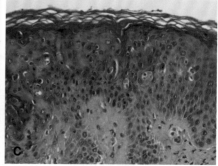

FIGURE 3-76. Juvenile idiopathic arthritis. A, Punch biopsy during the initial exanthematous phase of the disease. The superficial perivascular dermatitis with scattered neutrophils is shown. B, Dyskeratotic keratinocytes are evident within the cornified layer and the superficial epidermis. The neutrophils within the papillary dermis are shown. C, Dyskeratotic keratinocytes are present within the spinous, granular, and cornified layers. Adapted and obtained with permission, Woods MT, Gavino AC, Burford HN, et al. The evolution of histopathologic findings in adult Still disease. *Am J Dermatopathol.* 2011;33(7):736-739.

regulators as well as IL-6, IL-17F, IL-23A, IL-21, FOXP3, and STAT4.[378]

Clinical Presentation

Dermatomyositis is considered "juvenile" when presenting in a patient less than 18 years of age. Patients develop skeletal muscle myopathy with proximal muscle weakness and characteristic cutaneous manifestations. The cutaneous findings include heliotrope rash (faintly violaceous patches on sun-exposed areas of the upper face), Gottron papules (scaly papules over the knuckles and interphalangeal joints), and Gottron sign (pink to violaceous atrophic or scaly plaques over elbows and knees) (Figure 3-77).[373,377,379,380]

The European League Against Rheumatism and American College of Rheumatology developed new diagnostic classification criteria for dermatomyositis in 2017, which require that a pediatric patient with an inflammatory myopathy has a heliotrope rash, Gottron papules, or Gottron sign.[381] The heliotrope rash and Gottron papules are pathognomonic for dermatomyositis.[376,381] An uncommon manifestation is dermatomyositis *sine* myositis or amyopathic dermatomyositis.[372] This condition has the pathognomonic skin findings without clinical or laboratory findings of muscle involvement.[372]

The juvenile form of dermatomyositis is more likely than the adult form to have calcinosis cutis, present in 10% to 70% of patients, and nailfold capillaropathy.[380] Extracutaneous manifestations in the lungs, heart, gastrointestinal tract, and eyes have been reported.[376] In contrast to adults, pediatric patients with dermatomyositis are significantly less likely to have associated malignancies.[376] The current mortality of juvenile dermatomyositis is approximately 8%,[375] but prior to current treatment approaches was as high as 40%.[382]

Histologic Findings

The pathologic findings seen in juvenile dermatomyositis (JDM) are similar to those present in cutaneous lupus and adult dermatomyositis. The epidermis can be normal or atrophic. There is vacuolar alteration of the basal keratinocytes, which in some cases can be very subtle. There is a mostly superficial, perivascular, and sometimes vaguely lichenoid lymphohistiocytic infiltrate that also has scattered plasma cells (Figure 3-78). Increased interstitial dermal mucin is present. Some authors have suggested that chronic lesions of JDM have dermal fibrosis and thickened vascular walls, which can also be seen in scleroderma. Gottron papules have the pathologic findings that are similar to the poikilodermatous or erythematous lesions of dermatomyositis. The epidermis is acanthotic, with vague papillomatosis, and overlying hyperkeratosis, as opposed to the more atrophic pattern present in other conventional lesions of JDM. Interface changes are also present, including a superficial lymphocytic infiltrate and increased dermal mucin deposition (Figure 3-79).

A consequence of long-standing JDM in children is the presence of diffuse dermal calcinosis, also known as *calcinosis universalis*. In most of these cases, lymphocytes and

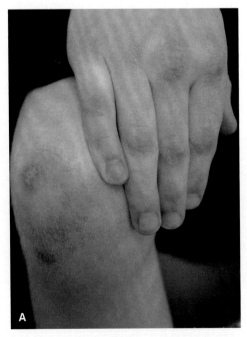 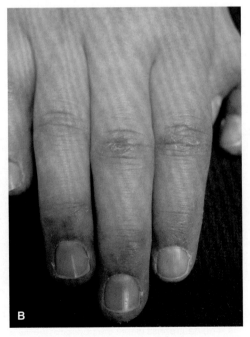

FIGURE 3-77. Juvenile dermatomyositis. A, Gottron sign (erythematous plaques over the knees) and Gottron papules (scaly papules over the knuckles). B, Periungual erythema and ragged cuticles.

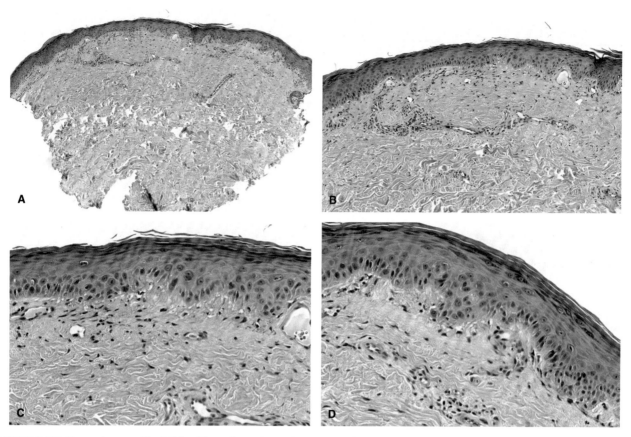

FIGURE 3-78. **Dermatomyositis.** Mild epidermal atrophy and subtle interface changes (A and B). The subtle interface pattern includes vacuolar alteration of the basal keratinocytes (C and D). Digital slides courtesy of Path Presenter.com.

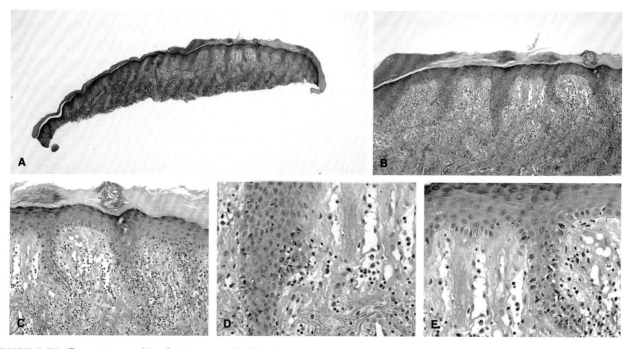

FIGURE 3-79. **Dermatomyositis. Gottron papule.** The changes present in the Gottron papules are characterized by epidermal acanthosis and hyperkeratosis (A and B). Interface changes are noted (C-E).

plasma cells are present, along with areas of dermal fibrosis. The elastic fibers show a granular blue appearance, consistent with calcium deposition. The other changes of JDM may or may not be seen.[383-389]

CAPSULE SUMMARY

JUVENILE DERMATOMYOSITIS

JDM is an idiopathic inflammatory in which patients develop proximal muscle weakness with cutaneous findings including Gottron papules, heliotrope rash, and periungal telangiectasias. The clinical diagnosis is supported by the presence of autoantibodies and signs of inflammation. The pathologic findings seen in JDM are similar to those present in lupus erythematosus and adult dermatomyositis.

REFERENCES

1. Eichenfield LF, Tom WL, Chamlin SL, et al. Guidelines of care for the management of atopic dermatitis: section 1. Diagnosis and assessment of atopic dermatitis. *J Am Acad Dermatol.* 2014;70(2):338-351. doi:10.1016/j.jaad.2013.10.010.
2. Eichenfield LF, Hanifin JM, Luger TA, Stevens SR, Pride HB. Consensus conference on pediatric atopic dermatitis. *J Am Acad Dermatol.* 2003;49(6):1088-1095.
3. Kay J, Gawkrodger DJ, Mortimer MJ, Jaron AG. The prevalence of childhood atopic eczema in a general population. *J Am Dermatol.* 1994;30(1):35-39.
4. Paternoster L, Savenije OEM, Heron J, et al. Identification of atopic dermatitis subgroups in children from 2 longitudinal birth cohorts. *J Allergy Clin Immunol.* 2018;141(3):964-971. doi:10.1016/j.jaci.2017.09.044.
5. Guttman-Yassky E, Waldman A, Ahluwalia J, Ong PY, Eichenfield LF. Atopic dermatitis: pathogenesis. *Semin Cutan Med Surg.* 2017;36(3):100-103. doi:10.12788/j.sder.2017.036.
6. Ferreira MA, Vonk JM, Baurecht H, et al. Shared genetic origin of asthma, hay fever and eczema elucidates allergic disease biology. *Nat Genet.* 2017;49(12):1752-1757. doi:10.1038/ng.3985.
7. Brunner PM, Guttman-Yassky E, Leung DYM. The immunology of atopic dermatitis and its reversibility with broad-spectrum and targeted therapies. *J Allergy Clin Immunol.* 2017;139(4S):S65-S76. doi:10.1016/j.jaci.2017.01.011.
8. Niebuhr M, Mamerow D, Heratizadeh A, Satzger I, Werfel T. Staphylococcal α-toxin induces a higher T cell proliferation and interleukin-31 in atopic dermatitis. *Int Arch Allergy Immunol.* 2011;156(4):412-415. doi:10.1159/000323905.
9. Tang C-S, Wang C-C, Huang C-F, Chen S-J, Tseng M-H, Lo W-T. Antimicrobial susceptibility of *Staphylococcus aureus* in children with atopic dermatitis. *Pediatrics International.* 2011;53(3):363-367. doi:10.1111/j.1442-200X.2010.03227.x.
10. Borkowski AW, Gallo RL. The coordinated response of the physical and antimicrobial peptide barriers of the skin. *J Invest Dermatol.* 2011;131(2):285-287. doi:10.1038/jid.2010.360.
11. Julián-Gónzalez RE, Orozco-Covarrubias L, Duran-McKinster C, Palacios-Lopez C, Ruiz-Maldonado R, Saez-de-Ocariz M. Less common clinical manifestations of atopic dermatitis: prevalence by age. *Pediatr Dermatol.* 2012;29(5):580-583. doi:10.1111/j.1525-1470.2012.01739.x.
12. Davis DM, Waldman A, Jacob S, et al. Diagnosis, comorbidity, and psychosocial impact of atopic dermatitis. *Semin Cutan Med Surg.* 2017;36(3):95-99. doi:10.12788/j.sder.2017.028.
13. Braathen LR, Forre O, Natvig JB, Eeg-Larsen T. Predominance of T lymphocytes in the dermal infiltrate of atopic dermatitis. *Br J Dermatol.* 1979;100(5):511-519.
14. Ofuji S, Uehara M. Follicular eruptions of atopic dermatitis. *Arch Dermatol.* 1973;107(1):54-55.
15. Uehara M, Miyauchi H. The morphologic characteristics of dry skin in atopic dermatitis. *Arch Dermatol.* 1984;120(9):1186-1190.
16. Paller AS, Mancini AJ. *Hurwitz Clinical Pediatric Dermatology.* New York: Elsevier Health Sciences; 2015.
17. Patil S, Maibach HI. Effect of age and sex on the elicitation of irritant contact dermatitis. *Contact Derm.* 1994;30(5):257-264.
18. Zhai H, Meier-Davis SR, Cayme B, Shudo J, Maibach H. Irritant contact dermatitis: effect of age. *Cutan Ocul Toxicol.* 2012;31(2):138-143. doi:10.3109/15569527.2011.618472.
19. Brancaccio RR, Alvarez MS. Contact allergy to food. *Dermatol Ther.* 2004;17(4):302-313. doi:10.1111/j.1396-0296.2004.04030.x.
20. Bolognia JL, Jorizzo JL, Schaffer JV. *Dermatology.* New York, NY: Elsevier Health Sciences; 2012.
21. Morris-Jones R, Robertson SJ, Ross JS, White IR, McFadden JP, Rycroft RJG. Dermatitis caused by physical irritants. *Br J Dermatol.* 2002;147(2):270-275.
22. Coughlin CC, Frieden IJ, Eichenfield LF. Clinical approaches to skin cleansing of the diaper area: practice and challenges. *Pediatr Dermatol.* 2014;31 suppl 1:1-4. doi:10.1111/pde.12461.
23. Coughlin CC, Eichenfield LF, Frieden IJ. Diaper dermatitis: clinical characteristics and differential diagnosis. *Pediatr Dermatol.* 2014;31 suppl 1:19-24. doi:10.1111/pde.12500.
24. Ortiz-Salvador J-M, Esteve-Martínez A, García-Rabasco A, Subiabre-Ferrer D, Martínez-Leboráns L, Zaragoza-Ninet V. Dermatitis of the foot: epidemiologic and clinical features in 389 children. *Pediatr Dermatol.* 2017;34(5):535-539. doi:10.1111/pde.13203.
25. Hill H, Jacob SE. Shin-guard dermatitis-detection and protection. *Pediatr Dermatol.* 2016;33(3):355-356. doi:10.1111/pde.12833.
26. Weston WL, Morelli JG. Dermatitis under soccer shin guards: allergy or contact irritant reaction? *Pediatr Dermatol.* 2006;23(1):19-20. doi:10.1111/j.1525-1470.2006.00162.x.
27. Ghali FE. "Car seat dermatitis": a newly described form of contact dermatitis. *Pediatr Dermatol.* 2011;28(3):321-326. doi:10.1111/j.1525-1470.2010.01213.x.
28. Isaacs MJ, Strausburg MB, Mousdicas N. Pediatric positional sitting dermatitis: a new form of pediatric contact dermatitis. *Pediatr Dermatol.* 2016;33(3):e226-e227. doi:10.1111/pde.12858.
29. Gulec AI, Albayrak H, Uslu E, Başkan E, Aliagaoglu C. Pustular irritant contact dermatitis caused by dexpanthenol in a child. *Cutan Ocul Toxicol.* 2015;34(1):75-76. doi:10.3109/15569527.2014.883405.
30. Cusano F, Mariano M. Fiberglass dermatitis microepidemic in a primary school. *Contact Derm.* 2007;57(5):351-352. doi:10.1111/j.1600-0536.2007.01147.x.
31. Warshaw EM, Paller AS, Fowler JF, Zirwas MJ. Practical management of cutaneous reactions to the methylphenidate transdermal system: recommendations from a dermatology expert panel consensus meeting. *Clin Ther.* 2008;30(2):326-337. doi:10.1016/j.clinthera.2008.01.022.
32. Kind F, Hofmeier KS, Bircher AJ. Irritant contact dermatitis from a black henna tattoo without sensitization to para-phenylendiamine. *Pediatrics.* 2013;131(6):e1974-e1976. doi:10.1542/peds.2012-2938.
33. Dong H, Kerl H, Cerroni L. EMLA cream-induced irritant contact dermatitis. *J Cutan Pathol.* 2002;29(3):190-192.
34. Neri I, Bianchi F, Giacomini F, Patrizi A. Acute irritant contact dermatitis due to Juglans regia. *Contact Dermatitis.* 2006;55(1):62-63. doi:10.1111/j.0105-1873.2006.0847h.x.
35. Gnanaraj P, Venugopal V, Mozhi MK, Pandurangan CN. An outbreak of Paederus dermatitis in a suburban hospital in South India: a report of 123 cases and review of literature. *J Am Acad Dermatol.* 2007;57(2):297-300. doi:10.1016/j.jaad.2006.10.982.

36. Veraldi S, Cuka E, Chiaratti A, Nazzaro G, Gianotti R, Süss L. Paederus fuscipes dermatitis: a report of nine cases observed in Italy and review of the literature. *Eur J Dermatol.* 2013;23(3):387-391. doi:10.1684/ejd.2013.2028.

37. Borroni G, Brazzelli V, Rosso R, Pavan M. Paederus fuscipes dermatitis. A histopathological study. *Am J Dermatopathol.* 1991;13(5): 467-474.

38. Lachapelle JM. Comparative histopathology of allergic and irritant patch test reactions in man. Current concepts and new prospects. *Arch Belg Dermatol Syphiligr.* 1973;29(1):83-92.

39. Koppes SA, Engebretsen KA, Agner T, et al. Current knowledge on biomarkers for contact sensitization and allergic contact dermatitis. *Contact Derm.* 2017;77(1):1-16. doi:10.1111/cod.12789.

40. Goldenberg A, Silverberg N, Silverberg JI, Treat J, Jacob SE. Pediatric allergic contact dermatitis: lessons for better care. *J Allergy Clin Immunol Pract.* 2015;3(5):661-667; quiz 668. doi:10.1016/j.jaip.2015.02. 007.

41. Martin SF. Immunological mechanisms in allergic contact dermatitis. *Curr Opin Allergy Clin Immunol.* 2015;15(2):124-130. doi:10.1097/ ACI.0000000000000142.

42. Fonacier LS, Dreskin SC, Leung DYM. Allergic skin diseases. *J Allergy Clin Immunol.* 2010;125(2 suppl 2):S138-S149. doi:10.1016/j. jaci.2009.05.039.

43. Jacob SE, McGowan M, Silverberg NB, et al. Pediatric contact dermatitis registry data on contact allergy in children with atopic dermatitis. *JAMA Dermatol.* 2017;153(8):765-770. doi:10.1001/ jamadermatol.2016.6136.

44. Friedmann PS, Sanchez-Elsner T, Schnuch A. Genetic factors in susceptibility to contact sensitivity. *Contact Derm.* 2015;72(5):263-274. doi:10.1111/cod.12362.

45. Goldenberg A, Admani S, Pelletier JL, Jacob SE. Belt buckles-increasing awareness of nickel exposure in children: a case report. *Pediatrics.* 2015;136(3):e691-e693. doi:10.1542/peds.2015-0794.

46. Schram SE, Willey A, Lee PK, Bohjanen KA, Warshaw EM. Black-spot poison ivy. *Dermatitis.* 2008;19(1):48-51.

47. Rashid RS, Shim TN. Contact dermatitis. *BMJ.* 2016;353:i3299.

48. Goldenberg A, Jacob SE. Paraphenylenediamine in black henna temporary tattoos: 12-year Food and Drug Administration data on incidence, symptoms, and outcomes. *J Am Acad Dermatol.* 2015;72(4):724-726. doi:10.1016/j.jaad.2014.11.031.

49. Chang MW, Nakrani R. Six children with allergic contact dermatitis to methylisothiazolinone in wet wipes (baby wipes). *Pediatrics.* 2014;133(2):e434-e438. doi:10.1542/peds.2013-1453.

50. Cotton CH, Admani SE, Jacob SE, Krakowski AC. "Mint" condition: contact dermatitis in an adolescent numismatist. *Pediatr Dermatol.* 2016;33(1):80-83. doi:10.1111/pde.12715.

51. Herro EM, Jacob SE. Systemic contact dermatitis—children and ketchup. *Pediatr Dermatol.* 2013;30(3):e32-e33. doi:10.1111/j .1525-1470.2011.01702.x.

52. Matiz C, Jacob SE. Systemic contact dermatitis in children: how an avoidance diet can make a difference. *Pediatr Dermatol.* 2011;28(4):368-374. doi:10.1111/j.1525-1470.2010.01130.x.

53. Mislankar M, Zirwas MJ. Low-nickel diet scoring system for systemic nickel allergy. *Dermatitis.* 2013;24(4):190-195. doi:10.1097/ DER.0b013e3182937e81.

54. Hamann CR, Hamann D, Egeberg A, Johansen JD, Silverberg J, Thyssen JP. Association between atopic dermatitis and contact sensitization: a systematic review and meta-analysis. *J Am Acad Dermatol.* 2017;77(1):70-78. doi:10.1016/j.jaad.2017.02.001.

55. Brancaccio RR, Cockerell CJ, Belsito D, Ostreicher R. Allergic contact dermatitis from color film developers: clinical and histologic features. *J Am Acad Dermatol.* 1993;28(5, pt 2):827-830.

56. Drut R, Peral CG, Garone A, Rositto A. Langerhans cell hyperplasia of the skin mimicking Langerhans cell histiocytosis: a report of two cases in children not associated with scabies. *Fetal Pediatr Pathol.* 2010;29(4):231-238.

57. Foley P, Zuo Y, Plunkett A, Merlin K, Marks R. The frequency of common skin conditions in preschool-aged children in Australia: seborrheic dermatitis and pityriasis capitis (cradle cap). *Arch Dermatol.* 2003;139(3):318-322.

58. Broberg A. Pityrosporum ovale in healthy children, infantile seborrhoeic dermatitis and atopic dermatitis. *Acta Derm Venereol Suppl (Stockh).* 1995;191:1-47.

59. Tollesson A, Frithz A, Stenlund K. Malassezia furfur in infantile seborrheic dermatitis. *Pediatr Dermatol.* 1997;14(6):423-425.

60. Yamamoto M, Umeda Y, Yo A, Yamaura M, Makimura K. Utilization of matrix-assisted laser desorption and ionization time-of-flight mass spectrometry for identification of infantile seborrheic dermatitis-causing Malassezia and incidence of culture-based cutaneous Malassezia microbiota of 1-month-old infants. *J Dermatol.* 2014;41(2):117-123. doi:10.1111/1346-8138.12364.

61. Moises-Alfaro CB, Caceres-Rios HW, Rueda M, Velazquez-Acosta A, Ruiz-Maldonado R. Are infantile seborrheic and atopic dermatitis clinical variants of the same disease? *Int J Dermatol.* 2002;41(6):349-351.

62. Alexopoulos A, Kakourou T, Orfanou I, Xaidara A, Chrousos G. Retrospective analysis of the relationship between infantile seborrheic dermatitis and atopic dermatitis. *Pediatr Dermatol.* 2014;31(2):125-130. doi:10.1111/pde.12216.

63. Fox BJ, Odom RB. Papulosquamous diseases: a review. *J Am Acad Dermatol.* 1985;12(4):597-624.

64. Miazek N, Michalek I, Pawlowska-Kisiel M, Olszewska M, Rudnicka L. Pityriasis alba—common disease, enigmatic entity: up-to-date review of the literature. *Pediatr Dermatol.* 2015;32(6):786-791. doi:10.1111/pde.12683.

65. Watkins DB. Pityriasis alba: a form of atopic dermatitis. A preliminary report. *Arch Dermatol.* 1961;83:915-919.

66. Brenninkmeijer EEA, Spuls PI, Legierse CM, Lindeboom R, Smitt JHS, Bos JD. Clinical differences between atopic and atopiform dermatitis. *J Am Acad Dermatol.* 2008;58(3):407-414. doi:10.1016/j.jaad.2007. 12.002.

67. Blessmann Weber M, Sponchiado de Avila LG, Albaneze R, Magalhães de Oliveira OL, Sudhaus BD, Cestari TF. Pityriasis alba: a study of pathogenic factors. *J Eur Acad Dermatol Venereol.* 2002;16(5):463-468.

68. Burkhart CG, Burkhart CN. Pityriasis alba: a condition with possible multiple etiologies. *Open Dermatol J.* 2009;3:7-8.

69. Galadari E, Helmy M, Ahmed M. Trace elements in serum of pityriasis alba patients. *Int J Dermatol.* 1992;31(7):525-526.

70. Jadotte YT, Janniger CK. Pityriasis alba revisited: perspectives on an enigmatic disorder of childhood. *Cutis.* 2011;87(2):66-72.

71. Lin RL, Janniger CK. Pityriasis alba. *Cutis.* 2005;76(1):21-24.

72. Diaz Urbe LH. Pitiriase alba: aspectos epidemiologicos, cliniocos e terpeuticos. *An Bras Dermatol.* 2000;75:359-367.

73. Zaynoun ST, Aftimos BG, Tenekjian KK, Bahuth N, Kurban AK. Extensive pityriasis alba: a histological histochemical and ultrastructural study. *Br J Dermatol.* 1983;108(1):83-90.

74. Di Lernia V, Ricci C. Progressive and extensive hypomelanosis and extensive pityriasis alba: same disease, different names? *J Eur Acad Dermatol Venereol.* 2005;19(3):370-372. doi:10.1111/j.1468-3083.2004.01170.x.

75. Toit du MJ, Jordaan HF. Pigmenting pityriasis alba. *Pediatr Dermatol.* 1993;10(1):1-5.

76. Alshahwan MA. Pigmenting pityriasis alba: case report and review of literature. *J Saudi Soc Dermatol Surg.* 2012;16:31-33.

77. Hacker SM. Common disorders of pigmentation: when are more than cosmetic cover ups required? *Postgrad Med.* 1996;99:177-186.

78. Dhar S, Kanwar AJ, Dawn G. Pigmenting pityriasis alba. *Pediatr Dermatol.* 1995;12(2):197-198.

79. In SI, Yi SW, Kang HY, Lee ES, Sohn S, Kim YC. Clinical and histopathological characteristics of pityriasis alba. *Clin Exp Dermatol.* 2009;34(5):591-597.

80. Martin RF, Lugo-Somolinos A, Sanchez JL. Clinicopathologic study on pityriasis alba. *Bol Asoc Med P R.* 1990;82(10):463-465.

81. Vargas-Ocampo F. Pityriasis alba: a histologic study. *Int J Dermatol.* 1993;32(12):870-873.

82. Renner ED, Rylaarsdam S, Anover-Sombke S, et al. Novel signal transducer and activator of transcription 3 (STAT3) mutations, reduced T(H)17 cell numbers, and variably defective STAT3 phosphorylation in hyper-IgE syndrome. *J Allergy Clin Immunol.* 2008;122(1):181-187. doi:10.1016/j.jaci.2008.04.037.

83. de Beaucoudrey L, Puel A, Filipe-Santos O, et al. Mutations in STAT3 and IL12RB1 impair the development of human IL-17-producing T cells. *J Exp Med.* 2008;205(7):1543-1550. doi:10.1084/jem.20080321.

84. Ma CS, Chew GYJ, Simpson N, et al. Deficiency of Th17 cells in hyper IgE syndrome due to mutations in STAT3. *J Exp Med.* 2008;205(7):1551-1557. doi:10.1084/jem.20080218.

85. Milner JD, Brenchley JM, Laurence A, et al. Impaired T(H)17 cell differentiation in subjects with autosomal dominant hyper-IgE syndrome. *Nature.* 2008;452(7188):773-776. doi:10.1038/nature06764.

86. Browne SK, Holland SM. Anti-cytokine autoantibodies explain some chronic mucocutaneous candidiasis. *Immunol Cell Biol.* 2010;88(6):614-615.

87. Puel A, Döffinger R, Natividad A, et al. Autoantibodies against IL-17A, IL-17F, and IL-22 in patients with chronic mucocutaneous candidiasis and autoimmune polyendocrine syndrome type I. *J Exp Med.* 2010;207(2):291-297. doi:10.1084/jem.20091983.

88. Kisand K, Bøe Wolff AS, Podkrajsek KT, et al. Chronic mucocutaneous candidiasis in APECED or thymoma patients correlates with autoimmunity to Th17-associated cytokines. *J Exp Med.* 2010;207(2):299-308. doi:10.1084/jem.20091669.

89. Conti HR, Baker O, Freeman AF, et al. New mechanism of oral immunity to mucosal candidiasis in hyper-IgE syndrome. *Mucosal Immunol.* 2011;4(4):448-455. doi:10.1038/mi.2011.5.

90. Minegishi Y, Saito M, Nagasawa M, et al. Molecular explanation for the contradiction between systemic Th17 defect and localized bacterial infection in hyper-IgE syndrome. *J Exp Med.* 2009;206(6):1291-1301. doi:10.1084/jem.20082767.

91. Nieminen P, Morgan NV, Fenwick AL, et al. Inactivation of IL11 signaling causes craniosynostosis, delayed tooth eruption, and supernumerary teeth. *Am J Hum Genet.* 2011;89(1):67-81. doi:10.1016/j.ajhg.2011.05.024.

92. Chamlin SL, McCalmont TH, Cunningham BB, et al. Cutaneous manifestations of hyper-IgE syndrome in infants and children. *J Pediatr.* 2002;141(4):572575. doi:10.1067/mpd.2002.127503.

93. Eberting CLD, Davis J, Puck JM, Holland SM, Turner ML. Dermatitis and the newborn rash of hyper-IgE syndrome. *Arch Dermatol.* 2004;140(9):1119-1125. doi:10.1001/archderm.140.9.1119.

94. Sowerwine KJ, Holland SM, Freeman AF. Hyper-IgE syndrome update. *Ann N Y Acad Sci.* 2012;1250:25-32. doi:10.1111/j.1749-6632.2011.06387.x.

95. Yong PFK, Freeman AF, Engelhardt KR, Holland S, Puck JM, Grimbacher B. An update on the hyper-IgE syndromes. *Arthritis Res Ther.* 2012;14(6):228. doi:10.1186/ar4069.

96. Grimbacher B, Holland SM, Gallin JI, et al. Hyper-IgE syndrome with recurrent infections—an autosomal dominant multisystem disorder. *N Engl J Med.* 1999;340(9):692-702. doi:10.1056/NEJM199903043400904.

97. Freeman AF, Davis J, Anderson VL, et al. Pneumocystis jiroveci infection in patients with hyper-immunoglobulin E syndrome. *Pediatrics.* 2006;118(4):e1271-e1275. doi:10.1542/peds.2006-0311.

98. Borges WG, Hensley T, Carey JC, Petrak BA, Hill HR. The face of Job. *J Pediatr.* 1998;133(2):303-305.

99. Freeman AF, Kleiner DE, Nadiminti H, et al. Causes of death in hyper-IgE syndrome. *J Allergy Clin Immunol.* 2007;119(5):1234-1240. doi:10.1016/j.jaci.2006.12.666.

100. Davis SD, Schaller J, Wedgwood RJ. Job's syndrome. Recurrent, 'cold', staphylococcal abscesses. *Lancet.* 1966;1(7445):1013-1015.

101. Gorin LJ, Jeha SC, Sullivan MP, Rosenblatt HM, Shearer WT. Burkitt's lymphoma developing in a 7-year-old boy with hyper-IgE syndrome. *J Allergy Clin Immunol.* 1989;83(1):5-10.

102. Leonard GD, Posadas E, Herrmann PC, et al. Non-Hodgkin's lymphoma in Job's syndrome: a case report and literature review. *Leuk Lymphoma.* 2004;45(12):2521-2525. doi:10.1080/10428190400004463.

103. Kumánovics A, Perkins SL, Gilbert H, Cessna MH, Augustine NH, Hill HR. Diffuse large B cell lymphoma in hyper-IgE syndrome due to STAT3 mutation. *J Clin Immunol.* 2010;30(6):886-893. doi:10.1007/s10875-010-9452-z.

104. Buckley RH. The hyper-IgE syndrome. *Clin Rev Allergy Immunol.* 2001;20(1):139-154. doi:10.1385/CRIAI:20:1:139.

105. Domingo DL, Freeman AF, Davis J, et al. Novel intraoral phenotypes in hyperimmunoglobulin-E syndrome. *Oral Dis.* 2008;14(1):73-81. doi:10.1111/j.1601-0825.2007.01363.x.

106. Shirafuji Y, Matsuura H, Sato A, Kanzaki H, Katayama H, Arata J. Hyperimmunoglobin E syndrome: a sign of TH1/TH2 imbalance? *Eur J Dermatol.* 1999;9(2):129-131.

107. Guenst BJ. Common pediatric foot dermatoses. *J Pediatr Health Care.* 1999;13(2):68-71. doi:10.1016/S0891-5245(99)90056-1.

108. Lemont H, Pearl B. Juvenile plantar dermatosis. *J Am Podiatr Med Assoc.* 1992;82(3):167-169. doi:10.7547/87507315-82-3-167.

109. Ashton RE, Jones RR, Griffiths A. Juvenile plantar dermatosis. A clinicopathologic study. *Arch Dermatol.* 1985;121(2):225-228.

110. Zagne V, Fernandes NC, Cuzzi T. Histopathological aspects of juvenile plantar dermatosis. *Am J Dermatopathol.* 2014;36(4):359-361.

111. Lynch PJ. Lichen simplex chronicus (atopic/neurodermatitis) of the anogenital region. *Dermatol Ther.* 2004;17(1):8-19.

112. Goh CL, Akarapanth R. Epidemiology of skin disease among children in a referral skin clinic in Singapore. *Pediatr Dermatol.* 1994;11(2):125-128.

113. Oza VS, Marco E, Frieden IJ. Improving the dermatologic care of individuals with autism: a review of relevant issues and a perspective. *Pediatr Dermatol.* 2015;32(4):447-454. doi:10.1111/pde.12548.

114. Gupta MA, Vujcic B, Gupta AK. Dissociation and conversion symptoms in dermatology. *Clin Dermatol.* 2017;35(3):267-272. doi:10.1016/j.clindermatol.2017.01.003.

115. Doyle JA, Connolly SM, Hunziker N, Winkelmann RK. Prurigo nodularis: a reappraisal of the clinical and histologic features. *J Cutan Pathol.* 1979;6(5):392-403.

116. Harris B, Harris K, Penneys NS. Demonstration by S-100 protein staining of increased numbers of nerves in the papillary dermis of patients with prurigo nodularis. *J Am Acad Dermatol.* 1992;26(1):56-58.

117. Mattila JO, Vornanen M, Katila ML. Histopathological and bacteriological findings in prurigo nodularis. *Acta Derm Venereol.* 1997;77(1):49-51.

118. Rowland Payne CM, Wilkinson JD, McKee PH, Jurecka W, Black MM. Nodular prurigo—a clinicopathological study of 46 patients. *Br J Dermatol.* 1985;113(4):431-439.

119. Weigelt N, Metze D, Stander S. Prurigo nodularis: systematic analysis of 58 histological criteria in 136 patients. *J Cutan Pathol.* 2010;37(5):578-586.

120. Stratigos AJ, Antoniou C, Katsambas AD. Polymorphous light eruption. *J Eur Acad Dermatol Venereol.* 2002;16(3):193-206.

121. Boonstra HE, van Weelden H, Toonstra J, van Vloten WA. Polymorphous light eruption: a clinical, photobiologic, and follow-up study of 110 patients. *J Am Dermatol.* 2000;42(2, pt 1):199-207. doi:10.1016/S0190-9622(00)90126-9.

122. Gruber-Wackernagel A, Byrne SN, Wolf P. Polymorphous light eruption: clinic aspects and pathogenesis. *Dermatol Clin.* 2014;32(3):315-334, viii. doi:10.1016/j.det.2014.03.012.

123. Wolf P, Gruber-Wackernagel A, Bambach I, et al. Photohardening of polymorphic light eruption patients decreases baseline epidermal Langerhans cell density while increasing mast cell numbers in the

papillary dermis. *Exp Dermatol.* 2014;23(6):428-430. doi:10.1111/exd.12427.

124. Isedeh P, Lim HW. Polymorphous light eruption presenting as pinhead papular eruption on the face. *J Drugs Dermatol.* 2013;12(11):1285-1286.

125. Molina-Ruiz AM, Sanmartín O, Santonja C, Kutzner H, Requena L. Spring and summer eruption of the elbows: a peculiar localized variant of polymorphous light eruption. *J Am Acad Dermatol.* 2013;68(2):306-312. doi:10.1016/j.jaad.2012.08.043.

126. Epstein JH. Polymorphous light eruption. *J Am Acad Dermatol.* 1980;3(4):329-343.

127. Epstein JH. Polymorphous light eruption. *Photodermatol Photoimmunol Photomed.* 1997;13(3):89-90.

128. Holzle E, Plewig G, von Kries R, Lehmann P. Polymorphous light eruption. *J Invest Dermatol.* 1987;88(3 suppl):32s 38s.

129. Honigsmann H. Polymorphous light eruption. *Photodermatol Photoimmunol Photomed.* 2008;24(3):155-161.

130. Hood AF, Elpern DJ, Morison WL. Histopathologic findings in papulovesicular light eruption. *J Cutan Pathol.* 1986;13(1):13-21.

131. Valbuena MC, Muvdi S, Lim HW. Actinic prurigo. *Dermatol Clin.* 2014;32(3):335-344, viii. doi:10.1016/j.det.2014.03.010.

132. McGregor JM, Grabczynska S, Vaughan R, Hawk JL, Lewis CM. Genetic modeling of abnormal photosensitivity in families with polymorphic light eruption and actinic prurigo. *J Invest Dermatol.* 2000;115(3):471-476. doi:10.1046/j.1523-1747.2000.00080.x.

133. Hojyo-Tomoka M-T, Vega-Memije M-E, Cortes-Franco R, Domínguez-Soto L. Diagnosis and treatment of actinic prurigo. *Dermatol Ther.* 2003;16(1):40-44.

134. Grabczynska SA, McGregor JM, Kondeatis E, Vaughan RW, Hawk JL. Actinic prurigo and polymorphic light eruption: common pathogenesis and the importance of HLA-DR4/DRB1*0407. *Br J Dermatol.* 1999;140(2):232-236.

135. Gómez A, Umana A, Trespalacios AA. Immune responses to isolated human skin antigens in actinic prurigo. *Med Sci Monit.* 2006;12(3):BR106-BR113.

136. Estrada-G I, Garibay-Escobar A, Núñez-Vázquez A, et al. Evidence that thalidomide modifies the immune response of patients suffering from actinic prurigo. *Int J Dermatol.* 2004;43(12):893-897. doi:10.1111/j.1365-4632.2004.02274.x.

137. Martínez-Luna E, Bologna-Molina R, Mosqueda-Taylor A, et al. Inmunohistochemical detection of mastocytes in tissue from patients with actinic prurigo. *J Clin Exp Dent.* 2015;7(5):e656-e659. doi:10.4317/jced.52823.

138. Plaza JA, Toussaint S, Prieto VG, et al. Actinic prurigo cheilitis: a clinicopathologic review of 75 cases. *Am J Dermatopathol.* 2016;38(6):418-422. doi:10.1097/DAD.0000000000000459.

139. Magaña M, Mendez Y, Rodriguez A, Mascott M. The conjunctivitis of solar (actinic) prurigo. *Pediatr Dermatol.* 2000;17(6):432-435.

140. Herrera-Geopfert R, Magana M. Follicular cheilitis. A distinctive histopathologic finding in actinic prurigo. *Am J Dermatopathol.* 1995;17(4):357-361.

141. Lane PR, Murphy F, Hogan DJ, Hull PR, Burgdorf WH. Histopathology of actinic prurigo. *Am J Dermatopathol.* 1993;15(4):326-331.

142. Dawe, Ibbotson. phototoxic.

143. Cacoub P, Musette P, Descamps V, et al. The DRESS syndrome: a literature review. *Am J Med.* 2011;124(7):588-597. doi:10.1016/j.amjmed.2011.01.017.

144. Fotiades J, Soter NA, Lim HW. Results of evaluation of 203 patients for photosensitivity in a 7.3-year period. *J Am Dermatol.* 1995;33(4):597-602.

145. Crouch RB, Foley PA, Baker CS. Analysis of patients with suspected photosensitivity referred for investigation to an Australian photodermatology clinic. *J Am Dermatol.* 2003;48(5):714-720. doi:10.1067/mjd.2003.219.

146. Khandpur S, Porter RM, Boulton SJ, Anstey A. Drug-induced photosensitivity: new insights into pathomechanisms and clinical variation through basic and applied science. *Br J Dermatol.* 2017;176(4):902-909. doi:10.1111/bjd.14935.

147. Sheu NH, Spielberg SP. Pharmacogenetics and adverse drug reactions in the skin. *Pediatr Dermatol.* 1983;1(2):165-173.

148. Carlsen K, Weismann K. Phytophotodermatitis in 19 children admitted to hospital and their differential diagnoses: child abuse and herpes simplex virus infection. *J Am Acad Dermatol.* 2007;57(5 suppl):S88-S91. doi:10.1016/j.jaad.2006.08.034.

149. Levy ML, Barron KS, Eichenfield A, Honig PJ. Naproxen-induced pseudoporphyria: a distinctive photodermatitis. *J Pediatr.* 1990;117(4):660-664.

150. De Silva B, Banney L, Uttley W, Luqmani R, Schofield O. Pseudoporphyria and nonsteroidal anti-inflammatory agents in children with juvenile idiopathic arthritis. *Pediatr Dermatol.* 2000;17(6):480-483.

151. Bryant P, Lachman P. Pseudoporphyria secondary to non-steroidal anti-inflammatory drugs. *Arch Dis Child.* 2003;88(11):961.

152. Bonvalet D, Baddoura R, Jeanmougin M. Value of the light-test histological study in photodermatoses [in French]. *Ann Dermatol Venereol.* 1986;113(12):1205-1212.

153. Su W, Hall BJ IV, Cockerell CJ. Photodermatitis with minimal inflammatory infiltrate: clinical inflammatory conditions with discordant histologic findings. *Am J Dermatopathol.* 2006;28(6):482-485.

154. Yoshikawa T, Takahashi Y, Kawaguchi H, et al. A dermal phototoxicity study following intravenous infusion administration of ciprofloxacin hydrochloride in the novel microminipigs. *Toxicol Pathol.* 2013;41(1):109-113.

155. Dibek Misirlioglu E, Guvenir H, Bahceci S, et al. Severe cutaneous adverse drug reactions in pediatric patients: a multicenter study. *J Allergy Clin Immunol Pract.* 2017;5(3):757-763. doi:10.1016/j.jaip.2017.02.013.

156. Newell BD, Moinfar M, Mancini AJ, Nopper AJ. Retrospective analysis of 32 pediatric patients with anticonvulsant hypersensitivity syndrome (ACHSS). *Pediatr Dermatol.* 2009;26(5):536-546. doi:10.1111/j.1525-1470.2009.00870.x.

157. Manuyakorn W, Mahasirimongkol S, Likkasittipan P, et al. Association of HLA genotypes with phenobarbital hypersensitivity in children. *Epilepsia.* 2016;57(10):1610-1616. doi:10.1111/epi.13509.

158. Musette P, Janela B. New insights into drug reaction with eosinophilia and systemic symptoms pathophysiology. *Front Med (Lausanne).* 2017;4:179. doi:10.3389/fmed.2017.00179.

159. Chen W-T, Wang C-W, Lu C-W, et al. The function of HLA-B*13:01 involved in the pathomechanism of dapsone-induced severe cutaneous adverse reactions. *J Invest Dermatol.* 2018;138(7):1546-1554. doi:10.1016/j.jid.2018.02.004.

160. Husain Z, Reddy BY, Schwartz RA. DRESS syndrome Part I. *J Am Acad Dermatol.* 2013;68(5):693.e1-693.e14. doi:10.1016/j.jaad.2013.01.033.

161. Cho Y-T, Yang C-W, Chu C-Y. Drug reaction with eosinophilia and systemic symptoms (DRESS): an interplay among drugs, viruses, and immune system. *Int J Mol Sci.* 2017;18(6). doi:10.3390/ijms18061243.

162. Choquet-Kastylevsky G, Intrator L, Chenal C, Bocquet H, Revuz J, Roujean JC. Increased levels of interleukin 5 are associated with the generation of eosinophilia in drug-induced hypersensitivity syndrome. *Br J Dermatol.* 1998;139(6):1026-1032.

163. Seishima M, Yamanaka S, Fujisawa T, Tohyama M, Hashimoto K. Reactivation of human herpesvirus (HHV) family members other than HHV-6 in drug-induced hypersensitivity syndrome. *Br J Dermatol.* 2006;155(2):344-349. doi:10.1111/j.1365-2133.2006.07332.x.

164. Chen Y-C, Chiang H-H, Cho Y-T, et al. Human herpes virus reactivations and dynamic cytokine profiles in patients with cutaneous adverse drug reactions—a prospective comparative study. *Allergy.* 2015;70(5):568-575. doi:10.1111/all.12602.

165. Shiohara T, Kano Y, Takahashi R, Ishida T, Mizukawa Y. Drug-induced hypersensitivity syndrome: recent advances in the

diagnosis, pathogenesis and management. *Chem Immunol Allergy.* 2012;97:122-138. doi:10.1159/000335624.

166. Ahluwalia J, Abuabara K, Perman MJ, Yan AC. Human herpesvirus 6 involvement in paediatric drug hypersensitivity syndrome. *Br J Dermatol.* 2015;172(4):1090-1095. doi:10.1111/bjd.13512.

167. Ang C-C, Wang Y-S, Yoosuff E-LM, Tay Y-K. Retrospective analysis of drug-induced hypersensitivity syndrome: a study of 27 patients. *J Am Acad Dermatol.* 2010;63(2):219-227. doi:10.1016/j.jaad.2009.08.050.

168. Kano Y, Ishida T, Hirahara K, Shiohara T. Visceral involvements and long-term sequelae in drug-induced hypersensitivity syndrome. *Med Clin North Am.* 2010;94(4):743-759, xi. doi:10.1016/j.mcna.2010.03.004.

169. Biesbroeck LK, Scott JD, Taraska C, Moore E, Falsey RR, Shinohara MM. Direct-acting antiviral-associated dermatitis during chronic hepatitis C virus treatment. *Am J Clin Dermatol.* 2013;14(6):497-502.

170. Borroni G, Torti S, Pezzini C, et al. Histopathologic spectrum of drug reaction with eosinophilia and systemic symptoms (DRESS): a diagnosis that needs clinico-pathological correlation. *G Ital Dermatol Venereol.* 2014;149(3):291-300.

171. Correa-de-Castro B, Paniago AM, Takita LC, Murback ND, Hans-Filho G. Drug reaction with eosinophilia and systemic symptoms: a clinico-pathological study of six cases at a teaching hospital in midwestern Brazil. *Int J Dermatol.* 2016;55(3):328-334.

172. Montaudie H, Passeron T, Cardot-Leccia N, Sebbag N, Lacour JP. Drug rash with eosinophilia and systemic symptoms due to telaprevir. *Dermatology.* 2010;221(4):303-305.

173. Walsh S, Diaz-Cano S, Higgins E, et al. Drug reaction with eosinophilia and systemic symptoms: is cutaneous phenotype a prognostic marker for outcome? A review of clinicopathological features of 27 cases. *Br J Dermatol.* 2013;168(2):391-401.

174. Browning JC. An update on pityriasis rosea and other similar childhood exanthems. *Curr Opin Pediatr.* 2009;21(4):481-485. doi:10.1097/MOP.0b013e32832db96e.

175. Chuh AA, Lee A, Molinari N. Case clustering in pityriasis rosea: a multicenter epidemiologic study in primary care settings in Hong Kong. *Arch Dermatol.* 2003;139(4):489-493. doi:10.1001/archderm.139.4.489.

176. Chuh A, Zawar V, Lee A. Atypical presentations of pityriasis rosea: case presentations. *J Eur Acad Dermatol Venereol.* 2005;19(1):120-126. doi:10.1111/j.1468-3083.2004.01105.x.

177. Chuh AA, Molinari N, Sciallis G, Harman M, Akdeniz S, Nanda A. Temporal case clustering in pityriasis rosea: a regression analysis on 1379 patients in Minnesota, kuwait, and diyarbakir, Turkey. *Arch Dermatol.* 2005;141(6):767-771. doi:10.1001/archderm.141.6.767.

178. Canpolat Kirac B, Adişen E, Bozdayi G, et al. The role of human herpesvirus 6, human herpesvirus 7, Epstein-Barr virus and cytomegalovirus in the aetiology of pityriasis rosea. *J Eur Acad Dermatol Venereol.* 2009;23(1):16-21. doi:10.1111/j.1468-3083.2008.02939.x.

179. Drago F, Broccolo F, Zaccaria E, et al. Pregnancy outcome in patients with pityriasis rosea. *J Am Acad Dermatol.* 2008;58(5 suppl 1):S78-S83. doi:10.1016/j.jaad.2007.05.030.

180. Drago F, Broccolo F, Rebora A. Pityriasis rosea: an update with a critical appraisal of its possible herpesviral etiology. *J Am Acad Dermatol.* 2009;61(2):303-318. doi:10.1016/j.jaad.2008.07.045.

181. Watanabe T, Kawamura T, Jacob SE, et al. Pityriasis rosea is associated with systemic active infection with both human herpesvirus-7 and human herpesvirus-6. *J Invest Dermatol.* 2002;119(4):793-797. doi:10.1046/j.1523-1747.2002.00200.x.

182. Chuh AA. Diagnostic criteria for pityriasis rosea: a prospective case control study for assessment of validity. *J Eur Acad Dermatol Venereol.* 2003;17(1):101-103.

183. Chuh A, Lee A, Zawar V, Sciallis G, Kempf W. Pityriasis rosea—an update. *Indian J Dermatol Venereol Leprol.* 2005;71(5):311-315.

184. Amer A, Fischer H, Li X. The natural history of pityriasis rosea in black American children: how correct is the "classic" description? *Arch Pediatr Adolesc Med.* 2007;161(5):503-506. doi:10.1001/archpedi.161.5.503.

185. Miranda SB, Lupi O, Lucas E. Vesicular pityriasis rosea: response to erythromycin treatment. *J Eur Acad Dermatol Venereol.* 2004;18(5):622-625.

186. Sasmaz S, Karabiber H, Boran C, Garipardic M, Balat A. Pityriasis rosea-like eruption due to pneumococcal vaccine in a child with nephrotic syndrome. *J Dermatol.* 2003;30(3):245-247.

187. Wilkinson SM, Smith AG, Davis MJ, Mattey D, Dawes PT. Pityriasis rosea and discoid eczema: dose related reactions to treatment with gold. *Ann Rheum Dis.* 1992;51(7):881-884.

188. Silverberg NB. Pediatric psoriasis: an update. *Ther Clin Risk Manag.* 2009;5:849-856.

189. Bronckers IM, Paller AS, van Geel MJ, van de Kerkhof PC, Seyger MM. Psoriasis in children and adolescents: diagnosis, management and comorbidities. *Paediatr Drugs.* 2015;17(5):373-384. doi:10.1007/s40272-015-0137-1.

190. Mercy K, Kwasny M, Cordoro KM, et al. Clinical manifestations of pediatric psoriasis: results of a multicenter study in the United States. *Pediatr Dermatol.* 2013;30(4):424-428. doi:10.1111/pde.12072.

191. Matusiewicz D, Koerber A, Schadendorf D, Wasem J, Neumann A. Childhood psoriasis—an analysis of German health insurance data. *Pediatr Dermatol.* 2014;31(1):8-13. doi:10.1111/pde.12205.

192. Tollefson MM, Crowson CS, McEvoy MT, Maradit Kremers H. Incidence of psoriasis in children: a population-based study. *J Am Acad Dermatol.* 2010;62(6):979-987. doi:10.1016/j.jaad.2009.07.029.

193. Raychaudhuri SP, Gross J. A comparative study of pediatric onset psoriasis with adult onset psoriasis. *Pediatr Dermatol.* 2000;17(3):174-178.

194. Takeichi T, Kobayashi A, Ogawa E, et al. Autosomal dominant familial generalized pustular psoriasis caused by a CARD14 mutation. *Br J Dermatol.* 2017;177(4):e133-e135. doi:10.1111/bjd.15442.

195. Cordoro KM, Hitraya-Low M, Taravati K, et al. Skin-infiltrating, interleukin-22-producing T cells differentiate pediatric psoriasis from adult psoriasis. *J Am Acad Dermatol.* 2017;77(3):417-424. doi:10.1016/j.jaad.2017.05.017.

196. Zhang L, Li Y, Yang X, et al. Characterization of Th17 and FoxP3(+) Treg cells in paediatric psoriasis patients. *Scand J Immunol.* 2016;83(3):174-180. doi:10.1111/sji.12404.

197. Krueger GG, Bergstresser PR, Lowe NJ, Voorhees JJ, Weinstein GD. Psoriasis. *J Am Acad Dermatol.* 1984;11(5, pt 2):937-947.

198. Ragaz A, Ackerman AB. Evolution, maturation, and regression of lesions of psoriasis. New observations and correlation of clinical and histologic findings. *Am J Dermatopathol.* 1979;1(3):199-214.

199. Werner B, Brenner FM, Boer A. Histopathologic study of scalp psoriasis: peculiar features including sebaceous gland atrophy. *Am J Dermatopathol.* 2008;30(2):93-100.

200. Yoon SY, Park HS, Lee JH, Cho S. Histological differentiation between palmoplantar pustulosis and pompholyx. *J Eur Acad Dermatol Venereol.* 2013;27(7):889-893.

201. Magro CM, Crowson AN. The clinical and histomorphological features of pityriasis rubra pilaris. A comparative analysis with psoriasis. *J Cutan Pathol.* 1997;24(7):416-424.

202. Griffiths WA. Pityriasis rubra pilaris. *Clin Exp Dermatol.* 1980;5(1):105-112.

203. Gelmetti C, Schiuma AA, Cerri D, Gianotti F. Pityriasis rubra pilaris in childhood: a long-term study of 29 cases. *Pediatr Dermatol.* 1986;3(6):446-451.

204. Allison DS, El-Azhary RA, Calobrisi SD, Dicken CH. Pityriasis rubra pilaris in children. *J Am Dermatol.* 2002;47(3):386-389.

205. Hong J-B, Chiu H-C, Wang S-H, Tsai TF. Recurrence of classical juvenile pityriasis rubra pilaris in adulthood: report of a case. *Br J Dermatol.* 2007;157(4):842-844. doi:10.1111/j.1365-2133.2007.08126.x.

206. Betlloch I, Ramón R, Silvestre JF, Carnero L, Albares MP, Bañuls J. Acute juvenile pityriasis rubra pilaris: a superantigen mediated disease? *Pediatr Dermatol.* 2001;18(5):411-414.

207. Martin KL, Holland KE, Lyon V, Chiu YE. An unusual cluster of circumscribed juvenile pityriasis rubra pilaris cases. *Pediatr Dermatol.* 2014;31(2):138-145. doi:10.1111/pde.12260.

208. Fuchs-Telem D, Sarig O, van Steensel MA, et al. Familial pityriasis rubra pilaris is caused by mutations in CARD14. *Am J Hum Genet.* 2012;91(1):163-170. doi:10.1016/j.ajhg.2012.05.010.

209. Takeichi T, Sugiura K, Nomura T, et al. Pityriasis rubra pilaris type V as an autoinflammatory disease by CARD14 mutations. *JAMA Dermatol.* 2017;153(1):66-70. doi:10.1001/jamadermatol.2016.3601.

210. Eytan O, Qiaoli L, Nousbeck J, et al. Increased epidermal expression and absence of mutations in CARD14 in a series of patients with sporadic pityriasis rubra pilaris. *Br J Dermatol.* 2014;170(5):1196-1198. doi:10.1111/bjd.12799.

211. Piamphongsant T, Akaraphant R. Pityriasis rubra pilaris: a new proposed classification. *Clin Exp Dermatol.* 1994;19(2):134-138.

212. Sehgal VN, Srivastava G. (Juvenile) Pityriasis rubra pilaris. *Int J Dermatol.* 2006;45(4):438-446. doi:10.1111/j.1365-4632.2006.02666.x.

213. Yang C-C, Shih I-H, Lin W-L, et al. Juvenile pityriasis rubra pilaris: report of 28 cases in Taiwan. *J Am Acad Dermatol.* 2008;59(6):943-948. doi:10.1016/j.jaad.2008.07.054.

214. Klein A, Landthaler M, Karrer S. Pityriasis rubra pilaris: a review of diagnosis and treatment. *Am J Clin Dermatol.* 2010;11(3):157-170. doi:10.2165/11530070-000000000-00000.

215. López-Gómez A, Vera-Casaño Á, Gómez-Moyano E, et al. Dermoscopy of circumscribed juvenile pityriasis rubra pilaris. *J Am Acad Dermatol.* 2015;72(1 Suppl):S58-S59. doi:10.1016/j.jaad.2014.07.053.

216. Thomson MA, Moss C. Pityriasis rubra pilaris in a mother and two daughters. *Br J Dermatol.* 2007;157(1):202-204. doi:10.1111/j.1365-2133.2007.07938.x.

217. Torrelo A, Mediero IG, Zambrano A. Keratosis lichenoides chronica in a child. *Pediatr Dermatol.* 1994;11(1):46-48.

218. Ruiz-Maldonado R, Duran-McKinster C, Orozco-Covarrubias L, Saez-de-Ocariz M, Palacios-Lopez C. Keratosis lichenoides chronica in pediatric patients: a different disease? *J Am Acad Dermatol.* 2007;56(2 suppl):S1-S5. doi:10.1016/j.jaad.2006.07.018.

219. Adişen E, Erdem O, Celepçi S, Gürer MA. Easy to diagnose, difficult to treat: keratosis lichenoides chronica. *Clin Exp Dermatol.* 2010;35(1):47-50. doi:10.1111/j.1365-2230.2008.03069.x.

220. Dubyk F, Smidt AC, Gifford LK, Stepenaskie S, Elwood HE. Histopathologic features of pediatric keratosis lichenoides chronica: a reports of four cases from New Mexico.

221. Geng S, Liu Y, Wang H, et al. Hypertrophic lichenoid eruption in a child successfully treated using acitretin and surgery: a case report and literature review. *Pediatr Dermatol.* 2015;32(6):e238-e241. doi:10.1111/pde.12658.

222. Keck LE, Padilla RS, Elwood H, Zlotoff BJ, Smidt AC. A dermatologic consequence of the Spanish conquest? Pediatric keratosis lichenoides chronica: a report of four cases from New Mexico.

223. Ghorpade A. Keratosis lichenoides chronica in an Indian child following erythroderma. *Int J Dermatol.* 2008;47(9):939-941.

224. Stefanato CM, Youssef EA, Cerio R, Kobza-Black A, Greaves MW. Atypical Nekam's disease—keratosis lichenoides chronica associated with porokeratotic histology and amyloidosis. *Clin Exp Dermatol.* 1993;18(3):274-276.

225. Kanwar AJ, Handa S, Ghosh S, Kaur S. Lichen planus in childhood: a report of 17 patients. *Pediatr Dermatol.* 1991;8(4):288-291.

226. Nnoruka EN. Lichen planus in African children: a study of 13 patients. *Pediatr Dermatol.* 2007;24(5):495-498. doi:10.1111/j.1525-1470.2007.00501.x.

227. Walton KE, Bowers EV, Drolet BA, Holland KE. Childhood lichen planus: demographics of a U.S. population. *Pediatr Dermatol.* 2010;27(1):34-38. doi:10.1111/j.1525-1470.2009.01072.x.

228. Pandhi D, Singal A, Bhattacharya SN. Lichen planus in childhood: a series of 316 patients. *Pediatr Dermatol.* 2014;31(1):59-67. doi:10.1111/pde.12155.

229. Nanda A, Al-Ajmi HS, Al-Sabah H, Al-Hasawi F, Alsaleh QA. Childhood lichen planus: a report of 23 cases. *Pediatr Dermatol.* 2001;18(1):1-4.

230. Limas C, Limas CJ. Lichen planus in children: a possible complication of hepatitis B vaccines. *Pediatr Dermatol.* 2002;19(3):204-209.

231. Laeijendecker R, Van Joost T, Tank B, Oranje AP, Neumann HAM. Oral lichen planus in childhood. *Pediatr Dermatol.* 2005;22(4):299-304. doi:10.1111/j.1525-1470.2005.22403.x.

232. Tosti A, Piraccini BM, Cambiaghi S, Jorizzo M. Nail lichen planus in children: clinical features, response to treatment, and long-term follow-up. *Arch Dermatol.* 2001;137(8):1027-1032.

233. Kabbash C, Laude TA, Weinberg JM, Silverberg NB. Lichen planus in the lines of Blaschko. *Pediatr Dermatol.* 2002;19(6):541-545.

234. Anuradha C, Reddy BV, Nandan SR, Kumar SR. Oral lichen planus. A review. *N Y State Dent J.* 2008;74(4):66-68.

235. Anuradha C, Reddy GS, Nandan SR, Kumar SR, Reddy BV. Oral mucosal lichen planus in nine-year-old child. *N Y State Dent J.* 2011;77(6):28-30.

236. Collgros H, Vicente A, Gonzalez-Ensenat MA, Azon-Masoliver A, Rovira-Zurriaga C. Childhood actinic lichen planus: four cases report in Caucasian Spanish children and review of the literature. *J Eur Acad Dermatol Venereol.* 2016;30(3):518-522.

237. Handa S, Sahoo B. Childhood lichen planus: a study of 87 cases. *Int J Dermatol.* 2002;41(7):423-427.

238. Kwee DJ, Dufresne RG, Ellis DL. Childhood bullous lichen planus. *Pediatr Dermatol.* 1987;4(4):325-327.

239. Sharma R, Maheshwari V. Childhood lichen planus: a report of fifty cases. *Pediatr Dermatol.* 1999;16(5):345-348.

240. Glorioso S, Jackson SC, Kopel AJ, Lewis V, Nicotri T. Actinic lichen nitidus in 3 African American patients. *J Am Acad Dermatol.* 2006;54(2 suppl):S48-S49. doi:10.1016/j.jaad.2005.06.018.

241. Di Lernia V, Piana S, Ricci C. Lichen planus appearing subsequent to generalized lichen nitidus in a child. *Pediatr Dermatol.* 2007;24(4):453-455. doi:10.1111/j.1525-1470.2007.00485.x.

242. Kanai C, Terao M, Tanemura A, Miyoshi Y, Ozono K, Katayama I. Generalized lichen nitidus in Russell-Silver syndrome. *Pediatr Dermatol.* 2013;30(1):150-151. doi:10.1111/j.1525-1470.2011.01613.x.

243. Henry M, Metry DW. Generalized lichen nitidus, with perioral and perinasal accentuation, in association with Down syndrome. *Pediatr Dermatol.* 2009;26(1):109-111. doi:10.1111/j.1525-1470.2008.00841.x.

244. Al-Mutairi N, Hassanein A, Nour-Eldin O, Arun J. Generalized lichen nitidus. *Pediatr Dermatol.* 2005;22(2):158-160. doi:10.1111/j.1525-1470.2005.22215.x.

245. Cakmak SK, Unal E, Gonul M, Yayla D, Ozhamam E. Lichen nitidus with involvement of the palms. *Pediatr Dermatol.* 2013;30(5):e100-e101. doi:10.1111/pde.12148.

246. Tay EY, Ho MS, Chandran NS, Lee JS, Heng YK. Lichen nitidus presenting with nail changes--case report and review of the literature. *Pediatr Dermatol.* 2015;32(3):386-388. doi:10.1111/pde.12425.

247. Eisen RF, Stenn J, Kahn SM, Bhawan J. Lichen nitidus with plasma cell infiltrate. *Arch Dermatol.* 1985;121(9):1193-1194.

248. Lapins NA, Willoughby C, Helwig EB. Lichen nitidus. A study of forty-three cases. *Cutis.* 1978;21(5):634-637.

249. Sanders S, Collier DA, Scott R, Wu H, MeNutt NS. Periappendageal lichen nitidus: report of a case. *J Cutan Pathol.* 2002;29(2):125-128.

250. Taniguchi Abagge K, Parolin Marinoni L, Giraldi S, Carvalho VO, de Oliveira Santini C, Favre H. Lichen striatus: description of 89 cases in children. *Pediatr Dermatol.* 2004;21(4):440-443. doi:10.1111/j.0736-8046.2004.21403.x.

251. Patrizi A, Neri I, Fiorentini C, Bonci A, Ricci G. Lichen striatus: clinical and laboratory features of 115 children. *Pediatr Dermatol.* 2004;21(3):197-204. doi:10.1111/j.0736-8046.2004.21302.x.

252. Racette AJ, Adams AD, Kessler SE. Simultaneous lichen striatus in siblings along the same Blaschko line. *Pediatr Dermatol.* 2009;26(1):50-54. doi:10.1111/j.1525-1470.2008.00821.x.

253. Mu EW, Abuav R, Cohen BA. Facial lichen striatus in children: retracing the lines of Blaschko. *Pediatr Dermatol.* 2013;30(3):364-366. doi:10.1111/j.1525-1470.2012.01844.x.

254. Yaosaka M, Sawamura D, Iitoyo M, Shibaki A, Shimizu H. Lichen striatus affecting a mother and her son. *J Am Acad Dermatol.* 2005;53(2):352-353. doi:10.1016/j.jaad.2005.02.010.

255. Keegan BR, Kamino H, Fangman W, Shin HT, Orlow SJ, Schaffer JV. "Pediatric blaschkitis": expanding the spectrum of childhood acquired Blaschko-linear dermatoses. *Pediatr Dermatol.* 2007;24(6):621-627. doi:10.1111/j.1525-1470.2007.00550.x.

256. Feely MA, Silverberg NB. Two cases of lichen striatus with prolonged active phase. *Pediatr Dermatol.* 2014;31(2):e67-e68. doi:10.1111/pde.12261.

257. Kavak A, Kutluay L. Nail involvement in lichen striatus. *Pediatr Dermatol.* 2002;19(2):136-138.

258. Batra P, Wang N, Kamino H, Possick P. Linear lichen planus. *Dermatol Online J.* 2008;14(10):16.

259. Reed RJ, Meek T, Ichinose H. Lichen striatus: a model for the histologic spectrum of lichenoid reactions. *J Cutan Pathol.* 1975;2(1):1-18.

260. Stewart WM, Lauret P, Pietrini P, Thiomine E. Lichen striatus; histologic features (author's transl) [in French]. *Ann Dermatol Venereol.* 1977;104(2):132-135.

261. Taieb A, el Youbi A, Grosshans E, Maleville J. Lichen striatus: a Blaschko linear acquired inflammatory skin eruption. *J Am Acad Dermatol.* 1991;25(4):637-642.

262. Zhang Y, McNutt NS. Lichen striatus. Histological, immunohistochemical, and ultrastructural study of 37 cases. *J Cutan Pathol.* 2001;28(2):65-71.

263. Jacobsohn DA. Acute graft-versus-host disease in children. *Bone Marrow Transplant.* 2008;41(2):215-221. doi:10.1038/sj.bmt.1705885.

264. Hymes SR, Alousi AM, Cowen EW. Graft-versus-host disease: part I. Pathogenesis and clinical manifestations of graft-versus-host disease. *J Am Acad Dermatol.* 2012;66(4):515.e1-515.e18, quiz 533-534. doi:10.1016/j.jaad.2011.11.960.

265. Feito-Rodríguez M, de Lucas-Laguna R, Gómez-Fernández C, et al. Cutaneous graft versus host disease in pediatric multivisceral transplantation. *Pediatr Dermatol.* 2013;30(3):335-341. doi:10.1111/j.1525-1470.2012.01839.x.

266. Filipovich AH, Weisdorf D, Pavletic S, et al. National Institutes of Health consensus development project on criteria for clinical trials in chronic graft-versus-host disease: I. Diagnosis and staging working group report. *Biol Blood Marrow Transplant.* 2005;11(12):945-956. doi:10.1016/j.bbmt.2005.09.004.

267. Higman MA, Vogelsang GB. Chronic graft versus host disease. *Br J Haematol.* 2004;125(4):435-454. doi:10.1111/j.1365-2141.2004.04945.x.

268. Baird K, Cooke K, Schultz KR. Chronic graft-versus-host disease (GVHD) in children. *Pediatr Clin North Am.* 2010;57(1):297-322. doi:10.1016/j.pcl.2009.11.003.

269. Tolland JP, Devereux C, Jones FC, Bingham EA. Sclerodermatous chronic graft-versus-host disease—a report of four pediatric cases. *Pediatr Dermatol.* 2008;25(2):240-244. doi:10.1111/j.1525-1470.2008.00643.x.

270. Akosa AB, Lampert IA. The sweat gland in graft versus host disease. *J Pathol.* 1990;161(3):261-266.

271. Castano E, Rodriguez-Peralto JL, Lopez-Rios F, Gomez C, Zimmermann M, Iglesias Diez L. Keratinocyte dysplasia: an usual finding after transplantation or chemotherapy. *J Cutan Pathol.* 2002;29(10):579-584.

272. Kim SJ, Choi JM, Kim JE, Cho BK, Kim DW, Park HJ. Clinicopathologic characteristics of cutaneous chronic graft-versus-host diseases: a retrospective study in Korean patients. *Int J Dermatol.* 2010;49(12):1386-1392.

273. Kohler S, Hendrickson MR, Chao NJ, Smoller BR. Value of skin biopsies in assessing prognosis and progression of acute graft-versus-host disease. *Am J Surg Pathol.* 1997;21(9):988-996.

274. Kohler S, Pascher A, Junge G, et al. Graft versus host disease after liver transplantation—a single center experience and review of literature. *Transpl Int.* 2008;21(5):441-451.

275. Massi D, Franchi A, Pimpinelli N, Laszlo D, Bosi A, Santucci M. A reappraisal of the histopathologic criteria for the diagnosis of cutaneous allogeneic acute graft-vs-host disease. *Am J Clin Pathol.* 1999;112(6):791-800.

276. Taguchi S, Kawachi Y, Fujisawa Y, Nakamura Y, Furuta J, Otsuka F. Psoriasiform eruption associated with graft-versus-host disease. *Cutis.* 2013;92(3):151-153.

277. Penas PF, Jones-Caballero M, Aragues M, Fernandez-Herrera J, Fraga J, Garcia-Diez A. Sclerodermatous graft-vs-host disease: clinical and pathological study of 17 patients. *Arch Dermatol.* 2002;138(7):924-934.

278. Huff JC, Weston WL, Tonnesen MG. Erythema multiforme: a critical review of characteristics, diagnostic criteria, and causes. *J Am Acad Dermatol.* 1983;8(6):763-775.

279. Karincaoğlu Y, Aki T, Erguvan-Onal R, Seyhan M. Erythema multiforme due to diphtheria-pertussis-tetanus vaccine. *Pediatr Dermatol.* 2007;24(3):334-335. doi:10.1111/j.1525-1470.2007.00423.x.

280. Ang-Tiu CU, Nicolas ME. Erythema multiforme in a 25-day old neonate. *Pediatr Dermatol.* 2013;30(6):e118-e120. doi:10.1111/j.1525-1470.2012.01873.x.

281. Schofield JK, Tatnall FM, Leigh IM. Recurrent erythema multiforme: clinical features and treatment in a large series of patients. *Br J Dermatol.* 1993;128(5):542-545.

282. Weston WL, Brice SL, Jester JD, Lane AT, Stockert S, Huff JC. Herpes simplex virus in childhood erythema multiforme. *Pediatrics.* 1992;89(1):32-34.

283. Keller N, Gilad O, Marom D, Marcus N, Garty BZ. Nonbullous erythema multiforme in hospitalized children: a 10-year survey. *Pediatr Dermatol.* 2015;32(5):701-703. doi:10.1111/pde.12659.

284. Nakai H, Sugata K, Usui C, et al. A case of erythema multiforme associated with primary Epstein-Barr virus infection. *Pediatr Dermatol.* 2011;28(1):23-25. doi:10.1111/j.1525-1470.2010.01217.x.

285. Aurelian L, Ono F, Burnett J. Herpes simplex virus (HSV)-associated erythema multiforme (HAEM): a viral disease with an autoimmune component. *Dermatol Online J.* 2003;9(1):1.

286. Pope E, Krafchik BR. Involvement of three mucous membranes in herpes-induced recurrent erythema multiforme. *J Am Acad Dermatol.* 2005;52(1):171-172. doi:10.1016/j.jaad.2004.06.048.

287. Bastuji-Garin S, Rzany B, Stern RS, Sheu NH, Naldi L, Roujeau JC. Clinical classification of cases of toxic epidermal necrolysis, Stevens-Johnson syndrome, and erythema multiforme. *Arch Dermatol.* 1993;129(1):92-96.

288. Canavan TN, Mathes EF, Frieden I, Shinkai K. Mycoplasma pneumoniae-induced rash and mucositis as a syndrome distinct from Stevens-Johnson syndrome and erythema multiforme: a systematic review. *J Am Acad Dermatol.* 2015;72(2):239-245. doi:10.1016/j.jaad.2014.06.026.

289. Wetter DA, Camilleri MJ. Clinical, etiologic, and histopathologic features of Stevens-Johnson syndrome during an 8-year period at Mayo Clinic. *Mayo Clin Proc.* 2010;85(2):131-138. doi:10.4065/mcp.2009.0379.

290. Hsu DY, Brieva J, Silverberg NB, Paller AS, Silverberg JI. Pediatric Stevens-Johnson syndrome and toxic epidermal necrolysis in the United States. *J Am Acad Dermatol.* 2017;76(5):811-817.e814. doi:10.1016/j.jaad.2016.12.024.

291. Finkelstein Y, Soon GS, Acuna P, et al. Recurrence and outcomes of Stevens-Johnson syndrome and toxic epidermal necrolysis in children. *Pediatrics.* 2011;128(4):723-728. doi:10.1542/peds.2010-3322.

292. Arca E, Köse O, Erbil AH, Nişanci M, Akar A, Gür AR. A 2-year-old girl with Stevens--Johnson syndrome/toxic epidermal necrolysis treated with intravenous immunoglobulin. *Pediatr Dermatol.* 2005;22(4):317-320. doi:10.1111/j.1525-1470.2005.22407.x.

293. Rizzo JA, Johnson R, Cartie RJ. Pediatric toxic epidermal necrolysis: experience of a tertiary burn center. *Pediatr Dermatol.* 2015;32(5):704-709. doi:10.1111/pde.12657.

294. Levi N, Bastuji-Garin S, Mockenhaupt M, et al. Medications as risk factors of Stevens-Johnson syndrome and toxic epidermal necrolysis in children: a pooled analysis. *Pediatrics.* 2009;123(2):e297-e304. doi:10.1542/peds.2008-1923.

295. Schwartz RA, McDonough PH, Lee BW. Toxic epidermal necrolysis: part II. Prognosis, sequelae, diagnosis, differential diagnosis,

prevention, and treatment. *J Am Acad Dermatol.* 2013;69(2):187.e1-187.e16, quiz 203-204. doi:10.1016/j.jaad.2013.05.002.

296. Dziuban EJ, Hughey AB, Stewart DA, et al. Stevens-Johnson syndrome and HIV in children in Swaziland. *Pediatr Infect Dis J.* 2013;32(12):1354-1358. doi:10.1097/INF.0b013e31829ec8e5.

297. Koh MJ, Tay YK. Stevens-Johnson syndrome and toxic epidermal necrolysis in Asian children. *J Am Acad Dermatol.* 2010;62(1):54-60. doi:10.1016/j.jaad.2009.06.085.

298. Quirke KP, Beck A, Gamelli RL, Mosier MJ. A 15-year review of pediatric toxic epidermal necrolysis. *J Burn Care Res.* 2015;36(1):130-136. doi:10.1097/BCR.0000000000000208.

299. Downey A, Jackson C, Harun N, Cooper A. Toxic epidermal necrolysis: review of pathogenesis and management. *J Am Acad Dermatol.* 2012;66(6):995-1003. doi:10.1016/j.jaad.2011.09.029.

300. Schwartz RA, McDonough PH, Lee BW. Toxic epidermal necrolysis: part I. Introduction, history, classification, clinical features, systemic manifestations, etiology, and immunopathogenesis. *J Am Acad Dermatol.* 2013;69(2):173.e1-173.e13, quiz 185-186. doi:10.1016/j.jaad.2013.05.003.

301. Frey N, Bircher A, Bodmer M, Jick SS, Meier CR, Spoendlin J. Antibiotic drug use and the risk of Stevens–Johnson syndrome and toxic epidermal necrolysis: a population-based case-control study. *J Invest Dermatol.* 2018;138(5):1207-1209. doi:10.1016/j.jid.2017.12.015.

302. Sassolas B, Haddad C, Mockenhaupt M, et al. ALDEN, an algorithm for assessment of drug causality in Stevens-Johnson syndrome and toxic epidermal necrolysis: comparison with case-control analysis. *Clin Pharmacol Ther.* 2010;88(1):60-68. doi:10.1038/clpt.2009.252.

303. Ichihara A, Wang Z, Jinnin M, et al. Upregulation of miR-18a-5p contributes to epidermal necrolysis in severe drug eruptions. *J Allergy Clin Immunol.* 2014;133(4):1065-1074. doi:10.1016/j.jaci.2013.09.019.

304. Maverakis E, Wang EA, Shinkai K, et al. Stevens–Johnson syndrome and toxic epidermal necrolysis standard reporting and evaluation guidelines: results of a National Institutes of Health Working Group. *JAMA Dermatol.* 2017;153(6):587-592. doi:10.1001/jamadermatol.2017.0160.

305. Léauté-Labrèze C, Lamireau T, Chawki D, Maleville J, Taïeb A. Diagnosis, classification, and management of erythema multiforme and Stevens–Johnson syndrome. *Arch Dis Child.* 2000;83(4):347-352.

306. Mayor-Ibarguren A, Feito-Rodríguez M, González-Ramos J, et al. Mucositis secondary to *Chlamydia pneumoniae* infection: expanding the mycoplasma pneumoniae-induced rash and mucositis concept. *Pediatr Dermatol.* 2017;34(4):465-472. doi:10.1111/pde.13140.

307. Sorrell J, Anthony L, Rademaker A, et al. Score of toxic epidermal necrosis predicts the outcomes of pediatric epidermal necrolysis. *Pediatr Dermatol.* 2017;34(4):433-437. doi:10.1111/pde.13172.

308. Olson D, Watkins LK, Demirjian A, et al. Outbreak of mycoplasma pneumoniae-associated Stevens–Johnson syndrome. *Pediatrics.* 2015;136(2):e386-e394. doi:10.1542/peds.2015-0278.

309. Prindaville B, Newell BD, Nopper AJ, Horii KA. Mycoplasma pneumonia–associated mucocutaneous disease in children: dilemmas in classification. *Pediatr Dermatol.* 2014;31(6):670-675. doi:10.1111/pde.12482.

310. Howland WW, Golitz LE, Weston WL, Huff JC. Erythema multiforme: clinical, histopathologic, and immunologic study. *J Am Acad Dermatol.* 1984;10(3):438-446.

311. Roujeau JC, Dubertret L, Moritz S, et al. Involvement of macrophages in the pathology of toxic epidermal necrolysis. *Br J Dermatol.* 1985;113(4):425-430.

312. Sebastian A, Patterson C, Zaenglein AL, Ioffreda MD, Helm KF. Histiocytic erythema multiforme. *J Cutan Pathol.* 2009;36(12):1323-1325.

313. Zohdi-Mofid M, Horn TD. Acrosyringeal concentration of necrotic keratinocytes in erythema multiforme: a clue to drug etiology. Clinicopathologic review of 29 cases. *J Cutan Pathol.* 1997;24(4):235-240.

314. Green M, Roy D. Rowell syndrome: targeting a true definition. *Cutis.* 2017;100(1):E8-E11.

315. Torrelo A, Zaballos P, Colmenero I, Mediero IG, de Prada I, Zambrano A. Erythema dyschromicum perstans in children: a report of 14 cases. *J Eur Acad Dermatol Venereol.* 2005;19(4):422-426. doi:10.1111/j.1468-3083.2005.01203.x.

316. Oiso N, Tsuruta D, Imanishi H, Kobayashi H, Kawada A. Erythema dyschromicum perstans in a Japanese child. *Pediatr Dermatol.* 2012;29(5):637-640. doi:10.1111/j.1525-1470.2011.01567.x.

317. Lee SJ, Chung KY. Erythema dyschromicum perstans in early childhood. *J Dermatol.* 1999;26(2):119-121.

318. Silverberg NB, Herz J, Wagner A, Paller AS. Erythema dyschromicum perstans in prepubertal children. *Pediatr Dermatol.* 2003;20(5):398-403.

319. Baranda L, Torres-Alvarez B, Cortes-Franco R, Moncada B, Portales-Perez DP, Gonzalez-Amaro R. Involvement of cell adhesion and activation molecules in the pathogenesis of erythema dyschromicum perstans (ashy dermatitis). The effect of clofazimine therapy. *Arch Dermatol.* 1997;133(3):325-329.

320. Lambert WC, Schwartz RA, Hamilton GB. Erythema dyschromicum perstans. *Cutis.* 1986;37(1):42-44.

321. Vasquez-Ochoa LA, Isaza-Guzman DM, Orozco-Mora B, Restrepo-Molina R, Trujillo-Perez J, Tapia FJ. Immunopathologic study of erythema dyschromicum perstans (ashy dermatosis). *Int J Dermatol.* 2006;45(8):937-941.

322. Petri M, Orbai A-M, Alarcón GS, et al. Derivation and validation of the Systemic Lupus International Collaborating Clinics classification criteria for systemic lupus erythematosus. *Arthritis Rheum.* 2012;64(8):2677-2686. doi:10.1002/art.34473.

323. Durosaro O, Davis MD, Reed KB, Rohlinger AL. Incidence of cutaneous lupus erythematosus, 1965-2005: a population-based study. *Arch Dermatol.* 2009;145(3):249-253. doi:10.1001/archdermatol.2009.21.

324. Wananukul S, Watana D, Pongprasit P. Cutaneous manifestations of childhood systemic lupus erythematosus. *Pediatr Dermatol.* 1998;15(5):342-346.

325. AlKharafi NN, Alsaeed K, AlSumait A, et al. Cutaneous lupus erythematosus in children: experience from a tertiary care pediatric dermatology clinic. *Pediatr Dermatol.* 2016;33(2):200-208. doi:10.1111/pde.12788.

326. Hiraki LT, Benseler SM, Tyrrell PN, Harvey E, Hebert D, Silverman ED. Ethnic differences in pediatric systemic lupus erythematosus. *J Rheumatol.* 2009;36(11):2539-2546. doi:10.3899/jrheum.081141.

327. Berry T, Walsh E, Berry R, DeSantis E, Smidt AC. Subacute cutaneous lupus erythematosus presenting in childhood: a case report and review of the literature. *Pediatr Dermatol.* 2014;31(3):368-372. doi:10.1111/pde.12007.

328. Schoch JJ, Peters MS, Reed AM, Tollefson MM. Pediatric subacute cutaneous lupus erythematosus: report of three cases. *Int J Dermatol.* 2015;54(5):e169-e174. doi:10.1111/ijd.12661.

329. Amato L, Coronella G, Berti S, Moretti S, Fabbri P. Subacute cutaneous lupus erythematosus in childhood. *Pediatr Dermatol.* 2003;20(1):31-34.

330. Camarillo D, McCalmont TH, Frieden IJ, Gilliam AE. Two pediatric cases of nonbullous histiocytoid neutrophilic dermatitis presenting as a cutaneous manifestation of lupus erythematosus. *Arch Dermatol.* 2008;144(11):1495-1498. doi:10.1001/archderm.144.11.1495.

331. Green JJ, Baker DJ. Linear childhood discoid lupus erythematosus following the lines of Blaschko: a case report with review of the linear manifestations of lupus erythematosus. *Pediatr Dermatol.* 1999;16(2):128-133.

332. Sampaio MC, de Oliveira ZN, Machado MC, dos Reis VM, Vilela MA. Discoid lupus erythematosus in children—a retrospective study of 34 patients. *Pediatr Dermatol.* 2008;25(2):163-167. doi:10.1111/j.1525-1470.2008.00625.x.

333. Requena C, Torrelo A, de Prada I, Zambrano A. Linear childhood cutaneous lupus erythematosus following Blaschko lines. *J Eur Acad Dermatol Venereol.* 2002;16(6):618-620.

334. Wimmershoff MB, Hohenleutner U, Landthaler M. Discoid lupus erythematosus and lupus profundus in childhood: a report of two cases. *Pediatr Dermatol.* 2003;20(2):140-145.

335. Arkin LM, Ansell L, Rademaker A, et al. The natural history of pediatric-onset discoid lupus erythematosus. *J Am Acad Dermatol.* 2015;72(4):628-633. doi:10.1016/j.jaad.2014.12.028.

336. Wieczorek IT, Propert KJ, Okawa J, Werth VP. Systemic symptoms in the progression of cutaneous to systemic lupus erythematosus. *JAMA Dermatol.* 2014;150(3):291-296. doi:10.1001/jamadermatol.2013.9026.

337. Bangert JL, Freeman RG, Sontheimer RD, Gilliam JN. Subacute cutaneous lupus erythematosus and discoid lupus erythematosus. Comparative histopathologic findings. *Arch Dermatol.* 1984;120(3):332-337.

338. Jerdan MS, Hood AF, Moore GW, Callen JP. Histopathologic comparison of the subsets of lupus erythematosus. *Arch Dermatol.* 1990;126(1):52-55.

339. Kettler AH, Bean SF, Duffy JO, Gammon WR. Systemic lupus erythematosus presenting as a bullous eruption in a child. *Arch Dermatol.* 1988;124(7):1083-1087.

340. Hsu S, Hwang LY, Ruiz H. Tumid lupus erythematosus. *Cutis.* 2002;69(3):227-230.

341. Ruiz H, Sanchez JL. Tumid lupus erythematosus. *Am J Dermatopathol.* 1999;21(4):356-360.

342. Thareja S, Paghdal K, Lien MH, Fenske NA. Reticular erythematous mucinosis—a review. *Int J Dermatol.* 2012;51(8):903-909.

343. Shirahama S, Furukawa F, Yagi H, Tanaka T, Hashimoto T, Takigawa M. Bullous systemic lupus erythematosus: detection of antibodies against noncollagenous domain of type VII collagen. *J Am Acad Dermatol.* 1998;38(5, pt 2):844-848.

344. Shirahama S, Yagi H, Furukawa F, Takigawa M. A case of bullous systemic lupus erythematosus. *Dermatology.* 1994;189 suppl 1:95-96.

345. Tincopa M, Puttgen KB, Sule S, Cohen BA, Gerstenblith MR. Bullous lupus: an unusual initial presentation of systemic lupus erythematosus in an adolescent girl. *Pediatr Dermatol.* 2010;27(4):373-376.

346. Hetem MB, Takada MH, Llorach Velludo MA, Foss NT. Neonatal lupus erythematosus. *Int J Dermatol.* 1996;35(1):42-44.

347. Lee LA. Neonatal lupus erythematosus. *J Invest Dermatol.* 1993;100(1):9S-13S.

348. Lee SH, Roh MR. Targetoid lesions and neutrophilic dermatosis: an initial clinical and histological presentation of neonatal lupus erythematosus. *Int J Dermatol.* 2014;53(6):764-766.

349. Penate Y, Lujan D, Rodriguez J, et al. Neonatal lupus erythematosus: 4 cases and clinical review [in Spanish]. *Actas Dermosifiliogr.* 2005;96(10):690-696.

350. Satter EK, High WA. Non-bullous neutrophilic dermatosis within neonatal lupus erythematosus. *J Cutan Pathol.* 2007;34(12):958-960.

351. Sitthinamsuwan P, Nitiyarom R, Chairatchaneeboon M, Wisuthsarewong W. Histiocytoid neutrophilic dermatitis, an unusual histopathology in neonatal lupus erythematosus. *J Cutan Pathol.* 2015;42(12):996-999.

352. Segal AR, Doherty KM, Leggott J, Barrett Z. Cutaneous reactions to drugs in children. *Pediatrics.* 2007;120(4):e1082-e1096. doi:10.1542/peds.2005-2321.

353. Sharma VK, Dhar S. Clinical pattern of cutaneous drug eruption among children and adolescents in North India. *Pediatr Dermatol.* 1995;12(2):178-183.

354. Morelli JG, Tay YK, Rogers M, Halbert A, Krafchik B, Weston WL. Fixed drug eruptions in children. *J Pediatr.* 1999;134(3):365-367.

355. Mahboob A, Haroon TS. Drugs causing fixed eruptions: a study of 450 cases. *Int J Dermatol.* 1998;37(11):833-838.

356. Shiohara T. Fixed drug eruption: pathogenesis and diagnostic tests. *Curr Opin Allergy Clin Immunol.* 2009;9(4):316-321. doi:10.1097/ACI.0b013e32832cda4c.

357. Savin JA. Current causes of fixed drug eruption in the UK. *Br J Dermatol.* 2001;145(4):667-668.

358. Nussinovitch M, Prais D, Ben-Amitai D, Amir J, Volovitz B. Fixed drug eruption in the genital area in 15 boys. *Pediatr Dermatol.* 2002;19(3):216-219.

359. Ozkaya-Bayazit E, Bayazit H, Ozarmagan G. Topical provocation in 27 cases of cotrimoxazole-induced fixed drug eruption. *Contact Dermatitis.* 1999;41(4):185-189.

360. Ozkaya-Bayazit E, Bayazit H, Ozarmagan G. Drug related clinical pattern in fixed drug eruption. *Eur J Dermatol.* 2000;10(4):288-291.

361. Petty RE, Southwood TR, Manners P, et al. International League of Associations for Rheumatology classification of juvenile idiopathic arthritis: second revision, Edmonton, 2001. *J Rheumatol.* 2004;31(2):390-392.

362. Abdwani R, Scuccumarri R, Duffy K, Duffy CM. Nodulosis in systemic onset juvenile idiopathic arthritis: an uncommon event with spontaneous resolution. *Pediatr Dermatol.* 2009;26(5):587-591. doi:10.1111/j.1525-1470.2009.00990.x.

363. Vastert SJ, Kuis W, Grom AA. Systemic JIA: new developments in the understanding of the pathophysiology and therapy. *Best Pract Res Clin Rheumatol.* 2009;23(5):655-664. doi:10.1016/j.berh.2009.08.003.

364. Frosch M, Metze D, Foell D, et al. Early activation of cutaneous vessels and epithelial cells is characteristic of acute systemic onset juvenile idiopathic arthritis. *Exp Dermatol.* 2005;14(4):259-265. doi:10.1111/j.0906-6705.2005.00271.x.

365. Prendiville JS, Tucker LB, Cabral DA, Crawford RI. A pruritic linear urticarial rash, fever, and systemic inflammatory disease in five adolescents: adult-onset still disease or systemic juvenile idiopathic arthritis sine arthritis? *Pediatr Dermatol.* 2004;21(5):580-588. doi:10.1111/j.0736-8046.2004.21513.x.

366. Fortna RR, Gudjonsson JE, Seidel G, et al. Persistent pruritic papules and plaques: a characteristic histopathologic presentation seen in a subset of patients with adult-onset and juvenile Still's disease. *J Cutan Pathol.* 2010;37(9):932-937. doi:10.1111/j.1600-0560.2010.01570.x.

367. Moon HR, Lee JH, Won CH, et al. A child with interstitial granulomatous dermatitis and juvenile idiopathic arthritis. *Pediatr Dermatol.* 2013;30(6):e272-e273. doi:10.1111/pde.12144.

368. Lee JY, Yang CC, Hsu MM. Histopathology of persistent papules and plaques in adult-onset Still's disease. *J Am Acad Dermatol.* 2005;52(6):1003-1008.

369. Suzuki K, Kimura Y, Aoki M, et al. Persistent plaques and linear pigmentation in adult-onset Still's disease. *Dermatology.* 2001;202(4):333-335.

370. Wolgamot G, Yoo J, Hurst S, Gardner G, Olerud J, Argenyi Z. Unique histopathologic findings in a patient with adult-onset Still disease. *Am J Dermatopathol.* 2007;29(2):194-196.

371. Chiu YE, Co DO. Juvenile dermatomyositis: immunopathogenesis, role of myositis-specific autoantibodies, and review of rituximab use. *Pediatr Dermatol.* 2011;28(4):357-367. doi:10.1111/j.1525-1470.2011.01501.x.

372. Huber AM, Kim S, Reed AM, et al. Childhood arthritis and rheumatology research alliance consensus clinical treatment plans for juvenile dermatomyositis with persistent skin rash. *J Rheumatol.* 2017;44(1):110-116. doi:10.3899/jrheum.160688.

373. Robinson AB, Reed AM. Clinical features, pathogenesis and treatment of juvenile and adult dermatomyositis. *Nat Rev Rheumatol.* 2011;7(11):664-675. doi:10.1038/nrrheum.2011.139.

374. Hussain A, Rawat A, Jindal AK, Gupta A, Singh S. Autoantibodies in children with juvenile dermatomyositis: a single centre experience from North-West India. *Rheumatol Int.* 2017;37(5):807-812. doi:10.1007/s00296-017-3707-4.

375. Okong'o LO, Esser M, Wilmshurst J, Scott C. Characteristics and outcome of children with juvenile dermatomyositis in Cape Town: a cross-sectional study. *Pediatr Rheumatol Online J.* 2016;14(1):60. doi:10.1186/s12969-016-0118-0.

376. Barut K, Aydin PO, Adrovic A, Sahin S, Kasapcopur O. Juvenile dermatomyositis: a tertiary center experience. *Clin Rheumatol.* 2017;36(2):361-366. doi:10.1007/s10067-016-3530-4.

377. Rider LG, Nistala K. The juvenile idiopathic inflammatory myopathies: pathogenesis, clinical and autoantibody phenotypes, and outcomes. *J Intern Med.* 2016;280(1):24-38. doi:10.1111/joim.12444.

378. López De Padilla CM, Crowson CS, Hein MS, et al. Gene expression profiling in blood and affected muscle tissues reveals differential activation pathways in patients with new-onset juvenile and adult dermatomyositis. *J Rheumatol.* 2017;44(1):117-124. doi:10.3899/jrheum.160293.

379. Kishi T, Miyamae T, Hara R, et al. Clinical analysis of 50 children with juvenile dermatomyositis. *Mod Rheumatol.* 2013;23(2):311-317. doi:10.1007/s10165-012-0647-4.

380. Hoeltzel MF, Oberle EJ, Robinson AB, Agarwal A, Rider LG. The presentation, assessment, pathogenesis, and treatment of calcinosis in juvenile dermatomyositis. *Curr Rheumatol Rep.* 2014;16(12):467. doi:10.1007/s11926-014-0467-y.

381. Lundberg IE, Tjärnlund A, Bottai M, et al. 2017 European League against rheumatism/American College of Rheumatology Classification Criteria for adult and juvenile idiopathic inflammatory myopathies and their major subgroups. *Arthritis Rheumatol.* 2017;69(12):2271-2282. doi:10.1002/art.40320.

382. Boccaletti V, Di Nuzzo S, Feliciani C, Fabrizi G, Pagliarello C. An update on juvenile dermatomyositis. *G Ital Dermatol Venereol.* 2014;149(5):519-524.

383. Woo TY, Callen JP, Voorhees JJ, Bickers DR, Hanno R, Hawkins C. Cutaneous lesions of dermatomyositis are improved by hydroxychloroquine. *J Am Acad Dermatol.* 1984;10(4):592-600.

384. Smith ES, Hallman JR, DeLuca AM, Goldenberg G, Jorizzo JL, Sangueza OP. Dermatomyositis: a clinicopathological study of 40 patients. *Am J Dermatopathol.* 2009;31(1):61-67.

385. Pachman LM, Veis A, Stock S, et al. Composition of calcifications in children with juvenile dermatomyositis: association with chronic cutaneous inflammation. *Arthritis Rheum.* 2006;54(10):3345-3350.

386. Nielsen AO, Johnson E, Hentzer B, Kobayasi T. Dermatomyositis with universal calcinosis. A histopathological and electron optic study. *J Cutan Pathol.* 1979;6(6):486-491.

387. Feldman BM, Rider LG, Reed AM, Pachman LM. Juvenile dermatomyositis and other idiopathic inflammatory myopathies of childhood. *Lancet.* 2008;371(9631):2201-2212.

388. Callen JP. Dermatomyositis. *Lancet.* 2000;355(9197):53-57.

389. Bowyer SL, Clark RA, Ragsdale CG, Hollister JR, Sullivan DB. Juvenile dermatomyositis: histological findings and pathogenetic hypothesis for the associated skin changes. *J Rheumatol.* 1986;13(4):753-759.

4

Vesiculobullous Disorders

Kristen P. Hook / Jonathan J. Davick / James W. Patterson

INTRODUCTION

Blistering diseases in infants can be a diagnostic challenge that requires consideration of age of onset, pattern of distribution, quality of blistering, and associated extracutaneous signs. They ultimately fall into one of several categories: benign, infectious, genetic, and autoimmune or hypersensitivity reactions. This chapter reviews key clinical signs, along with the pathologic and immunofluorescence findings of many infantile blistering conditions. Correlation among clinical, histologic, immunologic, and serologic data is crucial to establish the correct diagnosis. Genetic testing may be required, as treatments are available to certain mutations, and should be directed by clinical and pathologic data.

Inherited Blistering Diseases

EPIDERMOLYSIS BULLOSA

Epidermolysis bullosa (EB) is a collection of inherited blistering diseases. The main categories include epidermolysis bullosa simplex (EBS), junctional epidermolysis bullosa (JEB), dystrophic epidermolysis bullosa (DEB), and Kindler syndrome (KS).[1] Epidermolysis bullosa acquisita (EBA) is an acquired form of EB due to an antibody to collagen 7, and is therefore reviewed in the autoimmune section.

Patients with EB should be phenotypically and genetically categorized. Important phenotypic features include:

- The presence of localized or generalized involvement
- Mucous membrane involvement
- Other cutaneous/appendageal features (tooth enamel defects, hair abnormalities, nail abnormalities, hand/foot deformity)
- Extracutaneous features (anemia, esophageal strictures, pyloric atresia)

Skin biopsy for routine histologic analysis may yield minimal diagnostic data. Electron microscopy can provide added information but, because of technical and interpretive limitations, often proves difficult. Immunofluorescence may provide useful information about proteins to target for genetic testing and is quicker than genetic testing. However, with the high sensitivity of available genetic testing, and the high frequency of multiple mutations among affected individuals, genetic testing is recommended for every patient if possible.

When biopsy is used for diagnosis, a newly induced blister should be biopsied for immunofluorescence and electron microscopy. This can be purposefully produced by gently twisting a pencil eraser (or a Q-tip) on a region of skin that is subject to blister formation prior to biopsy. A well-formed blister may not be clinically perceptible, but the microscopic change is usually seen on biopsy.

EB has historically been characterized by eponymous names that indicated a clinical extent of involvement and sometimes diagnostic structural information. These names have been replaced by descriptive terms that state clearly the type, inheritance, and mutation involved. Each EB patient is truly unique. Not only may the specific mutation they carry be unique, but also the way a known mutation manifests phenotypically may vary among individuals, and many patients carry more than one mutation for varied types of EB that can result in unique phenotypic presentations.

EPIDERMOLYSIS BULLOSA SIMPLEX

Definition and Epidemiology

EBS is a group of inherited blistering disorders characterized by mechanical fragility and blister formation within the epidermis.[1] Historically, most cases were associated with mutations in the genes encoding keratin 5 (*KRT5*) and keratin 14 (*KRT14*). However, many other culprit genes have now been identified.[1,2]

EBS is a rare disease, with a prevalence of 6 per 1 million and the incidence of 7.9 per 1 million live births.[3] There are two major categories—basal and suprabasal—depending on the level of involvement in the epidermis.[1] Further subcategorizations are based on the affected gene/protein and other clinical features.[1] The most prevalent subtypes fall into the basal category and include localized EBS (66% of EBS cases), generalized severe EBS (7%), generalized intermediate EBS (6%), EBS with mottled pigmentation (0.4%), and EBS with muscular dystrophy (0.2%).[3] The remaining 21% include other rare subtypes, including those affecting suprabasal portions of the epidermis.[3]

Etiology

EBS is caused by a variety of mutations in genes encoding epidermal structural proteins leading to easy blistering of the skin.[1] *KRT5* and *KRT14* were the first proteins implicated in the pathogenesis of EBS. Many others have since been identified, including plectin, transglutaminase 5, desmoplakin, plakoglobin, plakophilin 1, exophilin, α6β4 integrin, and bullous pemphigoid (BP) antigen-1.[1] In one study of 76 patients, *KRT5* or *KRT14* mutations were identified in 75% of affected patients.[4] The most common mode of inheritance is autosomal dominant, with some unusual forms inherited in an autosomal recessive fashion.[5]

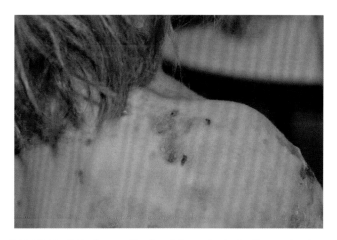
FIGURE 4-2. **Generalized epidermolysis bullosa simplex.** Flaccid blisters and erosions on an erythematous base. (Courtesy of Kristen Hook, MD.)

Clinical Presentation

Clinical presentations may include a localized disease of the palms and soles (see Figure 4-1) or generalized disease involving the entire body surface area. Blisters are typically well formed, but rupture easily on the body (see Figure 4-2). Nail dystrophy is a common associated feature (Figure 4-3). Brittle hair or tooth enamel defects may also be associated. Heat and warm weather can increase skin fragility, leading to increased blistering in warm climates or during summer months. Interventions to aid with cooling and drying the skin can be beneficial. Patients typically improve with age, with many young adults experiencing little to no blistering, blistering limited to the foot on warm days. Blisters may be uncomfortable, causing significant pain that precludes standing for long periods of time, which may affect work.

Histologic Findings

EBS is, by definition, an intraepidermal process, and intraepidermal blister formation is seen histologically (Figure 4-4).[6]

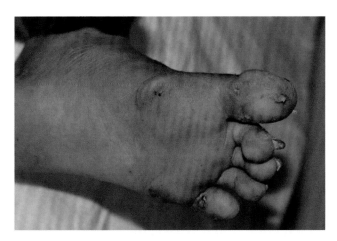
FIGURE 4-1. **Epidermolysis bullosa simplex.** Note well-formed bullae on the plantar surface. (Courtesy of Kristen Hook, MD.)

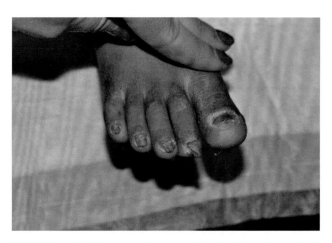
FIGURE 4-3. **Nail dystrophy associated with epidermolysis bullosa simplex.** (Courtesy of Kristen Hook, MD.)

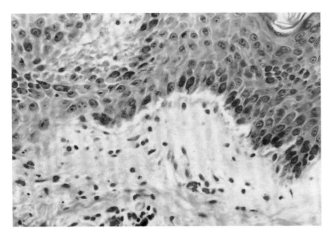

FIGURE 4-4. **Epidermolysis bullosa simplex.** This is an early lesion; similar changes can be obtained by applying mild trauma to intact skin prior to biopsy. Early clefting can be seen, with some attachment of basal keratinocyte fragments to the base of the separation.

In the most common basal types of EBS, a split in the epidermis just below the nuclei of the basal layer keratinocytes is most characteristic (Figure 4-4), although superficial layers of the epidermis can become involved with significant trauma.[6] Histologic sections for light microscopy may appear to demonstrate a subepidermal blister, as only a small portion of the basal layer keratinocyte cytoplasm may remain attached to the dermis. This is particularly true of older lesions.[6] Faint remnants of basal cell keratinocyte cytoplasm are often identified at the base of the blister, and the nucleated half of the split keratinocyte may be found in the blister cavity.[6] Blisters are often multiloculated, a feature most commonly seen in early lesions.[6] Very early lesions may show only prominent vacuolization (sometimes referred to as "cytolysis") of the basal layer keratinocyte cytoplasm just below the nucleus[6] (Figures 4-4 and 4-5).

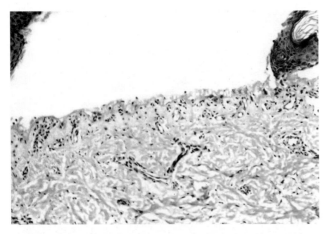

FIGURE 4-5. **Epidermolysis bullosa simplex.** A fully developed bulla may at first appear to be subepidermal, but the fragments of basal keratinocyte cytoplasm can be seen attached to the dermal side of the separation—indicating the degeneration of the infranuclear portions of basal keratinocytes that characterize this disease.

As the exact location of the blister may not be apparent on light microscopy alone (intraepidermal vs. subepidermal), immunohistochemical (IHC) stains, direct immunofluorescence (DIF), and electron microscopy (EM) are useful ancillary tests. While EM studies shaped our current understanding of the pathogenesis of EB,[7] IHC and DIF methods have largely supplanted ultrastructural examination of routine clinical specimens.

DIF or IHC studies show keratin(s), laminin, and type IV collagen along the floor of the blister. The presence of keratin, together with laminin and type IV collage, proves that small portions of the basal layer keratinocytes are present at the floor of the blister, confirming an intraepidermal process.[8]

Differential Diagnosis

The differential diagnosis for EBS includes other forms of EB, such as junctional EB or other subepidermal blistering processes. EBS may be distinguished by evidence of an intraepidermal blister. Evidence of cytolysis of the infranuclear portions of basal keratinocytes at the edge of blisters (or sometimes at specimen edges) can help in diagnosis.

CAPSULE SUMMARY

EPIDERMOLYSIS BULLOSA SIMPLEX

EBS is a diverse group of inherited blistering disorders that cause *intraepidermal* blisters. Inherited mutations in the structural proteins of the skin, the most common of which are *KRT5* and *KRT14*, lead to the clinical manifestations of the EBS diseases. Light microscopy sections show a very low intraepidermal split, most commonly just below the nuclei of the basal layer keratinocytes, although it may appear subepidermal in well-developed lesions. DIF or IHC studies demonstrate keratin(s) and type IV collagen and laminin along the floor of the blister.

JUNCTIONAL EPIDERMOLYSIS BULLOSA

Definition and Epidemiology

JEB is a group of inherited blistering disorders characterized by cleavage in the lamina lucida layer of the epidermis. Mutations in nine different culprit genes have been identified. The prevalence of JEB (all subtypes) is between 0.5 per 1 million and the incidence is 2.68 per 1 million live births.[1,3]

Etiology

The JEB cleavage plane is along the lamina lucida of the basement membrane zone and can involve many different structural proteins, including laminin-γ2 (*LAMC2*), laminin-β3 (*LAMB3*), collagen type 17-α1 (*COL17A1*), integrin-β4 (*ITGB4*), and laminin-α3 (*LAMA3*).

Clinical Presentation

Severe forms of this subtype can be lethal in the first days to months of life. Less severe forms may allow those affected to live for years, but typically with a limitation of some activities and considerable discomfort. Classic signs in the neonatal period include blistering in the diaper area or along the back (Figure 4-6). The blisters may have a "herpetiform" or raised appearance resulting from the granulation tissue. Mucous membranes are commonly involved. Fingernail and hair abnormalities may also be present (Figure 4-7).

Histologic Findings

JEB is caused by splitting of the skin at the layer of the lamida lucida, reflected by histologic sections demonstrating a subepidermal blister (Figure 4-8).[9] In contrast to EBS lesions, JEB lesions do not show cells or debris within the blister cavity (the so-called cell-free blister is characteristic).[9] There is typically no significant associated inflammatory infiltrate.[9] Absent or hypoplastic hemidesmosomes can be seen on ultrastructural examination, especially in more severe variants of the disease. IHC or DIF immunomapping identify BP antigen-1 on the roof of the blister, whereas laminin and type IV collagen are identified along the floor.

Differential Diagnosis

The differential diagnosis includes other pediatric blistering disorders discussed in this chapter. The key distinguishing feature is the level of splitting of the skin. Although EBS lesions may appear subepidermal, JEB blister cavities do not

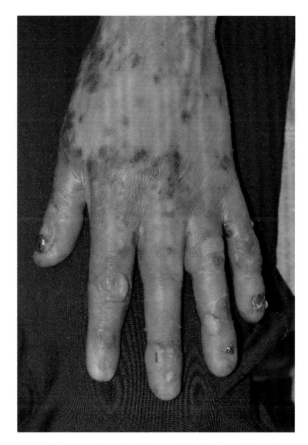

FIGURE 4-7. Junctional epidermolysis bullosa. Note fingernail involvement and dyspigmentation. (Courtesy of Kristen Hook, MD.)

typically contain cells or cellular debris as seen in EBS. The differential diagnosis also includes DEB, which can be distinguished by unique immunomapping profiles. Again, correlation with clinical features and molecular genetic studies can aid in the distinction of JEB from other disorders.

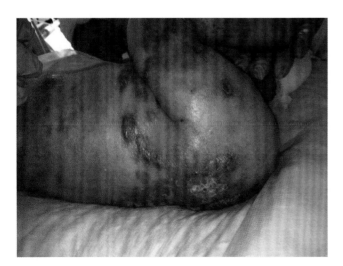

FIGURE 4-6. Junctional epidermolysis bullosa, generalized severe. Note the granulation tissue in wounds. (Courtesy of Kristen Hook, MD.)

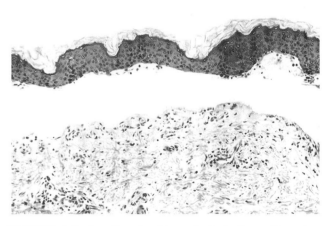

FIGURE 4-8. Junctional epidermolysis bullosa. There is a relatively "clean" subepidermal separation, with a smoothly contoured papillary dermis at the base. A few inflammatory cells are present in this example. Ultrastructural examination may show absent or reduced hypoplastic hemidesmosomes in this condition.

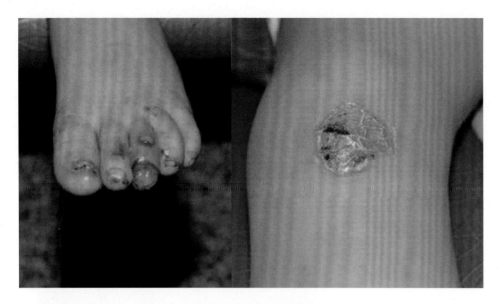

FIGURE 4-9. **Dominant dystrophic epidermolysis bullosa.** Blistering over knuckles, extensor joints, associated fingernail involvement is common. (Courtesy of Kristen Hook, MD.)

CAPSULE SUMMARY

JUNCTIONAL EPIDERMOLYSIS BULLOSA

JEB is a group of inherited blistering disorders characterized by blister formation in the lamina lucida of the dermal epidermal junction. Severe forms are lethal in infancy. Histologic sections show a subepidermal blistering without cells in the blister cavity. BP antigen-1 is generally identified on the roof of the blister, whereas laminin and type IV collagen are most often found on the floor of the blister.

DYSTROPHIC EPIDERMOLYSIS BULLOSA

Definition and Epidemiology

DEB is a group of inherited blistering disorders characterized by cleavage in the basement membrane, within the lamina densa.

The prevalence of dominant dystrophic epidermolysis bullosa (DDEB, all subtypes) is 1.5 per 1 million and the incidence is 2.12 per 1 million live births. The prevalence of recessive dystrophic epidermolysis bullosa (RDEB) is 1.4 per 1 million and the incidence is 3.05 per 1 million live births.[1,3]

Etiology

DEB is caused by many described mutations in collagen VII. Cleavage is below the lamina densa in the region of the anchoring fibrils. DEB is inherited in a dominant or recessive pattern.

Clinical Presentation

DDEB is characterized by blisters, atrophic papules, and milia. It most frequently affects the extensor surfaces (interphalangeal joints of the fingers and toes, elbows, knees) (Figures 4-9 and 4-10). Aplasia cutis (absence of the skin) may be a finding at birth (Figure 4-11). Blistering generally improves with age as injury to these areas becomes less frequent. RDEB is

characterized by widespread blistering and scarring, joint contractures, mitten deformity of the hands, microstomia, and tooth enamel defects (Figures 4-12 to 4-15). Generalized RDEB also has many systemic manifestations, including anemia, osteoporosis, and esophageal strictures. Patients with generalized severe subtype have a shortened life span and succumb to aggressive squamous cell carcinomas that form in the areas of frequent blistering. There is broad variation in phenotypic expression, and within these two variants there is much overlap. Patients may present with "mixed" mutations—for example, a collagen 7 mutation that may be associated with DDEB and another that may be associated with RDEB—which creates endless phenotypic heterogeneity.

Histologic Findings

DEB is caused by a split just below the lamida densa, with histologic sections demonstrating a subepidermal blister cavity (Figure 4-16). As with other forms of EB, the lesions

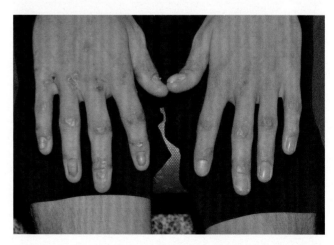

FIGURE 4-10. **Dominant dystrophic epidermolysis bullosa.** Note milia and scarring over extensor joints and associated nail dystrophy. (Courtesy of Kristen Hook, MD.)

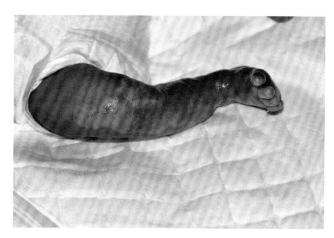

FIGURE 4-11. **Aplasia cutis.** Congenital absence of the skin can be present in multiple forms of epidermolysis bullosa. (Courtesy of Kristen Hook, MD.)

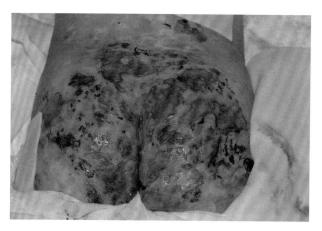

FIGURE 4-13. **Recessive dystrophic epidermolysis bullosa,** generalized intermediate subtype, involving the buttocks. (Courtesy of Kristen Hook, MD.)

usually lack an inflammatory infiltrate, although chronic inflammation and dermal scarring may accompany the lesions because of continuous skin damage over the course of the disease.[10] The numerous subtypes of DEB cannot be distinguished on histologic examination alone, and a specific diagnosis relies on correlation with the clinical and genetic features of the disorder.[1]

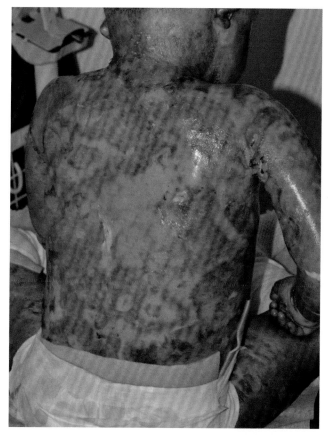

FIGURE 4-12. **Recessive dystrophic epidermolysis bullosa, generalized severe subtype.** Note generalized erosion, scarring, and dyspigmentation. (Courtesy of Kristen Hook, MD.)

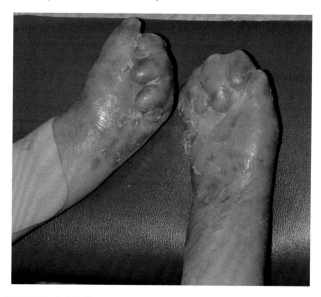

FIGURE 4-14. **Recessive dystrophic epidermolysis bullosa,** generalized severe subtype with associated mitten deformity. (Courtesy of Kristen Hook, MD.)

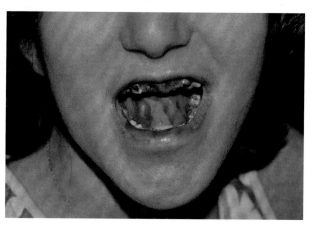

FIGURE 4-15. **Recessive dystrophic epidermolysis bullosa.** Note absent tongue papillae and enamel defects with associated tooth decay and concomitant microstomia. (Courtesy of Kristen Hook, MD.)

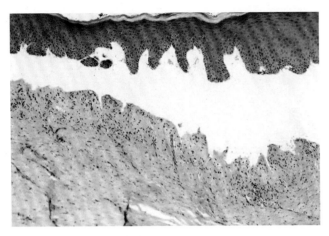

FIGURE 4-16. Dominant dystrophic epidermolysis bullosa. The subepidermal separation and scar are typical features. Some inflammation is present, suggesting that the bulla had been present for some time prior to biopsy.

Biopsies may be encountered from patients with known DEB to evaluate for squamous cell carcinoma (SCC). SCC is especially common in patients with RDEB (particularly the generalized severe variant), and may occur in adolescents.[11,12] Most cases associated with DEB are well-differentiated.[11] Despite this, SCCs in this disorder behave aggressively, and the majority of patients with RDEB, generalized severe subtype, die of metastatic SCC within 5 years of diagnosis.[11]

Milia formation is another well-known histopathologic finding associated with DEB. Milia are small dermal cysts lined by squamous epithelium and containing loose keratin (they are essentially miniaturized epidermal inclusion/epidermoid cysts) (Figure 4-17). In one case report, multiple milia was the presenting skin manifestation of DEB.[13] However, any disorder that causes repeated skin damage may result in milia formation, making the finding of milia nonspecific (the lesions of EBA, eg, also frequently show milia). Immunomapping studies show the presence of KRT5 and

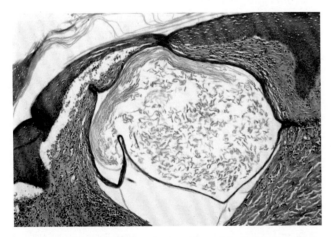

FIGURE 4-17. Recessive dystrophic epidermolysis bullosa. This image shows focal subepidermal separation, dermal scar, and milium formation—a characteristic feature of this form of epidermolysis bullosa.

KRT14, laminins, and type IV collagen along the roof of the blister. On ultrastructural examination, anchoring fibrils are often altered or reduced and may even be absent in severe recessive dystrophic forms of EB.

Differential Diagnosis

The histologic differential diagnosis of DEB includes other types of EB previously discussed. Milia formation and dermal scarring (features associated with DEB) may provide clues, although neither is specific for the disorder. A lack of cellular debris within the blister cavity can help distinguish DEB from EBS. Immunoreactants mapping to the roof of the blister distinguish DEB from JEB. Once again, correlation with the clinical and genetic features of the disorder is paramount in achieving a definitive diagnosis.

CAPSULE SUMMARY

DYSTROPHIC EPIDERMOLYSIS BULLOSA

DEB is a group of inherited blistering disorders caused by cleavage in the lamina densa of the basement membrane zone as a result of collagen VII mutations. Clinical manifestations include blister formation, milia formation, and scarring and joint contractures in some cases. Patients with generalized severe subtype of RDEB have a shortened life span because of the development of associated aggressive SCCs. Histologic features include subepidermal blister formation, milia, and dermal scarring. DIF and IHC studies will show KRT5/KRT14, laminins, and type IV collagen along the roof of the blister.

KINDLER SYNDROME

Definition and Epidemiology

KS is a rare subtype of inherited EB characterized by trauma-induced skin fragility, cutaneous atrophy, and progressive poikiloderma. Mucosal inflammation is often present. KS is extremely rare. Rare reports of patient cohorts are published.[14-16]

Etiology

KS results from mutations in the *FERMT1* (formerly *KIND-1*), which encodes fermitin family homolog 1 (FFH1) protein or Kindlin-1, a focal adhesion protein that binds the actin cytoskeleton to the underlying extracellular matrix. The protein regulates cell adhesion and motility by controlling lamellipodia formation in keratinocytes.

Clinical Presentation

KS is characterized by congenital acral blister formation and skin fragility. Photosensitivity, which manifests as progressive poikiloderma, is more prominent during childhood and usually improves with age.[15] Diffuse atrophic scarring and dyspigmentation continue to increase throughout life. Blistering occurs in photosensitive areas and associated atrophy may manifest as pseudosyndactyly (a fusion of the digits secondary to chronic scarring, as seen in the mitten deformity of RDEB). Palmoplantar hyperkeratosis and nail dystrophy are additional features. Mucosal manifestations are varied and can include hemorrhagic mucositis and gingivitis, periodontal disease, premature loss of teeth, and labial leukokeratosis. Severe long-term complications of KS include periodontitis and mucosal strictures (esophageal/laryngeal, anal, urethral, vaginal, and phimosis). Patients may have associated colitis. Patients have an increasing risk of developing SCC in acral skin and oral mucosa, and this risk increases with age.

Histologic Findings

Reported cases of KS describe hyperkeratosis, epidermal atrophy, vacuolar degeneration of the basal cell layer, telangiectasias (dilation of superficial dermal blood vessels), and pigment incontinence.[17,18] Vacuolar degeneration may extend into the areas of subepidermal cleft formation.[17,18] Colloid bodies have been described in the papillary dermis.[17] Ultrastructurally, multiple planes of cleavage in the dermal-epidermal junction may be seen, either in the lamina densa, the lamida lucida, or within the basal layer keratinocytes.[18] IHC or DIF studies using type IV or type VII collagen often show reduplication and interruptions of the basement membrane, although this finding is not entirely specific for KS.[18]

Differential Diagnosis

Because of skin fragility in the neonatal period, there can be clinical phenotypic overlap with DEB and EBS with mottled pigmentation. A diagnosis of KS cannot be made on histopathologic grounds alone as the findings of hyperkeratosis, epidermal atrophy, and vacuolar degeneration of the basement membrane frequently occur in other disorders (especially other poikilodermatous conditions). The finding of reduplication and disruption of the basement membrane on IHC/DIF studies can aid in making the diagnosis but is not diagnostic of KS. Correlation with clinical features, family history, and genetic studies is critical.

CAPSULE SUMMARY

KINDLER SYNDROME

KS is a rare subtype of EB in which patients develop acral blister formation which can progress to severe scarring. Mucosal involvement may be seen. Histologic findings include hyperkeratosis, epidermal atrophy, vacuolar degeneration of the basal cell layer, telangiectasias, and pigment incontinence. IHC or DIF studies show reduplication or interruptions of the basement membrane because of repeated blister formation and healing.

PORPHYRIA AND PSEUDOPORPHYRIA

Definition and Epidemiology

Porphyria is a group of nine inherited disorders caused by altered porphyrin production and characterized by variable photosensitivity and associated systemic signs and symptoms. Variants include acute intermittent porphyria (AIP), hereditary coproporphyria (HCP), variegate porphyria (VP), δ-aminolevulinic acid dehydratase deficiency porphyria (ADP), porphyria cutanea tarda (PCT), hepatoerythropoietic porphyria (HEP), congenital erythropoietic porphyria (CEP), erythropoietic protoporphyria (EPP), and X-linked protoporphyria (XLP). The most common form that presents in the pediatric population is EPP.

Pseudoporphyria demonstrates a photodistributed pattern of blistering but does not result from excessive porphyrin production.

Combined, all forms of porphyria affect roughly 200 000 people in the United States. European studies estimate the prevalence of the most common porphyria, PCT, at 1 in 10 000; the most common acute porphyria, AIP, at approximately 1 in 20 000; and the most common erythropoietic porphyria, EPP, at 1 in 50 000 to 75 000.[19] CEP is extremely rare, with prevalence estimates of 1 in 1 000 000 or less. ADP is even more rare, with only isolated case reports in the literature.[19] In the pediatric population, the forms most often diagnosed are EPP, AIP, and CEP.

Etiology

Porphyrias are a group of metabolic disorders resulting from abnormal function of the heme biosynthesis pathway and characterized by excessive accumulation and excretion of porphyrins and their precursors. Mutations in the enzymes of the pathway result in overproduction of heme precursors secondary to partial deficiency or, in XLP, increased activity. Each type of porphyria is identified by the enzyme affected and the resultant pattern of porphyrin accumulation. EPP is due to a defect in the enzyme ferrochelatase, which causes accumulation and excretion of protoporphyrin. Liver disease may be an attendant finding in EPP.[20]

Clinical Presentation

Children may report painful episodes in the sun resulting in severe sunburns. More chronic signs include ephelides, lentigines, and atrophic papules on the dorsal nose and cheeks. The lesions of EPP are usually not blisters, but consist of cobblestoned papules and scars (Figure 4-18). A review of acute porphyrias documented onset between the second and fourth decade of life, with abdominal pain as the most common symptom. Diagnosis is often delayed by more than a decade, and appendectomies and

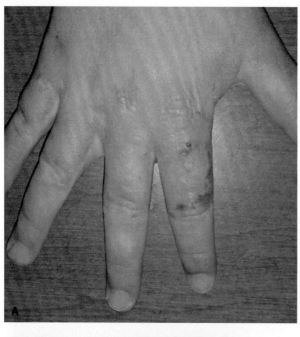

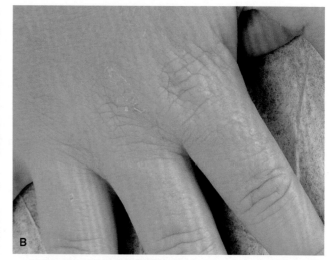

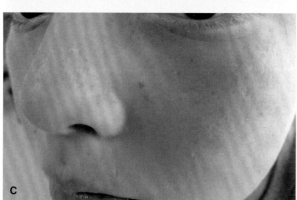

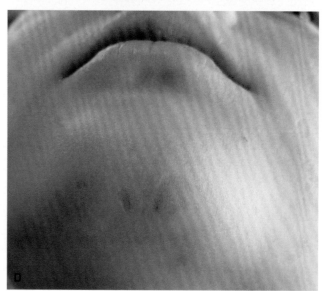

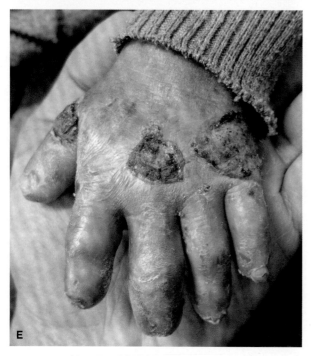

FIGURE 4-18. **Porphyria.** A, A boy with erythropoietic proto-porphyria with a small vesicle and erosions of the dorsal hand during an acute flare. B-D, The same patient after 2 years with subtle atrophic scarring in the sun-exposed areas of the nose, cheek, upper lip, chin, and dorsal hand. E, A child with congenital erythropoietic porphyria. There are erosions on the dorsal hand, and severe, mutilating scarring resulting in shortening of the dig-its and loss of fingernails.

cholecystectomies are common prior to diagnosis.[21] Serologic testing for EPP reveals an elevation of protoporphyrin in the erythrocytes, plasma, bile and feces due to a defect in ferrochelatase enzyme. The diagnosis of EPP is made by demonstrating increased total erythrocyte protoporphyrin and increased percentage of erythrocyte protoporphyrin rather than zinc protoporphyrin. In EPP, metal-free protoporphyrin generally represents more than 85% of the total porphyrins.

Histologic Findings

The different subtypes of porphyrias and pseudoporphyria appear histologically similar. When blister formation is present, histologic sections generally show a subepidermal blister that is free of cells or cellular debris (Figure 4-19). Lesions typically exhibit a small amount of associated chronic inflammation. The key histologic feature in the porphyrias is the presence of thick-walled, hyalinized vessels within the superficial (and sometimes deep) dermis. Periodic acid Schiff (PAS) staining highlights the material surrounding the blood vessels and may also demonstrate PAS-positive globules along the epidermal portion (roof) of the blister (sometimes referred to as "caterpillar bodies") (Figure 4-20).[22-24] The lesions may also show sclerosis of the dermis, and festooning (the presence of residual dermal papillae structures pushing into the blister cavity) is often a feature (Figure 4-21).[22-24] On the basis of ultrastructural studies and antigen mapping, the level of splitting in the blisters is variable, but most often involves the lamida lucida.[25] Accordingly, DIF or ICH antigen mapping studies most often demonstrate type IV collagen and laminin along the floor of the blister, and BP-1 antigen along the roof of the blister.[25] DIF testing also shows the deposition of C3, IgG, and IgM around vessels in the superficial dermis (sometimes described as

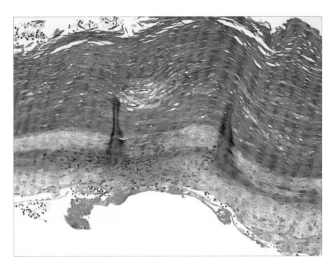

FIGURE 4-20. **Porphyria cutanea tarda.** The lesion is apparently from an acral location. Globular basement membrane material can be seen at the base of the epidermis; this material forms the so-called caterpillar bodies that are characteristic in this disease.

"doughnut-like" blood vessels, because of their thickened appearance).[26] Indirect immunofluorescence (IIF) is negative in these disorders.

Differential Diagnosis

The histologic differential diagnosis includes porphyria and pseudoporphyria. Distinction between these disorders is based on clinical and biochemical laboratory findings. Other disorders with cell-poor blister cavities including EBA, and some forms of EB may also be considered. DIF, IIF, and IHC studies are useful in distinguishing these disorders.

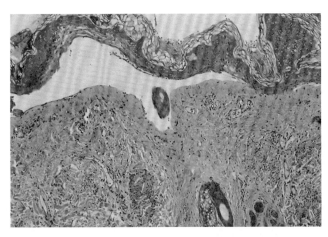

FIGURE 4-19. **Porphyria cutanea tarda.** There is an infiltrate-poor subepidermal bulla, with some degeneration of the separated epidermis.

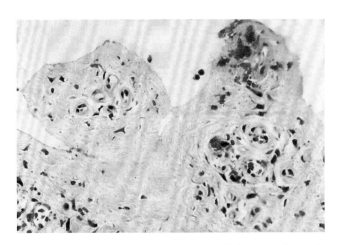

FIGURE 4-21. **Porphyria cutanea tarda.** This image shows the papillary dermis in another case. Note that the dermal papillae retain their shape ("festooning" of the blister base) and that the capillaries are thick-walled. Inflammation is sparse.

CAPSULE SUMMARY

PORPHYRIA

The porphyrias are a group of inherited defects in heme synthesis leading to the deposition of porphyrins in the skin and internal organs. Children may present with episodes of severe sunburns with resultant scarring of variable severity, depending on the subtype. Pseudoporphyria is an acquired disorder caused by medications, most commonly nonsteroidal anti-inflammatory drugs (NSAIDS). Histologic sections demonstrate a subepidermal blister with a festooning of the dermal papillae and thickened, hyalinized, "doughnut-shaped" vessels in the papillary dermis that are immunoreactive with antibodies to C3, IgG, and IgM.

Immune-Mediated Blistering Disorders

A review from a pediatric dermatology referral center for a population of 4 million people identified only 23 cases of immunobullous disease in patients less than 18 years of age over a 16-year period.[27] Autoimmune causes for blistering result from antibody formation to various proteins in the epidermis, dermis, or attachment proteins (desmosomes, etc). For these disorders, DIF is necessary for diagnosis. Most DIF labs can stain for basic epidermal proteins, but for more complex diagnoses, sendout to specialized labs may be required. IIF is also beneficial (diagnostic in some disorders) and can be used to assess treatment response in many cases.

EPIDERMOLYSIS BULLOSA ACQUISITA

Definition and Epidemiology

EBA results from antibody formation against collagen VII. This is in contrast to DEB, which is attributable to dysfunctional or absent collagen VII.

EBA is an acquired form of EB, most often affecting patients in the third to fourth decades of life, although transplacental passage in neonates has been reported. Involvement in children is rare, and the prognosis may be better than in adults.

Etiology

EBA is caused by an acquired autoantibody to collagen VII.

Clinical Presentation

EBA presents in one of two forms: generalized, well-formed blisters with an inflammatory component, or noninflammatory acral blistering with scarring and milia. Areas affected in DEB including scalp, mucous membranes (conjunctiva, esophagus, anogenital), and nails may also be involved.

Histologic Findings

The lesions of the noninflammatory/mechanobullous clinical subtype histologically demonstrate a cell-poor subepidermal blister (Figure 4-22). The other features of this variant include milia and scaring of the dermis. In contrast, the lesions of the inflammatory clinical subtype demonstrate a subepidermal separation with an associated mixed inflammatory infiltrate.[28] Occasionally, eosinophils may predominate the infiltrate, causing diagnostic confusion with BP.[28] In other instances, neutrophils predominate, and papillary neutrophilic microabscesses may resemble those seen in dermatitis herpetiformis (DH). In EBA, the basement membrane lines the roof of the blister. Fibrin is also frequently present along the floor of the blister. Ultrastructurally, the split is in the superficial dermis immediately below the lamina densa.[29,30] DIF or IHC studies will accordingly show type IV collagen along the roof of the blister.[29,30] DIF studies demonstrate linear IgG and C3 along the dermal-epidermal junction.[29,30] As EBA is caused by autoantibodies, IIF studies are useful in making the diagnosis, especially using salt-split skin IIF studies, which will demonstrate reactivity along the floor of the blister.[31] This same salt-split technique can be used on biopsies obtained for DIF.

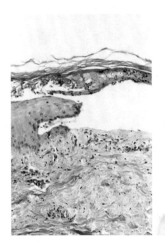 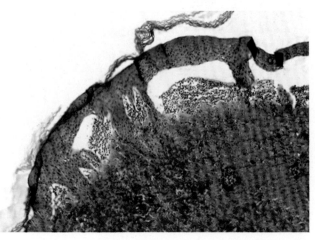

FIGURE 4-22. Epidermolysis bullosa acquisita. The left image shows a relatively infiltrate-poor subepidermal bulla; a few neutrophils can be seen within degenerated portions of the epidermis and in the papillary dermis. The right image shows papillary neutrophilic microabscesses—a feature in some examples of epidermolysis bullosa acquisita that can also be seen in other immunobullous diseases.

Differential Diagnosis

Histologically, inflammatory lesions may resemble BP, DH, or cicatricial pemphigoid (CP).[28] Other cell-poor, nonautoimmune blistering disorders discussed in this chapter may be considered in the differential diagnosis. DEB also demonstrates subepidermal blistering with associated scarring and milia formation. These can be distinguished by the presence of immunoreactants on DIF and split-skin IIF studies in EBA. As with all the disorders discussed in this chapter, establishing the diagnosis and excluding other disorders requires careful correlation with the clinical features of the disorder.

CAPSULE SUMMARY

EPIDERMOLYSIS BULLOSA ACQUISITA

EBA, a rare disease in children, is a structural skin disorder caused by autoantibodies to collagen VII. This is in contrast to DEB, which is often caused by mutations in the collagen VII gene. Histologically, lesions will demonstrate a subepidermal blister that may or may not have an associated inflammatory infiltrate. Milia and scarring may be seen in association with the lesions. Type IV collagen is seen along the roof of the blister. Linear IgG and C3 is seen along the dermal-epidermal junction in DIF studies. Split-skin IIF is useful in the diagnosis of EBA, and will show reactivity of the autoantibody along the floor of the blister.

Pemphigus—Overview

Pemphigus refers to a group of blistering diseases demonstrating suprabasilar cleavage resulting from autoantibodies (mostly IgG) directed against desmosomal antigens. Histologically, this manifests as acantholysis, or the loss of cell-cell adhesion. The overall incidence of pemphigus is estimated at 0.076 to 5 per 100 000 person years.[32]

Classic antigens implicated include desmogleins 1 and 3, but there is a growing body of evidence identifying pemphigus cases resulting from antibodies against desmocollin and other nondesmoglein antigens. Involvement in neonates should be considered from a transplacental passage of maternal autoantibodies.

PEMPHIGUS VULGARIS

Definition and Epidemiology

Pemphigus vulgaris (PV) is an immune-mediated blistering disorder that results from autoantibodies against the desmosomal protein desmoglein 3. PV is extremely rare in children, usually presenting in persons between 40 and 60 years old.[33] The incidence of PV is higher in women (male:female;

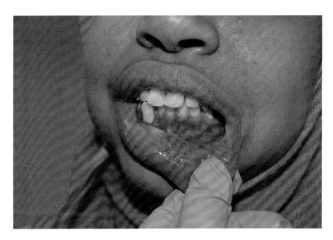

FIGURE 4-23. Pemphigus vulgaris with oral involvement. Erosions can be seen on the mucosal lip and the gingiva. (Photo courtesy of Sheilagh Maguiness, MD.)

1:1.1-2.25) and the Ashkenazi Jewish population. In a review of pediatric cases under 12 years of age, including 33 cases in 29 reports, mean age at onset was 8.3 years (range 1.5-12 years).

Etiology

Autoantibodies to desmoglein 3 are detected in the serum. Recently, *ST18*, a gene regulating apoptosis and inflammation, has been identified as an etiologic factor in populations predisposed to PV.[34]

Clinical Presentation

Classic presentation is characterized by flaccid vesicles or bullae, which may be associated with hemorrhagic crusting over the trunk, groin, extremities and can involve the oral mucosa. Mucosal involvement (97.0%) was more common than cutaneous involvement (84.8%). Oral mucosa was the most common site of mucosal involvement (93.9%), followed by genital (20.6%), ocular (11.8%), and nasal mucosa (2.9%)[35] (Figure 4-23).

Histologic Findings

Histologic sections from PV lesions demonstrate an intraepidermal blister with basal keratinocytes lining the floor of the blister cavity (the so-called "tombstone row") (Figure 4-24).[35] There is a marked suprabasal acantholysis of the epidermis with associated neutrophils[4] and/or eosinophils. Eosinophilic spongiosis can be a feature of early lesions. Follicular involvement helps distinguish PV from Hailey-Hailey disease.[36] DIF studies show IgG and C3 deposition between keratinocytes, conferring the characteristic "chicken-wire" pattern (Figure 4-25). IIF studies will demonstrate a deposition of the pemphigus autoantibody between keratinocytes in the epidermis.[37]

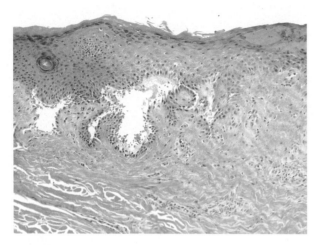

FIGURE 4-24. **Pemphigus Vulgaris.** Sections show an intraepidermal blister. Note the so-called tombstoning of basal layer keratinocytes along the floor of the blister.

Differential Diagnosis

The differential diagnosis of PV includes other acantholytic diseases such as Hailey-Hailey disease, Grover disease, and Darier disease. Clinical information and DIF/IIF studies are useful in distinguishing these disorders.

CAPSULE SUMMARY

PEMPHIGUS VULGARIS

PV is an intraepidermal blistering disease caused by autoantibodies to desmosomal proteins. It is extremely rare in children and presents as flaccid blisters and erosions on mucosal and cutaneous surfaces. Histologically, it is characterized by intraepidermal blister formation with splitting just above the basal layer keratinocytes. DIF and IIF studies demonstrate reactivity between keratinocytes (in a *chicken-wire* pattern).

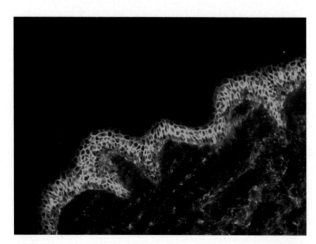

FIGURE 4-25. **Pemphigus.** Direct immunofluorescence studies show intracellular IgG in this photomicrograph. (Courtesy of Dr. Kim Yancey.)

PEMPHIGUS FOLIACEUS

Definition and Epidemiology

Pemphigus foliaceus (PF) is an immune-mediated blistering disorder that results from autoantibodies against the desmosomal protein desmoglein 1. It is rare in children, but can be seen as acquired disease or congenital disease from passive placental transfer of antibodies.

Etiology

PF is caused by autoantibodies against desmoglein 1. There is evidence that implicates nondesmoglein autoantibodies in the pathogenesis of PF.[38] Desmocollin-1 (Dsc1), which is expressed in the upper layers of the epidermis, also appears to play a role in the development of PF. Dsc1 knockout mice show a phenotype reminiscent of pemphigus foliaceus (PF).

Clinical Presentation

The disease may begin with crusted erosions on the scalp, which then spread to the trunk and extremities. They are characterized by a "cornflake"–like scale (Figure 4-26).

Fogo Selvagem: A form of PF known as fogo selvagem (FS) is endemic to Brazil. It shares clinical and histopathologic characteristics with PF, but has a unique epidemiologic history. Initial pockets of the disease were noted in Sao Paulo, but multiple other areas of incidence have been described as well, including neighboring countries such as Venezuela.[39] The occurrence of this disease diminishes as urbanization overcomes an area. Individuals exposed to hematophagous insects are more susceptible to developing the disease. It is postulated that insect bites release salivary proteins that initiate a pathogenic cross-reactive response in genetically prone individuals, leading to FS. Multiple human leukocyte antigen (HLA)-DRB1 alleles—*0404, *1402, *1406, or *0102—have been identified as risk factors.

Nonpathogenic anti-Dsg1 antibodies of the IgG1 subclass directed against the extracellular 5 domain of Dsg1 are detected in patients in the preclinical stage of the disease and also in healthy individuals living in endemic areas.

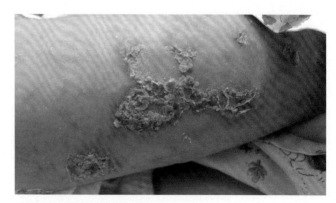

FIGURE 4-26. **Pemphigus foliaceus.** Erosions on the arm of a child with pemphigus foliaceus, with characteristic overlying "cornflake-like" scale.

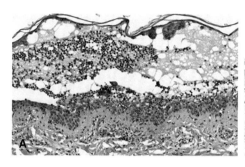
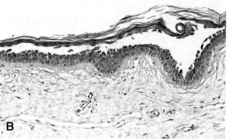

FIGURE 4-27. **Pemphigus foliaceus.** Suprabasilar acantholysis in the more superficial portions of the epidermis (A). The blister contains an abundance of neutrophils and eosinophils (B). Digital slides courtesy of Path Presenter.com.

Pathogenic anti-Dsg1 IgG4 autoantibodies that bind the pathogenic extracellular 1 and 2 domains of Dsg1 are found in patients with FS. Antigenic mimicry and epitope spreading are plausible hypotheses for these findings.[40]

Histologic Findings

As the autoantibody implicated in PF reacts with desmoglein 1 in the upper layers of the epidermis, the lesions of PF demonstrate acantholysis and blister formation just below the stratum corneum.[41] The blister cavities may contain neutrophils and acantholytic squamous cells (Figure 4-27).[41] DIF and IIF studies show similar findings to those seen in PV, with a deposition of IgG, C3, and the PF autoantibody between keratinocytes in the epidermis.

Differential Diagnosis

Clinically, impetigo and seborrheic dermatitis may initially be in the differential diagnosis. The histologic differential diagnosis may also include bullous impetigo, staphylococcal scalded skin syndrome, and IgA pemphigus. Ancillary DIF and IIF studies along with clinical features of the disorder and bacterial cultures aid in the distinction among these disorders.

CAPSULE SUMMARY

PEMPHIGUS FOLIACEUS

PF is rare in children. It is characterized by crusted erosions on the scalp which then spread to the trunk and extremities. Histologically, acantholysis and blister formation are seen in the upper layers of the epidermis just below the stratum corneum. DIF and IIF studies show reactivity between keratinocytes.

IGA PEMPHIGUS

Definition and Epidemiology

IgA pemphigus is a group of autoimmune blistering diseases characterized by vesiculopustular skin lesions, neutrophilic infiltrates, acantholysis, and bound and circulating IgA to cell surface keratinocyte antigens. Two main subtypes exist: subcorneal pustular dermatosis (SPD) and intraepidermal neutrophilic (IEN) types. IgA variants differ from normal variants as the immune-mediated attack is

through IgA rather than IgG, which is the case for PV, BP, and paraneoplastic pemphigus.

IgA pemphigus is rare in adults, and even more uncommon in children. A total of 6 pediatric cases of IgA pemphigus has been reported.[42]

Etiology

Desmocollin 1 has been implicated as the autoantigen for the SPD type.[43] Desmoglein 1 and 3 have been reported in the IEN variant.[43-47] Colonic involvement has been described, with desmoglein 2 implicated as a potential culprit autoantibody target.[42]

Clinical Presentation

Adults generally present with flaccid vesiculopustules on erythematous or normal skin, and involve the trunk, extremities, and skin folds of the axilla and groin. Impetigo-like lesions and vegetating plaques are also described in pediatric published cases. Mucosal involvement is not characteristic.[42]

Histologic Findings

The key histologic characteristic of IgA pemphigus lesions is the presence of neutrophils in the epidermis.[48] Figure 4-28 shows the characteristic histologic findings in IgA pemphigus.

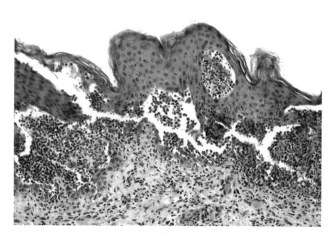

FIGURE 4-28. **IgA pemphigus.** This is the intraepidermal neutrophilic variant of IgA pemphigus (the other is the subcorneal pustular type). Note the partial preservation of the basilar layer.

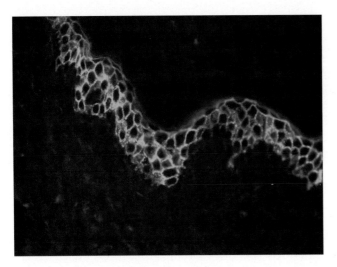

FIGURE 4-29. IgA pemphigus. Direct immunofluorescence shows intercellular IgA deposition within the epidermis.

Acantholysis may or may not be present in IgA pemphigus, and, if present, it is generally milder than in other forms of pemphigus.[48] In IEN-type IgA pemphigus, these findings occur in the mid-epidermis.[48] DIF studies demonstrate the presence of IgA deposition within the epidermis between keratinocytes (Figure 4-29). Occasionally, intercellular deposition of IgG or complement is also seen, although this is rare.[49] The IgA autoantibody titer in patients with IgA pemphigus is low, yielding limited sensitivity of IIF.[49]

Differential Diagnosis

The histologic differential diagnosis of IgA pemphigus includes other disorders with epidermal neutrophilic infiltrates. Intraepidermal neutrophils and blister formation should prompt a consideration of infectious processes, especially bullous impetigo. SPD and PF may also enter the histologic differential diagnosis, although clinical features may help distinguish these disorders. Other considerations may include pustular psoriasis, acute generalized exanthematous pustulosis, dermatitis herpetiformis, bullous pemphigoid, and bullous systemic lupus erythematosus. Stains for infectious organisms and correlation with microbial cultures are crucial. DIF studies aid in the distinction between different

---

CAPSULE SUMMARY

IGA PEMPHIGUS

IgA pemphigus is caused by an IgA autoantibody to skin structural proteins (desmocollin 1 or desmoglein 1 and 3). Clinically, it manifests as flacid vesiculopustules. Biopsies show neutrophils within the epidermis. Acantholysis may or may not be present. There are two subtypes, SPD (where neutrophils are seen beneath the stratum corneum) and IEN (where neutrophils are seen in the mid-epidermis).

---

types of pemphigus and other blistering disorders discussed in this chapter.

PARANEOPLASTIC PEMPHIGUS

Definition and Epidemiology

Paraneoplastic pemphigus (PNP) is an immune-mediated blistering disorder that develops in the setting of underlying malignancy. Skin and serum tests—as well as evaluation for malignancy—are needed for precise diagnosis. Autoantibody targets include desmogleins and plakins.

Approximately 10 publications exist describing PNP in the pediatric population.[50-57] It presents most commonly in adults, most often affecting those between 45 and 70 years of age, but may present in children, particularly when associated with Castleman disease. There is no known correlation between incidence of the disease and specific sex, race, or place of origin.[58]

Etiology

Interactions between the immune system and a concomitant neoplasm seem to be the basis of pathogenesis, with autoantibodies directed against both desmosomal and hemidesmosomal antigens. The vast majority of patients with PNP have autoantibodies to periplakins and envoplakins. PNP is characterized by the presence of autoantibodies against antigens such as desmoplakin I (250 kD), BP antigen I (230 kD), desmoplakin II (210 kD), envoplakin (210 kD), periplakin (190 kD), plectin (500 kD), and a 170 kD protein. Unlike other forms of pemphigus, PNP can affect other types of epithelia, such as gastrointestinal and respiratory tract. In the pediatric population, PNP is most often associated with Castleman disease. A transplacental passage of maternal autoantibodies has also been described.[57]

Clinical Presentation

Clinical presentation classically involves the mucous membranes, with severe, hemorrhagic stomatitis being the most consistent finding. Cutaneous involvement has been described as erythema multiforme-like, dermatitis, or blistering.

Histologic Findings

The majority of PNP lesions in children and adolescents include both lichenoid dermatitis and acantholysis, although some cases will demonstrate only one of the two patterns. Occasional keratinocyte necrosis is seen (Figure 4-30). DIF studies typically show an intercellular deposition of complement and IgG. IIF studies likewise show the deposition of IgG on cellular surfaces.[7] Common target antigens include 250 kDa (desmoplakin 1), 230 kDa (BP antigen), 210 kDa (envoplakin), and 190 kDa (periplakin) antigens. Positive indirect IF using murine (rat) bladder epithelium shows intercellular staining,

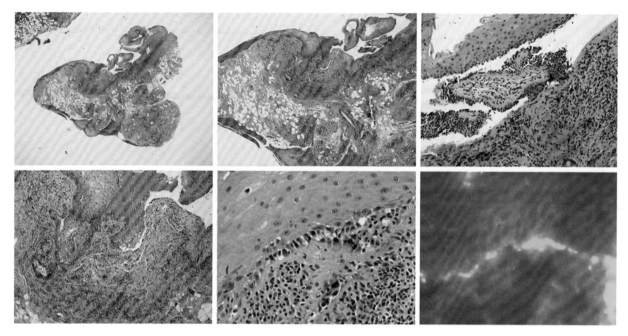

FIGURE 4-30. Paraneoplastic pemphigus. In paraneoplastic pemphigus, there is typically a combination of the suprabasilar acantholytic changes present in pemphigus vulgaris, and interface changes with keratinocyte necrosis. This biopsy is taken from the oral cavity of a patient with a history of myasthenia gravis. Direct immunofluorescence shows both intercellular IgG deposition in the epidermis and linear staining along the dermal-epidermal junction.

a characteristic but not particularly sensitive finding (negative in 25% of cases), and not entirely specific, as positive results have sometimes been found in both PV and PF.

Differential Diagnosis

The histologic differential diagnosis of PNP depends on whether lichenoid or acantholytic patterns are seen histologically. Other lichenoid/interface processes such as lichenoid drug eruption or lichen planus may be considered. Single-cell necrosis in the epidermis may also raise concern for erythema multiforme or graft versus host disease (GVHD). In cases where histologic sections show predominantly acantholysis, the other forms of pemphigus may enter the differential. Achieving the correct diagnosis requires correlation with the clinical features of the disorder as well as immunofluorescence studies.[58]

CAPSULE SUMMARY

PARANEOPLASTIC PEMPHIGUS

PNP is rare in children and is most often associated with Castleman disease. Clinically, patients present with severe, erosive, hemorrhagic mucositis with variable cutaneous involvement. The histologic sections of lesions generally show acantholysis and lichenoid inflammation, although either may be present in isolation. DIF studies show the deposition of IgG and complement between keratinocytes in the epidermis.

BULLOUS PEMPHIGOID

Definition and Epidemiology

BP is the most common immune-mediated acquired blistering disorder. It is characterized characterized by tense bullae on the skin. In infants, acral surfaces are most often involved. In older children and adults, the presentation may be more generalized. Skin and serum tests are required for precise diagnosis. BP is most often a disease of the elderly, but of the immune-mediated blistering disorders that can present in children, BP is the most common.

Etiology

BP is due to autoantibodies to BP230 (BP antigen 1 or BPAg1), and/or BP180 (BPAg2), which are found along the basement membrane. BP180 is thought to be the direct antibody target because of its location along the basement membrane, and antibodies to BP230 may be produced secondarily. One case of antilaminin 332 mucous membrane pemphigoid has been described in the literature following diptheria tetanus vaccination.[59]

BP can also be seen in other blistering disorders and GVHD. This is thought to be attributed to increased antigen presentation and "secondary sensitization" to bystander antibodies. For example, primary injury to the skin may expose previously hidden antigens to the immune system leading to secondary sensitization and autoimmune disease. Affected patients may also have pemphigus antibodies present. Occasionally, patients with EB can develop BP.

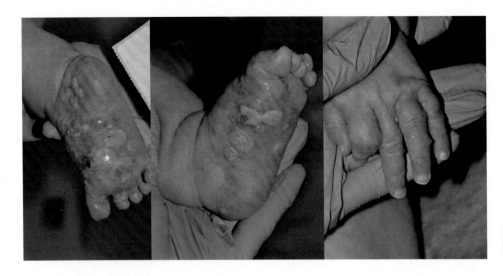

FIGURE 4-31. Infantile bullous pemphigoid. There are tense bullae on the feet, soon after vaccination. (Courtesy of Kristen Hook, MD.)

Finally, both BP and EBA have both been associated with IPEX (*Immune Dysregulation, Polyendocrinopathy, Enteropathy, X-linked*) syndrome because of abnormalities in Treg cells.[60,61]

Clinical Presentation

BP in childhood most often presents as acral, tense, well-formed bullae (Figure 4-31). Generalized BP is also characterized by tense, well-formed bullae that may occur on any cutaneous surface. Erosions, pruritus, and urticaria may be associated findings (Figures 4-32 and 4-33). It presents most often following vaccination, but is not considered a contraindication to further vaccination.[59,62] It has also been described following viral infections. Most children respond well to treatment (topical or systemic) and their disease enters remission. Vaccination or illness may also uncover a genetic predisposition to the autoimmune disorder, which may lead to a longer, more chronic course.

Histologic Findings

The histologic features of BP in children are identical to those seen in the adult population.[63] Biopsies classically demonstrate subepidermal blister formation containing numerous eosinophils (Figure 4-34). In rare cases, neutrophils may predominate, causing confusion with DH.[63] DIF studies demonstrate a linear deposition of IgG and C3 along the basement membrane.[60] IIF studies likewise demonstrate an antibasement membrane IgG antibody.[63]

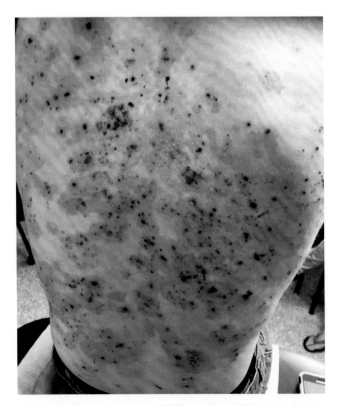

FIGURE 4-32. Bullous pemphigoid with associated urticaria. This patient also had epitope spreading with positive pemphigus autoantibodies. (Courtesy of Kristen Hook, MD.)

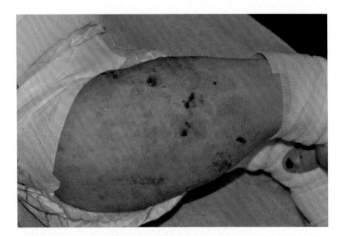

FIGURE 4-33. Bullous pemphigoid (BP). Tense blisters of BP in a patient with epidermolysis bullosa. (Courtesy of Kristen Hook, MD.)

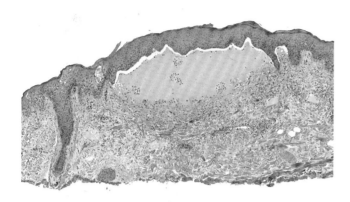

FIGURE 4-34. **Bullous pemphigoid.** Scanning power shows a subepidermal blister containing eosinophils.

Differential Diagnosis

The differential diagnosis of BP includes DH, especially in cases where neutrophils predominate. Other considerations include linear IgA disease, EBA, and bullous systemic lupus erythematosus (BSLE). IIF, DIF, and western blot studies are useful in distinguishing among these disorders. IHC for type IV collagen is also useful in distinguishing BP from these disorders and is particularly beneficial as it can be performed on formalin-fixed paraffin-embedded tissue; type IV collagen lines the floor of the blister in BP and the roof of the blister in EBA and BSLE.[64]

CAPSULE SUMMARY

BULLOUS PEMPHIGOID

BP in children usually presents as tense, well-formed blisters on acral surfaces. The classic histologic feature is the presence of an eosinophil-rich subepidermal blister. DIF studies demonstrate linear IgG deposition along the basement membrane, and IHC for type IV collagen demonstrates reactivity along the floor of the blister (in contrast to EBA and BSLE, where it lines the roof of the blister).

CICATRICIAL PEMPHIGOID

Definition and Epidemiology

CP is a group of immune-mediated blistering disorders that fall under the larger designation of mucous membrane pemphigoid. The cicatricial variants produce scarring that can result in blindness and laryngeal stenosis. CP is rare in children.

Less than 20 cases of pediatric CP have been published in the literature.[65-68]

Clinical Presentation

Unlike BP in children, CP has a more chronic course and can lead to adhesions (synechia) of the nasal mucosa and conjunctiva, blindness, and laryngeal stenosis. CP with solely mucous membrane involvement has been described, without cutaneous lesions.[68]

Histologic Findings

Blister formation occurs in the lamina lucida. Histologic sections from lesions demonstrate separation between the stratified squamous epithelium and the underlying submucosa. The submucosa often demonstrates a mixed inflammatory infiltrate (Figure 4-35). CP features linear deposits of immunoglobulin and complement (especially C3). Older lesions demonstrate scar formation. Three forms have been described: 1) a variant seemingly identical to adult pemphigoid, that has linear deposits of IgG and C3 above the lamina densa (demonstrable with salt-splitting techniques). 2) Another form, seemingly indistinguishable from linear IgA disease (chronic bullous disease of childhood [CBDC]), shows linear IgA as the predominant reactant along the basement membrane zone. 3) A variant resembling a mucous membrane variety of EBA, shows linear IgG or C3 deposition below the lamina densa. IIF may reveal antibodies to several target antigens in the basement membrane zone.

Differential Diagnosis

The diagnosis is largely based on clinical features and the distribution of lesions. In some cases, CP may be indistinguishable from BP.

CAPSULE SUMMARY

CICATRICIAL PEMPHIGOID

CP is very rare in children and presents with a scarring of mucous membranes and conjunctiva. The separation occurs in the lamida lucida, between the mucosa and submucosa, resulting in histologic sections that demonstrate a submucosal split. A linear deposition of complement is characteristic.

DERMATITIS HERPETIFORMIS

Definition and Epidemiology

DH is an extremely pruritic blistering disorder that classically affects the extensor elbows, knees, and buttocks. It is regarded as the cutaneous representation of celiac disease

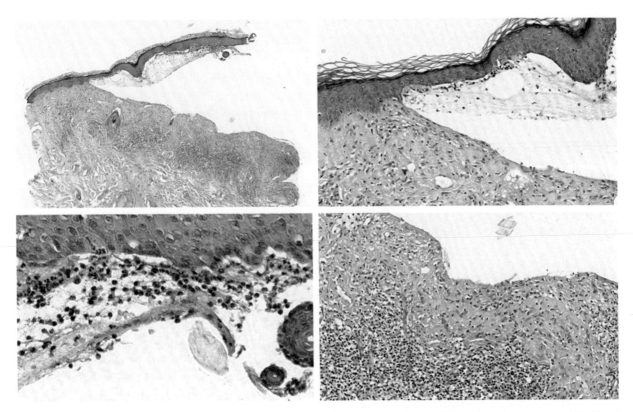

FIGURE 4-35. Cicatricial pemphigoid. There is a subepidermal blister containing neutrophils and scattered eosinophils. The dermis shows fibrosis and a lichenoid lymphoplasmacytic infiltrate. Digital slides courtesy of Path Presenter.com.

or gluten sensitivity. Although it is most commonly a disease of adults, children may be affected. Studies from the United States and Europe estimate that the incidence of celiac disease is 3 to 13 cases per 1000, with a higher prevalence among first-degree relatives of patients with CD.[69-71]

Etiology

Most experts feel DH represents the cutaneous representation of celiac disease, or gluten sensitivity. Both diseases are correlated with HLADR3 and DQw2. The ingestion of gluten in genetically susceptible individuals leads to the production of antibodies against gut-specific tissue transglutaminase. Cross-reactivity leads to the production of serum IgA antitransglutaminase 3 antibodies that are specific to DH and correlate with disease activity.

Clinical Presentation

Intensely pruritic, well-formed vesicles on the extensor elbows and buttocks with associated excoriation are the quintessential clinical finding for DH. Lesions are characteristically grouped with symmetric distribution. Vesicles are notably monomorphic, small (<0.5 cm), and rupture easily, leaving mostly erythematous, excoriated papules and plaques.

Histologic Findings

The characteristic histologic finding in DH is the presence of neutrophil microabscesses at the tips of the dermal papillae (Figure 4-36). However, identifying microabscesses sometimes requires a careful examination of multiple tissue levels. Leukocytoclasis is also often a feature

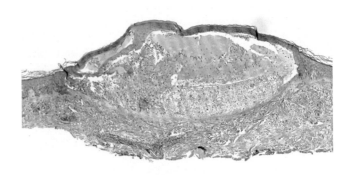

FIGURE 4-36. Dermatitis herpetiformis. Low-power view showing a subepidermal blister.

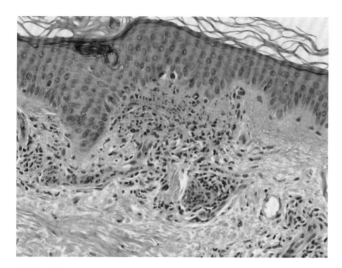

FIGURE 4-37. **Dermatitis herpetiformis.** High-power view showing an infiltrate composed predominantly of neutrophils. Note that the collection of neutrophils centers around vessels and the dermal papillae.

(Figure 4-37).[72] Biopsies may show clefting between the papillary dermal changes and the overlying epidermis and fibrin deposition above the collections of neutrophils in the papillary dermis.[72] DIF studies demonstrate granular IgA deposition in the papillary dermis (Figure 4-38).

Differential Diagnosis

A diagnosis of DH is based on the clinical presentation, histopathology, and immunofluorescence findings, as well as serologic testing and treatment response. The differential diagnosis includes other blistering disorders discussed in this chapter—in particular, BSLE and linear IgA disease. Some cases of BP may show a predominance of neutrophils rather

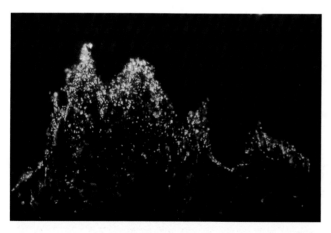

FIGURE 4-38. **Dermatitis herpetiformis direct immunofluorescence** Granular IgA deposits are seen here at the dermal-epidermal junction. Reprinted with permission from Barnadas MA. Dermatitis herpetiformis: A review of direct immunofluorescence findings. *Am J Dermatopathol.* 2016;38(4):283-288. doi:10.1097/DAD.0000000000000420.

than eosinophils, which may cause confusion with DH. Correlation with ancillary studies (especially IF) and the clinical presentation help differentiate among these disorders.

CAPSULE SUMMARY

DERMATITIS HERPETIFORMIS

DH is generally considered to be a cutaneous manifestation of celiac disease. Intensely pruritic, well-formed vesicles on the extensor elbows, buttocks with associated excoriation are the quintessential clinical finding. The characteristic histologic finding is the presence of neutrophil microabscesses at the tips of the dermal papillae. However, this finding is not entirely specific and should prompt a consideration of other etiologies, especially infectious disorders. DIF studies demonstrate a granular deposition of IgA in the papillary dermis.

LINEAR IGA BULLOUS DERMATOSIS OF CHILDHOOD

Definition and Epidemiology

Linear IgA bullous dermatosis of childhood is a rare acquired autoimmune blistering disorder for which there are two variants (adult and childhood forms).[73] In children, this disorder is also referred to as chronic bullous dermatosis of childhood (CBDC).

CBDC usually presents in preschool years (before age 5) and remits by puberty. The eruption can persist for around 5 years.[74] An incidence ranging between 0.2 and 1.0 cases in 1 million cases per year was estimated in different regions and seems to be higher in developing countries.[75]

Etiology

Linear IgA bullous dermatosis (LABD) has been triggered by medications and viruses in children (amoxicillin-clavulanic acid, vancomycin, and NSAIDS are best described in the literature[76-79]). Most cases are idiopathic. Linear IgA deposition is seen along the basement membrane, with associated IgM, IgG, and C3 in some cases, with IgA showing the strongest fluorescence staining pattern. LABD-causing antibodies target a cleavage product of the extracellular domain of BP180 (LABD-97 and LAD-1).[80,81]

Clinical Presentation

Bullae form in characteristic annular or rosette-like plaques with "string of pearls" well-formed vesicles/bullae surrounding central crust (Figure 4-39). Blisters may occur on any area of the body but may more prominently involve the lower abdomen, medial thighs, genitalia, and buttocks. Mucosal involvement is noted in half of the patients. Dapsone is the treatment of choice, but occasionally, steroids may be indicated. If the disease is drug-induced, withdrawal of

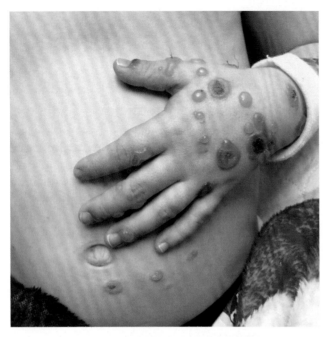

FIGURE 4-39. **Chronic bullous disease of childhood**. Tense annular bullae in a "string of pearls distribution". (Courtesy of Kristen Hook, MD.)

the offending agent is usually successful. LABD has been associated with ulcerative colitis in the adult population.[82]

Histologic Findings

The biopsies of linear IgA lesions show subepidermal blister formation. The blister often contains collections of neutrophils or rarely, eosinophils. As the name of the disorder implies, DIF studies demonstrate linear IgA deposition along the basement membrane (Figure 4-40).[77]

Differential Diagnosis

Subepidermal blister formation with associated neutrophils most often raises the differential consideration of DH. Histologically, linear IgA disease may also be indistinguishable from BP, as both disorders may have an associated neutrophilic or eosinophilic infiltrate. Clinical distinction between BP and linear IgA is also sometimes difficult. Bullous lupus may also enter the histologic differential diagnosis. DIF and IIF studies as well as careful correlation with clinical history and response to treatment are critical.

CAPSULE SUMMARY

LINEAR IGA BULLOUS DERMATOSIS IN CHILDHOOD

CBD Linear IgA bullous dermatosis in childhood (also known as chronic bullous disease of childhood [CBDC]) usually present in preschool years and remits by puberty. Bullae may occur on any area of the body and form in characteristic annular or rosette-like plaques. The biopsies of linear IgA lesions show subepidermal blister formation. The blister often contains collections of neutrophils or, rarely, eosinophils. DIF studies show a linear deposition of IgA along the basement membrane.

BULLOUS SYSTEMIC LUPUS ERYTHEMATOSUS

Definition and Epidemiology

Bullous lupus is a vesiculopustular dermatosis that is extremely rare in children. The diagnosis is based on American College of Rheumatology criteria including: (1) fulfillment of criteria for systemic lupus erythematosus, (2) vesicles and bullae arising upon but not limited to sun-exposed skin,

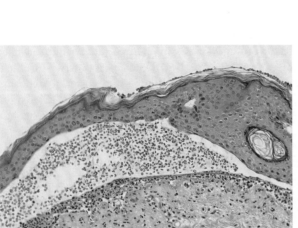

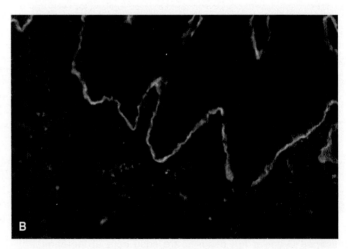

FIGURE 4-40. **Linear IgA disease.** A, Neutrophils appear to "line up" along the basement membrane zone in confluent fashion, although papillary neutrophilic microabscesses can be identified in other areas. This results in the formation of a subepidermal bulla. (Photomicrograph by Jessica Kwock, MD, University of Virginia.) B, Direct immunofluorescence shows a linear deposition of IgA along the dermal-epidermal junction.

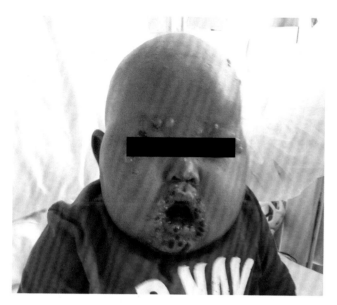

FIGURE 4-41. **Bullous lupus erythematosus**. Tense bullae present on the face. (Courtesy of Kristen Hook, MD.)

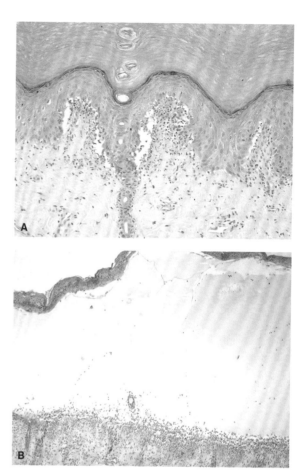

(3) histopathology showing a subepidermal blister with a neutrophilic infiltrate, (4) direct immunofluorescence that revealing IgG or IgM and often IgA at the BMZ, and (5) evidence of antibodies to type VII collagen.[83]

BSLE commonly presents in the second to third decades and most often affects young women, especially African Americans. It rarely affects children.

Etiology

Similar to EBA, patients with bullous lupus demonstrate antibodies directed against collagen VII. Many medications have been linked to bullous lupus, including methimazole.[84]

Clinical Presentation

Clinical exam demonstrates well-formed fluid-filled vesicles and bullae most predominantly on sun-exposed surfaces of the scalp, face, and neck (Figure 4-41). Other areas of the body may be involved as well, including oral mucosa. Bullous lupus may be the presenting sign of SLE, or may develop in a patient with known SLE.

Histologic Findings

The histologic features of BSLE lesions show significant overlap with those of DH. Bullous lupus lesions show a subepidermal blister with associated neutrophils or neutrophil microabscesses (Figure 4-42A). The lesions may also demonstrate associated fibrin deposition and karyorrhectic debris (Figure 4-42B).[85,86] By DIF, the lesions demonstrate a deposition of immunoglobulins and complement along the basement membrane. Cases may either show linear (more common) or granular deposition of multiple immunoreactants (the so-called lupus band).[85]

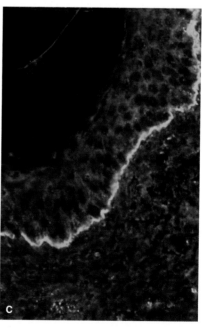

FIGURE 4-42. **Bullous lupus erythematosus.** A, An acral lesion shows papillary neutrophilic microabscesses and early subepidermal clefting. B, This is a fully developed subepidermal bulla. Note the numerous neutrophils accumulated along the blister base. C, Direct immunofluorescence shows linear IgG staining along the dermal-epidermal junction. With saline splitting methods, the deposits can be shown to occur below the lamina densa of the basement membrane zone.

Differential Diagnosis

The main histologic differential diagnosis for BSLE includes EBA and DH. In contrast to EBA, the lesions of BSLE generally do not show scarring. DH and BSLE may be histologically indistinguishable, and correlation with clinical and IF studies is necessary.

CAPSULE SUMMARY

BULLOUS SYSTEMIC LUPUS ERYTHEMATOSUS

BSLE is very rare in children. It may be seen as a presenting sign of SLE or occur in patients with known SLE. Clinical exam demonstrates well-formed fluid-filled vesicles and bullae most predominantly on sun-exposed surfaces of the scalp, face, and neck. Histologically, lesions show a subepidermal blister with associated neutrophils or neutrophil microabscesses. DIF shows deposition of multiple immunoglobulins and complement along the basement membrane.

ACUTE GENERALIZED EXANTHEMATOUS PUSTULOSIS

Definition and Epidemiology

Acute generalized exanthematous pustulosis (AGEP) is a severe cutaneous drug hypersensitivity reaction occurring in children and adults. The appearance is rapid following drug exposure, usually within 1 week. The incidence is estimated at 1 to 5 cases per million per year in the general population.[87] It is rare in children, but has been observed following medication administration and viral infection.

Etiology

AGEP is most often caused by medications in the adult population. In children, it is typically associated with viral etiologies such as Parvovirus, Coxsackie virus, and cytomegalovirus, although bacterial infections (*Chlamydia pneumoniae* and *Mycoplasma pneumoniae*) and medications have also been implicated. Eruption after exposure to aminopenicillins, cefixime, clindamycin, paracetamol, bufexamac, cytarabine, vancomycin, and possibly labetalol has been documented in children.[88-91]

Clinical Presentation

The reaction presents within 1 week of drug exposure. Erythema or erythroderma may precede the formation of blistering, and may be more prominent in skin folds. Diffuse, monomorphic, nonfollicular, subepidermal, sterile pustules and vesicles form shortly thereafter, and may involve

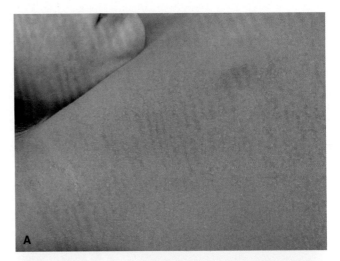

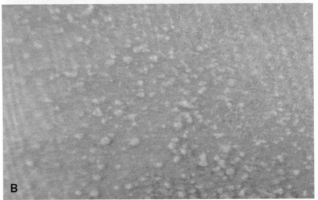

FIGURE 4-43. A, **Acute generalized exanthematous pustulosis.** Monomorphic superficial vesiculopustules. (Photo courtesy of Sheilagh Maguiness, MD.) B, Close-up clinical photograph of AGEP lesions (Photo courtesy of Sheilagh Maguiness, MD.)

scalp, ears, face, trunk, and extremities (Figure 4-43A and B). Associated signs may include fever, a mild nonerosive enanthem, and peripheral leukocytosis. Overlapping cutaneous exanthems are possible (ie, AGEP and drug reaction with eosinophilia and systemic symptoms [DRESS], or AGEP and erythema multiforme). Biopsy is necessary to confirm diagnosis in these cases. AGEP is self-limited and will resolve with diffuse desquamation and no scarring within 2 weeks. For severe cases, topical or oral corticosteroids may be indicated in addition to withdrawal of the offending drug in all cases.[92]

Histologic Findings

Histologic sections from AGEP lesions demonstrate subcorneal or intraepidermal pustules with a mild degree of spongiform pustulation, scattered apoptotic keratinocytes, papillary dermal edema, changes suggestive of a small vessel vasculitis, and a dermal infiltrate containing eosinophils (Figure 4-44).[93] Direct immunofluorescence findings are typically negative or nonspecific.

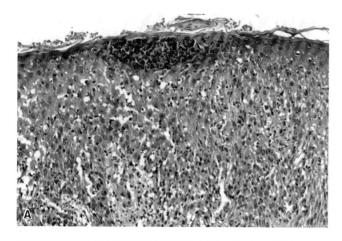

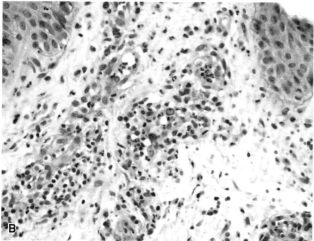

FIGURE 4-44. **Acute generalized exanthematous pustulosis.** A, A small neutrophilic pustule can be seen near the epidermal surface. In this example, there is also a considerable exocytosis of neutrophils along with keratinocyte apoptosis. B, Neutrophils are identified in and around the walls of superficial dermal vessels. These changes can sometimes be sufficiently developed to suggest leukocytoclastic vasculitis.

Differential Diagnosis

The histologic differential diagnosis of AGEP lesions importantly includes impetigo (and other infectious disorders), infantile acropustulosis, PF, DH, pustular psoriasis, and Sneddon-Wilkinson disease (SPD).[94] Pustular psoriasis and SPD show significant overlap with AGEP, and may require clinical correlation to differentiate. The differentiation of AGEP from infectious disorders is critical and requires correlation with special stains and cultures for microorganisms. DIF studies are useful in the differentiation between AGEP, PF, and DH. As always, clinical history, especially a history of beginning a new medication preceding the eruption (supporting AGEP), is useful in distinguishing between these disorders.

CAPSULE SUMMARY

ACUTE GENERALIZED EXANTHEMATOUS PUSTULOSIS

AGEP is a severe cutaneous reaction to drugs or infection. The reaction usually presents within 1 week of drug exposure. Diffuse monomorphic nonfollicular subepidermal sterile pustules and vesicles may involve scalp, ears, face, trunk, and extremities. Histologic sections from AGEP lesions demonstrate a subcorneal separation containing neutrophils.

INFANTILE ACROPUSTULOSIS

Definition and Epidemiology

Infantile acropustulosis is a benign, recurrent vesiculopustular eruption occurring most often on the hands and feet of infants. The reaction is recurrent but self-limited and tends to resolve in 1 to 2 years. Scabies infection often precedes this eruption. The exact prevalence is unknown, but it may be more prevalent in international adoptees.[95] Onset is usually between birth and age 2.

Etiology

Although the exact etiology of infantile acropustulosis is not known, some experts feel that it may represent a post-scabetic hypersensitivity reaction.[96]

Clinical Presentation

Infantile acropustulosis is characterized by recurrent crops of acral, well-formed vesicles and bullae that are extremely pruritic and recur every few weeks to months. These most often affect the palms and soles, notably the interdigital spaces and outer edges of the lateral foot and heel (Figure 4-45).

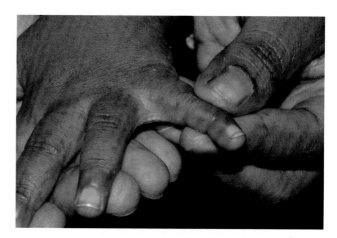

FIGURE 4-45. **Infantile acropustulosis.** Vesiculopustules in interdigital spaces. (Courtesy of Kristen Hook, MD.)

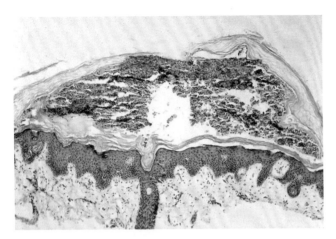

FIGURE 4-46. **Infantile acropustulosis.** A neutrophilic pustule is seen within the stratum corneum in this example.

Treatment can shorten the duration of each eruption and increase the time frame between eruptions. Usually, the eruption remits after a period of months to years.

Histologic Findings

Similar to AGEP, the biopsies of infantile acropustulosis demonstrate collections of subcorneal neutrophils (Figure 4-46). Cases with numerous eosinophils have also been described, but the exact classification of cases with eosinophils is controversial.[97]

Differential Diagnosis

The differential diagnosis importantly includes infectious etiologies (impetigo, herpes simplex infection, dermatophytes, and Candida). Children are often misdiagnosed with scabies infections because of the predominance of acral blistering. Appropriate viral, fungal, and bacterial stains should be performed in all biopsies demonstrating epidermal collections of neutrophils. Pustular psoriasis and AGEP may also be included in the histopathologic differential diagnosis.

CAPSULE SUMMARY

INFANTILE ACROPUSTULOSIS

Infantile acropustulosis is a benign, recurrent vesiculopustular eruption occurring most often on the hands and feet of young children. The reaction is self-limited and tends to resolve in 1 to 2 years. The disease is often preceded by scabies infection. Biopsies demonstrate collections of subcorneal neutrophils.

STAPHYLOCOCCAL *SCALDED SKIN* SYNDROME AND BULLOUS IMPETIGO

Definition and Epidemiology

Staphylococcal *scalded skin* syndrome (SSSS) and bullous impetigo are toxin-mediated blistering diseases caused by exfoliative toxins released by specific strains of *Staphylococcus aureus*. They can occur in any age group, although they are more common in infants and young children. In adults, SSSS is more common in those with impaired renal status.[98]

In a recent review of the Nationwide Inpatient Sample 2008-2012 (which includes a 20% sample of US hospitalizations and 589 cases of SSSS), the mean annual incidence of SSSS was 7.67 (range 1.83-11.88) per million US children, with 45.1 cases per million US infants of age less than 2 years. It was significantly associated with female sex, younger age, black race/ethnicity, and summer season.[99]

Etiology

Bullous impetigo is caused by localized infection with *S. aureus*. About 5% of *S. aureus* strains produce exfoliative toxin A or B (ETA/ETB), that cleave desmoglein 1 and induce epidermal blistering. ETA is linked more often with SSSS in the United States and Europe.[100]

SSSS results from a systemic distribution of ETA or ETB and are produced from a distant source such as the nares, throat, umbilicus, circumcision site, or a pustule.[101]

Clinical Presentation

Bullous impetigo most often presents with thin, well-formed or already ruptured bullae that may leave a collarette of desquamated skin or postinflammatory hyperpigmentation. It can be solitary or multiple, and organisms may be cultured from lesional skin.

SSSS is characterized by widespread, thin desquamation often preceded by erythroderma. Erythema may be more prominent in the skin fold areas: neck, axillae, inguinal folds. Perioral fissuring is also a common clinical finding (Figures 4-47 and 4-48) but notably without

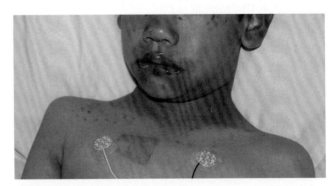

FIGURE 4-47. **Staphylococcal scalded skin syndrome.** Erythema in skin folds with perioral fissuring. Note the denuded skin at the site of adhesive lead.

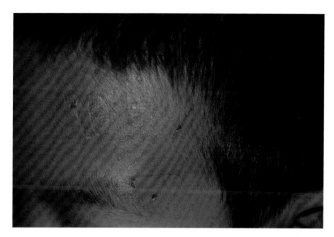

FIGURE 4-48. **Staphylococcal scalded skin syndrome.** Superficial desquamation seen with Nikolsky's sign.

mucosal involvement. Association with other infections is common, including upper respiratory infection and skin infection.[99] If the nidus of infection can be identified, culture may be helpful. However, unlike bullous impetigo, a culture of lesional skin will not yield organisms. Blood cultures may be positive. Associated fevers and leukocytosis are common.

Histologic Findings

Biopsies from SSSS and bullous impetigo lesions characteristically demonstrate a cleft in the granular cell layer of the epidermis (Figure 4-49). Adjacent acantholysis may be seen. There is usually only a sparse-associated inflammatory infiltrate.[102] Gram stain is typically negative in SSSS, but may show cocci in bullous impetigo.

Differential Diagnosis

Although uncommon in children, the most important entity in the clinical differential diagnosis of SSSS is toxic epidermal necrolysis (TEN). TEN, however, demonstrates a subepidermal blister, whereas SSSS demonstrates splitting of the epidermis through the granular layer. TEN also generally shows a lymphocytic infiltrate, whereas the inflammatory infiltrate in SSSS is usually sparse.[102]

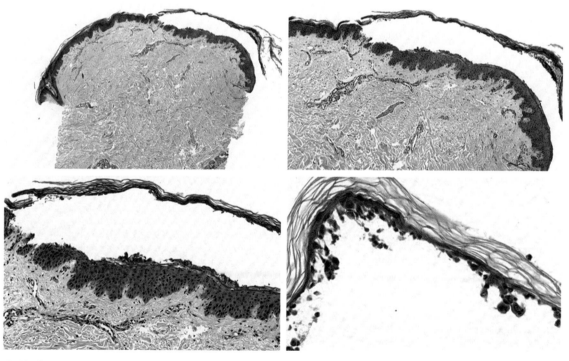

FIGURE 4-49. **Staphylococcal scalded skin syndrome (SSSS).** In this biopsy of SSSS, there is a cleft in the granular cell layer of the epidermis. Adjacent acantholysis is also seen. There is only a sparse-associated inflammatory infiltrate. Digital slide courtesy of Path Presenter.

CAPSULE SUMMARY

STAPHYLOCOCCAL *SCALDED SKIN* SYNDROME AND BULLOUS IMPETIGO

SSSS and bullous impetigo are toxin-mediated blistering diseases caused by exfoliative toxins (ETA/ETB) released by specific strains of staph aureus. SSSS is characterized by widespread thin desquamation often preceded by erythroderma, while bullous impetigo produces only localized flaccid bullae or erosions. Biopsies characteristically demonstrate a cleft in the granular cell layer of the epidermis without significant associated inflammation.

REFERENCES

1. Fine JD, Bruckner-Tuderman L, Eady RA, et al. Inherited epidermolysis bullosa: Updated recommendations on diagnosis and classification. *J Am Acad Dermatol.* 2014;70(6):1103-1126. doi:10.1016/j.jaad.2014.01.903.
2. Fine JD, Eady RA, Bauer EA, et al. The classification of inherited epidermolysis bullosa (EB): report of the third international consensus meeting on diagnosis and classification of EB. *J Am Acad Dermatol.* 2008;58(6):931-950. doi:10.1016/j.jaad.2008.02.004.
3. Fine JD. Epidemiology of inherited epidermolysis bullosa based on incidence and prevalence estimates from the national epidermolysis bullosa registry. *JAMA Dermatol.* 2016;152(11):1231-1238. doi:10.1001/jamadermatol.2016.2473.
4. Bolling MC, Lemmink HH, Jansen GH, Jonkman MF. Mutations in *KRT5* and *KRT14* cause epidermolysis bullosa simplex in 75% of the patients. *Br J Dermatol.* 2011;164(3):637-644. doi:10.1111/j.1365-2133.2010.10146.x.
5. Intong LR, Murrell DF. Inherited epidermolysis bullosa: New diagnostic criteria and classification. *Clin Dermatol.* 2012;30(1):70-77. doi:10.1016/j.clindermatol.2011.03.012.
6. Pearson RW. Histopathologic and ultrastructural findings in certain genodermatoses. *Clin Dermatol.* 1985;3(1):143-174.
7. Pearson RW. Studies on the pathogenesis of epidermolysis bullosa. *J Invest Dermatol.* 1962;39:551-575. doi:10.1038/jid.1962.156.
8. Prieto VG, McNutt NS. Immunohistochemical detection of keratin with the monoclonal antibody MNF116 is useful in the diagnosis of epidermolysis bullosa simplex. *J Cutan Pathol.* 1994;21(2):118-122.
9. Fine JD. Epidermolysis bullosa: clinical aspects, pathology, and recent advances in research *Int J Dermatol.* 1986;25(3):143-157.
10. Cianfarani F, Zambruno G, Castiglia D, Odorisio T. Pathomechanisms of altered wound healing in recessive dystrophic epidermolysis bullosa. *Am J Pathol.* 2017;187(7):1445-1453. doi:10.1016/j.ajpath.2017.03.003.
11. Fine JD, Johnson LB, Weiner M, Li KP, Suchindran C. Epidermolysis bullosa and the risk of life-threatening cancers: the national EB registry experience, 1986-2006. *J Am Acad Dermatol.* 2009;60(2):203-211. doi:10.1016/j.jaad.2008.09.035.
12. Mittapalli VR, Madl J, Loffek S, et al. Injury-driven stiffening of the dermis expedites skin carcinoma progression. *Cancer Res.* 2016;76(4):940-951. doi:10.1158/0008-5472.CAN-15-1348.
13. Akasaka E, Nakano H, Takagi Y, Toyomaki Y, Sawamura D. Multiple milia as an isolated skin manifestation of dominant dystrophic epidermolysis bullosa: evidence of phenotypic variability. *Pediatr Dermatol.* 2017;34(2):e106-e108. doi:10.1111/pde.13047.
14. Youssefian L, Vahidnezhad H, Barzegar M, et al. The Kindler syndrome: a spectrum of FERMT1 mutations in Iranian families. *J Invest Dermatol.* 2015;135(5):1447-1450.
15. Youssefian, L, Vahidnezhad, H, Uitto, J. Kindler Syndrome (Congenital Bullous Poikiloderma). *GeneReviews.* https://www.ncbi.nlm.nih.gov/books/NBK349072/. Updated December 1, 2016. Accessed June 21, 2018.
16. Ashton GH. Kindler syndrome. *Clin Exp Dermatol.* 2004;29(2):116-121. doi: 1465 [pii].
17. Mendes L, Nogueira L, Vilasboas V, Talhari C, Talhari S, Santos M. Kindler syndrome: Report of two cases *An Bras Dermatol.* 2012;87(5):779-781. doi:10.1111/j.1365-2230.2004.01465.x.
18. Lai-Cheong JE, McGrath JA. Kindler syndrome. *Dermatol Clin.* 2010;28(1):119-124. doi:10.1016/j.det.2009.10.013.
19. Ramanujam VM, Anderson KE. Porphyria diagnostics—Part 1: a brief overview of the porphyrias. *Curr Protoc Hum Genet.* 2015;86:17.20.1-17.20.26.
20. Bloomer JR, Wang Y, Singhal A, Risheg H. Biochemical abnormality in erythropoietic protoporphyria: cause and consequences. *J Pediatr Gastroenterol Nutr.* 2006;43(Suppl 1):S36-S40.
21. Bonkovsky HL, Maddukuri VC, Yazici C, et al. Acute porphyrias in the USA: features of 108 subjects from porphyrias consortium. *Am J Med.* 2014;127(12):1233-1241. doi:10.1016/j.amjmed.2014.06.036.
22. Epstein JH, Tuffanelli DL, Epstein WL. Cutaneous changes in the porphyrias. A microscopic study. *Arch Dermatol.* 1973;107(5):689-698.
23. Cormane RH, Szabo E, Hoo TT. Histopathology of the skin in acquired and hereditary porphyria cutanea tarda. *Br J Dermatol.* 1971;85(6):531-539.
24. Wolff K, Honigsmann H, Rauschmeier W, Schuler G, Pechlaner R. Microscopic and fine structural aspects of porphyrias. *Acta Derm Venereol Suppl (Stockh).* 1982;100:17-28.
25. Dabski C, Beutner EH. Studies of laminin and type IV collagen in blisters of porphyria cutanea tarda and drug-induced pseudoporphyria. *J Am Acad Dermatol.* 1991;25(1 Pt 1):28-32.
26. Maynard B, Peters MS. Histologic and immunofluorescence study of cutaneous porphyrias. *J Cutan Pathol.* 1992;19(1):40-47.
27. Weston WL, Morelli JG, Huff JC. Misdiagnosis, treatments, and outcomes in the immunobullous diseases in children. *Pediatr Dermatol.* 1997;14:264-272.
28. Gammon WR, Briggaman RA, Woodley DT, Heald PW, Wheeler CE Jr. Epidermolysis bullosa acquisita—a pemphigoid-like disease. *J Am Acad Dermatol.* 1984;11(5 Pt 1):820-832.
29. Nieboer C, Boorsma DM, Woerdeman MJ, Kalsbeek GL. Epidermolysis bullosa acquisita. immunofluorescence, electron microscopic and immunoelectron microscopic studies in four patients. *Br J Dermatol.* 1980;102(4):383-392.
30. Yaoita H, Briggaman RA, Lawley TJ, Provost TT, Katz SI. Epidermolysis bullosa acquisita: ultrastructural and immunological studies. *J Invest Dermatol.* 1981;76(4):288-292. doi:10.1111/1523-1747.ep12526124.
31. Ghohestani RF, Nicolas JF, Rousselle P, Claudy AL. Diagnostic value of indirect immunofluorescence on sodium chloride-split skin in differential diagnosis of subepidermal autoimmune bullous dermatoses *Arch Dermatol.* 1997;133(9):1102-1107.
32. Gupta VK, Kelbel TE, Nguyen D et al. A globally available internet-based patient survey of pemphigus vulgaris: epidemiology and disease characteristics. *Dermatol Clin.* 2011;29:393-404.
33. Chen IH, Mu SC, Tsai D, Chou YY, Wang LF, Wang LJ. Oral ulcers as an initial presentation of juvenile pemphigus: a case report. *Pediatr Neonatol.* 2016;57(4):338-342. doi:10.1016/j.pedneo.2013.08.008.
34. Sarig O, Bercovici S, Zoller L, et al. Population-specific association between a polymorphic variant in ST18, encoding a pro-apoptotic molecule, and pemphigus vulgaris. *J Invest Dermatol.* 2012;132:1798-1805.
35. Mabrouk D, Ahmed AR. Analysis of current therapy and clinical outcome in childhood pemphigus vulgaris. *Pediatr Dermatol.* 2011;28(5):485-493. doi:10.1111/j.1525-1470.2011.01514.x.
36. Mahalingam M. Follicular acantholysis: a subtle clue to the early diagnosis of pemphigus vulgaris. *Am J Dermatopathol.* 2005;27(3):237-239. doi:10.1097/01.dad.0000138656.86095.f4.
37. Beutner EH, Lever WF, Witebsky E, Jordon R, Chertock B. Autoantibodies in pemphigus vulgaris: response to an intercellular substance of epidermis. *JAMA.* 1965;192:682-688.

38. Geller S, Gat A, Harel A, et al. Childhood pemphigus foliaceus with exclusive immunoglobulin G autoantibodies to desmocollins. *Pediatr Dermatol.* 2016;33(1):e10-e13. doi:10.1111/pde.12729.

39. González F, Sáenz AM, Cirocco A, Tacaronte IM, Fajardo JE, Calebotta A. Endemic pemphigus foliaceus in Venezuela: report of two children. *Pediatr Dermatol.* 2006;23(2):132-135.

40. Aoki V, Rivitti EA, Diaz LA; Cooperative Group on Fogo Selvagem Research. Update on fogo selvagem, an endemic form of pemphigus foliaceus. *J Dermatol.* 2015;42(1):18-26.

41. Matsuo K, Komai A, Ishii K, et al. Pemphigus foliaceus with prominent neutrophilic pustules *Br J Dermatol.* 2001;145(1):132-136. doi:10.1046/j.1365-2133.2001.04297.x.

42. Bruckner AL, Fitzpatrick JE, Hashimoto T, Weston WL, Morelli JG. Atypical IgA/IgG pemphigus involving the skin, oral mucosa, and colon in a child: a novel variant of IgA pemphigus? *Pediatr Dermatol.* 2005;22(4):321-327.

43. Hashimoto T, Kiyokawa C, Mori O, et al. Human desmocollin 1 (Dsc 1) is an autoantigen for the subcorneal pustular dermatosis type of IgA pemphigus. *J Invest Dermatol.* 1997;109:127-131.

44. Hasimoto T, Komai A, Futei Y, Nishikawa T, Amagai M. Detection of IgA autoantibodies to desmogleins by an enzyme-linked immunosorbent assay: the presence of new minor subtypes of IgA pemphigus. *Arch Dermatol.* 2001;137:735-738.

45. Karpati S, Amagai M, Liu WL, Dmochowski M, Hashimoto T, Horváth A. Identification of desmoglein 1 as autoantigen in a patient with intraepidermal neutrophilic IgA dermatosis type of IgA pemphigus. *Exp Dermatol.* 2000;9:224-228.

46. Prost C, Intrator L, Wechsler J, et al. IgA autoantibodies bind to pemphigus vulgaris antigen in a case of intraepidermal neutrophilic IgA dermatosis. *J Am Acad Dermatol.* 1991;25:846-848.

47. Wang J, Kwon J, Ding X, Fairley JA, Woodley DT, Chan LS. Nonsecretory IgA1 autoantibodies targeting desmosomal component desmoglein 3 in intraepidermal neutrophilic IgA dermatosis. *Am J Pathol.* 1997;150:1901-1907.

48. Tsuruta D, Ishii N, Hamada T, et al. IgA pemphigus. *Clin Dermatol.* 2011;29(4):437-442. doi:10.1016/j.clindermatol.2011.01.014.

49. Hodak E, David M, Ingber A, et al. The clinical and histopathological spectrum of IgA-pemphigus—report of two cases. *Clin Exp Dermatol.* 1990;15(6):433-437.

50. Daneshpazhooh M, Moeineddin F, Kiani A, et al. Fatal paraneoplastic pemphigus after removal of Castleman's disease in a child. *Pediatr Dermatol.* 2012;29(5):656-657. doi:10.1111/j.1525-1470.2011.01670.x.

51. Jindal T, Meena M, Kumar A, Khaitan BK. Paraneoplastic pemphigus with Castleman's disease and bronchiolitis obliterans. *Pediatr Int.* 2011;53(6):1108-1109. doi:10.1111/j.1442-200X.2011.03507.x.

52. Koch LH, Layton CJ, Pilichowska M, Stadecker MJ, Barak O. Paraneoplastic pemphigus and Castleman's disease in the setting of herpes simplex virus infection. *Pediatr Dermatol.* 2012;29(5):629-632. doi:10.1111/j.1525-1470.2011.01557.x.

53. Hung IJ, Lin JJ, Yang CP, Hsueh C. Paraneoplastic syndrome and intrathoracic Castleman disease. *Pediatr Blood Cancer.* 2006;47(5):616-620.

54. Mar WA, Glaesser R, Struble K, Stephens-Grott S, Bangert J, Hansen RC. Paraneoplastic pemphigus with bronchiolitis obliterans in a child. *Pediatr Dermatol.* 2003;20(3):238-242.

55. Chin AC, Stich D, White FV, Radhakrishnan J, Holterman MJ. Paraneoplastic pemphigus and bronchiolitis obliterans associated with a mediastinal mass: A rare case of Castleman's disease with respiratory failure requiring lung transplantation. *J Pediatr Surg.* 2001;36(12):E22.

56. Mimouni D, Anhalt GJ, Lazarova Z, et al. Paraneoplastic pemphigus in children and adolescents. *Br J Dermatol.* 2002;147(4):725-732. doi:10.1046/j.1365-2133.2002.04992.x.

57. Schoch JJ, Boull CL, Camilleri MJ, Tollefson MM, Hook KP, Polcari IC. Transplacental transmission of pemphigus herpetiformis in the setting of maternal lymphoma. *Pediatr Dermatol.* 2015;32(6):e234-e237. doi:10.1111/pde.12649.

58. Czernik A, Camilleri M, Pittelkow MR, Grando SA. Paraneoplastic autoimmune multiorgan syndrome: 20 years after. *Int J Dermatol.* 2011;50:905-914.

59. Sezin T, Egozi E, Hillou W, Avitan-Hersh E, Bergman R. Anti-laminin-332 mucous membrane pemphigoid developing after a diphtheria tetanus vaccination. *JAMA Dermatol.* 2013;149(7):858-862. doi:10.1001/jamadermatol.2013.741.

60. McGinness JL, Bivens MM, Greer KE, Patterson JW, Saulsbury FT. Immune dysregulation, polyendocrinopathy, enteropathy, X-linked syndrome (IPEX) associated with pemphgioid nodularis: a case report and review of the literature. *J Am Acad Dermatol.* 2006;55:143-148.

61. Bis S, Maguiness SM, Gellis SE, et al. Immune dysregulation, polyendocrinopathy, enteropathy, X-linked syndrome associated with neonatal epidermolysis bullosa acquisita. *Pediatr Dermatol.* 2015;32(3):e74-e77. doi:10.1111/pde.12550.

62. Baroero L, Coppo P, Bertolino L, Maccario S, Savino F. Three case reports of post immunization and post viral Bullous Pemphigoid: looking for the right trigger. *BMC Pediatr.* 2017;17(1):60. doi:10.1186/s12887-017-0813-0.

63. Fisler RE, Saeb M, Liang MG, Howard RM, McKee PH. Childhood bullous pemphigoid: a clinicopathologic study and review of the literature. *Am J Dermatopathol.* 2003;25(3):183-189.

64. Nemeth AJ, Klein AD, Gould EW, Schachner LA. Childhood bullous pemphigoid. clinical and immunologic features, treatment, and prognosis. *Arch Dermatol.* 1991;127(3):378-386.

65. Oranje AP, van Joost T. Pemphigoid in children. *Pediatr Dermatol.* 1989;6(4):267-274.

66. Kharfi M, Khaled A, Anane R, Fazaa B, Kamoun MR. Early onset childhood cicatricial pemphigoid: a case report and review of the literature. *Pediatr Dermatol.* 2010;27(2):119-124.

67. Schoeffler A, Roth B, Causeret A, Kanaitakis J, Faure M, Claudy A. Vulvar cicatricial pemphigoid of childhood. *Pediatr Dermatol.* 2004;21(1):51-53.

68. Kahn E, Spence Shishido A, Yancey KB, Lawley LP. Anti-laminin-332 mucous membrane pemphigoid in a 9-year old girl. *Pediatr Dermatol.* 2014;31(3):e76-e79.

69. Guandalini S, Assiri A. Celiac disease: a review. *JAMA Pediatr.* 2014;168(3):272-278. doi:10.1001/jamapediatrics.2013.3858.

70. Hill ID, Dirks MH, Liptak GS, et al; North American Society for Pediatric Gastroenterology, Hepatology and Nutrition. Guideline for the diagnosis and treatment of celiac disease in children: recommendations of the North American Society for Pediatric Gastroenterology, Hepatology and Nutrition. *J Pediatr Gastroenterol Nutr.* 2005;40(1):1-19.

71. Lionetti E, Castellaneta S, Pulvirenti A, et al; Italian Working Group of Weaning and Celiac Disease Risk. Prevalence and natural history of potential celiac disease in at-family-risk infants prospectively investigated from birth. *J Pediatr.* 2012;161(5):908-914.

72. Blenkinsopp WK, Haffenden GP, Fry L, Leonard JN. Histology of linear IgA disease, dermatitis herpetiformis, and bullous pemphigoid. *Am J Dermatopathol.* 1983;5(6):547-554.

73. Antiga E, Caproni M, Fabbri P. Linear immunoglobulin a bullous dermatosis: need for an agreement on diagnostic criteria. *Dermatology.* 2013;226:329-332.

74. Lara-Corrales I, Pope E. Autoimmune blistering diseases in children. *Semin Cutan Med Surg.* 2010;29:85-91.

75. Kridin K. Subepidermal autoimmune bullous diseases: overview, epidemiology, and associations. *Immunol Res.* 2018;66(1):6-17. doi:10.1007/s12026-017-8975-2.

76. Gouveia AI, Teixeira A, Freitas JP, Soares-de-Almeida L, Filipe P, Sacramento-Marques M. Linear immunoglobulin A bullous dermatosis. *J Pediatr.* 2016;170:338-338.e1. doi:10.1016/j.jpeds.2015.11.078.

77. Kuechle MK, Stegemeir E, Maynard B, Gibson LE, Leiferman KM, Peters MS. Drug-induced linear IgA bullous dermatosis: report of six cases and review of the literature. *J Am Acad Dermatol.* 1994;30(2, pt 1):187-192.

78. Nousari HC, Kimyai-Asadi A, Caeiro JP, Anhalt GJ. Clinical, demographic, and immunohistologic features of vancomycin-induced linear IgA bullous disease of the skin: report of 2 cases and review of the literature. *Medicine (Baltimore)*. 1999;78(1):1-8.

79. Ho JC, Ng PL, Tan SH, Giam YC. Childhood linear IgA bullous disease triggered by amoxicillin-clavulanic acid. *Pediatr Dermatol*. 2007;24(5):E40-E43.

80. Ishiko A, Shimizu H, Masunaga T, et al. 97 kDa linear IgA bullous dermatosis antigen localizes in the lamina lucida between the NC16A and carboxyl terminal domains of the 180 kDa bullous pemphigoid antigen. *J Invest Dermatol*. 1998;111:93-96.

81. Pas HH, Kloosterhuis GJ, Heeres K, van der Meer JB, Jonkman MF. Bullous pemphigoid and linear IgA dermatosis sera recognize a similar 120-kDa keratinocyte collagenous glycoprotein with antigenic cross-reactivity to BP180. *J Invest Dermatol*. 1997; 108:423-429.

82. Paige DG, Leonard JN, Wojnarowska F, Fry L. Linear IgA disease and ulcerative colitis. *Br J Dermatol*. 1997;136(5):779-782.

83. Camisa C, Sharma HM. Vesiculobullous systemic lupus erythematosus: report of two cases and a review of the literature. *J Am Acad Dermatol*. 1983;9:924-933.

84. Seo JY, Byun HJ, Cho KH, Lee EB. Methimazole-induced bullous systemic lupus erythematosus: a case report. *J Korean Med Sci*. 2012;27(7):818-821. doi:10.3346/jkms.2012.27.7.818.

85. Gammon WR, Briggaman RA. Bullous SLE: a phenotypically distinctive but immunologically heterogeneous bullous disorder. *J Invest Dermatol*. 1993;100(1):S28-S34. doi:10.1038/jid.1993.20.

86. Su WP, Alegre VA. Bullous lesions in cutaneous lupus erythematosus. *Changgeng Yi Xue Za Zhi*. 1991;14(1):15-21.

87. Sidoroff A, Halevy S, Bavinck JN, Vaillant L, Roujeau JC. Acute generalized exanthematous pustulosis (AGEP)—a clinical reaction pattern. *J Cutan Pathol*. 2001;28(3):113-119.

88. Roujeau JC, Bioulac-Sage P, Bourseau C, et al. Acute generalized exanthematous pustulosis: analysis of 63 cases. *Arch Dermatol*. 1991;127(9): 1333-1338.

89. Meadows KP, Egan CA, Vanderhooft S. Acute generalized exanthematous pustulosis (AGEP), an uncommon condition in children: case report and review of the literature. *Pediatr Dermatol*. 2000;17(5):399-402.

90. Ersoy S, Paller AS, Mancini AJ. Acute generalized exanthematous pustulosis in children. *Arch Dermatol*. 2004;140(9):1172-1173.

91. Fernando SL. Acute generalised exanthematous pustulosis. *Australas J Dermatol*. 2012;53(2):87-92.

92. Heelen K, Shear N. Cutaneous drug reactions in children: an update. *Pediatr Drugs*. 2013;15:493-503.

93. Wick MR. Bullous, pseudobullous, & pustular dermatoses. *Semin Diagn Pathol*. 2017;34(3):250-260. doi:10.1053/j.semdp.2016.12.001.

94. Cheng S, Edmonds E, Ben-Gashir M, Yu RC. Subcorneal pustular dermatosis: 50 years on. *Clin Exp Dermatol*. 2008;33(3):229-233. doi:10.1111/j.1365-2230.2008.02706.x.

95. Good LM1, Good TJ, High WA. Infantile acropustulosis in internationally adopted children. *J Am Acad Dermatol*. 2011;65(4):763-771. doi:10.1016/j.jaad.2010.06.047.

96. Paller A, Mancini, AJ. *Hurwitz: Clinical Pediatric Dermatology*. 3rd ed. Philadelphia, PA: Elsevier Saunders;2006:482.

97. Falanga V. Infantile acropustulosis with eosinophilia. *J Am Acad Dermatol*. 1985;13(5, pt 1):826-828.

98. Cribbier B, Piemont Y, Grosshans E. Staphylococcal scalded skin syndrome in adults: a clinical review illustrated with a case. *J Am Acad Dermatol*. 30:319-324.

99. Staiman A, Hsu DY, Silverberg JI. Epidemiology of staphylococcal scalded skin syndrome in U.S. children. *Br J Dermatol*. 2017;178(3):704-708. doi:10.1111/bjd.16097.

100. Ladhani S, Joannou CL, Lochrie DP, Evans RW, Poston SM. Clinical, microbial and biochemical aspects of the exfoliative toxins causing staphylococcal scalded skin syndrome. *Clin Microbiol. Rev*. 1999;12:224-242.

101. Hussain S, Venepally M, Treat JR. Vesicles and pustules in the neonate. *Semin Perinatol*. 2013;37(1):8-15.

102. Amon RB, Dimond RL. Toxic epidermal necrolysis: rapid differentiation between staphylococcal- and drug-induced disease. *Arch Dermatol*. 1975;111(11):1433-1437.

5

Panniculitis, Granulomatous, and Fibrosing Disorders

Thomas Stringer / Lori D. Prok / Vikash S. Oza

ERYTHEMA NODOSUM

Definition and Epidemiology

Erythema nodosum (EN), one of the best-recognized panniculitides, is believed to be a delayed-type hypersensitivity reaction in response to a wide variety of stimuli. In the pediatric population, EN is most common among adolescents. EN in children less than 2 years of age is infrequently encountered. In contrast to the far greater incidence of EN in adult females relative to adult males, no such pattern has been found in children.[1]

Etiology

Approximately 50% of cases of EN are not associated with an underlying etiology and are, therefore, deemed idiopathic. The most common established cause in children is beta-hemolytic *Streptococcus* infection. In a recent case series of 35 pediatric EN patients, half of the patients were found to have a streptococcal infection of the pharynx.[2] Other infectious etiologies include *Mycoplasma pneumonia*, Epstein-Barr virus (EBV), mycobacteria, and *Coccidioides* spp. Systemic inflammatory disorders may also give rise to these lesions including sarcoidosis, inflammatory bowel disorder, Behcet disease, pregnancy, drug reaction, or malignancy.[3]

Clinical Presentation

Similar to adults, EN within children classically presents as pretibial red, tender nodules measuring 1 to 5 cm in diameter (Figure 5-1). Nodules evolve to adopt a reddish-brown or ecchymotic appearance and may persist for 4 to 8 weeks.[1]

Less common locations include the thighs, arms, trunk, and face. EN should not suppurate or ulcerate and such findings should prompt an evaluation for an alternative diagnosis. Fever, malaise, and arthralgias may precede the development of EN and accompanying lower extremity edema and pain can lead to difficulty with ambulation. Most cases can be managed with supportive care, including bedrest, leg elevation, and nonsteroidal anti-inflammatory drugs. In cases complicated by severe pain, treatment with potassium iodide or colchicine can hasten resolution. Although recurrent cases of pediatric EN have been documented, recrudescence is uncommon.[2]

Histologic Findings

EN is the prototypical septal panniculitis, characterized histologically by a widening of, and inflammation in, the subcutaneous fat septae, with associated septal fibrosis. One often appreciates "spill-over" inflammation into the surrounding fat lobules as well, but low-power microscopic examination usually clearly demonstrates septal involvement as the primary process. The inflammatory cell infiltrate is composed of lymphocytes and histiocytes (Figure 5-2). In acute disease, a varying number of neutrophils and eosinophils are often present, and vasculitis may rarely be noted. Small granulomas formed by the aggregates of histiocytes surrounding a central cleft (so-called Miescher's radial granulomas) are often present; they are common in, but not pathognomonic for, EN, and can be seen in other forms of panniculitis, as well as in neutrophilic dermatoses and necrobiosis lipoidica (NL) diabeticorum.[4,5]

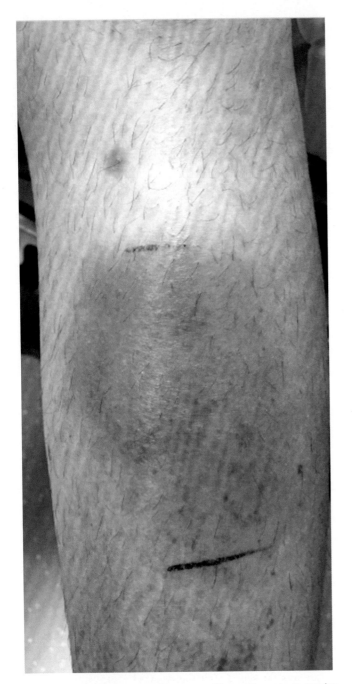

FIGURE 5-1. Erythema nodosum on shin: erythematous, tender plaque on the pretibial shins.

Differential Diagnosis

In children, EN is, by far, the most common septal panniculitis a pathologist will encounter. Occasionally, the specimen submitted may be suboptimal, or the degree of lobular inflammation may make the identification of the septal-focused process difficult. Chronic EN (subacute nodular migratory panniculitis) demonstrates more impressive septal fibrosis and granulomas. If vasculitis is prominent, thrombophlebitis and cutaneous polyarteritis nodosa should be considered. Occasionally, morphea profunda,

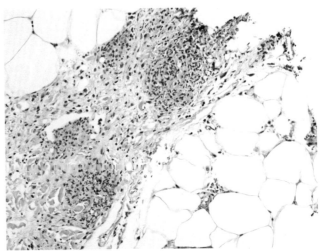

FIGURE 5-2. Erythema nodosum histopathology: widening and chronic inflammation of the subcutaneous fat septae.

deep granuloma annulare (GA), or cutaneous Crohn disease may involve, widen, and/or inflame the fat septae; these entities can usually be distinguished by their characteristic dermal features overlying the foci of panniculitis.

CAPSULE SUMMARY

ERYTHEMA NODOSUM

EN demonstrates a septal (or mixed septal/lobular) panniculitis with a mixed lymphohistiocytic infiltrate, septal fibrosis, and granuloma formation.

ERYTHEMA INDURATUM (NODULAR VASCULITIS)

Definition and Epidemiology

Erythema induratum (EI) was first coined in the mid-19th century to describe an inflammatory panniculitis related to the tuberculosis infection. Since then, identical clinical and histologic patterns have also been documented with other infectious or inflammatory diseases or have been idiopathic. The term "nodular vasculitis" has often been used to describe this EI-like pattern without underlying tuberculosis. Both the clinical and histopathologic presentation of EI and nodular vasculitis are identical. Both EI and nodular vasculitis are exceedingly rare in children and most commonly described in middle-aged adults.

Etiology

Although PCR detection of tuberculosis organisms has substantiated the role of *M. tuberculosis* in the pathogenesis of EI, the precise etiology is controversial and variably

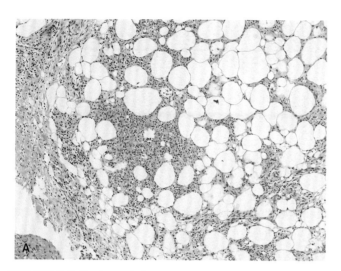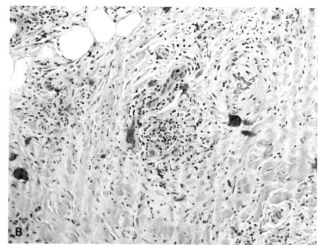

FIGURE 5-3. Erythema induratum histopathology: mixed lobular inflammation (**A**) and early vasculitis in lobular panniculitis (**B**).

considered to be a Type III or IV hypersensitivity reaction to bacterial antigen. Nodular vasculitis has been documented with various infections or inflammatory disorders, including sarcoidosis, chronic hepatitis C infection, inflammatory bowel disease, nontuberculosis mycobacterial infections (*Mycobacterium chelonae*, *Mycobacterium avium*, and *Mycobacterium monacense*), and bacteria (*Nocardia*, *Pseudomonas*, *Fusarium*, *Chlamydophila pneumonia*).[6-9]

Clinical Presentation

EI manifests as symmetrical, tender, deep-seated nodules that may progress to ulceration and heal with atrophic scarring. EI most commonly affects the lower extremities, particularly the calves. Treatment should be carried out expediently with antituberculosis drugs, to which the cutaneous manifestations respond well. Although spontaneous resolution can occur, most cases of EI are chronic and/or recurrent if not treated.

Histologic Findings

EI is histologically identical to nodular vasculitis. Because mycobacteria is not consistently identified in cases of EI, and because numerous inflammatory and other triggers are known to result in the clinical and histologic features of nodular vasculitis, this distinction in nomenclature between the two entities has fallen out of favor within dermatopathology as well, with many authors preferring a unified description.[10] EI-nodular vasculitis is characterized histologically by a primarily lobular panniculitis, with lymphohistiocytic granuloma formation and variable necrosis (Figure 5-3A). Vasculitis is the most reliable finding and may present as a necrotizing form in early lesions (Figure 5-3B).[11] Careful search for mycobacterial organisms should be done, using special stains (AFB [acid-fast bacilli], FITE) or immunohistochemistry for tuberculosis.

Differential Diagnosis

EI-nodular vasculitis usually involves several adjacent fat lobules, in contrast to polyarteritis nodosa, where the vasculitis involves one large vessel with variable surrounding and associated panniculitis. The other forms of lobular panniculitis are usually excluded by the presence of vasculitis.

CAPSULE SUMMARY

ERYTHEMA INDURATUM (NODULAR VASCULITIS)

EI-nodular vasculitis is a lobular panniculitis with characteristic vasculitis, granuloma formation, and necrosis.

ALPHA-1 ANTITRYPSIN DEFICIENCY PANNICULITIS

Definition and Epidemiology

Alpha-1 antitrypsin deficiency is an inborn error of metabolism leading to variably low blood serum concentrations of the protease inhibitor alpha-1 antitrypsin. Excessive protease activity predisposes patients to chronic obstructive pulmonary disease, hepatic cirrhosis, and panniculitis. Between 80 000 and 100 000 individuals in the United States are thought to suffer from its symptoms.[12,13]

Etiology

Alpha-1 antitrypsin is an acute-phase reactant that can modulate proteases, most notably neutrophil elastase, as well as the activity of neutrophils, monocytes, macrophages, and mast cells. Its deficiency allows excessive protease activity, leading to tissue damage and the manifestations of the disease. The genes that encode the protein are inherited in

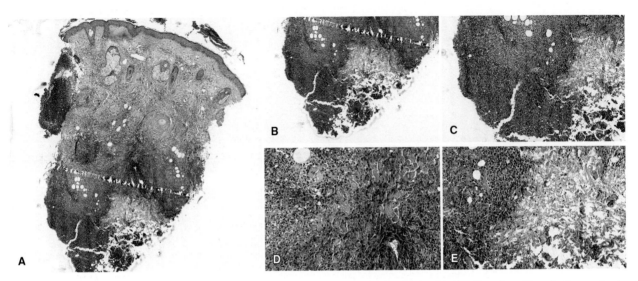

FIGURE 5-4. Alpha-1 antitrypsin deficiency panniculitis. There is mostly lobular panniculitis (**A**). Prominent liquefactive and subcutaneous necrosis is present. The infiltrate is composed of lymphocytes and histiocytes (**B-E**). Digital slides courtesy of Path Presenter.com.

autosomal codominant fashion. The most common deficiency alleles are termed S or Z, whereas the normal allele is designated M. Broadly speaking, MS heterozygotes and SS homozygotes are at low risk for clinically significant disease, MZ and SZ heterozygotes are at greater risk, and ZZ homozygotes develop the most severe symptoms.[14]

Clinical Presentation

In both pediatric and adult patients, alpha-1 antitrypsin deficiency can present with panniculitis manifesting as purple, tender nodules or plaques, most commonly on the lower trunk, buttocks, and proximal extremities. Lesions can be precipitated by minor trauma and therefore may be misdiagnosed as factitial or artifactual panniculitis. The panniculitis can progress to develop deep, necrotic ulcers that exude oily material. No specific treatment is indicated for the cutaneous findings of this condition—the amelioration of the process with enzyme replacement therapy is sufficient to effect its resolution.

The most common presenting symptom of alpha-1 antitrypsin deficiency in pediatric patients is intrahepatic cholestasis, which in rare cases results in cirrhosis requiring liver transplantation.[14] The other extracutaneous manifestations include pulmonary emphysema, pancreatitis, pulmonary embolism or effusion, angioedema, arthritis, or vasculitis.[14]

Histologic Findings

Alpha-1 antitrypsin deficiency presents as a lobular panniculitis, classically neutrophil-predominant in early lesions, and demonstrating lymphocytes and histiocytes in more long-standing nodules. Liquefactive necrosis of dermal collagen and lipocytes is characteristic, and correlates clinically with oily drainage from ulcerated plaques (Figure 5-4).[15] Collagenolysis of fat septae is also common. In the liver, cirrhosis is typical, with the presence of globular inclusions in the periportal areas (Figure 5-5).

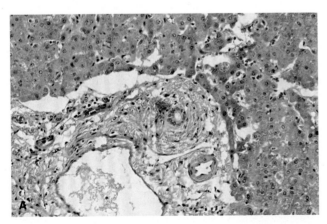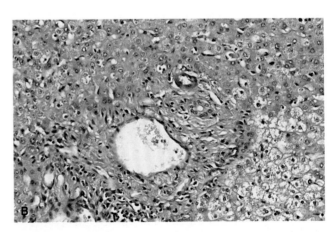

FIGURE 5-5. Alpha-1 antitrypsin deficiency liver abnormalities. A characteristic finding is the presence of periportal globules within the hepatocytes, demonstrated on hematoxylin and eosin (**A**) and periodic acid-Schiff (**B**) stains.

Differential Diagnosis

Alpha-1 antitrypsin deficiency is a rare form of panniculitis in childhood. The more common forms of neutrophilic panniculitis should be excluded in the evaluation, including infection, Sweet syndrome and other neutrophilic dermatoses, and foreign objects or injected substances (eg, factitial disorder).[16] Special stains for microorganisms and polarized light examination are recommended when evaluating neutrophilic panniculitis. BRAF-inhibitors are becoming more widely used in the pediatric age group for brain and other solid organ tumors and have been associated with drug-induced neutrophilic panniculitis.[17,18] This type of panniculitis is not associated with liquefactive necrosis.

CAPSULE SUMMARY

ALPHA-1 ANTITRYPSIN DEFICIENCY PANNICULITIS

Neutrophilic panniculitis in childhood should prompt a consideration of alpha-1 antitrypsin deficiency, although infection is a more common cause of lobular neutrophilic panniculitis, particularly in hospitalized or immunocompromised patients. A medication reaction should also be considered.

LIPOATROPHIC PANNICULITIS

Definition and Epidemiology

Known variously as annular lipoatrophic panniculitis and lipophagic panniculitis, lipoatrophic panniculitis is loosely defined as a panniculitis that heals with fat atrophy accompanied by constitutional symptoms. This entity presents most often in infants and young children 3 to 13 years of age.[19]

Etiology

The etiology of lipoatrophic panniculitis is poorly understood, although it is likely autoinflammatory in nature, given that cases have been reported with Hashimoto's thyroiditis, Graves' disease, juvenile rheumatoid arthritis, and alopecia areata.[19]

Clinical Presentation

Lipoatrophic panniculitis is characterized by the episodic development of inflamed subcutaneous nodules that expand radially and are followed by permanent lipoatrophy, which is often circumferential around the ankle (Figure 5-6). Lipoatrophic panniculitis follows a relapsing course, with multiple bouts of inflammation and atrophic resolution occurring over the course of months.[20] Lesions most often occur on the extremities, and their onset may

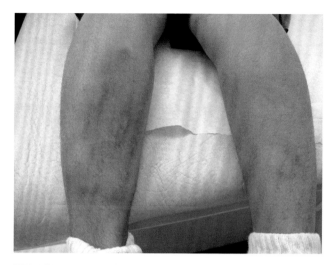

FIGURE 5-6. Lipoatrophic panniculitis: large annular plaque on the medial shin with central atrophy and peripheral erythema and induration.

be preceded by an upper respiratory infection. The clinical differential diagnosis includes deep GA, deep erythema annulare centrifugum, EN, lupus panniculitis, erythema migrans, and morphea. Systemic symptoms associated with this disease include constitutional symptoms, particularly fever, hepatosplenomegaly, arthralgias, and abdominal pain.[20,21]

Histologic Findings

In early lesions, this disorder presents with lipophagic panniculitis, characterized by a dense mixed inflammatory infiltrate centered on the subcutaneous fat lobules, with numerous foamy lipophages (Figure 5-7A and B).[22] Neutrophils are often present in early disease, with histiocytes predominating in later lesions. There is no vasculitis. In very established lesions where clinical atrophy is longstanding, the infiltrate may be sparse, with notable atrophy and fibrosis of the fat lobules.[20]

Differential Diagnosis

Infection and trauma may both demonstrate lipophagic changes and should be excluded in the evaluation of lipoatrophic panniculitis. The various forms of neutrophilic panniculitis may be considered in early lesions. Once atrophy predominates, the findings may not be distinguishable from other forms of lipoatrophy and lipodystrophy; these disorders are usually able to be excluded on the basis of clinical history. Several reports have described lymphocytes rimming adipocytes as well as mildly atypical lymphocytes infiltrating subcutaneous vessels; these findings may prompt a consideration of subcutaneous panniculitis-like T-cell lymphoma, which can be excluded by the lack of necrosis or lymphocyte phagocytosis by histiocytes.[23]

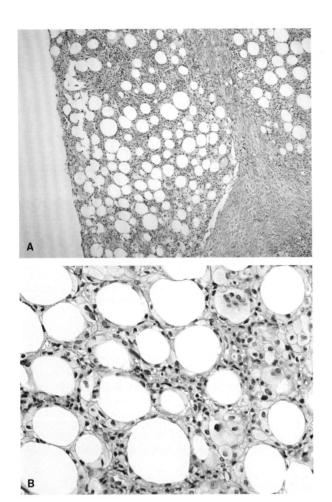

FIGURE 5-7. Lipoatrophic panniculitis histopathology: lobular panniculitis with fat necrosis (**A**). High-power view highlighting lipophagic fat necrosis and foamy histiocytes (**B**).

CAPSULE SUMMARY

LIPOATROPHIC PANNICULITIS

Lipoatrophic or lipophagic panniculitis presents histologically with a mixed lobular infiltrate, with lipid-laden macrophages, and lobular atrophy, likely triggered by an autoimmune or inflammatory process.

COLD-INDUCED PANNICULITIS

Definition and Epidemiology

Cold-induced panniculitis is an eruption of subcutaneous nodules in response to prolonged cold exposure. Although cold panniculitis may present well into adulthood, most cases, including the initial reports, tend to occur in young children.[24]

Etiology

The predilection of cold-induced panniculitis for younger patients is thought to arise because of a higher ratio of unsaturated to saturated fatty acids in the subcutaneous fat, the former of which have a higher freezing point.

Clinical Presentation

Cold-induced panniculitis presents with painful, poorly defined erythematous plaques or subcutaneous nodules (Figure 5-8). The lesions often persist for hours to days post exposure and resolve spontaneously. The sources of exposure include cold ambient temperatures, ice packs, or cooling blankets.[25] The phenomenon known as "popsicle panniculitis" is a well-described presentation in teething children given frozen substances as an analgesic and the subsequent development of panniculitis involving the cheeks or submental area.[26]

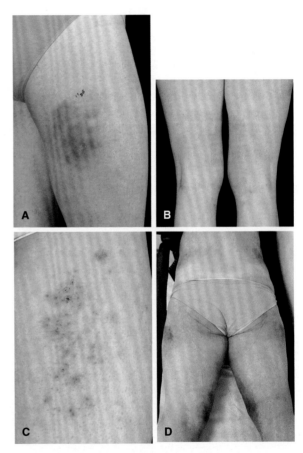

FIGURE 5-8. **Cold panniculitis.** Clinical aspects of cold-associated perniosis of the thighs. **A**, Typical presentation with livid-red, infiltrated lesions on the lateral aspect of the thigh; **B**, similar clinical presentation but lesions located on the posterior aspect of both thighs; **C**, partly eroded lesions located on the lateral aspect of the thigh; **D**, widespread involvement with lesions located on the lateral and medial aspects of both thighs as well as both flanks. Reprinted with permission from Ferrara G, Cerroni L. Cold-associated perniosis of the thighs ("equestrian-type" chilblain): a reappraisal based on a clinicopathologic and immunohistochemical study of 6 cases. *Am J Dermatopathol.* 2016;38(10):726-731.

Histologic Findings

A histologic hallmark of cold panniculitis is the presence of edema in the papillary dermis; as such, incisional specimens that do not include overlying superficial dermis are not ideal when evaluating for this entity. Cold panniculitis presents with mixed acute and chronic lobular inflammation, with characteristic adipocyte necrosis (Figures 5-9 and 5-10). A clinical history of cold exposure is helpful in evaluation.[27]

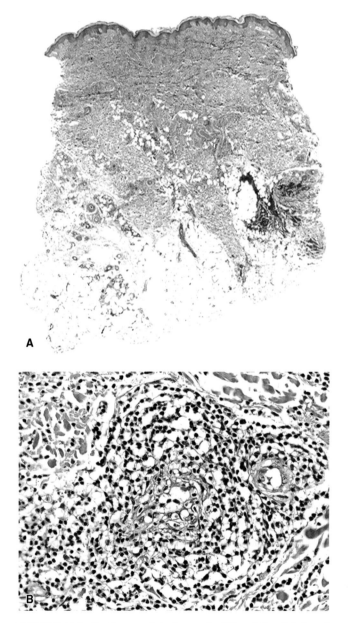

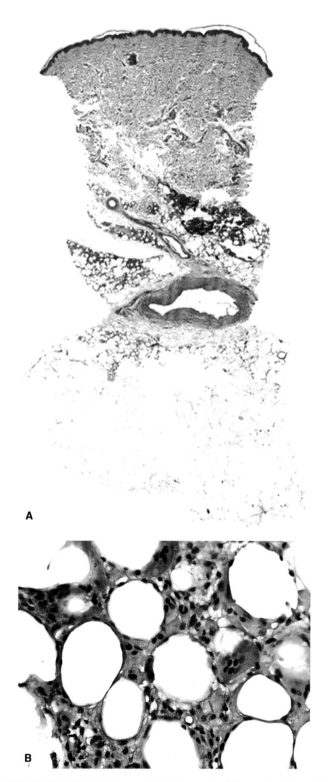

FIGURE 5-9. Cold-associated panniculitis of the thighs. A, Dense inflammatory infiltrates predominantly located within the dermis and only superficial portion of subcutaneous fat. **B,** Prominent involvement of a vessel with features of lymphocytic venulitis. Reprinted with permission from Ferrara G, Cerroni L. Cold-associated perniosis of the thighs ("equestrian-type" chilblain): a reappraisal based on a clinicopathologic and immunohistochemical study of 6 cases. *Am J Dermatopathol.* 2016;38(10):726-731.

FIGURE 5-10. Cold-associated panniculitis. Late stage of cold-associated perniosis of the thighs with lipophagic features in the upper part of the subcutaneous fat (**B**); only minimal dermal and subcutaneous inflammatory infiltrate present (**A**). Reprinted with permission from Ferrara G, Cerroni L. Cold-associated perniosis of the thighs ("equestrian-type" chilblain): a reappraisal based on a clinicopathologic and immunohistochemical study of 6 cases. *Am J Dermatopathol.* 2016;38(10):726-731.

Differential Diagnosis

Other "physical" causes of panniculitis can show similar histologic features to cold panniculitis, including traumatic and factitial panniculitis. All can present with acute inflammation and necrosis. Clinical-pathologic correlation is required in most cases. Polarized light examination should be performed to exclude foreign material.

CAPSULE SUMMARY

COLD-INDUCED PANNICULITIS

Cold panniculitis demonstrates a lobular panniculitis with mixed inflammation and marked papillary dermal edema. Clinical-pathologic correlation is helpful in making the correct diagnosis.

LUPUS PANNICULITIS

Definition and Epidemiology

Lupus erythematosus panniculitis (LEP) represents a subcutaneous variant of cutaneous lupus erythematosus. LEP is an uncommon diagnosis in children, believed to represent only 2% of pediatric patients with cutaneous systemic lupus erythematosus (SLE). The mean age of onset of LEP is 8 years.[28]

Etiology

LEP can occur independently or in association with discoid lupus erythematosus or SLE. In 70% of cases of LEP, the overlying lesions of discoid lupus erythematosus are seen, and half have symptoms of SLE, most commonly fever, arthritis, and lymphadenopathy.[25,29]

Clinical Presentation

LEP often presents with firm, asymptomatic, sharply demarcated, rubbery dermal plaques or nodules most commonly on the face and/or upper arms in children.[30] As inflammation subsides, lipoatrophy typically develops, placing patients at risk for permanent disfigurement. LEP should be distinguished from EN, another common form of panniculitis in patients with SLE. Unlike EN, LEP does not typically involve the shins, is chronic in duration, and is typically painless. The diagnosis of LEP is best established by a skin biopsy, and laboratory workup is infrequently helpful. A positive antinuclear antibody (ANA) is inconsistently found in children with LEP.[30]

Histologic Findings

Lupus panniculitis is characterized by dense lobules of lymphocytes often centered at the periphery of the fat lobules in association with marked fibrosis. A mixed lobular and

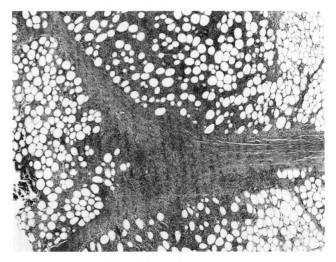

FIGURE 5-11. Lupus panniculitis: dense lymphocytic lobular panniculitis and hyalinized fat septae.

septal panniculitis may be seen. Histiocytes and plasma cells are usually also present. Lymphoid follicles are typical. There is reliable hyaline necrosis of the fat lobules, with associated edema, mucin deposition, and variable calcification (Figure 5-11).[5,31] The overlying epidermis frequently demonstrates classic interface changes of lupus, with basal vacuolar change, dyskeratosis, and lymphocytic inflammation at the dermo-epidermal junction and follicles.[32]

Differential Diagnosis

Panniculitis associated with dermatomyositis demonstrates identical histologic features to lupus panniculitis and must be distinguished clinically. The other forms of lobular panniculitis can be excluded on the basis of hyaline necrosis, mucin deposition, and overlying epidermal and papillary dermal changes.

CAPSULE SUMMARY

LUPUS PANNICULITIS

Lupus panniculitis demonstrates dense mixed but lymphocyte-predominant lobular panniculitis with hyaline fat necrosis. The overlying epidermis and papillary dermis should always be examined for evidence of interface changes and lichenoid inflammation.

SUBCUTANEOUS PANNICULITIS-LIKE T-CELL LYMPHOMA

Definition and Epidemiology

Subcutaneous panniculitis-like T-cell lymphoma (SPTCL) is a panniculitis of neoplastic origin driven by cytotoxic T-cells with the α/β lineage.[33] The former cases with a γ/δ phenotype are now designated as primary cutaneous γ/δ

T-cell lymphoma. SPTCL may present in a broad age range. A review of 83 cases found a mean age of 36, with a range extending from 9 to 79 years of age.[34]

Etiology

It is unclear whether or to what extent SPTCL is a reactive T-cell lymphoproliferative syndrome, as opposed to a primary malignancy in its own right. SPTCL is well described as occurring in patients previously diagnosed with LEP, and there is a striking histopathologic similarity between the two.[35,36]

Clinical Presentation

SPTCL presents in similar fashion to LEP, rendering the distinction between the two on clinical grounds difficult, although case series indicate that the latter disease often possesses more prominent constitutional symptoms, leukopenia, and increased erythrocyte sedimentation rate.[36] The cases with associated hemophagocytosis have a more aggressive clinical course.

Much ambiguity exists regarding the clinical separation of SPTCL, LEP, and the entity cytophagic histiocytic panniculitis (CHP), the latter an idiopathic febrile panniculitis in the setting of hemophagocytosis, also considered to represent a reactive lymphocytic process. The symptomatology of these disorders, which often includes constitutional symptoms, cytopenias, hepatosplenomegaly, and other end organ involvement, makes them difficult to distinguish. Moreover, it is an open question whether or not CHP and SPTCL fall onto a continuum of neoplastic disease or whether they represent their own separate disorders with unique clinical spectra of presentation.[37-39]

Histologic Findings

A dense, monotonous infiltrate of small- to medium-sized atypical lymphocytes infiltrate the subcutaneous fat lobules, giving the appearance of a lobular panniculitis. Tumor cells demonstrate karyorrhexis and pleomorphism. Mixed inflammation and granulomatous foci may be present, and fat necrosis is common. "Rimming" of individual adipocytes by tumor cells is a characteristic feature, although not specific.[40] Vascular invasion is variably present. Immunohistochemistry highlights cytotoxic T-cells, with a CD8 predominant phenotype (CD3+, CD4−, CD8+, CD56−). All SPTCL are BF1+ (TCR alpha/beta phenotype). Ki67 shows frequent increased proliferation among the neoplastic cells.

Differential Diagnosis

SPTCL may be mistaken for a benign or reactive lobular panniculitis, particularly lupus panniculitis. Cytologic atypia, rimming of adipocytes, lack of any dermal involvement, and the absence of interface changes in the overlying epidermis help distinguish SPTCL. LEP typically has pronounced

fibrosis and lymphoid follicles. Other lymphomas may be excluded on the basis of immunohistochemistry.

CAPSULE SUMMARY

SUBCUTANEOUS PANNICULITIS-LIKE T-CELL LYMPHOMA

SPTCL presents histologically as an atypical lymphocytic infiltrate confined to the subcutis, mimicking a lobular panniculitis.

NEUTROPHILIC LOBULAR PANNICULITIS

Definition and Epidemiology

Neutrophilic lobular panniculitis is a neutrophil-driven, principally lobular panniculitis often presenting alongside relapsing fevers and other constitutional symptoms. Neutrophilic lobular panniculitis is best described as a histopathologic reaction pattern and not as a distinct clinical entity, which can be associated with various cutaneous and systemic disorders.

Etiology

Infection, Sweet syndrome and other neutrophilic dermatoses, foreign objects or injected substances, trauma, early lipophagic panniculitis, alpha-1 antitrypsin deficiency, and autoimmune diseases (particularly rheumatoid arthritis and inflammatory bowel disease) may all be associated with neutrophilic panniculitis.[16] A special consideration in the pediatric age group is neutrophilic panniculitis as a reaction to BRAF inhibitor medications, the use of which are becoming more frequent in the treatment of cutaneous and solid organ malignancies.[18]

Clinical Presentation

Any of the aforementioned etiologies may manifest with subcutaneous nodules in concert with recurrent fevers. Patients with this clinical presentation and histologic features of a neutrophilic panniculitis must undergo a thorough infectious disease workup.

The term Weber-Christian disease, which denotes a febrile panniculitis of unknown origin, has fallen out of favor in the dermatologic literature following a 1998 study in which alternative clinicopathologic diagnoses were found in all 30 examined adult cases previously diagnosed as Weber-Christian. It is now considered a placeholder for the panniculitis of etiology yet to be uncovered.[41]

Histologic Findings

As the name indicates, neutrophilic panniculitis is characterized by a neutrophil-predominant inflammatory cell

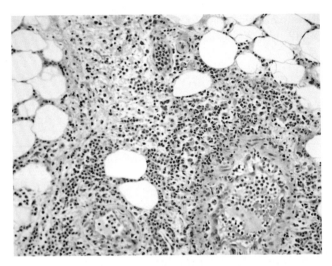

FIGURE 5-12. Neutrophilic lobular panniculitis histopathology: neutrophil-predominant lobular infiltrate in a patient treated with BRAF inhibitor therapy for glioblastoma.

infiltrate of the fat lobules with a relative sparing of the septi (Figure 5-12). Leukocytoclasis can be very prominent in the absence of frank vasculitis.

Differential Diagnosis

Some cases of neutrophilic panniculitis may demonstrate variable septal inflammation. In these cases, EN and Sweet syndrome involving the subcutis should be excluded. Special stains for microorganisms and polarized light examination are always recommended when evaluating neutrophilic panniculitis.

CAPSULE SUMMARY

NEUTROPHILIC LOBULAR PANNICULITIS

Neutrophilic panniculitis is a reaction pattern characterized by neutrophilic lobular or mixed lobular and septal inflammation. Medication reaction to BRAF inhibitor is a well-documented cause of neutrophilic panniculitis in children. Several other cutaneous and systemic disorders can present with similar histologic features.

TRAUMATIC/FACTITIAL PANNICULITIS

Definition and Epidemiology

Factitial, or traumatic, panniculitides are produced by adventitious injury. Factitial panniculitides are most often described in young adults and middle-aged women.

Etiology

The causes of these injuries are commonly grouped into mechanical (eg, traumatic), physical (eg, arising from application of cold or heat), and chemical. It is important to note that panniculitides arising from iatrogenic sources are considered to be factitial. The most salient agents for pediatric purposes are vaccination, particularly antihepatitis vaccination or antitetanus toxoid, and phytonadione, or vitamin K. A subcutaneous reaction pattern can be induced by penetrating or blunt trauma, the injection of foreign substances, or persistent local pressure. Surreptitiously injected substances may include mineral or vegetable oils, which induce subcutaneous inflammation.

Clinical Presentation

The morphology of the lesions may vary depending upon the nature of the insult. Panniculitis ensuing from penetrating trauma may be well demarcated and/or sharply angulated, whereas nodules induced by blunt trauma may appear ecchymotic, often arising on the arm or hand. The diagnosis is made more difficult by the idiosyncratic reactions of injected agents, such as Texier disease in the context of vitamin K injections. Early in the course, these may appear as robust eczematous reactions, whereas late presentations may resemble sclerotic lesions with a lilac border. Careful evaluation of the clinical history and distribution must be undertaken to arrive at the proper diagnosis.

Histologic Features

Acute or chronic trauma of the fat presents histologically as a lobular panniculitis, with chronic mixed inflammation and foci of fat necrosis and lipomembranous change. Low-power examination often reveals cystic spaces in the fat lobules. Hemorrhage and hemosiderosis are common, and fibrosis is usually present in chronic lesions. Clinical hypertrichosis has been reported overlying plaques of traumatic panniculitis, but is not associated with histologic changes of the hair follicles.[42] A "mobile encapsulated lipoma" is a discrete focus of traumatized and necrotic fat that has been isolated in the skin (Figure 5-13A). It is often surprisingly mobile beneath the skin surface. It demonstrates identical histologic features, but in a small, encapsulated deep dermal nodule (Figure 5-13B).[43]

Differential Diagnosis

Cold panniculitis, foreign material, and other forms of factitial panniculitis may all present with mixed lobular inflammation and fat necrosis. Clinical history is critical in distinguishing these entities. Histologic features that may be helpful include dermal edema (frequent in cold panniculitis), foreign material demonstrated on polarized light examination, and the presence of irregular "Swiss cheese-like" cystic spaces in forms of factitial panniculitis.

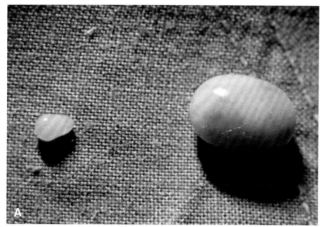

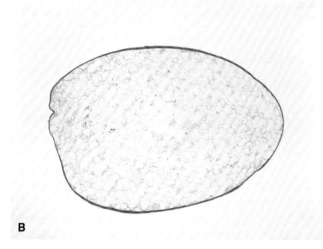

FIGURE 5-13. **A**, Mobile encapsulated lipoma gross: shiny, encapsulated, soft nodule; easily excised intact. **B**, Mobile encapsulated lipoma histopathology: well-circumscribed and encapsulated aggregate of necrotic lipocytes.

CAPSULE SUMMARY

TRAUMATIC/FACTITIAL PANNICULITIS

Traumatic panniculitis demonstrates mixed lobular inflammation with necrosis, hemorrhage, and fibrosis.

GRANULOMA ANNULARE

Definition and Epidemiology

GA is a noninfectious granulomatous skin condition presenting with variable clinical morphologies. In general, GA is most common in school-aged children. The subcutaneous variant preferentially occurs in young children, with the most number of children being less than 6 years of age.

Etiology

GA is believed to be caused by a delayed-type hypersensitivity reaction due to unknown stimulating antigens.[44] Most cases of childhood GA occur in the absence of an underlying medical condition. Risk factors associated with GA include diabetes mellitus, tetanus or BCG vaccination, Hepatitis B viral infection, *Borrelia* infection, Hodgkin's lymphoma, and acute lymphocytic leukemia.[25]

Clinical Presentation

The lesions of GA are comprised of small skin colored to pink/violaceous individual papules coalescing to form an annular or circinate plaque without scale (Figure 5-14). The four most common clinical variants are localized, generalized, subcutaneous, and perforating GA. Localized GA typically involves the extremities, specifically the wrists, ankles, and the dorsal surface of the hands and feet. By definition, generalized GA must involve the trunk and at least one set of extremities and may follow a more protracted course than other variants.[45] The perforating morphology may present as grouped papules with central umbilication, crusting, and scaling. Subcutaneous GA presents with subcutaneous nodules on the feet, anterior tibial surface, fingers, hands, or scalp. This variant can appear clinically similar to rheumatoid or pseudorheumatoid nodules, but both of these diagnoses are much less common in children than in adults.[46]

GA is a self-limited disorder with 50% of lesions resolving in 2 years, and therefore, observation is a reasonable management approach.[47] Potent topical corticosteroids, intralesional corticosteroids, and cryotherapy have all been used to treat individual lesions. Occasionally, severe and generalized disease may require systemic medication, and isotretinoin, antimalarial (plaquenil), and dapsone have been used in this setting.[25]

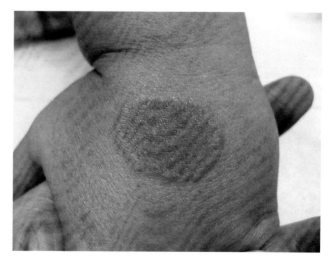

FIGURE 5-14. Granuloma annulare: erythematous, annular plaque with a raised border of monomorphous papules. Courtesy of Anna Bruckner, MD.

Histologic Findings

Classic GA is characterized histologically by necrobiotic granulomas in the superficial and mid dermis. These demonstrate altered, eosinophilic, and thickened collagen at the center, with lymphocytes and histiocytes surrounding in a palisaded manner (Figure 5-15). Eosinophils may be present, and scattered multinucleate histiocytes are frequent. Mucin deposition is present in the necrobiotic foci, a feature that helps distinguish GA from other granulomatous infiltrates. The mucin can be demonstrated with the use of Alcian blue or colloidal iron stains. A perivascular lymphocytic infiltrate is usually noted in the surrounding dermis. In the interstitial form of GA, histiocytes intercalate between dermal collagen bundles, giving a "busy" appearance to the dermis at low-power examination, without distinct necrobiotic foci. Interstitial mucin is present.

Differential Diagnosis

NL diabeticorum can appear similar to GA histologically, but generally shows pandermal granulomas rather than discrete foci and a lack of mucin deposition. Rheumatoid nodules are larger, demonstrate more fiery pink collagen with fibrin deposition and necrosis, and are present deeper in the dermis. The presence of numerous multinucleate histiocytes and/or acute inflammation should prompt the consideration of a foreign body granuloma and the performance of polarized light examination. Infection should also be considered if granulomas and neutrophilic inflammation are present. Occasionally, the presence of dense and well-formed granulomas without definitive necrobiosis may mimic features of cutaneous sarcoidosis.[48] The interstitial form of GA demonstrates histologic features similar to an interstitial drug eruption and some forms of

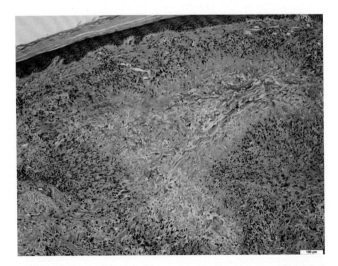

FIGURE 5-15. Granuloma annulare histopathology: necrobiotic granuloma, demonstrating central eosinophilic collagen and mucin, with surrounding palisaded lymphohistiocytic inflammation.

scleromyxedema.[49,50] If neutrophils are present in association with interstitial granulomatous inflammation, "palisaded neutrophilic and granulomatous dermatitis" (which may be associated with a variety of underlying diseases including rheumatoid arthritis, lupus and other connective tissue disorders, inflammatory bowel disease, myeloproliferative disorders, infection, and medications) should be considered.[51,52]

CAPSULE SUMMARY

GRANULOMA ANNULARE

GA is common in children and shows diagnostic histologic features of necrobiotic, palisaded granulomas with central mucin.

NECROBIOSIS LIPODICA

Definition and Epidemiology

Necrobiosis lipoidica NL is a chronic granulomatous condition with a predilection for the shins. Although an association between NL and diabetes mellitus exists, its magnitude may be less significant than previously estimated, such that many clinicians advocate striking "diabeticorum" from its name.[53] The condition occurs in fewer than 1% of diabetes mellitus patients, and one series has reported a 15% rate of DM upon presentation with NL. A female predilection of 3:1 has been noted.[25,54] NL is exceedingly rare in children, and its reportage is largely limited to isolated cases and small series.[55,56]

Etiology

NL is classically associated with diabetes mellitus, most commonly type I. Historically, this condition has been described as NL diabeticorum. Among patients with diabetes, patients with NL are at a higher risk for other diabetes-related complications such as peripheral neuropathy and retinopathy, but NL is not clearly associated with poorer glycemic control.[57,58]

Clinical Presentation

NL most often presents as asymptomatic, slowly enlarging, irregularly bordered red to yellow-brown plaques, appearing most often on the pretibial surface. Most patients have multiple, symmetric plaques, whereas less common sites of involvement include the upper extremities, face, and scalp (Figure 5-16). Occasionally, NL plaques can be complicated by ulceration, decreased pinprick sensation, hypohidrosis, and alopecia. Asymptomatic lesions may be treated with watchful waiting, whereas a symptomatic rash can be treated with intralesional versus topical corticosteroids, psoralen + UVA (PUVA), chloroquine, and, in certain cases, oral corticosteroids.[25]

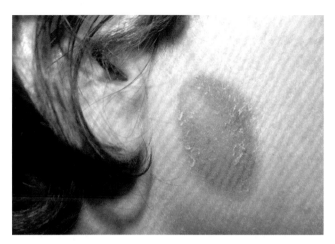

FIGURE 5-16. Necrobiosis lipoidica: Pink-yellow plaque on the cheek of a young girl. Courtesy James E. Fitzpatrick, MD from the Fitzsimons Army Medical Center Collection.

Histologic Findings

Although rare, NL has been reported in children and demonstrates similar histologic features to those seen in adult patients.[55] Pandermal necrobiotic granulomas that frequently extend into the subcutis are the histologic hallmark of NL (Figure 5-17). Eosinophilic degenerated collagen is surrounded by palisaded lymphocytes, histiocytes, and frequent plasma cells, in an arrangement that involves the dermis "top to bottom" and "side to side", often covering

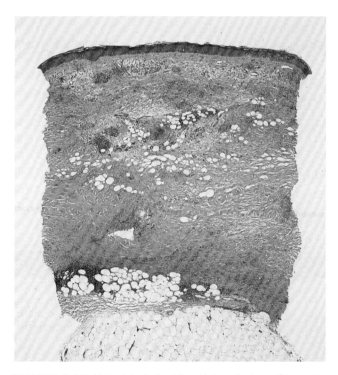

FIGURE 5-17. Necrobiosis lipoidica histopathology: Characteristic "layered cake" architecture, with bands of necrobiosis and palisaded inflammation involving the entire dermis.

the entirety of punch specimens, and giving a tiered or layered appearance to the dermis. Dermal vessels demonstrate thick walls, luminal narrowing, and chronic inflammation, features reflective of the diabetic microangiopathy frequent in patients with NL.[59]

Differential Diagnosis

GA is the most important histologic mimic to NL in children and is characterized by more discrete, superficial granulomas that do not coalesce or involve the entire dermis, and demonstrate central mucin.

CAPSULE SUMMARY

NECROBIOSIS LIPODICA

NL is distinguished by necrobiotic granulomas throughout the dermis and subcutis, with plasma cell inflammation and characteristic vascular changes.

SARCOIDOSIS

Definition and Epidemiology

Sarcoidosis is a chronic inflammatory disease resulting in noncaseating granulomas affecting multiple organ systems, most commonly the lung. Sarcoidosis is an uncommon diagnosis in children. Sarcoidosis is more commonly seen in adolescents and is exceedingly rare in prepubertal children. National registry data from Denmark estimate an incidence of 0.29 per 100 000 children with a median age of 13 years at diagnosis.[60]

Etiology

The etiology of sarcoidosis is not known.

Clinical Presentation

Cutaneous manifestations appear in 25% of adults diagnosed with sarcoidosis; the incidence of skin findings has not been demonstrated in children.[61,62] Sarcoidosis of the skin often presents as yellow-brown to red flat-topped papules, infiltrated plaques, and/or nodules. Lesions adopt a classic "apple-jelly" color on diascopy, and may or may not present with scale. The distribution of the rash favors the face, nares, lips, and eyelids, but may also occur in sites of trauma. Older children and adolescents are most commonly affected by these classic findings.[25]

Systemic findings, such as fever and weight loss, may precede the development of the rash. Of note, 50% of pediatric patients experience ophthalmologic involvement (eg, anterior segment chorioretinitis, uveitis, or keratitis).[63]

Children younger than school age experience a relapsing-remitting course and have been found to exhibit polyarthritis, severe uveitis, parotid gland involvement,

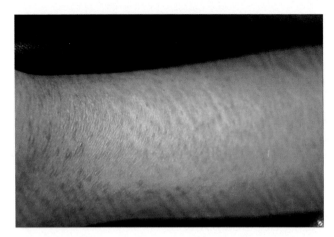

FIGURE 5-18. Blau syndrome: Monomorphous red-brown papules widespread on a forearm. Courtesy of Lisa Arkin, MD.

peripheral neuropathy, synovial thickening of the wrists and fingers, and an absence of pulmonary findings.

Blau syndrome, or early-onset sarcoidosis, is an autosomal dominant autoinflammatory disorder instigated by a mutation in the *CARD15* gene. Blau syndrome typically manifests prior to 4 years of age. It presents as generalized erythematous papules and plaques, iritis, arthritis, synovial cysts, and camptodactyly (ie, congenital flexural contractures) (Figure 5-18). Because of its generalized, erythematous papular morphology, Blau syndrome is frequently misdiagnosed as atopic dermatitis or ichthyosis depending on the extent of desquamation. The classic triad of skin eruption, arthritis, and uveitis is seen in only 42% of these patients.[64] Children with this syndrome carry an increased risk for the development of Crohn syndrome. As such, special care should be taken to elicit new-onset gastrointestinal symptoms. Erythromycin, used for its anti-inflammatory properties, constitutes first-line treatment. Therapeutic escalation to methotrexate or tumor necrosis factor α inhibitors can be considered for refractory patients.[25]

Histologic Findings

The granulomas of cutaneous sarcoidosis are characterized by dense, uniform, discrete aggregates of epithelioid histiocytes with minimal surrounding lymphocytic inflammation (Figure 5-19A). They present in the superficial and deep dermis, and may involve the subcutis (Figure 5-19B). Multinucleate giant cells are often present, and may demonstrate calcium inclusions (Schaumann bodies), PAS-positive inclusions (Hamazaki-Wesenberg bodies), or pink star-shaped intracytoplasmic "asteroid" bodies, the latter of which is not specific for sarcoid, and can be seen in granulomatous infections.[65,66] An interstitial granulomatous form of cutaneous sarcoidosis has also been reported in the pediatric age group.[67]

Differential Diagnosis

Foreign body granulomas, particularly silica granulomas or tattoo reactions, may mimic sarcoidal granulomas

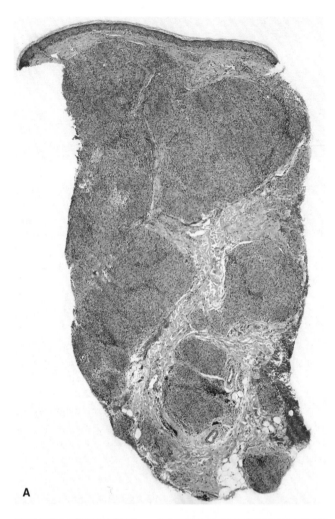

A

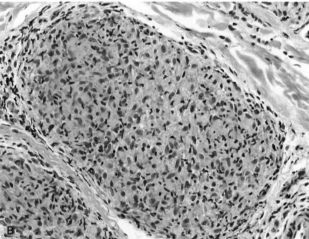

B

FIGURE 5-19. Sarcoidosis histopathology: well-formed granulomas, without significant surrounding or interstitial inflammation (**A**). High-power view of dense lymphohistiocytic granuloma (**B**).

histologically, but foreign material may also be a nidus for cutaneous granuloma formation in cases of sarcoidosis.[68] Infection from tuberculosis, leprosy, and fungus must be excluded, as all can present with granulomatous reactions.

Crohn disease, granulomatous rosacea, and granulomatous drug reactions should also be considered in the histologic differential diagnosis of sarcoidosis.

CAPSULE SUMMARY

SARCOIDOSIS

Sarcoidal granulomas present as discrete aggregates dermal of histiocytes, with minimal surrounding inflammation. An evaluation for infection and foreign material should be performed.

IDIOPATHIC FACIAL ASEPTIC GRANULOMA

Definition and Epidemiology

A new and incompletely understood clinical entity, idiopathic facial aseptic granuloma (IFAG) presents as an inflammatory nodule on the cheek of a young child. Case series indicate that IFAG is a disease of early childhood with an average age of onset of 4 years. IFAG typically affects otherwise healthy children and has not been associated with any medical conditions.[69]

Etiology

The underlying etiology for IFAG is controversial. Hypotheses include an inflammatory reaction to an arthropod bite, granulomatous response to an embryologic remnant, or a presentation of childhood rosacea. In a prospective series of 38 children with IFAG, 42% had other signs of rosacea including flushing, papulopustular eruption, or recurrent chalazions.[69]

Clinical Presentation

IFAG classically presents as a solitary, nontender, erythematous to violaceous nodule measuring 0.5 to 2 cm in diameter most commonly found on the cheeks or eyelids (Figure 5-20). Most nodules are minimally inflamed and nontender. The nonspecific clinical morphology often prompts a broad differential diagnosis including pilomatricoma, epidermoid or dermoid cyst, infection (bacterial, fungal or atypical mycobacterium), Spitz nevi, or an infantile hemangioma. IFAGs typically resolve over many months without residual scarring. Ultrasounds are frequently obtained during the diagnostic workup. Although the classic sonographic appearance of this condition is of a well-demarcated, cystic, hypoechoic lesion without calcium deposits, other cases have been found to have ill-defined and irregular appearances.[70,71]

Histologic Findings

The histologic features of IFAG are generally nonspecific, with most cases demonstrating a dense mixed dermal infiltrate of lymphocytes, multinucleate histiocytes, and plasma

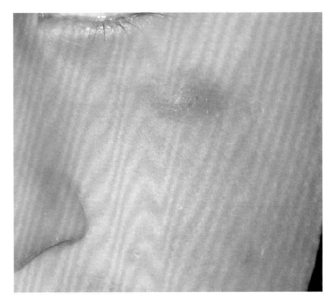

FIGURE 5-20. Idiopathic facial aseptic granuloma: pink to violaceous subcutaneous nodule on the cheek of a young boy. Courtesy of Anna Bruckner, MD.

cells, with variable acute neutrophilic and eosinophilic inflammation (Figure 5-21).[71] Lymphocytic folliculitis and perifolliculitis are often noted. True granulomas may be present, and there is occasionally frank abscess formation. Special stains and culture for microorganisms are negative, and no polarizable foreign material is present.

Differential Diagnosis

Granulomatous rosacea is the major histologic mimic; indeed, many authors consider IFAG to be a variant of childhood rosacea.[72] Ruptured cyst and infectious abscess can be excluded by histologic examination and special staining, respectively.

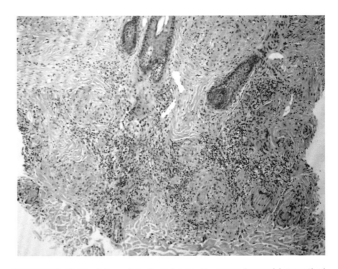

FIGURE 5-21. Idiopathic facial aseptic granuloma histopathology: Granulomatous inflammation in the superficial and middermis, with focal perifollicular inflammation.

CAPSULE SUMMARY

IDIOPATHIC FACIAL ASEPTIC GRANULOMA

IFAG is likely a variant of granulomatous rosacea in childhood and demonstrates variable nonspecific histologic features of mixed lymphohistiocytic inflammation, folliculitis, and granuloma formation.

CHILDHOOD GRANULOMATOUS PERIORIFICIAL DERMATITIS

Definition

Childhood granulomatous periorificial dermatitis (CGPD), previously termed "facial Afro-Caribbean childhood eruption," is a self-limited papular eruption of facial granulomatous lesions.

Etiology

CGPD is believed to be an uncommon variant of perioral dermatitis and may exist on a continuum with rosacea. Topical fluorinated corticosteroids are the most well-known triggers, but allergic or irritant contactants such as essential oils and formaldehyde have also been associated.[73,74]

Epidemiology

CGPD tends to occur in prepubertal children and slightly favors male over female patients.[75]

Clinical Presentation

Initially described in 1970,[75] CGPD is a self-limited eruption best characterized by erythematous papules, pustules, or papulovesicles in conjunction with diffuse facial erythema (Figure 5-22). The lesions tend to concentrate around the mouth, nares, and eyes and may heal with scarring. Extrafacial lesions are known to occur in severe cases.[76] Patients should be questioned on topical or inhaled corticosteroid use since it is a known precipitating factor.

Histologic Features

Periorificial dermatitis presents histologically with perivascular and perifollicular chronic inflammation, dilation of dermal blood vessels, papillary dermal edema, and follicular hyperkeratosis.[73] In the granulomatous form, the perifollicular inflammation is more pronounced and granulomatous, with lymphocytes and multinucleate histiocytes forming aggregates or small nodules in the dermis (Figure 5-23).[77] The stains for microorganisms are negative.

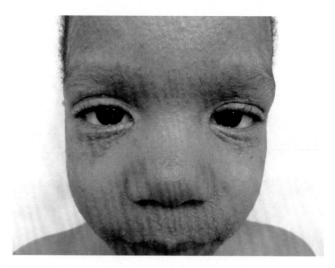

FIGURE 5-22. Childhood granulomatous periorificial dermatitis: Numerous erythematous monomorphous papules widespread on the face and concentrated around the mouth, alar creases, and eyes.

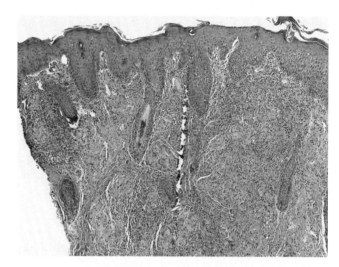

FIGURE 5-23. Childhood granulomatous periorificial dermatitis histopathology: Intradermal granulomatous infiltrate associated with lymphocytes and scattered multinucleated giant cells. The epidermis exhibits acanthosis, spongiosis, and confluent parakeratosis.

Differential Diagnosis

Granulomatous rosacea and IFAG present with similar histologic features to granulomatous periorificial dermatitis. Some authors consider granulomatous periorificial dermatitis to represent a manifestation of childhood lupus miliaris disseminatus faciei.[78] Clinical correlation is necessary to make a definitive diagnosis, as these entities likely have similar pathogeneses.[74] Other granulomatous inflammatory infiltrates, including foreign body reactions, ruptured cysts or follicles, cutaneous sarcoidosis, drug reactions, and infection should also be considered.

CHILDHOOD GRANULOMATOUS PERIORIFICIAL DERMATITIS

The histologic features of granulomatous periorificial dermatitis are similar to those seen in granulomatous rosacea and IFAG, with perifollicular granulomatous and chronic inflammation, and lack of infectious organisms.

FOREIGN BODY GRANULOMA

Definition and Epidemiology

Foreign body granuloma is an inflammatory response to an exogenous or endogenous element. A foreign body granuloma may occur at any stage of life.

Etiology

A foreign body granuloma represents a chronic inflammatory reaction as activated macrophages attempt to sequester indigestible inorganic or persistent organic material. In children, common provoking materials include keratin, suture, arthropod parts, graphite, tattoo ink, or organic plant materials such as wood splinters.[79]

Clinical Presentation

Foreign body granulomas can develop at any body site. Red to brown papules, nodules or plaques can develop at the site of the foreign material weeks to years later. Lesions may be firm to palpation as surrounding fibrosis develops; occasionally, ulceration or tracking fistulas can arise. The clinical differential diagnosis may include insect bite hypersensitivity reaction, cutaneous pseudolymphoma, or implantable infection such as atypical mycobacterium or subcutaneous (deep) fungus.

Histologic Features

Foreign body granulomas demonstrate foci of dense mixed inflammation, usually with numerous, multinucleate "giant cell" histiocytes (Figure 5-24). In foreign body granulomas from acute follicular or cyst rupture, neutrophilic inflammation may be prominent. Fragments of loose keratin or broken hair shafts are often present, and may be best visualized by dropping the microscope condenser. All granulomas should be examined with polarized light, although the offending foreign object may not be present in the planes of section submitted. An examination of deeper tissue levels may be revealing.

Differential Diagnosis

Dense acute inflammation should prompt a consideration of, and examination for, microorganisms. Acneiform

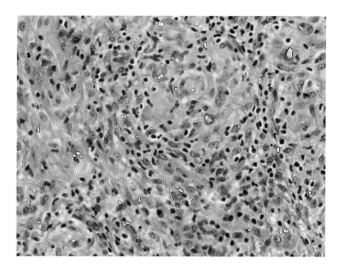

FIGURE 5-24. Foreign body granuloma histopathology: Granulomatous inflammation with multinucleate giant cells, and refractile-angulated foreign material (melamine particles used in ink from an "invisible" tattoo).

lesions, ruptured folliculitis, acne keloidalis nuchae, and other inflammatory disorders often present with small foreign body granulomas to the involved hair. In the case of injected or inoculated foreign material, the granulomatous inflammation may be present in the deep dermis or subcutis. GA, granulomatous drug eruptions, and sarcoidosis can present with similar features, but generally lack the prominent multinucleate forms classic in foreign body granulomas.

FOREIGN BODY GRANULOMA

Foreign body granulomas show dense mixed acute and chronic inflammation with multinucleate histiocytes, and variable findings on polarized light examination.

MELKERSSON-ROSENTHAL SYNDROME, GRANULOMATOUS CHEILITIS, AND CUTANEOUS CROHN DISEASE

Definition

First described in 1931, Melkersson-Rosenthal syndrome (MRS) denotes the triad of recurrent facial nerve palsy, granulomatous cheilitis and facial swelling, and tongue plication (fissured tongue).[80]

Etiology

The etiology of MRS is unknown; there is no known genetic, infectious, or allergic origin, although some argue that the presence of orofacial herpes in some cases points to a role for herpes simplex virus in the development of the disease.[81]

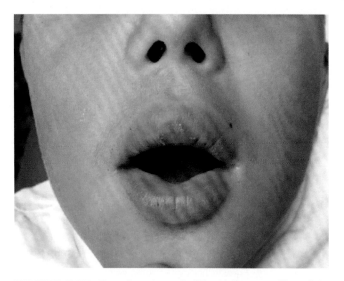

FIGURE 5-25. Granulomatous cheilitis: Uniform swelling of the upper and lower lip with mild swelling of the cheeks.

Epidemiology

Most cases of granulomatous cheilitis occur in isolation and without the other features of MRS. MRS is uncommon in childhood and more commonly occurs in the second and third decades of life, appearing rarely in childhood.[82]

Clinical Presentation

Of MRS's three defining symptoms, the most common is painless, uncommonly pruritic swelling of the upper lip, which occurs in 75% of cases.[83] Granulomatous cheilitis, in which labial swelling is attributed to nonnecrotizing granulomas, is considered to be a *forme fruste* of MRS (Figure 5-25). Corticosteroids in either oral, topical, or intralesional form are the first-line therapy for MRS.

Granulomatous cheilitis is also considered to be one presentation of orofacial granulomatosis (OFG), a clinical entity in which facial and/or labial swelling ensue from granulomatous inflammation in these areas. OFG can occur during

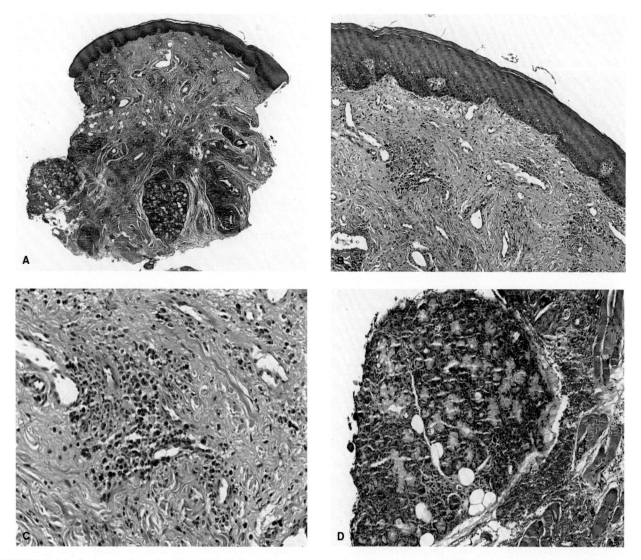

FIGURE 5-26. Granulomatous cheilitis: Early findings show a chronic lymphoplasmacytic infiltrate of the submucosa (**A**). Superficial telangiectasia is noted (**B**), in addition to a rich plasma cell infiltrate (**C**). Chronic inflammation of salivary gland tissue is also seen (**D**). Digital slides courtesy of Path Presenter.com.

both childhood and adolescence. Swelling to the lips may start intermittent but then becomes persistent. Importantly, granulomatous cheilitis maybe a cutaneous manifestation of Crohn disease or can predate the development of intestinal Crohn disease by years. An estimated 40% of children with OFG either have or go on to develop Crohn disease, necessitating an evaluation for underlying Crohn disease in children diagnosed with OFG.[84] Corticosteroids are again the first-line agent in the management of OFG, and alternative treatments include azathioprine, infliximab, and thalidomide.

Histologic Features

Granulomatous cheilitis often demonstrates subtle histologic features, with submucosal edema, telangiectasia, and chronic perivascular inflammation. Noncaseating lymphohistiocytic granulomas are usually present but may be sparse; as such, serial sectioning of tissue is recommended in cases where clinical suspicion for granulomatous cheilitis is high. The well-developed lesions of MRS typically have large, loosely formed granulomas, with an intralymphatic distribution (Figures 5-26 and 5-27).

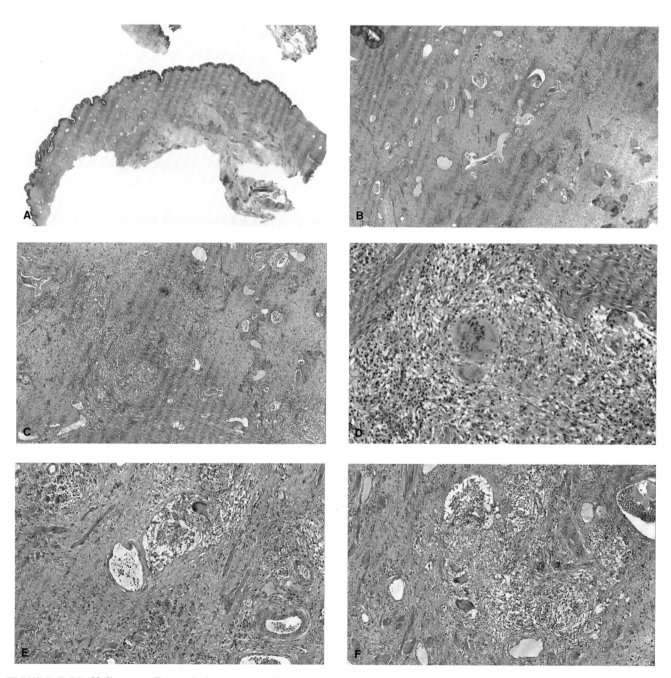

FIGURE 5-27. Melkersson-Rosenthal syndrome. There is a granulomatous dermatitis with telangiectasis (**A** and **B**). The poorly formed granulomata have frequent multinucleated giant cells (**C** and **D**). Many of them have an intralymphatic distribution (**E** and **F**).

Differential Diagnosis

Other granulomatous infiltrates, particularly those associated with granulomatous rosacea, cutaneous sarcoidosis, and cutaneous Crohn disease, may mimic the histologic features of granulomatous cheilitis.[85] These can usually be distinguished with appropriate clinical history, although it should be noted that granulomatous cheilitis may be an early clinical sign of both sarcoidosis and Crohn disease. Infections, including mucocutaneous leishmaniasis, and drug reactions should be excluded.[86]

CAPSULE SUMMARY

GRANULOMATOUS CHEILITIS

Granulomatous cheilitis presents histologically with edema and granulomatous inflammation of the mucosa, although granulomas may be sparse in some cases. Clinical correlation is required to exclude cutaneous sarcoidosis and Crohn disease.

CHRONIC GRANULOMATOUS DISEASE

Definition

Chronic granulomatous disease (CGD) is an immunodeficiency in phagocyte function typically inherited in X-linked recessive fashion.[87]

Etiology

CGD can be due to a mutation in one of the five genes (*p91phox, p47phox, p22phox, p67phox,* and *p40phox*) that make up the phagocytic NADPH-oxidase complex. A loss of function of this complex results in a dysfunctional respiratory burst, hampering intracellular killing of pathogens, most notably catalase-positive organisms that include many bacterial and fungal organisms. The most severe infections are due to *Aspergillus, S. aureus, Burkholderia (Pseudomonas) cepacia, Serratia marcescens,* and *Nocardia* species.[88]

Epidemiology

CGD is thought to affect roughly 1 in 500 000 individuals.[89] Because of its X-linked recessive inheritance pattern, it typically affects males. Most patients are diagnosed prior to 5 years of age, but CGD can present at any point between infancy and adulthood.

Clinical Presentation

CGD patients have a lifetime risk of recurrent infections typically affecting the skin, lung, liver, and lymph nodes (Figures 5-28 and 5-29). Cutaneous manifestations of CGD can be infectious or inflammatory in etiology. Early in life,

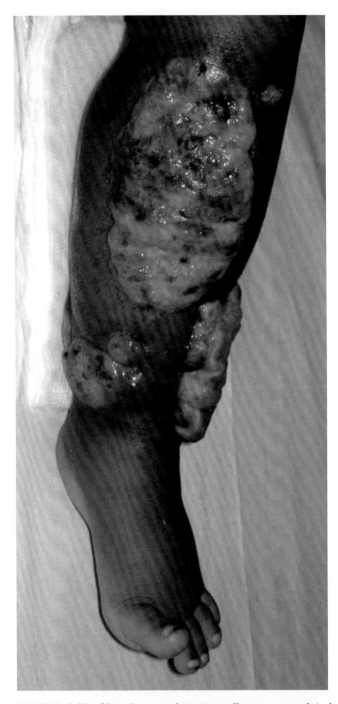

FIGURE 5-28. Chronic granulomatous disease–associated infection with aspergillus. Left leg, 2 burgeoning and suppurative tumors. Reprinted with permission from Khemiri M, El fekih N, Borgi A, Kharfi M, Boubaker S, Barsaoui S. Pseudotumoral cutaneous aspergillosis in chronic granulomatous disease, report of a pediatric case. *Am J Dermatopathol.* 2012;34(7):749-752.

cutaneous infections may present as recurrent or persistent furuncles or abscesses involving the face and perianal area, pyoderma overlying infected lymph nodes, impetigo, and ecthyma. Inflammatory cutaneous manifestations in CGD include seborrheic dermatitis-like eruptions, discoid

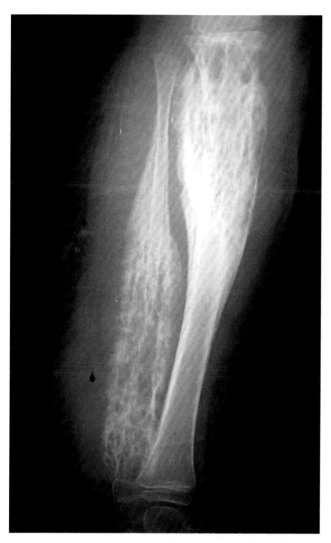

FIGURE 5-29. Chronic granulomatous disease–associated infection with aspergillus. Left leg radiograph, multiple lytic lesions of fibula and tibia. Reprinted with permission from Khemiri M, El fekih N, Borgi A, Kharfi M, Boubaker S, Barsaoui S. Pseudotumoral cutaneous aspergillosis in chronic granulomatous disease, report of a pediatric case. *Am J Dermatopathol.* 2012;34(7):749-752.

lupus-like rashes, and Sweet syndrome.[90] Cutaneous findings in CGD appear to be attenuated by prophylaxis with trimethoprim-sulfamethoxazole.[91]

Histologic Findings

The cutaneous lesions of CGD demonstrate similar histologic features to those seen in other organs, with noncaseating granuloma formation, mixed chronic inflammation, and variable abscess formation. Pigment-laden macrophages, a hallmark feature in the gastrointestinal tract and other organs, are also often present in cutaneous lesions.[92] Biopsies from affected patients may also demonstrate other cutaneous lesions associated with CGD, including pyoderma gangrenosum, lupus-like lesions, and infectious abscesses.[93,94]

Differential Diagnosis

Infectious organisms, particularly unusual bacterial species or fungus, may be present in the skin lesions of CGD, with or without granulomas. Cutaneous Crohn disease may also demonstrate similar histologic features, with dermal granulomatous and mixed chronic inflammation. The presence of pigment-laden macrophages is helpful in distinguishing CGD, but may not be present in all cases.

CAPSULE SUMMARY

CHRONIC GRANULOMATOUS DISEASE

CGD commonly manifests with a variety of cutaneous lesions and may demonstrate infectious and granulomatous features histologically.

SYSTEMIC SCLEROSIS AND MORPHEA

Definition and Epidemiology

Juvenile systemic sclerosis (JSSc) and morphea (localized scleroderma) are sclerotic disorders of the skin. JSSc is an uncommon diagnosis in childhood. Its localized counterpart, morphea, is more commonly encountered in children. Morphea is estimated to affect 2.7 cases per million children in the United Kingdom and Ireland.[95] A predilection for females was reported, and the mean age of onset was 8 years, whereas mean age at presentation was 10 years.

Etiology

The precise etiology of JSSc and morphea is unknown. The disease process appears to hinge on uncontrolled extracellular matrix synthesis and deposition, immune activation, and endothelial trauma.[96]

Clinical Presentation

Morphea is differentiated from systemic sclerosis on principally clinical grounds. The former process tends not to present with such characteristic SS symptoms as sclerodactyly, Raynaud's phenomenon, and nailfold capillary changes, and evinces localized, as opposed to diffuse, cutaneous involvement.[97] Lesions typically begin in inflammatory fashion, presenting with erythematous or violaceous patches or plaques, the center of which whiten and thicken over time. As the lesions evolve, the plaques become completely sclerotic, effacing adnexal structures in the area of involvement, with variable pigmentary changes.[98]

Morphea is classically divided into five subclassifications: plaque-type (circumscribed), generalized, bullous, linear, and deep.[99] Linear morphea occurs at higher rates in children than adults, and often presents in a horizontal orientation on the trunk and vertical on extremities.

Linear morphea involving the face, most commonly the forehead, is termed *"en coup de sabre"* (Figure 5-30). The segmental patterning of linear morphea can be reminiscent of a Blaschkoid distribution. Sequelae of linear morphea include an atrophy of underlying muscle and bone, growth defects of affected extremities, and contractures if the process traverses a joint space. Progressive hemifacial atrophy, or Parry-Romberg syndrome, occurs within the first two decades of life and with or without the cutaneous changes of localized scleroderma. The atrophy of Parry-Romberg may extend to the bone and cartilage, and it is associated with a wide variety of neurologic sequelae, including paresthesias, epilepsy, and trigeminal neuralgia.[100]

In plaque morphea, patients present with up to three indurate plaques of variable depth most commonly affecting the trunk.[97] Generalized disease represents a progression of plaque morphea, in which patients present with more than four lesions involving less than two body sites excluding the face and hands. This variant is less common in children than adults. Pansclerotic morphea is a disabling, rapidly progressive subtype that most commonly occurs in females aged 1 to 14 and commonly involves tissue layers from the epidermis to the bone. The distribution of cutaneous lesions may

be similar to generalized morphea, whereas visceral involvement has been reported in the esophagus, muscles, lymph nodes, heart, and lungs. Prognosis is poor, and the disease is often refractory to treatment.[101]

Deep morphea is defined by sclerosis involving the deep dermis and subcutaneous fat. Patients may present with hard, bound-down plaques. Bullous morphea is the rarest variant, characterized by bullae within plaques of morphea. As the morphea subtypes occur on a continuum, an overlap of different subtypes within the same patient is not uncommon.

In general, morphea is an inflammatory sclerotic disease that typically lasts several years. Treatment focuses on targeting active inflammation to minimize disease progression. Limited disease involvement may be treated with topical or intralesional corticosteroids, topical calcineurin inhibitors, or calcipotriene. Severe disease with a risk of disfigurement or functional limitation may be treated with phototherapy (NB-UVB, UVA), systemic corticosteroids, methotrexate, and mycophenolate mofetil.

JSSc is a multisystem connective tissue disease in which sclerosis can impact the skin, lung, esophagus, intestine, heart, and kidneys. JSSc is typically diagnosed on clinical grounds; proximal skin sclerosis/induration is required, and may be attended by a number of cutaneous (sclerodactyly, Raynaud's phenomenon, digital ulcers) and extracutaneous (dysphagia, gastroesophageal reflux, pulmonary fibrosis or hypertension, neuropathy, carpal tunnel syndrome, arthritis, myositis) symptoms. Constitutional symptoms such as fatigue and weight loss may predominate during the first 3 to 5 years of the patient's course, which are often the most severe. Serologic markers for the disease include antinuclear antigen, anticentromere, antitopoisomerase-I (Scl-70), antifibrillarin, anti-PMScl, antifibrillin, or anti-RNA polymerase I or III antibodies.[102] A recent study characterized by the subtle clinical differences between JSSc patients and their adult-onset counterparts, finding a significantly higher incidence of overlap syndromes and rate of survival in the latter group, along with a significantly lower propensity for diffuse cutaneous disease.[103]

Histologic Findings

The cutaneous lesions of systemic sclerosis and localized cutaneous sclerosis (morphea) are histologically indistinguishable. Both are characterized by a sclerosis of collagen throughout the dermis. Collagen bundles appear thickened, eosinophilic, and densely packed (Figure 5-31). There is a paucity of normal adnexal structures, and those present appear "trapped" in the sclerotic collagen bundles. Eccrine units are often noted high in the dermis, with loss of their normal peri-eccrine fat "pads". There is sharp demarcation at the dermal-subcutaneous junction, with an infiltrate of plasma cells in this area. In deep morphea or "morphea profunda", the sclerosis involves the subcutaneous fat septae, with variable amounts of sclerosis in the dermis. In early or

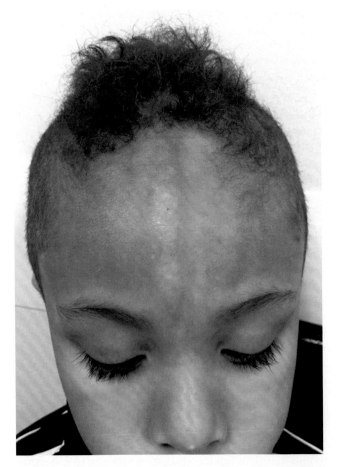

FIGURE 5-30. En coup de sabre: Linear shiny, white, firm plaque extending from frontal scalp to glabella with violaceous rim.

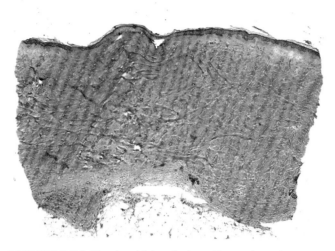

FIGURE 5-31. Morphea histopathology: Dense dermal sclerosis with a loss of adnexal structures and sharp demarcation at the dermal-subcutaneous junction.

inflammatory morphea, perivascular lymphocytic inflammation is present in the superficial dermis.[104] Many cases of morphea demonstrate features of lichen sclerosus (LS) in the overlying epidermis and papillary dermis.[105]

Differential Diagnosis

Scars and other fibrotic disorders may be mistaken for morphea, but usually show more fascicled collagen bundles with associated arcuate and vertically aligned vessels along with reactive interstitial fibroblasts. In contrast, the specimens of morphea demonstrate more striking dense sclerosis without interstitial inflammation. Chronic EN may also be considered in the differential diagnosis of morphea profunda, but demonstrates more septal inflammation, often with some associated inflammation in the adjacent fat lobule. Eosinophilic fasciitis (EF) may be difficult to distinguish from morphea profunda histologically, but has been reported to demonstrate more eosinophilic inflammation (in both the peripheral blood and lesional tissue) and focal loss of CD34 staining.[106]

CAPSULE SUMMARY

SYSTEMIC SCLEROSIS AND MORPHEA

Morphea demonstrates thick sclerotic collagen throughout the dermis, with a lack of adnexal structures, sharp dermal-subcutaneous demarcation, and variable plasma cells in the deep dermis.

EOSINOPHILIC FASCIITIS

Definition and Epidemiology

EF is characterized by initial inflammation and subsequent sclerosis of the deep subcutaneous tissue and fascia.[107]

Etiology

The pathogenesis of EF is unknown, although it has been reported in response to a wide variety of triggers, including exercise, infection, or autoimmune/hematologic disorders. The majority of cases are idiopathic.[108]

EF is exceedingly rare in childhood, with less than 50 reported cases. A comparison between EF's childhood and adult forms shows a female predilection in the latter (75% as opposed to 37%).[109,110]

Clinical Presentation

EF commonly presents as acute, symmetric induration of the extremities generally sparing the hands and feet. The overlying skin may be erythematous and adopt a puckered or "*peau d'orange texture*". As the disease progresses, the skin becomes bound down and a "groove sign", indentation along veins due to underlying deep sclerosis, becomes apparent (Figure 5-32). Sclerodactyly, a characteristic feature of systemic sclerosis, is notably absent in EF. Patients commonly complain of myalgias or arthralgias, and contractures can develop. A polyclonal gammopathy can be present along with peripheral eosinophilia in the early phase of the disease. Magnetic resonance imaging (MRI) can be useful to confirm fascial inflammation. A deep incisional biopsy extending down to the fascia is typically needed for histopathologic confirmation.[111,112] Common first-line treatments include systemic glucocorticoids, although recent literature in adult patients indicate improved rates of clinical improvement with the combination of systemic steroids and methotrexate.[113,114]

Histologic Findings

Markedly thickened and sclerotic fascia is the hallmark histologic feature of EF. In early disease, edema and mixed inflammation with lymphocytes, histiocytes, plasma cells, and eosinophils are present, and the fascia may demonstrate degenerative changes and necrosis. In more established

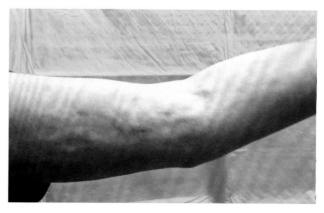

FIGURE 5-32. Eosinophilic fasciitis: Bound down thickening of the upper arm with a pseudo-cellulite appearance and depressions along veins consistent with the groove sign.

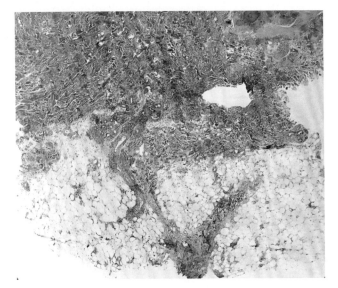

FIGURE 5-33. Eosinophilic fasciitis histopathology: Thickened and hylanized collagen bundles throughout the reticular dermis and a perivascular infiltrate of lymphocytes and plasma cells at the junction between the lower reticular dermis and subcutis.

lesions, sclerosis is prominent, and dense lymphocytic inflammation resembling lymphoid follicles is common. The sclerotic changes extend to involve the subcutaneous fat septae, causing the entrapment of aggregates of lipocytes at the subcutaneous-fascial junction (Figure 5-33). Dense fibrosis and/or sclerosis, eccrine gland atrophy, and other morphea-like changes are often present in the dermis.

Differential Diagnosis

The dermal and subcutaneous changes may mimic morphea or morphea profunda, although the presence of eosinophils and the focal loss of CD34 staining has been reported to be more supportive of EF.[106] If eosinophilic inflammation is prominent, an arthropod bite reaction or reaction to injected medication should be considered.

CAPSULE SUMMARY

EOSINOPHILIC FASCIITIS

EF is characterized by prominent fascial thickening and sclerosis, associated with mixed inflammation, fascial necrosis, and characteristic changes of the overlying dermis and subcutis.

NEPHROGENIC SYSTEMIC FIBROSIS

Definition and Epidemiology

Nephrogenic systemic fibrosis (NSF) is a multisystem fibrosing disorder occurring in patients with renal failure, most often in the context of gadolinium-based contrast administration during MRI procedures. NSF is an exceedingly rare entity in children, with only 10 extant cases in the English-language literature.[115] There is no known gender, ethnic, or age predilection.[116]

Etiology

The pathogenesis of NSF is not known; it is theorized that gadolinium-based agents provoke an aberrant, exuberant wound-healing response in patients unable to clear the drug characterized by myofibroblast dysregulation.[117,118]

Clinical Presentation

NSF presents as symmetric indurated to bound down nodules and plaques typically involving the distal extremities and advancing proximally. Similar to other deep cutaneous sclerosing disorders, the skin may adopt a "cobblestone" or *peau d'orange* appearance. Contractures can subsequently develop. Fibrotic changes to the lungs, pleura, pericardium and myocardium, and dura mater have been described. Most cases of NSF start 2 to 4 weeks after gadolinium exposure, but NSF has been reported years afterward.

NSF often takes a chronic and unremitting course, and there is no known medical therapy of proven efficacy. UVA phototherapy, extracorporeal photopheresis, and renal transplantation have all been utilized in the treatment of this disease, although a strong evidence of efficacy remains forthcoming.[119]

Histologic Findings

Few cases of NSF have been reported in children, but they appear to demonstrate similar histologic features to those seen in adults.[116,120] The most reproducible findings are thickened collagen bundles with surrounding clefts, a proliferation of CD34-positive dermal spindle cells, and increased stromal mucin. In early lesions, the spindle cells are numerous and diffuse, intercalating between thickened dermal collagen bundles. In later lesions, the spindle cells are sparse, and the mucin deposition and collagen clefting less pronounced. Increased numbers of elastic fibers, oriented parallel to the epidermal surface, may be highlighted with elastic fiber staining. Inflammation is usually minimal in NSF, although cases demonstrating more impressive inflammation, multinucleate histiocytes, unique sclerotic bodies, and granulomatous inflammation have been reported.[121,122] Iron deposition within dermal fibrocytes is also considered a useful diagnostic tool.[123]

Differential Diagnosis

The spindle cell proliferation present in NSF may prompt a consideration of CD34-positive dermal tumors of the pediatric age group, including giant cell fibroblastoma, CD34+ dermal dendrocytic hamartoma (so-called medallion tumor), and dermatofibrosarcoma protuberans. These tumors lack the characteristic mucin deposition and collagen clefting seen in NSF.

LICHEN SCLEROSUS

Definition and Epidemiology

LS is a chronic inflammatory disorder resulting in epithelial thinning, principally involving the anogenital area. LS is known for bimodal peaks of incidence in prepubertal girls and postmenopausal women, with a mean age of onset of 5.4 years in the former group.[124]

Etiology

The etiology of LS is not known—mechanisms ranging from local vulvar factors, low estrogen levels, autoimmune dysregulation, and infection (ie, *Borrelia burgdorferi*) have been variously implicated.

Clinical Presentation

The majority of patients with LS are young girls with involvement of the genitalia; extragenital involvement may occur, but is uncommon. Vulvar LS presents with ivory-white, atrophic papules coalescing to plaques frequently involving the labia and occasionally extending down the perineum and around the anus in a "figure of 8 pattern." Vulvar LS in young girls often results in chronic vulvar pruritus, burning, dysuria, or constipation because of stool-withholding behavior.[125] Vulvar LS can occasionally present with bullae, erosions, or hemorrhagic purpura and in these cases may be mistaken for physical signs of sexual abuse. Extragenital LS occurs in a minority of patients with vulvar LS and is very uncommon in children. The common sites of extragenital LS include the back, shoulders, neck, thighs, and inframammary areas (Figure 5-34). Neoplastic transformation in pediatric vulvar LS is exceedingly uncommon, but rare reports of vulvar melanoma have been described.[126] It is important to emphasize that melanocytic nevi in association with LS can be easily confused with melanoma (Figure 5-35).

Ultra-high potency topical corticosteroids constitute first-line therapy. Recent guidelines from the European Academy of Dermatology and Venerology underscore the need for maintenance therapy, such as lower potency

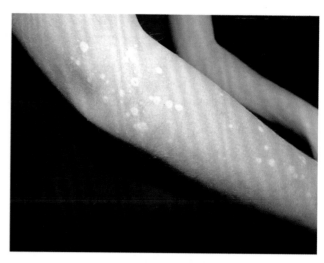

FIGURE 5-34. Lichen sclerosus, clinical findings. The presence of numerous 2 to 4 mm, mostly perifollicular, hypopigmented, slightly atrophic papules on the bilateral upper extremities. A central hyperkeratotic plug is noted in some of the lesions. Reprinted with permission from El Habr C, Mannava K, Koch S, et al. Folliculocentric lichen sclerosus et atrophicus in a 10-year-old girl. *Am J Dermatopathol.* 2017;39(1):59-61.

topical corticosteroids or topical calcineurin inhibitors, to prevent long-term complications.[127-129]

Histologic Findings

LS has very distinct and diagnostic histologic features. The hallmark of this disorder histologically is homogenized and often pallorous papillary dermal collagen associated with epidermal atrophy and overlying compact hyperkeratosis (Figure 5-36). The hyperkeratosis is often much thicker than the entire epidermis. Follicular plugging is a common feature. A perivascular band-like lymphocytic infiltrate is present in the superficial dermis, just beneath the focus of homogenized collagen. Telangiectatic vessels are also present. Bullous and folliculocentric variants are less common presentations.[130,131] Genital melanocytic nevi arising in a background of LS are very difficult to interpret because of the extent of atypia that such lesions can manifest including stromal changes misinterpreted as representing regression (Figure 5-37).

Differential Diagnosis

The biopsies of localized scleroderma (morphea) may demonstrate LS changes of the epidermis and superficial dermis, with more classic features of morphea in the deep dermis. As such, the conditions may be difficult to distinguish in superficial skin samples. Scar and other fibrotic disorders can be confused with LS; they are distinguished by the presence of dermal fibrosis rather than pallor and edema of the collagen, vertically aligned rather than dilated vessels, and the presence of reactive fibroblasts and chronic interstitial inflammation in the former.

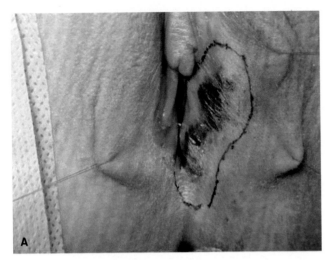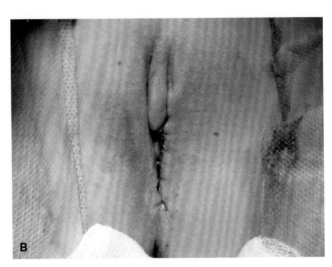

FIGURE 5-35. Lichen sclerosus (LS) and atypical melanocytic nevus in the genital area. A, Preoperative aspect of the vulvar lesion: variegated tan-brown to speckled black nevus on a background of LS. The lesion measured approximately 4 × 2 cm, started on the left inner labia, and had grown significantly over 3 months. It extended inferiorly, crossed over the vaginal introitus, and incorporated the inferior third of the right labia minora. **B,** Two-month follow-up visit showing a near-complete healing of surgery site, no evidence of local recurrence, and no signs of LS. Reprinted with permission from Pinto A, Mclaren SH, Poppas DP, Magro CM. Genital melanocytic nevus arising in a background of lichen sclerosus in a 7-year-old female: the diagnostic pitfall with malignant melanoma. A literature review. *Am J Dermatopathol.* 2012;34(8):838-843.

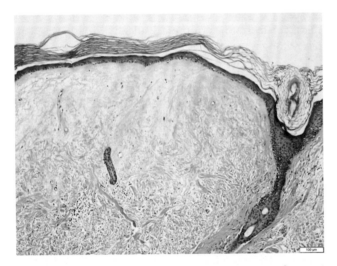

FIGURE 5-36. Lichen sclerosus histopathology: Compact hyperkeratosis, follicular plugging, epidermal atrophy, papillary dermal pallor, and homogenization. There is only scant dermal inflammation in this case.

CAPSULE SUMMARY

LICHEN SCLEROSUS

LS presents histologically with thick compact hyperkeratosis, follicular plugging, epidermal atrophy, homogenized papillary dermal collagen, band-like dermal lymphocytic inflammation, and telangiectatic vessels.

CYTOPHAGIC HISTIOCYTIC PANNICULITIS

Definition and Epidemiology

CHP was originally described by Crotty and Winkelmann in 1981[38] as a form of panniculitis with the infiltration of subcutaneous adipose tissue by benign-appearing T-cells and phagocytic histiocytes ("bean bag cells"). Only on rare occasions has this disease been reported in children.[132,133]

Etiology

CHP may be an isolated skin disease or associated with nonmalignant conditions, such as infections, as well as malignancies, including SPTCL, a rare form of non-Hodgkin lymphoma infiltrating into the subcutaneous adipose tissue. Subcutaneous panniculitis has been reported in a small number of patients with hemophagocytic lymphohistiocytosis (HLH), a life-threatening condition characterized by uncontrolled activation and proliferation of T-cells resulting in hypercytokinemia, proliferation of histiocytes, and hemophagocytosis.[134,135] The familial form of HLH (FHL) is a genetically heterogeneous disorder caused by mutations in genes involved in the granule-dependent exocytosis pathway.[136] The association between HLH and viral infections, such as EBV and cytomegalovirus, has been strongly established.[137,138]

Clinical Presentation

The lesions are more commonly plaques or nodules of varying sizes, discrete or that coalesce to form large indurates plaques of up to 20 cm in diameter. The lesions are present

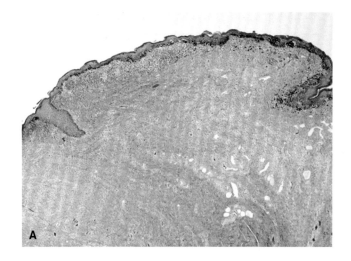
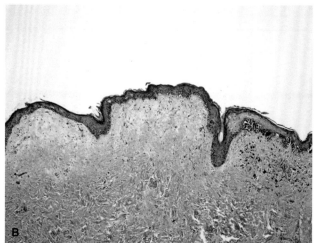
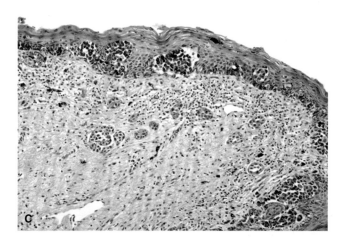
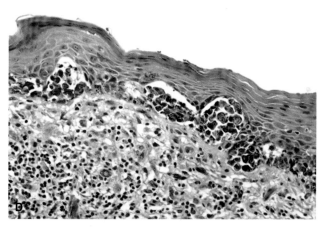

FIGURE 5-37. Lichen sclerosus (LS) and atypical melanocytic nevus in the genital area. Low-power view of the lesion showing zones of intermediate to high-density lentiginous and nested growth of melanocytes, with concomitant epidermal attenuation. There is a supervening band-like lymphocytic infiltrate. This low-power architecture is very worrisome for a significantly atypical melanocytic proliferation based on the alteration of the epidermal architecture, the density of proliferation, and supervening inflammation (**A**). Subepidermal fibrosis with patchy lymphocytic infiltration is seen, characteristic of LS (**B**). The cells are disposed singly and in nests along the attenuated epidermis. Pagetoid ascent of rare atypical melanocytes can be seen (**C** and **D**). Reprinted with permission from Pinto A, Mclaren SH, Poppas DP, Magro CM. Genital melanocytic nevus arising in a background of lichen sclerosus in a 7-year-old female: the diagnostic pitfall with malignant melanoma. a literature review. *Am J Dermatopathol.* 2012;34(8):838-843.

in the extremities, trunk, breasts, shoulders, neck, and face. The skin can be pink-colored, or erythematous, violaceous, bluish purple, purpuric, ecchymotic, or hyperpigmented. The lesions can be flat or raised, discrete or ill-defined, and can be soft or indurated. The lesions can be single or in crops, and persist for a few weeks to months (Figure 5-38).

Patients with systemic HLH can have a variety of clinical manifestations that range from fever, generalized malaise, weight loss, hepatosplenomegaly, lymphadenopathy, multiple effusions, etc. The characteristic laboratory data is the presence of anemia (with a marked elevation of ferritin levels), liver dysfunction, a coagulopathy, and hypertriglyceridemia.[39,139]

Histologic Findings

There is a mixed septal and lobular panniculitis containing a rich infiltrate of histiocytes and lymphocytes.[39,134,139] Plasma cells, eosinophils, and neutrophils can also be present. The more characteristic features are the histiocytes between and around the adipocytes with a variable amount of fat necrosis. Extravasation of erythrocytes, frank hemorrhage, erythrophagocytosis (or a phagocytosis of leukocytes, platelets, and nuclear debris) by histiocytes, and vascular changes (edema, intimal proliferation, thickened arterioles, fibrinoid necrosis, etc) are typical of CHP. The erythrophagocytosis is more prominent in the adipose tissue, particularly within the edematous stroma or septal

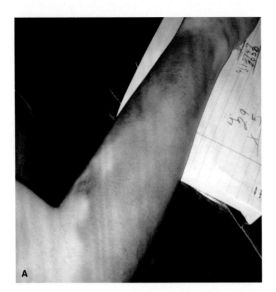
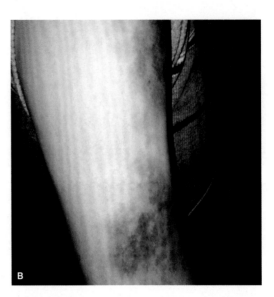

FIGURE 5-38. **Cytophagic histiocytic panniculitis. A** and **B,** The clinical findings in this case include the presence of indurated plaques with marked hemorrhage. In this particular case, presenting in an adolescent, the clinical concern was of familial abuse.

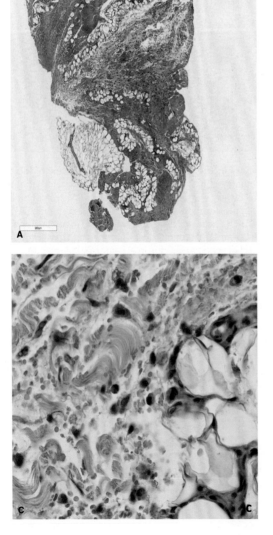
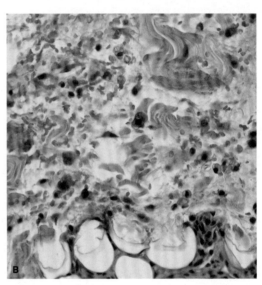

FIGURE 5-39. **Cytophagic histiocytic panniculitis (CHP)—histopathology.** There is a mixed septal and lobular chronic inflammatory infiltrate with edema and hemorrhage (**A**). The classic finding in CHP is the presence of histiocytes engulfing red blood cells ('bean bag cells') (**B** and **C**).

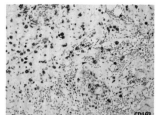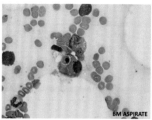

FIGURE 55-40. Cytophagic histiocytic panniculitis—histopathology. CD163 is positive among the histiocytes with erythrophagocytosis. The bone marrow (BM) aspirate slide shows the typical presence of hemophagocytosis in a case associated with hemophagocytic lymphohistiocytosis.

areas. The "bean bag cells" are stuffed histiocytes with cells and nuclear debris. With time, the infiltrate becomes more chronic, with a predominance of lymphocytes (Figures 5-39A–C and 5-40) CHP. The histiocytes can be highlighted by a CD68 and CD163 IHC. Some cases can show a clonal population of T-cells.[132,140]

Differential Diagnosis

The differential diagnosis includes other forms of panniculitis (septal and lobular). However, a careful approach should be done to exclude the possibility of SPTCL and primary cutaneous gamma-delta T-cell lymphoma (both lymphoma subtypes with a predominant panniculitic appearance). SPTCL usually shows a dense atypical lymphocytic infiltrate with "rimming" of the adipocytes by the neoplastic cells. Its association with connective tissue disorders is quite characteristic. PCGDTCL is exceedingly rare in children. It is an aggressive lymphoma with a marked atypia of the neoplastic cells and the presence of malignant T-cells with a gamma/delta phenotype.

CAPSULE SUMMARY

CYTOPHAGIC HISTIOCYTIC PANNICULITIS

CHP is a form of panniculitis with an infiltration of subcutaneous adipose tissue by benign-appearing T-cells and phagocytic histiocytes ("bean bag cells").

REFERENCES

1. Labbé L, Perel Y, Maleville J, Taïeb A. Erythema nodosum in children: a study of 27 patients. *Pediatr Dermatol.* 1996;13(6):447-450.
2. Kakourou T, Drosatou P, Psychou F, Aroni K, Nicolaidou P. Erythema nodosum in children: a prospective study. *J Am Acad Dermatol.* 2001;44(1):17-21.
3. Requena L, Requena C. Erythema nodosum. *Dermatol Online J.* 2002;8(1):4.
4. Blaustein A, Moreno A, Noguera J, de Moragas JM. Septal granulomatous panniculitis in Sweet's syndrome: report of two cases. *Arch Dermatol.* 1985;121(6):785-788.
5. Wick MR. Panniculitis: A summary. *Semin Diagn Pathol.* 2017;34(3): 261-272.
6. Sakuma H, Niiyama S, Amoh Y, Katsuoka K. *Chlamydophila pneumoniae* infection induced nodular vasculitis. Case Rep Dermatol. 2011;3(3):263-267.
7. Campbell SM, Winkelmann RR, Sammons DL. Erythema induratum caused by Mycobacterium chelonei in an immunocompetent patient. *J Clin Aesthet Dermatol.* 2013;6(5):38.
8. Hattori M, Shimizu A, Hisada T, Fukumoto T, Ishikawa O. Erythema induratum in a patient with pulmonary Mycobacterium avium infection. *Acta Derm Venereol.* 2016;96(5):705-706.
9. Romero JJ, Herrera P, Cartelle M, Barba P, Tello S, Zurita J. Panniculitis caused by Mycobacterium monacense mimicking erythema induratum: a case in Ecuador. *New Microbes New Infect.* 2016;10:112-115.
10. Yus ES, Simon P. About the histopathology of erythema induratum-nodular vasculitis. *Am J Dermatopathol.* 1999;21:301-303.
11. Ferrara G, Stefanato CM, Gianotti R, Kubba A, Annessi G. Panniculitis with vasculitis. *G Ital Dermatol Venereol.* 2013;148(4):387-394.
12. Stoller JK, Sandhaus RA, Turino G, Dickson R, Rodgers K, Strange C. Delay in diagnosis of α1-antitrypsin deficiency. *Chest.* 2005;128(4):1989-1994.
13. Campos MA, Wanner A, Zhang G, Sandhaus RA. Trends in the diagnosis of symptomatic patients with α1-antitrypsin deficiency between 1968 and 2003. *Chest.* 2005;128(3):1179-1186.
14. de Serres F, Blanco I. Role of alpha-1 antitrypsin in human health and disease. *J Intern Med.* 2014;276(4):311-335
15. Hendrick SJ, Silverman AK, Solomon AR, Headington JT. Alpha 1-antitrypsin deficiency associated with panniculitis. *J Am Acad Dermatol.* 1988;18(4, pt 1):684-692.
16. Chan MP. Neutrophilic panniculitis: algorithmic approach to a heterogeneous group of disorders. *Arch Pathol Lab Med.* 2014;138(10):1337-1343.
17. Maldonado-Seral C, Berros-Fombella JP, Vivanco-Allende B, Coto-Segura P, Vazquez-Lopez F, Perez-Oliva N. Vemurafenib-associated neutrophilic panniculitis: an emergent adverse effect of variable severity. *Dermatol Online J.* 2013;19(4):16.
18. West ES, Williams VL, Morelli JG. Vemurafenib-induced neutrophilic panniculitis in a child with a brainstem glioma. *Pediatr Dermatol.* 2015;32(1):153-154.
19. Dimson OG, Esterly NB. Annular lipoatrophy of the ankles. *J Am Acad Dermatol.* 2006;54(2):S40-S42.
20. Torrelo A, Noguera-Morel L, Hernández-Martín A, et al. Recurrent lipoatrophic panniculitis of children. *J Eur Acad Dermatol Venereol.* 2017;31(3):536-543.
21. Ng SY, D'Arcy C, Orchard D. Acquired idiopathic lipoatrophic panniculitis in a 12-month-old infant. *Australas J Dermatol.* 2015;56(4):e102-e104.
22. Levy J, Burnett ME, Magro CM. Lipophagic panniculitis of childhood: a case report and comprehensive review of the literature. *Am J Dermatopathol.* 2017;39(3):217-224.
23. Santonja C, Gonzalo I, Feito M, Beato-Merino M, Requena L. Lipoatrophic panniculitis of the ankles in childhood: differential diagnosis with subcutaneous panniculitis-like T-cell lymphoma. *Am J Dermatopathol.* 2012;34(3):295-300.
24. Saenz BI, Meeker J, Jalali O, Lynch MC. Cold-induced dermatoses: case report and review of literature. *Am J Dermatopathol.* 2018;40(4):291-294.
25. Paller AS, Mancini AJ. *Hurwitz Clinical Pediatric Dermatology E-Book: A Textbook of Skin Disorders of Childhood and Adolescence.* Philadelphia, PA: Elsevier Health Sciences; 2015.
26. Huang FW, Berk DR, Bayliss SJ. Popsicle panniculitis in a 5-month-old child on systemic prednisolone therapy. *Pediatr Dermatol.* 2008;25(4):502-503.
27. Lipke MM, Cutlan JE, Smith AC. Cold panniculitis: delayed onset in an adult. *Cutis.* 2015;95(1):21-24.
28. Park HS, Choi JW, Kim BK, Cho KH. Lupus erythematosus panniculitis: clinicopathological, immunophenotypic, and molecular studies. *Am J Dermatopathol.* 2010;32(1):24-30.

29. Fraga J, García-Díez A. Lupus erythematosus panniculitis. *Dermatol Clin*. 2008;26(4):453-463.

30. Weingartner JS, Zedek DC, Burkhart CN, Morrell DS. Lupus erythematosus panniculitis in children: report of three cases and review of previously reported cases. *Pediatr Dermatol*. 2012;29(2):169-176.

31. Shiau CJ, Abi Daoud MS, Wong SM, Crawford RI. Lymphocytic panniculitis: an algorithmic approach to lymphocytes in subcutaneous tissue. *J Clin Pathol*. 2015;68(12):954-962.

32. Zhao YK, Wang F, Chen WN, et al. Lupus panniculitis as an initial manifestation of systemic lupus erythematosus: a case report. *Medicine (Baltimore)*. 2016;95(16):e3429.

33. Quintanilla-Martinez L, Jansen PM, Kinney MC, Swerdlow SH, Willemze R. Non-mycosis fungoides cutaneous T-cell lymphomas. *Am J Clin Pathol*. 2013;139(4):491-514.

34. Willemze R, Jansen PM, Cerroni L, et al; EORTC Cutaneous Lymphoma Group. Subcutaneous panniculitis-like T-cell lymphoma: definition, classification, and prognostic factors: an EORTC Cutaneous Lymphoma Group Study of 83 cases. *Blood*. 2008;111(2):838-845.

35. Michonneau D, Petrella T, Ortonne N, et al. Subcutaneous panniculitis-like T-cell lymphoma: immunosuppressive drugs induce better response than polychemotherapy. *Acta Derm Venereol*. 2017;97(3):358-364.

36. Magro CM, Crowson AN, Kovatich AJ, Burns F. Lupus profundus, indeterminate lymphocytic lobular panniculitis and subcutaneous T-cell lymphoma: a spectrum of subcuticular T-cell lymphoid dyscrasia. *J Cutan Pathol*. 2001;28(5):235-547.

37. Craig AJ, Cualing H, Thomas G, Lamerson C, Smith R. Cytophagic histiocytic panniculitis—a syndrome associated with benign and malignant panniculitis: case comparison and review of the literature. *J Am Acad Dermatol*. 1998;39(5, pt 1):721-736.

38. Marzano AV, Berti E, Paulli M, Caputo R. Cytophagic histiocytic panniculitis and subcutaneous panniculitis-like T-cell lymphoma: report of 7 cases. *Arch Dermatol*. 2000;136(7):889-896.

39. Winkelmann RK, Bowie EJ. Hemorrhagic diathesis associated with benign histiocytic, cytophagic panniculitis and systemic histiocytosis. *Arch Intern Med*. 1980;140(11):1460.

40. Parveen Z, Thompson K. Subcutaneous panniculitis-like T-cell lymphoma: redefinition of diagnostic criteria in the recent World Health Organization-European Organization for Research and Treatment of Cancer classification for cutaneous lymphomas. *Arch Pathol Lab Med*. 2009;133(2):303-308.

41. White JW, Winkelmann RK. Weber-Christian panniculitis: a review of 30 cases with this diagnosis. *J Am Acad Dermatol*. 1998;39(1):56-62.

42. Lee JH, Jung KE, Kim HS, Kim HO, Park YM, Lee JY. Traumatic panniculitis with localized hypertrichosis: two new cases and considerations. *J Dermatol*. 2013;40(2):139-141.

43. Santos-Juanes J, Coto P, Galache C, Sánchez del Río J, Soto de Delás J. Encapsulated fat necrosis: a form of traumatic panniculitis. *J Eur Acad Dermatol Venereol*. 2007;21(3):405-406.

44. Keimig EL. Granuloma annulare. *Dermatol Clin*. 2015;33(3):315-329.

45. Yun JH, Lee JY, Kim MK, et al. Clinical and pathological features of generalized granuloma annulare with their correlation: a retrospective multicenter study in Korea. *Ann Dermatol*. 2009;21(2):113-119.

46. Patrizi A, Gurioli C, Neri I. Childhood granuloma annulare: a review. *G Ital Dermatol Venereol*. 2014;149(6):663-674.

47. Rosenbach MA, Wanat KA, Reisenauer A, et al. Non-infectious granulomas. In: Bolognia JL, Jorizzo JL, Schaffer JV, et al, eds. *Dermatology*. Vol. 2. New York, NY: Mosby; 2012:1557.

48. Cohen PR, Carlos CA. Granuloma annulare mimicking sarcoidosis: report of patient with localized granuloma annulare whose skin lesions show 3 clinical morphologies and 2 histology patterns. *Am J Dermatopathol*. 2015;37(7):547-550.

49. Rongioletti F, Cozzani E, Parodi A. Scleromyxedema with an interstitial granulomatous-like pattern: a rare histologic variant mimicking granuloma annulare. *J Cutan Pathol*. 2010;37(10):1084-1087.

50. Coutinho I, Pereira N, Gouveia M, Cardoso JC, Tellechea O. Interstitial granulomatous dermatitis: a clinicopathological study. *Am J Dermatopathol*. 2015;37(8):614-619.

51. Nguyen TA, Celano NJ, Matiz C. Palisaded neutrophilic granulomatous dermatitis in a child with juvenile idiopathic arthritis on etanercept. *Pediatr Dermatol*. 2016;33(2):e156-e157.

52. Rosenbach M, English JC 3rd. Reactive granulomatous dermatitis: a review of palisaded neutrophilic and granulomatousdermatitis, interstitial granulomatous dermatitis, interstitial granulomatous drug reaction, and a proposed reclassification. *Dermatol Clin*. 2015;33(3):373-387.

53. O'toole EA, Kennedy U, Nolan JJ, Young MM, Rogers S, Barnes L. Necrobiosis lipoidica: only a minority of patients have diabetes mellitus. *Br J Dermatol*. 1999;140(2):283-286.

54. Muller SA, Winkelmann RK. Necrobiosis lipoidica diabeticorum. *Arch Dermatol*. 1966;93(3):272.

55. Bonura C, Frontino G, Rigamonti A, et al. Necrobiosis lipoidica diabeticorum: A pediatric case report. *Dermatoendocrinol*. 2014;6(1):e983683.

56. Nascimento J, Machado S. Pediatric-onset necrobiosis lipoidica. *Pediatr Int*. 2016;58(2):165-166.

57. Boateng B, Hiller D, Albrecht HP, Hornstein OP. Cutaneous microcirculation in pretibial necrobiosis lipoidica. Comparative laser Doppler flowmetry and oxygen partial pressure determinations in patients and healthy probands [in German]. *Hautarzt*. 1993;44(9):581-586.

58. Ngo B, Wigington G, Hayes K, et al. Skin blood flow in necrobiosis lipoidica diabeticorum. *Int J Dermatol*. 2008;47(4):354-358.

59. Ngo BT, Hayes KD, DiMiao DJ, Srinivasan SK, Huerter CJ, Rendell MS. Manifestations of cutaneous diabetic microangiopathy. *Am J Clin Dermatol*. 2005;6(4):225-237.

60. Hoffmann AL, Milman N, Byg KE. Childhood sarcoidosis in Denmark 1979-1994: incidence, clinical features and laboratory results at presentation in 48 children. *Acta Paediatr*. 2004;93(1):30-36.

61. Mañá J, Marcoval J, Graells J, Salazar A, Peyrí J, Pujol R. Cutaneous involvement in sarcoidosis. Relationship to systemic disease. *Arch Dermatol*. 1997;133(7):882-888.

62. Mishra P, Mishra S, Agarwalla SK, Mohanty N, Das RR. An adolescent with extensive cutaneous sarcoidosis without lung involvement. *Indian J Pediatr*. 2017;84(6):479-480.

63. Nathan N, Marcelo P, Houdouin V, et al. Lung sarcoidosis in children: update on disease expression and management. *Thorax*. 2015;70(6):537-542.

64. Rose CD. Blau syndrome: a systemic granulomatous disease of cutaneous onset and phenotypic complexity. *Pediatr Dermatol*. 2017;34(2):216-218.

65. Ishak R, Kurban M, Kibbi AG, Abbas O. Cutaneous sarcoidosis: clinicopathologic study of 76 patients from Lebanon. *Int J Dermatol*. 2015;54(1):33-41.

66. Esteves TC, Aparicio G, Ferrer B, Garcia-Patos V. Prognostic value of skin lesions in sarcoidosis: clinical and histopathological clues. *Eur J Dermatol*. 2015;25(6):556-562.

67. Kwon EJ, Hivnor CM, Yan AC, et al. Interstitial granulomatous lesions as part of the spectrum of presenting cutaneous signs in pediatric sarcoidosis. *Pediatr Dermatol*. 2007;24(5):517-524.

68. Tanner SL, Menzies S. Cutaneous sarcoid granulomas within a cosmetic tattoo. *BMJ*. 2017;356:i6324.

69. Prey S, Ezzedine K, Mazereeuw-Hautier J, et al. IFAG and childhood rosacea: a possible link?. *Pediatr Dermatol*. 2013;30(4):429-432.

70. Boralevi F, Léauté-Labrèze C, Lepreux S, et al. Idiopathic facial aseptic granuloma: a multicentre prospective study of 30 cases. *Br J Dermatol*. 2007;156(4):705-708.

71. Zitelli KB, Sheil AT, Fleck R, Schwentker A, Lucky AW. Idiopathic facial aseptic granuloma: review of an evolving clinical entity. *Pediatr Dermatol*. 2015;32(4):e136-e139. doi:10.1111/pde.12571.

72. Satta R, Montesu MA, Biondi G, Lissia A. Idiopathic facial aseptic granuloma: case report and literature review. *Int J Dermatol*. 2016;55(12):1381-1387.

73. Kim YJ, Shin JW, Lee JS, Park Y-L, Whang K-U, Lee SY. Childhood granulomatous periorificial dermatitis. *Ann Dermatol.* 2011;23(3):386-388.

74. Lucas CR, Korman NJ, Gilliam AC. Granulomatous periorificial dermatitis: a variant of granulomatous rosacea in children? *J Cutan Med Surg.* 2009;13(2):115-118.

75. Gianotti F, Ermacora E, Bennelli MG, Caputo R. Particuliere dermatite peri-orale infantile. Observations sur 5 cas. *Bull Soc Fr Dermatol Syphiligr.* 1970;77:341.

76. Gutte R, Holmukhe S, Garg G, Kharkar V, Khopkar U. Childhood granulomatous periorificial dermatitis in children with extra-facial involvement. *Indian J Dermatol, Venereol Leprol.* 2011;77(6):703-706.

77. Smith KW. Perioral dermatitis with histopathologic features of granulomatous rosacea: successful treatment with isotretinoin. *Cutis.* 1990;46(5):413-415.

78. Misago N, Nakafusa J, Narisawa Y. Childhood granulomatous periorificial dermatitis: lupus miliaris disseminatus faciei in children?. *J Eur Acad Dermatol Venereol.* 2005;19(4):470-473.

79. Hirsh BC, Johnson WC. Pathology of granulomatous diseases. *Int J Dermatol.* 1984;23(9):585-597.

80. Ang KL, Jones NS. Melkersson-Rosenthal syndrome. *J Laryngol Otol.* 2002;116(5):386-388.

81. Ziem PE, Pfrommer C, Goerdt S, Orfanos CE, Blume-Peytavi U. Melkersson-Rosenthal syndrome in childhood: a challenge in differential diagnosis and treatment. *Br J Dermatol.* 2000;143(4):860-863.

82. Zimmer WM, Rogers RS, Reeve CM, Sheridan PJ. Orofacial manifestations of Melkersson-Rosenthal syndrome: a study of 42 patients and review of 220 cases from the literature. *Oral Surg Oral Med Oral Pathol.* 1992;74(5):610-619.

83. van der Waal R, Schulten E, van de Scheur M, Wauters I, Starink T, van der Waal I. Cheilitis granulomatosa. *J Eur Acad Dermatol Venereol.* 2001;15(6):519-523.

84. Lazzerini M, Bramuzzo M, Ventura A. Association between orofacial granulomatosis and Crohn's disease in children: systematic review. *World J Gastroenterol.* 2014;20(23):7497-7504.

85. Oliveira AM, Martins M, Martins A, Ramos de Deus J. Granulomatous cheilitis associated with crohn's disease. *Am J Gastroenterol.* 2016;111(4):456.

86. Serarslan G, Aksakal M. Cutaneous leishmaniasis mimicking granulomatous cheilitis and treated successfully with oral fluconazole in a boy. *Ann Parasitol.* 2015;61(3):197-199.

87. Naveen KN, Pradeep AV. Chronic granulomatous disease. *Indian Dermatol Online J.* 2015;6(1):64-65.

88. Marciano BE, Spalding C, Fitzgerald A, et al. Common severe infections in chronic granulomatous disease. *Clin Infect Dis.* 2015;60(8):1176-1183.

89. Curnutte JT. Chronic granulomatous disease: the solving of a clinical riddle at the molecular level. *Clin Immunol Immunopathol.* 1993;67(3):S2.

90. Dohil M, Prendiville JS, Crawford RI, Speert DP. Cutaneous manifestations of chronic granulomatous disease: a report of four cases and review of the literature. *J Am Acad Dermatol.* 1997;36(6):899-907.

91. Forrest CB, Forehand JR, Axtell RA, Roberts RL, Johnston RB. Clinical features and current management of chronic granulomatous disease. *Hematol Oncol Clin North Am.* 1988;2(2):253-266.

92. Beghin A, Comini M, Soresina A, et al. Chronic granulomatous disease in children: a single center experience. *Clin Immunol.* 2018;188:12-19

93. Nanoudis S, Tsona A, Tsachouridou O, et al. Pyoderma gangrenosum in a patient with chronic granulomatous disease: a case report. *Medicine (Baltimore).* 2017;96(31):e7718.

94. Carvalho S, Machado S, Sampaio R, et al. Chronic granulomatous disease as a risk factor for cutaneous lupus in childhood. *Dermatol Online J.* 2017;23(3).

95. Herrick AL, Ennis H, Bhushan M, Silman AJ, Baildam EM. Incidence of childhood linear scleroderma and systemic sclerosis in the UK and Ireland. *Arthritis Care Res (Hoboken).* 2010;62(2):213-218.

96. Denton CP, Black CM, Abraham DJ. Mechanisms and consequences of fibrosis in systemic sclerosis. *Nat Clin Pract Rheumatol.* 2006;2(3):134-144.

97. Browning JC. Pediatric morphea. *Dermatol Clin.* 2013;31(2):229-237.

98. Fett N, Werth VP. Update on morphea: part I. Epidemiology, clinical presentation, and pathogenesis. *J Am Acad Dermatol.* 2011;64(2):217-228.

99. Peterson LS, Nelson AM, Su WD. Classification of morphea (localized scleroderma). *Mayo Clin Proc.* 1995;70(11):1068-1076.

100. Deshingkar SA, Barpande SR, Bhavthankar JD, Humbe JG. Progressive hemifacial atrophy (Parry-Romberg Syndrome). *Contemp Clin Dent.* 2012;3(suppl 1):S78-S81.

101. Odhav A, Hoeltzel MF, Canty K. Pansclerotic morphea with features of eosinophilic fasciitis: distinct entities or part of a continuum? *Pediatr Dermatol.* 2014;31(2):e42-e47.

102. Zulian F, Woo P, Athreya BH, et al. The Pediatric Rheumatology European Society/American College of Rheumatology/European League against rheumatism provisional classification criteria for juvenile systemic sclerosis. *Arthritis Rheum.* 2007;57(2):203-212.

103. Foeldvari I, Nihtyanova SI, Wierk A, Denton CP. Characteristics of patients with juvenile onset systemic sclerosis in an adult single-center cohort. *J Rheumatol.* 2010;37(11):2422-2426.

104. Pickert AJ, Carpentieri D, Price H, Hansen RC. Early morphea mimicking acquired port-wine stain. *Pediatr Dermatol.* 2014;31(5):591-594.

105. Carneiro S, Ramos-e-Silva M, Russi DC, Albuquerque EM, Sousa MA. Coexistence of generalized morphea and lichen sclerosus et atrophicus mimicking systemic disease. *Skinmed.* 2011;9(2):131-133.

106. Onajin O, Wieland CN, Peters MS, Lohse CM, Lehman JS.Clinicopathologic and immunophenotypic features of eosinophilic fasciitis and morphea profunda: A comparative study of 27 cases. *J Am Acad Dermatol.* 2018;78(1):121-128.

107. Shulman LE. Diffuse fasciitis with hypergammaglobulinemia and eosinophilia: a new syndrome? *J Rheumatol.* 1984;11(5):569-570.

108. Long H, Zhang G, Wang L, Lu Q. Eosinophilic skin diseases: a comprehensive review. *Clin Rev Allergy Immunol.* 2016;50(2):189-213.

109. Farrington ML, Haas JE, Nazar-Stewart V, Mellins ED. Eosinophilic fasciitis in children frequently progresses to scleroderma-like cutaneous fibrosis. *J Rheumatol.* 1993;20(1):128-132.

110. Grisanti MW, Moore TL, Osborn TG, Haber PL. Eosinophilic fasciitis in children. *Semin Arthritis Rheum.* 1989;19(3):151-157.

111. Moulton SJ, Kransdorf MJ, Ginsburg WW, Abril A, Persellin S. Eosinophilic fasciitis: spectrum of MRI findings. *Am J Roentgenol.* 2005;184(3):975-978.

112. Chan V, Soans B, Mathers D. Ultrasound and magnetic resonance imaging features in a patient with eosinophilic fasciitis. *Australas Radiol.* 2004;48(3):414-417.

113. Wright NA, Mazori DR, Patel M, Merola JF, Femia AN, Vleugels RA. Epidemiology and treatment of eosinophilic fasciitis. *JAMA Dermatol.* 2016;152(1):97.

114. Mertens JS, Zweers MC, Kievit W, et al. High-dose intravenous pulse methotrexate in patients with eosinophilic fasciitis. *JAMA Dermatol.* 2016;152(11):1262.

115. Mendichovszky IA, Marks SD, Simcock CM, Olsen ØE. Gadolinium and nephrogenic systemic fibrosis: time to tighten practice. *Pediatr Radiol.* 2008;38(5):489-496.

116. Weller A, Barber JL, Olsen ØE. Gadolinium and nephrogenic systemic fibrosis: an update. *Pediatr Nephrol.* 2014;29(10):1927-1937.

117. Mendoza FA, Artlett CM, Sandorfi N, Latinis K, Piera-Velazquez S, Jimenez SA. Description of 12 cases of nephrogenic fibrosing dermopathy and review of the literature. *Semin Arthritis Rheum.* 2006;35(4):238-249.

118. Jiménez SA, Artlett CM, Sandorfi N, et al. Dialysis-associated systemic fibrosis (nephrogenic fibrosing dermopathy): study of inflammatory cells and transforming growth factor β1 expression in affected skin. *Arthritis Rheum.* 2004;50(8):2660-2666.

119. Scheinfeld N. Nephrogenic fibrosing dermopathy: a comprehensive review for the dermatologist. *Am J Clin Dermatol.* 2006;7(4):237-247.

120. Foss C, Smith JK, Ortiz L, Hanevold C, Davis L. Gadolinium-associated nephrogenic systemic fibrosis in a 9-year-old boy. *Pediatr Dermatol.* 2009;26(5):579-582.

121. Bhawan J, Swick BL, Koff AB, Stone MS. Sclerotic bodies in nephrogenic systemic fibrosis: a new histopathologic finding. *J Cutan Pathol.* 2009;36(5):548-552.

122. Wilford C, Fine JD, Boyd AS, Sanyal S, Abraham JL, Kantrow SM. Nephrogenic systemic fibrosis: report of an additional case with granulomatous inflammation. *Am J Dermatopathol.* 2010;32(1):71-75.

123. Miyamoto J, Tanikawa A, Igarashi A, et al. Detection of iron deposition in dermal fibrocytes is a useful tool for histologic diagnosis of nephrogenic systemic fibrosis. *Am J Dermatopathol.* 2011;33(3):271-276.

124. Dinh H, Purcell SM, Chung C, Zaenglein AL. Pediatric lichen sclerosus: a review of the literature and management recommendations. *J Clin Aesthet Dermatol.* 2016;9(9):49-54.

125. Maronn ML, Esterly NB. Constipation as a feature of anogenital lichen sclerosus in children. *Pediatrics.* 2005;115(2):e230-e232.

126. La Spina M, Meli MC, De Pasquale R, et al. Vulvar melanoma associated with lichen sclerosus in a child: case report and literature review. *Pediatr Dermatol.* 2016;33(3):e190-e194.

127. Patrizi A, Gurioli C, Medri M, Neri I. Childhood lichen sclerosus: a long-term follow-up. *Pediatr Dermatol.* 2010;27(1):101-103.

128. Nerantzoulis I, Grigoriadis T, Michala L. Genital lichen sclerosus in childhood and adolescence—a retrospective case series of 15 patients: early diagnosis is crucial to avoid long-term sequelae. *Eur J Pediatr.* 2017;176(10):1429-1432.

129. Kirtschig G, Becker K, Günthert A, et al. Evidence-based (S3) guideline on (anogenital) lichen sclerosus. *J Eur Acad Dermatology Venereol.* 2015;29(10):e1-e43.

130. Vukicevic J. Extensive bullous lichen sclerosus et atrophicus. *An Bras Dermatol.* 2016;91(5)(suppl 1):81-83.

131. El Habr C, Mannava K, Koch S, et al. Folliculocentric lichen sclerosus et atrophicus in a 10-year-old girl. *Am J Dermatopathol.* 2017;39(1):59-61.

132. Bader-Meunier B, Fraitag S, Janssen C, et al. Clonal cytophagic histiocytic panniculitis in children may be cured by cyclosporine A. *Pediatrics.* 2013;132(2):e545-e549.

133. Pauwels C, Livideanu CB, Maza A, Lamant L, Paul C. Cytophagic histiocytic panniculitis after H1N1 vaccination: a case report and review of the cutaneous side effects of influenza vaccines. *Dermatology.* 2011;222(3):217-220.

134. Pasqualini C, Jorini M, Carloni I, et al. Cytophagic histiocytic panniculitis, hemophagocytic lymphohistiocytosis and undetermined autoimmune disorder: reconciling the puzzle. *Ital J Pediatr.* 2014;40(1):17.

135. Aronson IK, Worobec SM. Cytophagic histiocytic panniculitis and hemophagocytic lymphohistiocytosis: an overview. *Dermatol Ther.* 2010;23:389-402.

136. Gupta S, Weitzman S. Primary and secondary hemophagocytic lymphohistiocytosis: clinical features, pathogenesis and therapy. *Expert Rev Clin Immunol.* 2010;6:137-154.

137. Cetica V, Pende D, Griffiths GM, Aricò M. Molecular basis of familial hemophagocytic lymphohistiocytosis. *Haematologica.* 2010;95:538-541.

138. Ahn JS, Rew SY, Shin MG, et al. Clinical significance of clonality and Epstein-Barr virus infection in adult patients with hemophagocytic lymphohistiocytosis. *Am J Hematol.* 2010;85:719-722.

139. Wick MR, Patterson JW. Cytophagic histiocytic panniculitis—a critical reappraisal. *Arch Dermatol.* 2000;136:922-924.

140. Hytiroglou P, Phelps RG, Wattenberg DJ, Strauchen JA. Histiocytic cytophagic panniculitis: molecular evidence for a clonal T-cell disorder. *J Am Acad Dermatol.* 1992;27(2, pt 2):333-336.

6

Vasculopathic, Vasculitic, and Neutrophilic Dermatosis

Ines Wu Soukoulis / Alejandro A. Gru

URTICARIA AND URTICARIAL VASCULITIS

Definition and Epidemiology

Urticaria generally represents a type 1 hypersensitivity reaction that can be triggered by a wide variety of factors, both immunologic and nonimmunologic. Acute and chronic forms exist, with the chronic form lasting more than 6 weeks. The great majority of urticaria cases resolve within a few weeks. This disease process can occur anytime from infancy to adulthood. Overall, it is estimated to occur in about 20% of people in their lifetime.[1]

Etiology

This type 1 hypersensitivity reaction can be caused by immunologic triggers or nonimmunologic factors that lead to mast cell release. Acute urticaria resolves within 6 weeks. In young children, common causes are infections such as a viral illness, medications such as anticonvulsants and antibiotics, and foods. Chronic urticaria recurs for more than 6 weeks and is less common in children than in adults; idiopathic and autoimmune causes are most common.[2] Children with chronic urticaria may have a higher rate of autoimmune thyroid disease.[3] Chronic urticaria can also be caused by foods, medications, and parasitic infections.[4,5] Cold urticaria is a type of physical urticarial that is induced by cold exposure; in children, one-third of patients can have anaphylactic reactions.[6] Cholinergic urticaria results from activities such as exercise and hot water that raise core body temperature.[2]

Clinical Presentation

Lesions are erythematous, edematous wheals frequently with central clearing that are very pruritic. They range in size from pinpoint papules to large plaques (Figure 6-1).

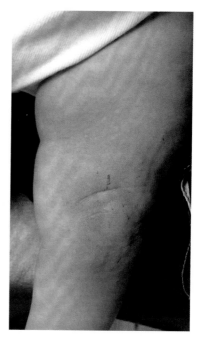

FIGURE 6-1. Acute urticarial papules and plaques with excoriation on the knee of a 7-month-old infant secondary to peanut allergy.

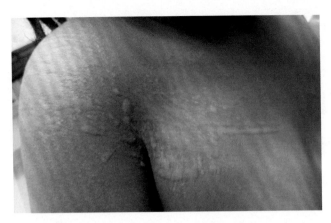

FIGURE 6-2. Dermatographism in a young child.

They are characteristically transient, with each individual lesion resolving within 24 hours. Lesions resolve without dyspigmentation or scarring. Dermatographism is common (Figure 6-2).

Urticaria multiforme, also called "acute annular urticarial," occurs in pediatric patients and presents with characteristic annular, serpiginous, and polycyclic urticarial plaques and is often associated with acral or facial edema (Figure 6-3).

Lesions can be centrally dusky and can resemble ecchymosis. This condition is more common in children ranging from ages 2 months to 4 years.[7] Children may have fever but are overall well appearing; they can have symptoms of concurrent illness such as upper respiratory infection, otitis media, or other viral symptoms.[7] This rash is self-limited and generally resolves in 1 to 2 weeks. Clinical findings can often be confused for erythema multiforme and serum sickness–like reactions (SSLR).[7,8] Papular urticaria is typically seen in children, but can also be present in adolescents and young adults. It is characterized clinically by pruritic, edematous, and erythematous papules and wheals of variable size (3-10 mm). The lesions are located on the extremities and face, with sparing of the axillae and groin. The lesions can last for days to weeks, and leave residual hyperpigmentation at the affected sites. Recurrence following exposure to the causative agent is very frequent, although hyposensitization to the antigen can occur upon multiple reexposures.[9]

Histologic Findings

Urticaria is one of the conditions where the clinical finding can be quite drastic, but the histologic aspects are very underwhelming (Figure 6-4). Urticaria is one of the conditions that enter the pathologic diagnosis of "normal skin." Early lesions of urticaria show intravascular clusters of neutrophils within the lumen, without much inflammation extravasated outside the vessels. Later on, there is a superficial and deep, or superficial to mid dermal, perivascular and interstitial mixed inflammatory infiltrate. The inflammatory cells include neutrophils, eosinophils, lymphocytes, and histiocytes. Papillary dermal edema and vascular congestion can

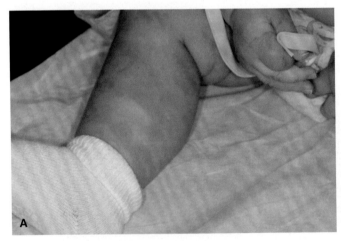

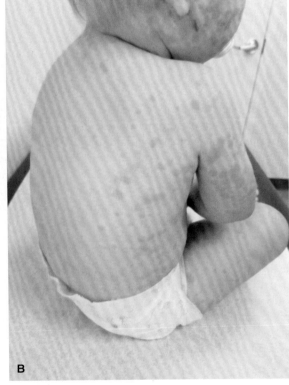

FIGURE 6-3. **Urticaria multiforme.** Annular, serpiginous, and polycyclic urticarial plaques are present (A,B).

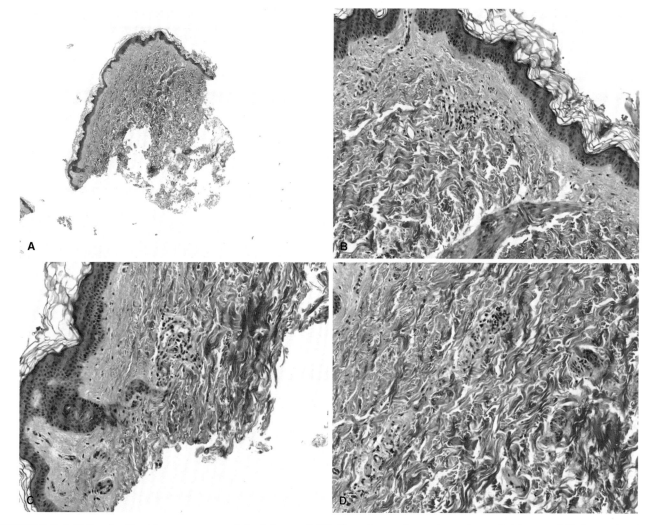

FIGURE 6-4. Urticaria. The biopsy appears relatively "normal" (A). There is a perivascular and superficial very mild inflammatory infiltrate with slight dermal edema (B). Intravascular collections of neutrophils and eosinophils are seen (C,D).

also be present. Chronic or resolving lesions of urticaria can show a slightly increased number of mast cells.[10-17]

Papular urticaria is not a well-characterized pathologic term, but show features that are similar and indistinguishable from a dermal hypersensitivity reaction to a medication or arthropod bite reaction.[9,18] In some cases, there might be a mild degree of spongiosis, but most of the time the epidermis is relatively unremarkable. There is a superficial and deep, perivascular and interstitial dense inflammatory infiltrate, composed of lymphocytes, histiocytes, eosinophils, and neutrophils. In cases where there is an abundance of eosinophils, degranulated cells and occasional "flame figures" can be seen. The inflammation can also extend into the subcutaneous tissue.

Differential Diagnosis

It is important when evaluating a biopsy for urticaria to obtain multiple levels of section to search for evidence of leukocytoclastic vasculitis (LCV), hence excluding the diagnosis

of urticarial vasculitis. Frequently, early lesions of urticarial vasculitis show a brisk perivascular neutrophilic infiltrate with leukocytoclasis (nuclear dust), but without significant fibrinoid necrosis or endothelial swelling. Other disorders that present with a clinical and histologic urticarial pattern can also be considered in the differential diagnosis of urticaria. Bullous pemphigoid (BP), although more common in adults, has also been described in the pediatric population. The early phases of BP present with an urticarial pattern. One of the main differences between the urticarial BP and urticaria is the aggregation of eosinophils in the papillary dermis, near the dermal-epidermal junction. Additionally, eosinophilic spongiosis can be present, a feature that is not typical of urticaria. Later on, BP shows a subepidermal blister with eosinophils and neutrophils (in the classic form), and sometimes a pauci-inflammatory subepidermal bulla (in the cell poor variant). Invariably, direct immunofluorescence reveals linear deposits of C3 and IgG along the dermal-epidermal junction. Other considerations included in the differential diagnosis are dermal hypersensitivity reactions (from a medication), telangiectasia macularis eruptive perstans (TMEP), arthropod bite reactions, and gyrate erythemas. Dermal hypersensitivity reactions typically lack the edema of urticaria and the vascular collections of neutrophils. TMEP is uncommonly seen in children and has a blaschkoid distribution. Performing special stains (Giemsa, Leder) or immunohistochemistry for mast cells (CD117, mast cell tryptase) is capital to establishing the diagnosis of this condition. Arthropod bite reactions and popular urticaria show identical findings. Gyrate erythemas can also have dermal edema, but the infiltrate is mostly lymphocytic, and the number of eosinophils is low, if present.

CAPSULE SUMMARY

URTICARIA

Urticaria generally represents a type 1 hypersensitivity reaction that can be triggered by a wide variety of factors, both immunologic and nonimmunologic. Acute and chronic forms exist, with the chronic form lasting more than 6 weeks. The great majority of urticaria cases resolve within a few weeks. Lesions are erythematous, edematous wheals frequently with central clearing that are very pruritic. They range in size from pinpoint papules to large plaques. Urticaria is one of the conditions where the clinical finding can be quite drastic, but the histologic aspects are very underwhelming. Urticaria is one of the conditions that enter the pathologic diagnosis of "normal skin." Early lesions of urticaria show intravascular clusters of neutrophils within the lumen, without much inflammation extravasated outside the vessels. Later on, there is a superficial and deep, or superficial to mid dermal, perivascular and interstitial mixed inflammatory infiltrate with the presence of frequent eosinophils.

URTICARIAL VASCULITIS

Definition and Epidemiology

Urticarial vasculitis (UV) is a small-vessel vasculitis that is frequently associated with an underlying condition such as connective tissue disease. It is distinguished into two main groups: normocomplementemic and hypocomplementemic. Systemic disease is more commonly associated with the hypocomplementemic form.[19] This condition is more commonly seen in adults and is rare in children.[20]

Etiology

UV is known to be triggered by underlying conditions including autoimmune conditions, infections, medications, and

malignancy. In children, it is frequently preceded by an upper respiratory infection.[19,21] It can also be an idiopathic condition.

Clinical Presentation

Clinical lesions of UV can be distinguished from urticaria by their persistence past 24 hours and their dusky and purpuric appearance (Figure 6-5).[19] Lesions can be painful in addition to pruritic and can resolve with hyperpigmentation. They tend to be on the trunk and proximal extremities. Angioedema and joint pains can also occur.[21] Confirmation of diagnosis often requires a biopsy, because it can present very similarly to urticaria. If confirmed, physical exam and labs are indicated to evaluate for underlying trigger. Hypocomplementemia, ANA, and anti-C1q antibodies are associated with a poor prognosis of the disease and with a systemic involvement. Nevertheless, these findings are exceptional in childhood.

Histologic Findings

The pathologic criteria for the diagnosis of UV are less rigorous than for other LCV, because the infiltrates are sparser, and the vasculitic changes can be focal and subtle. Pathologically, there is a perivascular and interstitial neutrophilic and eosinophilic infiltrate, with either focal small-vessel neutrophilic vasculitis (evidence of fibrinoid necrosis) or focal perivascular leukocytoclasis without fibrin deposition, and with or without extravasated red blood cells (Figure 6-6). Therefore, the minimal histologic criteria for the diagnosis of UV include the presence

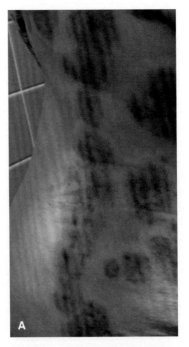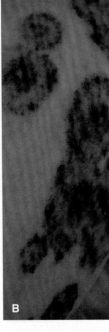

FIGURE 6-5. Urticarial vasculitis. Annular erythematous patches and plaques with dusky and purpuric appearance (A,B).

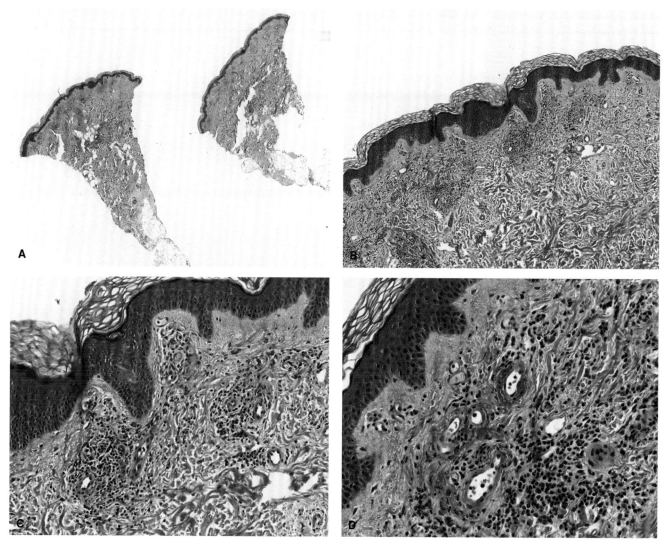

FIGURE 6-6. Urticarial vasculitis. In addition to the typical changes of urticaria, there is a leukocytoclastic vasculitis with fibrinoid changes, karyorrhectic debris, and a rich background of dermal eosinophils (A-D).

of perivascular leukocytoclasis, or fibrin deposits, with or without extravasated red blood cells. In hypocomplementemic UV, diffuse dermal neutrophilic infiltrates can be seen. Dermal eosinophils are more typical of the normocomplementemic forms of UV.[22]

CAPSULE SUMMARY

URTICARIAL VASCULITIS

UV is a small-vessel vasculitis that is frequently associated with an underlying condition such as connective tissue disease. It is distinguished into two main groups: normocomplementemic and hypocomplementemic.

Systemic disease is more commonly associated with the hypocomplementemic form. This condition is more commonly seen in adults and is rare in children. Clinical lesions of UV can be distinguished from urticaria by their persistence past 24 hours and their dusky and purpuric appearance. The pathologic criteria for the diagnosis of UV are less rigorous than for other LCV, because the infiltrates are sparser, and the vasculitic changes can be focal and subtle. Pathologically, there is a perivascular and interstitial neutrophilic and eosinophilic infiltrate, with either focal small-vessel neutrophilic vasculitis (evidence of fibrinoid necrosis) or focal perivascular leukocytoclasis without fibrin deposition, and with or without extravasated red blood cells.

SERUM SICKNESS AND SERUM SICKNESS–LIKE REACTIONS

Definition and Epidemiology

True serum sickness (SS) is a type 3 hypersensitivity reaction that was more frequently seen in the past after the administration of horse or rabbit serum. SSLR are more common and can present with similar symptoms, but do not involve immune complex formation. SS is rarely seen in the pediatric population; in recent years, it has been reported in relation to rituximab.[23] SSLR can occur occasionally in children. It is classically seen most often with cefaclor; however, other medications such as antibiotics, antifungals, psychiatric medications, and vaccinations have also been reported.[24-27] Interestingly, children who develop SSLR to cefaclor usually do not have a similar reaction with other cephalosporin medications.[28,29]

Etiology

True SS involves deposition of immune complexes that are formed between host antibody and foreign protein, leading to an inflammatory cascade that includes the activation of complement. Deposition of these immune complexes in target tissues such as the vascular endothelial and glomerular basement membrane leads to damage of these areas.[30,31] SSLR is thought to be caused by an inflammatory response to metabolites of the offending medication.[30]

Clinical Presentation

Classic symptoms of both diseases include fever, rash, and joint pains. The skin eruption in SS develops about one week after exposure and is generally morbilliform, with or without an urticarial component on the trunk before spreading to the extremities; the rash resolves within 2 weeks (Figure 6-7). A characteristic serpiginous erythema develops on the sides of the hands and feet.[31,32] Patients can also have systemic manifestations including vasculitis, arthralgias/arthritis, gastrointestinal (GI) symptoms, nephritis causing proteinuria, and lymphadenopathy. SSLR presents with a rash about 1 to 2 weeks after the triggering medication that tends to be more urticarial and polycyclic; centrally, the lesions may have a violaceous discoloration. Joint swelling can occur, especially around the knees. Children can have facial swelling, myalgias, and headache. Nephritis and vasculitis do not happen because there are no immune complexes involved. This disease is generally self-limited and subsides within 2 to 3 weeks of discontinuing the medication.[30,33]

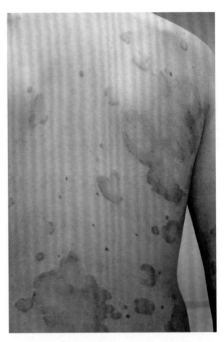

FIGURE 6-7. Serum sickness–like reaction. Urticarial and morbilliform eruption in the trunk.

Histologic Findings

Because of the rare circumstances when a biopsy is performed, the pathologic findings are poorly characterized. Skin biopsies of these patients reveal limited lymphocytic and histiocytic perivascular infiltrates with only rare neutrophils. Fibrinoid necrosis is not typically seen, although there have been subsequent reports of true small-vessel vasculitis in SS. Some have documented the presence of abundant neutrophils and eosinophils in this condition.[34,35]

CAPSULE SUMMARY

SERUM SICKNESS AND SS-LIKE REACTIONS

True SS is a type 3 hypersensitivity reaction that was more frequently seen in the past after the administration of horse or rabbit serum. SS is rarely seen in the pediatric population; in recent years, it has been reported in relation to rituximab. Classic symptoms of both diseases include fever, rash, and joint pains. The skin eruption in SS develops about one week after exposure and is generally morbilliform, with or without an urticarial component on the trunk before spreading to the extremities; the rash resolves within 2 weeks.

ARTHROPOD BITE REACTIONS

Definition and Epidemiology

Arthropod reactions can occur in reaction to various bites, including by mites, ticks spiders, lice mosquitoes, fleas, bees, and bedbugs. This section focuses on two common distinct arthropod reactions in children: scabies and papular urticaria.

SCABIES

Scabies infestation is caused by the *Sarcoptes scabiei* mite and presents as a very pruritic rash. It is most often transmitted by direct human contact with an infested individual, although it can also be spread by contact with infested clothing and bedding. This infestation occurs in all ages, from infancy to adulthood, with the highest prevalence under age 2.[36] Women and children appear to be infested more often, as well as immunocompromised individuals and those with mental or physical handicap.

Etiology

This infestation is caused by the *S. scabiei* mite, which is an obligated human parasite. The female mite burrows into the stratum corneum and causes a hypersensitivity reaction.

Clinical Presentation

The clinical presentation of scabies infestation varies according to age. Newborns and infants present shortly after infestation with very inflamed papulovesicles and nodules that can be crusted and serpiginous.[36] Scabies nodules are primarily seen in infants. Lesions are reddish-brown and most commonly occur on the trunk, genital region, and axillae. They represent a hypersensitivity response and may persist for months.

In infants, the scalp is frequently affected, which is rarely involved in older children and adults; the trunk is also more likely to be affected. In addition, infants and younger children are more likely to present with lesions that are vesiculated. In older children and adults, the incubation period is approximately 3 weeks.[37] Skin lesions include papules, papulovesicles, and nodules and are most commonly seen in the web spaces of the hands and feet, wrists, ankles, axillae, inguinal areas, and palms and soles. There are frequently linear and curvilinear burrows on the palms and soles (Figure 6-8A and B). Excoriations are commonly seen, and secondary bacterial infection is common. In older children and adults who are healthy, the number of mites during an infestation averages around 10 to 12.[37]

Crusted or Norwegian scabies occurs primarily in immunocompromised patients and is extremely contagious, given the much higher mite load compared with classic scabies infection. Skin findings can mimic eczema and psoriasis and can be hyperkeratotic.[37] This form of scabies can be the source for epidemic involvement in hospitals.

CAPSULE SUMMARY

SCABIES

Scabies infestation is caused by the *S. scabiei* mite and presents as a very pruritic rash. This infection occurs in all ages, from infancy to adulthood, with the highest prevalence under age 2. Newborns and infants present shortly after infestation with very inflamed papulovesicles and nodules that can be crusted and serpiginous. Scabies nodules are primarily seen in infants. Lesions are reddish-brown and most commonly occur on the trunk, genital region, and axillae.

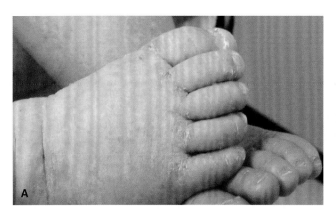
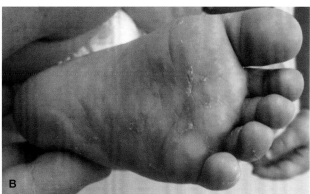

FIGURE 6-8. (A) Erythematous papules with scaling and crusting on the foot of a scabies-infested infant. (B) Linear burrows and erythematous papules on the sole of an infant's foot with scabies infection.

The pathologic findings and differential diagnosis are discussed in detail in Chapter 21 about parasitic infestations.

PAPULAR URTICARIA

Definition and Epidemiology

This is a common rash in childhood that presents with pruritic erythematous urticarial papules that are most commonly caused by a hypersensitivity reaction to arthropod bites. This can be seen in children and adults of all ages, but is most prevalent in children ages 2 to 10 years.[1]

Etiology

This can be caused by a number of different bites, including mosquitoes, fleas, bedbugs, and mites.

Clinical Presentation

Lesions are typically urticarial and clustered erythematous papules; they are often in a linear array and can vesiculate. They can occur anywhere on the body, although they frequently spare intertriginous areas.[1] Excoriation and crusting can be seen, and a central punctum is often visible (Figure 6-9). Each individual lesion resolves over 1 to 2 weeks. Recurrence is common, especially if there is reexposure.

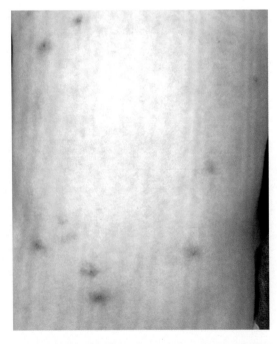

FIGURE 6-9. Urticarial papules on the trunk secondary to blea bites on a young child with central punctum, vesiculation, and scabbed excoriation.

Histologic Findings

The histopathologic findings present in association with arthropod bite reactions/papular urticaria are variable (Figure 6-10): those depend on the arthropod subtype, the duration of the clinical lesion, the immunologic reaction, the presence or absence of arthropod parts, and the discharge of toxins. Changes caused by tick bites involve both the epidermis and the dermis. In the epidermis, there is variable acanthosis, which in some cases can be exuberant and have a pseudoepitheliomatous appearance. Epidermal spongiosis can also be seen, particularly in the acute phases. The spongiotic reaction can be localized to the site of the bite, or more extensive, with multiple intraepidermal vesicles and sometimes frank necrosis. Eosinophilic spongiosis can be a particular feature seen in arthropod bites. The dermal reaction is characterized by wedge-shaped dense foci of inflammatory cells consisting of lymphocytes, histiocytes, plasma cells, and eosinophils especially in the periappendageal region. Secondary lymphoid follicles with germinal centers are formed in some lesions. Mouth parts of the tick can be present sometimes, typically in the mid dermis and covered by a down-growth of the epidermis. The arthropod parts can be polarizable. Reactions to fleas, fire ants, mosquitoes, and spider envenomation show a predominance of neutrophils with vasculitic foci. Hemorrhage and edema can also be prominent.

Pseudolymphomatous changes can also be seen: the pleomorphism of the mononuclear infiltrate may simulate mycosis fungoides or other lymphomas of the skin including Hodgkin disease, especially when accompanied by eosinophils. Cells resembling those of Sternberg-Reed may sometimes be present. Usually, the clinical history and the

---

CAPSULE SUMMARY

PAPULAR URTICARIA

This is a common rash in childhood that presents with pruritic erythematous urticarial papules that are most commonly caused by a hypersensitivity reaction to arthropod bites. Lesions are typically urticarial and clustered erythematous papules; they are often in a linear array and can vesiculate. They can occur anywhere on the body, although they frequently spare intertriginous areas. The dermal reaction is characterized by wedge-shaped dense foci of inflammatory cells consisting of lymphocytes, histiocytes, plasma cells, and eosinophils, especially in the periappendageal region. Secondary lymphoid follicles with germinal centers are formed in some lesions.

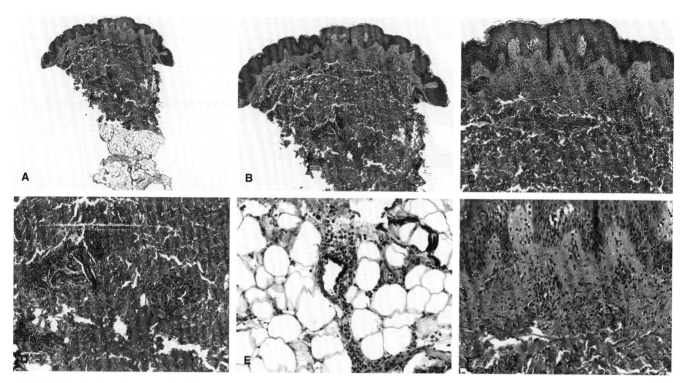

FIGURE 6-10. **Papular urticaria.** There is a superficial and deep, perivascular and interstitial inflammatory infiltrate (A-C). The interstitial inflammation has numerous eosinophils (D). The eosinophilic infiltrate extends deep into the subcutis (E). Mild epidermal spongiosis is present (F).

presence of a single lesion help exclude lymphoma, but, when lesions are numerous, differentiation may be difficult. The abundance of plasma cells in the insect bite may aid in the differentiation.

ANNULAR (GYRATE) ERYTHEMAS

This reactive group of skin conditions is characterized by serpiginous and annular eruptions, including erythema annulare centrifugum (EAC), annular erythema of infancy, and erythema chronicum migrans (ECM). These are entities that need to be differentiated from other annular conditions such as erythema multiforme, tinea corporis, and SSLR.

ERYTHEMA ANNULARE CENTRIFUGUM

Epidemiology and Etiology

This rash can vary widely in age from infancy to adulthood. Many cases are thought to represent a hypersensitivity to medications, foods, fungal infections elsewhere on the skin,

autoimmune processes, and malignancies.[38,39] Some cases are idiopathic.

Clinical Presentation

Skin lesions are annular plaques with central clearing and often have a fine raised trailing scale and can extend peripherally rapidly. They are usually asymptomatic and tend to be on the trunk and buttocks. Lesions can last weeks to months, and some can have recurrent lesions over the course of years.[40]

Histologic Findings

The biopsies of EAC show the prototypic findings of a gyrate erythema, a lymphocytic vasculitis: there is a superficial to mid dermal, very tight, perivascular mostly lymphocytic infiltrate (Figure 6-11). The epidermis is relatively normal. However, the superficial variant of EAC can have spongiosis, exocytosis of lymphocytes, and areas of parakeratosis. Papillary dermal edema can be sometimes present. The tight perivascular character of the lymphocytic infiltrate has also been described to as having a "coat sleeve" or "pipe stem" appearance. As opposed to other types of vasculitis, fibrinoid changes and extravasated red blood cells are not seen. In a small number of cases, scattered dermal eosinophils are present. A "deep" form of gyrate erythema has been described, in which the inflammatory infiltrate extends to involve the deep vessels in the reticular dermis. The latter form lacks epidermal changes.[41-44]

Differential Diagnosis

Other gyrate erythemas (described in the following paragraphs: annular erythema of infancy, erythema marginatum, and ECM) should always be included in the differential diagnosis of EAC. Arthropod bite reactions can also be considered in the differential diagnosis. As opposed to EAC, they typically have both a superficial and deep character of inflammation, a wedge-shaped appearance, sometimes a punctum (site of arthropod bite), and an abundance of dermal eosinophils. Tumid lupus, reticular erythematous mucinosis, and Jessner's lymphocytic infiltrate can also have a tight perivascular lymphocytic inflammation. As opposed to EAC, there is a significant amount of interstitial dermal mucin. Polymorphous light eruptions also have a tight lymphocytic perivascular inflammation. However, the latter shows a significant amount of edema, and sometimes epidermal changes. The superficial form of EAC can have a similar differential diagnoses to subacute and chronic spongiotic dermatitis (eczema, contact dermatitis, id reactions, atopic dermatitis, spongiotic drug reactions).

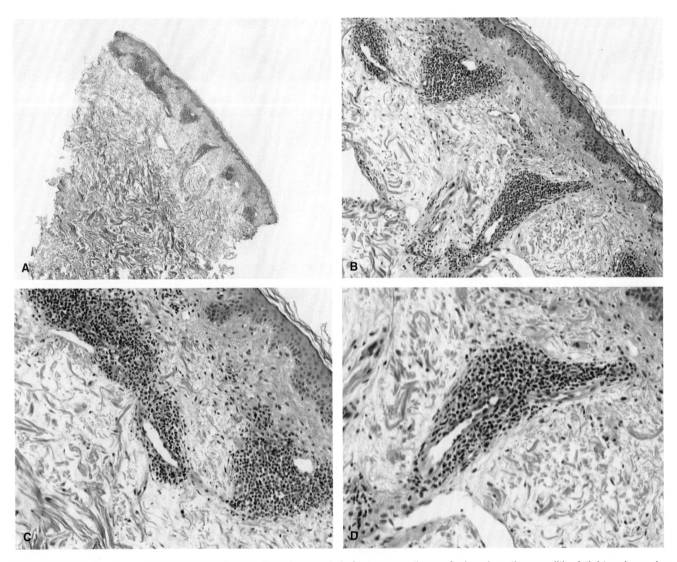

FIGURE 6-11. Erythema annulare centrifugum. The characteristic features are those of a lymphocytic vasculitis. A tight perivascular infiltrate in the superficial to mid dermis is noted, without significant epidermal changes (A,B). The infiltrate has also been described to as having a "coat sleeve" appearance (C,D).

CAPSULE SUMMARY

ERYTHEMA ANNULARE CENTRIFUGUM

Skin lesions are annular plaques with central clearing and often have a fine raised trailing scale and can extend peripherally rapidly. They are usually asymptomatic and tend to be on the trunk and buttocks. The biopsies of EAC show the prototypic findings of a gyrate erythema, a lymphocytic vasculitis: there is a superficial to mid dermal, very tight, perivascular mostly lymphocytic infiltrate.

ANNULAR ERYTHEMA OF INFANCY

Epidemiology and Etiology

This annular erythema usually starts shortly after birth and is thought to be a hypersensitivity reaction to an unknown antigen.[45]

Clinical Presentation

Infants develop an asymptomatic 2 to 3 cm arcuate and annular eruptions with raised borders that classically last a few days, but frequently can recur for months to rarely years (Figure 6-12). Lesions resolve without hyperpigmentation or scarring, and there are no systemic symptoms.[46,47]

Histologic Finding

It is important to emphasize that a variety of histopathologic patterns have been linked to this condition. It appears likely that more than one process is grouped into this particular disease category. The majority of the pathologic reports describe a dense perivascular inflammatory infiltrate composed of lymphocytes, with scattered eosinophils and

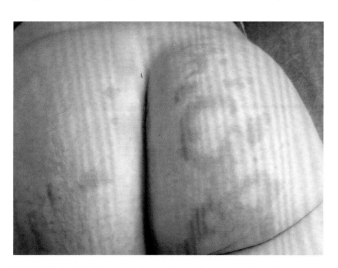

FIGURE 6-12. Recurrent erythematous annular plaques on the buttocks of an infant representing annular erythema of infancy. No definitive cause was identified.

plasma cells. Others have documented a more interstitial pattern of inflammation with a predominance of eosinophils. An additional case report describes a case with perivascular leukocytoclasis[45,46,48,49]

CAPSULE SUMMARY

ANNULAR ERYTHEMA OF INFANCY

This annular erythema usually starts shortly after birth and is thought to be a hypersensitivity reaction to an unknown antigen. Infants develop an asymptomatic 2 to 3 cm arcuate and annular eruptions with raised borders that classically last a few days, but frequently can recur for months to rarely years. A variety of histopathologic patterns have been linked to this condition. The majority of the pathologic reports describe a dense perivascular inflammatory infiltrate composed of lymphocytes, with scattered eosinophils and plasma cells.

ERYTHEMA CHRONICUM MIGRANS

Epidemiology and Etiology

This is the earliest sign of Lyme disease, which is caused by a tick bite from the spirochete Borrelia burgdorferi. Both children and adults can be affected. Cases have been reported in North America, Europe, and Asia. In the United States, the majority of cases are in the northeastern, north-central, and western states.[50]

Clinical Presentation

Localized erythema migrans presents as an annular erythematous lesion with central clearing that expands to be several centimeters over days; this is the typical bull's eye rash that appears between 1 and 30 days after the tick bite.[50] Sometimes, the center of the lesion can vesiculate or ulcerate. Without treatment, the lesion can last for 1 to 4 weeks. In early disseminated disease, multiple lesions are seen and can be accompanied by fever and joint pains.[50]

Histologic Findings

The pathologic findings are similar to those of other gyrate erythemas (Figure 6-13). This condition is also referred to as Borrelia-induced lymphocytoma cutis. There is a superficial and deep, mostly perivascular tight lymphocytic infiltrate with the presence of plasma cells. The biopsies typically lack epidermal changes. Scattered eosinophils can also be present. A particular perineural infiltration of lymphocytes and plasma cells has been described in some cases of ECM. An interstitial pattern of inflammation has also been documented in some cases. Special stains for microorganisms (Warthin-Starry stain) and polymerase chain reaction analysis for Lyme can help in establishing the diagnosis. Other

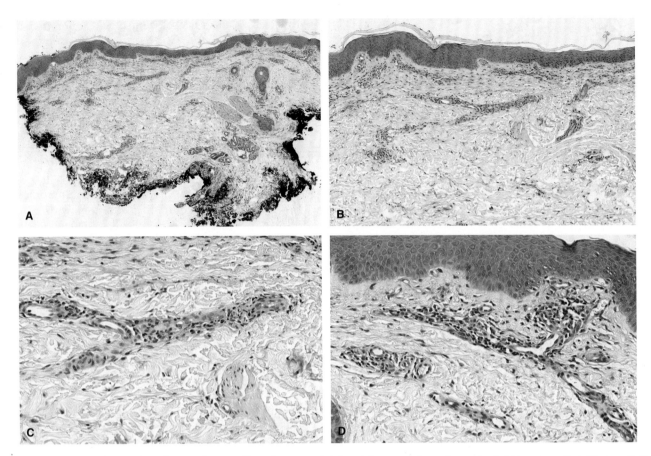

FIGURE 6-13. Erythema chronicum migrans. There is a superficial and deep, mostly perivascular tight lymphocytic infiltrate with the presence of plasma cells. The biopsies typically lack epidermal changes (A-D). Digital slides courtesy of Path Presenter.com.

findings that can be seen in association with Lyme disease include acrodermatitis chronica atrophicans and cutaneous lymphoid hyperplasia.[51-54]

Differential Diagnosis

Other gyrate erythemas typically lack the plasma cell infiltrate typical of ECM. Tumid lupus/Jessner's/reticular erythematous mucinosis can also share the presence of plasma cells. However, ECM lacks the significant amount of mucin present in those conditions.

CAPSULE SUMMARY

ERYTHEMA CHRONICUM MIGRANS

ECM is the earliest sign of Lyme disease, caused by a tick bite from the spirochete Borrelia burgdorferi. Both children and adults can be affected. Localized erythema migrans presents as an annular erythematous lesion with central clearing that expands to be several centimeters over days; this is the typical bull's eye rash that appears between 1 and 30 days after the tick bite. Pathologically, there is a superficial and deep, mostly perivascular tight lymphocytic infiltrate with the presence of plasma cells.

ERYTHEMA MARGINATUM

Definition and Etiology

This is a form of annular erythema that occurs in approximately 2% to 4% of patients with rheumatic fever. It is seen more frequently in children than in adults. The pathogenesis remains unknown. A study documenting the accumulation of bradykinin in the stromal tissue and endothelial cells in the skin biopsy of erythema marginatum has been reported. Bradykinin appears to be important in the pathogenesis of erythema marginatum associated with hereditary angioedema.[55-58]

Clinical Presentation

The lesions appear on the trunk (particularly the abdomen) and proximal extremities as pink macules and papules that often have an annular and polycyclic pattern.

Histologic Findings

The biopsies of this condition show a neutrophilic infiltrate within the dermal papillae and around the superficial vessels. There is no definitive evidence of vasculitis. Leukocytoclasis is present. Scattered apoptotic keratinocytes in the epidermis can be present. A rare case report of an urticarial presentation of this form of gyrate erythema has been described (with similar pathologic changes to those seen in urticaria). Neutrophilic figurate erythema of infancy may have identical pathologic findings, but is not associated with rheumatic fever.[11,49,56-58]

CAPSULE SUMMARY

ERYTHEMA MARGINATUM

This is a form of annular erythema that occurs in approximately 2% to 4% of patients with rheumatic fever. It is seen more frequently in children than in adults. The lesions appear on the trunk (particularly the abdomen) and proximal extremities as pink macules and papules that often have an annular and polycyclic pattern. The biopsies of this condition show a neutrophilic infiltrate within the dermal papillae and around the superficial vessels. There is no definitive evidence of vasculitis.

PERNIOSIS (CHILBLAINS)

Definition and Epidemiology

Pernio is an inflammatory process that occurs because of an abnormal exuberant response to cold temperatures in predisposed individuals. It is more common in colder climates such as the northern United States and northern Europe and is most common in young women aged 15 to 30.[59] Within the pediatric population, it occurs most in teenagers, but can also occur in younger ages.[60] In children, the presence of cryoproteins can be associated with pernio.[61] In adolescents, it has been reported in the context of anorexia and may be related to impaired thermoregulation.[62] Thin habitus was also noted in one series to be a common characteristic, and in one pediatric patient, weight loss secondary to celiac disease was speculated to contribute to the development of pernio lesions.[59,63]

Etiology

Some studies have suggested that pernio may be caused by vasospasm, which in turn is caused by cold temperatures, leading to inflammatory changes secondary to ischemia.[64] Others postulate that it may be caused by endothelial cell injury leading to abnormally persistent vasoconstriction of the deep cutaneous arterioles with dilation of the smaller superficial vessels.[60]

Clinical Presentation

Typical acute lesions occur on the fingers, toes, and nose and appear several hours after exposure to cold and typically resolve within 1 to 3 weeks. They appear as blanching macules in its mild form and progress to firmer edematous nodules that can be pink to violaceous; lesions can be painful,

pruritic, or burning (Figures 6-14 and 6-15).[59] Lesions can blister or ulcerate. The condition tends to begin in the fall and winter and resolve by the spring and summer, although in chronic cases with repeated exposure to cold, the lesions can become persistent through the warmer months as well.[59] Dorsal fingers and toes, heels, lower legs, nose, and ears can be affected as well. If lesions occur in unusual circumstances or are persistent, then evaluation for other possible causes is warranted. Possible underlying conditions include connective tissue disease and hematologic disorders.[65] Bloodwork checked includes complete blood count, antinuclear antibody, cryoglobulin, cryofibrinogen, and cold agglutinin. In adults, serum protein electrophoresis is often checked for monoclonal gammopathy, but this is much less likely in children. Genetic disorders have also been associated with perniosis, including Aicardi-Goutieres syndrome (particularly those with dominant type *TREX1* mutation) and familial chilblain lupus (heterozygous mutation in *TREX1*).[66]

Histologic Findings

Biopsies from perniosis show a superficial and deep, perivascular and periadnexal lymphocytic infiltrate in an acral location (Figure 6-16). Marked papillary dermal edema is also seen. Sometimes, small vascular thrombi and fibrinoid changes of the vascular walls are present. Some cases can also have increased dermal mucin, and interface changes. In most cases, the epidermis is relatively unremarkable.[59,61,67,68]

Differential Diagnosis

Lupus erythematosus should always be considered in the differential diagnosis. The clinical, serologic findings, and the presence of increased dermal mucin can help in establishing a diagnosis of lupus. Other forms of gyrate erythemas can also be considered in the differential diagnosis. But, the acral location of perniosis can easily discern between such diagnostic possibilities. A small-vessel vasculitis (LCV) can also be considered in the differential diagnosis.

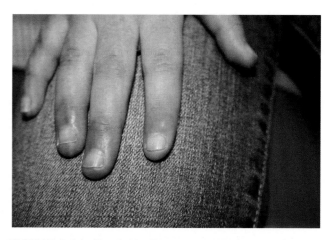

FIGURE 6-14. **Perniosis.** Edematous nodules on the fingers.

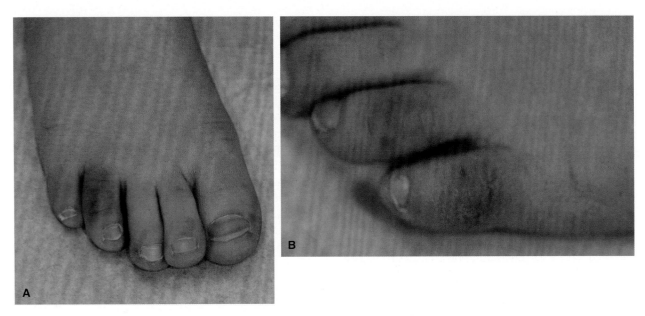

FIGURE 6-15. Firm, indurated nodules, with a dusky and hemorrhagic appearance are seen on the toes (A,B).

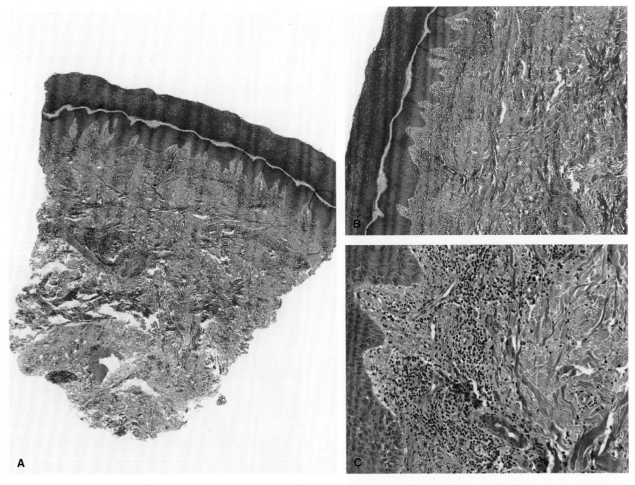

FIGURE 6-16. **Perniosis.** There is a superficial and deep, perivascular and periadnexal lymphocytic infiltrate in an acral location (A). Marked papillary dermal edema is also seen (B,C).

However, LCV shows a neutrophilic infiltrate with leukocytoclasis, features usually missing in cases of perniosis.

CAPSULE SUMMARY

PERNIOSIS (CHILBLAINS)

Pernio is an inflammatory process that occurs because of an abnormal exuberant response to cold temperatures in predisposed individuals. Within the pediatric population, it occurs most in teenagers but can also occur in younger ages. Typical acute lesions occur on the fingers, toes, and nose and appear several hours after exposure to cold and typically resolve within 1 to 3 weeks. They appear as blanching macules in its mild form and progress to firmer edematous nodules that can be pink to violaceous; lesions can be painful, pruritic, or burning. Biopsies from perniosis show a superficial and deep, perivascular and periadnexal lymphocytic infiltrate in an acral location. Marked papillary dermal edema is also seen.

PITYRIASIS LICHENOIDES

Definition and Epidemiology

This a spectrum of skin diseases that is broken down into the acute and chronic forms, called PLEVA (pityriasis lichenoides et varioliformis acuta or Mucha–Habermann disease) and PLC (pityriasis lichenoides chronica). PLEVA occurs more acutely and presents with papulovesicles that can become necrotic and ulcerated; PLC presents with recurrent scaly lichenoid papules that tend to be recurrent.[69]

Pityriasis lichenoides is relatively frequent in the pediatric population. In one study, almost 20% of cases were seen in the pediatric age group.[70] Most cases are reported in kids under the age of 10, with peaks in the preschool and early school years in one study of 124 children.[69] It generally does not occur under age 2, although rare cases can occur in infancy.[71,72] Winter and fall were the most common seasons for this disorder to occur.[69]

Etiology

Pityriasis lichenoides is considered an interface dermatitis with an associated lymphocytic vasculitis, that is likely triggered by an antigenic stimulus.[73] There is frequently history of a preceding infection such as a viral illness, medication, or vaccination in children.[74,75] Most PLEVA samples in one study were found to be monoclonal, which differed from the PLC cases that were mostly polyclonal. It is hypothesized that host immune response determines the clinical presentation and histology of this condition.[76] Although its potential evolution to malignancy is unclear, there are rare reports of cutaneous T-cell lymphoma in patients with a history of PLEVA/PLC.[77,78] In the author's perspective, such reports are biased by a selection of cases, and in most circumstances, MOST patients with PLEVA or PLC DO NOT progress to a cutaneous T-cell lymphoma, such as mycosis fungoides or lymphomatoid papulosis.

Clinical Presentation

One study reported equal frequencies of occurrence between PLEVA and PLC, with many cases having an overlap presentation.[74] In both forms, the distribution of lesions was mostly diffuse in the majority of patients (75%) and localized (in about 20%).[69]

PLEVA begins suddenly as 2 to 3 mm reddish-brown macules and papules on the trunk and proximal extremities that appear in crops and quickly develop vesicles, purpura, and sometimes necrosis (Figure 6-17). They can be asymptomatic or pruritic. In this stage, lesions can appear similar to varicella, bug bites, and impetigo. Lesions then develop fine scaling and can resolve with a small scar as well as transient hyperpigmentation or hypopigmentation. The time to resolution ranges anywhere from weeks to many months.[69]

The febrile ulceronecrotic form is rare and presents with ulceronecrotic nodules and plaques with fever; half of all cases have been in children.[79,80]

PLC lesions are scaly lichenoid papules that resolve with hypopigmentation (Figure 6-18A). At times in

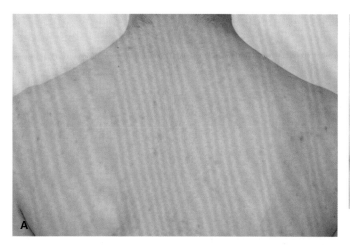
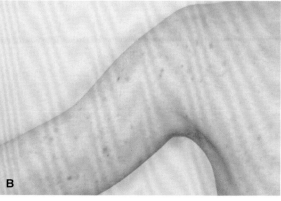

FIGURE 6-17. Two- to three-millimeter reddish-brown macules and papules on the trunk and proximal extremities (A,B).

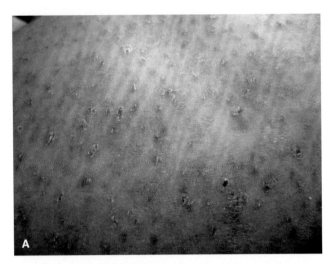 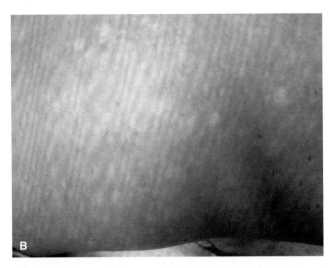

FIGURE 6-18. (A) Multiple scaly erythematous papules in a child with pityriasis lichenoides chronica. (B) Hypopigmentation is prominent in this darker-skinned child with pityriasis lichenoides chronica. Small scaly erythematous papules are seen as well.

darker-skinned patients, hypopigmentation may be the most prominent finding (Figure 6-18B).

The course of PLC tends to be more prolonged than PLEVA and lasts several months, often with recurrence.[81]

Histologic Findings

Biopsies of PLEVA and PLC show a range in severity, density, and pattern of lichenoid and interface changes.[76,82,83] Biopsies of PLEVA classically show variable thickness of the epidermis, depending upon the developmental stage

of the lesion, which is being biopsied. Lesions with chronic evidence of trauma may show psoriasiform changes. Thick parakeratosis is present. There is an interface tissue reaction with numerous dyskeratotic and apoptotic keratinocytes, in addition to vacuolar degeneration of the basal keratinocytes (Figures 6-19 and 6-20). In some cases, extensive and diffuse epidermal necrosis can be seen. A superficial to deep, lymphocytic infiltrate in the dermis is present, with a wedge-shaped appearance. The infiltrate shows extension into the surface epidermis. A lymphocytic vasculitis is also

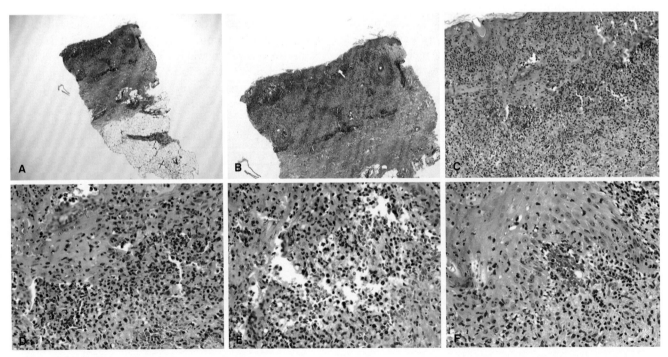

FIGURE 6-19. Pityriasis lichenoides et varioliformis acuta. A localized area of epidermal necrosis with surface ulceration is noted (A-C). Closer inspection shows numerous necrotic and apoptotic keratinocytes at all layers of the epidermis (D), vacuolar degeneration of the basal keratinocytes (E and F), and prominent lymphoid exocytosis.

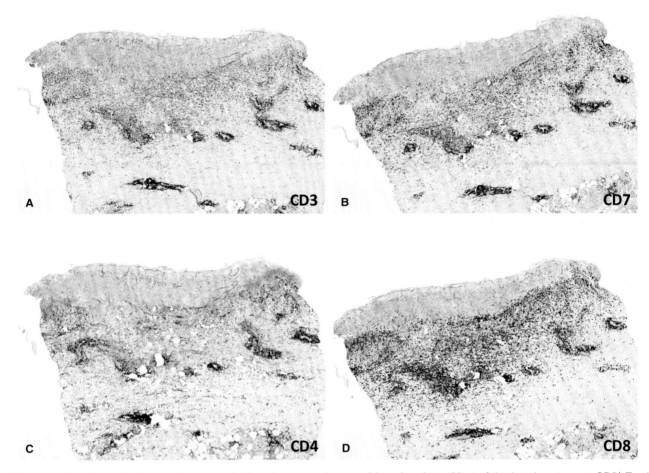

FIGURE 6-20. **Pityriasis lichenoides et varioliformis acuta—immunohistochemistry.** Most of the lymphocytes are CD3$^+$ T-cells (A) with retained expression of CD7 (B). The CD4:CD8 ratio is markedly inverted, with a large predominance of cytotoxic T-cells (C,D).

seen, in the form of tight perivascular collections of lymphocytes with dermal edema and extravasated red blood cells. Eosinophils are not frequently seen.

Under the microscope, PLC displays both interface lichenoid changes and mild spongiosis in the epidermis (Figure 6-21). Lymphocytes approximate the dermal-epidermal junction, accompanied by basovacuolar change and scattered dyskeratotic keratinocytes in the epidermis. Small intraepidermal lymphocytes with regular nuclear contours are seen. There is variable ortho-and parakeratosis. The dermis typically shows a superficial perivascular lymphocytic infiltrate. Eosinophils are rarely present. Fibrin deposition may be observed within vessel walls, but frank vasculitis is not seen. Other common histologic findings include the presence of extravasated red blood cells and/or melanophages in the upper dermis.

Although PLEVA and PLC are thought to be closely related conditions, or even different manifestations of a single disorder by some, they may manifest different immunophenotypes. The infiltrate of PLEVA has been found to more

often display an elevated CD8:CD4 ratio (Figure 6-20), whereas the T lymphocytes in PLC show a predominance of CD4$^+$ cells rather than CD8$^+$ cells. Moreover, T-cell intracellular antigen-1 (TIA-1) is more likely to be expressed in the T lymphocytes of PLEVA, compared with PLC which shows increased expressed of FOXP3, a marker of T-regulatory cells. Interestingly, one recent study found that 4 out of 23 cases diagnosed as PLC with a benign clinical course showed a predominantly γδ T-cell phenotype, even though γδ T-cells have more traditionally been associated with aggressive lymphomas.

Clonal rearrangement of the T-cell receptor gene may be observed in PLC; on the basis of this finding PLC has been classified as a T-cell dyscrasia. A study by Magro and colleagues found evidence of T-cell clonality in 33/35 patients with pityriasis lichenoides. The patients studied were interpreted to have either PLEVA or PLC considering both clinical and histopathologic findings, with the majority of the patients classified as having PLC. Two other studies have found occasional clonal TCR-γ gene rearrangement in their

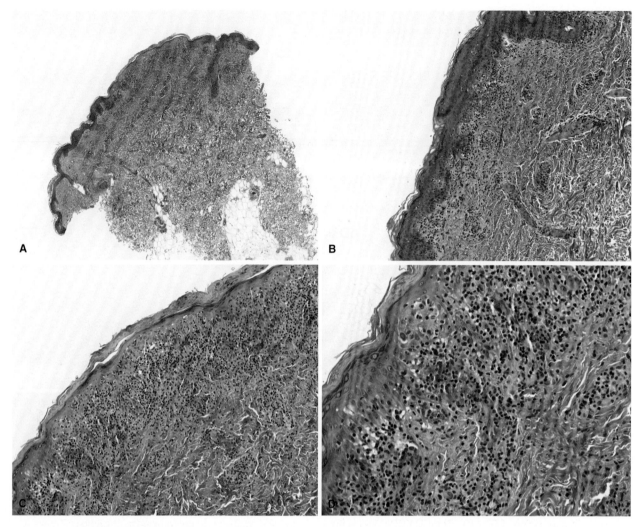

FIGURE 6-21. Pityriasis lichenoides chronica (PLC). The findings in PLC are similar to those of pityriasis lichenoides et varioliformis acuta (PLEVA), but milder. There is a lichenoid and interface process (A,B). The lymphoid population also extends to the epidermis, but there is no extensive keratinocyte apoptosis as seen in PLEVA (C,D). Extravasated red blood cells are also present (D).

PLC patients, in 1/13 and 3/16 patients, respectively. By contrast, Kim et al. did not detect clonal TCR-γ gene rearrangement in any of the 13 PLC patients. The differences in these studies may reflect some of the difficulties in differentiating PLC from early lesions of mycosis fungoides.[73,76,83-86]

Differential Diagnosis

The histopathologic changes of PLC closely resemble those of PLEVA, because both show lymphocyte exocytosis, interface dermatitis with basovacuolar alteration, mild spongiosis, a superficial lymphocytic infiltrate, and papillary dermal hemorrhage. However, the microscopic findings in PLC are typically more subtle than in PLEVA; the lymphocytic infiltrate of the latter is more intense in both the epidermal and dermal compartments, with a wedge-shaped perivascular lymphocytic inflammation extending into the reticular dermis. In addition, ulceration is not a characteristic

observation in PLC but is seen with some frequency in more severe cases of PLEVA, often in conjunction with a serum crust containing neutrophils.

Some variants of mycosis fungoides may be difficult to distinguish from PLC, both clinically and histologically. A recent study detailed four patients with eventual diagnoses of papular mycosis fungoides, all of whom had small reddish-brown papules present between 5 and 25 years.[87] On the basis of initial clinical-pathologic correlation, three of the four patients were initially felt to have pityriasis lichenoides, but additional biopsies in each case demonstrated characteristic findings of mycosis fungoides on histology, including epidermotropism with lymphocyte atypia and elevated CD4:CD8 ratios. Hypopigmented mycosis fungoides often demonstrates overlapping histologic findings with PLC, and in these cases, clinical-pathologic correlation is essential.

Other diagnostic considerations include pityriasis rosea, guttate psoriasis, small plaque parapsoriasis (digitate dermatosis), arthropod bite reactions, and lymphomatoid papulosis. As opposed to the more confluent pattern of parakeratosis, pityriasis rosea only shows mounds of it In addition, the "tilting" phenomenon of the parakeratotic mounds is typical of pityriasis rosea (PR), but not of pityriasis lichenoides (PL). PR also differs on the spongiotic pattern, as opposed to the interface changes seen in both PLEVA and PLC. Guttate psoriasis has a very different histologic appearance, with only mild or very modest pathologic changes, which include vascular telangiectasia, mild acanthosis, and few scattered neutrophils in the epidermis or corneal layer. Digitate dermatosis lacks the interface changes of PLC/PLEVA and the red cell extravasation. Although arthropod reactions can share the wedge-shaped dense inflammation in the dermis, they have an abundance of dermal eosinophils, a feature not present in PLC/PLEVA. Lymphomatoid papulosis has different histologic patterns, all of which are based on the finding of atypical CD30⁺ large cells. The lesions can also have the scarring seen in PLC/PLEVA.

CAPSULE SUMMARY

PITYRIASIS LICHENOIDES

This is a spectrum of skin diseases that is broken down into the acute and chronic forms, called PLEVA and PLC. PLEVA occurs more acutely and presents with papulovesicles that can become necrotic and ulcerated; PLC presents with recurrent scaly lichenoid papules that tend to be recurrent. Biopsies of PLEVA and PLC show a range in severity, density, and pattern of lichenoid and interface changes.

SWEET SYNDROME (ACUTE FEBRILE NEUTROPHILIC DERMATOSIS)

Definition and Epidemiology

Sweet syndrome, also known as acute febrile neutrophilic dermatosis, presents with painful edematous lesions along with fever and leukocytosis. It is estimated that about 5% of cases are seen in the pediatric population.[88,89] The mean age is reported to be just over 5 years old, and cases can present in infancy with the youngest presentation at 3 days old.[90-92] There is a male predominance in patients under age 3 and an equal gender distribution in cases over age 3.[90] Most patients who present before age 6 weeks tend to have a serious underlying condition such as immunodeficiency or malignancy.[91,93]

Etiology

Etiology is not known, and this condition is thought to represent a hypersensitivity response to triggers. The classic pediatric case presents with a history of an upper respiratory infection or GI illness about 1 to 3 weeks prior to the onset of skin lesions.[90,91] Other associated diseases in children include autoimmune conditions such as systemic lupus erythematosus (SLE),[94,95] immunodeficiencies,[96] and other infectious processes such as otitis media[40] and HIV.[97] Medications including trimethoprim-sulfamethoxazole and granulocyte colony-stimulating factor have also been reported.[98-100] In children, about one-quarter of cases are linked with an underlying malignancy, usually hematologic. In addition, cases of Sweet syndrome with malignancy tend to occur in older age.[90,91,101]

Clinical Presentation

Classic lesions are erythematous to violaceous edematous painful papules, plaques, and nodules that are most commonly on the face, upper trunk, and upper arms (Figures 6-22 and 6-23**).** More edematous lesions can develop a mamillated appearance. Mucosal lesions can rarely be seen.[91] Pathergy is noted in about 20% to 30% of pediatric patients.[91] It is common to have high fevers early in the course or even preceding the skin eruption; leukocytosis and elevated inflammatory markers are common lab findings. Muscle aches, joint pains, and conjunctivitis can occur. Extracutaneous disease has been reported in almost every organ, including the liver, lungs, and kidneys. Skin lesions generally resolve without scarring, although a significant number of pediatric cases can resolve with atrophic dyspigmented scarring and acquired cutis laxa.[91] It should be noted that patients with acquired cutis laxa can develop severe cardiac complications.[91,102]

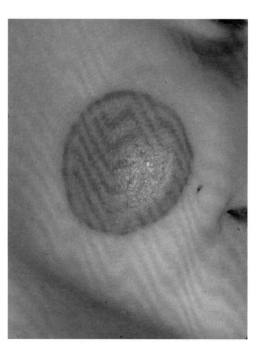

FIGURE 6-22. **Sweet syndrome.** Large, erythematous, plaque on the cheek.

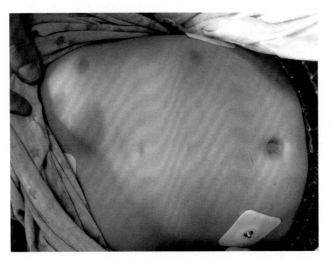

FIGURE 6-23. Sweet syndrome, histiocytoid variant. Erythematous nodules and plaques on the trunk, identical in character to the conventional variant of Sweet syndrome.

Histologic Findings

The main pathologic finding of classic lesions of Sweet syndrome is the presence of a neutrophilic dermatosis (Figure 6-24). Hence, the epidermis is somewhat normal, but a subepidermal blister can be present, usually a result of edema in the dermis. There is a superficial and deep, mostly interstitial neutrophilic infiltrate with marked leukocytoclasis. The leukocytoclasis reflects the presence of

nuclear fragments, remnants of neutrophils undergoing degeneration. The dermis also has prominent edema. Although the neutrophils can be seen around vascular spaces, true vasculitic changes are not typical of Sweet's. The early lesions of Sweet's lack a significant neutrophilic infiltrate and can be more lymphocytic in nature. Scattered eosinophils are present, but an abundance of them is not frequent. Recent data have shown that a pathologic overlap between Sweet's and some cases of cutaneous lupus can be seen. The neutrophilic inflammation can also extend into the adipose tissue, and sometimes be the epicenter of the process (subcutaneous Sweet syndrome). Resolving lesions may show elastolysis, and clinically manifest with slack skin. The finding appears to be secondary to the enzymatic degradation of the elastic fibers.[91,92,103-112]

A *histiocytoid variant* of Sweet's has been reported more recently (Figure 6-25).[113-115] Approximately 30% of such cases are associated with a hematologic malignancy, and many of them were seen in the pediatric age group. The clinical appearance of the lesions is similar to the conventional Sweet's variant. Pathologically, the epidermis is spared and this variant shares the prominent dermal edema seen in cases of conventional Sweet syndrome. There is a superficial and deep, perivascular and interstitial mononuclear cell infiltrate in the dermis. These mononuclear cells showed large, elongated, twisted or kidney-shaped vesicular nuclei, inconspicuous nucleoli, and scant eosinophilic cytoplasm mimicking small

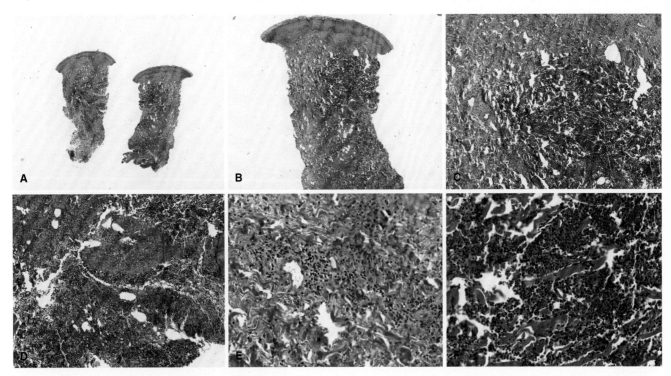

FIGURE 6-24. Sweet syndrome. There is a diffuse, mostly interstitial, superficial and deep dermal infiltrate (A,B). The infiltrate is composed of mostly neutrophils with a remarkable degree of leukocytoclasis (C-F). Although the inflammation is present around the blood vessel walls, definitive vasculitis is not seen (E).

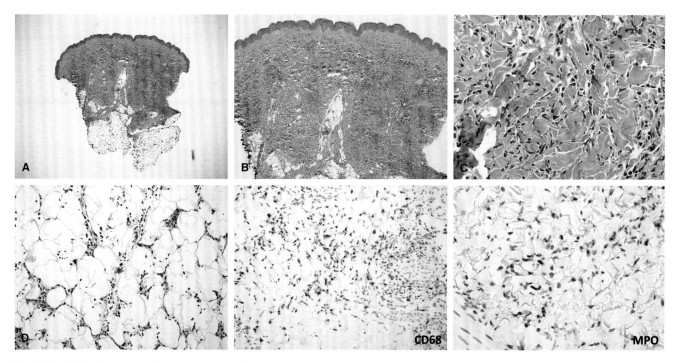

FIGURE 6-25. **Sweet syndrome, histiocytoid variant.** Diffuse, superficial, and deep infiltrate with extension into the adipose tissue (A,B). The infiltrate is composed of mononuclear cells with a histiocytoid appearance (C). Many of the cells also extend to the adipose tissue (D). The infiltrate is positive for CD68 and myeloperoxidase.

histiocytes. By immunohistochemistry, the mononuclear cells are positive with histiocytic markers (CD68, CD163, Lysozyme) and show characteristic expression of myeloperoxidase (MPO). Many have argued that the population of immature cells could represent in some cases neoplastic myeloid precursors.[116] These cells lack immature marker expression (CD123, CD34, TdT, CD117, CD1a).

Differential Diagnosis

The first pathologic differential, when encountering a dense neutrophilic infiltrate, often in the setting of a hematologic condition, and possibly immunodeficiency, is an infectious process. Therefore, routine use of special stains for bacterial organisms, fungus, and mycobacteria should be performed in all cases (Gram, GMS, PAS, AFB, FITE). In general, the edema seen in infectious processes tend to be more significant than the degree of inflammation, whereas Sweet syndrome typically shows the opposite. Pyoderma gangrenosum (PG) is the second form of neutrophilic dermatosis that should be included in the differential diagnosis. The lesions of PG are frequently ulcerated and can start with a follicular-based pattern. Regardless, distinguishing both conditions on a pure histopathologic assessment is virtually impossible. The evanescent macular eruption associated with juvenile rheumatoid arthritis (Still disease) is

more prominent when the patient is febrile and is pathologically characterized by superficial perivascular neutrophilic infiltration and papillary dermal edema. LCV can also be included in the differential diagnosis. LCV can be distinguished on the basis of vascular damage, with fibrinoid necrosis, endothelial damage, and a perivascular character of leukocytoclasis. Pathologically, erythema elevatum diutinum shares many of the histologic findings of LCV and can also be included in the differential diagnosis.

In the case of a histiocytoid form of Sweet syndrome, a diagnosis of leukemia cutis appears to be the most important and challenging condition to exclude. Indeed, given the fact that many cases of leukemia cutis show a monocytic phenotype, the use of immature markers is of limited value (because most of these cases lack expression of CD34, TdT, or CD117). Therefore, one should make a rational clinicopathologic approach to determine whether the infiltrate is "mature" or "immature." Acute hemorrhagic edema of infancy is also in the differential diagnosis of Sweet syndrome, and can be frequently excluded on the basis of the clinical findings.

Cases of subcutaneous Sweet Syndrome may resemble other forms of lobular neutrophilic panniculitis, including alpha-1-antitrypsin deficiency, factitial panniculitis, infection, and even lupus panniculitis.

CAPSULE SUMMARY

SWEET SYNDROME

Sweet syndrome, also known as acute febrile neutrophilic dermatosis, presents with painful edematous lesions along with fever and leukocytosis. It is estimated that about 5% of cases are seen in the pediatric population. In children, about one-quarter of cases are linked with an underlying malignancy, usually hematologic. Classic lesions are erythematous to violaceous edematous painful papules, plaques, and nodules that are most commonly on the face, upper trunk, and upper arms. More edematous lesions can develop a mamillated appearance. The main pathologic finding of classic lesions of Sweet syndrome is the presence of a neutrophilic dermatosis. A more recent histiocytoid variant has also been documented of late.

BOWEL-ASSOCIATED DERMATOSIS–ARTHRITIS SYNDROME (BADAS)

Definition and Epidemiology

This neutrophilic dermatosis presents with recurrent episodes of arthritis and skin lesions in the context of bowel disease. It was originally described in adult patients after jejunoileal bypass surgery, but is now recognized to occur in the context of other GI disorders. It is rare in the pediatric population.

Etiology

This is thought to result from inflammation and abnormal circulating immune complexes against bacterial peptidoglycan, which are produced as a result of intestinal bacterial overgrowth related to bowel stasis.[117,118]

Clinical Presentation

Classic lesions present as crops of erythematous macules that quickly morph into inflammatory papules and purpuric vesiculopustules on the upper extremities and trunk that can be necrotic and then heal without scarring.[119] The lesions last about one week and can recur for weeks to months. Lesions are generally asymptomatic or slightly pruritic, although acral lesions can be painful. Acral lesions can mimic gonococcemia and shin and ankle lesions can mimic erythema nodosum. The skin eruptions can present with flu-like symptoms such as fever and myalgias, as well as peripheral joint pains that leave no long-term sequelae.[119,120]

Histologic Findings

Histologically, BADAS has been described as identical to Sweet syndrome (acute febrile dermatosis), a mature

neutrophilic infiltrate in the dermis with papillary dermal edema. BADAS characteristically does not result in vessel destruction. On biopsy, vessels are patent and there is no evidence for fibrinoid necrosis or infarction, and early reports suggesting such findings have been dismissed in later literature. This distinguishes BADAS from LCV. In addition, multiple staining techniques confirm the absence of microorganisms. Several studies have suggested that the histopathology of cutaneous lesions is temporally dependent on disease progression: The macular stage produces a perivascular mononuclear cell infiltrate; the papular stage produces edema of the papillary and reticular dermis. Neutrophils are concentrated in dermal venules in the former, and present diffusely in the dermis in the latter stage. In older papules and vesicles, the neutrophilic infiltrate is denser, incorporating nuclear debris and few eosinophils. Massive edema of the papillary dermis contributes to vesicle formation, whereas expulsion of neutrophilic debris through the epidermis results in pustules.[121-124]

CAPSULE SUMMARY

BOWEL-ASSOCIATED DERMATOSIS–ARTHRITIS SYNDROME

This neutrophilic dermatosis presents with recurrent episodes of arthritis and skin lesions in the context of bowel disease. It was originally described in adult patients after jejunoileal bypass surgery, but is now recognized to occur in the context of other GI disorders. It is rare in the pediatric population. Classic lesions present as crops of erythematous macules that quickly morph into inflammatory papules and purpuric vesiculopustules on the upper extremities and trunk that can be necrotic and then heal without scarring. Histologically, BADAS has been described as identical to Sweet syndrome (acute febrile dermatosis), a mature neutrophilic infiltrate in the dermis with papillary dermal edema. BADAS characteristically does not result in vessel destruction.

ECCRINE HIDRADENITIS

PALMOPLANTAR HIDRADENITIS

Definition and Epidemiology

This benign self-limited skin eruption occurs mainly on the soles and sometimes on the palms of healthy children and is associated with vigorous physical activity.

This condition happens in healthy children from toddler years to adolescence who have often engaged in intense physical activity. Examples of intense physical activity included dancing, mountain climbing, having a sport day at school, and crawling on the hands and knees on aluminum bleachers.[125,126] One series showed a mean age of 6 years and suggested seasonal peaks in the spring and fall seasons.[127] Excessive sweating and prolonged exposure to moisture such as with wet footwear are thought to be triggers as well.[128]

Etiology

Mechanical and/or thermal trauma is thought to result in rupture of the eccrine glands in the affected soles and palms, leading to the activation of a cytokine cascade that attracts neutrophils and results in tender inflamed lesions.[127]

Clinical Presentation

Painful erythematous macules and nodules develop abruptly on the palmar and plantar surfaces soon after intense exercise (Figure 6-26). The soles of the feet are most commonly involved, which leads to difficulty walking. Lesions generally resolve spontaneously generally within 1 to 4 weeks with rest, although it recurs in about half of cases.[125,127] Clinically, other conditions to consider include chilblains, insect bite reaction, erythema nodosum, and cellulitis.

Histologic Findings

Typical histologic findings include a neutrophilic perieccrine infiltrate in the setting of varying degrees of superficial and deep perivascular infiltrates of neutrophils, lymphocytes, and histiocytes as well as septal panniculitis.[125,129]

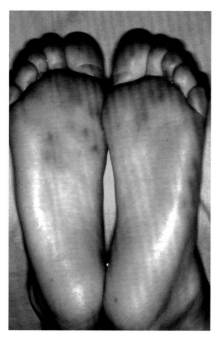

FIGURE 6-26. Palmoplantar hidradenitis. Painful erythematous macules and nodules develop abruptly on the palmar and plantar surfaces soon after intense exercise.

CAPSULE SUMMARY

PALMOPLANTAR HIDRADENITIS

This benign self-limited skin eruption occurs mainly on the soles and sometimes on the palms of healthy children and is associated with vigorous physical activity. Painful erythematous macules and nodules develop abruptly on the palmar and plantar surfaces soon after intense exercise. The soles of the feet are most commonly involved, which leads to difficulty walking. Typical histologic findings include a neutrophilic perieccrine infiltrate in the setting of varying degrees of superficial and deep perivascular infiltrates of neutrophils.

NEUTROPHILIC ECCRINE HIDRADENITIS

Definition and Epidemiology

Neutrophilic eccrine hidradenitis (NEH) is a neutrophilic dermatosis that usually occurs as result of chemotherapy toxicity to eccrine glands. It was initially described in association with induction chemotherapy for acute myelogenous leukemia.[130] Lesions develop about 1 to 2 weeks after starting chemotherapy, most commonly cytarabine and anthracyclines, but have also been described in the setting of cancer and infection.[131]

Etiology

Lesions are thought to occur as a result of direct toxicity of chemotherapy to the eccrine glands.

Clinical Presentation

Erythematous papules and plaques occur on the trunk and extremities about 1 to 2 weeks after starting chemotherapy, often accompanied by fever. Lesions can be asymptomatic or painful.

Histologic Findings

Histologic examination of NEH shows a degeneration of eccrine glands in association with an inflammatory infiltrate replete with neutrophils. Secretory coils of the eccrine glands are variably damaged by vacuolar alteration and necrosis of cells. In some cases, the ductal epithelia are unaffected, whereas in others, squamous metaplasia with dyskeratosis, spongiosis, vacuolization, and necrosis have been reported (Figure 6-27). The lower dermis is edematous and contains a perivascular, sometimes more diffuse and dense, infiltrate of neutrophils, lymphocytes, and macrophages, and rarely eosinophils. The epidermis and pilosebaceous units are usually normal.[132-134]

Differential Diagnosis

Sweat gland necrosis in drug-and carbon monoxide-induced coma differs from that in NEH by a less dense inflammatory reaction and by the additional presence of necrosis

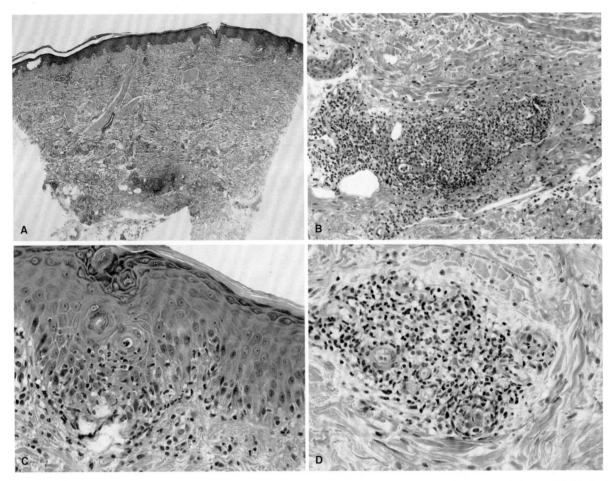

FIGURE 6-27. **Neutrophilic eccrine hidradenitis.** There is a superficial and deep, perieccrine inflammatory infiltrate (A). Marked acute inflammation extends around and infiltrates into the sweat gland epithelium (B,D). Some degenerated sweat ducts are seen. The inflammation also follows the areas of entrance of the sweat duct into the surface epidermis (C).

in the pilosebaceous apparatus and the epidermis. Other neutrophilic disorders, such as LCV, Sweet syndrome, PG, hidradenitis suppurativa, and miliaria profunda, can be distinguished clearly by the fact that they do not show degeneration and necrosis of the secretory parts of the sweat glands in areas devoid of inflammation.

CAPSULE SUMMARY

NEUTROPHILIC ECCRINE HIDRADENITIS

NEH is a neutrophilic dermatosis that usually occurs as result of chemotherapy toxicity to eccrine glands. It was initially described in association with induction chemotherapy for acute myelogenous leukemia. Erythematous papules and plaques occur on the trunk and extremities about 1 to 2 weeks after starting chemotherapy, often accompanied by fever. Histologic examination of NEH shows a degeneration of eccrine glands in association with an inflammatory infiltrate replete with neutrophils. Secretory coils of the eccrine glands are variably damaged by vacuolar alteration and necrosis of cells.

WELLS SYNDROME

Definition and Epidemiology

This is a benign dermatosis, also called "eosinophilic cellulitis with flame figures," that can range from a localized inflammatory plaque resembling cellulitis to rarely a widespread blistering eruption. Most cases occur in adults, and this condition happens occasionally in the pediatric population.

Etiology

This is considered to be a hypersensitivity reaction to a variety of possible triggers, including insect bites,[135] medications, infections including parvovirus B19,[136] and hematologic disorders. A trigger is not identified in about half of cases.[137] Elevated IL-5, which plays a role in eosinophil mobilization and homing, have been correlated with disease activity.[137,138]

Clinical Presentation

Lesions are very pruritic erythematous plaques that evolve quickly over 2 to 3 days; they are often confused for bacterial cellulitis and can vesiculate (Figure 6-28A and B).[137] Bullous

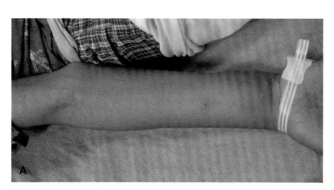 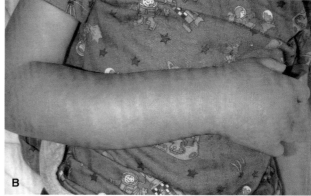

FIGURE 6-28. (A and B) Characteristic erythematous, edematous plaques seen in Wells syndrome. Obtained with permission from Gru AA, Schaffer A, eds. *Hematopathology of the Skin: Clinical and Pathological Approach*. 1st ed. Philadelphia, PA: Wolters Kluwer; 2016.

lesions can rarely be quite severe.[135] The lower extremities are most commonly affected, although other areas of the body can have lesions as well. Lesions generally resolve in 2 weeks to 2 months with discolored patches and atrophic skin; on the scalp, scarring alopecia can occur.[135] Episodes frequently recur, sometimes over years.[137] Leukocytosis and peripheral eosinophilia occurs in up to 50% of cases during the active inflammatory phase. The disease usually runs a benign course, but sometimes systemic symptoms such as fever, malaise, and joint pains can occur.[136] Overall, the diagnosis should be considered in a child with a cellulitis-like presentation and elevated peripheral eosinophils who does not improve with antibiotics.

Histologic Findings

The pathologic findings seen in Wells syndrome include a dense, superficial and deep, perivascular and interstitial infiltrate that is rich in dermal eosinophils. Dermal edema is also typical of this condition (Figure 6-29). The dermal eosinophils show marked degranulation, and eosinophilic material is present surrounding degenerated collagen fibers, a pathologic finding that is called "flame figures." It is important to emphasize that, although flame figures are typical of this entity, they are not specific. Flame figures can be seen in a variety of inflammatory dermatoses that contain a large number of dermal eosinophils.

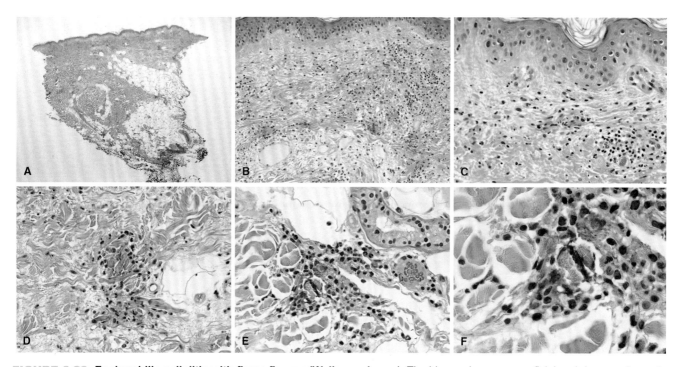

FIGURE 6-29. Eosinophilic cellulitis with flame figures (Wells syndrome). The biopsy shows a superficial and deep, perivascular and interstitial infiltrate (A,B). Many eosinophils are present, in the absence of significant changes in the epidermis (C). The classic flame figures are present (D-F).

Differential Diagnosis

The differential includes other inflammatory disorders with an abundance of eosinophils: those include urticaria, dermal hypersensitivity reactions, arthropod bite reactions, UV, eosinophilic pustular folliculitis, mastocytic proliferations, and papular urticaria. A high degree of clinicopathologic correlation is necessary for the diagnosis of Wells syndrome.[139-142]

CAPSULE SUMMARY

WELLS SYNDROME

This is a benign dermatosis, also called "eosinophilic cellulitis with flame figures," that can range from a localized inflammatory plaque resembling cellulitis to rarely a widespread blistering eruption. Most cases occur in adults and occurs only occasionally in the pediatric population. Lesions are very pruritic erythematous plaques that evolve quickly over 2 to 3 days; they are often confused for bacterial cellulitis and can vesiculate. The pathologic findings seen in Wells syndrome include a dense, superficial and deep, perivascular and interstitial infiltrate that is rich in dermal eosinophils. The dermal eosinophils show marked degranulation and "flame figures."

VASCULITIS

HENOCH-SCHÖNLEIN PURPURA

Definition and Epidemiology

Henoch-Schönlein Purpura (HSP) is the most common acute vasculitis affecting children; it is a small-vessel vasculitis that presents with a classic tetrad of symptoms involving the skin, kidneys, GI tract, and joints. The disease is generally self-limited with good prognosis; renal involvement is the biggest cause of possible long-term morbidity.[143] The vast majority of patients are between ages 2 and 10 with a male predominance. There does appear to be a seasonal variation, with the least number of cases occurring in the summer.[144] Children younger than age 2 tend to have milder disease.

Etiology

This is thought to be a hypersensitivity reaction and patients often have a history of preceding infection, such as upper respiratory tract infection and GI infection. One study reported positive throat culture for group A beta-hemolytic streptococcus in 20% of patients.[145] Vaccination has also been linked.[144] Molecularly, abnormal Immunoglobulin A (IgA) immune complexes deposit in small-vessel walls and trigger an inflammatory reaction.[146]

Clinical Presentation

In addition to skin, systemic involvement happens in 80% of HSP cases, with the kidney, GI tract, and joints being the most common. Episodes last a few weeks. Single episodes and recurrent episodes over weeks to months have both been reported.[144,145]

- **Palpable purpura**: Palpable purpura occurs in almost all children and is the presenting sign in about 70% of cases. Most lesions appear on the buttocks and lower extremities and are initially urticarial before quickly evolving to become the characteristic palpable purpura. Lesion size can range from petechial to large ecchymoses (Figure 6-30).[144] Other morphologies such as vesicular and bullous lesions as well as eroded and ulcerated lesions can also occur.[147] Lesions resolve with hyperpigmentation within a few days.
- **Renal**: Of the systemic involvement with HSP, renal involvement is most common. More than half of patients have findings, ranging from mild proteinuria to severe nephropathy, leading to impaired renal function. Most patients with severe nephropathy were older than 4 years. Renal abnormalities presented within the first 2 weeks in 75% of patients. The majority of renal abnormalities presented within 3 months after disease onset which was after skin lesions had resolved.[144,148] Risk factors for renal disease include age more than 4, severe abdominal pain, persistent purpura, and decreased coagulation factor 13 activity.[149,150] Initial renal insufficiency at disease onset may be the best predictor of the clinical course for HSP-related nephritis.[151,152]
- **GI**: Half of patients have vasculitis of the bowel wall, causing symptoms such as nausea and vomiting and GI bleeding.[144] Intussusception can occur in a small percentage of patients, more commonly in boys; this is a condition that generally occurs under the age of 2, so if seen in an older age, the diagnosis of HSP should be considered.
- **Joints:** Joint involvement occurs in about 75% of patients, with knees and ankles being commonly affected.[144] This generally does not result in long-term effects.
- **Edema:** Swelling of the feet, ankles, and hands can occur in half of patients.[144]
- **Other:** Twenty percent of male patients develop acute scrotal swelling that can be painful and represents vasculitis of the vessels in the scrotum; clinically, symptoms can be difficult to differentiate from testicular torsion.[153] Central nervous system (CNS) involvement and pulmonary involvement can also occur.[154]

Histologic Findings

The pathologic findings seen in HSP are those of a classic LCV (Figure 6-31). There is a rich acute inflammatory infiltrate in the dermis with a perivascular distribution. The infiltrate is composed of neutrophils and scattered eosinophils. In most cases, the postcapillary venules are the most affected sites. In addition to the transmural extension of

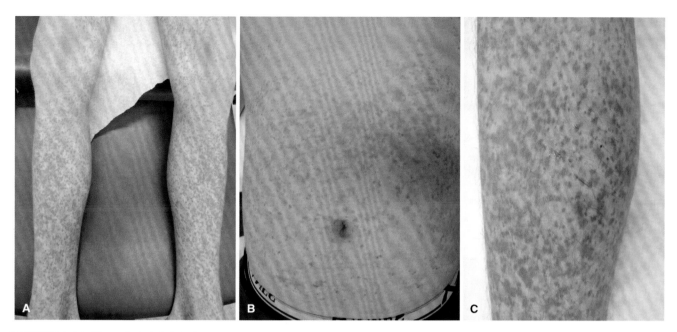

FIGURE 6-30. **Henoch-Schönlein Purpura.** Palpable purpura is present in the trunk and extremities (A-C).

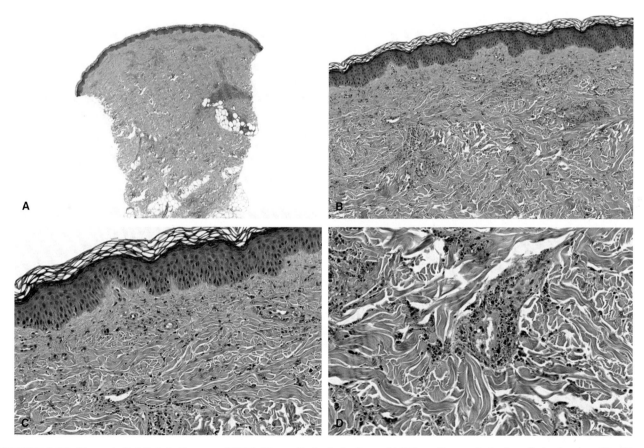

FIGURE 6-31. **Henoch-Schönlein Purpura (HSP).** The pathologic findings of HSP are those of a leukocytoclastic vasculitis. There is a superficial to mid-dermal, brisk perivascular infiltrate (A,B). Fibrinoid changes in the blood vessel walls and leukocytoclasis are evidence (C,D). Digital slides courtesy of Path Presenter.com.

neutrophils, endothelial swelling and destruction, fibrin thrombi, and extravasated erythrocytes are present. Leukocytoclasis is also typical. Infarction with necrosis, ulceration, and diffuse dermal inflammation can be seen in florid cases. HSP is associated with IgA deposition in blood vessel walls, both in the dermis and in the glomeruli. Fibrinogen and C3 are also frequently positive in the vascular walls. The finding of IgA deposition by direct immunofluorescence is not equivalent to a diagnosis of HSP (Figure 6-32). A vasculitis with the presence of IgA deposits in patients lacking other features of HSP has clinically been described in association with cancer, granulomatosis with polyangiitis (GPA), and inflammatory bowel disease. In a single study, only 24% of patients with vascular IgA deposits had HSP.[155-158]

CAPSULE SUMMARY

HENOCH-SCHÖNLEIN PURPURA

HSP is the most common acute vasculitis affecting children; it is a small-vessel vasculitis that presents with a classic tetrad of symptoms involving the skin, kidneys, GI tract, and joints. The disease is generally self-limited with good prognosis; renal involvement is the biggest cause of possible long-term morbidity. Palpable purpura occurs in almost all children and is the presenting sign in about 70% of cases. Most lesions appear on the buttocks and lower extremities and are initially urticarial before quickly evolving to become the characteristic palpable purpura. The pathologic findings seen in HSP are those of a classic LCV. HSP is associated with IgA deposition in blood vessel walls, both in the dermis and in the glomeruli. Fibrinogen and C3 are also frequently positive in the vascular walls. The finding of IgA deposition by direct immunofluorescence is not equivalent to a diagnosis of HSP.

ACUTE HEMORRHAGIC EDEMA OF INFANCY

Definition and Epidemiology

This is a small-vessel LCV that presents with dramatic targetoid large purpuric lesions on the cheeks, ears, and extremities associated with extremity edema in an overall well-appearing young child.[159] It has various other clinical names, including cockade purpura and edema. It is thought by some to represent a benign infantile form of HSP, although many advocate acute hemorrhagic edema (AHE) to be a separate entity.[160] The majority (80%) of cases occur between 6 and 24 months of age.[159]

Etiology

The majority of patients have skin eruptions occurring in the setting of infection, with most of these being an upper respiratory infection; diarrhea and urinary tract infection were also seen. Medications are thought to possibly trigger some cases, and a small subset of patients developed the eruption about 2 weeks after vaccination.[159,161]

Clinical Presentation

Skin lesions are prominent and characteristic; large round red to purple plaques ("cockade purpura"), sometimes with central clearing, appear on the cheeks, ears, and extremities (Figure 6-33). The trunk tends to be relatively spared. Painful nonpitting edema is another frequent manifestation affecting the face and distal extremities. Purpuric lesions and edema can sometimes affect the scrotum in boys. Low-grade fever is common, although children overall appear nontoxic.[162] Lesions resolve within 1 to 3 weeks, and systemic involvement generally does not occur.[159] (94) Differential diagnosis of the skin lesions includes urticaria/urticaria multiforme, erythema multiforme, HSP, and Kawasaki disease (KD).[163]

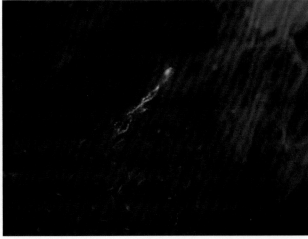

FIGURE 6-32. **Henoch-Schönlein Purpura—direct immunofluorescence.** Granular deposits of Immunoglobulin A are seen in the blood vessel walls of the papillary dermis (A,B).

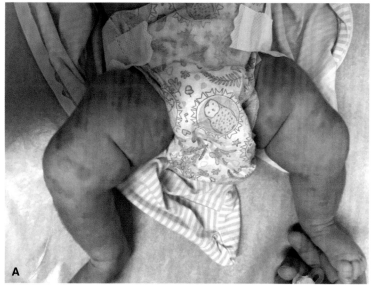
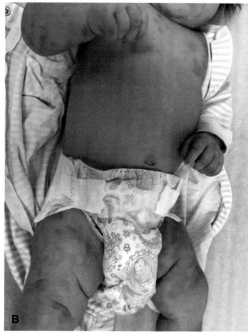

FIGURE 6-33. **Acute hemorrhagic edema.** Skin lesions are prominent and characteristic; large round red to purple plaques ("cockade purpura"), sometimes with central clearing, are seen (A,B).

Histologic Findings

In 150 children (boys, 77%), the diagnosis of acute hemorrhagic edema of young children was supported by the findings of a skin biopsy, which demonstrated a characteristic LCV involving small blood vessels in the dermis. A direct immunofluorescence study was performed in 67 of the mentioned children and disclosed depositions of IgA in 16 (24%).[164]

CAPSULE SUMMARY

ACUTE HEMORRHAGIC EDEMA OF INFANCY

This is a small-vessel LCV that presents with dramatic targetoid large purpuric lesions on the cheeks, ears, and extremities associated with extremity edema in an overall well-appearing young child. Skin lesions are prominent and characteristic; large round red to purple plaques ("cockade purpura"), sometimes with central clearing, appear on the cheeks, ears, and extremities. The trunk tends to be relatively spared. Pathologic changes are those of a LCV.

LEUKOCYTOCLASTIC/HYPERSENSITIVITY VASCULITIS

Definition and Epidemiology

This form of vasculitis consists of leukocytoclastic vasculitides that do not fall into another subgroup of vasculitis such as IgA vasculitis, UV, or antineutrophil cytoplasmic

antibody (ANCA)-associated vasculitis.[165] This occurs in both children and adults.

Etiology

In one study, most cases were due to autoimmune connective tissue disease, infection, drug reaction, and idiopathic.[165]

Clinical Presentation

Lesions tend to occur in crops with palpable purpura, often on the lower extremities (Figure 6-34).[165] Lesions may be burning or painful and resolve with dyspigmentation. Systemic involvement is uncommon.

Histologic Findings

The pathologic findings have been previously described with HSP (Figure 6-35).

HYPOCOMPLEMENTEMIC URTICARIAL VASCULITIS SYNDROME

Definition and Epidemiology

This form of UV presents with recurrent urticarial lesions in association with systemic symptoms, including eye inflammation, glomerulonephritis, and arthritis. This is an uncommon disease that is generally seen in the third and fourth decade of life, but has rarely been reported in children as well.[166]

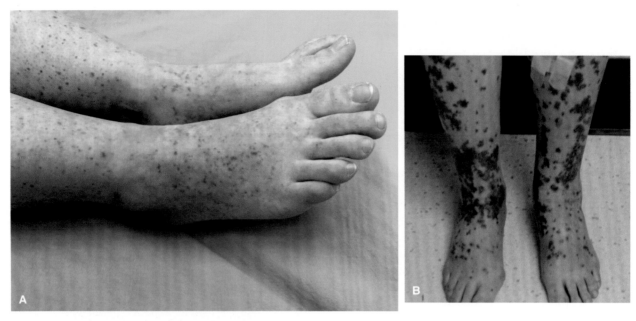

FIGURE 6-34. Leukocytoclastic vasculitis. Palpable purpura (A,B).

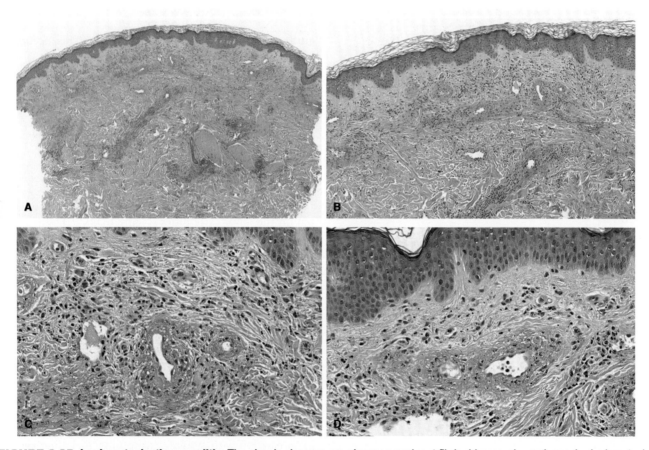

FIGURE 6-35. Leukocytoclastic vasculitis. The classic changes are shown: prominent fibrinoid necrosis, perivascular leukocytoclasis, and a mixed infiltrate of neutrophils and eosinophils (A-D). Red blood cell extravasation is also shown. Digital slides courtesy of Path Presenter.com.

Etiology

This is an immune complex–medicated disease of unknown etiology. It is associated with a lowered C1q level in most with an autoantibody against this factor. There is one report of three siblings, which suggests a possible genetic component.[166]

Clinical Presentation

Lesions are urticarial on the trunk and proximal extremities. There is often an element of purpura and lesions persist longer than allergic urticaria. There can be pain and burning, along with resolution with hyperpigmentation. Renal involvement in hypocomplementemic UV syndrome is more common and severe than in adults and may lead to end-stage renal disease more often than in adults.[167] Some have suggested a possible progression to SLE.[168]

Histologic Findings

The pathologic findings of this entity are poorly characterized but appear to be similar to those of classic LCV.

CRYOGLOBULINEMIA

Definition and Epidemiology

Cryoglobulins (CG) are separated into three groups on the basis of whether there is monoclonality and whether there is association with rheumatoid factor. Type 1 CG involve monoclonal antibodies and is associated with hematologic malignancies. Types 2 and 3 involve a mixed antibody response and is most commonly associated with hepatitis C. This can happen in all ages and is overall rare in children.

Etiology

When circulating immunoglobulins precipitate below body temperature and deposit in blood vessel walls, complement is activated and cryoglobulinemia vasculitis occurs. It has been associated with a number of conditions, most commonly essential cryoglobulinemia, infection, and autoimmune conditions.[169] Hepatitis C is associated with mixed cryoglobulinemia.

Clinical Presentation

This condition can present with a variety of skin manifestations, including purpura, Raynaud syndrome, ulcers on the skin, and livedo reticularis. Fever, arthralgia, peripheral neuropathy, and liver and renal involvement can also occur.[169]

Histologic Findings

The pathologic findings seen in cryoglobulinemia depend on the nature of the circulating CG. Type I CG manifests as thromboocclusive vasculopathy (Figure 6-36). Superficial

dermal vessels are occluded by PAS-positive homogeneous eosinophilic material. There is no vasculitis, but a scant perivascular lymphocytic infiltrate can be present. Mixed CG manifests as acute vasculitis, typically in the form of LCV that involves both the superficial and deep dermal vessels. Endothelial swelling, fibrinoid changes of the vessel walls, and leukocytoclasis are the main microscopic findings. The intensity of the inflammatory infiltrate and degree of leukocytoclasis varies and depends on the age of the lesion.[170-172]

Differential Diagnosis

Clinically, lesions of CG can resemble perniosis. However, in perniosis, no hyaline vascular thrombi or LCV is noted. A diagnosis of CG is usually based on the presence of the CG in the patient's serum. Therefore, when CG is present in the blood and the appropriate clinical and histopathologic findings are noted, a diagnosis of CG can be easily established.

CAPSULE SUMMARY

CRYOGLOBULINS

CG are separated into three groups on the basis of whether there is monoclonality and whether there is association with rheumatoid factor. Type 1 CG involve monoclonal antibodies and is associated with hematologic malignancies. Types 2 and 3 involve a mixed antibody response and are most commonly associated with hepatitis C. This can happen for people of all ages but is rare in children. This condition can present with a variety of skin manifestations, including purpura, Raynaud syndrome, ulcers on the skin, and livedo reticularis. Type I CG presents as a thrombotic vasculopathy, whereas type II does as an LCV.

GRANULOMATOSIS WITH POLYANGIITIS (WEGENER'S GRANULOMATOSIS)

Definition and Epidemiology

This is a necrotizing granulomatous vasculitis of the small and medium vessels that affect the upper and lower respiratory tracts as well as the kidneys. Other organs may be affected as well. This condition is rare in children, although among the primary systemic vasculitis disorders, this is one of the most common.[173] Disease onset is most common in adolescence.[174] Different than adults, pediatric Wegener syndrome has a female predominance.[174]

Etiology

Etiology is unclear. There has been a suggestion that *staphylococcus aureus* bacteria may be a trigger for disease.[175,176]

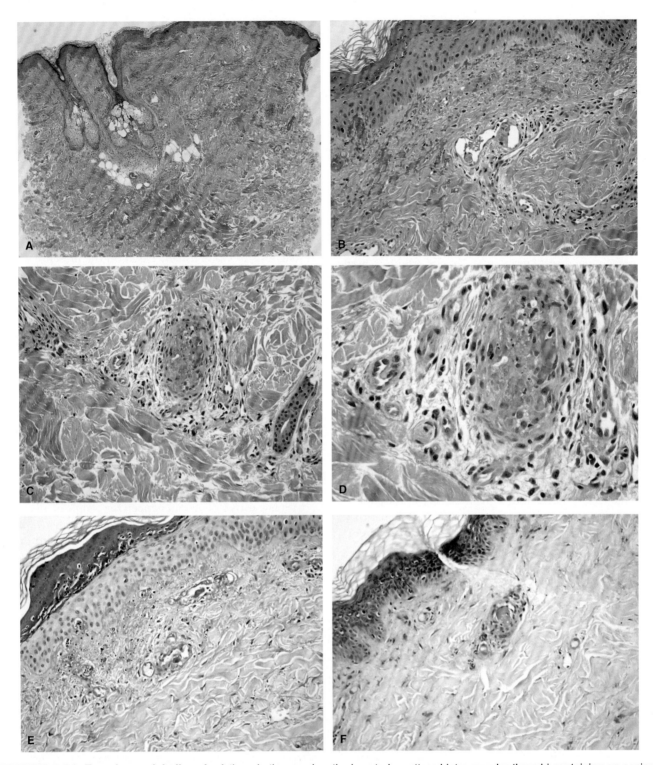

FIGURE 6-36. Type 1 cryoglobulinemia. A thrombotic vasculopathy is noted: scattered intravascular thrombi containing an eosinophilic material are seen (A-D). The material is positive with Periodic acid–Schiff stain (E,F). Obtained with permission from Gru AA, Schaffer A, eds. *Hematopathology of the Skin: Clinical and Pathological Approach.* 1st ed. Philadelphia, PA: Wolters Kluwer; 2016.

Clinical Presentation

Upper and lower airway symptoms are very common, including cough, rhinitis, and sinusitis, which can be difficult to differentiate initially from infectious or allergic presentations.[177] Otitis media can be a presenting symptom.[178] Subglottic stenosis and nasal deformity can occur and are thought to be more common than the adult population.[177-179] Patients have systemic symptoms such as

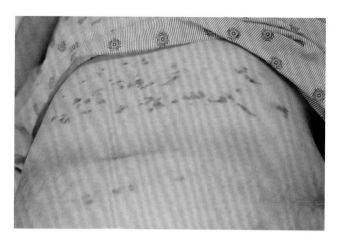

FIGURE 6-37. **Granulomatosis with polyangiitis (GPA).** A classic presentation of GPA is one of a common leukocytoclastic vasculitis, palpable purpura on the abdomen.

fatigue, fever, and weight loss. Renal involvement is common, affecting almost 90% of patients.[180] Other systemic findings can be pulmonary involvement, conjunctivitis, gingivitis, venous thrombotic disease, and cerebral vasculitis, which can include intracerebral hemorrhage.[180,181] About 80% of patients have positive c-ANCA with negative p-ANCA.

About half of patients with GPA present with skin lesions throughout the course of disease, with about 10% presenting at onset.[174,177,182,183] Palpable purpura is most common (Figure 6-37); there can be a necrotic quality that can be more common on the extremities, especially the elbows, but also on the scalp and face.[182] Lesions can also present as ulcers and as subcutaneous nodules.[174,175,182] Oral mucosal lesions can develop as well. Some children can present with eyelid swelling that can represent an orbital pseudotumor.[175,184]

Histologic Findings

Most often, LCV is the corresponding histopathologic pattern for GPA in the majority of patients, especially in those with palpable purpura (Figure 6-38). LCV may also be the histopathologic correlate to ulcerations and nodules. In LCV, there is a robust neutrophilic inflammatory infiltrate that is associated with vascular destruction and extravascular inflammation. The vascular involvement is not only restricted to the superficial dermal vessels but also affected the mid-dermal vasculature. The histopathologic pattern of pyoderma-like facial lesions of GPA is characterized by foci of palisaded neutrophilic and granulomatous dermatitis, prominent granulomatous and neutrophilic necrotizing vasculitis, and basophilic collagen degeneration.[185]

Differential Diagnosis

Numerous other causes of LCV should be included in the differential diagnosis. In general, 75% to 90% of patients with active, systemic GPA will have positive cANCA/PR3-ANCA test results at some point during their disease course. However, in 10% to 25% of patients with active, systemic disease and 40% of those with limited disease, ANCA serologies may be negative. Other conditions that are associated with cANCA/PR3-ANCA positivity include microscopic polyangiitis (10%-50%), Churg-Strauss syndrome, drug-induced ANCA-associated vasculitis, collagen vascular disease (rare), and subacute bacterial endocarditis. In contrast to PG, which shows a striking neutrophilic epidermal and dermal necrosis with mononuclear cell dominant vascular inflammation, it occurs away from the zones of marked extravascular inflammation and does not have luminal or mural fibrin deposition. Histopathologic differences between pyoderma-like ulcerations of GPA and PG may be more subtle in the early phases of disease, when follicular and perifollicular inflammation with intradermal abscess formation is present.

CAPSULE SUMMARY

GRANULOMATOSIS WITH POLYANGIITIS

This is a necrotizing granulomatous vasculitis of the small and medium vessels that affects the upper and lower respiratory tracts as well as the kidneys. Other organs may be affected as well. This condition is rare in children, although among the primary systemic vasculitis disorders, this is one of the most common. Most often, LCV is the corresponding histopathologic pattern for GPA in the majority of patients, especially in those with palpable purpura.

CHURG-STRAUSS SYNDROME (ALLERGIC GPA)

Definition and Epidemiology

This is a rare small- and medium-vessel vasculitis in children and presents with atopic findings with significant eosinophilia along with systemic vasculitis. This condition occurs most often in males between ages 30 and 40. It is uncommon in children.

Etiology

Etiology is unclear. It is thought to involve the activation of eosinophils that release enzymes and cause damage in vascular and perivascular tissues.[186]

Clinical Presentation

Three stages of clinical disease are described in adults.[187] Many patients present initially with allergic rhinitis and

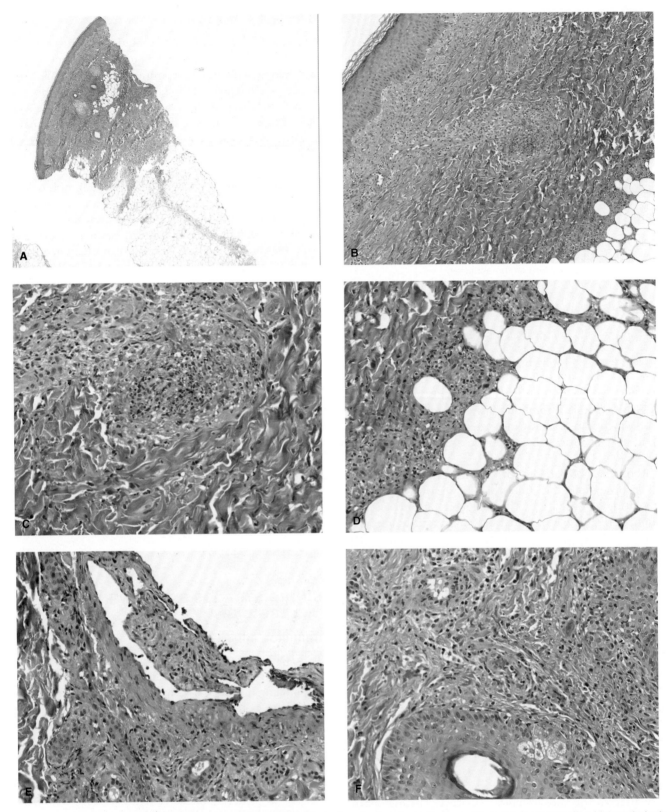

FIGURE 6-38. Granulomatosis with polyangiitis (GPA). Most often, leukocytoclastic vasculitis is the corresponding histopathologic pattern for GPA in the majority of patients, especially in those with palpable purpura. Close inspection shows a robust neutrophilic inflammatory infiltrate that is associated with vascular destruction and extravascular inflammation. The vascular involvement is not only restricted to the superficial dermal vessels but also affects the mid-dermal vasculature (A-F).

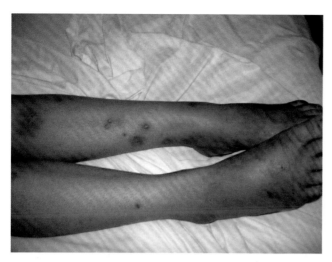

FIGURE 6-39. **Allergic granulomatosis with polyangiitis (Churg-Strauss syndrome).** Multiple nodular erythematous skin lesions of the lower extremities with a tender, edematous, and erythematous surrounding skin with a foot drop of the left leg. Reprinted with permission from Basak RB, Narchi H, Bakir M, Joshi S, Conca W. Churg–Strauss syndrome without respiratory symptoms in a child. *Indian J Dermatol.* 2011;56(1):84-86.

asthma that can last for years. In adults, one distinguishing difference is that the asthma presents later in life, usually with a mean age in the 30s. After years, patients develop worsening of their asthma along with peripheral eosinophilia and eosinophilic tissue infiltration. The final phase is systemic vasculitis including fever, weight loss, and widespread vasculitis and inflammation. The skin is involved in 70% of patients; lesions can be similar to Wegener's and include palpable purpura, subcutaneous nodules (Figure 6-39), and papulonecrotic lesions.[187] Urticarial lesions can sometimes be seen. Cardiac involvement includes pericarditis, myocarditis, and tamponade. Eosinophils and serum Ig E are elevated. In adults, most patients have positive p-ANCA, but this is somewhat less common in children; one study showed about 25% of patients with positive p-ANCA.[186] In one large series, children tended to have more cardiopulmonary involvement and less common peripheral neuropathy; mortality was higher.[186] This disease is fatal if not treated.

Histologic Findings

Histopathologically, there is a pronounced perivascular inflammatory infiltrate dominated by eosinophils, but also macrophages and lymphocytes that pervade the vessel wall of arterioles, venules, and capillaries. Flame figures caused by degranulating eosinophils are also a typical feature. The strong inflammation leads to fibrinoid necrosis in medium- to small-sized vessels and subsequently to necrosis within the connective tissue with characteristic granuloma formation (Figure 6-40).

CAPSULE SUMMARY

CHURG-STRAUSS SYNDROME

This is a rare small- and medium-vessel vasculitis in children and presents with atopic findings with significant eosinophilia along with systemic vasculitis. This condition occurs most often in males between ages 30 and 40. It is uncommon in children. The skin is involved in 70% of patients; lesions can be similar to Wegener's and include palpable purpura, subcutaneous nodules, and papulonecrotic lesions.

POLYARTERITIS NODOSA (PAN), INFANTILE PAN, AND BENIGN CUTANEOUS PAN

PAN is a necrotizing vasculitis of the small- and medium-sized vessels that is uncommon in children. Prognosis is dependent on the level of systemic involvement. Systemic PAN has poor prognosis. The most common form of PAN in children is benign cutaneous PAN, which has a good prognosis, because there is limited systemic involvement despite often having a recurrent chronic course.

PEDIATRIC PAN

Epidemiology and Etiology

This form is uncommon in children. The etiology is unknown but is thought to involve immunocomplexes. Group A streptococcal infection and hepatitis B virus have been thought to be linked.[188]

Clinical Presentation

Clinical presentation is similar to that of adults with systemic PAN. Constitutional symptoms are common with fever and malaise. Involvement of the skin, musculoskeletal system, and GI system are most common, along with renal and CNS involvement.[189-191] Pulmonary involvement is uncommon. Skin lesions include purpura, skin nodules, livedo reticularis, as well as superficial and deep skin infarctions that can heal with atrophic stellate scars.[192] This form of PAN can cause death related to renal failure, intracranial or intraabdominal hemorrhage, and cardiac reasons.

INFANTILE PAN

Epidemiology and Etiology

This condition occurs in children younger than age 2 and is a systemic disease with poor prognosis. There is some suggestion that infantile PAN and Kawasaki disease (KD) may represent diseases on the same spectrum.[193]

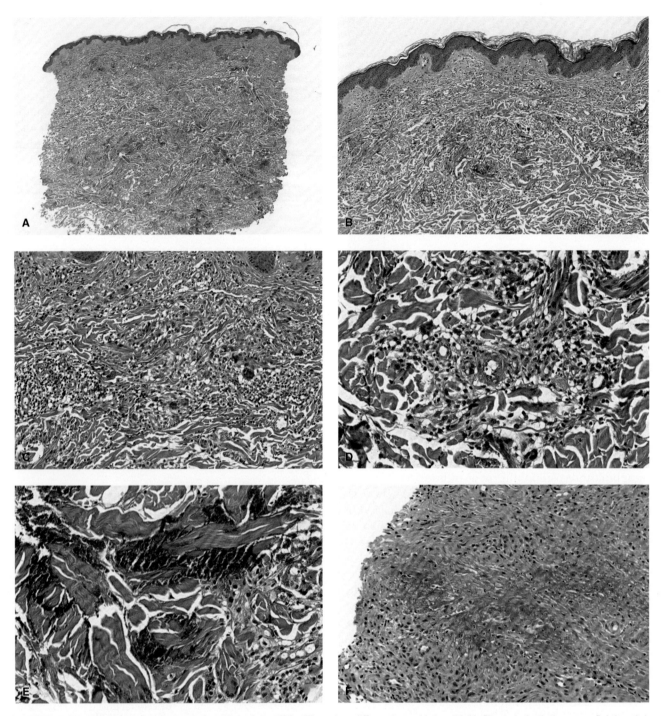

FIGURE 6-40. Allergic granulomatosis with polyangiitis. There is a diffuse dermal interstitial infiltrate in both the superficial and deep portions of the biopsy (A). The infiltrate shows granulomatous changes with the presence of multinucleated giant cells (B,C). Areas of vasculitis are seen (D). Flame figures (E) and necrobiosis are also shown (F). Digital slides courtesy of Path Presenter.com.

Clinical Presentation

Progression of this form tends to be faster than pediatric PAN in older age groups. Infantile PAN appears to preferentially affect the coronary arteries.[194] Skin features tend to be morbilliform instead of petechial and purpuric. Skin nodules are not as common in this form of PAN. Patients can present with hypertension, myocardial infarction, coronary artery aneurysms, and chronic heart failure. The nervous system can be involved as well with paralysis and seizures. Some infants have rapidly declining courses and are diagnosed only afterward by autopsy, when the findings of coronary artery disease and vasculitis are seen.[194]

BENIGN CUTANEOUS PDA PAN

Epidemiology and Etiology

This is the most common form of PAN in children that presents with vasculitis affecting the skin, muscle, and joints. Overall prognosis is good because there is no visceral involvement.[195] The etiology is unknown, although it is thought to involve immunocomplexes. It has been associated most commonly with streptococcal infection and has also been reported in the context of diphtheria-tetanus-pertussis immunizations, medications, and wasp stings.[39,196,197]

Clinical Presentation

The disease is primarily on the skin with little to no systemic involvement. Skin lesions are painful erythematous nodules with ulcers on the lower extremities (Figure 6-41).[198] Livedo reticularis and urticaria can be seen. Peripheral gangrene and autoamputation has been reported in children in their first decade of life.[39] The disease can have chronic recurrent flares that follow a benign course. In addition to skin findings, patients can have fever, malaise, arthralgias, and neuropathy.[199] In general, the cutaneous form does not tend to progress to systemic PAN.[189]

Histologic Findings of PAN

The pathologic findings in PAN include a vasculitis of small- to medium-sized caliber vessels. The vasculitis is mostly neutrophilic, and has swelling of the endothelium, fibrinoid necrosis, leukocytoclasis, red blood cell extravasation, and fibrin thrombi in the lumen of the vessels. Although small vessels can be affected, the classic diagnostic finding is the

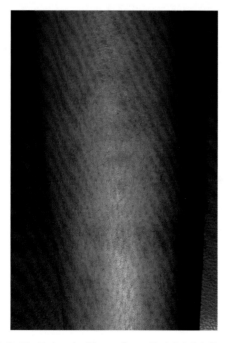

FIGURE 6-41. **Polyarteritis nodosa.** Painful, faintly erythematous and hyperpigmented nodules on the lower extremities of a 15-year-old girl.

involvement of the muscular arteries in the deep dermis and adipose tissue. The pathologic findings in PAN have also been divided into stages (Figures 6-42 to 6-44): the first stage (acute) shows small-sized muscular arteries affected at the dermal-epidermal junction, with a predominance of neutrophils with leukocytoclasis around the vessel walls. The intima shows partial loss or damage of the lining endothelium, and the vascular lumen contains fibrin thrombi. An elastic stain lacks disruption of the internal elastic lamina. The second stage (subacute) also has the luminal thrombi and fibrinoid necrosis of the intima. Focal fibrinoid depositions are appadepositsrent in the disrupted areas of the media. Some cases can show a target-like appearance with subendothelial concentric fibrinoid necrosis lined by an inner layer of remaining endothelial cells and an outer layer of the internal elastic lamina. The elastic stain shows disruption of the internal elastic lamina. The third stage (reparative or healing) has vascular thrombi, and there is an intimal fibroblastic proliferation. Neoangiogenesis with the formation of small vessels in the perivascular area is noted. The final stage (healed) has marked thickening of the intima with resultant luminal obliteration. Minimal inflammation is present at this stage. The coexistence of different stages of arteritis is seen in 50% of cases.[191,200-204]

Differential Diagnosis

Subcutaneous small- to medium-sized muscular vessel vasculitis including nodular vasculitis, thrombophlebitis, Sneddon syndrome, and GPA will be incorporated into the differential diagnosis of PAN. Thrombophlebitis is not common in children. In thrombophlebitis, the medial layers comprise haphazard smooth muscle bundles and are rich in elastic and collagen fibers, rather than the continuous wreath of concentric muscular layers with minimal elastic fibers seen in an artery. In Sneddon syndrome, there is a lymphocytic arteriolitis and arteritis that is different from the neutrophilic pattern seen in PAN. Nodular vasculitis (erythema induratum) shows a lobular panniculitis and a venulitis. Most cases of GPA show a pattern typical of LCV that differs from PAN. Additionally, some cases can have a granulomatous arteritis with a predominance of histiocytic inflammation. The large-caliber vessel vasculitides (temporal arteritis and Takayasu arteritis) also have granuloma formation in the affected vessel wall.

Macular arteritis (MA) and lymphocytic thrombophilic arteritis (LTA) are two recently described novel cutaneous arteritis syndromes that are believed to be clinically similar but histologically distinct from PAN. Macular hyperpigmented lesions are typical of MA, and plaques and nodules are characteristic of LTA and PAN, respectively. However, many believe that MA–LTA–PAN may be a unique spectrum of changes that follow a chronologic progression from one to another. Under this observation, it appears plausible that MA represents a latent, nonnodule–forming variant of PAN. Conversely, the frequency of symptoms such as pain, arthralgias, fever, muscle pain, ulcers, livedo racemosa, neuropathy,

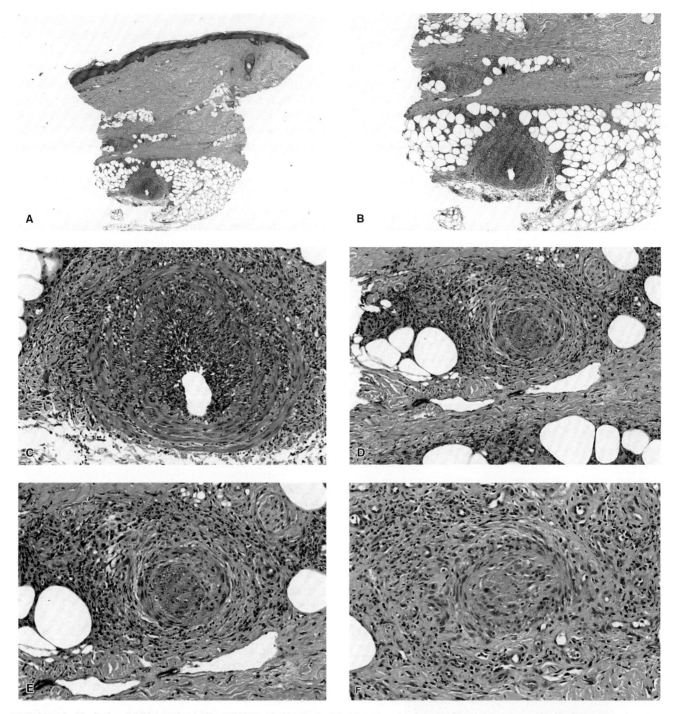

FIGURE 6-42. Polyarteritis nodosa. Two stages are shown in this biopsy, subacute (A-C) and reparative (D-F). The subacute stage shows the luminal thrombi, and fibrinoid necrosis of the intima. Focal fibrinoid depositions are apparent in the disrupted areas of the media. Leukocytoclasis is also present. The reparative stage has vascular thrombi, and there is an intimal fibroblastic proliferation. Neo-angiogenesis with the formation of small vessels in the perivascular area is noted. Digital slides courtesy of Path Presenter.com.

and serologic markers of inflammation are increased from MA to LTA to CPA. Histologically, MA displays a predominant lymphocytic vessel wall infiltrate, with no polymorphonuclear cells, a typical hyalinized fibrin ring in the vessel lumen, and usually the absence of internal elastic lamina disruption. LTA is characterized by a temporally heterogeneous subcutaneous arteritis targeting the endothelium and

intima with changes ranging from incipient intimal expansion by hyaluronic acid to concentric intimal fibrin deposition to one of an end-stage acellular intraluminal obliterative fibrous arteriopathy. The infiltrate is predominated by lymphocytes and histiocytes. The intimal elastic lamina is intact in most cases. Numerous studies have shown that it is currently not possible to separate MA and LTA from PAN.[206-210]

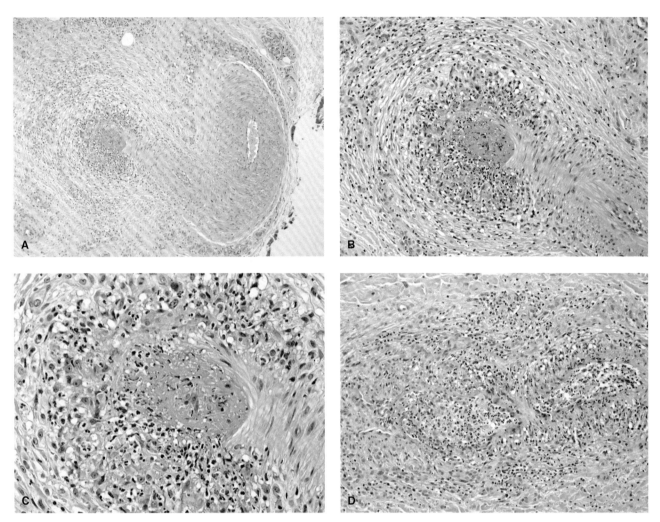

FIGURE 6-43. **Polyarteritis nodosa (PAN).** Another characteristic feature of PAN is the segmental and focal involvement of the muscular vessels, in this biopsy of a subacute stage (A-D).

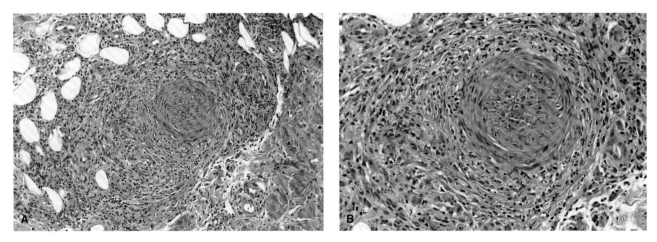

FIGURE 6-44. **The final stage (healed) has a marked thickening of the intima with resultant luminal obliteration.** Minimal inflammation is present at this stage (A,B).

POLYARTERITIS NODOSA

PAN is a necrotizing vasculitis of the small- and medium-sized vessels that is uncommon in children. Prognosis is dependent on the level of systemic involvement. Systemic PAN has poor prognosis. The most common form of PAN in children is benign cutaneous PAN, which has a good prognosis, because there is limited systemic involvement despite often having a recurrent chronic course. The disease is primarily on the skin with little to no systemic involvement. Skin lesions are painful erythematous nodules with ulcers on the lower extremities.

Livedo reticularis and urticaria can be seen. The pathologic findings in PAN include a vasculitis of small- to medium-sized caliber vessels. The vasculitis is mostly neutrophilic, and has swelling of the endothelium, fibrinoid necrosis, leukocytoclasis, red blood cell extravasation, and fibrin thrombi in the lumen of the vessels. Although small vessels can be affected, the classic diagnostic finding is the involvement of the muscular arteries in the deep dermis and adipose tissue.

KAWASAKI DISEASE

Definition and Epidemiology

KD is also called "acute febrile mucocutaneous lymph node syndrome." It is a small- and medium-sized vasculitis of the arteries that preferentially targets the coronary vessels. Worldwide, it is now one of the top causes of acquired heart disease.[211] Coronary artery disease is the most significant cause of morbidity in this disease. Clinically, this disease can be similar to infantile PAN.

The disease has been reported in all ages, but it is most common between 6 months and 5 years.[212] It is most common in patients with Asian descent, with incidence rates highest in Japan, Korea, and Taiwan. In the United States, Asian and Pacific Islanders are more commonly affected; because of this, Hawaii is the state with the highest incidence.[213] The peak age in Japan is 6 months, whereas in the United States, the peak age is around 13 months. Males are more commonly affected, and there appears to be seasonal clusters in the winter and from spring to summer.[213,214]

Etiology

Etiology remains unknown. The observation that the disease is most common in those of Japanese descendance regardless of the area they live suggests a genetic susceptibility to the disease; one study identified association of an *ORAI1* gene variation.[213,215] In addition, seasonal clusters and community-wide outbreaks suggest that there might

be an infectious component that has yet to be elucidated.[213] Newer studies have also suggested a link between allergic diseases and KD; atopic diseases may increase the risk for KD or may share common pathogenetic factors.[216,217]

Clinical Presentation

Approximately 90% of patients present with mucocutaneous symptoms. Fever, rash, and red eyes in a young child are features that should prompt a consideration of KD. Prolonged, unexplained fever in an infant should also bring up a consideration of KD. There is no reliable confirmatory testing that can be done, and diagnosis can sometimes be challenging because of incomplete and atypical presentations.[212,218-221]

The clinical course can be described in three phases: acute, subacute, and convalescent. The acute phase is marked by an onset of fever until resolution (about 1-2 weeks). The subacute phase lasts until all clinical features have resolved (about 2 weeks), and the convalescent phase is complete once erythrocyte sedimentation rate and platelet count are normal (4-8 weeks).

Fevers in KD are high (<39) and last 1 to 2 weeks if untreated. The fevers generally do not respond to antipyretic medications.[212] Centers for Disease Control and Prevention defines the fever as lasting for more than 5 days, although if other symptoms are seen, diagnosis can be made sooner than this period.

Diagnostic criteria include **fever** for at least 5 days in addition to at least four of the following five clinical signs:

- Bilateral conjunctival injection with no exudate. This occurs in 80% to 90% of patients.
- Oral mucous membrane findings: injected pharynx, injected or fissured lips, strawberry tongue
- Peripheral extremity changes. Erythema or edema in the acute phase can be painful and is often well demarcated on the wrists and ankles. Desquamation of the periungual skin of the fingers and toes is one of the most common skin findings in the subacute phase, typically following erythema and edema of the hands and feet.[212]
- Polymorphous rash. The rash is a nonspecific diffuse macular and papular erythematous eruption (Figure 6-45). One distinguishing characteristic is that there is often accentuation of the eruption in intertriginous areas, especially the groin. In one series, an erythematous desquamating perineal eruption was seen in 67% of patients, usually within the first week.[222] In addition, psoriasiform rash has been reported in the acute to convalescent phases.[223]
- Cervical lymphadenopathy that is usually unilateral. This is the least commonly seen feature in KD (50%-75%) and is usually obvious.

KD can sometimes be confused with acute adenoviral infection, but major distinguishing features of acute adenovirus infection are purulent conjunctivitis and lack of perineal accentuation.

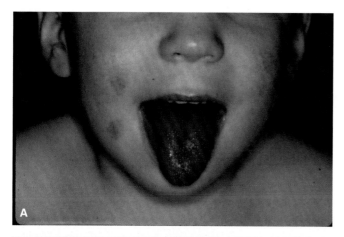
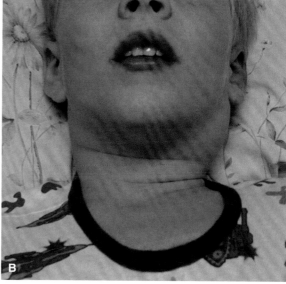
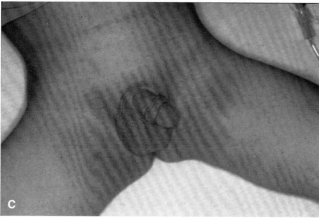

FIGURE 6-45. **Kawasaki disease.** Strawberry tongue, unilateral cervical lymphadenopathy, and macular erythematous rage accentuated in the intertriginous areas (A-C).

Histologic findings

The pathologic changes seen in KD are those of a LCV. In most cases, the postcapillary venules are the affected vascular structures. However, the involvement of medium-sized muscular arteries has been reported and correlates clinically with a nodule, similar to what is present in PAN. A subset of patients can show spongiform pustules. An additional report of cases with features of psoriasis has also been described in children.[224-226]

CAPSULE SUMMARY

KAWASAKI DISEASE

KD is also called "acute febrile mucocutaneous lymph node syndrome." It is a small- and medium-sized vasculitis of the arteries that preferentially targets the coronary vessels. Worldwide, it is now one of the top causes of acquired heart disease. Approximately 90% of patients present with mucocutaneous symptoms. Fever, rash, and red eyes in a young child are features that should prompt a

consideration of KD. Prolonged, unexplained fever in an infant should also bring up a consideration of KD. The rash is a nonspecific diffuse macular and papular erythematous eruption. One distinguishing characteristic is that there is often accentuation of the eruption in intertriginous areas, especially the groin. The more typical pathologic findings are those of an LCV.

ANTIPHOSPHOLIPID SYNDROME

Definition and Epidemiology

This syndrome is an autoimmune thrombotic disorder that presents with clots in the vasculature; blood tests show persistent antiphospholipid antibodies. This is a rare syndrome in the pediatric population and can occur as early as the neonatal period. In a registry of 121 pediatric patients, about half of cases were primary and the remaining were secondary to an autoimmune process; one patient had underlying Hodgkin's lymphoma.[227] Within the cases of APS associated with autoimmune processes, SLE was most common. In addition, about 30% of patients with SLE were initially diagnosed with primary APS before presenting with SLE symptoms. Primary APS patients were younger (8.7 years old vs. 12.7 years old) and tended to have more arterial thrombosis leading to ischemic stroke. Secondary APS patients with autoimmune conditions were older and tended to have more venous thrombosis, hematologic manifestations, and skin involvement. In addition, almost half of patients had an inherited prothrombotic disorder. Pediatric APS is less frequently associated with malignancy, compared with the adult population.

Etiology

Antiphospholipid antibodies (anticardiolipin, lupus anticoagulant, and anti-beta2 glycoprotein I antibodies) are thought to not only be serum markers of disease but also actually play a role in the process of inducing a thrombophilic state.[228] There has been noted to be a high frequency of antiphospholipid antibody–related thrombosis at the time of SLE onset, and it is thought that the inflammatory state of SLE works additively with antiphospholipid antibodies in increasing thrombotic risk.[227,229]

Clinical Presentation

The major presentation of pediatric APS is vascular thrombosis, particularly in the leg veins (40%), followed by ischemic stroke secondary to arterial thrombosis (26%).[227,230] Recurrent thrombosis is common. Skin manifestations are more common in secondary APS patients and overall occur in roughly 20% of patients; findings can include livedo reticularis which appears as a network pattern of violaceous to dusky discoloration (Figure 6-46), Raynaud phenomenon, skin ulcers, pseudovasculitic lesions, chronic urticaria, and Degos-like lesions.

Hematologic disorders can also be seen as well as migraines, chorea, and epilepsy.[227,228] In addition, neurodevelopmental issues with attention and memory related to APS can be difficult to differentiate from more common developmental problems and so it is important to consider these symptoms as potential clues to diagnosis as well.[231] A small subset of patients develop catastrophic APS who develop thrombosis of at least three organs over the course of days to weeks; it is fatal in roughly a quarter of patients.[232]

Histologic Findings

Thrombotic disorders can produce widespread damage secondary to thrombosis, mimicking cutaneous and systemic vasculitis. These disorders include Coumadin-induced skin necrosis, purpura fulminans, antiphospholipid syndrome (APS), and livedoid vasculopathy. All of these disorders are characterized histologically by noninflammatory small-vessel fibrin-platelet thrombi associated with variable hemorrhage and when thrombi extensively occlude vascular beds, ulceration, and infarction (Figure 6-47). There is no significant perivascular inflammation or evidence of vascular wall damage. Older lesions can show epidermal necrosis, ulceration, and a reactive inflammatory infiltrate.

Multiple deep biopsies are often required to show vascular thrombi with partial or complete obstruction (often associated with lymphocytes) affecting small-to medium-sized arteries localized at the dermal-subcutis junction or within the subcutis in patients with livedo reticularis. Disruption of the elastic lamina, suggesting coexisting inflammation, has been described in APS. Small-vessel thrombi are found in patients' purpuric and/or necrotic skin lesions. Reactive angioendotheliomatosis (intravascular proliferation of endothelial cells with associated microthrombi formation) can be a presenting or associated histologic sign of APS.[228,233-235] A catastrophic presentation of APS has been reported in the pediatric setting in association with trisomy 21: the case shows numerous and disseminated fibrin thrombi in multiple organs and sites.[236]

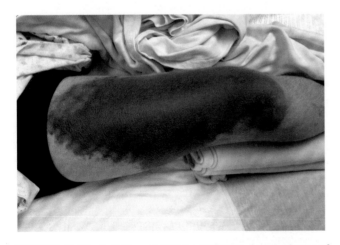

FIGURE 6-46. Antiphospholipid syndrome. Large plaque of epidermal necrosis, with purple and dusky pigmentation.

CAPSULE SUMMARY

ANTIPHOSPHOLIPID SYNDROME

This syndrome is an autoimmune thrombotic disorder that presents with clots in the vasculature; blood tests show persistent antiphospholipid antibodies. This is a rare syndrome in the pediatric population and can occur as early as the neonatal period. Thrombotic disorders can produce widespread damage secondary to thrombosis, mimicking cutaneous and systemic vasculitis. These disorders include Coumadin-induced skin necrosis, purpura fulminans, APS, and livedoid vasculopathy. All of these disorders are characterized histologically by noninflammatory small-vessel fibrin-platelet thrombi associated with variable hemorrhage and when thrombi extensively occlude vascular beds, ulceration, and infarction.

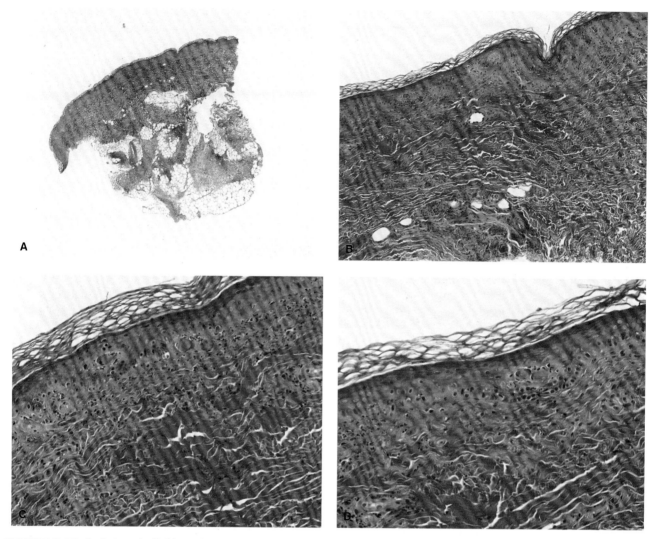

FIGURE 6-47. **Antiphospholipid syndrome.** The low-power view shows a very red-appearing dermis. The epidermis is atrophic and shows ischemic features (A,B). Numerous fibrin thrombi are seen in the superficial dermal vessels in the absence of vasculitis (C,D).

DEGOS DISEASE (MALIGNANT ATROPHIC PAPULOSIS)

Definition and Epidemiology

This vasoocclusive disease is also referred to as malignant atrophic papulosis. Typical skin lesions are small porcelain white macules representing multiple areas of infarct. Patients with internal involvement have poor prognosis, usually dying from GI or CNS involvement. However, there is a subset of patients who follow a benign course.[237] This condition generally occurs in middle-aged adults and is rare in children; congenital onset has been reported.[238]

Etiology

Pathogenesis is unknown, although some patients have been found to have dysfunctional platelets. Familial cases are described.[239,240] Degos-like lesions can be seen in APL and/or SLE.[241]

Clinical Presentation

Skin lesions are small atrophic, porcelain white papules with an erythematous telangiectatic border on the trunk and extremities (Figure 6-48); this can precede systemic involvement by months to years. GI involvement can lead to peritonitis, perforation, and infection. Intracranial involvement can include headache, hemorrhage, or ischemic strokes, seizures, and polyneuropathy.[242] Other organ systems that can be affected include the lungs, heart, eyes, and kidney. When internal disease occurs, patients die within 2 to 3 years from GI or CNS involvement.[237,243] One review of the pediatric literature of Degos disease found that 60% of reported cases were fatal, with death occurring on average 3.6 years after presentation.[244]

Histologic Findings

Skin biopsies of Degos disease show a wedge-shaped area of cutaneous ischemia, the apex of which extends into the deep dermis (Figure 6-49). The dermal area is uniformly

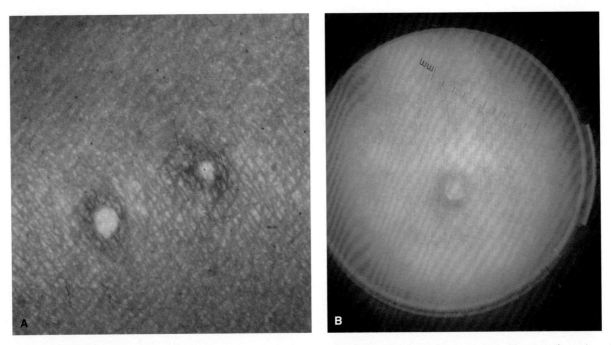

FIGURE 6-48. Malignant atrophic papulosis (Degos disease). Small atrophic, porcelain white papules with an erythematous telangiectatic border (A). Closer magnification using dermoscopy (B).

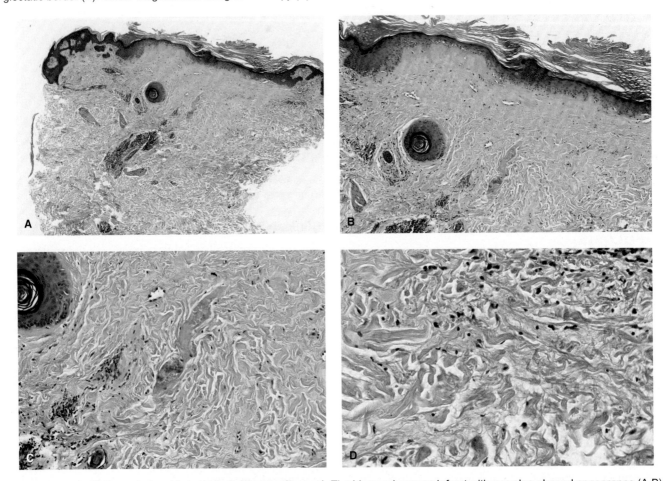

FIGURE 6-49. Malignant atrophic papulosis (Degos disease). The biopsy shows an infarct with a wedge-shaped appearance (A,B). At the apex, fibrin thrombi are seen (C). Marked increased interstitial dermal mucin is also present (D). Digital slides courtesy of Path Presenter.com.

hypereosinophilic and relatively acellular. Vessels at the apex show endothelial swelling and proliferation with partial or complete obliteration of the lumen with thrombus. A mild to moderately dense perivascular lymphocytic infiltrate is often but not invariably present. The overlying epidermis is atrophic with variable hyperkeratosis. Alcian blue staining of early lesions reveals abundant mucopolysaccharide deposition throughout the dermis. In established lesions, mucin is seen only at the edges of the infarcted area.[245-248]

CAPSULE SUMMARY

DEGOS DISEASE (MALIGNANT ATROPHIC PAPULOSIS)

This vasoocclusive disease is also referred to as "malignant atrophic papulosis." Typical skin lesions are small porcelain white macules representing multiple areas of infarct. Patients with internal involvement have poor prognosis, usually dying from GI or CNS involvement. Skin biopsies of Degos disease show a wedge-shaped area of cutaneous ischemia, the apex of which extends into the deep dermis. Vessels at the apex show endothelial swelling and proliferation with partial or complete obliteration of the lumen with thrombus. Increased dermal mucin is noted.

REFERENCES

1. Langley EW, Gigante J. Anaphylaxis, urticaria, and angioedema. *Pediatr Rev.* 2013;34(6):247-257.
2. Bailey E, Shaker M. An update on childhood urticaria and angioedema. *Curr Opin Pediatr.* 2008;20(4):425-430.
3. Levy Y, Segal N, Weintrob N, Danon YL. Chronic urticaria: association with thyroid autoimmunity. *Arch Dis Child.* 2003;88(6):517-519.
4. Chansakulporn S, Pongpreuksa S, Sangacharoenkit P, et al. The natural history of chronic urticaria in childhood: a prospective study. *J Am Dermatol.* 2014;71(4):663-668.
5. Choi SH, Baek HS. Approaches to the diagnosis and management of chronic urticaria in children. *Korean J Pediatr.* 2015;58(5):159-164.
6. Alangari AA, Twarog FJ, Shih MC, Schneider LC. Clinical features and anaphylaxis in children with cold urticaria. *Pediatrics.* 2004;113(4):e313-e317.
7. Shah KN, Honig PJ, Yan AC. "Urticaria multiforme": a case series and review of acute annular urticarial hypersensitivity syndromes in children. *Pediatrics.* 2007;119(5):e1177-e1183.
8. Emer JJ, Bernardo SG, Kovalerchik O, Ahmad M. Urticaria multiforme. *J Clin Aesthet Dermatol.* 2013;6(3):34-39.
9. Steen CJ, Carbonaro PA, Schwartz RA. Arthropods in dermatology. *J Am Acad Dermatol.* 2004;50(6):819-842, quiz 842-814.
10. Amaya D, Sanchez A, Sanchez J. Inducible urticaria: case series and literature review. *Biomedica.* 2016;36(1):10-21.
11. Nousari HC, Kimyai-Asadi A, Ketabchi N, Cohen BA. Urticarial eruption associated with rheumatic fever in a child. *Pediatr Dermatol.* 1999;16(4):288-291.
12. Peteiro C, Toribio J. Incidence of leukocytoclastic vasculitis in chronic idiopathic urticaria. Study of 100 cases. *Am J Dermatopathol.* 1989;11(6):528-533.
13. Raigosa M, Toro Y, Sanchez J. Solar urticaria. Case report and literature review [in Spanish]. *Rev Alerg Mex.* 2017;64(3):371-375.

14. Sanchez J, Amaya E, Acevedo A, Celis A, Caraballo D, Cardona R. Prevalence of inducible urticaria in patients with chronic spontaneous urticaria: associated risk factors. *J Allergy Clin Immunol Pract.* 2017;5(2):464-470.
15. Sanchez JL, Benmaman O. Clinicopathological correlation in chronic urticaria. *Am J Dermatopathol.* 1992;14(3):220-223.
16. Toyoda M, Maruyama T, Morohashi M, Bhawan J. Free eosinophil granules in urticaria: a correlation with the duration of wheals. *Am J Dermatopathol.* 1996;18(1):49-57.
17. Zembowicz A, Mastalerz L, Setkowicz M, Radziszewski W, Szczeklik A. Histological spectrum of cutaneous reactions to aspirin in chronic idiopathic urticaria. *J Cutan Pathol.* 2004;31(4):323-329.
18. Jordaan HF, Schneider JW. Papular urticaria: a histopathologic study of 30 patients. *Am J Dermatopathol.* 1997;19(2):119-126.
19. Imbernón-Moya A, Vargas-Laguna E, Burgos F, Fernández-Cogolludo E, Aguilar-Martínez A, Gallego-Valdés MÁ. Urticaria vasculitis in a child: a case report and literature review. *Clin Case Rep.* 2017;5(8):1255-1257.
20. Soylu A, Kavukçu S, Uzuner N, Olgaç N, Karaman O, Ozer E. Systemic lupus erythematosus presenting with normocomplementemic urticarial vasculitis in a 4-year-old girl. *Pediatr Int.* 2001;43(4):420-422.
21. Loricera J, Calvo-Río V, Mata C, et al. Urticarial vasculitis in Northern Spain: clinical study of 21 cases. *Medicine.* 2014;93(1):53-60.
22. Sanchez NP, Winkelmann RK, Schroeter AL, Dicken CH. The clinical and histopathologic spectrums of urticarial vasculitis: study of forty cases. *J Am Acad Dermatol.* 1982;7(5):599-605.
23. Goto S, Goto H, Tanoshima R, et al. Serum sickness with an elevated level of human anti-chimeric antibody following treatment with rituximab in a child with chronic immune thrombocytopenic purpura. *Int J Hematol.* 2009;89(3):305-309.
24. Harel L, Amir J, Livni E, Straussberg R, Varsano I. Serum-sickness-like reaction associated with minocycline therapy in adolescents. *Ann Pharmacother.* 1996;30(5):481-483.
25. Chiong FJ, Loewenthal M, Boyle M, Attia J. Serum sickness-like reaction after influenza vaccination. *BMJ Case Rep.* 2015;2015. doi:10.1136/bcr-2015-211917.
26. Arkachaisri T. Serum sickness and hepatitis B vaccine including review of the literature. *J Med Assoc Thai.* 2002;85(suppl 2):S607-S612.
27. Colton RL, Amir J, Mimouni M, Zeharia A. Serum sickness-like reaction associated with griseofulvin. *Ann Pharmacother.* 2004;38(4):609-611.
28. Kearns GL, Wheeler JG, Rieder MJ, Reid J. Serum sickness-like reaction to cefaclor: lack of in vitro cross-reactivity with loracarbef. *Clin Pharmacol Ther.* 1998;63(6):686-693.
29. Kearns GL, Wheeler JG, Childress SH, Letzig LG. Serum sickness-like reactions to cefaclor: role of hepatic metabolism and individual susceptibility. *J Pediatr.* 1994;125(5 pt 1):805-811.
30. Yorulmaz A, Akın F, Sert A, Ağır MA, Yılmaz R, Arslan Ş. Demographic and clinical characteristics of patients with serum sickness-like reaction. *Clin Rheumatol.* 2018;37(5):1389-1394.
31. Lawley TJ, Bielory L, Gascon P, Yancey KB, Young NS, Frank MM. A prospective clinical and immunologic analysis of patients with serum sickness. *N Engl J Med.* 1984;311(22):1407-1413.
32. Bielory L, Yancey KB, Young NS, Frank MM, Lawley TJ. Cutaneous manifestations of serum sickness in patients receiving antithymocyte globulin. *J Am Dermatol.* 1985;13(3):411-417.
33. King BA, Geelhoed GC. Adverse skin and joint reactions associated with oral antibiotics in children: the role of cefaclor in serum sickness-like reactions. *J Paediatr Child Health.* 2003;39(9):677-681.
34. Nguyen CV, Miller DD. Serum sickness-like drug reaction: two cases with a neutrophilic urticarial pattern. *J Cutan Pathol.* 2017;44(2):177-182.
35. Tolpinrud WL, Bunick CG, King BA. Serum sickness-like reaction: histopathology and case report. *J Am Acad Dermatol.* 2011;65(3):e83-e85.
36. Hill TA, Cohen B. Scabies in babies. *Pediatr Dermatol.* 2017;34(6):690-694.

37. Chosidow O. Scabies and pediculosis. *Lancet*. 2000;355(9206):819-826.

38. Kruse LL, Kenner-Bell BM, Mancini AJ. Pediatric erythema annulare centrifugum treated with oral fluconazole: a retrospective series. *Pediatr Dermatol*. 2016;33(5):501-506.

39. Kumar L, Thapa BR, Sarkar B, Walia BN. Benign cutaneous polyarteritis nodosa in children below 10 years of age—a clinical experience. *Ann Rheum Dis*. 1995;54(2):134-136.

40. Kumar P, Savant SS. Erythema annulare centrifugum. *Indian Pediatr*. 2015;52(4):356-357.

41. Kim KJ, Chang SE, Choi JH, Sung KJ, Moon KC, Koh JK. Clinicopathologic analysis of 66 cases of erythema annulare centrifugum. *J Dermatol*. 2002;29(2):61-67.

42. Weyers W, Diaz-Cascajo C, Weyers I. Erythema annulare centrifugum: results of a clinicopathologic study of 73 patients. *Am J Dermatopathol*. 2003;25(6):451-462.

43. Ziemer M, Eisendle K, Zelger B. New concepts on erythema annulare centrifugum: a clinical reaction pattern that does not represent a specific clinicopathological entity. *Br J Dermatol*. 2009;160(1):119-126.

44. Ziemer M, Eisendle K, Zelger B. Erythema annulare centrifugum. A clinical reaction pattern [in German]. *Hautarzt*. 2010;61(11):967-972.

45. Helm TN, Bass J, Chang LW, Bergfeld WF. Persistent annular erythema of infancy. *Pediatr Dermatol*. 1993;10(1):46-48.

46. Hebert AA, Esterly NB. Annular erythema of infancy. *J Am Dermatol*. 1986;14(2 pt 2):339-343.

47. Pfingstler LF, Miller KP, Pride H. Recurring diffuse annular erythematous plaques in a newborn. *JAMA Dermatol*. 2014;150(5):565.

48. Cox NH, McQueen A, Evans TJ, Morley WN. An annular erythema of infancy. *Arch Dermatol*. 1987;123(4):510-513.

49. Patrizi A, Savoia F, Varotti E, Gaspari V, Passarini B, Neri I. Neutrophilic figurate erythema of infancy. *Pediatr Dermatol*. 2008;25(2):255-260.

50. Athreya BH, Rose CD. Lyme disease. *Curr Probl Pediatr*. 1996;26(6):189-207.

51. Asbrink E, Brehmer-Andersson E, Hovmark A. Acrodermatitis chronica atrophicans—a spirochetosis. Clinical and histopathological picture based on 32 patients; course and relationship to erythema chronicum migrans Afzelius. *Am J Dermatopathol*. 1986;8(3):209-219.

52. Boer A, Bresch M, Dayrit J, Falk TM. Erythema migrans: a reassessment of diagnostic criteria for early cutaneous manifestations of borreliosis with particular emphasis on clonality investigations. *Br J Dermatol*. 2007;156(6):1263-1271.

53. Moreno C, Kutzner H, Palmedo G, Goerttler E, Carrasco L, Requena L. Interstitial granulomatous dermatitis with histiocytic pseudorosettes: a new histopathologic pattern in cutaneous borreliosis. Detection of Borrelia burgdorferi DNA sequences by a highly sensitive PCR-ELISA. *J Am Acad Dermatol*. 2003;48(3):376-384.

54. Seidel MF, Domene AB, Vetter H. Differential diagnoses of suspected Lyme borreliosis or post-Lyme-disease syndrome. *Eur J Clin Microbiol Infect Dis*. 2007;26(9):611-617.

55. Bitar FF, Hayek P, Obeid M, Gharzeddine W, Mikati M, Dbaibo GS. Rheumatic fever in children: a 15-year experience in a developing country. *Pediatr Cardiol*. 2000;21(2):119-122.

56. Carvalho SM, Dalben I, Corrente JE, Magalhaes CS. Rheumatic fever presentation and outcome: a case-series report. *Rev Bras Reumatol*. 2012;52(2):241-246.

57. Troyer C, Grossman ME, Silvers DN. Erythema marginatum in rheumatic fever: early diagnosis by skin biopsy. *J Am Acad Dermatol*. 1983;8(5):724-728.

58. Starr JC, Brasher GW, Rao A, Posey D. Erythema marginatum and hereditary angioedema. *South Med J*. 2004;97(10):948-950.

59. Simon TD. Pernio in pediatrics. *Pediatrics*. 2005;116(3):e472-e475.

60. Verma P, Singal A, Yadav P. Perniosis in an infant treated with topical nitroglycerine. 2013;30(5):623-624.

61. Weston WL, Morelli JG. Childhood pernio and cryoproteins. *Pediatr Dermatol*. 2000;17(2):97-99.

62. White KP, Rothe MJ, Milanese A, Grant-Kels JM. Perniosis in association with anorexia nervosa. *Pediatr Dermatol*. 1994;11(1):1-5.

63. St Clair NE, Kim CC, Semrin G, et al. Celiac disease presenting with chilblains in an adolescent girl. *Pediatr Dermatol*. 2006;23(5):451-454.

64. Shahi V, Wetter DA, Cappel JA, Davis MD, Spittell PC. Vasospasm is a consistent finding in pernio (chilblains) and a possible clue to pathogenesis. *Dermatology*. 2015;231(3):274-279.

65. Cappel JA, Wetter DA. Clinical characteristics, etiologic associations, laboratory findings, treatment, and proposal of diagnostic criteria of pernio (chilblains) in a series of 104 patients at Mayo Clinic, 2000 to 2011. *Mayo Clin Proc*. 2014;89(2):207-215.

66. Abe J, Nakamura K, Nishikomori R, et al. A nationwide survey of Aicardi-Goutières syndrome patients identifies a strong association between dominant TREX1 mutations and chilblain lesions: Japanese cohort study. *Rheumatology*. 2014;53(3):448-458.

67. Boada A, Bielsa I, Fernandez-Figueras MT, Ferrandiz C. Perniosis: clinical and histopathological analysis. *Am J Dermatopathol*. 2010;32(1):19-23.

68. Crowson AN, Magro CM. Idiopathic perniosis and its mimics: a clinical and histological study of 38 cases. *Hum Pathol*. 1997;28(4):478-484.

69. Ersoy-Evans S, Greco MF, Mancini AJ, Subaşı N, Paller AS. Pityriasis lichenoides in childhood: a retrospective review of 124 patients. *J Am Acad Dermatol*. 2007;56(2):205-210.

70. Romaní J, Puig L, Fernández-Figueras MT, de Moragas JM. Pityriasis lichenoides in children: clinicopathologic review of 22 patients. *Pediatr Dermatol*. 1998;15(1):1-6.

71. Chand S, Srivastava N, Khopkar U, Singh S. Pityriasis lichenoides chronica: onset at birth. *Pediatr Dermatol*. 2008;25(1):135-136.

72. López-Villaescusa MT, Hernández-Martín A, Colmenero I, Torrelo A. Pityriasis lichenoides in a 9-month-old boy. *Actas Dermosifiliogr*. 2013;104(9):829-830.

73. Magro C, Crowson AN, Kovatich A, Burns F. Pityriasis lichenoides: a clonal T-cell lymphoproliferative disorder. *Hum Pathol*. 2002;33(8):788-795.

74. Geller L, Antonov NK, Lauren CT, Morel KD, Garzon MC. Pityriasis lichenoides in childhood: review of clinical presentation and treatment options. *Pediatr Dermatol*. 2015;32(5):579-592.

75. Cho E, Jun HJ, Cho SH, Lee JD. Varicella-zoster virus as a possible cause of pityriasis lichenoides et varioliformis acuta. *Pediatr Dermatol*. 2014;31(2):259-260.

76. Weinberg JM, Kristal L, Chooback L, Honig PJ, Kramer EM, Lessin SR. The clonal nature of pityriasis lichenoides. *Arch Dermatol*. 2002;138(8):1063-1067.

77. Fortson JS, Schroeter AL, Esterly NB. Cutaneous T-cell lymphoma (parapsoriasis en plaque). An association with pityriasis lichenoides et varioliformis acuta in young children. *Arch Dermatol*. 1990;126(11):1449-1453.

78. Lam J, Pope E. Pediatric pityriasis lichenoides and cutaneous T-cell lymphoma. *Curr Opin Pediatr*. 2007;19(4):441-445.

79. Nanda A, Alshalfan F, Al-Otaibi M, Al-Sabah H, Rajy JM. Febrile ulceronecrotic Mucha-Habermann disease (pityriasis lichenoides et varioliformis acuta fulminans) associated with parvovirus infection. *Am J Dermatopathol*. 2013;35(4):503-506.

80. Tsuji T, Kasamatsu M, Yokota M, Morita A, Schwartz RA. Mucha-Habermann disease and its febrile ulceronecrotic variant. *Cutis*. 1996;58(2):123-131.

81. Clayton R, Warin A. Pityriasis lichenoides chronica presenting as hypopigmentation. *Br J Dermatol*. 1979;100(3):297-302.

82. Kim JE, Yun WJ, Mun SK, et al. Pityriasis lichenoides et varioliformis acuta and pityriasis lichenoides chronica: comparison of lesional T-cell subsets and investigation of viral associations. *J Cutan Pathol*. 2011;38(8):649-656.

83. Magro CM, Crowson AN, Morrison C, Li J. Pityriasis lichenoides chronica: stratification by molecular and phenotypic profile. *Hum Pathol*. 2007;38(3):479-490.

84. Jang MS, Kang DY, Park JB, et al. Pityriasis lichenoides-like mycosis fungoides: clinical and histologic features and response to phototherapy. *Ann Dermatol.* 2016;28(5):540-547.

85. Martinez-Escala ME, Sidiropoulos M, Deonizio J, Gerami P, Kadin ME, Guitar J. gammadelta T-cell-rich variants of pityriasis lichenoides and lymphomatoid papulosis: benign cutaneous disorders to be distinguished from aggressive cutaneous gammadelta T-cell lymphomas. *Br J Dermatol.* 2015;172(2):372-379.

86. Shieh S, Mikkola DL, Wood GS. Differentiation and clonality of lesional lymphocytes in pityriasis lichenoides chronica. *Arch Dermatol.* 2001;137(3):305-308.

87. de Unamuno Bustos B, Ferriols AP, Sanchez RB, et al. Adult pityriasis lichenoides-like mycosis fungoides: a clinical variant of mycosis fungoides. *Int J Dermatol.* 2014;53(11):1331-1338.

88. Fitzgerald RL, McBurney EI, Nesbitt LT. Sweet's syndrome. *Int J Dermatol.* 1996;35(1):9-15.

89. Berk DR, Bayliss SJ. Neutrophilic dermatoses in children. *Pediatr Dermatol.* 2008;25(5):509-519.

90. Halpern J, Salim A. Pediatric sweet syndrome: case report and literature review. *Pediatr Dermatol.* 2009;26(4):452-457.

91. Uihlein LC, Brandling-Bennett HA, Lio PA, Liang MG. Sweet syndrome in children. *Pediatr Dermatol.* 2011;29(1):38-44.

92. Mohr MR, Torosky CM, Hood AF, Cunnion KM, Fisher RG, Williams JV. Sweet syndrome in infancy. *Pediatr Dermatol.* 2010;27(2):208-209.

93. Gray PE, Bock V, Ziegler DS, Wargon O. Neonatal sweet syndrome: a potential marker of serious systemic illness. *Pediatrics.* 2012;129(5):e1353-e1359.

94. Herron MD, Coffin CM, Vanderhooft SL. Sweet syndrome in two children. *Pediatr Dermatol.* 2005;22(6):525-529.

95. Burnham JM, Cron RQ. Sweet syndrome as an initial presentation in a child with systemic lupus erythematosus. *Lupus.* 2005;14(12):974-975.

96. Haliasos E, Soder B, Rubenstein DS, Henderson W, Morrell DS. Pediatric sweet syndrome and immunodeficiency successfully treated with intravenous immunoglobulin. *Pediatr Dermatol.* 2005;22(6):530-535.

97. Brady RC, Morris J, Connelly BL, Boiko S. Sweet's syndrome as an initial manifestation of pediatric human immunodeficiency virus infection. *Pediatrics.* 1999;104(5 pt 1):1142-1144.

98. Khaled A, Kharfi M, Fazaa B, et al. A first case of trimethoprim-sulfamethoxazole induced Sweet's syndrome in a child. *Pediatr Dermatol.* 2009;26(6):744-746.

99. Garty BZ, Levy I, Nitzan M, Barak Y. Sweet syndrome associated with G-CSF treatment in a child with glycogen storage disease type Ib. *Pediatrics.* 1996;97(3):401-403.

100. Shimizu T, Yoshida I, Eguchi H, Takahashi K, Inada H, Kato H. Sweet syndrome in a child with aplastic anemia receiving recombinant granulocyte colony-stimulating factor. *J Pediatr Hematol Oncol.* 1996;18(3):282-284.

101. García-Romero MT, Ho N. Pediatric sweet syndrome. A retrospective study. *Int J Dermatol.* 2015;54(5):518-522.

102. Hospach T, den Driesch von P, Dannecker GE. Acute febrile neutrophilic dermatosis (Sweet's syndrome) in childhood and adolescence: two new patients and review of the literature on associated diseases. *Eur J Pediatr.* 2008;168(1):1-9.

103. Abbas O, Kibbi AG, Rubeiz N. Sweet's syndrome: retrospective study of clinical and histologic features of 44 cases from a tertiary care center. *Int J Dermatol.* 2010;49(11):1244-1249.

104. Bi XL, Gu J, Yan M, Gao CF. A case of Sweet's syndrome with slack skin and pathergy phenomenon. *Int J Dermatol.* 2008;47(8):842-844.

105. Callen JP. Cutaneous vasculitis and other neutrophilic dermatoses. *Curr Opin Rheumatol.* 1993;5(1):33-40.

106. Camarillo D, McCalmont TH, Frieden IJ, Gilliam AE. Two pediatric cases of nonbullous histiocytoid neutrophilic dermatitis presenting as a cutaneous manifestation of lupus erythematosus. *Arch Dermatol.* 2008;144(11):1495-1498.

107. Cohen PR. Sweet's syndrome—a comprehensive review of an acute febrile neutrophilic dermatosis. *Orphanet J Rare Dis.* 2007;2:34.

108. Guhamajumdar M, Agarwala B. Sweet syndrome, cutis laxa, and fatal cardiac manifestations in a 2-year-old girl. *Tex Heart Inst J.* 2011;38(3):285-287.

109. Lee SH, Roh MR. Targetoid lesions and neutrophilic dermatosis: an initial clinical and histological presentation of neonatal lupus erythematosus. *Int J Dermatol.* 2014;53(6):764-766.

110. Malone JC, Slone SP, Wills-Frank LA, et al. Vascular inflammation (vasculitis) in sweet syndrome: a clinicopathologic study of 28 biopsy specimens from 21 patients. *Arch Dermatol.* 2002;138(3):345-349.

111. Morgan KW, Callen JP. Sweet's syndrome in acute myelogenous leukemia presenting as periorbital cellulitis with an infiltrate of leukemic cells. *J Am Acad Dermatol.* 2001;45(4):590-595.

112. Satter EK, High WA. Non-bullous neutrophilic dermatosis within neonatal lupus erythematosus. *J Cutan Pathol.* 2007;34(12):958-960.

113. Kitamura H, Kaneko T, Nakano H, Terui K, Ito E, Sawamura D. Juvenile myelomonocytic leukemia presenting multiple painful erythematous lesions diagnosed as Sweet's syndrome. *J Dermatol.* 2008;35(6):368-370.

114. Peroni A, Colato C, Schena D, Rongioletti F, Girolomoni G. Histiocytoid sweet syndrome is infiltrated predominantly by M2-like macrophages. *J Am Acad Dermatol.* 2015;72(1):131-139.

115. Alegria-Landa V, Cerroni L, Requena L. Histiocytoid Sweet syndrome and myelodysplastic syndrome-reply. *JAMA Dermatol.* 2017;153(8):836-837.

116. Kasuya A, Fujiyama T, Hashizume H, Inuzuka M, Tokura Y. Histiocytoid Sweet's syndrome associated with t(9;22)(q34;q11)-positive chronic myelogenous leukemia: immature granulocytic origin of histiocytic cells. *Int J Dermatol.* 2013;52(12):1577-1579.

117. Pereira E, Estanqueiro P, Almeida S, Ferreira R, Tellechea O, Salgado M. Bowel-associated dermatosis-arthritis syndrome in an adolescent with short bowel syndrome. *J Clin Rheumatol.* 2014;20(6):322-324.

118. Carubbi F, Ruscitti P, Pantano I, et al. Jejunoileal bypass as the main procedure in the onset of immune-related conditions: the model of BADAS. *Expert Rev Clin Immunol.* 2013;9(5):441-452.

119. Thrash B, Patel M, Shah KR, Boland CR, Menter A. Cutaneous manifestations of gastrointestinal disease: part II. *J Am Acad Dermatol.* 2013;68(2):211.e1-211.e33; quiz 244-246.

120. Oldfield CW, Heffernan-Stroud LA, Buehler-Bota TS, Williams JV. Bowel-associated dermatosis-arthritis syndrome (BADAS) in a pediatric patient. *JAAD Case Rep.* 2016;2(3):272-274.

121. Dicken CH. Bowel-associated dermatosis-arthritis syndrome: bowel bypass syndrome without bowel bypass. *Mayo Clin Proc.* 1984;59(1):43-46.

122. Dicken CH. Bowel-associated dermatosis-arthritis syndrome: bowel bypass syndrome without bowel bypass. *J Am Acad Dermatol.* 1986;14(5 pt 1):792-796.

123. Dicken CH, Seehafer JR. Bowel bypass syndrome. *Arch Dermatol.* 1979;115(7):837-839.

124. Ely PH. The bowel bypass syndrome: a response to bacterial peptidoglycans. *J Am Acad Dermatol.* 1980;2(6):473-487.

125. Rubinson R, Larralde M, Santos-Muñoz A, Parra V, de Parra NP. Palmoplantar eccrine hidradenitis: seven new cases. *Pediatr Dermatol.* 2004;21(4):466-468.

126. Shehan JM, Clowers-Webb HE, Kalaaji AN. Recurrent palmoplantar hidradenitis with exclusive palmar involvement and an association with trauma and exposure to aluminum dust. *Pediatr Dermatol.* 2004;21(1):30-32.

127. Simon M, Cremer H, den Driesch von P. Idiopathic recurrent palmoplantar hidradenitis in children. Report of 22 cases. *Arch Dermatol.* 1998;134(1):76-79.

128. Naimer SA, Zvulunov A, Ben-Amitai D, Landau M. Plantar hidradenitis in children induced by exposure to wet footwear. *Pediatr Emerg Care.* 2000;16(3):182-183.

129. Esler-Brauer L, Rothman I. Tender nodules on the palms and soles: palmoplantar eccrine hidradenitis. *Arch Dermatol.* 2007;143(9):1201-1206.

130. Harrist TJ, Fine JD, Berman RS, Murphy GF, Mihm MC. Neutrophilic eccrine hidradenitis. A distinctive type of neutrophilic dermatosis associated with myelogenous leukemia and chemotherapy. *Arch Dermatol.* 1982;118(4):263-266.

131. Lee GL, Chen AYY. Neutrophilic dermatoses: kids are not just little people. *Clin Dermatol.* 2017;35(6):541-554.

132. Fitzpatrick JE, Bennion SD, Reed OM, Wilson T, Reddy VV, Golitz L. Neutrophilic eccrine hidradenitis associated with induction chemotherapy. *J Cutan Pathol.* 1987;14(5);272-278.

133. Flynn TC, Harrist TJ, Murphy GF, Loss RW, Moschella SL. Neutrophilic eccrine hidradenitis: a distinctive rash associated with cytarabine therapy and acute leukemia. *J Am Acad Dermatol.* 1984;11(4 pt 1):584-590.

134. Greenbaum BH, Heymann WR, Reid CS, Travis SF, Donaldson MH. Chemotherapy-associated eccrine hidradenitis: neutrophilic eccrine hidradenitis reevaluated: the role of neutrophilic infiltration. *Med Pediatr Oncol.* 1988;16(5):351-355.

135. Anderson CR, Jenkins D, Tron V, Prendiville JS. Wells' syndrome in childhood: case report and review of the literature. *J Am Dermatol.* 1995;33(5 pt 2):857-864.

136. Barreiros H, Matos D, Furtado C, Cunha H, Bártolo E. Wells syndrome in a child triggered by parvovirus B19 infection? *J Am Acad Dermatol.* 2012;67(4):e166-e167.

137. Gilliam AE, Bruckner AL, Howard RM, Lee BP, Wu S, Frieden IJ. Bullous "cellulitis" with eosinophilia: case report and review of Wells' syndrome in childhood. *Pediatrics.* 2005;116(1):e149-e155.

138. España A, Sanz ML, Sola J, Gil P. Wells' syndrome (eosinophilic cellulitis): correlation between clinical activity, eosinophil levels, eosinophil cation protein and interleukin-5. *Br J Dermatol.* 1999;140(1):127-130.

139. Fisher GB, Greer KE, Cooper PH. Eosinophilic cellulitis (Wells' syndrome). *Int J Dermatol.* 1985;24(2):101-107.

140. Garty BZ, Feinmesser M, David M, Gayer S, Danon YL. Congenital Wells syndrome. *Pediatr Dermatol.* 1997;14(4):312-315.

141. Schorr WF, Tauscheck AL, Dickson KB, Melski JW. Eosinophilic cellulitis (Wells' syndrome): histologic and clinical features in arthropod bite reactions. *J Am Acad Dermatol.* 1984;11(6):1043-1049.

142. Wood C, Miller AC, Jacobs A, Hart R, Nickoloff BJ. Eosinophilic infiltration with flame figures. A distinctive tissue reaction seen in Wells' syndrome and other diseases. *Am J Dermatopathol.* 1986;8(3):186-193.

143. Davin JC, Coppo R. Henoch-Schönlein purpura nephritis in children. *Nat Rev Nephrol.* 2014;10(10):563-573.

144. Trapani S, Micheli A, Grisolia F, et al. Henoch Schonlein purpura in childhood: epidemiological and clinical analysis of 150 cases over a 5-year period and review of literature. *Semin Arthritis Rheum.* 2005;35(3):143-153.

145. Saulsbury FT. Henoch-Schönlein purpura in children. Report of 100 patients and review of the literature. *Medicine* [Internet]. 2011;78(6):395-409.

146. Trnka P. Henoch-Schönlein purpura in children. *J Paediatr Child Health.* 2013;49(12):995-1003.

147. Trapani S, Mariotti P, Resti M, Nappini L, De Martino M, Falcini F. Severe hemorrhagic bullous lesions in Henoch Schonlein purpura: three pediatric cases and review of the literature. *Rheumatol Int.* 2009;30(10):1355-1359.

148. Narchi H. Risk of long term renal impairment and duration of follow up recommended for Henoch-Schönlein purpura with normal or minimal urinary findings: a systematic review. *Arch Dis Child.* 2005;90(9):916-920.

149. Sano H, Izumida M, Shimizu H, Ogawa Y. Risk factors of renal involvement and significant proteinuria in Henoch-Schönlein purpura. *Eur J Pediatr.* 2002;161(4):196-201.

150. Mao Y, Yin L, Huang H, Zhou Z, Chen T, Zhou W. Henoch-Schönlein purpura in 535 Chinese children: clinical features and risk factors for renal involvement. *J Int Med Res.* 2014;42(4):1043-1049.

151. Schärer K, Krmar R, Querfeld U, Ruder H, Waldherr R, Schaefer F. Clinical outcome of Schönlein-Henoch purpura nephritis in children. *Pediatr Nephrol.* 1999;13(9):816-823.

152. Limpongsanurak W, Kietkajornkul C, Singalavanija S. Predictive factor of severe renal involvement in children with Henoch-Schoenlein purpura. *J Med Assoc Thai.* 2011;94(suppl 3):S204-S208.

153. Ha TS, Lee JS. Scrotal involvement in childhood Henoch-Schönlein purpura. *Acta Paediatr.* 2007;96(4):552-555.

154. Chen SY, Chang KC, Yu MC, Asueh S, Ou LS. Pulmonary hemorrhage associated with Henoch Schönlein purpura in pediatric patients: case report and review of the literature. 2011;41(2):305-312.

155. Calvo-Rio V, Loricera J, Mata C, et al. Henoch-Schonlein purpura in northern Spain: clinical spectrum of the disease in 417 patients from a single center. *Medicine (Baltimore).* 2014;93(2):106-113.

156. Farhadian JA, Castilla C, Shvartsbeyn M, Meehan SA, Neimann A, Pomeranz MK. IgA vasculitis (Henoch-Schonlein purpura). *Dermatol Online J.* 2015;21(12). pii:13030/qt72p3m3q2.

157. Kedia PP, Tirumalae R, Puttegowda D, Antony M. "Joining the spots in adults and young tots": a clinicopathological study of Henoch-Schonlein purpura (IgA Vasculitis). *Am J Dermatopathol.* 2017;39(8):587-592.

158. Lava SA, Milani GP, Fossali EF, Simonetti GD, Agostoni C, Bianchetti MG. Cutaneous manifestations of small-vessel leukocytoclastic vasculitides in childhood. *Clin Rev Allergy Immunol.* 2017;53(3):439-451.

159. Fiore E, Rizzi M, Ragazzi M, et al. Acute hemorrhagic edema of young children (cockade purpura and edema): a case series and systematic review. *J Am Acad Dermatol.* 2008;59(4):684-695.

160. Caksen H, Odabaş D, Kösem M, et al. Report of eight infants with acute infantile hemorrhagic edema and review of the literature. *J Dermatol.* 2002;29(5):290-295.

161. Karremann M, Jordan AJ, Bell N, Witsch M, Dürken M. Acute hemorrhagic edema of infancy: report of 4 cases and review of the current literature. *Clin Pediatr (Phila).* 2008;48(3):323-326.

162. Ferrarini A, Benetti C, Camozzi P, et al. Acute hemorrhagic edema of young children: a prospective case series. *Eur J Pediatr.* 2015;175(4):557-561.

163. Homme JL, Block JM. Acute hemorrhagic edema of infancy and common mimics. *Am J Emerg Med.* 2016;34(5):936.e3-936.e6.

164. Fiore E, Rizzi M, Simonetti GD, Garzoni L, Bianchetti MG, Bettinelli A. Acute hemorrhagic edema of young children: a concise narrative review. *Eur J Pediatr.* 2011;170(12):1507-1511.

165. Johnson EF, Wetter DA, Lehman JS, Hand JL, Davis DM, Tollefson MM. Leukocytoclastic vasculitis in children: clinical characteristics, subtypes, causes and direct immunofluorescence findings of 56 biopsy-confirmed cases. *J Eur Acad Dermatol Venereol.* 2016;31(3):544-549.

166. Özçakar ZB, Yalçınkaya F, Altugan FŞ, Kavaz A, Ensari A, Ekim M. Hypocomplementemic urticarial vasculitis syndrome in three siblings. *Rheumatol Int.* 2010;33(3):763-766.

167. Pasini A, Bracaglia C, Aceti A, et al. Renal involvement in hypocomplementaemic urticarial vasculitis syndrome: a report of three paediatric cases. *Rheumatology.* 2014;53(8):1409-1413.

168. Al Mosawi ZS, Al Hermi BE. Hypocomplementemic urticarial vasculitis syndrome in an 8-year-old boy: a case report and review of literature. *Oman Med J.* 2013;28(4):275-277.

169. Liou YT, Huang JL, Ou LS, et al. Comparison of cryoglobulinemia in children and adults. *J Microbiol Immunol Infect.* 2013;46(1):59-64.

170. Berliner S, Weinberger A, Ben-Bassat M, et al. Small skin blood vessel occlusions by cryoglobulin aggregates in ulcerative lesions in IgM-IgG cryoglobulinemia. *J Cutan Pathol.* 1982;9(2):96-103.

171. Resnik KS. Intravascular eosinophilic deposits-when common knowledge is insufficient to render a diagnosis. *Am J Dermatopathol.* 2009;31(3):211-217.

172. Schwartzenberg S, Levo Y, Averbuch M. Generalized vasculitis, thrombocytopenia, and transient lymphoproliferative disorder caused by idiopathic mixed cryoglobulinemia. *Am J Med Sci*. 2003;326(1):47-50.

173. Cabral DA, Uribe AG, Benseler S, et al. Classification, presentation, and initial treatment of Wegener's granulomatosis in childhood. *Arthritis Rheum*. 2009;60(11):3413-3424.

174. Stein SL, Miller LC, Konnikov N. Wegener's granulomatosis: case report and literature review. *Pediatr Dermatol*. 1998;15(5):352-356.

175. Gajic-Veljic M, Nikolic M, Peco-Antic A, Bogdanovic R, Andrejevic S, Bonaci-Nikolic B. Granulomatosis with polyangiitis (Wegener's granulomatosis) in children: report of three cases with cutaneous manifestations and literature review. *Pediatr Dermatol*. 2012;30(4):e37-e42.

176. Popa ER, Tervaert JW. The relation between Staphylococcus aureus and Wegener's granulomatosis: current knowledge and future directions. *Intern Med*. 2003;42(9):771-780.

177. Rottem M, Fauci AS, Hallahan CW, et al. Wegener granulomatosis in children and adolescents: clinical presentation and outcome. *J Pediatr*. 1993;122(1):26-31.

178. Atula T, Honkanen V, Tarkkanen J, Jero J. Otitis media as a sign of Wegener's granulomatosis in childhood. *Acta Otolaryngol Suppl*. 2000;543:48-50.

179. White JB, Shah RK. Wegener's granulomatosis of the pediatric airway: a case demonstrating a conservative management approach. *Am J Otolaryngol*. 2009;30(3):212-215.

180. Akikusa JD, Schneider R, Harvey EA, et al. Clinical features and outcome of pediatric Wegener's granulomatosis. *Arthritis Rheum*. 2007;57(5):837-844.

181. Ulinski T, Martin H, Mac Gregor B, Dardelin R, Cochat P. Fatal neurologic involvement in pediatric Wegener's granulomatosis. *Pediatr Neurol*. 2005;32(4):278-281.

182. Fiorentino DF. Cutaneous vasculitis. *J Am Dermatol*. 2003;48(3):311-340.

183. Chyu JY, Hagstrom WJ, Soltani K, Faibisoff B, Whitney DH. Wegener's granulomatosis in childhood: cutaneous manifestations as the presenting signs. *J Am Dermatol*. 1984;10(2 pt 2):341-346.

184. Parelhoff ES, Chavis RM, Friendly DS. Wegener's granulomatosis presenting as orbital pseudotumor in children. *J Pediatr Ophthalmol Strabismus*. 1985;22(3):100-104.

185. Comfere NI, Macaron NC, Gibson LE. Cutaneous manifestations of Wegener's granulomatosis: a clinicopathologic study of 17 patients and correlation to antineutrophil cytoplasmic antibody status. *J Cutan Pathol*. 2007;34(10):739-747.

186. Zwerina J, Eger G, Englbrecht M, Manger B, Schett G. Churg-Strauss syndrome in childhood: a systematic literature review and clinical comparison with adult patients. 2009;39(2):108-115.

187. Boyer D, Vargas SO, Slattery D, Rivera-Sanchez YM, Colin AA. Churg-Strauss syndrome in children: a clinical and pathologic review. *Pediatrics*. 2006;118(3):e914-e920.

188. Ozen S, Pistorio A, Iusan SM, et al. EULAR/PRINTO/PRES criteria for Henoch-Schonlein purpura, childhood polyarteritis nodosa, childhood Wegener granulomatosis and childhood Takayasu arteritis: Ankara 2008. Part II: final classification criteria. *Ann Rheum Dis*. 2010;69(5):798-806.

189. Ozen S, Antón J, Arisoy N, et al. Juvenile polyarteritis: results of a multicenter survey of 110 children. *J Pediatr*. 2004;145(4):517-522.

190. Rodrigues M, Amaral D, Barreira JL, Brito I. Childhood polyarteritis nodosa presenting as stroke and arterial hypertension. *BMJ Case Rep*. 2014;2014. doi:10.1136/bcr-2014-207866.

191. Eleftheriou D, Dillon MJ, Tullus K, et al. Systemic polyarteritis nodosa in the young: a single-center experience over thirty-two years. *Arthritis Rheum*. 2013;65(9):2476-2485.

192. Ruperto N, Ozen S, Pistorio A, et al. EULAR/PRINTO/PRES criteria for Henoch-Schonlein purpura, childhood polyarteritis nodosa, childhood Wegener granulomatosis and childhood Takayasu

arteritis: Ankara 2008. Part I: overall methodology and clinical characterisation. *Ann Rheum Dis*. 2010;69(5):790-797.

193. Kelly PC, Pearl WR, Weir MR. Infantile polyarteritis nodosa with mucocutaneous lymph node syndrome treated with long-term corticosteroids. *South Med J*. 1987;80(8):1045-1048.

194. Ettlinger RE, Nelson AM, Burke EC, Lie JT. Polyarteritis nodosa in childhood a clinical pathologic study. *Arthritis Rheum*. 1979;22(8):820-825.

195. Fathalla BM, Miller L, Brady S, Schaller JG. Cutaneous polyarteritis nodosa in children. *J Am Acad Dermatol*. 2005;53(4):724-728.

196. Till SH, Amos RS. Long-term follow-up of juvenile-onset cutaneous polyarteritis nodosa associated with streptococcal infection. *Br J Rheumatol*. 1997;36(8):909-911.

197. Sheth AP, Olson JC, Esterly NB. Cutaneous polyarteritis nodosa of childhood. *J Am Dermatol*. 1994;31(4):561-566.

198. Mocan H, Mocan MC, Peru H, Ozoran Y. Cutaneous polyarteritis nodosa in a child and a review of the literature. *Acta Paediatr*. 1998;87(3):351-353.

199. Morgan AJ, Schwartz RA. Cutaneous polyarteritis nodosa: a comprehensive review. *Int J Dermatol*. 2010;49(7):750-756.

200. Bansal NK, Houghton KM. Cutaneous polyarteritis nodosa in childhood: a case report and review of the literature. *Arthritis*. 2010; 2010:687547.

201. Daoud MS, Hutton KP, Gibson LE. Cutaneous periarteritis nodosa: a clinicopathological study of 79 cases. *Br J Dermatol*. 1997;136(5):706-713.

202. Minkowitz G, Smoller BR, McNutt NS. Benign cutaneous polyarteritis nodosa. Relationship to systemic polyarteritis nodosa and to hepatitis B infection. *Arch Dermatol*. 1991;127(10):1520-1523.

203. Reimold EW, Weinberg AG, Fink CW, Battles ND. Polyarteritis in children. *Am J Dis Child*. 1976;130(5):534-541.

204. Ishibashi M, Chen KR. A morphological study of evolution of cutaneous polyarteritis nodosa. *Am J Dermatopathol*. 2008;30(4):319-326.

205. Buffiere-Morgado A, Battistella M, Vignon-Pennamen MD, et al. Relationship between cutaneous polyarteritis nodosa (cPAN) and macular lymphocytic arteritis (MLA): blinded histologic assessment of 35 cPAN cases. *J Am Acad Dermatol*. 2015;73(6):1013-1020.

206. Macarenco RS, Galan A, Simoni PM, et al. Cutaneous lymphocytic thrombophilic (macular) arteritis: a distinct entity or an indolent (reparative) stage of cutaneous polyarteritis nodosa? Report of 2 cases of cutaneous arteritis and review of the literature. *Am J Dermatopathol*. 2013;35(2):213-219.

207. Magro CM, Saab J. Lymphocytic thrombophilic arteritis: a distinct inflammatory type I interferon and C5b-9 mediated subcutaneous endovasculitis. *Ann Diagn Pathol*. 2017;31:23-29.

208. Morimoto A, Chen KR. Reappraisal of histopathology of cutaneous polyarteritis nodosa. *J Cutan Pathol*. 2016;43(12):1131-1138.

209. Taconet S, Vignon-Pennamen MD, Fouchard N. Macular lymphocytic arteritis and periarteritis nodosa: a case report showing diagnostic and nosological challenges posed by these two entities [in French]. *Ann Dermatol Venereol*. 2015;142(10):567-571.

210. Wee E, Nikpour M, Balta S, Williams RA, Kelly RI. Lymphocytic thrombophilic arteritis complicated by systemic involvement. *Australas J Dermatol*. 2018. doi:10.1111/ajd.12798.

211. Bayers S, Shulman ST, Paller AS. Kawasaki disease. *J Am Dermatol*. 2013;69(4):513.e1-513.e8.

212. Bayers S, Shulman ST, Paller AS. Kawasaki disease. *J Am Dermatol*. 2013;69(4):501.e1-501.e11.

213. Uehara R, Belay ED. Epidemiology of Kawasaki disease in Asia, Europe, and the United States. *J Epidemiol*. 2012;22(2):79-85.

214. Ha S, Seo GH, Kim KY, Kim DS. Epidemiologic study on Kawasaki disease in Korea, 2007-2014: based on Health Insurance Review & Assessment Service claims. *J Korean Med Sci*. 2016;31(9):1445-1449.

215. Onouchi Y, Fukazawa R, Yamamura K, et al. Variations in ORAI1 gene associated with Kawasaki disease. *PLoS One*. 2016;11(1):e0145486.

216. Wei CC, Lin CL, Kao CH, et al. Increased risk of Kawasaki disease in children with common allergic diseases. *Ann Epidemiol.* 2014;24(5):340-343.

217. Liew WK, Lim CWT, Tan TH, et al. The effect of Kawasaki disease on childhood allergies-a sibling control study. *Pediatr Allergy Immunol.* 2011;22(5):488-493.

218. Pucci A, Martino S, Tibaldi M, Bartoloni G. Incomplete and atypical Kawasaki disease: a clinicopathologic paradox at high risk of sudden and unexpected infant death. *Pediatr Cardiol.* 2012;33(5):802-805.

219. Manlhiot C, Christie E, McCrindle BW, Rosenberg H, Chahal N, Yeung RS. Complete and incomplete Kawasaki disease: two sides of the same coin. *Eur J Pediatr.* 2012;171(4):657-662.

220. Kallada S. A 5-year-old boy with fever and rash. *Pediatr Ann.* 2011;40(4):185-187.

221. Fradin KN, Rhim HJ. An Adolescent with fever, jaundice, and abdominal pain: an unusual presentation of Kawasaki disease. *J Adolesc Health.* 2013;52(1):131-133.

222. Friter BS, Lucky AW. The perineal eruption of Kawasaki syndrome. *Arch Dermatol.* 1988;124(12):1805-1810.

223. Eberhard BA, Sundel RP, Newburger JW, et al. Psoriatic eruption in Kawasaki disease. *J Pediatr.* 2000;137(4):578-580.

224. Amano S, Hazama F, Hamashima Y. Pathology of Kawasaki disease: I. Pathology and morphogenesis of the vascular changes. *Jpn Circ J.* 1979;43(7):633-643.

225. Haddock ES, Calame A, Shimizu C, Tremoulet AH, Burns JC, Tom WL. Psoriasiform eruptions during Kawasaki disease (KD): a distinct phenotype. *J Am Acad Dermatol.* 2016;75(1):69.e2-76.e2.

226. Kimura T, Miyazawa H, Watanabe K, Moriya T. Small pustules in Kawasaki disease. A clinicopathological study of four patients. *Am J Dermatopathol.* 1988;10(3):218-223.

227. Avcin T, Cimaz R, Silverman ED, et al. Pediatric Antiphospholipid syndrome: clinical and immunologic features of 121 patients in an international registry. *Pediatrics.* 2008;122(5):e1100-e1107.

228. Gibson GE, Su WP, Pittelkow MR. Antiphospholipid syndrome and the skin. *J Am Dermatol.* 1997;36(6 pt 1):970-982.

229. Driest KD, Sturm MS, O'Brien SH, et al. Factors associated with thrombosis in pediatric patients with systemic lupus erythematosus. *Lupus.* 2015;25(7):749-753.

230. Ma J, Song H, Wei M, He Y. Clinical characteristics and thrombosis outcomes of paediatric antiphospholipid syndrome: analysis of 58 patients. *Clin Rheumatol.* 2018;37(5):1295-1303.

231. Rumsey DG, Myones B, Massicotte P. Diagnosis and treatment of antiphospholipid syndrome in childhood: a review. *Blood Cells Mol Dis.* 2017;67:34-40.

232. Berman H, Rodríguez-Pintó I, Cervera R, et al. Pediatric catastrophic antiphospholipid syndrome: descriptive analysis of 45 patients from the "CAPS Registry." *Autoimmun Rev.* 2014;13(2):157-162.

233. Frances C, Niang S, Laffitte E, Pelletier F, Costedoat N, Piette JC. Dermatologic manifestations of the antiphospholipid syndrome: two hundred consecutive cases. *Arthritis Rheum.* 2005;52(6):1785-1793.

234. Thai KE, Barrett W, Kossard S. Reactive angioendotheliomatosis in the setting of antiphospholipid syndrome. *Australas J Dermatol.* 2003;44(2):151-155.

235. McMenamin ME, Fletcher CD. Reactive angioendotheliomatosis: a study of 15 cases demonstrating a wide clinicopathologic spectrum. *Am J Surg Pathol.* 2002;26(6):685-697.

236. Gru A, Dehner LP. Catastrophic antiphospholipid syndrome in a child with trisomy 21. An acquired thrombopathy with a discussion of thrombopathies in childhood. *Pediatr Dev Pathol.* 2010;13(3):178-183.

237. Theodoridis A, Konstantinidou A, Makranfonaki E, Zouboulis CC. Malignant and benign forms of atrophic papulosis (Köhlmeier-Degos disease): systemic involvement determines the prognosis. *Br J Dermatol.* 2014;170(1):110-115.

238. Calderón-Castrat X, Castro R, Peceros-Escalante J, Villate Caballero M, Chian C, Ballona R. Congenital Degos disease: case report and dermoscopic findings. *Pediatr Dermatol.* 2017;34(3):e109-e115.

239. Powell J, Bordea C, Wojnarowska F, Farrell AM, Morris PJ. Benign familial Degos disease worsening during immunosuppression. *Br J Dermatol.* 1999;141(3):524-527.

240. Katz SK, Mudd LJ, Roenigk HH. Malignant atrophic papulosis (Degos' disease) involving three generations of a family. *J Am Dermatol.* 1997;37(3 pt 1):480-484.

241. Jang MS, Park JB, Yang MH, et al. Degos-like lesions associated with systemic lupus erythematosus. *Ann Dermatol.* 2017;29(2):215.

242. Karaoğlu P, Topçu Y, Bayram E, et al. Severe neurologic involvement of Degos disease in a pediatric patient. *J Child Neurol.* 2013;29(4):550-554.

243. Ahmadi M. A fatal case of Degos' disease which presented with recurrent intestinal perforation. *World J Gastrointest Surg.* 2011;3(10):156.

244. Wilson J, Walling HW, Stone MS. Benign cutaneous Degos disease in a 16-year-old girl. *Pediatr Dermatol.* 2007;24(1):18-24.

245. Zouboulis CC, Theodoridis A, Brunner M, Magro CM. Benign atrophic papulosis (Kohlmeier-Degos disease): the wedge-shaped dermal necrosis can resolve with time. *J Eur Acad Dermatol Venereol.* 2017;31(10):1753-1756.

246. Magro CM, Poe JC, Kim C, et al. Degos disease: a C5b-9/interferon-alpha-mediated endotheliopathy syndrome. *Am J Clin Pathol.* 2011;135(4):599-610.

247. Ball E, Newburger A, Ackerman AB. Degos' disease: a distinctive pattern of disease, chiefly of lupus erythematosus, and not a specific disease per se. *Am J Dermatopathol.* 2003;25(4):308-320.

248. Chave TA, Varma S, Patel GK, Knight AG. Malignant atrophic papulosis (Degos' disease): clinicopathological correlations. *J Eur Acad Dermatol Venereol.* 2001;15(1):43-45.

7

Genetic Disorders of Epidermal Maturation and Cornification

Jennifer A. Day / Adnan Mir

ICHTHYOSIS

Definition and Epidemiology

The ichthyoses are a large, heterogeneous group of heritable disorders characterized by abnormal epidermal differentiation and resulting in generalized scaling of the skin. They range from mild to severe and may occur in isolation or as a part of a broader syndrome. The nonsyndromic ichthyoses will be discussed in this chapter. These include ichthyosis vulgaris, X-linked recessive ichthyosis, the autosomal recessive congenital ichthyoses (ARCI, including lamellar ichthyosis, congenital ichthyosiform erythroderma, and Harlequin ichthyosis), and epidermolytic ichthyosis. The ichthyoses, the most common of which is ichthyosis vulgaris, are highly variable in incidence.

Etiology and Clinical Presentation

Table 7-1 highlights the genetic defects and clinical features of several common and uncommon ichthyoses. In general, the genetic defects in ARCI result in abnormal lipid metabolism, which in turn results in abnormalities of cornification. Ichthyosis vulgaris is caused by mutation in *profilaggrin*, which also results in abnormal formation of the stratum corneum. The epidermolytic ichthyosis is caused by mutations in *keratins 1* and *10*, leading to epidermolysis and superficial blister formation early in life.[1]

Several of these disorders present at birth with a collodion membrane—a taut, shiny membrane covering the infant's entire body, derived from thickened stratum corneum. The tightness results in eclabium, ectropion, and in severe cases, restrictive pulmonary dysfunction. The membrane is shed over the first weeks of life, eventually revealing the life-long phenotype.

Histologic Findings

Histopathologic changes are often subtle in ichthyotic conditions, except in certain disorders with characteristic findings (Table 7-2).[8] Isolated hypogranulosis is suggestive of ichthyosis vulgaris, and epidermolytic hyperkeratosis is diagnostic of epidermolytic ichthyosis in the correct clinical context. This change can be seen in epidermal nevi that are caused by somatic mutations in *KRT-1* and *KRT-10*. In general, a definitive diagnosis of the ichthyoses relies on molecular testing with multigene panels to determine a causative genetic mutation.

Collodion membranes, a shared finding in several ichthyotic disorders, demonstrate histologic findings of compact orthokeratotic hyperkeratosis of the stratum corneum.[22]

Differential Diagnosis

There is broad overlap in the clinical and histopathologic findings of the ichthyoses. They can be distinguished by the character and distribution of scale, as well as genetic evaluation. Orthokeratotic hyperkeratosis with a diminished granular layer is characteristic of ichthyosis vulgaris, but can also be seen in the syndromic ichthyoses Refsum syndrome, trichothiodystrophy, and Conradi-Hünermann–Happle Syndrome. Epidermolytic hyperkeratosis, present in epidermolytic ichthyoses, can also be found in epidermal nevi, ichthyosis bullosa of Siemens, or as an incidental finding.

223

TABLE 7-1. Selected nonsyndromic ichthyoses

Diagnosis	Epidemiology	Etiology	Clinical Presentation
Ichthyosis vulgaris[2-7] (Figure 7-1)	1:100-1:250	Autosomal semidominant mutation in *profilaggrin*, resulting in the abnormal development of the cornified cell envelope	**Cutaneous Manifestations:** Fine, white scales on trunk and extremities; spares flexures; hyperlinear palms **Onset:** Develops in infancy or early childhood, rarely present at birth with severe mutation, tends to improve in adolescence/adulthood **Associations:** Atopic dermatitis and keratosis pilaris
X-linked recessive ichthyosis (steroid sulfatase deficiency)[4,8,9] (Figure 7-2)	1:2000-1:9500 males	X-linked recessive mutation in steroid sulfatase, resulting in the accumulation of cholesterol metabolites in the epidermis and subsequent inhibition of transglutaminase 1 (TGM1)	**Cutaneous Manifestation:** Large, brown scales accentuated at neck; relative sparing of flexures **Other Manifestations:** Asymptomatic corneal opacities, cryptorchidism, prolonged labor with affected fetuses due to insufficient cervical dilation **Associations:** Mental retardation, Kallman syndrome, and/or chondrodysplasia punctata
Epidermolytic ichthyosis[10,11] (Figure 7-3)	1:300 000	Usually autosomal dominant mutation in KRT1 or KRT10	**Cutaneous Manifestations:** *At birth:* Superficial blistering *Childhood/adulthood:* Progressive predominance of hyperkeratosis, classically described as corrugated, accentuated on flexure surfaces and over joints
ARCI—Lamellar ichthyosis[11-13]	1:300 000	Usually autosomal recessive Transglutaminase 1 (TGM1)	**Cutaneous Manifestations:** *At birth:* Collodion membrane *Childhood/adulthood:* Large, plate-like scales in generalized distribution; ectropion, alopecia, nail dystrophy
ARCI—Congenital ichthyosiform erythroderma[11,14-17] (Figures 7-4 and 7-5)	1:300 000	Autosomal recessive mutation in several genes: TGM1 CYP4F22 ALOXE3 PNPLA1 ALOX12B LIPM NIPAL4 CerS3 ABCA12	**Cutaneous Manifestations:** *At birth:* Collodion membrane *Childhood/adulthood:* Fine white scaling overlying generalized erythema, ectropion, alopecia **Other Manifestations:** Neurologic abnormalities
ARCI—Harlequin ichthyosis18-21 (Figure 7-6)	Rare	Autosomal recessive mutation ABCA12 (B61)—truncating mutations or deletions (B62)	**Cutaneous Manifestations:** *At birth:* Harlequin fetus—thick, yellow/brown plates of scale interspersed with large, deep, bright red fissures; ectropion; eclabium; ear abnormalities; prematurity common *Childhood/adulthood:* CIE (congenital ichthyosiform erythroderma)-like presentation Mortality in the neonatal period is high, typically because of sepsis or respiratory failure

Abbreviations: ABCA12, ABC lipid transporter; ARCI, autosomal recessive congenital ichthyosis; FLG, profillagrin; KRT1/10, keratins 1/10; STS, steroid sulfatase; TGM1, transglutaminase 1.

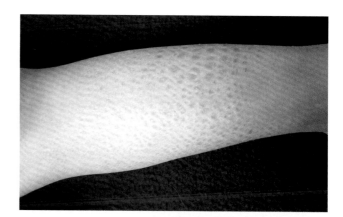

FIGURE 7-1. A child with ichthyosis vulgaris. The lower leg shows dry, polygonal, hyperpigmented scaling.

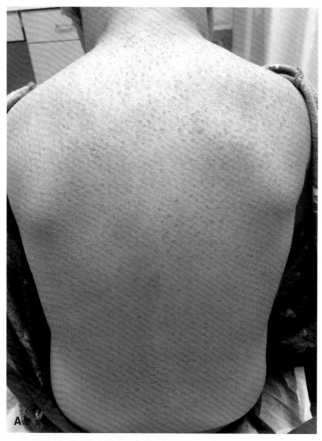

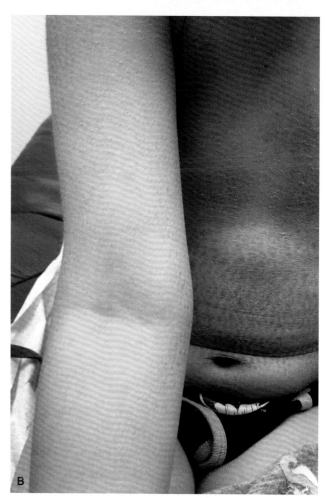

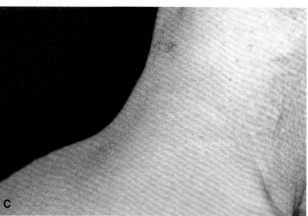

FIGURE 7-2. X-linked recessive ichthyosis with characteristic hyperpigmented scale on the back extending onto the neck (**A** and **B**) and conspicuous sparing of the antecubital fossa (**C**).

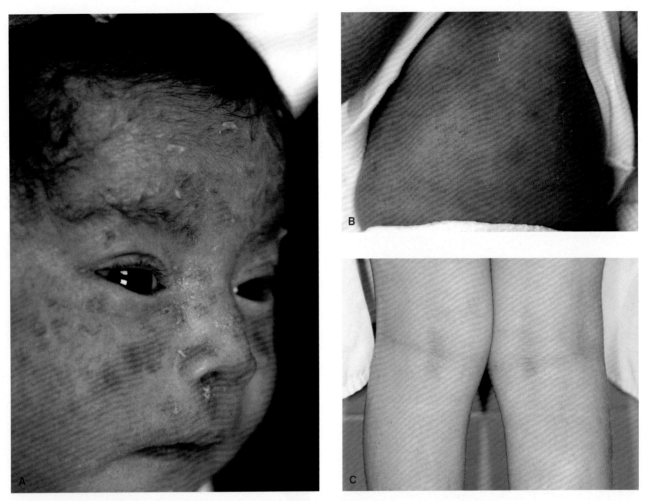

FIGURE 7-3. Epidermolytic ichthyosis. A baby showing blisters in the face, nose (**A**), and trunk (**B**). Progressive corrugated hyperkeratosis is seen in olden children, in association with a pattern of accentuation in flexural sites (**C**).

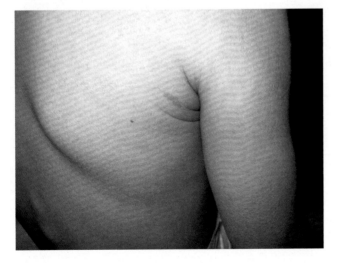

FIGURE 7-4. Autosomal recessive congenital ichthyosis with a congenital ichthyosiform erythroderma phenotype, showing fine, diffuse scale with mild underlying erythema.

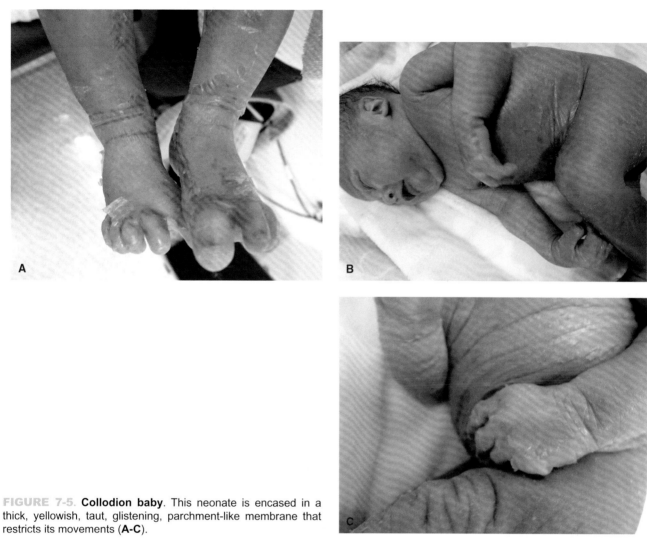

FIGURE 7-5. **Collodion baby**. This neonate is encased in a thick, yellowish, taut, glistening, parchment-like membrane that restricts its movements (**A-C**).

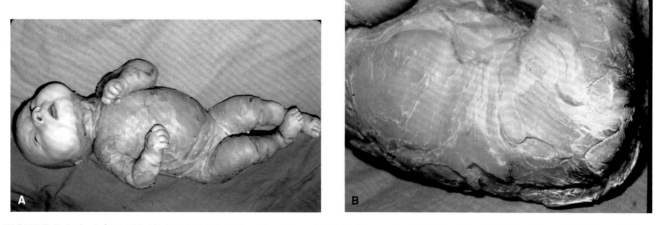

FIGURE 7-6. An infant with Harlequin ichthyosis with extremely thick, fissured scaled skin (**A** and **B**). Courtesy of Dr Kenneth Greer. Department of Dermatology. University of Virginia.

TABLE 7-2.	Histopathologic findings for selected nonsyndromic ichthyoses		
Diagnosis	**Histopathology**	**Electron Microscopy**	**Other**
Ichthyosis vulgaris[11,23-25] (Figure 7-7)	SC: Mild hyperorthokeratosis SG: ± Diminished	Absent or abnormal keratohyalin granules	Absent or diminished filaggrin staining by IHC
X-linked recessive ichthyosis (steroid sulfatase deficiency)[11,23,25,26] (Figure 7-8)	SC: Ortho- or parakeratosis; melanosomes and desmosomes retained SG: Normal or thickened ± Acanthosis Hyperkeratosis of follicular and sweat duct orifices	Increased size and number of keratohyalin granules	
Epidermolytic ichthyosis[11,27,28] (Figure 7-9)	Epidermolytic hyperkeratosis: SC: thick hyperorthokeratosis SG: hypergranulosis Acantholysis of suprabasal layers, leading to intraepidermal blisters Mild perivascular lymphohistiocytic infiltrate Clumped keratin intermediate filaments can be seen in keratinocytes	Clumped, fragmented keratin intermediate filaments in lower epidermis	Epidermolytic hyperkeratosis can also be seen in epidermolytic acanthomas (solitary papule) and epidermal nevi
ARCI— Congenital ichthyosiform erythroderma[11,27,29]	SC: Parakeratosis SG: Thickened Acanthosis	Increased number of lamellar bodies Variable translucent lipid droplets in SC Disorganized intercellular lamellae	Markedly increased epidermal proliferation
ARCI—Lamellar ichthyosis[11,23,27,29,30] (Figure 7-10)	SC: Massive hyperorthokeratosis, Acanthosis (can be psoriasiform or papillomatous)	Elongated cholesterol clefts Variable translucent lipid droplets in SC Thin or absent cornified envelope	Epidermal proliferation rate normal or mildly elevated. Diminished staining of transglutaminase-1 on IHC Diminished transglutaminase-1 activity in cultured keratinocytes Other transglutaminase assays, not widely available.
ARCI—Harlequin ichthyosis[31]	SC: Massive hyperorthokeratosis ± parakeratosis Hyperkeratotic plugging of follicles and sweat ducts Hair follicles: concentric accumulation of hyperkeratotic material around hair shaft	Absent or abnormal lamellar bodies in SG Absent extracellular lipid lamellae Variable translucent lipid droplets in SC	

Abbreviations: ARCI, autosomal recessive congenital ichthyosis; IHC, immunohistochemistry; SC, stratum corneum; SG, stratum granulosum.

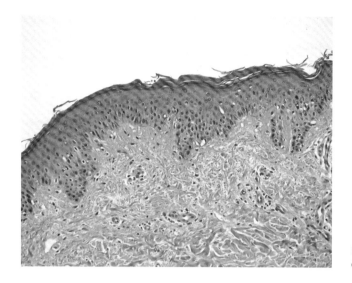

FIGURE 7-7. Ichthyosis vulgaris. Compact orthokeratosis and a diminished granular layer.

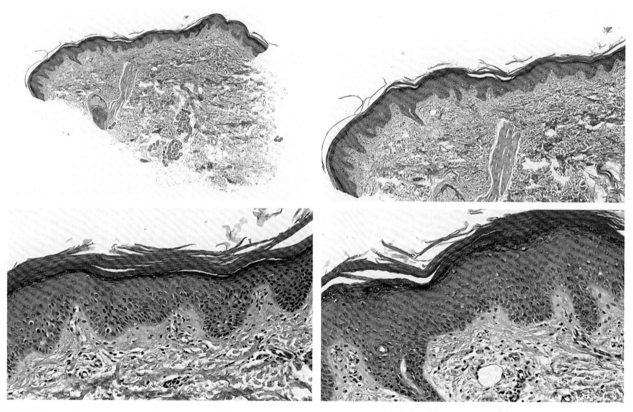

FIGURE 7-8. X-linked recessive ichthyosis. Mild epidermal acanthosis and hyperorthokeratosis. The granular cell layer is preserved (as opposed to ichthyosis vulgaris). There is mild hyperkeratosis around the sweat gland orifices. Digital slides courtesy of Path Presenter.com.

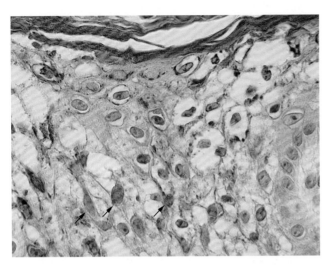

FIGURE 7-9. Epidermolytic hyperkeratosis with cytolysis of keratinocytes in the upper spinous layer and eosinophilic inclusions. Reprinted with permission from Bergman R, Khamaysi Z, Sprecher E. A Unique pattern of dyskeratosis characterizes epidermolytic hyperkeratosis and epidermolytic palmoplantar keratoderma. *Am J Dermatopathol.* 2008;30(2):101-105.

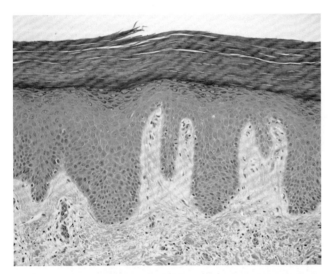

FIGURE 7-10. **Lamellar ichthyosis.** Thick hyperkeratosis with acanthosis and mild hypergranulosis.

CAPSULE SUMMARY

ICHTHYOSIS

Ichthyoses are a diverse group of heritable disorders characterized by a generalized scaling of the skin. They are caused by mutations in a heterogeneous group of genes, eventually resulting in an abnormal formation or a thickening of the stratum corneum. Histopathologic analysis can be subtle and may include orthohyperkeratosis and a variably diminished granular layer.

NETHERTON SYNDROME

Definition and Epidemiology

Netherton syndrome (NS) is an autosomal recessive inherited disorder featuring congenital ichthyosiform erythroderma, characteristic hair abnormalities, severe atopic diathesis, and immune dysregulation. NS is thought to affect approximately 1:50 000 to 1:200 000 patients worldwide.[32-34]

Etiology

NS is caused by a mutation in the serine protease inhibitor Kazal type 5 (*SPINK5*) that encodes the protein lymphoepithelial Kazal-type-related inhibitor (LEKTI).[33,34] LEKTI is primarily expressed in epidermal lamellar granules as well as lymphoid tissue. The causative mutation results in an overactivity of serine proteases, leading to disrupted regulation of lipid-processing enzymes and abnormal stratum corneum lipid envelope.[35,36] Additionally, there is an enhanced degradation of desmoglein 1, contributing to impaired cellular cohesion in the stratum corneum.[37,38]

Clinical Presentation

Patients present at birth with congenital erythroderma and skin peeling.[39] Within the neonatal period, potential complications include abnormal temperature regulation, electrolyte abnormalities, pneumonia, and sepsis.[34,40,41] In childhood, patients tend to develop one of two phenotypes: ichthyosis linearis circumflexa (Figure 7-11) or congenital ichthyosiform erythroderma-like scale (Figure 7-12). The former is more common, characterized by migratory, circinate, scaly, erythematous plaques with a border of double-edged scale.[42] In both presentations, pruritus and eczematous plaques are ubiquitous. Hair findings include trichorrhexis invaginata (Figure 7-13), giving the phenotype of dry, fragile, and poorly manageable hair.[43] The distribution of affected hair within an individual is variable, but is often concentrated on lateral eyebrows. Thick, adherent scalp scale can also be seen.

Immune manifestations include severely elevated immunoglobulin E ([IgE] up to 10 000 IU/mL), impaired B- and NK-cell function, reduced response to vaccination, and increased levels of proinflammatory cytokines.[44] Patients experience recurrent infections, particularly involving the respiratory tract and skin. The common microbes involved in skin infections include *Staphylococcus aureus* and human papillomavirus,[45] the latter of which can predispose patients to squamous cell carcinoma.[46] Food and environmental allergies are common.

Histologic Findings

The biopsy specimens of ichthyosis linearis circumflexa show hyperkeratosis, a normal granular cell layer, and

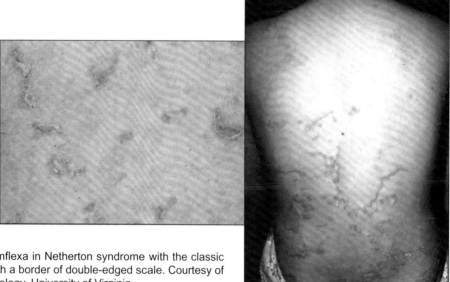

FIGURE 7-11. Ichthyosis linearis circumflexa in Netherton syndrome with the classic circinate, scaly, erythematous plaques with a border of double-edged scale. Courtesy of Dr Kenneth Greer. Department of Dermatology. University of Virginia.

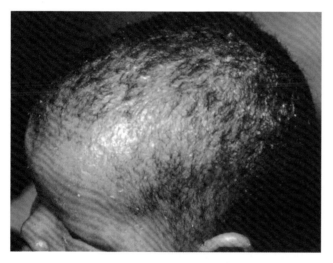

FIGURE 7-12. **Congenital ichthyosiform erythroderma-like scale in Netherton syndrome**. Diffuse scalp erythema and mild thin scaling is present. Courtesy of Dr Kenneth Greer. Department of Dermatology. University of Virginia.

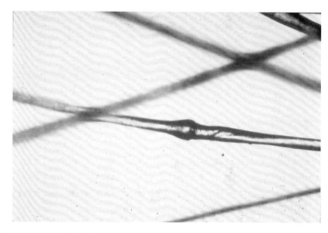

FIGURE 7-13. Trichorrhexis invaginata (Bamboo hair), typical of Netherton syndrome. Courtesy of Dr Kenneth Greer. Department of Dermatology. University of Virginia.

acanthosis. Focal parakeratosis, hypogranulosis, and exocytosis of neutrophils are variably present (Figure 7-14).[47-49] In erythrodermic cases, parakeratosis can be confluent. A perivascular lymphohistiocytic infiltrate may be present in the superficial dermis.[50] Periodic acid–Schiff staining demonstrates densely staining granules in upper epidermal layers.[8] A microscopic evaluation of affected hair shafts reveals trichorrhexis invaginata, with a telescoping of the distal hair shaft into the proximal shaft.[43] Other hair shaft findings, such as trichorrhexis nodosa, pili torti, and "matchstick" abnormality, can also be seen.

The electron microscopic findings of premature secretion of lamellar bodies within the epidermis, electron-dense accumulations between corneocytes, and atypical splitting within the stratum corneum are fairly specific for NS.[49]

Differential Diagnosis

The clinical differential diagnosis of erythroderma in a neonate includes congenital ichthyosiform erythroderma, psoriasis, peeling skin syndrome, or another primary immunodeficiency. Features favoring NS include elevated serum IgE and characteristic trichorrhexis invaginata, although this often does not develop until after infancy. Immunodeficiency syndromes that may present with erythematous, eczematous eruption and high-serum IgE include autosomal dominant hyper IgE-syndrome, Wiskott Aldrich syndrome, Omenn syndrome, and IPEX (immune dysregulation, polyendocrinopathy, enteropathy, X-linked) syndrome. The main histopathologic differential diagnosis of ichthyosis linearis circumflexa is psoriasis, which may appear virtually identical. Differentiation is based on clinical history and physical findings. Additional considerations include other

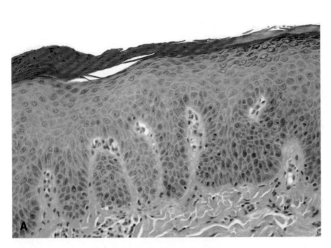 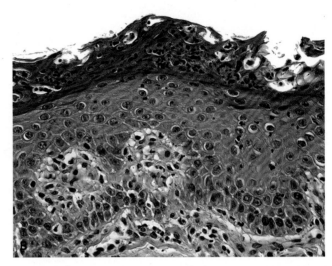

FIGURE 7-14. Skin biopsies from Netherton syndrome show psoriasiform hyperplasia and may have overlying parakeratosis (**A**) and neutrophils within the epidermis and stratum corneum (**B**). Differentiation from psoriasis must be made on a clinical basis. Reprinted with permission from Leclerc-Mercier S, Bodemer C, Furio L, et al. Skin biopsy in Netherton syndrome: a histological review of a large series and new findings. *Am J Dermatopathol.* 2016;38(2):83-91.

syndromic and nonsyndromic ichthyoses, eczematous dermatitis, and dermatophytosis.

CAPSULE SUMMARY

NETHERTON SYNDROME

This syndrome is an inherited disorder due to autosomal dominant mutation in *SPINK5*. It is characterized by ichthyosis, hair abnormalities, severe eczematous dermatitis, and immune deficiency. Patients present with neonatal erythroderma and subsequently develop either ichthyosis linearis circumflexa or an ichthyosiform erythroderma-like chronic dermatosis. The hallmark microscopic finding is trichorrhexis invaginata. Ichthyosis linearis circumflexa features parakeratosis and hypogranulosis and must be distinguished from psoriasis on the basis of history and clinical findings.

REFSUM DISEASE

Definition and Epidemiology

Refsum disease (RD) is an autosomal recessive inherited disorder caused by mutations in peroxisomal metabolism, leading to deficient oxidation of phytanic acid. Patients present with ichthyosis and progressive neurologic dysfunction. RD is rare, with fewer than 100 cases reported in the literature.[51]

Etiology

Causative mutations have been identified in phytanoyl-CoA hydroxylase (*PHYH*, Type 1) and peroxisomal targeting signal 2 receptor (*PEX7*, Type 2).[52] Both genes are involved in the function of peroxisomes, and abnormalities lead to the inability to oxidize phytanic acid, resulting in aberrantly elevated serum levels.[53] Phytanic acid, a branched, long-chain fatty acid, is derived from chlorophyll; thus, circulating levels in humans are delivered via dietary intake.[54] Abnormally high levels interfere with cholesterol metabolism, leading to deficiencies in essential fatty acids, which in turn results in ichthyosis.

Clinical Presentation

Cutaneous findings include fine, white scaling on the trunk and extremities and hyperlinear palmoplantar markings, similar to those seen in ichthyosis vulgaris.[53,54] This generally begins with or after neurologic symptoms.

The onset of neurologic abnormalities is typically in late childhood or adolescence. Prominent features include sensorineural deafness, anosmia, visual disturbance (reduced visual acuity and night blindness due to retinitis pigmentosa, with classic "salt and pepper" retinal pigmentation), and sensorimotor neuropathy leading to weakness and poor balance.[51,53,54] Neurologic findings are typically insidious in onset and slowly progressive. Reduction in the dietary intake of sources of phytanic acid (green vegetables, dairy) may delay the progression of neurologic abnormalities. Additional manifestations developing over time include cataracts, renal tubular dysfunction, and cardiomyopathy.[54,55]

CAPSULE SUMMARY

REFSUM DISEASE

RD is a rare, autosomal recessive disorder of abnormal peroxisomal metabolism of phytanic acid, leading to progressive neurologic abnormalities and mild ichthyosis. Symptoms and progression are mitigated by a diet low in phytols. Skin biopsy specimens show hyperorthokeratosis and a diminished granular layer and can be differentiated from ichthyosis vulgaris by the presence of lipid accumulation on electron microscopy and by clinical history.

Histologic Findings

Skin biopsy specimens from patients with RD may show mild hyperorthokeratosis and a diminished granular layer. The accumulation of lipid droplets can be appreciated in specimens fixed in alcohol with lipid stains such as Sudan black or ultrastructural analysis with electron microscopy.[55]

Differential Diagnosis

The clinical differential diagnosis of the cutaneous manifestations of RD includes ichthyosis vulgaris and vitamin B deficiency. Mild ichthyosis in association with hearing loss can be seen in other peroxisomal deficiency disorders as well as neutral lipid storage disease. Prominent neurologic abnormalities are also seen in Sjögren–Larsson syndrome (SLS). The cutaneous histopathologic changes in RD are virtually identical to those seen in ichthyosis vulgaris. However, the accumulation of epidermal lipid is absent, and these patients lack neurologic symptoms.

SJÖGREN-LARSSON SYNDROME

Definition and Epidemiology

SLS is an autosomal recessive inherited disorder characterized by ichthyosis, progressive di- or tetraplegia, and intellectual disability. It is caused by mutation in the fatty aldehyde dehydrogenase *ALDH3A2*. SLS has an incidence of fewer than 1 in 100 000, with highest incidence in Sweden.[56] It has been reported worldwide.

Etiology

Mutations in *ALDH3A2*, encoding fatty aldehyde dehydrogenase (FALDH), lead to a reduced oxidation of long-chain fatty acids. FALDH is normally involved in the recycling of cell membrane components, including ceramides in the epidermis and sphingolipids in the brain.[57] Chronic pruritus is attributed to the accumulation of high levels of leukotriene B4.

Clinical Presentation

SLS presents at birth with variable degrees of erythema, scaling, and hyperkeratosis (Figure 7-15).[58] Later, erythema fades and gives way to fine to plate-like scaling or nonscaling

hyperkeratosis, predominantly on abdomen, neck, and flexures.[58-60] The face tends to be spared. There is associated pruritus, accounting for commonly seen lichenification. Approximately 70% of affected patients have palmoplantar keratoderma.[59,60] Hair and nails are normal.

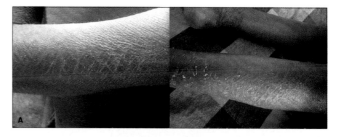

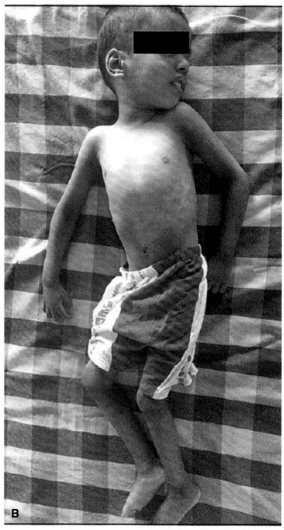

FIGURE 7-15. **Marked ichthyosis in a patient with Sjögren–Larsson syndrome. A,** Brown color diamond-shaped adherent scales on the upper limb and peeling of skin on the lower limb. **B,** Kyphoscoliosis of the trunk is present. Obtained with permission from Subramanian V, Hariharan P, Balaji J. Sjögren-Larsson syndrome: a rare neurocutaneous disorder. *J Pediatr Neurosci.* 2016;11(1):68-70, Figure 1 and 2.

Neurologic complications typically manifest by 1 year of age. Characteristic findings include delayed motor development, ultimately leading to gradually progressive spastic di- and tetraplegia, spasticity, and contractures.[56,59] The other findings include intellectual disability, white matter abnormalities, and seizures.[56,59,60]

Ocular findings include perifoveal glistening white dots, a nearly pathognomonic feature. Photophobia is a common symptom.

Histologic Findings

The histologic features of SLS include hyperorthokeratosis with scattered parakeratosis, a mildly papillated surface, and variable changes in the granular layer. Ultrastructural analysis reveals lamellar inclusions in the upper layers of the epidermis.[61]

Differential Diagnosis

The clinical differential diagnosis of SLS includes X-linked recessive ichthyosis, severe ichthyosis vulgaris, or mild ARCI. Similar cutaneous and neurologic findings have been described in a large kindred identified to have mutations in elongase-4 (*EVOVL4*).[62]

Histologically, SLS can be differentiated from other ichthyoses by the presence of focal parakeratosis, papillomatosis, and occasionally a thickened granular layer.

CAPSULE SUMMARY

SJÖGREN–LARSSON SYNDROME

SLS is an autosomal recessive disorder caused by mutation in *ALDH3A2/FALDH*, leading to ichthyosis and neurologic abnormalities, including spastic paraplegia and intellectual disability. Histologically, the skin is characterized by papillomatosis, hyperkeratosis, focal parakeratosis, and occasional hypergranulosis.

MEDNIK SYNDROME

Definition and Epidemiology

MEDNIK syndrome (Erythrokeratodermia Variabilis 3) is an autosomal recessive disorder with a constellation of symptoms including *M*ental retardation, *E*nteropathy, *D*eafness, *N*europathy, *I*chthyosis, and *K*eratoderma. It is caused by mutation in adapter protein complex subunit a1 (*AP1S1*).[63,64]

MEDNIK syndrome is rare—the majority of reported cases are individuals sharing common ancestors in Canada.

Etiology

AP1S1 encodes adapter protein complex subunit 1a, which is involved in vesicular trafficking during skin and spinal cord development.[63]

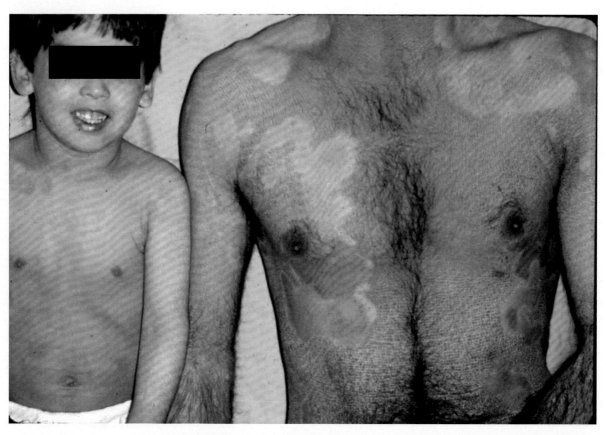

FIGURE 7-16. **Father and son with erythrokeratoderma variabilis.** Multiple circinated patches and plaques with erythema, hyperkeratosis, variable pigmentation, and hair distribution. Courtesy of Dr Kenneth Greer. Department of Dermatology. University of Virginia.

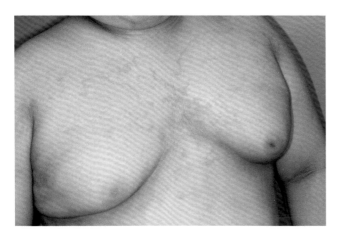

FIGURE 7-17. Erythrokeratoderma variabilis. Slightly erythematous patches in the trunk.

Clinical Presentation

Infants present at birth or within the first few weeks of life. Cutaneous manifestations include erythematous patches and hyperkeratotic plaques of variable size (Figures 7-16 and 7-17).[65] Mucosal and nail involvement are common. The other findings include sensorineural deafness, delayed psychomotor development, growth retardation, and peripheral neuropathy.[63] A chronic and life-threatening complication is severe congenital diarrhea.[1]

Histologic Findings

The histologic changes in MEDNIK syndrome have not specifically been described. In general, the erythrokeratodermas have nonspecific findings including hyperkeratosis, gentle papillomatosis, and focal parakeratosis.

Differential Diagnosis

The other forms of erythrokeratoderma variabilis should be considered. These are relatively rare disorders caused by mutations in gap junction genes *GJA1, GJB3,* or *GJB4.*

CAPSULE SUMMARY

MEDNIK SYNDROME

MEDNIK syndrome is a rare, autosomal recessive disorder resulting in an erythrokeratoderma-type phenotype, caused by mutation in *AP1S1.*

ARTHROGRYPOSIS–RENAL DYSFUNCTION–CHOLESTASIS SYNDROME

Definition

*A*rthrogryposis–*r*enal dysfunction–*c*holestasis (ARC) syndrome is a multisystem, life-threatening, autosomal recessive disorder arising from mutations in *VPS33B* or *VIPAR*.[66]

Only scattered cases have been reported from Europe and Asia, with most reports from Saudi Arabia and Pakistan.[67]

Etiology

Vacuolar protein sorting 33 homolog B (VPS33B) regulates SNARE protein-mediated fusion of membrane vesicles.[66] VPS33B-interacting protein, apical-basolateral polarity regulatory (VIPAR) is a protein that complexes with VPS33B and is involved in orienting cells to apical-basolateral polarity. The pathogenic role in ichthyosis is related to altered lamellar body secretion.[66,67]

Clinical Presentation

Cutaneous findings, seen in about 50% of affected patients, are evident within the first few days or weeks of life. Infants develop generalized scaling on trunk, extremities. There is relative sparing of skin folds (Figure 7-18).[66,68,69]

Affected infants present with arthrogryposis (congenital joint contracture) and develop renal tubular acidosis as well as cholestasis because of intrahepatic bile duct hypoplasia. Aminoaciduria can be seen. The hallmark neuromuscular findings are arthrogryposis or severe congenital contractures. The other findings include failure to thrive, sensorineural hearing loss, central nervous system anomalies, congenital heart defects, and platelet abnormalities leading to hemorrhage. Mortality tends to occur within the first year of life, although attenuated phenotypes with longer life expectancy have also been described.

Histologic Findings and Differential Diagnosis

Although the cutaneous findings of ARC syndrome are classified as ichthyosiform, no specific histologic findings have been reported.

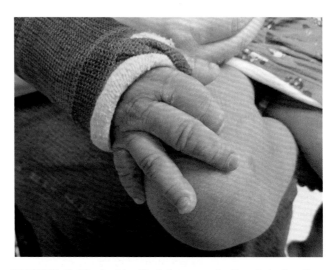

FIGURE 7-18. A girl with Arthrogryposis–Renal dysfunction–Cholestasis syndrome, with generalized ichthyosis and flexion contractures of multiple joints, including the knees. Courtesy of Dr. Nnenna Agim. Department of Dermatology. University of Texas Southwestern Medical Center.

Arthrogryposis is a congenital feature with a broad differential diagnosis ranging from genetic syndromes to intrauterine growth restriction or maternal exposures.[70] ARC syndrome may be differentiated on the basis of the presence of cholestasis and ichthyosis.

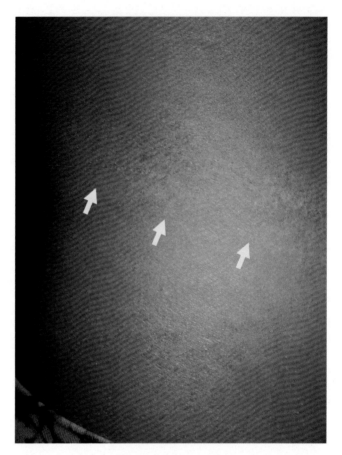

FIGURE 7-19. Conradi-Hunermann-Happle syndrome, showing generalized fine scaling and larger scales in a Blaschkolinear pattern (arrows). Courtesy of Dr. Nnenna Agim. Department of Dermatology. University of Texas Southwestern Medical Center.

CAPSULE SUMMARY

ARTHROGRYPOSIS–RENAL DYSFUNCTION–CHOLESTASIS SYNDROME

ARC syndrome is a multisystem, life-threatening, autosomal recessive disorder due to mutations in vesicular trafficking proteins. Patients may develop ichthyosis.

CONRADI-HÜNERMANN-HAPPLE SYNDROME

Definition and Epidemiology

Conradi-Hünermann-Happle syndrome (CHHS, chondrodysplasia punctata type 2) is a rare, X-linked dominant disorder caused by mutations in emopamil-binding protein (EBP), with characteristic ichthyosiform dermatosis, skeletal abnormalities, and cataracts. CHHS is almost exclusively seen in female patients because of its X-linked dominant inheritance, as the typical mutations are lethal in male fetuses.[71] When present in males, it is usually the result of postzygotic somatic mutation.

Etiology

EBP is a ubiquitously expressed integral membrane protein with Δ8-Δ7-sterol isomerase activity. Mutations cause the accumulation of abnormal sterols in tissue and plasma.[72]

Clinical Presentation

Affected infants present at birth with erythroderma and overlying feathery, adherent scale along Blaschko's likes (Figures 7-19 and 7-20). This ichthyosiform erythroderma resolves over time and older children develop linear plaques of follicular atrophoderma in the same distribution. Affected plaques demonstrate patulous follicular openings, ice-pick-like scarring, and scaling. Additional cutaneous findings include linear dyspigmentation, patchy scarring alopecia, course hair, and onychoschizia.[71]

The characteristic skeletal finding is chondrodysplasia punctata, or epiphyseal stippling seen on radiographs, during infancy. Stippling represents premature calcification of long bones, tracheal cartilage, and vertebrae.[73] Premature calcification results in a rhizomelic shortening of limbs, in which the proximal bones are disproportionately shorter than the distal bones. Additional bony findings include frontal bossing, malar hypoplasia, and a flat nasal bridge.

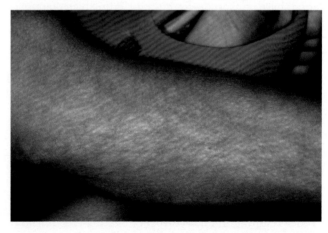

FIGURE 7-20. Conradi-Hunermann-Happle syndrome. Linear plaques of follicular atrophoderma.

Affected patients may develop unilateral cataracts within the first several months of life, which may be associated with microphthalmia or microcornea.[71] The other associations include congenital heart defects, sensorineural hearing loss, central nervous system anomalies, and congenital renal abnormalities. Life expectancy is normal.

Histologic Findings

Biopsy specimens from ichthyotic plaques in patients with CHHS display dilated follicular ostia, hyperorthokeratosis, and occasional hypergranulosis. Early lesions show calcification within corneocytes, which can be demonstrated by Von Kossa staining.[74,75]

Differential Diagnosis

Epiphyseal stippling may be seen in congenital hemidysplasia with ichthyosiform erythroderma and limb defects syndrome, which is differentiated by the unilateral involvement of radiologic stippling and ichthyotic plaques. The Blaschkoid distribution of follicular atrophoderma in CHHS is distinguished from pigmentary mosaicism, incontinentia pigmenti, and epidermal nevi by the characteristic features of dilated follicular openings and scarring.

As with many syndromic ichthyoses, there is significant histologic overlap with ichthyosis vulgaris. CHHS may be differentiated by epidermal calcification, which is highlighted by Von Kossa staining.

CAPSULE SUMMARY

CONRADI-HÜNERMANN-HAPPLE SYNDROME

CHHS is a rare, X-linked dominant disorder caused by mutations in *EBP*. Affected patients are born with feathery, hyperkeratotic linear and whorled plaques with underlying erythroderma. Childhood cutaneous involvement includes follicular atrophoderma along Blaschko's lines. Characteristic skeletal findings include chondrodysplasia punctata and shortened bones in the proximal limbs. Skin biopsies show hyperorthokeratosis, hypogranulosis, dilated follicular ostia, and the deposition of calcium within the epidermis.

CHILD SYNDROME

Definition and Epidemiology

CHILD syndrome is an X-linked dominant disorder characterized by Congenital Hemidysplasia, Ichthyosiform erythroderma, and Limb Defects; caused by mutation in the *NSDHL* gene (NAD[P]H steroid dehydrogenase-like protein). Fewer than 100 cases have been reported worldwide. The majority of cases occur in female patients, as this mutation is typically lethal in male fetuses.[76,77]

Etiology

The NSDHL protein is located on the membranes of endoplasmic reticulum and lipid-containing organelles. Mutations lead to dysfunction in the cholesterol biosynthetic pathway. This in turn leads to embryologic signaling defects and the clinical findings discussed in the next section.[78]

Clinical Presentation

Affected patients present at or soon after birth with striking unilateral musculoskeletal, cutaneous, and visceral abnormalities. Cutaneous manifestations include thick, scaly, erythematous plaques that are Blaschkoid to nearly confluent in nature, and are unilateral with a sharp midline demarcation (Figure 7-21)[76,79]. As patients age, hyperkeratosis predominates over erythema. The face is spared, and findings are often accentuated within body folds and on the vulva. Patients may also have unilateral alopecia and onychorrhexis of the affected side.

Ipsilateral limb abnormalities are present at birth. These include unilateral mandibular hypoplasia, pelvic

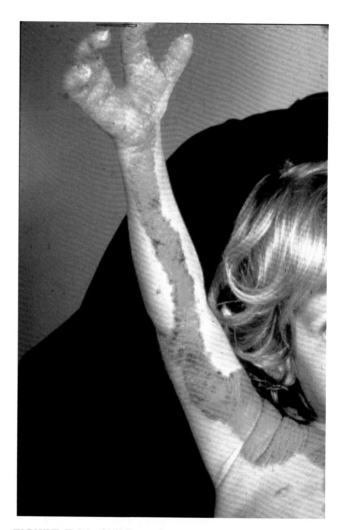

FIGURE 7-21. CHILD syndrome. Thick, scaly, erythematous plaques that are Blaschkoid to nearly confluent in nature are present and are unilateral with a sharp midline demarcation. CHILD, Congenital Hemidysplasia with Ichthyosiform erythroderma and Limb Defects. Courtesy of Dr Kenneth Greer. Department of Dermatology. University of Virginia.

hypoplasia, hypomelia, joint contractures, and epiphyseal stippling. Internal abnormalities are also frequent, including unilateral brain, lung, renal, and endocrine gland hypoplasia; as well as cardiovascular defects. Sensorineural hearing loss and mild intellectual impairment are also seen.

Histologic Findings

The CHILD nevus is characterized by verrucous epidermal hyperplasia with hyperkeratosis and focal parakeratosis. Neutrophils are often present within the zones of parakeratosis. A characteristic feature is the presence of foamy histiocytes within the dermal papillae, as are seen in verruciform xanthomas.[80]

Differential Diagnosis

The clinical findings in CHILD syndrome leave little doubt as to the diagnosis, but cases have been reported with mild skin findings, or absent limb findings. The histologic features of the CHILD nevus show significant overlap with psoriasis and inflammatory verrucous epidermal nevus (ILVEN), but can often be distinguished by the presence of foamy histiocytes in the dermal papillae. This change can be seen on any affected area. Nonsyndromic verruciform xanthomas are typically perioral or genital in origin.

CAPSULE SUMMARY

CHILD SYNDROME

CHILD syndrome (Congenital *Hemidysplasia, Ichthyosiform erythroderma, and Limb Defects*) presents with a striking constellation of unilateral features including a thick, scaly, erythematous, plaque with a midline demarcation, shortened limbs, and visceral hypoplasia. It is inherited in an X-linked dominant manner, and almost always seen in girls. The histology of skin lesions shows verrucous hyperkeratosis with focal parakeratosis, and foamy histiocytes within the dermal papillae.

DARIER DISEASE

Definition and Epidemiology

Darier disease (keratosis follicularis) is a rare genetic disorder of epidermal maturation and adhesion that presents with an eruption of erythematous to brown papules in a seborrheic distribution. It is caused by mutations in *ATP2A2*, which encodes the calcium pump SERCA2, which can be inherited in an autosomal dominant manner or occur sporadically.[81,82] European studies have found an incidence of 1 in 30 000 to 20 000.[83,84] Males and females are equally affected.

Etiology

SERCA2 is responsible for maintaining the cytosolic levels of Ca^{2+} by pumping ions into the endoplasmic reticulum. In vitro studies suggest that this results in the retention of desmosomal cadherins in the endoplasmic reticulum, which in

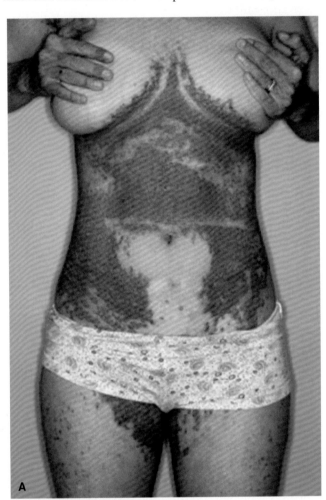

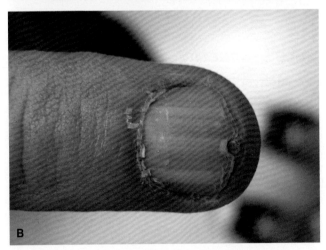

FIGURE 7-22. Darier disease with coalescing plaques of red-brown papules (**A**) and classic nail findings of longitudinal erythronychia and V-shaped nicking at the distal-free margin (**B**).

turn leads to a loss of keratinocyte adhesion and aberrant keratinization.[85] Abnormal cellular stress responses mediated by low ER levels of CA^{2+} lead to a reduced level of apoptosis, allowing the retention of dissociated keratinocytes.[86] Darier disease is caused by haploinsufficiency, with patients having one normal copy of the *ATP2A2* gene, and one mutant copy. Sun exposure has been shown to reduce the expression of normal SERCA2, resulting in ultraviolet (UV)-related exacerbation in sun-exposed areas.[87]

Clinical Presentation

Darier disease typically presents in the second decade of life, with pruritic, red-brown to yellowish papules on the scalp, forehead, alar creases, ears, and upper trunk. Mild axillary involvement is common, although there is a small subset of patients in which flexural disease predominates. Flexural involvement often results in vegetative lesions with maceration and superinfection that can lead to distressing malodor. Acral involvement is also common, with skin-colored, warty keratotic papules on the dorsa of the hands, punctate palmoplantar depressions, and the characteristic nail findings of red longitudinal bands and distal nail margin V-shaped nicking (Figure 7-22).

Segmental cases have been described, caused by postzygotic mutations.[88] Acrokeratosis Verruciformis of Hopf is often considered to be a forme fruste of Darier disease, and a specific *ATP2A2* mutation has been detected in affected patients.[89]

Histologic Findings

The primary histologic features of Darier disease include loss of keratinocyte adhesion (acantholysis) and abnormal keratinization (dyskeratosis). Acantholysis occurs in the suprabasilar layers of the epidermis and can result in intraepidermal vesicle formation. Dyskeratosis results in the formation of corps ronds (large, brightly eosinophilic cells with eccentric nuclei and pericellular halos) in the upper spinous and granular layers of the epidermis, and corps grains (oval cells with dark, cigar-shaped nuclei resembling grains of rice) in the granular layer which can extend into the corneum as well (Figure 7-23).[82] There are often overlying hyperkeratosis and parakeratosis which form a keratinous plug. Notably, the lesions of Darier disease are not folliculocentric, as the name keratosis follicularis implies.

Differential Diagnosis

The clinical differential diagnosis of Darier disease includes Hailey-Hailey disease (HHD), seborrheic dermatitis, and Grover disease (transient acantholytic dermatosis). HHD can be differentiated by predominance in flexural areas, but

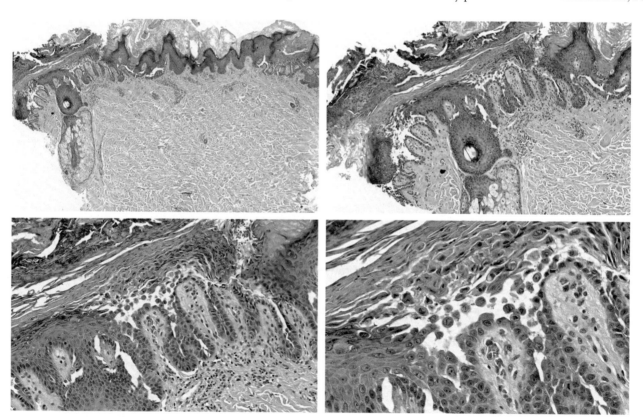

FIGURE 7-23. Darier disease. Suprabasilar acantholysis and dyskeratosis are present, with typical corps ronds (large, brightly eosinophilic cells with eccentric nuclei and pericellular halos) and corps grains (oval cells with dark, cigar-shaped nuclei resembling grains of rice). There is overlying hyperkeratosis. Digital slides courtesy of Path Presenter.com.

may require histopathologic confirmation. Grover Disease is a self-limited benign condition that favors the chest and upper back.

A significant histopathologic overlap exists between Darier and Grover diseases, but the latter tends to result in smaller, more localized lesions, and can be easily differentiated on a clinical basis. HHD lacks significant dyskeratosis. Warty dyskeratomas feature corps ronds and grains, but present as solitary lesions. Finally, pemphigus vulgaris (PV) presents with suprabasilar acantholysis, with the preservation of the basal layer along the dermoepidermal junction, which can also be seen in Darier disease. However, PV is an immunoblistering condition that lacks corps ronds and grains, has variable dermal inflammation that includes eosinophils, and can be differentiated by direct immunofluorescence studies.

CAPSULE SUMMARY

DARIER DISEASE (KERATOSIS FOLLICULARIS)

Darier disease is caused by an autosomal dominant mutation in the *SERCA2* calcium pump and is characterized by pruritic, erythematous to brown-yellow papules in a seborrheic distribution beginning during adolescence. Histopathologic findings include acantholysis and dyskeratosis with prominent corps ronds and corps grains and overlying hyperkeratosis.

HAILEY–HAILEY DISEASE

Definition and Epidemiology

HHD (familial benign chronic pemphigus) is an autosomal dominant genetic disorder of keratinocyte adhesion caused by mutations in *ATP2C1*, which encodes secretory pathway Ca^{2+}/Mn^{2+} ATPase (SPCA1).[90] Patients present with macerated plaques within intertriginous areas. Onset is typically during the 3rd and 4th decades of life, but symptoms may appear during the teenage years.

Although the true incidence of HHD has not been established, it appears to have a similar incidence to Darier disease. Males and females are equally affected, and although a family history is present in the majority of patients, sporadic cases are also common.[91]

Etiology

Like Darier disease, HHD appears to be caused by perturbations in intracellular calcium homeostasis and subsequent loss of intercellular adhesion. SPCA1 is expressed on the golgi membrane and is responsible for pumping Ca^{2+} and Mn^{2+} from the cytosol into the golgi apparatus. Although the exact mechanism of adhesion defects is not clear, it may

be caused by abnormalities in posttranslational desmosomal processing within the golgi.[92]

Clinical Presentation

Patients present in the 3rd and 4th decades of life with grouped flaccid vesicles and erosions forming erythematous, macerated plaques on the lateral neck, in the axillae, groin, and perianal areas (Figure 7-24). The scalp, chest, antecubital fossae, and popliteal fossae are less commonly involved. Mucosal involvement is rare. Plaques may be burning and/or pruritic in nature, and are often malodorous. Secondary staphylococcal, candidal, and herpetic infection is not uncommon.

The disease follows a chronic relapsing and remitting course, and can be triggered by factors such as trauma, sweating, infection, pregnancy, and UV exposure.[91,93]

Histologic Findings

Skin biopsies of HHD show suprabasilar epidermal acantholysis that may be subtle in early lesions, and extensive in well-established lesions. Acantholysis is often

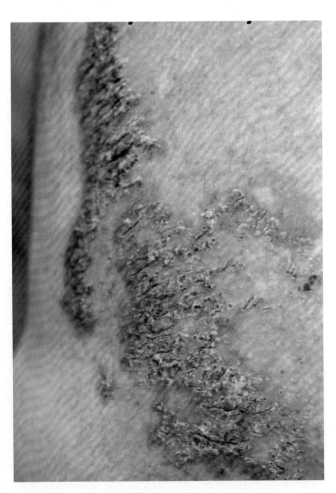

FIGURE 7-24. Hailey-Hailey disease. Grouped flaccid vesicles and erosions form erythematous, macerated plaques.

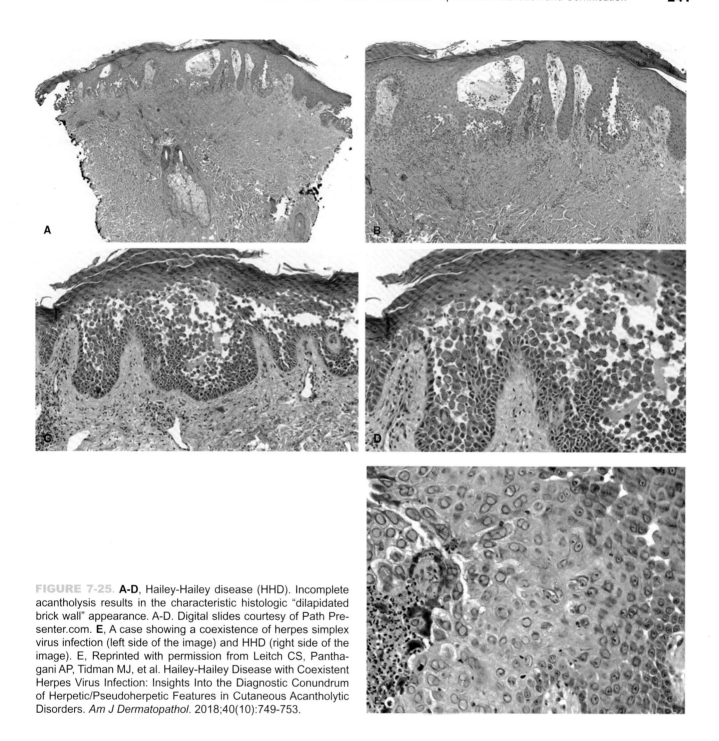

FIGURE 7-25. **A-D**, Hailey-Hailey disease (HHD). Incomplete acantholysis results in the characteristic histologic "dilapidated brick wall" appearance. A-D. Digital slides courtesy of Path Presenter.com. **E**, A case showing a coexistence of herpes simplex virus infection (left side of the image) and HHD (right side of the image). E, Reprinted with permission from Leitch CS, Panthagani AP, Tidman MJ, et al. Hailey-Hailey Disease with Coexistent Herpes Virus Infection: Insights Into the Diagnostic Conundrum of Herpetic/Pseudoherpetic Features in Cutaneous Acantholytic Disorders. *Am J Dermatopathol.* 2018;40(10):749-753.

incomplete, leading to some residual intercellular connection and the classic "dilapidated brick wall" appearance (Figure 7-25A-D). Epidermal hyperplasia is common. Unlike Darier disease, adnexal involvement is uncommon. Interestingly, microscopic findings of acantholysis can be seen even in clinically uninvolved skin in affected patients.[94,95] The coexistence of HHD and HSV infection has been previously documented and can create histopathologic challenges (Figure 7-25E**)**.

Differential Diagnosis

The clinical differential diagnosis of HHD includes immune-mediated subtypes of pemphigus including vulgaris, vegetans, and foliaceus; infections such as erythrasma and intertrigo with candidiasis; and extramammary Paget disease.

Histologically, HHD can be differentiated from Darier disease by the presence of dyskeratotic corps ronds and corps grains in the latter, and the involvement of adnexal structures. PV tends to have a more well-defined suprabasilar split with less acantholysis, and is character-ized by an intercellular deposition of immunoreactants on direct immunofluorescence.

CAPSULE SUMMARY

HAILEY-HAILEY DISEASE

HHD is an uncommon genodermatosis characterized by the recurrent development of macerated, vesicular plaques on the neck and in intertriginous areas. It is caused by mutation in the calcium-transporter-encod-ing *ATP2C1*. Histopathologic features include supra-basilar acantholysis, which can appear as a cleft in early lesions, or in the classic "dilapidated brick wall" config-uration in more well-developed lesions.

POROKERATOSIS

Definition and Epidemiology

Porokeratosis is a disorder of keratinization character-ized by the presence of annular lesions with a distinctive, thread-like scale that projects at an angle toward the center of the lesion and corresponds to the histologic finding of a cornoid lamella. There are many different forms of poro-keratosis, which can be solitary or multiple, congenital or acquired, and occur on virtually any body surface.

Porokeratoses are common lesions, although the exact incidence has not been studied. The most common type, disseminated superficial actinic porokeratosis, is rarely en-countered in children. This review will focus on porokera-tosis of Mibelli, linear porokeratosis, and porokeratosis palmaris et plantaris disseminata, which are the subtypes most commonly seen in children.

Etiology

Porokeratosis can be caused by several different somatic mutations that result in a clonal proliferation of kera-tinocytes with abnormal maturation. Among the genes implicated are *PMVK* (phosphomevalonate kinase), *MVD* (mevalonate phosphate decarboxylase), *MVK* (mevalonate kinase), and *SLC17A9*.[96-98] The mechanisms by which these mutations lead to the clinical phenotype are unclear.

Porokeratosis may occur sporadically or through auto-somal dominant familial inheritance. Familial cases have incomplete expressivity. Postzygotic mosaicism is likely re-sponsible for porokeratosis of Mibelli and linear porokerato-sis.[99] The known risk factors for the sporadic development of porokeratosis include UV exposure and immunosuppression.

Clinical Presentation

Porokeratosis of Mibelli is the classic type, typically pre-senting early in childhood as a small, variably pruritic,

skin-colored to brown papule that slowly expands over the course of several years. The periphery of the lesion is marked by the characteristic thread-like porokeratotic scale, but the center of the lesion can vary in appearance from atrophic to scaly, with dyspigmentation, alopecia, anhidrosis, or a com-bination of features (Figure 7-26). Lesions tend to occur on the extremities, but may appear anywhere.[100] They typically reach a few centimeters in diameter, but can grow as large as 20 cm.[101] Although they are usually solitary in nature, multiple lesions may be present.

Linear porokeratosis also arises during infancy or early childhood, but presents as one or multiple lesions in a Blaschkoid distribution. It is typically unilateral and lim-ited in distribution, but generalized linear porokeratosis has been reported.[102] Porokeratotic eccrine ostial and der-mal duct nevus is a linear form of porokeratosis that in-volves adnexal structures and presents as linearly arranged hyperkeratotic papules and keratin-filled pits.[103]

Porokeratosis palmaris et plantaris disseminata presents during adolescence as papules or small plaques, initially on the palms and soles with occasional subsequent proximal spread. Disseminated involvement has been reported.[104] Punctate porokeratosis also occurs primarily on the palms and soles, but presents as multiple very small, keratotic papules.

Squamous cell carcinoma may develop within long-standing lesions of porokeratosis. Linear porokerato-sis is the highest risk subtype.[105]

Histologic Findings

The hallmark histologic finding in porokeratosis is the cor-noid lamella, which is composed of a column of parakera-tosis with underlying hypogranulosis and dyskeratosis/keratinocytic atypia. The column of parakeratosis typically

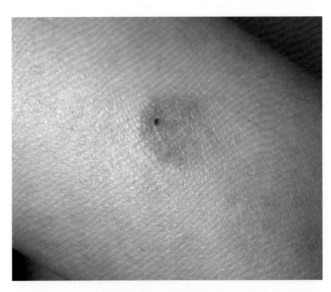

FIGURE 7-26. Porokeratosis of Mibelli in a child. There is an annular thin plaque with a thread-like border.

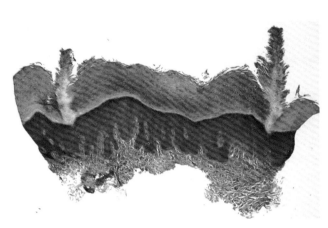
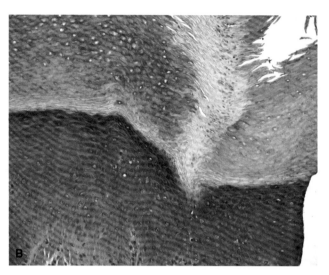

FIGURE 7-27. **Porokeratosis. A**, At scanning magnification, cornoid lamellae are seen at either end of the specimen. There is psoriasiform hyperplasia in the middle of the lesion, but other patterns may occur. **B**, High-power image of a cornoid lamella with a column of parakeratosis overlying a zone of hypogranulosis and dyskeratosis.

points toward the center of the lesion, corresponding to the angled scale that can be seen clinically (Figure 7-27). If the edge of the lesion is not sampled, or if the specimen is oriented parallel to the plane of section, diagnostic features may be missed. The center of the lesion may have any number of findings, including epidermal atrophy or hyperplasia, alopecia, and variable inflammation, or be completely unremarkable.

Differential Diagnosis

The clinical differential diagnosis of porokeratosis includes other annular dermatoses such as tinea corporis, erythema annulare centrifugum, lichen planus, and psoriasis. Linear porokeratosis may resemble other Blaschkoid dermatoses such as linear psoriasis or ILVEN.

Histologically, cornoid lamellae may occur incidentally in a number of other skin conditions such as psoriasis, actinic keratoses, or even basal cell carcinoma. These can typically be differentiated on the basis of surrounding histologic and clinical findings.

CAPSULE SUMMARY

POROKERATOSIS

Porokeratoses are a group of annular, clonal keratinocytic lesions characterized by the histologic finding of a cornoid lamella that corresponds to the clinical presence of a thread-like scale at the periphery of the lesion. The cornoid lamella is characterized by a parakeratotic column over a zone of hypogranulosis with dyskeratosis.

PALMOPLANTAR KERATODERMAS

Definition, Etiology, and Clinical Presentation

The palmoplantar keratodermas (PPK) are a diverse group of rare hereditary disorders characterized by hyperkeratosis of the palms and soles.

The PPKs are categorized on the basis of pattern (diffuse, focal/striate, or punctate), and the presence or absence of other cutaneous or internal findings. PPK may be isolated to the palmoplantar surfaces (nontransgradient) or extend onto the dorsal surfaces of the hands and feet (transgradient).

The most common diffuse PPK, epidermolytic PPK, is caused by mutations in keratins 1 and 9 (*KRT-1* and *KRT-9*). Defects in these cytoskeletal elements lead to intraepidermal blistering and subsequent hyperkeratosis (Figure 7-28). Affected patients present during infancy with thick, yellow

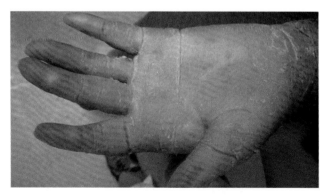

FIGURE 7-28. **Epidermolytic palmoplantar keratoderma (EPPK).** Thick, yellowish hyperkeratosis on the palm of a patient with EPPK. There is fissuring over the ventral surface of the wrist.

hyperkeratosis of the palms and soles that is sharply demarcated at the borders with peripheral erythema and does not extend onto the dorsa of the hands and feet (nontransgradient).[106,107] Epidermolytic PPK can be seen in association with epidermolytic ichthyosis when caused by mutation in *KRT-1*, which is expressed on all skin surfaces, including the palms and soles. Mutations in *KRT-9* present with isolated PPK, as this protein is expressed only on the palms and soles.

Tables 7-3 and 7-4 review the clinical and histologic features of various syndromic and nonsyndromic diseases which feature PPK.

TABLE 7-3.	**Features of isolated hereditary keratodermas**			
	Diagnosis	**Mutation/Inheritance**	**Clinical Findings**	**Histopathologic Changes**
Diffuse	Epidermolytic PPK (Figure 7-28)	KRT-1 (Unna–Thost syndrome; Figure 7-29) *and* KRT-9/AD	Erythema followed by thick, well-demarcated, yellow PPK with red borders Painful fissuring Nontransgradient	Hyperorthokeratosis, papillomatosis, acanthosis, epidermolytic hyperkeratosis with irregular eosinophilic granules
	Bothnia NEPPK[108]	Aquaporin 5/AD	Waxy, thick PPK Hyperhidrosis common Spongy, white swelling with water exposure Nontransgradient, but with thickening of the dorsa of the digits and hyperkeratosis over MCP joints	Hyperorthokeratosis, variable papillomatosis and hypergranulosis, acanthosis.
	Kimonis NEPPK[109]	KRT-1/AD	Moderate to severe PPK Slight transgradient with extension along Achilles tendon Hyperkeratosis over MCP joints	
	Nagashima NEPPK[110]	SERPINB7/AR	Mild, erythematous PPK Hyperhidrosis common Transgradient extension	
	Mal de Maleda NEPPK[111]	SLURP1/AR	Thick, mutilating PPK with transgradient spread Constricting bands of the digits that may lead to autoamputation Hyperhidrosis and secondary infections common Periorbital/perioral erythema, subungual hyperkeratosis, hair on volar skin	
Focal	Striate PPK[112] (Figure 7-30)	Desmoglein 1, Desmoplakin, KRT-1/ASD	Variable severity, linear PPK over pressure points and areas of friction May be painful	Hyperorthokeratosis, hypergranulosis, acanthosis, and slight keratinocyte separation.[113]
	Punctate PPK[114] (Figure 7-31)	AAGAB/AD	Small papules with central hyperkeratotic cores that become verrucous Can aggregate to form larger plaques over pressure points over time May be present only in the creases of volar skin in the patients of African descent	Column of hyperorthokeratosis over a central epidermal depression
	Spiny PPK112 (Figure 7-32)	Unknown/AD	Tiny keratotic spines on the palms and soles Tends to start during puberty	Column of parakeratosis over a small central dell. Normal granular layer, no dyskeratosis.

Abbreviations: AD, autosomal dominant; ASD, autosomal semidominant; MCP, metacarpal-phalangeal; NEPPK, nonepidermolytic palmoplantar keratoderma; PPK, palmoplantar keratoderma.

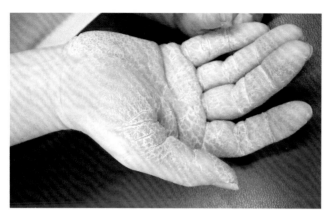

FIGURE 7-29. Diffuse hereditary palmoplantar keratoderma of Unna-Thost syndrome (associated with *KRT-1* mutation).

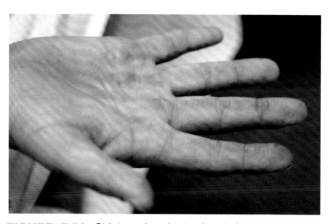

FIGURE 7-30. Striate palmoplantar keratoderma caused by desmoglein 1 mutation. Note the slight acantholysis.

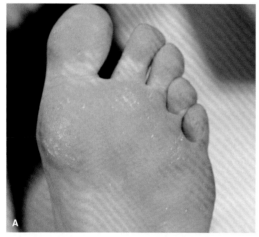

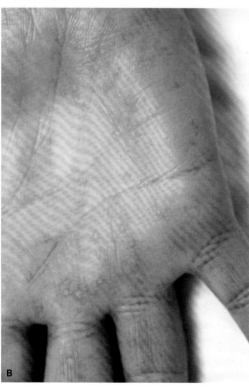

FIGURE 7-31. Punctate palmoplantar keratoderma. Small papules with central hyperkeratotic cores that become verrucous in the sole (**A**) and palms (**B**).

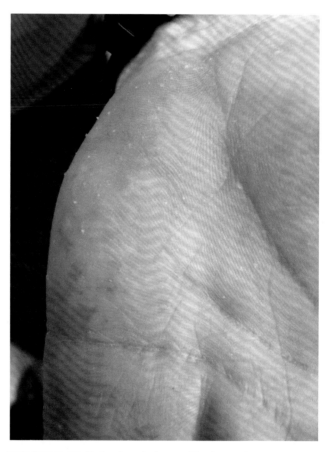

FIGURE 7-32. Spiny keratoderma. Tiny keratotic spiny papules on the palms. Reprinted with permission from Jorge EA. "Gloves Cling to My Hands": a case report of spiny keratoderma. *J Dermatol Nurses Assoc.* 2017;9(6):308-311.

Histologic Findings

The hallmark feature of PPKs is massive hyperkeratosis (Figures 7-34 and 7-35). A few specific patterns are recognizable. Epidermolytic PPK is characterized by the classic features of epidermolytic hyperkeratosis, with vacuolated suprabasilar keratinocytes with irregular eosinophilic

TABLE 7-4. Features of selected syndromic hereditary keratodermas

	Diagnosis	Mutation/Inheritance	Clinical Findings	Syndromic Features	Histopathologic Changes
Diffuse	Vohwinkel syndrome[115]	GJB2/AD	Pitted "honeycomb" PPK	Sensorineural hearing loss Starfish-shaped keratoses over MCP, feet, elbows, knees Constricting digital bands with autoamputation (pseudoainhum)	Hyperkeratosis, nonspecific Fibrosis in areas of pseudoainhum
	Loricrin keratoderma/variant Vohwinkel syndrome[116]	Loricrin/AD	Vohwinkel-type, honeycomb PPK	Congenital ichthyosis Pseudoainhum Starfish keratoses	Hyperkeratosis with parakeratosis, hypergranulosis
	Keratosis linearis with ichthyosis congenita and sclerosing keratoderma[117,118]	POMP/AR	Transgradient PPK	Congenital ichthyosis Linear keratotic contractures over flexor surfaces Occasional pseudoainhum	Hyperkeratosis, acanthosis, irregular hypergranulosis
	Huriez syndrome	Unknown/AD	Mild PPK	Sclerodactyly and adermatoglyphia and hypoplastic nails Increased risk of SCC	Hyperkeratosis, acanthosis, absence of Langerhans cells[119]
Focal	Dilated cardiomyopathy with wolly hair and keratoderma/Carvajal syndrome	Desmoplakin/AR	Mild to moderate PPK over weight-bearing points	Wooly hair Dilated cardiomyopathy (left>right/both)	Epidermolytic hyperkeratosis with ultrastructural loosening of desmosomal attachments
	Howel-Evans syndrome[120]	RHBDF2/AD	PPK over weight-bearing points	Oral leukokeratosis Esophageal SCC	Hyperkeratosis, hypergranulosis, acanthosis Buccal lesions with hyperkeratosis, parakeratosis, and vacuolated/spongiotic spinous layer
	Pachyonychia Congenita Types 1 and 2 (Figure 7-33)	KRT-6a, 6b, 16, 17	PPK over weight-bearing points with fissuring Plantar pain Thickened toenails	Variable based on type: oral leukokeratosis, fingernail dystrophy, steatocystomas, vellous hair cysts, natal teeth	Hyperkeratosis with parakeratosis Persistence of K14 in suprabasilar layers by immunochemistry

Abbreviations: AD, autosomal dominant; AR, autosomal recessive; KLICK, keratosis linearis with ichthyosis congenita and sclerosing keratoderma; MCP, metacarpal-phalangeal; NEPPK, nonepidermolytic palmoplantar keratoderma, PPK, palmoplantar keratoderma; SCC, squamous cell carcinoma.

granules. Punctate PPK features columns of massive hyperkeratosis over depressions in the underlying epidermis. Various diseases and syndromes that feature PPK may sometimes be differentiated by subtle histologic or ultrastructural clues, and many of these are addressed in Tables 7-3 and 7-4.

Differential Diagnosis

The clinical and histopathologic differential diagnosis for PPKs includes many heritable and acquired conditions. Careful history, family history, and physical examination can help differentiate these conditions, and genetic testing is often confirmatory.

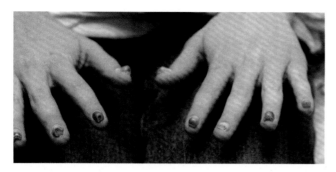

FIGURE7-33. **Pachyonychia Congenita**. Fingernail dystrophy.

CAPSULE SUMMARY

PALMOPLANTAR KERATODERMAS

PPK are a diverse group of inherited disorders featuring diffuse or focal thickening of the skin of the palms and soles. These findings may occur in isolation or with associated syndromes, and their differentiation often depends on clinical presentation and the results of genetic testing. All of these conditions share a common histologic finding of massive epidermal hyperkeratosis.

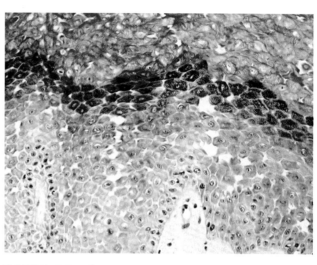

FIGURE 7-35. **Striate palmoplantar keratoderma.** Hyperorthokeratosis, hypergranulosis, acanthosis, and slight keratinocyte separation is present.

ECTODERMAL DYSPLASIAS

Definition and Epidemiology

The ectodermal dysplasias (ED) are a diverse group of nearly 200 genetic development disorders characterized by abnormalities in ectodermally derived structures. To qualify as an

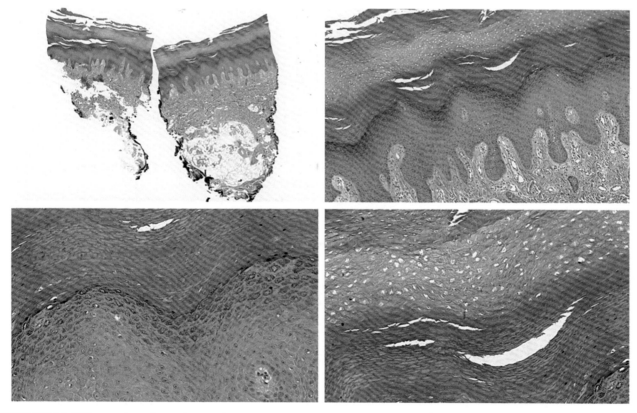

FIGURE 7-34. **Diffuse palmoplantar keratoderma.** Massive hyperkeratosis and early changes of epidermolytic hyperkeratosis. Digital slides courtesy of Path Presenter.com.

ED, at least two of the four major ectodermal derivatives must be affected—hair, teeth, nails, and eccrine glands. Disorders are classified on the basis of which of these are affected, and the presence or absence of associated immune dysregulation. EDs are caused by mutations in genes encoding signaling pathway components, adhesion molecules, and transcription factors important during embryologic development.[121]

Each of the forms of ectodermal dysplasia is rare, with the most common being X-linked hypohidrotic ED caused by Ectodysplasin A (EDA) mutation. This form occurs almost exclusively in males, although mild or rare severe cases have been reported in females. The other forms of ED are primarily autosomal, and occur equally in males and females.

Etiology

Many of the causative mutations for ectodermal dysplasias have been identified, and can be divided into the following general categories of defect that lead to an abnormal development of ectodermal structures:[122]

- Genes encoding cell signaling and communication molecules
  - *EDA, EDAR, EDARADD* (hypohidrotic ED)
  - *GJB2, GJB6* (PPK with deafness and hidrotic ED/ Clouston syndrome, respectively)
  - *NEMO* (incontinentia pigmenti type 2; hypohidrotic ectodermal dysplasia with immunodeficiency; and osteopetrosis, lymphedema, EDA, and immunodeficiency/OLEDAID syndrome)
- Adhesion-related molecules
  - *Plakophilin 1* (ED with skin fragility syndrome)
  - *TP63* (ectodermal dysplasia, ectrodactyly, and clefting (EEC) syndrome; ankyloblepharon, ectodermal dysplasia, and clefting (AEC)/Hay-Wells syndrome; and Rapp-Hodgkin syndrome)
- Developmental signaling molecules
  - *Hox 7* (Withkop syndrome)
  - *Sonic Hedgehog* (Solitary median maxillary central incisor syndrome)
- Other
  - *Dyskerin* (Dyskeratosis congenita)
  - *RecQL4* (Rothmund-Thomson syndrome)

Clinical Presentation

The clinical presentations of the ectodermal dysplasias are varied on the basis of causative mutation and affected structures. Hypohidrotic ectodermal dysplasias are characterized by the triad of sparse hair, absent/abnormal teeth, and hypo-/anhidrosis. Anhidrosis results in core temperature dysregulation, which may lead to seizures or fatal hyperthermia in undetected cases.[123] Characteristic facies feature frontal bossing, saddle nose, thickened lips, and

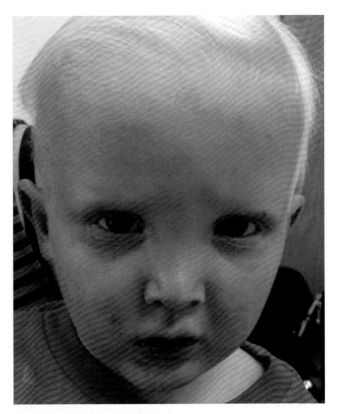

FIGURE 7-36. Hypohidrotic ectodermal dysplasia. Characteristic facies with saddle nose and thickened lips.

large ears. Patients often develop troublesome atopic dermatitis (Figures 7-36 to 7-38).

Patients with hidrotic ectodermal dysplasia (Clouston syndrome) present with brittle, sparse hair to complete alopecia and hypoplastic, dystrophic nails. They may have thickened palmar skin, clubbed digits, and eye abnormalities including cataracts and photophobia. The teeth and sweat glands are normal.

Patients with AEC syndrome present at birth with ankyloblepharon (strands of tissue connecting the upper and lower eyelids), cleft lip and palate, sparse hair, nail dystrophy, reduced sweating, and frequent erosive scalp dermatitis.[124] EEC syndrome presents with pale, brittle hair, nail abnormalities, cleft lip and palate, hypodontia, and ectrodactyly (split hand/foot). Sweating is typically normal.

Hypohidrotic ectodermal dysplasia with immune deficiency is caused by *NEMO* mutation, which causes a disruption in the NFκB signaling pathway. These patients present with immune dysfunction characterized by recurrent bacterial and mycobacterial infections of the skin and respiratory tract, with a few reports of serious viral and fungal infections.[125]

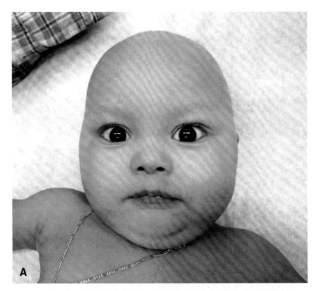

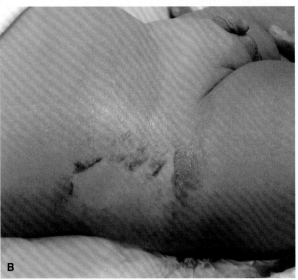

FIGURE 7-37. **Hypohidrotic ectodermal dysplasia.** Another example showing a marked reduction in scalp hair (**A**) and associated skin fragility (**B**).

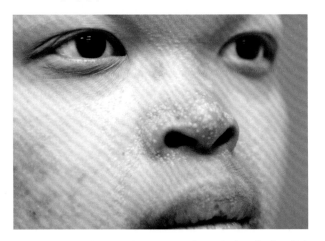

FIGURE 7-38. **Hypohidrotic ectodermal dysplasia.** Sebaceous gland hyperplasia.

Histologic Findings

There are few characteristic histologic findings in the skin biopsies of affected patients. A lack of eccrine glands can be detected in patients with hypohidrotic forms of ED.

Differential Diagnosis

The clinical differential diagnosis for each component of each condition is quite broad. Alopecia areata is a consideration for sparse hair, as is aplasia cutis congenita. Incontinentia pigmenti may have overlapping features with hypohidrotic ED. Nail abnormalities can occur in a number of conditions, or may even be normal in infants and young children. A complete history and physical examination, with targeted genetic testing, is essential for accurate diagnosis.

CAPSULE SUMMARY

ECTODERMAL DYSPLASIAS

ED are a heterogeneous group of developmental anomalies of structures derived from the ectoderm. The development of hair, nails, teeth, and sweat glands may be affected by a number of mutations in a diverse group of genes. Patients with hypohidrotic forms of ectodermal dysplasia may present with hyperthermia, and skin biopsies from these patients demonstrate a paucity of eccrine glands.

GRANULAR PARAKERATOSIS

Definition and Epidemiology

Granular parakeratosis (GP) is an acquired, benign disorder of keratinization that typically occurs in the axilla and presents as a coalescing, pruritic plaque. It is characterized and named for its unique histologic findings. GP occurs most commonly in adult women, but adolescents and infants may also be affected.

Etiology

Initial reports linked the development of GP to the use of mineral underarm deodorants, salts, and other personal care products. This is supported by improvement in many cases when the offending agent is discontinued. Nevertheless, it may occur in areas not exposed to these products and in patients with no history of relevant exposures.

The underlying pathophysiology of GP is not well understood. It has been suggested that an acquired defect in profilaggrin processing results in failure to break down keratohyaline granules and subsequent defects in keratinization.[126]

Clinical Presentation

In adolescents and adults, GP occurs most commonly in the axilla, but may also occur in other intertriginous sites.

It presents as yellow to red-brown keratotic papules that coalesce into plaques that may be pruritic in nature. Maceration is common. In infants, the diaper area is most often affected, and it may appear as keratotic linear plaques in the inguinal folds or as plaques over pressure points (Figure 7-39).[127]

GP may follow a chronic, relapsing course, or it may resolve with discontinuation of the offending agent and the use of topical corticosteroids.

Histologic Findings

The histologic hallmark of granular parakeratosis is thick hyperparakeratosis with retained keratohyaline granules in the corneal layer (Figure 7-40). There is variable underlying epidermal hyperplasia and an occasional mild superficial perivascular lymphocytic inflammation.

Differential Diagnosis

The clinical differential diagnosis includes candidiasis, psoriasis, seborrheic dermatitis, allergic contact dermatitis, Fox

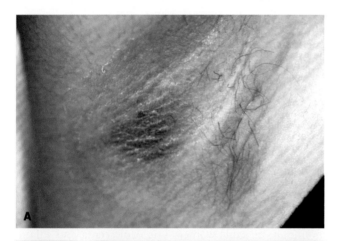

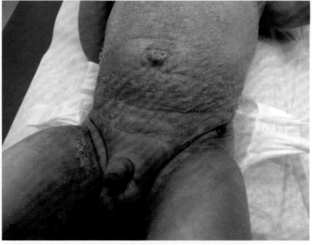

FIGURE 7-39. **Granular parakeratosis. A,** Typical axillary location in an adolescent. **B,** Severe diaper area involvement in an infant. Courtesy of Dr. Seth Orlow. Ronald O. Perelman Department of Dermatology. New York University.

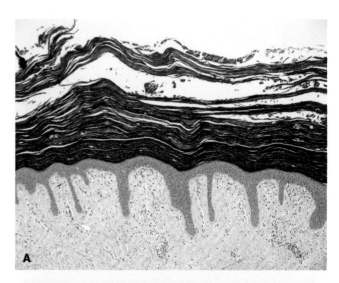

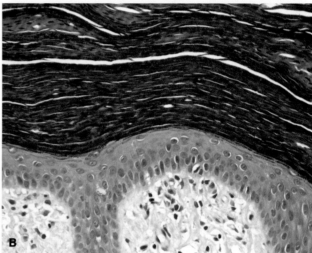

FIGURE 7-40. **Granular parakeratosis.** Low- (**A**) and high-power (**B**) images showing hyperparakeratosis and conspicuous retention of keratohyaline granules in the stratum corneum. There is underlying epidermal atrophy in this case.

Fordyce disease, and erythrasma, among other entities that cause intertrigo.

The histologic finding of granular parakeratosis may be seen as an incidental finding in a number of other conditions from molluscum to squamous cell carcinoma. These are easily differentiated on the basis of clinical findings and other histologic findings.[128-130]

CAPSULE SUMMARY

GRANULAR PARAKERATOSIS

Granular parakeratosis is a benign, acquired disorder of keratinization in which presents most often in the axillae of adult women, but also occurs in the diaper area of infants. The typical clinical finding is of hyperkeratotic yellow to red-brown papules that coalesce into larger plaques. The diagnosis is confirmed by the characteristic histologic finding of hyperkeratosis with parakeratosis and retained keratohyaline granules in the stratum corneum.

REFERENCES

1. Schmuth M, Martinz V, Janecke AR, et al. Inherited ichthyoses/generalized Mendelian disorders of cornification. *Eur J Hum Genet.* 2013;21(2):123-133.
2. Palmer CN, Irvine AD, Terron-Kwiatkowski A, et al. Common loss-of-function variants of the epidermal barrier protein filaggrin are a major predisposing factor for atopic dermatitis. *Nat Genet.* 2006;38(4):441-446.
3. Thyssen JP, Godoy-Gijon E, Elias PM. Ichthyosis vulgaris: the filaggrin mutation disease. *Br J Dermatol.* 2013;168(6):1155-1166.
4. Traupe H, Fischer J, Oji V. Nonsyndromic types of ichthyoses: an update. *J Dtsch Dermatol Ges.* 2014;12(2):109-121.
5. Weidinger S, O'Sullivan M, Illig T, et al. Filaggrin mutations, atopic eczema, hay fever, and asthma in children. *J Allergy Clin Immunol.* 2008;121(5):1203-1209.e1.
6. Wells RS, Kerr CB. Clinical features of autosomal dominant and sex-linked ichthyosis in an English population. *Br Med J.* 1966;1(5493):947-950.
7. Ziprkowski L, Feinstein A. A survey of ichthyosis vulgaris in Israel. *Br J Dermatol.* 1972;86(1):1-8.
8. Bonifas JM, Morley BJ, Oakey RE, Kan YW, Epstein EH Jr. Cloning of a cDNA for steroid sulfatase: frequent occurrence of gene deletions in patients with recessive X chromosome-linked ichthyosis. *Proc Natl Acad Sci U S A.* 1987;84(24):9248-9251.
9. Richard G, Ringpfeil F. Ichthyoses, erythrokeratodermas, and related disorders. In: Bolognia JL, Schaffer JV, Cerroni L, eds. *Dermatology.* 4th ed. Philadelphia, PA: Elsevier; 2018:888-923.
10. Irvine AD, McLean WH. Human keratin diseases: the increasing spectrum of disease and subtlety of the phenotype-genotype correlation. *Br J Dermatol.* 1999;140(5):815-828.
11. Vahlquist A, Fischer J, Torma H. Inherited nonsyndromic ichthyoses: an update on pathophysiology, diagnosis and treatment. *Am J Clin Dermatol.* 2018;19(1):51-66.
12. Akiyama M. Severe congenital ichthyosis of the neonate. *Int J Dermatol.* 1998;37(10):722-728.
13. Herman ML, Farasat S, Steinbach PJ, et al. Transglutaminase-1 gene mutations in autosomal recessive congenital ichthyosis: summary of mutations (including 23 novel) and modeling of TGase-1. *Hum Mutat.* 2009;30(4):537-547.
14. Israeli S, Goldberg I, Fuchs-Telem D, et al. Non-syndromic autosomal recessive congenital ichthyosis in the Israeli population. *Clin Exp Dermatol.* 2013;38(8):911-916.
15. Kihara A. Synthesis and degradation pathways, functions, and pathology of ceramides and epidermal acylceramides. *Prog Lipid Res.* 2016;63:50-69.
16. Akiyama M. ABCA12 mutations and autosomal recessive congenital ichthyosis: a review of genotype/phenotype correlations and of pathogenetic concepts. *Hum Mutat.* 2010;31(10):1090-1096.
17. Brown VL, Farrant PB, Turner RJ, Price ML, Burge SM. Multiple aggressive squamous skin cancers in association with nonbullous congenital ichthyosiform erythroderma. *Br J Dermatol.* 2008;158(5):1125-1128.
18. Rajpopat S, Moss C, Mellerio J, et al. Harlequin ichthyosis: a review of clinical and molecular findings in 45 cases. *Arch Dermatol.* 2011;147(6):681-686.
19. Roberts LJ. Long-term survival of a harlequin fetus. *J Am Acad Dermatol.* 1989;21(2 Pt 2):335-339.
20. Unamuno P, Pierola JM, Fernandez E, Roman C, Velasco JA. Harlequin foetus in four siblings. *Br J Dermatol.* 1987;116(4):569-572.
21. Chan YC, Tay YK, Tan LK, Happle R, Giam YC. Harlequin ichthyosis in association with hypothyroidism and juvenile rheumatoid arthritis. *Pediatr Dermatol.* 2003;20(5):421-426.
22. Van Gysel D, Lijnen RL, Moekti SS, de Laat PC, Oranje AP. Collodion baby: a follow-up study of 17 cases. *J Eur Acad Dermatol Venereol.* 2002;16(5):472-475.
23. DiLeonardo M. Ichthyosis vulgaris vs. X-linked ichthyosis vs. lamellar ichthyosis. *Dermatopathol Pract Concep.* 1997;2:132.
24. Fleckman P, Brumbaugh S. Absence of the granular layer and keratohyalin define a morphologically distinct subset of individuals with ichthyosis vulgaris. *Exp Dermatol.* 2002;11(4):327-336.
25. Scheimberg I, Harper JI, Malone M, Lake BD. Inherited ichthyoses: a review of the histology of the skin. *Pediatr Pathol Lab Med.* 1996;16(3):359-378.
26. De Unamuno P, Martin-Pascual A, Garcia-Perez A. X-linked ichthyosis. *Br J Dermatol.* 1977;97(1):53-58.
27. Ghadially R, Williams ML, Hou SY, Elias PM. Membrane structural abnormalities in the stratum corneum of the autosomal recessive ichthyoses. *J Invest Dermatol.* 1992;99(6):755-763.
28. Ackerman AB. Histopathologic concept of epidermolytic hyperkeratosis. *Arch Dermatol.* 1970;102(3):253-259.
29. Hohl D, Aeschlimann D, Huber M. In vitro and rapid in situ transglutaminase assays for congenital ichthyoses: a comparative study. *J Invest Dermatol.* 1998;110(3):268-271.
30. Kanerva L, Lauharanta J, Niemi KM, Lassus A. New observations on the fine structure of lamellar ichthyosis and the effect of treatment with etretinate. *Am J Dermatopathol.* 1983;5(6):555-568.
31. Fleck RM, Barnadas M, Schulz WW, Roberts LJ, Freeman RG. Harlequin ichthyosis: an ultrastructural study. *J Am Acad Dermatol.* 1989;21(5 Pt 1):999-1006.
32. Traupe H. *The Ichthyoses: A Guide to Clinical Diagnosis, Genetic Counseling, and Therapy.* 1st ed. Berlin: Springer Verlag; 1989.
33. Chavanas S, Bodemer C, Rochat A, et al. Mutations in SPINK5, encoding a serine protease inhibitor, cause Netherton syndrome. *Nat Genet.* 2000;25(2):141-142.
34. Sprecher E, Chavanas S, DiGiovanna JJ, et al. The spectrum of pathogenic mutations in SPINK5 in 19 families with Netherton syndrome: implications for mutation detection and first case of prenatal diagnosis. *J Invest Dermatol.* 2001;117(2):179-187.
35. Descargues P, Deraison C, Prost C, et al. Corneodesmosomal cadherins are preferential targets of stratum corneum trypsin- and chymotrypsin-like hyperactivity in Netherton syndrome. *J Invest Dermatol.* 2006;126(7):1622-1632.
36. Hachem JP, Houben E, Crumrine D, et al. Serine protease signaling of epidermal permeability barrier homeostasis. *J Invest Dermatol.* 2006;126(9):2074-2086.
37. Descargues P, Deraison C, Bonnart C, et al. Spink5-deficient mice mimic Netherton syndrome through degradation of desmoglein 1 by epidermal protease hyperactivity. *Nat Genet.* 2005;37(1):56-65.
38. Ishida-Yamamoto A, Deraison C, Bonnart C, et al. LEKTI is localized in lamellar granules, separated from KLK5 and KLK7, and is secreted in the extracellular spaces of the superficial stratum granulosum. *J Invest Dermatol.* 2005;124(2):360-366.
39. Pruszkowski A, Bodemer C, Fraitag S, Teillac-Hamel D, Amoric JC, de Prost Y. Neonatal and infantile erythrodermas: a retrospective study of 51 patients. *Arch Dermatol.* 2000;136(7):875-880.
40. Stoll C, Alembik Y, Tchomakov D, et al. Severe hypernatremic dehydration in an infant with Netherton syndrome. *Genet Couns.* 2001;12(3):237-43.
41. Van Gysel D, Koning H, Baert MR, Savelkoul HF, Neijens HJ, Oranje AP. Clinico-immunological heterogeneity in Comel-Netherton syndrome. *Dermatology.* 2001;202(2):99-107.

42. Paller AS, Mancini AJ. Hereditary disorders of cornification. In: Paller AS, Mancini AJ, eds. *Hurwitz Clinical Pediatric Dermatology*. 5th ed. Philadelphia, PA: Elsevier; 2016:95-118.

43. Powell J, Dawber RP, Ferguson DJ, Griffiths WA. Netherton's syndrome: increased likelihood of diagnosis by examining eyebrow hairs. *Br J Dermatol*. 1999;141(3):544-546.

44. Renner ED, Hartl D, Rylaarsdam S, et al. Comel-Netherton syndrome defined as primary immunodeficiency. *J Allergy Clin Immunol*. 2009;124(3):536-543.

45. Folster-Holst R, Swensson O, Stockfleth E, Monig H, Mrowietz U, Christophers E. Comel-Netherton syndrome complicated by papillomatous skin lesions containing human papillomaviruses 51 and 52 and plane warts containing human papillomavirus 16. *Br J Dermatol*. 1999;140(6):1139-1143.

46. Natsuga K, Akiyama M, Shimizu H. Malignant skin tumours in patients with inherited ichthyosis. *Br J Dermatol*. 2011;165(2):263-268.

47. Yoshiike T, Manabe M, Negi M, Ogawa H. Ichthyosis linearis circumflexa: morphological and biochemical studies. *Br J Dermatol*. 1985;112(3):277-283.

48. Mizuno Y, Suga Y, Haruna K, et al. A case of a Japanese neonate with congenital ichthyosiform erythroderma diagnosed as Netherton syndrome. *Clin Exp Dermatol*. 2006;31(5):677-680.

49. Leclerc-Mercier S, Bodemer C, Furio L, et al. Skin biopsy in Netherton syndrome: a histological review of a large series and new findings. *Am J Dermatopathol*. 2016;38(2):83-91.

50. Fartasch M, Williams ML, Elias PM. Altered lamellar body secretion and stratum corneum membrane structure in Netherton syndrome: differentiation from other infantile erythrodermas and pathogenic implications. *Arch Dermatol*. 1999;135(7):823-832.

51. Wanders RJ, Jansen GA, Skjeldal OH. Refsum disease, peroxisomes and phytanic acid oxidation: a review. *J Neuropathol Exp Neurol*. 2001;60(11):1021-1031.

52. Jansen GA, Waterham HR, Wanders RJ. Molecular basis of Refsum disease: sequence variations in phytanoyl-CoA hydroxylase (PHYH) and the PTS2 receptor (PEX7). *Hum Mutat*. 2004;23(3):209-218.

53. Menon GK, Orso E, Aslanidis C, Crumrine D, Schmitz G, Elias PM. Ultrastructure of skin from Refsum disease with emphasis on epidermal lamellar bodies and stratum corneum barrier lipid organization. *Arch Dermatol Res*. 2014;306(8):731-737.

54. Wanders RJA, Waterham HR, Leroy BP. Refsum disease. In: Adam MP, Ardinger HH, Pagon RA, et al., eds. *GeneReviews*. Seattle, WA: University of Washington; 1993.

55. Davies MG, Marks R, Dykes PJ, Reynolds D. Epidermal abnormalities in Refsum's disease. *Br J Dermatol*. 1977;97(4):401-406.

56. Sjogren T, Larsson T. Oligophrenia in combination with congenital ichthyosis and spastic disorders; a clinical and genetic study. *Acta Psychiatr Neurol Scand Suppl*. 1957;113:1-112.

57. Rizzo WB, Craft DA. Sjogren-Larsson syndrome. Deficient activity of the fatty aldehyde dehydrogenase component of fatty alcohol:NAD+ oxidoreductase in cultured fibroblasts. *J Clin Invest*. 1991;88(5):1643-1648.

58. Jagell S, Liden S. Ichthyosis in the Sjogren-Larsson syndrome. *Clin Genet*. 1982;21(4):243-252.

59. Rizzo WB. Sjogren-Larsson syndrome: molecular genetics and biochemical pathogenesis of fatty aldehyde dehydrogenase deficiency. *Mol Genet Metab*. 2007;90(1):1-9.

60. Brandling-Bennett HA, Liang MG. What syndrome is this? Sjogren-Larsson syndrome. *Pediatr Dermatol*. 2005;22(6):569-571.

61. Ito M, Oguro K, Sato Y. Ultrastructural study of the skin in Sjogren-Larsson syndrome. *Arch Dermatol Res*. 1991;283(3):141-148.

62. Cadieux-Dion M, Turcotte-Gauthier M, Noreau A, et al. Expanding the clinical phenotype associated with ELOVL4 mutation: study of a large French-Canadian family with autosomal dominant spinocerebellar ataxia and erythrokeratodermia. *JAMA Neurol*. 2014;71(4):470-475.

63. Montpetit A, Cote S, Brustein E, et al. Disruption of AP1S1, causing a novel neurocutaneous syndrome, perturbs development of the skin and spinal cord. *PLoS Genet*. 2008;4(12):e1000296.

64. Martinelli D, Travaglini L, Drouin CA, et al. MEDNIK syndrome: a novel defect of copper metabolism treatable by zinc acetate therapy. *Brain*. 2013;136(Pt 3):872-881.

65. Saba TG, Montpetit A, Verner A, et al. An atypical form of erythrokeratodermia variabilis maps to chromosome 7q22. *Hum Genet*. 2005;116(3):167-171.

66. Smith H, Galmes R, Gogolina E, et al. Associations among genotype, clinical phenotype, and intracellular localization of trafficking proteins in ARC syndrome. *Hum Mutat*. 2012;33(12):1656-1664.

67. Cullinane AR, Straatman-Iwanowska A, Zaucker A, et al. Mutations in VIPAR cause an arthrogryposis, renal dysfunction and cholestasis syndrome phenotype with defects in epithelial polarization. *Nat Genet*. 2010;42(4):303-312.

68. Zhou Y, Zhang J. Arthrogryposis-renal dysfunction-cholestasis (ARC) syndrome: from molecular genetics to clinical features. *Ital J Pediatr*. 2014;40:77.

69. Choi HJ, Lee MW, Choi JH, Moon KC, Koh JK. Ichthyosis associated with ARC syndrome: ARC syndrome is one of the differential diagnoses of ichthyosis. *Pediatr Dermatol*. 2005;22(6):539-542.

70. Hall JG. Arthrogryposis (multiple congenital contractures): diagnostic approach to etiology, classification, genetics, and general principles. *Eur J Med Genet*. 2014;57(8):464-472.

71. Hoang MP, Carder KR, Pandya AG, Bennett MJ. Ichthyosis and keratotic follicular plugs containing dystrophic calcification in newborns: distinctive histopathologic features of x-linked dominant chondrodysplasia punctata (Conradi-Hunermann-Happle syndrome). *Am J Dermatopathol*. 2004;26(1):53-58.

72. Derry JM, Gormally E, Means GD, et al. Mutations in a delta 8-delta 7 sterol isomerase in the tattered mouse and X-linked dominant chondrodysplasia punctata. jderry@immunex.com. *Nat Genet*. 1999;22(3):286-290.

73. Hamaguchi T, Bondar G, Siegfried E, Penneys NS. Cutaneous histopathology of Conradi-Hunermann syndrome. *J Cutan Pathol*. 1995;22(1):38-41.

74. Braverman N, Lin P, Moebius FF, et al. Mutations in the gene encoding 3 beta-hydroxysteroid-delta 8, delta 7-isomerase cause X-linked dominant Conradi-Hunermann syndrome. *Nat Genet*. 1999;22(3):291-294.

75. Happle R. X-linked dominant chondrodysplasia punctata. Review of literature and report of a case. *Hum Genet*. 1979;53(1):65-73.

76. Happle R, Koch H, Lenz W. The CHILD syndrome. Congenital hemidysplasia with ichthyosiform erythroderma and limb defects. *Eur J Pediatr*. 1980;134(1):27-33.

77. Hummel M, Cunningham D, Mullett CJ, Kelley RI, Herman GE. Left-sided CHILD syndrome caused by a nonsense mutation in the NSDHL gene. *Am J Med Genet A*. 2003;122A(3):246-251.

78. Bornholdt D, Konig A, Happle R, et al. Mutational spectrum of NSDHL in CHILD syndrome. *J Med Genet*. 2005;42(2):e17.

79. Happle R, Mittag H, Kuster W. The CHILD nevus: a distinct skin disorder. *Dermatology*. 1995;191(3):210-216.

80. Gantner S, Rutten A, Requena L, Gassenmaier G, Landthaler M, Hafner C. CHILD syndrome with mild skin lesions: histopathologic clues for the diagnosis. *J Cutan Pathol*. 2014;41(10):787-790.

81. Sakuntabhai A, Ruiz-Perez V, Carter S, et al. Mutations in ATP2A2, encoding a Ca2+ pump, cause Darier disease. *Nat Genet*. 1999;21(3):271-277.

82. Takagi A, Kamijo M, Ikeda S. Darier disease. *J Dermatol*. 2016;43(3):275-279.

83. Tavadia S, Mortimer E, Munro CS. Genetic epidemiology of Darier's disease: a population study in the west of Scotland. *Br J Dermatol*. 2002;146(1):107-109.

84. Svendsen IB, Albrectsen B. The prevalence of dyskeratosis follicularis (Darier's disease) in Denmark: an investigation of the heredity in 22 families. *Acta Derm Venereol*. 1959;39:256-269.

85. Li N, Park M, Xiao S, Liu Z, Diaz LA. ER-to-Golgi blockade of nascent desmosomal cadherins in SERCA2-inhibited keratinocytes: Implications for Darier's disease. *Traffic*. 2017;18(4):232-241.

86. Savignac M, Edir A, Simon M, Hovnanian A. Darier disease: a disease model of impaired calcium homeostasis in the skin. *Biochim Biophys Acta*. 2011;1813(5):1111-1117.

87. Mayuzumi N, Ikeda S, Kawada H, Fan PS, Ogawa H. Effects of ultraviolet B irradiation, proinflammatory cytokines and raised extracellular calcium concentration on the expression of ATP2A2 and ATP2C1. *Br J Dermatol*. 2005;152(4):697-701.

88. Sakuntabhai A, Dhitavat J, Burge S, Hovnanian A. Mosaicism for ATP2A2 mutations causes segmental Darier's disease. *J Invest Dermatol*. 2000;115(6):1144-1147.

89. Ronan A, Ingrey A, Murray N, Chee P. Recurrent ATP2A2 p.(Pro602Leu) mutation differentiates Acrokeratosis verruciformis of Hopf from the allelic condition Darier disease. *Am J Med Genet A*. 2017.

90. Hu Z, Bonifas JM, Beech J, et al. Mutations in ATP2C1, encoding a calcium pump, cause Hailey-Hailey disease. *Nat Genet*. 2000;24(1):61-65.

91. Burge SM. Hailey-Hailey disease: the clinical features, response to treatment and prognosis. *Br J Dermatol*. 1992;126(3):275-282.

92. Deng H, Xiao H. The role of the ATP2C1 gene in Hailey-Hailey disease. *Cell Mol Life Sci*. 2017;74(20):3687-3696.

93. Engin B, Kutlubay Z, Celik U, Serdaroglu S, Tuzun Y. Hailey-Hailey disease: a fold (intertriginous) dermatosis. *Clin Dermatol*. 2015;33(4):452-425.

94. Burge SM, Millard PR, Wojnarowska F. Hailey-Hailey disease: a widespread abnormality of cell adhesion. *Br J Dermatol*. 1991;124(4):329-332.

95. Michel B. "Familial benign chronic pemphigus" by Hailey and Hailey, April 1939. Commentary: Hailey-Hailey disease, familial benign chronic pemphigus. *Arch Dermatol*. 1982;118(10):774-783.

96. Cui H, Li L, Wang W, et al. Exome sequencing identifies SLC17A9 pathogenic gene in two Chinese pedigrees with disseminated superficial actinic porokeratosis. *J Med Genet*. 2014;51(10):699-704.

97. Zhang SQ, Jiang T, Li M, et al. Exome sequencing identifies MVK mutations in disseminated superficial actinic porokeratosis. *Nat Genet*. 2012;44(10):1156-1160.

98. Zhang Z, Li C, Wu F, et al. Genomic variations of the mevalonate pathway in porokeratosis. *Elife*. 2015;4:e06322.

99. Happle R. Mibelli revisited: a case of type 2 segmental porokeratosis from 1893. *J Am Acad Dermatol*. 2010;62(1):136-138.

100. Leow YH, Soon YH, Tham SN. A report of 31 cases of porokeratosis at the National Skin Centre. *Ann Acad Med Singapore*. 1996;25(6):837-841.

101. Avhad G, Jerajani H. Porokeratosis of Mibelli: giant variant. *Indian Dermatol Online J*. 2013;4(3):262-263.

102. Dervis E, Demirkesen C. Generalized linear porokeratosis. *Int J Dermatol*. 2006;45(9):1077-1079.

103. Goddard DS, Rogers M, Frieden IJ, et al. Widespread porokeratotic adnexal ostial nevus: clinical features and proposal of a new name unifying porokeratotic eccrine ostial and dermal duct nevus and porokeratotic eccrine and hair follicle nevus. *J Am Acad Dermatol*. 2009;61(6):1060 e1-14.

104. Patrizi A, Passarini B, Minghetti G, Masina M. Porokeratosis palmaris et plantaris disseminata: an unusual clinical presentation. *J Am Acad Dermatol*. 1989;21(2 Pt 2):415-418.

105. Sasson M, Krain AD. Porokeratosis and cutaneous malignancy. A review. *Dermatol Surg*. 1996;22(4):339-342.

106. Kelsell DP, Stevens HP. The palmoplantar keratodermas: much more than palms and soles. *Mol Med Today*. 1999;5(3):107-113.

107. Ratnavel RC, Griffiths WA. The inherited palmoplantar keratodermas. *Br J Dermatol*. 1997;137(4):485-490.

108. Wennerstrand LM, Lind LK, Hofer PA, Lundstrom A. Homozygous palmoplantar keratoderma type bothnia improved by erythromycin: a case report. *Acta Derm Venereol*. 2004;84(5):405-406.

109. Kimonis V, DiGiovanna JJ, Yang JM, Doyle SZ, Bale SJ, Compton JG. A mutation in the V1 end domain of keratin 1 in non-epidermolytic palmar-plantar keratoderma. *J Invest Dermatol*. 1994;103(6):764-769.

110. Mizuno O, Nomura T, Suzuki S, et al. Highly prevalent SERPINB7 founder mutation causes pseudodominant inheritance pattern in Nagashima-type palmoplantar keratosis. *Br J Dermatol*. 2014;171(4):847-853.

111. Fischer J, Bouadjar B, Heilig R, Fizames C, Prud'homme JF, Weissenbach J. Genetic linkage of Meleda disease to chromosome 8qter. *Eur J Hum Genet*. 1998;6(6):542-547.

112. Sakiyama T, Kubo A. Hereditary palmoplantar keratoderma "clinical and genetic differential diagnosis." *J Dermatol*. 2016;43(3):264-274.

113. Hunt DM, Rickman L, Whittock NV, et al. Spectrum of dominant mutations in the desmosomal cadherin desmoglein 1, causing the skin disease striate palmoplantar keratoderma. *Eur J Hum Genet*. 2001;9(3):197-203.

114. Pohler E, Mamai O, Hirst J, et al. Haploinsufficiency for AAGAB causes clinically heterogeneous forms of punctate palmoplantar keratoderma. *Nat Genet*. 2012;44(11):1272-1276.

115. Sensi A, Bettoli V, Zampino MR, Gandini E, Calzolari E. Vohwinkel syndrome (mutilating keratoderma) associated with craniofacial anomalies. *Am J Med Genet*. 1994;50(2):201-203.

116. Maestrini E, Monaco AP, McGrath JA, et al. A molecular defect in loricrin, the major component of the cornified cell envelope, underlies Vohwinkel's syndrome. *Nat Genet*. 1996;13(1):70-77.

117. Dahlqvist J, Klar J, Tiwari N, et al. A single-nucleotide deletion in the POMP 5' UTR causes a transcriptional switch and altered epidermal proteasome distribution in KLICK genodermatosis. *Am J Hum Genet*. 2010;86(4):596-603.

118. Vahlquist A, Ponten F, Pettersson A. Keratosis linearis with ichthyosis congenita and sclerosing keratoderma (KLICK-syndrome): a rare, autosomal recessive disorder of keratohyaline formation? *Acta Derm Venereol*. 1997;77(3):225-227.

119. Hamm H, Traupe H, Brocker EB, Schubert H, Kolde G. The scleroatrophic syndrome of Huriez: a cancer-prone genodermatosis. *Br J Dermatol*. 1996;134(3):512-518.

120. Stevens HP, Kelsell DP, Bryant SP, et al. Linkage of an American pedigree with palmoplantar keratoderma and malignancy (palmoplantar ectodermal dysplasia type III) to 17q24. Literature survey and proposed updated classification of the keratodermas. *Arch Dermatol*. 1996;132(6):640-651.

121. Visinoni AF, Lisboa-Costa T, Pagnan NA, Chautard-Freire-Maia EA. Ectodermal dysplasias: clinical and molecular review. *Am J Med Genet A*. 2009;149A(9):1980-2002.

122. Lamartine J. Towards a new classification of ectodermal dysplasias. *Clin Exp Dermatol*. 2003;28(4):351-355.

123. Clarke A, Phillips DI, Brown R, Harper PS. Clinical aspects of X-linked hypohidrotic ectodermal dysplasia. *Arch Dis Child*. 1987;62(10):989-996.

124. Rinne T, Hamel B, van Bokhoven H, Brunner HG. Pattern of p63 mutations and their phenotypes: update. *Am J Med Genet A*. 2006;140(13):1396-1406.

125. Fusco F, Pescatore A, Conte MI, et al. EDA-ID and IP, two faces of the same coin: how the same IKBKG/NEMO mutation affecting the NF-kappaB pathway can cause immunodeficiency and/or inflammation. *Int Rev Immunol*. 2015;34(6):445-459.

126. Metze D, Rutten A. Granular parakeratosis: a unique acquired disorder of keratinization. *J Cutan Pathol*. 1999;26(7):339-352.

127. Chang MW, Kaufmann JM, Orlow SJ, Cohen DE, Mobini N, Kamino H. Infantile granular parakeratosis: recognition of two clinical patterns. *J Am Acad Dermatol*. 2004;50(5 suppl):S93-S96.

128. Pock L, Hercogova J. Incidental granular parakeratosis associated with dermatomyositis. *Am J Dermatopathol*. 2006;28(2):147-149.

129. Pock L, Cermakova A, Zipfelova J, Hercogova J. Incidental granular parakeratosis associated with molluscum contagiosum. *Am J Dermatopathol*. 2006;28(1):45-47.

130. Resnik KS, DiLeonardo M. Incidental granular parakeratotic cornification in carcinomas. *Am J Dermatopathol*. 2007;29(3):264-269.

8

Genetic Disorders of Pigmentation

Jennifer A. Day / Travis Vandergriff / Adnan Mir

VITILIGO

Definition and Epidemiology

Vitiligo is an acquired pigmentary dermatosis character-ized by a loss of cutaneous melanocytes resulting in de-pigmented patches on the skin. It is relatively common, with a frequency of 1% to 2% in the United States. There is variation in the occurrence worldwide, with a frequency of nearly 9% reported in one part of India.[1] A family history is common, as is the coexistence of other autoimmune con-ditions. Concordance between monozygotic twins is 23%. Males and females appear to be equally affected. About 50% of patients experience onset prior to age 20, and those who experience childhood onset are more likely to have affected family members.[2-4]

Etiology

Although vitiligo occurs at a high frequency in patients with a family history of the disease, it is likely a polygenic trait that results in autoimmune destruction of melano-cytes. Early linkage analyses and more recent genome-wide association studies have identified a number of associa-tions, including immune mediators, melanocyte compo-nents, and regulators of apoptosis.[5,6] Complex interactions of these pathways, likely coupled with environmental fac-tors, lead to the development of the clinical phenotype seen in vitiligo.

The autoimmune nature of vitiligo is supported by genetic studies as well as several key pieces of evidence:

(1) There are circulating antibodies targeting melanocyte proteins.[7] (2) The clinical development of vitiligo in pa-tients with melanoma has long been known to be a posi-tive prognostic factor, suggesting that the antimelanocyte immune reaction evident in the skin depigmentation of these patients also targets malignant melanocytes.[8] (3) Vitiligo often coexists in patients or families with other autoimmune conditions such as Hashimoto thyroiditis and Graves' disease, type 1 diabetes mellitus, alopecia areata, and pernicious anemia.[9,10] (4) Finally, vitiligo is among the autoimmune phenomena that occur in pa-tients with rheumatologic and gastrointestinal inflam-matory diseases treated with tumor necrosis factor-alpha inhibitors.[11] Other hypotheses that have been put forth for the pathogenesis of vitiligo include dysregulation of the nervous system, cytotoxic mechanisms, oxidative stress-induced depigmentation, reduced melanocyte ad-hesion and survival, and others. Although each of these may play a role in individual patients, evidence is mount-ing that the underlying factor allowing or promoting me-lanocyte targeting is autoimmune in nature.

Clinical Presentation

The clinical presentation of vitiligo is varied, but almost always includes depigmented, white patches and macules. Classically, it presents as symmetric, well-demarcated, de-pigmented patches that favor the scalp, face, neck, fore-arms, waist, genitalia, knees, and dorsal hands and feet (Figure 8-1A-C). It favors areas of repetitive stress or trauma

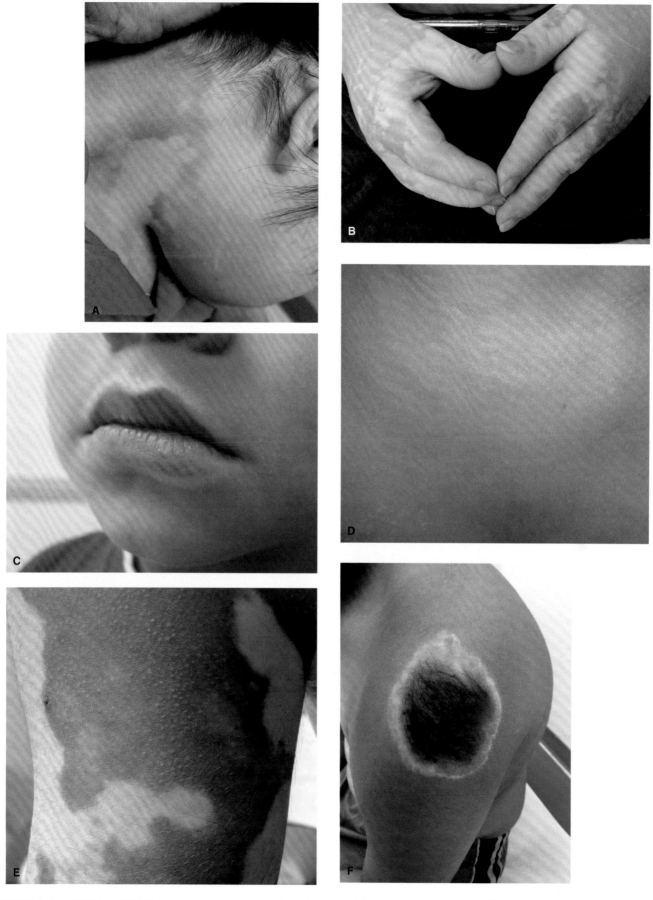

FIGURE 8-1. Vitiligo. (A) Well-demarcated, depigmented, coalescing patches on the neck of a boy with Down syndrome. (B) Symmetric patches on the hands. Note linear depigmentation on the wrist, representing trauma-induced vitiligo, or Koebner phenomenon. Rough nails (trachyonychia) are also seen. (C) Perioral depigmentation. (D) Marginal inflammatory vitiligo with an erythematous, raised border. (E) Trichrome vitiligo, with three distinct shades of pigmentation. (F) A halo congenital nevus, with a depigmented patch around a typical, medium-sized congenital nevus. The patient had patches of vitiligo on his knees as well.

like joints or backs of the hands and can manifest the Koebner phenomena. Widespread cases may affect any surface, and in severe cases, near-total depigmentation may occur. In patients with light skin, depigmented patches may be subtle and difficult to detect without the aid of a Wood's lamp.

Segmental vitiligo, typically unilateral and confined to a single segment of the body with a sharp midline demarcation, shares many clinical features of nonsegmental vitiligo, but is likely predisposed by somatic mutation in a susceptibility gene, as described earlier. It is not typically associated with other autoimmune conditions, but may respond to standard therapies.

Inflammatory vitiligo may present with a raised, thread-like rim of linear erythema at the border (Figure 8-1D), which may indicate active spread, but often remains stable for many months. Trichrome vitiligo (Figure 8-1E), in which three distinct shades of pigmentation are visible within a body area, and vitiligo with confetti-like depigmented macules sometimes occur, and may portend a poor prognosis with rapid progression.[12] Patches of vitiligo on hair-bearing areas may present with poliosis, or depigmented, white hair. Halo nevi (Figure 8-1F), which are melanocytic nevi with a surrounding depigmented patch, are often associated with vitiligo and are sometimes the first sign of disease.[13]

Spontaneous repigmentation sometimes occurs and can be hastened by a number of immunosuppressive treatment modalities. This repigmentation may be from peripheral extension (as occurs with topical steroid treatment) or may appear as perifollicular pigmented macules (as occurs with phototherapy) within the lesion from a follicular source of melanocytes.

The morbidity of vitiligo is primarily evident in its impact on the quality of life. Affected children and adults often suffer from significant psychosocial stress, depression, and anxiety.[14,15]

Histologic Findings

Although vitiligo is primarily a clinical diagnosis, biopsy may sometimes be necessary to differentiate it from other diseases of hypo-or depigmentation. At scanning magnification, biopsy specimens may appear completely unremarkable. Well-developed lesions are characterized by a complete absence of melanocytes and pigment (Figure 8-2). The absence of pigment may be confirmed by negative

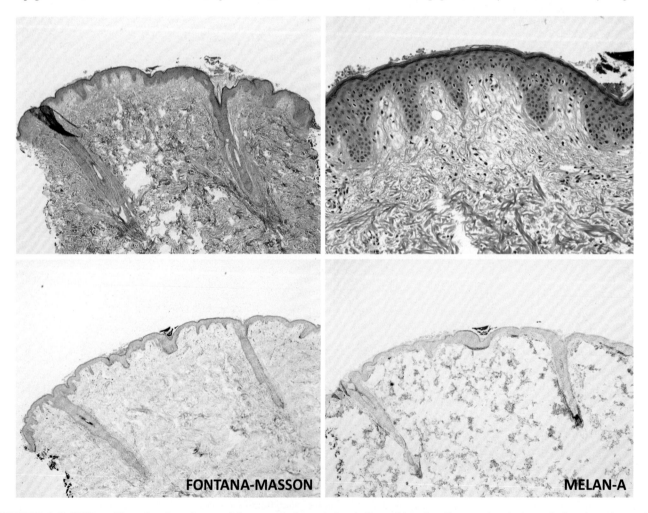

FONTANA-MASSON

MELAN-A

FIGURE 8-2. Vitiligo. There is a broad area of decreased pigmentation in the epidermis with occasional pigmented melanophages in the dermis. A Fontana–Masson stain highlights the marked reduced presence of melanin pigment in the epidermis. A Melan-A immunostain shows a marked reduction in the density of melanocytes throughout the lesion.

Fontana–Masson staining, and a lack of melanocytes may be evident by immunohistochemical studies. Inflammation is sometimes present, both in specimens that appear clinically inflammatory and in those that do not, in the form of a mild superficial lymphohistiocytic infiltrate. A more exuberant, lichenoid interface dermatitis is sometimes seen, and can appear in clinically inflamed areas, depigmented areas, and even distant, clinically uninvolved skin.[16]

Differential Diagnosis

There is a broad clinical differential diagnosis for vitiligo. Hypopigmented lesions may sometimes be difficult to differentiate from depigmented lesions, and can be present in many conditions, including nevus depigmentosus/pigmentary mosaicism, pityriasis alba, and tinea versicolor (Figure 8-3). Postinflammatory hypo-and depigmentation should be preceded by inflammation, although a history of skin inflammation is not always elicited. Chemical leukoderma may present with a strikingly similar pattern to that of vitiligo and is often occupational in nature.

Conditions of congenital depigmentation, such as Waardenburg syndrome or piebaldism, should be considered for midline patches affecting the face and trunk. These patches may sometimes be present on the extremities as well. Syndromic vitiligo may be seen in Vogt-Koyanagi-Harada, Alezzandrini syndrome, and autoimmune polyendocrinopathy candidiasis-ectodermal dystrophy syndromes.

The histologic differential diagnosis includes chemical leukoderma, piebaldism, and nevus depigmentosus. These may be indistinguishable from vitiligo and require clinical history to differentiate. In inflammatory lesions, vitiligo may mimic lichenoid dermatoses such as lichen planus and its subtypes. These conditions lack clinical depigmentation, although hypopigmented lesions may appear similar to early lesions of vitiligo. Finally, patch-stage mycosis fungoides (MF) and inflammatory lesions of vitiligo may share clinical and histopathologic findings. MF, however, should have some degree of

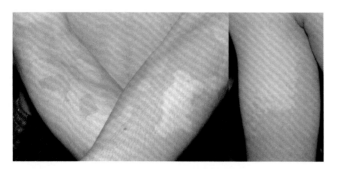

FIGURE 8-3. Tinea versicolor. Widespread tinea versicolor mimicking vitiligo. Note the peripheral, scalloped border indicating coalescing macules. Clinically, the presence of fine scale and the retention of some pigment differentiates tinea versicolor from vitiligo, and the two can be easily distinguished by histology.

lymphocytic atypia, and Pautrier microabscesses may be present. In some cases, multiple biopsies may be necessary to distinguish the two entities.

CAPSULE SUMMARY

VITILIGO

Vitiligo is a common, multifactorial, polygenic condition of autoimmune melanocyte loss. Patients often present in childhood with well-demarcated, depigmented macules and patches. The histologic findings include loss of epidermal melanocytes and pigment, as well as occasional inflammation, which is sometimes quite intense.

OCULOCUTANEOUS ALBINISM

Definition and Epidemiology

Oculocutaneous albinism (OCA) is a group of autosomal dominant, inherited disorders of melanin synthesis. Patients present at birth with variable hypopigmentation of skin, hair, and eyes. There are seven subtypes of nonsyndromic OCA, with types 1 to 4 accounting for the majority of reported cases.[17,18]

The incidence of OCA is estimated at 1 in 17 000 live births in the United States. Incidence in some worldwide populations is as high as 1 in 500 to 1 in 100 including in some areas of Africa and in native populations in North and South America (as high as 1 in 92).[19] The most common form is OCA2, with prevalence estimated at 1 in 36 000 for Caucasian individuals and 1 in 3900 to 10 000 for those of African descent.[20] OCA4 is the most common type in Japan, and OCA5-7 are rare, having been described in only one to a few families each.[21-25]

Etiology

Several genes-encoding proteins crucial for melanin synthesis have been identified as etiologic factors in OCA. Tyrosinase (TYR) is a key enzyme in the melanin production pathway, catalyzing the conversion of tyrosine to dopaquinone, a precursor of melanin. Absence or deficiency of TYR activity, as seen in OCA1a and OCA1b, results in diffuse depigmentation. P protein is a factor in the synthesis of melanosomes as well as typical processing and transport of TYR and Tyrosinase-related protein 1 (TYRP1). TYRP1 is a catalyst for the oxidation of 5,6-dihydroxyindole-2-carboxylic acid, another melanin precursor. TYRP1 and membrane-associated transporter protein are involved in the transport of TYR from the endoplasmic reticulum into melanosomes.

Clinical Presentation

Clinically, OCA is characterized by variable degrees of congenital pigmentary dilution of skin, eyes, and hair (Table 8-1). The lifetime development of pigmentation in affected patients is variable, with some patients devoid of pigment throughout life (as in OCA1a) and others able to create lentigines and melanocytic nevi. Ocular involvement includes characteristic translucent blue irides, hypopigmented retinal fundus, and nystagmus. In young adulthood, accelerated photoaging (telangiectasias, rhytids) are seen, in addition to actinic cheilitis, actinic keratoses, and skin malignancies.[26] Squamous cell carcinoma and basal cell carcinoma are more common than melanoma, which, when present, is often amelanotic.[26,27] OCA can be associated

with significant psychosocial stress and, in some areas of the world, physical threat of assault or death caused by cultural conceptions surrounding albinism.[28]

Histologic Findings

Melanocytes are normal in number and morphology, but there is reduced or absent melanin, as can be seen with Fontana–Masson staining. Hair follicle melanin may be preserved in some forms of OCA.

Differential Diagnosis

The primary clinical differential diagnoses include syndromic causes of OCA, such as Hermansky-Pudlak,

TABLE 8-1.	Causes and clinical features of oculocutaneous albinism.	
Variant	**Gene/Etiology**	**Clinical Manifestations**
OCA1A[26,27,29-32]	TYR mutation—lack of protein *tyrosinase-negative OCA*	**Cutaneous:** White skin and hair, blue irises. Hair may develop yellowish discoloration with age. Highest risk of premature photoaging and cutaneous malignancies. **Ocular:** Photophobia, nystagmus, strabismus, and reduced visual acuity (often legally blind) **Associations:** ADHD
OCA1B[29,30]	TYR—reduced activity of protein *tyrosinase-negative OCA*	**Cutaneous:** Yellow Mutant Variant: Hair turns yellow in first few years; gradually pigments to blonde/light brown. Platinum Variant: Small amounts of pigment with metallic tinge in childhood Minimal Pigment Variant: Pigment develops in eyes only.
OCA1—Temperature Sensitive[29,30]	TYR—high temperature-dependent reduced activity of protein	**Cutaneous:** Born with white skin and hair, blue eyes. During the second decade of life, develop pigmentation at extremities and acral sites.
OCA2[33]	P protein	**Cutaneous:** Brown albinism: Slight to moderate pigmentary dilution in skin, hair, and eyes. Increased pigmentation including lentigines and nevi develop at sun-exposed sites. Lower risk of skin cancer. **Ocular:** Less severe ocular manifestations **Associations:** ~1% of patients with Angelman or Prader-Willi syndromes due to contiguous deletions on chromosome 15
OCA3 (Rufous OCA)[34,35]	Tyrosinase-related protein 1 TRYP1	Red hair, reddish-bronze skin, and blue or brown irises.
OCA4[36]	MATP	Similar to OCA2
OCA5[22]	Unknown (mutation at 4q24)	**Cutaneous:** Golden hair and white skin **Ocular:** Nystagmus, photophobia, foveal hypoplasia, and reduced visual acuity
OCA6[23,24]	SLC24A5	**Cutaneous:** Blond hair that darkens with age, white skin **Ocular:** Translucent light eyes (brown, green, or blue), nystagmus, photophobia, foveal hypoplasia
OCA7[25]	c10orf11	**Cutaneous:** Light skin, pale blond to light brown hair **Ocular:** Light blue or green eyes, nystagmus, mild photophobia

Abbreviations: ADHD, attention deficit disorder; MATP, membrane-associated transporter protein; OCA, oculocutaneous albinism; TYR, tyrosinase; TYRP1, tyrosinase-related protein 1.

Griscelli, and Chédiak-Higashi syndromes, which are discussed later in this chapter.

Histologically, other dermatoses with subtle findings of dyspigmentation may be considered. Vitiligo lacks melanocytes, and tinea versicolor has conspicuous fungal elements in the stratum corneum that should be seen on routine hematoxylin and eosin-stained sections.

CAPSULE SUMMARY

OCULOCUTANEOUS ALBINISM

This is a group of heritable disorders of melanin synthesis that presents with variable hypopigmentation and depigmentation of the skin, hair, and eyes. Patients are often at markedly increased risk of cutaneous and ocular malignancy. Histologically, OCA is characterized by a lack of melanin, but a normal number of melanocytes.

HERMANSKY-PUDLAK SYNDROME

Definition and Epidemiology

Hermansky-Pudlak syndrome (HPS) is a group of autosomal recessive heritable disorders characterized by pigmentary dilution, platelet abnormalities, and accumulation of ceroid-lipofuscin within internal organs.[37-39]

HPS is common among Puerto Ricans, occurring in approximately 1 in 1800 to 1 in 400 people.[37,39] There is also a high incidence among people of Dutch descent and East Indians from Madras. Males and females are equally affected.

Etiology and Clinical Presentation

The genes involved in all subtypes of HPS encode proteins involved in the regulation of vesicular trafficking within lysosome-related organelles, including platelet dense granules and melanosomes.[40-43] Table 8-2 lists gene associations and unique clinical features of the ten described variants of HPS. With the exceptions of HPS2 and 10, the involved genes are organized into functional structures of interacting proteins that participate in vesicular trafficking, known as BLOCs (biogenesis of lysosome-related organelles complex). Specific features of each HPS subtype depend on where each component is expressed: BLOC1 is present in melanosomes and platelet dense granules, BLOC2 is present in melanosomes alone and co-localizes with TYR and TYRP1, and biogenesis of lysosome-related organelles complex 3 (BLOC3) is present in melanosomes, dense granules, and lamellar bodies of type 2 pneumocytes. HPS2 is a subunit of AP-3, which mediates trafficking into lysosomal transport vesicles in multiple tissue types. HPS10 interacts with AP-3.

Patients with HPS exhibit variable pigmentary dilution of the skin and eyes, nystagmus, photophobia, and reduced visual acuity. Many experience systemic manifestations, the most common of which is pulmonary fibrosis, which may be life-threatening.

Hematologic manifestations include bleeding diathesis caused by defective dense granules in platelets.[39] Patients may present with ecchymoses, epistaxis, and menometrorrhagia, but may not be apparent without the use of aspirin or prostaglandin inhibitors. Other rare complications include granulomatous colitis, cardiomyopathy, and renal failure.[44-46] Life expectancy is 30 to 50 years.[37]

TABLE 8-2.	Hermansky-Pudlak syndrome.		
Variant	**Gene**	**Etiology**	**Unique Features**
HPS-1[44]	HPS1	Component of BLOC3	Nystagmus, reduced visual acuity, prolonged bleeding, pulmonary fibrosis, granulomatous colitis (up to 1/3 of patients)
HPS-2	AP3B1	Subunit of AP-3	Nystagmus, reduced visual acuity, prolonged bleeding, neutropenia, recurrent bacterial and viral infections, conductive hearing loss.
HPS-3	HPS3	Component of BLOC2	Nystagmus, reduced visual acuity, mild extraocular manifestation
HPS-4	HPS4	Component of BLOC3	
HPS-5[42]	HPS5	Component of BLOC2	Hypercholesterolemia and hypertriglyceridemia
HPS-6	HPS6	Component of BLOC2	
HPS-7[41]	DTNBP1	Subunits of BLOC1,	
HPS-8[42]	BLOC1S	Subunit of BLOC1	Nystagmus, reduced visual acuity, prolonged bleeding
HPS-9[47]	HPS9/PLDN	Subunit of BLOC1	Nystagmus, immunodeficiency, no bleeding diathesis described to date.
HPS-10	AP3D1	Component of AP-3	Severe neurologic disease with developmental delay and refractory seizures, immunodeficiency.

Abbreviations: AP-3, adaptor protein; BLOC, biogenesis of lysosome-related organelles complex; DNTBP1, dystrobrevin binding protein 1; HPS, Hermansky-Pudlak syndrome; PLDN, Pallidin.

Histologic Findings

There are no specific histologic findings in HPS. Ultrastructural studies reveal a reduction in mature melanosomes.

Differential Diagnosis

The clinical differential diagnosis includes OCA, Chédiak-Higashi syndrome, Griscelli syndrome, and ectrodactyly, ectodermal dysplasia, and clefting. HPS can be differentiated by the presence of bleeding diathesis in most patients, as well as other systemic findings such as pulmonary fibrosis and colitis.

CAPSULE SUMMARY

HERMANSKY-PUDLAK SYNDROME

This is a group of genetic diseases that feature pigmentary dilution of the skin, hair, and eyes, as well as bleeding diathesis in most subtypes. It is a disorder of lysosomal vesicular trafficking.

CHÉDIAK-HIGASHI SYNDROME

Definition and Epidemiology

Chédiak-Higashi Syndrome (CHS) is an autosomal recessive, heritable disorder characterized by silvery hair, grayish skin pigmentary dilution, and immunodeficiency caused by mutations in LYST, a lysosomal transport protein.[37,48,49] It is a rare condition that has been described in patients worldwide. There is no gender predilection.

Etiology

LYST regulates fusion of primary lysozyme-like structures within cells, and its dysfunction results in an inability to properly target and transfer lysosomal vesicles.[48] Giant granules accumulate within the cells of affected tissues, represented by giant melanosomes in melanocytes, dense granules in platelets, and abnormal peroxidase-positive granules in neutrophils.[50] The functional result is an inability to transfer melanosomes to keratinocytes and to degranulate platelets and neutrophils.

Clinical Presentation

The primary cutaneous findings are congenital pigmentary dilution and silver hair that is relatively gray in comparison with other pigmentary dilution syndromes (Figure 8-4).[49] In darkly pigmented patients, hyperpigmentation may be present on acral sites.[51,52] Ocular findings include photophobia, strabismus, and nystagmus, whereas visual acuity tends to be normal.

The primary morbidity of CHS results from hematologic and immunologic defects that result from defective lysosomal function and manifest as recurrent skin,

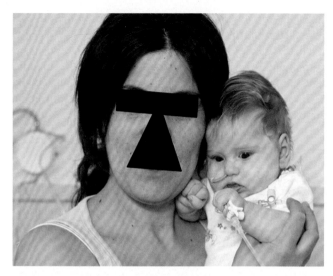

FIGURE 8-4. **Chédiak-Higashi syndrome.** Fair hair and skin in an affected patient. From Nielsen C, Agergaard CN, Jakobsen MA, Møller MB, Fisker N, Barington T. Infantile hemophagocytic lymphohistiocytosis in a case of Chediak-Higashi syndrome caused by a mutation in the LYST/CHS1 Gene presenting with delayed umbilical cord detachment and diarrhea. *J Pediatr Hematol Oncol.* 2015;37(2):e73-e79.

upper respiratory, and pulmonary infections, primarily by *Staphylococcal* and *Streptococcal* species. The majority of patients eventually suffer from a life-threatening "accelerated phase" in the first decade of life, involving diffuse visceral infiltration with lymphoid and histiocytic cells.[50,53] This represents an inherited form of hemophagocytic lymphohistiocytosis (HLH) that is triggered by infection with Epstein–Barr virus, and is associated with anemia, bleeding, and overwhelming infection that typically leads to death at a mean age of 6 years. A minority of patients have less severe mutations and survive into adulthood.[54] These patients experience progressive neurologic deterioration including gait change, paresthesias, and dysesthesias.

Histologic Findings

The primarily microscopic finding in CHS is clumping of melanin in hair (Figure 8-5). The clumping is regularly spaced in contrast to Griscelli syndrome. There is no specific skin histologic finding, although giant melanosomes can sometimes be seen in affected patients.

Differential Diagnosis

The primary differential diagnoses are the other so-called silvery hair syndromes including Griscelli syndrome. Griscelli syndrome type 2 also manifests with an HLH-like phenotype that is very similar to the accelerated phase of CHS.[55] Table 8-3 compares salient differences among selected pigmentary dilution syndromes.

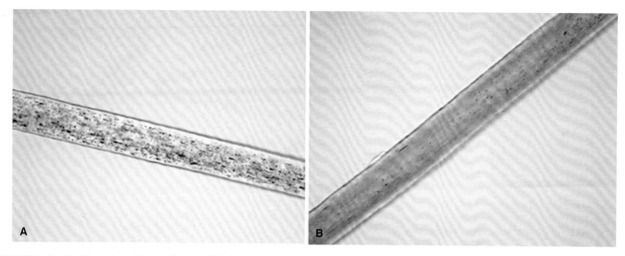

FIGURE 8-5. Chédiak-Higashi syndrome. (A) Clumped melanin granules in the hair shaft of an affected patient. (B) Normal hair shaft with homogenous pigmentation. From Nielsen C, Agergaard CN, Jakobsen MA, Møller MB, Fisker N, Barington T. Infantile hemophagocytic lymphohistiocytosis in a case of Chediak-Higashi syndrome caused by a mutation in the LYST/CHS1 Gene presenting with delayed umbilical cord detachment and diarrhea. *J Pediatr Hematol Oncol.* 2015;37(2):e73-e79.

CAPSULE SUMMARY

CHÉDIAK-HIGASHI SYNDROME

CHS is an autosomal recessive genodermatosis featuring gray-silvery skin and hair, light eyes, and immunodeficiency due to granulocyte dysfunction. It is caused by a lysosomal trafficking defect. Patients often succumb to a HLH syndrome during the first decade of life. Microscopic findings include clumped melanin in hair, occasionally enlarged melanosomes in the skin, and giant granules in neutrophils on peripheral smear.

GRISCELLI SYNDROME

Definition and Epidemiology

Griscelli syndrome (GS) is a group of rare, autosomal recessive genetic disorders with common cutaneous findings of silvery hair and pigmentary dilution.[57] Type 1 GS, including the variant Elejalde syndrome, is associated with neurologic deficits, Type 2 GS with immunodeficiency and risk for HLH,[55] and Type 3 GS with pigmentary changes only.[57]

GS is quite rare, with fewer than 100 cases reported worldwide, with the majority from Turkey and India. Males and females are equally affected.

Etiology

GS is caused by mutations in vesicular trafficking-associated proteins. Type 1 is caused by mutation in myosin Va (MYO5A), which is expressed in melanocytes and the nervous system, and binds melanosomes to actin filaments for transport throughout the cell. Type 2 results from mutation in RAB27A, a GTP-binding protein involved in melanosome transfer. It is also expressed in hematopoietic cells and is required for exocytosis of cytolytic granules. Type 3 is caused by mutations in melanophilin, which is found only in the skin, and interacts with MYO5A and RAB27A to facilitate melanosome transport.[58] Ultimately, the inability to efficiently traffic melanosomes leads to accumulation within melanocytes and pigmentary dilution.

Clinical Presentation

The cutaneous features of grayish pigmentary dilution, blue irides, and silvery hair are common to all three types of

TABLE 8-3.	Comparison of pigmentary dilution syndromes	
Syndrome	Hematologic Findings	Hair Shaft
Hermansky-Pudlak Syndrome	Abnormal platelet dense granules leading to bleeding diathesis in most types	Hypertrichosis of the lashes and trichomegaly in some types[56]
Chédiak-Higashi Syndrome	Lymphohistiocytic infiltration within first decade, pancytopenia present, giant inclusions in circulating neutrophils	Giant melanosomes (smaller than in Griscelli) at evenly spaced intervals
Griscelli Syndrome[55]	Lymphohistiocytic infiltration tends to occur within first year in Type 2, pancytopenia present	Larger, irregularly spaced giant melanosomes

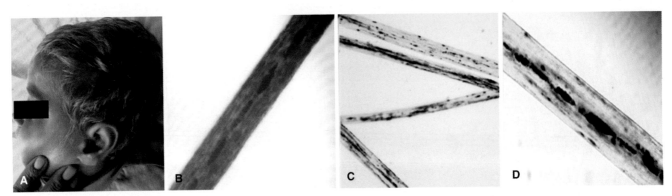

FIGURE 8-6. **Griscelli syndrome.** (A) Silvery hair and light skin in an affected patient. (B) Normal hair with uniform pigmentation. (C and D) Clumped melanin granules in a hair shaft from an affected patient. Reprinted with permission from Saini AG, Nagaraju S, Sahu JK, et al. Teaching NeuroImages: Griscelli syndrome and CNS lymphohistiocytosis. *Neurology.* 2014;82(14):e122-e123.

GS and are similar to those seen in CHS (Figure 8-6). Granulomatous skin lesions can also be seen in types 1 and 2.[59,60] Additional clinical features are related to extracutaneous sites of gene expression. Type 1 GS demonstrates neurologic findings of developmental delay, hypotonia, and seizures. Elejalde syndrome presents with the most severe findings, including profound psychomotor delay.[57,61-63] Type 2 GS presents with immune deficiency (reduced T-cell mediated cytotoxicity and exocytosis of cytolytic granules), as well as severe, life-threatening HLH after Epstein-Barr virus infection.[55] Type 3 GS features pigmentary changes only; there is no associated immunologic or neurologic deficit.

Histologic Findings

The characteristic microscopic finding in GS is clumped melanin within hair shafts. It tends to be finer and more irregular than that seen in CHS. Histologically, melanin is absent in keratinocytes, but mature melanosomes may be seen within melanocytes.

Differential Diagnosis

Other cutaneous pigmentary dilution syndromes such as CHS and HPS should be considered. There is significant overlap between type 2 GS and CHS, and they may be difficult to differentiate with a trichogram. Thus, genetic testing may be required for definitive diagnosis.

CAPSULE SUMMARY

GRISCELLI SYNDROME

GS is a group of three disorders caused by a failure of cellular vesicle transport that results in pigmentary dilution and silvery hair. Neurologic manifestations and immune deficiency are type-specific and may be severe and life-threatening. Histologic findings are subtle, with mature melanosomes in melanocytes and absence in keratinocytes. Trichogram shows characteristic melanin clumping.

PIEBALDISM

Definition and Epidemiology

Piebaldism is an autosomal dominant congenital disorder featuring congenital patterned depigmented patches on the skin and focal patches of white hair caused by an absence of melanosomes. The exact frequency is not known, but it is an uncommon disorder that occurs in all races, equally in males and females.

Etiology

Causative mutations have been identified in the protooncogene KIT as well as Snail homolog 2 (SNAI2/SLUG).[64,65] KIT encodes a cell surface receptor for stem cell growth factor and mast cell growth factor and is essential for normal neural crest cell migration during embryogenesis. These neural crest cells, from which melanocytes are derived, migrate during fetal development from the dorsal side where they originate, to the ventral side. Failure of cells to complete migration to the anterior midline likely results in the characteristic pattern of involvement. The interaction between KIT and its ligand may also be required for survival of melanocytes, which may also play a role in this phenotype.[66]

Clinical Presentation

The characteristic feature, present in approximately 80% to 90% of affected patients, is a white forelock.[67,68] (Figure 8-7A) Well-demarcated, leukoderma is also seen in the midline on the face (primarily forehead, eyebrows, nose, and chin), on the anterior trunk, and on the ventral extremities (Figure 8-7B and C). Islands of normal pigment or even hyperpigmentation may occasionally be seen within depigmented patches, and these patches are concave at the border. This is in contrast to the lack of islands of sparing and the convex borders of most vitiligo patches. Depigmentation tends to persist throughout life.

Histologic Findings

Melanocytes are absent in skin and hair follicles of affected skin. Perilesional hyperpigmented skin can be seen

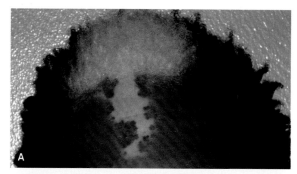
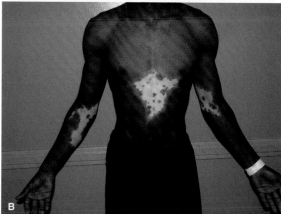
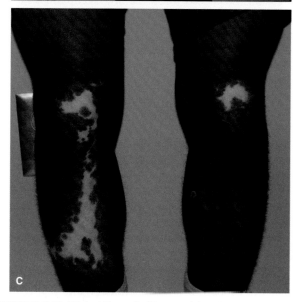

FIGURE 8-7. **Piebaldism.** A 17-year-old male with piebaldism, with (A) a white forelock and leukoderma of the forehead and anterior trunk and extremities. (B and C) Note poliosis of the affected area on the legs as well. Multiple male and female family members were affected.

histologically as hyperpigmentation of melanocytes and keratinocytes as well.

Differential Diagnosis

The primary differential diagnoses for piebaldism include vitiligo, an acquired autoimmune destruction of melanocytes. These may appear histologically identical and require clinical correlation for differentiation. Waardenburg syndrome may present with piebaldism-type pigmentary abnormalities as an associated feature, but patients present with characteristic facies, sensorineural hearing loss, and other systemic findings.

CAPSULE SUMMARY

PIEBALDISM

Piebaldism is a congenital, autosomal dominant condition that presents with leukoderma along the midline and ventral extremities. It is caused by mutation in KIT and tends to persist throughout life. Histologically, it is characterized by a complete lack of melanocytes in affected skin.

WAARDENBURG SYNDROME

Definition and Epidemiology

Waardenburg syndrome (WS) is a group of autosomal dominant disorders characterized by heterochromia irides, piebald depigmentation, and often congenital deafness.[69] The most common form is WS1.[70] Initially described in the Netherlands, WS has been reported worldwide. Males and females are equally affected.

Etiology and Clinical Presentation

There are four major types of WS, described in Table 8-4. The presentation is highly variable, even within family members and monozygotic twins.[71] In general, WS is caused by abnormalities in the development of neural crest derivatives. These abnormalities may manifest as failure to migrate and localize to the appropriate tissue, failure of survival signals, and failure of proper differentiation (Figure 8-8).

Histologic Findings and Differential Diagnosis

Skin biopsy specimens show a lack of melanocytes, which can be confirmed with immunohistochemical studies. The differential diagnosis includes vitiligo and piebaldism, which can be easily differentiated by clinical history.

CAPSULE SUMMARY

WAARDENBURG SYNDROME

WS is a group of genetic disorders characterized by a dysgenesis of neural crest derivatives in multiple tissues. Patients with type 1 WS, the most common type, may present with a white forelock. Heterochromia irides and dysmorphic facies may also be seen in some types.

TABLE 8-4.	Features and causes of Waardenburg syndrome					
WS Type	Gene	Etiology	White Forelock/Cutaneous Depigmentation	Congenital Deafness	Unique Clinical Features
WS1[72,73]	PAX3	Loss of function of PAX3 gene involved in melanocyte migration and facial embryogenesis	30-45%	47-58%	Atypical facies: broad nasal root, dystopia canthorum, *heterochromia irides, spina bifida*
WSII[74-76]	MITF—15-21% SOX10—15% SNAI/SLUG	Transcription factors involved in neural crest development and migration		80%	Normal facies; heterochromic irides, strabismus
WSIII[75]	PAX3	See WSI			Musculoskeletal abnormalities, neural tube defects
WSIV[77-82]	EDN3 EDNRB SOX10				Normal facies; Hirschsprung disease

Abbreviations: EDN3, endothelin-3; EDNRB, endothelin B receptor; MITF, microphthalmia-associated transcription factor; SOX10, sex-determining region Y-box10; WS, Waardenburg syndrome.

CHEMICALLY INDUCED PIGMENTATION

Definition

A wide variety of chemicals and drugs can result in changes in skin pigmentation. Patients may present with hyper- or hypopigmentation, or even depigmentation. Causative agents include topical and systemic medications, home products, foods, and occupational exposures.

Etiology, Clinical Presentation, and Histologic Findings

Dyspigmentation may occur by a number of mechanisms, including deposition of exogenous pigment, external

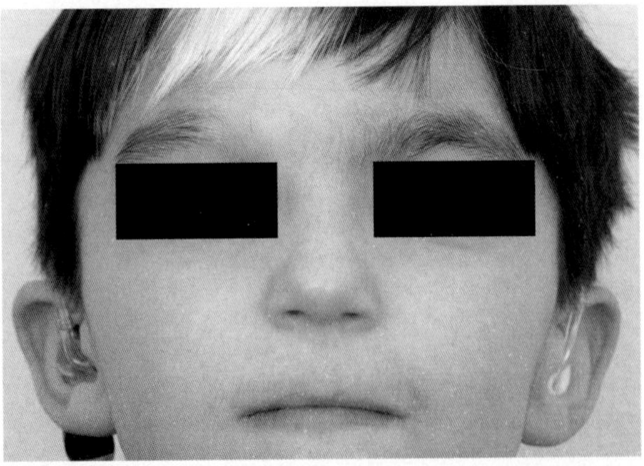

FIGURE 8-8. **Waardenburg syndrome.** An affected boy with white forelock and dystopia canthorum. From Kontorinis G, Lenarz T, Giourgas A, Durisin M, Lesinski-Schiedat A. Outcomes and special considerations of cochlear implantation in Waardenburg syndrome. *Otol Neurotol.* 2011;32(6):951-955.

binding to the skin and staining, and destruction of melanocytes through chemical or immune processes. For some chemicals, exposure to the offending agent must be followed by sun exposure for development of the dermatosis (Figures 8-9 and 8-10). The pattern of pigmentation depends on the mechanism, route, and means of exposure to the chemical, as well as the mechanism of deposition in the skin (hematogenous, eccrine sweat, etc) (Figures 8-11 and 8-12). Table 8-5 outlines a number of different chemicals and their clinical presentations.

The histopathologic features vary widely on the basis of chemical reaction and the mechanism of dyspigmentation. Salient features are listed in Table 8-5.

IDIOPATHIC GUTTATE HYPOMELANOSIS

Definition and Epidemiology

Idiopathic guttate hypomelanosis (IGH) is a common condition characterized by the development of white macules on sun-exposed areas. It occurs in males and females equally, and the incidence increases with age. IGH is traditionally a condition of middle-aged and elderly individuals, although in one study of 47 Korean patients, 30% were affected before the age of 20.[88]

Etiology

As implied by the name, the causes of IGH are not well understood. HLA-DQ3 has been shown to be associated with IGH in patients with renal transplants, suggesting an autoimmune cause.[89] Other proposed factors include senescence, trauma, and sun damage.

TABLE 8-5.	Chemically induced pigmentation			
Chemical/Dermatosis	**Source**	**Route of Exposure**	**Clinical Presentation**	**Histologic Findings**
Furocoumarins/ Phytophotodermatitis	Plants—lime, parsley, celery, parsnip, hogweed, fennel, fig	Topical with photoactivation and resultant inflammation	Phytophotodermatitis— Bizarre, linear, or geometric arrays of erythema, vesicles, or hyperpigmentation (Figure 8-9A)	Phototoxic pattern—Apoptotic keratinocytes with variable spongiosis and superficial dermal lymphohistiocytic inflammation, occasional neutrophils and eosinophils (Figure 8-9B)
p-Phenylenediamine	Dyes, black henna	Topical staining, allergic contact dermatitis	Black staining, eczematous dermatitis, postinflammatory dyspigmentation	For contact dermatitis, spongiotic dermatitis with eosinophils
Minocycline hyperpigmentation	Minocycline	Ingestion	Three types: 1) Blue-black in scars 2) Blue-gray over the shins 3) Diffuse brown in sun-exposed areas	1. Iron deposition 2. Iron and melanin deposition 3. Melanin deposition[83]
Antimalarial hyperpigmentation	Chloroquine, hydroxychloroquine,	Ingestion	Gray-blue over the shins, face, nails	Yellow-brown granules within histiocytes, stain with Fontana–Masson[84]
Hydroquinone/ Ochronosis	Hydroquinone	Topical application	Blue-black on areas of exposure	Yellow-brown, amorphous deposition in dermis
Phenols, Chatecols[85]/ Chemical leukoderma	Anticorrosive agents, varnishes, adhesives, disinfectants, rubber items	Cytotoxic effect, possibly competition with tyrosine in melanocytes	White macules and patches in exposed areas, typically hands, arms, and sometimes face (Figure 8-10)	Loss of melanocytes
Silver/Argyria	Silver salts, amalgam fillings	Topical (mining, silverwork), consumption of colloidal silver	Gray to blue to silver patches, frequently on sun-exposed sites, mucosal surfaces	Small, black granules on elastic fibers and around eccrine glands (Figure 8-11)
Carotenemia[86,87]	Carrots, squash, sweet potatoes	Excessive consumption, diabetes, thyroid disease	Diffuse orange/yellow pigmentation, concentrated on acral sites	Occasional epidermal intercellular autofluorescence
Juglone[85]	Fresh walnuts	Topical, binding/ staining	Brown-black pigmentation on hands (Figure 8-12)	

Clinical Presentation

Patients present with sharply demarcated, discrete hypopigmented to depigmented macules in sun-exposed areas. They are relatively small (<5 mm) and may be few or number in the hundreds. They anterior legs and dorsal arms are most commonly affected, but other sun-exposed sites may also be involved (Figure 8-13). The face is typically spared.

Histologic Features

The main histologic finding in IGH is a loss of melanin, with a reduction in the normal number of melanocytes (Figure 8-13).

Melanin content may be highlighted by Fontana–Masson staining, but it is often difficult to interpret without an area of normal skin for comparison.[90] The epidermal rete may be flattened, and hyperkeratosis is often present.[88]

Differential Diagnosis

The clinical differential diagnosis includes postinflammatory pigmentary change, vitiligo, atrophy blanche, lichen sclerosis, scar, and tinea versicolor. Postinflammatory hypopigmentation may be difficult to distinguish from IGH on a histologic basis, but should retain a normal number of

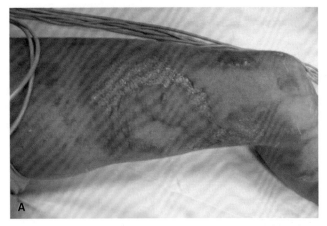

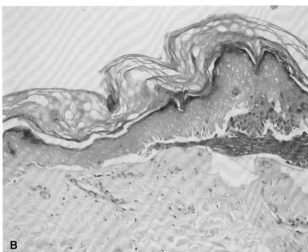

FIGURE 8-9. **Phytophotodermatitis.** (A) A child with geographic blistering and ulceration, with linear erythema and hyperpigmentation after contact with lime juice and concurrent sun exposure. (B) Histologic image of a severe case showing confluent epidermal necrosis with formation of a subepidermal blister. From Darracq MA, Heppner J, Lee H, Armenian P. Backyard pool party: not your typical sunburn. *Pediatr Emerg Care.* 2017;33(6):440-442.

melanocytes, and should be preceded by a history of an inflammatory lesion. Vitiligo will lack melanocytes in affected skin. Atrophie blanche, lichen sclerosis, scar, and tinea versicolor are easily differentiated on routine histology.

CAPSULE SUMMARY

IDIOPATHIC GUTTATE HYPOMELANOSIS

IGH is a common, acquired dermatosis characterized by the appearance of white macules on sun-exposed areas. It is most common in adults, but may be seen in children and adolescents. Histologically, it is characterized by a reduction in epidermal melanin and in the total number of melanocytes, with variable flattening of the epidermal rete and hyperkeratosis.

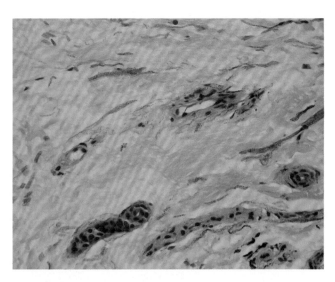

FIGURE 8-11. **Argyria.** Small black granules are deposited on elastic fibers within the dermis and are concentrated around vessels and eccrine coils.

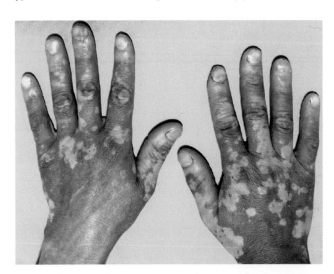

FIGURE 8-10. **Chemical leukoderma.** Depigmented macules on the hands of an adult after the use of rubber gloves. From Bonamonte D, Foti C, Romita P, Vestita M, Angelini G. Colors and contact dermatitis. *Dermatitis.* 2014; 25(4):155-162.

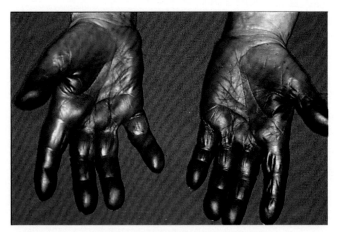

FIGURE 8-12. **Juglone dermatitis.** Black staining of the hands after exposure to fresh walnuts. From Bonamonte D, Foti C, Romita P, Vestita M, Angelini G. Colors and contact dermatitis. *Dermatitis.* 2014; 25(4):155-162.

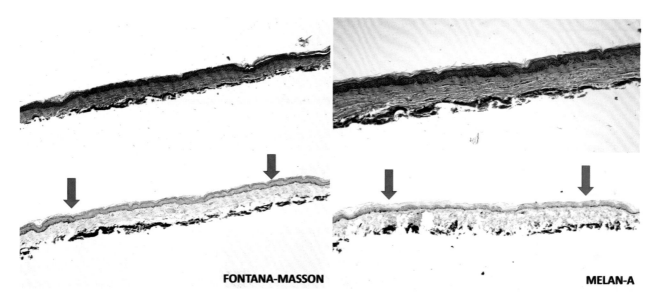

FONTANA-MASSON   MELAN-A

FIGURE 8-13. **Idiopathic guttate hypomelanosis.** In this particular case, the hematoxylin and eosin-stained section is relatively normal, and the most notorious findings can be appreciated only with the use of special stains and immunohistochemistry (IHC). There is a focal and small localized area of reduced pigmentation, present in the Fontana–Masson stain and contained within the arrows. The same area shows a reduced density of melanocytes by a Melan-A immunostain. As opposed to vitiligo, the density is reduced, but not absent.

OCHRONOSIS

Definition and Epidemiology

Ochronosis is pigment deposition in the skin, sclerae, and cartilage in patients with alkaptonuria, an inborn error of metabolism that results in a buildup of homogentisic acid within tissues. Exogenous ochronosis may occur in any individual and is caused by long-term, topical exposure to a number of chemicals, the most common of which is hydroquinone.

Alkaptonuria is rare worldwide, with a frequency of about 1 in 100 000 to 250 000, but reaches 1 in 19 000 in Slovakia.[91] Males and females are equally affected. Exogenous ochronosis is highest in cultures in which lightening creams containing phenols and hydroquinone are used.

Etiology

Alkaptonuria is caused by mutation in homogentisic acid oxidase. The resultant buildup of homogentisic acid in tissues leads to oxidation to benzoquinone acetic acid. This then binds to collagen in the skin, sclerae, and cartilage irreversibly to produce the brown-black pigment that is characteristic of this disease.

The underlying pathophysiology of exogenous ochronosis is not well understood. Exposure to hydroquinone, phenol, benzene, resorcinol, and mercury lead to a similar deposition of pigment on collagen fibers. In both alkaptonuria and exogenous ochronosis, findings are most dramatic on sun-exposed surfaces.

Clinical Presentation

The first sign of alkaptonuria is dark coloration of urine after prolonged exposure of wet diapers to air. Sweat and cerumen may also be affected in the first decade of life. The pigmentary changes of alkaptonuria are typically seen first in the sclerae (Figure 8-14A) in the fifth decade of life, and subsequently on the face, ears, buccal mucosa, nail beds, and within intertriginous regions (Figure 8-14B and C). Cutaneous pigmentation appears as indistinct blue-black, deep macules and patches.

The tympanic membranes, tendons, and cartilage are also affected.[92] Cartilaginous involvement eventually leads to arthritis and degenerative disc disease.[93] Involvement of the tympanic membrane and cartilaginous structures of the inner ear may lead to hearing impairment, tinnitus, or otalgia.[94] Cardiac involvement has rarely been reported to result in valvular dysfunction, and kidney stones may develop.[95]

Exogenous ochronosis is localized to the area of chemical exposure and occurs after prolonged use. The development of ochronosis has led to the banning of high potency hydroquinone-containing over-the-counter products in the United States.

Histologic Findings

Skin biopsies from patients with ochronosis show characteristic yellow-brown, or ochre, deposits within the dermis, often referred to as "banana bodies." Pigment may be seen in the basement membrane at the dermoepidermal junction and surrounding adnexal structures (Figure 8-15).[96]

Differential Diagnosis

The clinical differential diagnosis includes argyria; hyperpigmentation caused by medications such as minocycline,

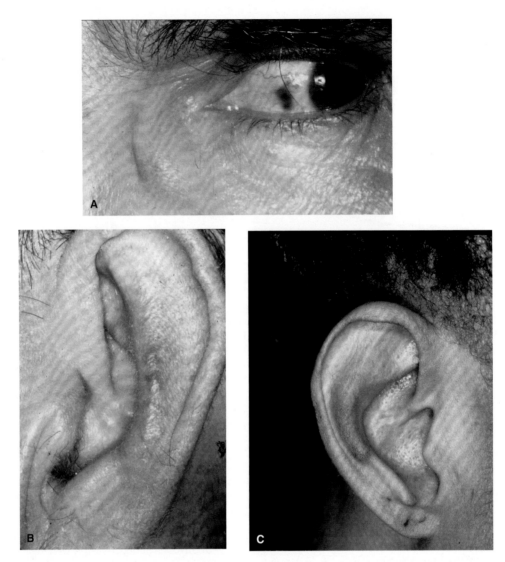

FIGURE 8-14. (A) Scleral pigment in alkaptonuria (B) and (C) blue-black discoloration of cartilaginous ear in alkaptonuria (all three photos: Courtesy of Ken Greer).

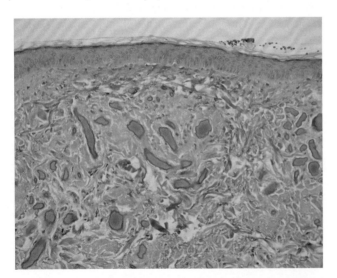

FIGURE 8-15. Ochronosis. Yellow-brown, banana-shaped inclusions within the dermis. Reactive granulomatous inflammation is present in this case.

amiodarone, and bleomycin; and postinflammatory hyperpigmentation. In hydroquinone-induced ochronosis, hyperpigmentation often mimics that seen in melasma or other pigmentary disorders. The distinctive histopathologic findings in ochronosis make diagnosis relatively straightforward on routine histology.

CAPSULE SUMMARY

OCHRONOSIS

Ochronosis is caused by deposition of pigment on collagen fibers in the dermis in patients with alkaptonuria or who have been exposed to hydroquinone or other skin-lightening agents. Patients present with blue-black hyperpigmentation in sun-exposed areas. Alkaptonuria is first indicated by dark discoloration of urine in infants. Histologically, ochronosis is characterized by yellow-brown, well-demarcated, banana-shaped dermal inclusions.

REFERENCES

1. Taieb A, Picardo M, Members V. The definition and assessment of vitiligo: a consensus report of the Vitiligo European Task Force. *Pigment Cell Res.* 2007;20(1):27-35.

2. Prcic S, Djuran V, Mikov A, Mikov I. Vitiligo in children. *Pediatr Dermatol.* 2007;24(6):666.

3. Alkhateeb A, Fain PR, Thody A, Bennett DC, Spritz RA. Epidemiology of vitiligo and associated autoimmune diseases in Caucasian probands and their families. *Pigment Cell Res.* 2003;16(3):208-214.

4. Ezzedine K, Diallo A, Leaute-Labreze C, et al. Pre-vs. post-pubertal onset of vitiligo: multivariate analysis indicates atopic diathesis association in pre-pubertal onset vitiligo. *Br J Dermatol.* 2012;167(3):490-495.

5. Spritz RA. The genetics of generalized vitiligo. *Curr Dir Autoimmun.* 2008;10:244-257.

6. Jin Y, Andersen G, Yorgov D, et al. Genome-wide association studies of autoimmune vitiligo identify 23 new risk loci and highlight key pathways and regulatory variants. *Nat Genet.* 2016;48(11):1418-1424.

7. Ongenae K, Van Geel N, Naeyaert JM. Evidence for an autoimmune pathogenesis of vitiligo. *Pigment Cell Res.* 2003;16(2):90-100.

8. Bystryn JC, Rigel D, Friedman RJ, Kopf A. Prognostic significance of hypopigmentation in malignant melanoma. *Arch Dermatol.* 1987;123(8):1053-1055.

9. Oiso N, Suzuki T, Fukai K, Katayama I, Kawada A. Nonsegmental vitiligo and autoimmune mechanism. *Dermatol Res Pract.* 2011;2011:518090.

10. Handa S, Dogra S. Epidemiology of childhood vitiligo: a study of 625 patients from north India. *Pediatr Dermatol.* 2003;20(3):207-210.

11. Bae JM, Kim M, Lee HH, et al. Increased risk of vitiligo following anti-tumor necrosis factor therapy: a 10-year population-based cohort study. *J Invest Dermatol.* 2018;138(4):768-774.

12. Goh BK, Pandya AG. Presentations, signs of activity, and differential diagnosis of vitiligo. *Dermatol Clin.* 2017;35(2):135-144.

13. Stierman SC, Tierney EP, Shwayder TA. Halo congenital nevocellular nevi associated with extralesional vitiligo: a case series with review of the literature. *Pediatr Dermatol.* 2009;26(4):414-424.

14. Silverberg JI, Silverberg NB. Quality of life impairment in children and adolescents with vitiligo. *Pediatr Dermatol.* 2014;31(3):309-318.

15. Manzoni AP, Weber MB, Nagatomi AR, Pereira RL, Townsend RZ, Cestari TF. Assessing depression and anxiety in the caregivers of pediatric patients with chronic skin disorders. *An Bras Dermatol.* 2013;88(6):894-899.

16. Attili VR, Attili SK. Lichenoid inflammation in vitiligo—a clinical and histopathologic review of 210 cases. *Int J Dermatol.* 2008;47(7):663-669.

17. Gronskov K, Brondum-Nielsen K, Lorenz B, Preising MN. Clinical utility gene card for: oculocutaneous albinism. *Eur J Hum Genet.* 2014;22(8). doi:10.1038/ejhg.2013.307.

18. Montoliu L, Gronskov K, Wei AH, et al. Increasing the complexity: new genes and new types of albinism. *Pigment Cell Melanoma Res.* 2014;27(1):11-18.

19. Woolf CM. Albinism (OCA2) in Amerindians. *Am J Phys Anthropol.* 2005;suppl 41:118-140.

20. Paller AS, Mancini, A. J. Disorders of pigmentation In: Paller AS, Mancini AJ, eds. *Hurwitz Clinical Pediatric Dermatology.* 5th ed. Philadelphia, PA: Elsevier; 2016:245-278.

21. Inagaki K, Suzuki T, Shimizu H, et al. Oculocutaneous albinism type 4 is one of the most common types of albinism in Japan. *Am J Hum Genet.* 2004;74(3):466-471.

22. Kausar T, Bhatti MA, Ali M, Shaikh RS, Ahmed ZM. OCA5, a novel locus for non-syndromic oculocutaneous albinism, maps to chromosome 4q24. *Clin Genet.* 2013;84(1):91-93.

23. Wei AH, Zang DJ, Zhang Z, et al. Exome sequencing identifies SLC24A5 as a candidate gene for nonsyndromic oculocutaneous albinism. *J Invest Dermatol.* 2013;133(7):1834-1840.

24. Morice-Picard F, Lasseaux E, Francois S, et al. SLC24A5 mutations are associated with non-syndromic oculocutaneous albinism. *J Invest Dermatol.* 2014;134(2):568-571.

25. Gronskov K, Dooley CM, Ostergaard E, et al. Mutations in c10orf11, a melanocyte-differentiation gene, cause autosomal-recessive albinism. *Am J Hum Genet.* 2013;92(3):415-421.

26. Kiprono SK, Chaula BM, Beltraminelli H. Histological review of skin cancers in African Albinos: a 10-year retrospective review. *BMC Cancer.* 2014;14:157.

27. Terenziani M, Spreafico F, Serra A, Podda M, Cereda S, Belli F. Amelanotic melanoma in a child with oculocutaneous albinism. *Med Pediatr Oncol.* 2003;41(2):179-180.

28. Ladizinski B, Cruz-Inigo AE, Sethi A. The genocide of individuals with albinism in Africa. *Arch Dermatol.* 2012;148(10):1151.

29. Toyofuku K, Wada I, Spritz RA, Hearing VJ. The molecular basis of oculocutaneous albinism type 1 (OCA1): sorting failure and degradation of mutant tyrosinases results in a lack of pigmentation. *Biochem J.* 2001;355(Pt 2):259-269.

30. King RA, Pietsch J, Fryer JP, et al. Tyrosinase gene mutations in oculocutaneous albinism 1 (OCA1): definition of the phenotype. *Hum Genet.* 2003;113(6):502-513.

31. Russell-Eggitt I. Albinism. *Ophthalmol Clin North Am.* 2001;14(3):533-546.

32. Kutzbach BR, Summers CG, Holleschau AM, MacDonald JT. Neurodevelopment in children with albinism. *Ophthalmology.* 2008;115(10):1805-1808,e1-e2.

33. Brilliant MH. The mouse p (pink-eyed dilution) and human P genes, oculocutaneous albinism type 2 (OCA2), and melanosomal pH. *Pigment Cell Res.* 2001;14(2):86-93.

34. Sarangarajan R, Boissy RE. Tyrp1 and oculocutaneous albinism type 3. *Pigment Cell Res.* 2001;14(6):437-444.

35. Manga P, Kromberg JG, Box NF, Sturm RA, Jenkins T, Ramsay M. Rufous oculocutaneous albinism in southern African Blacks is caused by mutations in the TYRP1 gene. *Am J Hum Genet.* 1997;61(5):1095-1101.

36. Newton JM, Cohen-Barak O, Hagiwara N, et al. Mutations in the human orthologue of the mouse underwhite gene (uw) underlie a new form of oculocutaneous albinism, OCA4. *Am J Hum Genet.* 2001;69(5):981-988.

37. Huizing M, Gahl WA. Disorders of vesicles of lysosomal lineage: the Hermansky-Pudlak syndromes. *Curr Mol Med.* 2002;2(5):451-467.

38. Dessinioti C, Stratigos AJ, Rigopoulos D, Katsambas AD. A review of genetic disorders of hypopigmentation: lessons learned from the biology of melanocytes. *Exp Dermatol.* 2009;18(9):741-749.

39. Huizing M, Helip-Wooley A, Westbroek W, Gunay-Aygun M, Gahl WA. Disorders of lysosome-related organelle biogenesis: clinical and molecular genetics. *Annu Rev Genomics Hum Genet.* 2008;9:359-86.

40. Wei AH, Li W. Hermansky-Pudlak syndrome: pigmentary and non-pigmentary defects and their pathogenesis. *Pigment Cell Melanoma Res.* 2013;26(2):176-192.

41. Li W, Zhang Q, Oiso N, et al. Hermansky-Pudlak syndrome type 7 (HPS-7) results from mutant dysbindin, a member of the biogenesis of lysosome-related organelles complex 1 (BLOC-1). *Nat Genet.* 2003;35(1):84-89.

42. Huizing M, Hess R, Dorward H, et al. Cellular, molecular and clinical characterization of patients with Hermansky-Pudlak syndrome type 5. *Traffic.* 2004;5(9):711-722.

43. Morgan NV, Pasha S, Johnson CA, et al. A germline mutation in BLOC1S3/reduced pigmentation causes a novel variant of Hermansky-Pudlak syndrome (HPS8). *Am J Hum Genet.* 2006;78(1):160-166.

44. Mahadeo R, Markowitz J, Fisher S, Daum F. Hermansky-Pudlak syndrome with granulomatous colitis in children. *J Pediatr.* 1991;118(6):904-906.

45. Salvaggio HL, Graeber KE, Clarke LE, Schlosser BJ, Orlow SJ, Clarke JT. Mucocutaneous granulomatous disease in a patient with Hermansky-Pudlak syndrome. *JAMA Dermatol.* 2014;150(10):1083-1087.

46. Harada T, Ishimatsu Y, Nakashima S, et al. An autopsy case of Hermansky-Pudlak syndrome: a case report and review of the literature on treatment. *Intern Med.* 2014;53(23):2705-2709.

47. Cullinane AR, Curry JA, Carmona-Rivera C, et al. A BLOC-1 mutation screen reveals that PLDN is mutated in Hermansky-Pudlak Syndrome type 9. *Am J Hum Genet.* 2011;88(6):778-787.

48. Ward DM, Shiflett SL, Kaplan J. Chediak-Higashi syndrome: a clinical and molecular view of a rare lysosomal storage disorder. *Curr Mol Med.* 2002;2(5):469-477.

49. Kaplan J, De Domenico I, Ward DM. Chediak-Higashi syndrome. *Curr Opin Hematol.* 2008;15(1):22-29.

50. Dinauer MC. Disorders of neutrophil function: an overview. *Methods Mol Biol*. 2007;412:489-504.

51. Anderson LL, Paller AS, Malpass D, Schmidt ML, Berger TG. Chediak-Higashi syndrome in a black child. *Pediatr Dermatol*. 1992;9(1):31-36.

52. Al-Khenaizan S. Hyperpigmentation in Chediak-Higashi syndrome. *J Am Acad Dermatol*. 2003;49(5 suppl):S244-S246.

53. Ahluwalia J, Pattari S, Trehan A, Marwaha RK, Garewal G. Accelerated phase at initial presentation: an uncommon occurrence in Chediak-Higashi syndrome. *Pediatr Hematol Oncol*. 2003;20(7):563-567.

54. Karim MA, Suzuki K, Fukai K, et al. Apparent genotype-phenotype correlation in childhood, adolescent, and adult Chediak-Higashi syndrome. *Am J Med Genet*. 2002;108(1):16-22.

55. Menasche G, Pastural E, Feldmann J, et al. Mutations in RAB27A cause Griscelli syndrome associated with haemophagocytic syndrome. *Nat Genet*. 2000;25(2):173-176.

56. Toro J, Turner M, Gahl WA. Dermatologic manifestations of Hermansky-Pudlak syndrome in patients with and without a 16-base pair duplication in the HPS1 gene. *Arch Dermatol*. 1999;135(7):774-780.

57. Sanal O, Ersoy F, Tezcan I, et al. Griscelli disease: genotype-phenotype correlation in an array of clinical heterogeneity. *J Clin Immunol*. 2002;22(4):237-243.

58. Fukuda M, Kuroda TS, Mikoshiba K. Slac2-a/melanophilin, the missing link between Rab27 and myosin Va: implications of a tripartite protein complex for melanosome transport. *J Biol Chem*. 2002;277(14):12432-12436.

59. Navarrete CL, Aranibar L, Mardones F, Avila R, Velozo L. Cutaneous granulomas in Griscelli type 2 syndrome. *Int J Dermatol*. 2016;55(7):804-805.

60. Eyer D, Petiau P, Finck S, Heid E, Grosshans E, Lutz P. [Granulomatous skin lesions in Griscelli disease]. *Ann Dermatol Venereol*. 1998;125(10):727-728.

61. Anikster Y, Huizing M, Anderson PD, et al. Evidence that Griscelli syndrome with neurological involvement is caused by mutations in RAB27A, not MYO5A. *Am J Hum Genet*. 2002;71(2):407-414.

62. Duran-McKinster C, Rodriguez-Jurado R, Ridaura C, de la Luz Orozco-Covarrubias M, Tamayo L, Ruiz-Maldonado R. Elejalde syndrome—a melanolysosomal neurocutaneous syndrome: clinical and morphological findings in 7 patients. *Arch Dermatol*. 1999;135(2):182-186.

63. Sanal O, Yel L, Kucukali T, et al. An allelic variant of Griscelli disease: presentation with severe hypotonia, mental-motor retardation, and hypopigmentation consistent with Elejalde syndrome (neuroectodermal melanolysosomal disorder). *J Neurol*. 2000;247(7):570-572.

64. Sanchez-Martin M, Perez-Losada J, Rodriguez-Garcia A, et al. Deletion of the SLUG (SNAI2) gene results in human piebaldism. *Am J Med Genet A*. 2003;122A(2):125-132.

65. Spritz RA. The molecular basis of human piebaldism. *Pigment Cell Res*. 1992;5(5 Pt 2):340-343.

66. Hornyak TJ. The developmental biology of melanocytes and its application to understanding human congenital disorders of pigmentation. *Adv Dermatol*. 2006;22:201-218.

67. Oiso N, Fukai K, Kawada A, Suzuki T. Piebaldism. *J Dermatol*. 2013;40(5):330-335.

68. Ward KA, Moss C, Sanders DS. Human piebaldism: relationship between phenotype and site of kit gene mutation. *Br J Dermatol*. 1995;132(6):929-935.

69. Cambiaghi S, Cavalli R, Legnani C, Gelmetti C. What syndrome is this? Waardenburg syndrome. *Pediatr Dermatol*. 1998;15(3):235-237.

70. Nayak CS, Isaacson G. Worldwide distribution of Waardenburg syndrome. *Ann Otol Rhinol Laryngol*. 2003;112(9 Pt 1):817-820.

71. Suyugul Z, Tuysuz B, Tukenmez F, Basaran M, Cenani A. Waardenburg syndrome: variable phenotypic expression in monozygotic twins. *Clin Dysmorphol*. 1998;7(1):77-78.

72. Wollnik B, Tukel T, Uyguner O, et al. Homozygous and heterozygous inheritance of PAX3 mutations causes different types of Waardenburg syndrome. *Am J Med Genet A*. 2003;122A(1):42-45.

73. Pingault V, Ente D, Dastot-Le Moal F, Goossens M, Marlin S, Bondurand N. Review and update of mutations causing Waardenburg syndrome. *Hum Mutat*. 2010;31(4):391-406.

74. Yang S, Dai P, Liu X, et al. Genetic and phenotypic heterogeneity in Chinese patients with Waardenburg syndrome type II. *PLoS One*. 2013;8(10):e77149.

75. Nye JS, Balkin N, Lucas H, Knepper PA, McLone DG, Charrow J. Myelomeningocele and Waardenburg syndrome (type 3) in patients with interstitial deletions of 2q35 and the PAX3 gene: possible digenic inheritance of a neural tube defect. *Am J Med Genet*. 1998;75(4):401-408.

76. Leger S, Balguerie X, Goldenberg A, et al. Novel and recurrent non-truncating mutations of the MITF basic domain: genotypic and phenotypic variations in Waardenburg and Tietz syndromes. *Eur J Hum Genet*. 2012;20(5):584-587.

77. Vinuela A, Morin M, Villamar M, et al. Genetic and phenotypic heterogeneity in two novel cases of Waardenburg syndrome type IV. *Am J Med Genet A*. 2009;149A(10):2296-2302.

78. Arimoto Y, Namba K, Nakano A, Matsunaga T. Chronic constipation recognized as a sign of a SOX10 mutation in a patient with Waardenburg syndrome. *Gene*. 2014;540(2):258-262.

79. Hofstra RM, Osinga J, Tan-Sindhunata G, et al. A homozygous mutation in the endothelin-3 gene associated with a combined Waardenburg type 2 and Hirschsprung phenotype (Shah-Waardenburg syndrome). *Nat Genet*. 1996;12(4):445-447.

80. Boardman JP, Syrris P, Holder SE, Robertson NJ, Carter N, Lakhoo K. A novel mutation in the endothelin B receptor gene in a patient with Shah-Waardenburg syndrome and Down syndrome. *J Med Genetics*. 2001;38(9):646-647.

81. Pingault V, Girard M, Bondurand N, et al. SOX10 mutations in chronic intestinal pseudo-obstruction suggest a complex physiopathological mechanism. *Hum Genet*. 2002;111(2):198-206.

82. Inoue K, Shilo K, Boerkoel CF, et al. Congenital hypomyelinating neuropathy, central dysmyelination, and Waardenburg-Hirschsprung disease: phenotypes linked by SOX10 mutation. *Ann Neurol*. 2002;52(6):836-842.

83. Okada N, Sato S, Sasou T, Aoyama M, Nishida K, Yoshikawa K. Characterization of pigmented granules in minocycline-induced cutaneous pigmentation: observations using fluorescence microscopy and high-performance liquid chromatography. *Br J Dermatol*. 1993;129(4):403-407.

84. Puri PK, Lountzis NI, Tyler W, Ferringer T. Hydroxychloroquine-induced hyperpigmentation: the staining pattern. *J Cutan Pathol*. 2008;35(12):1134-1137.

85. Bonamonte D, Foti C, Romita P, Vestita M, Angelini G. Colors and contact dermatitis. *Dermatitis*. 2014;25(4):155-162.

86. Sale TA, Stratman E. Carotenemia associated with green bean ingestion. *Pediatr Dermatol*. 2004;21(6):657-659.

87. Stawiski MA, Voorhees JJ. Cutaneous signs of diabetes mellitus. *Cutis*. 1976;18(3):415-421.

88. Kim SK, Kim EH, Kang HY, Lee ES, Sohn S, Kim YC. Comprehensive understanding of idiopathic guttate hypomelanosis: clinical and histopathological correlation. *Int J Dermatol*. 2010;49(2):162-166.

89. Arrunategui A, Trujillo RA, Marulanda MP, et al. HLA-DQ3 is associated with idiopathic guttate hypomelanosis, whereas HLA-DR8 is not, in a group of renal transplant patients. *Int J Dermatol*. 2002;41(11):744-747.

90. Falabella R, Escobar C, Giraldo N, et al. On the pathogenesis of idiopathic guttate hypomelanosis. *J Am Acad Dermatol*. 1987;16(1 Pt 1):35-44.

91. Zatkova A, de Bernabe DB, Polakova H, et al. High frequency of alkaptonuria in Slovakia: evidence for the appearance of multiple mutations in HGO involving different mutational hot spots. *Am J Hum Genet*. 2000;67(5):1333-1339.

92. Ranganath LR, Cox TF. Natural history of alkaptonuria revisited: analyses based on scoring systems. *J Inherit Metab Dis*. 2011;34(6):1141-1151.

93. Cetinus E, Cever I, Kural C, Erturk H, Akyildiz M. Ochronotic arthritis: case reports and review of the literature. *Rheumatol Int*. 2005;25(6):465-468.

94. Steven RA, Kinshuck AJ, McCormick MS, Ranganath LR. ENT manifestations of alkaptonuria: report on a case series. *J Laryngol Otol*. 2015;129(10):1004-1008.

95. Butany JW, Naseemuddin A, Moshkowitz Y, Nair V. Ochronosis and aortic valve stenosis. *J Card Surg*. 2006;21(2):182-184.

96. Helliwell TR, Gallagher JA, Ranganath L. Alkaptonuria—a review of surgical and autopsy pathology. *Histopathology*. 2008;53(5):503-512.

9

Genetic Disorders of Dermal Connective Tissue

Adnan Mir / Kevin Y. Shi

EHLERS-DANLOS SYNDROME

Definition and Epidemiology

Ehlers-Danlos syndrome (EDS) is a heterogeneous group of diseases caused by hereditable anomalies of the extracellular matrix (ECM) resulting in skin hyperextensibility, fragility, and abnormal wound healing.[1] EDS is currently classified into 13 subtypes on the basis of genetic defects and clinical features (Table 9-1).[2]

The incidence of EDS is approximately 1 in 5000 worldwide.[3] The hypermobility and classical types account for 90% of the cases, whereas the vascular type accounts for another approximately 5%.[4] Several subtypes have only been described in limited case reports. EDS may be inherited in autosomal dominant and/or recessive manner on the basis of subtype.

Etiology

The majority of EDS-associated mutations involve the biosynthesis of collagens I, III, and V.[5] Because of the complex nature of collagen fibril assembly, assorted dominant negative, haploinsufficient, or biallelic null mutations account for the variable inheritance pattern of EDS.

EDS mutations other than those responsible for collagen assembly highlight the phenotypic convergence of heterogeneous genotypes. Classic-like and hypermobile EDS result from the loss of tenascin-X expression.[1] Although its exact function is not well characterized, tenascin-X deficiency results in an aberrant organization of collagen subunits and morphologically irregular elastic fibers.[6] Mutations in the C1r and C1s protease subunits of complement component 1 cause the periodontal type, which likely leads to

abnormal intracellular protease activation.[7] Perturbations in glycosaminoglycan biosynthesis (*B4GALT7, B3GALT6*), zinc homeostasis (*SLC39A13*), the transcription factors of ECM constituents (*ZNF469* and *PRDM5*), and the catalysis of protein folding/chaperoning in the ER (*FKBP14I*) have all been linked to the subtypes of EDS.[5,8,9]

Clinical Presentation

EDS subtypes are characterized by varied clinical features, but they all present with some degree of skin hyperextensibility and fragility[1] (Tables 9-1 and 9-2, Figure 9-1A). Patients also frequently exhibit wound expansion, dehiscence, and eventual formation of irregular, atrophic scars. Generalized joint flexibility is prominent in most types, except vascular and dermatosparaxis EDS (Figure 9-1B). Severe joint hyperflexibility is associated with chronic pain and poor functional status. Frequent bruising due to fragile small vessels is seen in all types of EDS. Benign cutaneous findings can be seen at the sites of frequent trauma such as spheroid nodules of calcified fat and molluscoid pseudotumor, which are nodules of skin and fibrous tissues found on the knees and elbows.

Histologic Findings

EDS is diagnosed on the basis of clinical and laboratory evaluation, without specific histopathologic findings.[1,10] The epidermis is unremarkable, and loose dermal collagen bundles are seen in a few subtypes, but these findings are likely nonspecific. Transmission electron microscopy may show single collagen fibrils with irregular cross-sectional

TABLE 9-1. Categorization and features of Ehlers-Danlos syndrome

Type (Historic Category)	Genetic Mutations	Major Features	Inheritance Pattern	Salient Histologic/ Ultrastructural Features
Classic (I, II)	COL5A1, COL5A2. COL1A1	Skin hyperextensibility with atrophic scarring, GJH	AD	Flower-like collagen fibrils
Classic-like	TNXB	Skin hyperextensibility without atrophic scarring, easy bruising, GJH	AR	
Cardiac valvular	COL1A2	Cardiac valvular disease, classic skin involvement, joint hypermobility	AR	
Hypermobile (III)	Mostly unknown, partially due to TNXB heterozygous	Joint hypermobility, less skin involvement, abdominal hernia, pelvic organ prolapse, aortic root dilatation	AD	Calcified deposits within an amorphous matrix of elastic fibers and clusters of hyaluronic acid
Vascular (IV)	COL3A1	Early arterial rupture, sigmoid colon perforation, gestational uterine rupture, peripartum perineum laceration, carotid-cavernous sinus fistula, family history of vascular Ehlers-Danlos syndrome (vEDS)	AD	Thin dermis, irregular thickness of dermal–epidermal junction, fibroblasts with lysosome
Kyphoscoliotic (VIA)	PLOD1. FKBP14	Congenital hypotonia, congenital or early-onset kyphoscoliosis, GJH	AR	Subtle irregularities in collagen fibril contour and spacing
Musculocontractural (VIB)	CHST14. DSE	Characteristic congenital contractures, characteristic facies, classic skin involvement with palmar wrinkling	AR	Dispersal of collagen fibrils
Arthrochalasia (VIIA, VIIB)	COL1A1, COL1A2	Congenital bilateral hip dislocation, severe GJH, skin hyperextensibility	AD	Collagen fibrils with variable diameter and highly irregular contour
Dermatosparaxis (VIIC)	ADAMTS2	Extreme congenital skin fragility, characteristic facies, lax skin with palmar wrinkling, severe bruisability, umbilical hernia, growth retardation, short appendages, perinatal complications	AR	Hieroglyphic collagen fibrils
Periodontal (VIII)	C1R, C1S	Severe periodontitis, detached gingiva, pretibial plaques, family history of periodontal Ehlers-Danlos syndrome (pEDS)	AD	
Spondylodysplastic	B4GALT7. B3GALT6. SLC39A13	Short stature, congenital hypotonia, limb bowing	AR	
Brittle cornea syndrome	ZNF469. PRDM5	Thin cornea, keratoconus, keratoglobus, blue sclera	AR	
Myopathic	COL12A1	Congenital hypotonia with/without atrophy, joint contractures, hypermobility of distal joints	AD or AR	

Abbreviations: AD, autosomal dominant; AR, autosomal recessive; GJH, generalized joint hypermobility. Roman numerals in parentheses represent former numerical designations. Adapted from Malfait F, Francomano C, Byers P, et al. The 2017 international classification of the Ehlers-Danlos syndromes. *Am J Med Genet C Semin Med Genet.* 2017;175(1):8-26; Byers PH, Murray ML. Ehlers-Danlos syndrome: a showcase of conditions that lead to understanding matrix biology. *Matrix Biol.* 2014;33:10-15; Ong K-T, Plauchu H, Peyrol S, et al. Ultrastructural scoring of skin biopsies for diagnosis of vascular Ehlers–Danlos syndrome. *Virchows Arch.* 2012;460(6): 637-649; Rohrbach M, Vandersteen A, Yiş U, et al. Phenotypic variability of the kyphoscoliotic type of Ehlers-Danlos syndrome (EDS VIA): clinical, molecular and biochemical delineation. *Orphanet J Rare Dis.* 2011;6:46; Janecke AR, Li B, Boehm M, et al. The phenotype of the musculocontractural type of Ehlers-Danlos syndrome due to CHST14 mutations. *Am J Med Genet A.* 2016;170A(1):103-115.

TABLE 9-2.	Pediatric findings in Ehlers-Danlos syndrome
Clinical Features	**Ehlers-Danlos Syndrome Subtypes**
Characteristic facies	Vascular, *Plod1*-associated dermatosparaxis, periodontal, kyphosclerotic, brittle cornea syndrome, spondylodysplastic, musculocontractural[11]
Congenital hearing loss	*FKBP14*-associated kyphoscoliotic
Severe neonatal skin tearing	Dermatosparaxis
Blue sclera	Brittle cornea syndrome, dermatosparaxis, kyphoscoliosis, spondylodysplastic, musculocontractural
Generalized hypotonia	Kyphoscoliotic, arthrochalasia, spondylodysplastic, myopathic
In utero and congenital hip dysplasia	Arthrochalasia[12]
Congenital or early-onset kyphoscoliosis	Kyphoscoliotic, arthrochalasia, *B3GALT6*-associated spondylodysplastic
Joint contractures	Musculocontractural, *B3GALT6*-associated spondylodysplastic

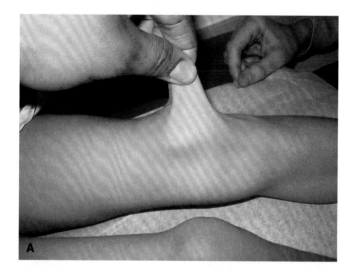
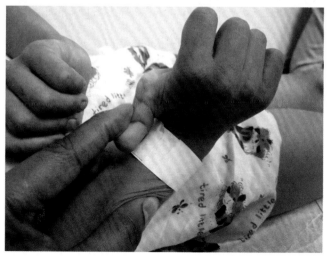

FIGURE 9-1. **Ehlers-Danlos syndrome.** Skin hyperextensibility (**A**) and joint hypermobility (**B**).

contours, significant variability in diameters, and disorganized packing into larger fibers.

A few subtype-specific findings have been consistently reported. Significantly thinned dermis distinguishes vascular EDS. Gross fragmentation of elastic fibers has been seen in hypermobile EDS, which is associated with morphologic abnormalities of the amorphous elastin matrix. Distinctive cross-sectional contours of single collagen fibrils are seen in classic (flower like), vascular (hieroglyphic), and arthrochalasia (stellate) types.

Differential Diagnosis

The clinical differential diagnosis for EDS includes Marfan syndrome due to marfanoid habitus of kyphoscoliotic and periodontal subtypes. Cutis laxa features loose and doughy skin, which is seen in dermatosparaxis EDS. Loeys-Dietz syndrome (LDS; caused by TGF-β receptor mutations) presents with similar cutaneous and vascular complications to those found in vascular EDS, but presents with characteristic facies. Osteogenesis imperfecta type I can be distinguished by its significant bone pathology. Benign

CAPSULE SUMMARY

EHLERS-DANLOS SYNDROME

Ehlers-Danlos is a group of genetically and clinically heterogeneous diseases of the ECM, which features skin hyperextensibility and fragility and poor wound healing. Pathologic joint laxity is a prominent feature of most of the 13 subtypes. Diagnosis requires careful clinical evaluation, and genetic and laboratory testing. There are no consistent skin histopathologic features in this condition.

joint hypermobility syndrome should be easily excluded by the lack of cutaneous findings of hypermobile EDS and, if uncertain, by the strict application of diagnostic criteria.

MARFAN SYNDROME

Definition and Epidemiology

Marfan syndrome (MFS) is caused by mutations in *FBN1*, resulting in connective tissue defects in the skeletal, cardiovascular, ocular systems.[13,14] Diagnosis is based on the 2010 revised Ghent nosology, which requires information on family history, syndromic features, and the identification of genetic mutations. The reported prevalence of MFS is approximately between 1/5000 and 1/15 000 without gender predilection.[15]

Etiology

Mutation in the *FBN1* gene is identified in more than 90% of Marfan patients. Because of the gene's extremely large size, more than 1800 different mutations have been identified to date in *FBN1*.[16] Although most specific mutations do not predict organ system involvement, mutations located in exons 24 to 32 frequently result in neonatal MFS, the most severe form of the disease.[17] About 25% of MFS-associated mutations are sporadic, but the majority are inherited in an autosomal dominant manner. Mutations in *FBN1* cause reduced expression and misassembled microfibrils, leading to errors in elastic fiber formation and a compromise of the mechanical integrity of connective tissues.[13] FBN1 has also been strongly implicated in the regulation of TGF-β signaling. Functional protein sequesters and inactivates TGF-β cytokine in the ECM. The loss of FBN1 results in an increase in TGB-β signaling, which likely accounts for some phenotypic elements (eg, cardiac valvular myxoma).

Clinical Presentation

The classic signs of MFS are reduced upper to lower segment ratio, severe pectus excavatum, scoliosis, ectopia lentis, dilatation and dissection of the ascending aorta, and lumbosacral dural ectasia.[14] These features are not always present in childhood.[18] Aortic root dilatation and ectopia lentis are the most constant features, and are, therefore, the most useful diagnostic criteria in the pediatric population.[19] Patients present with a typical habitus characterized by tall, thin stature with long arms, legs, fingers, and toes (Figure 9-2).

Although the cutaneous findings of striae atrophicae and incisional hernias are found in MFS, they are not major diagnostic criteria.[14] The prevalence of striae increases with age and is present in the vast majority of adult Marfan patients, appearing as atrophic, linear plaques ranging from erythematous to white in color.[20,21] Presence in locations other than the thighs, buttocks, and hips occurs significantly more frequently in affected patients than in the general population. Infantile striae have been reported in the neonatal form of MFS.[22] Abnormal wound healing is

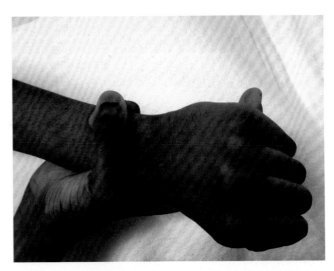

FIGURE 9-2. Marfan syndrome. Long fingers result in the thumb sign, in which the thumb protrudes from a closed fist, and the wrist sign, in which the thumb and fifth finger overlap when encircling the opposite wrist. Reprinted with permission from Bitterman AD, Sponseller PD. Marfan syndrome: a clinical update. *J Am Acad Orthop Surg.* 2017;25(9):603-609, Figure 2.

a common finding, with wide or atrophic scarring, dyspigmentation, and recurrent incisional hernias.

Histologic Findings

Clinically normal-appearing skin of patients with MFS may have characteristic histologic dermal findings. Elastic fibers appear fragmented with some scattering in orientation.[23] Immunohistochemical evaluation for fibrillin protein shows discontinuous staining of the dermoepidermal junction, attenuation in the papillary dermis, and near-absence in the reticular dermis.[24] The epidermis and dermal collagen appear normal. Ultrastructural studies show thinned elastic fibers that are randomly packed into large tortuous strands.[23] Cross-sectional evaluation shows peripheral fragmentation of the elastin matrix, rendering a cobweb-like appearance.

As in striae from normal patients, biopsies from MFS patients show thinning of the epidermis with attenuation of the rete.[25] The dermis is also thin, with hypertrophied collagen and elastic fibers run in parallel with the surface. Atrophic scars in a patient with incomplete MFS (ie, mitral valve prolapse, aortic enlargement, skin and skeletal findings syndrome [MASS]) show short, broken elastic fibers in the papillary dermis, which formed large aggregates in older lesions.[26]

Differential Diagnosis

LDS, a primary disorder of TGF-β signaling, and EDS share some clinical features with MFS.[27] The distinct features of LDS include hypertelorism, bifid uvula or cleft palate, aortic aneurysm, and arterial tortuosity. Although some subtypes of EDS can have a marfanoid habitus, they are distinguished by skin hyperextensibility and atrophic wound healing in EDS, which are absent in MFS. Mutations in

FBN2 cause congenital contractural arachnodactyly (CCA), which is characterized by contractures, arachnodactyly, scoliosis, and crumpled ears. These findings can be seen in neonatal MFS, but aortic root involvement and valvular disease is not typical of CCA.[28] MFS-spectrum disorders (mitral valve prolapse syndrome, ectopia lentis syndrome, and MASS) can all be diagnosed under the current guidelines.[14]

CAPSULE SUMMARY

MARFAN SYNDROME

MFS is caused by genetic defects in the elastic fiber network, which can lead to significant complications in the skeletal, cardiovascular, and ocular systems. Although their presence can support the diagnosis, the cutaneous findings of striae atrophicae and recurrent incisional hernias are not specific to MFS. Careful clinical and genetic evaluations are required to secure the diagnosis.

CUTIS LAXA

Definition and Epidemiology

Cutis laxa (CL), or generalized elastolysis, is a group of disorders characterized by loose, hypoelastic skin folds caused by the disruption of dermal elastic fibers.[29,30] Autosomal dominant, recessive, and X-linked inheritance patterns have all been reported with a number of implicated genes and associated systemic features. Acquired forms may be associated with inflammatory dermatoses and other systemic diseases. CL is rare, and there is no known predilection for specific populations.

Etiology

Heritable CL is subtyped on the basis of causal mutation that disrupts the synthesis and function of elastic fibers (Table 9-3).[29] Mutation in *ELN*, which encodes for elastin, leads to an autosomal dominant version of CL. Recessive

TABLE 9-3.	Causes and features of cutis laxa			
Disorder	**Inheritance**	**Gene**	**Distribution**	**Associated Features**
ADCL type 1	AD	*ELN*	Generalized	Aortic dilatation, emphysema, GI diverticula.[40]
ADCL type 2		*FBLN5*		
ARCL type 1A	AR	*FBLN5*	Generalized	Aortic dilatation, supravalvular aortic stenosis, pulmonary artery stenosis, arterial tortuosity, emphysema, GI/GU diverticula, growth retardation, joint laxity, congenital hip dysplasia.[30]
ARCL type 1B		*FBLN4*		
ARCL type 1C (Urban-Rifkin-Davis syndrome)	AR	*LTBP4*	Generalized	Emphysema, pulmonary artery stenosis, valvular insufficiency, GI/GU diverticula, dysmorphic facial features
ARCL type 2A (Debré type)	AR	*ATP6V0A2*	Generalized. Improves in childhood[41]	• Intrauterine growth restriction, joint laxity, congenital hip dysplasia, growth retardation, scoliosis, dysmorphic facial features, • De Barsy phenotype: mental retardation, athetosis, corneal clouding.[42] • Wrinkly skin syndrome is a phenotypic variant of ARCL 2A without GU involvement and milder facial and skin defects.
ARCL type 2B	AR	*PYCR1*	Generalized. Dorsal acral and abdomen (2B).	
De Barsy syndrome B (ARCL type 3B)				
ADCL type 3[43]	AD	*ALDH18A1*		
De Barsy syndrome A (ARCL type 3A)	AR			
ARCL type 2C	AR	*ATP6V1E1*	Generalized with sparse subcutaneous fat[44]	Hypotonia, cardiac abnormalities, aortic dilation, hip dysplasia, "mask-like" triangular face (2C), marfanoid habitus (2D), neurodevelopmental abnormalities (2D)
ARCL type 2D		*ATP6V1A*		
Geroderma osteodysplasticum	AR	*GORAB*	Cheeks, hands, feet, abdomen	Labial frenulum hypoplasia, malar hypoplasia, prognathism, oblique furrows on the lateral aspect of the face, osteoporosis, dwarfism
MACS	AR	*RIN2*	Generalized[45]	Macrocephaly, sparse hair, facial coarsening, gingival hypertrophy, scoliosis, osteoporosis, joint laxity
Occipital horn syndrome	X-linked recessive	*ATP7A*	Generalized	Occipital horn, coarse hair, arterial tortuosity, bladder diverticula, mental retardation, delayed motor development, joint laxity, osteoporosis, scoliosis. Allelic to Menke syndrome.

Abbreviations: AD, autosomal dominant; ADCL, autosomal dominant cutis laxa; AR, autosomal recessive; ARCL, autosomal recessive cutis laxa; GI, gastrointestinal; GU, genitourinary; MACS, Macrocephaly, Alopecia, Cutis Laxa, and Scoliosis.

disease is caused by mutations in elastin support proteins (*FBLN4* and *FBLN5*), the TGF-β pathway (*LTBP4*), vesicular ATPase (*ATP6V0A2, ATP6V1E1, ATP6V1A*), vesicular trafficking proteins (*GORAB, RIN2*), and mitochondrial components (*PYCR1, ALDH18A1*). Occipital horn syndrome, previously categorized as a subtype of EDS, is caused by an X-linked defect in cooper transport (*ATP7A*). Many other congenital syndromes also feature hypoelastic skin.

Postinflammatory reactions that cause the enzymatic degradation of the elastin network can cause acquired CL. It may be associated with conditions such as Sweet syndrome, infections, inflammatory connective tissue disease, plasma cell dyscrasias, and others.[31] D-penicillamine, a cooper chelator that abrogates elastin cross-linking by inhibiting lysyl oxidase activity, is a cause of drug-induced CL.[32]

Clinical Presentation

The redundant skin in CL is hyperextensible but lacks the elastic recoil seen in EDS (with the exception of dermatosparaxis EDS). Pendulous skin folds around the cheeks, periorbital area, and neck create a progeroid appearance (Figure 9-3). Recessive forms of CL usually manifest in

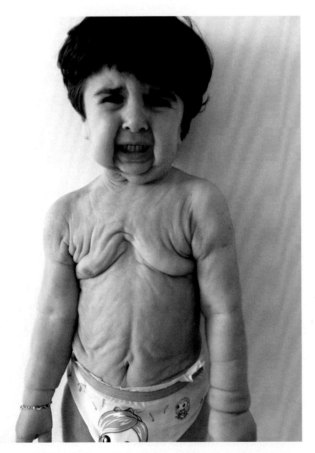

FIGURE 9-3. Cutis laxa. Pendulous skin folds confer a progeroid appearance. Reprinted with permission from Duz MB, Kirat E, Coucke PJ, et al. A novel case of autosomal dominant cutis laxa in a consanguineous family: report and literature review. *Clin Dysmorphol.* 2017;26(3):142-147.

neonates and have a more aggressive phenotype, whereas autosomal and acquired forms can be adult-onset. Although skin findings are mostly generalized, more localized findings can be features of the autosomal recessive ARCL type 2B, geroderma osteodysplasticum, and acquired CL. Many recessive subtypes also have severe extracutaneous features such as neonatal emphysema, cardiovascular malformations, and developmental issues involving the neurologic, skeletal, gastrointestinal, and genitourinary systems. These associated findings overlap significantly between subtypes, and diagnosis can be difficult on clinical grounds alone.

Histologic Findings

For all forms of CL, elastic fibers found throughout the dermis can appear granular, clumped, or nearly absent.[29] The epidermis appears normal. Dermal inflammation specific to particular dermatoses may be found in dermatosis-associated CL.[33,34] Concurrent dermal immunoglobulin deposits can be detected in systemic diseases.[35]

Ultrastructural analysis demonstrates poorly organized clumps of elastin matrix around abnormal microfibrils.[30] Immunoglobulin deposition along the edge of elastic fiber borders has been reported in patients with acquired CL.[36,37]

Differential Diagnosis

EDS is a disease of defective collagen and features hyperextensible skin that retains its elastic quality.[2] In contrast to CL, joint hypermobility, skin fragility, and abnormal wound healing are dominant features of the disease. Elastic fiber loss and fragmentation are not seen on histology in EDS. Pseudoxanthoma elasticum (PXE) can lead to secondary CL, but primary papular lesions should precede the appearance of saggy skin. The presence of calcified elastic fibers in PXE is a distinct histologic finding.[38] Mid-dermal elastolysis has the pathognomonic finding of a band-like loss of mid-dermal elastic fibers.[39]

CAPSULE SUMMARY

CUTIS LAXA

CL presents with redundant, hypoelastic skin folds, and has numerous genetic and secondary causes. Primary causes can have significant associated congenital defects. A histologic evaluation of the skin shows the loss of normal elastic fiber network of the dermis.

APLASIA CUTIS CONGENITA

Definition and Epidemiology

Aplasia cutis congenita (ACC) is a neonatal finding of scarred or absent skin.[46,47] Associated defects of the underlying bone and meninges are not uncommon. There is no single cause of ACC, which can be categorized on the basis of the number and location of lesions and associated clinical features (Table 9-4). The estimated incidence of ACC is approximately 3 in 10 000 births with a predominance in females.[48,49]

Etiology

ACC is a finding associated with a number of pathologic conditions.[46] Developmental defects in skin morphogenesis are seen mostly in syndrome-associated ACC. For example, Adams-Oliver syndrome (AOS) features scalp ACC with frequent underlying skull defects, cutis marmorata telangiectatica congenita, transverse terminal limb defects, central nervous system (CNS) anomalies, and cardiac malformations.[50] Loss-of-function mutations in Notch signaling and actin regulation pathways, both critical for general tissue morphogenesis, are known causes of AOS. ACC is also seen in focal dermal hypoplasia, a disorder of mesoectodermal development.[51] A heterozygous missense mutation of *BMS1* (a ribosomal GTPase) causes isolated, autosomal dominant ACC.[52] BMS1 likely plays a role in cell cycle progression, critical for the rapidly proliferating cells of the developing scalp. In patients with epidermolysis bullosa, intrauterine trauma causes lesions localized to the extremities (Bart syndrome). Extrinsic factors that cause intrauterine insult, such as teratogens, infections, amniotic band sequence, and ischemic events, can also cause ACC.

TABLE 9-4.	Causes of aplasia cutis congenita		
Group	**Clinical Features**	**Inheritance**	**Associated Anomalies**
1. Scalp ACC, nonsyndromic	Vertex. Membranous or scar-like	AD (*BMS1*) or sporadic	Midline defects, tracheoesophageal fistula, patent ductus arteriosus, polycystic kidneys
2. Scalp ACC associated with Adams–Oliver syndrome	Scalp. Irregular borders and hemorrhagic to healing base	AD (*ARHGAP31*, *RBPJ*, *NOTCH1*, *DLL4*) or AR (*DOCK6*, *EOGT*)	Terminal transverse limb defect, cutis marmorata telangiectatica congenita, cardiac malformations, CNS abnormalities
3. Scalp ACC with skin/organoid nevi	Scalp. Membranous base	Sporadic	Epidermal nevi, congenital melanocytic nevi, ocular abnormalities, seizures.
4. ACC overlying embryologic malformations	Scalp, chest, abdomen, lumbosacral	Variable	Cranial malformations, spinal malformations, abdominal wall defect, sternal cleft, or combination
5. ACC with fetus papyraceus or placental infarcts	Scalp, trunk, extremity. Can be symmetric with irregular borders	Sporadic	Single umbilical artery, gastrointestinal atresia
6. ACC associated with epidermolysis bullosa	Trunk, extremity (Bart syndrome). Eroded or ulcerated	Varies on the basis of the type of epidermolysis bullosa (See Chapter 4)	Blistering of skin and/or mucous membranes, dystrophic nails, pyloric or duodenal atresia, abnormal ears and nose, ureteral stenosis, renal anomalies, amniotic bands
7. ACC localized to extremities without blistering	Extensor and dorsal surfaces of extremities	Autosomal dominant or recessive	Radial dysplasia
8. ACC caused by teratogens	Scalp (drugs), variable (infections)	Not inherited	Methimazole (with imperforate anus, urachal malformation), misoprostol low-molecular-weight heparin, valproic acid, intrauterine infection with varicella, herpes simplex, rubella.
9. ACC associated with congenital syndromes	Variable	Variable	Trisomy 13, Wolf-Hirschhorn syndrome, focal dermal hypoplasia, focal facial dermal dysplasia, amniotic band sequence, microphthalmia with linear skin defects syndrome, Johanson-Blizzard syndrome, scalp–ear–nipple syndrome, oculocerebrocutaneous syndrome, oculoectodermal syndrome.

Abbreviations: ACC, aplasia cutis congenita; AD, autosomal dominant; AR, autosomal recessive; CNS, central nervous system Reprinted from Frieden IJ. Aplasia cutis congenita: a clinical review and proposal for classification. *J Am Acad Dermatol*. 1986;14(4):646-660. Copyright © 1986 Mosby, Inc. With permission. From Evers ME, Steijlen PM, Hamel BC. Aplasia cutis congenita and associated disorders: an update. *Clin Genet*. 1995;47(6):295-301. Copyright © 1995, John Wiley and Sons. Reprinted by permission of John Wiley & Sons, Inc.

Clinical Presentation

ACC predominantly occurs on the scalp (>85% of single lesions), usually on the vertex.[47] The initial appearance of ACC is highly variable, with the typical end result being an atrophic or hypertrophic scar. The complete absence of skin presents as a translucent membrane overlying a punched out-appearing defect. A ring of coarse hair is sometimes present surrounding the membranous defect, the "hair collar sign," and may indicate an underlying CNS malformation (Figure 9-4).[53] Exposure and injury of the sagittal sinus has been reported for exceptionally deep lesions that involve the dura.[54] Bullous ACC is a variant presenting with a serous fluid-filled vesicle with surface telangectasias.[55] Patients may also present with lesions featuring ragged, stellate borders with a granulated or hemorrhagic base. This finding likely represents in utero wound healing and

is usually secondary to intrauterine ischemic events, AOS, or the erosions of epidermolysis bullosa. Three cases of systemic ACC (>90% total body involvement) have been reported, in which cutaneous structures down to the subcutis were missing.[56]

Histologic Features

The diagnosis of ACC is clinical, and histologic features most likely reflect various stages of tissue regeneration. Deeply ulcerated lesions may show a complete absence of cutaneous structures.[47] As the lesion heals, the epidermis is flattened and may be remarkably thin at 1 to 2 cell layers thick.[51] The underlying dermis takes on the appearance of granulation tissue or an atrophic scar.[57,58] Adnexal structures are uniformly missing, and elastic fibers are sparse if present (Figure 9-5). For bullous ACC, the unremarkable

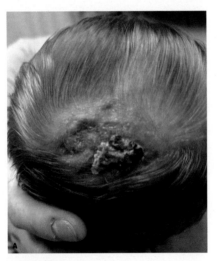

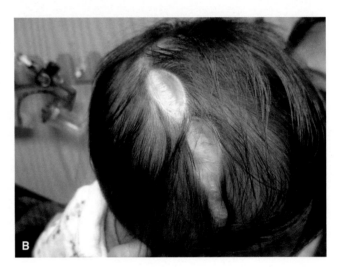

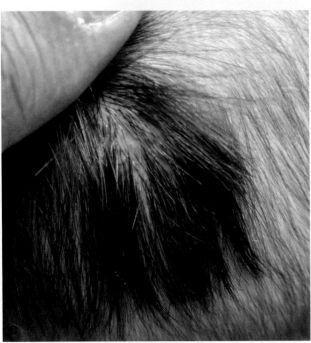

FIGURE 9-4. Aplasia cutis congenital. A, A crusted, healing erosion on the vertex of the scalp in a newborn infant. **B**, Extensive, well-healed aplasia cutis with resultant atrophic plaques. **C**, Aplasia cutis with hair collar sign—a rim of dark hair that may indicate underlying skull or central nervous system defects.

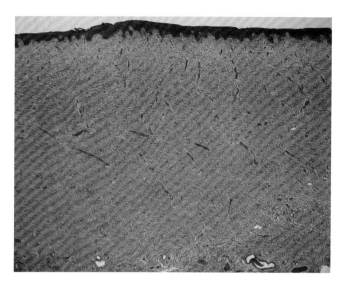

FIGURE 9-5. **Aplasia cutis congenital.** Thin epidermis overlies a dermal scar that lacks adnexal structures.

epidermis overlies an edematous dermis with very loose connective tissue.

Differential Diagnosis

ACC should be distinguishable from perinatal injury through a careful clinical evaluation. Neural tube defects should be ruled out with imaging. Congenital Volkmann ischemic contracture is a compressive intrauterine injury to the upper limb that can produce necrotic lesions similar to ACC. Neuromuscular defect can be present, and histologic findings are consistent with ischemic necrosis.[59] Congenital varicella may be considered, but a dermatomal distribution of lesions is frequently seen.[60]

CAPSULE SUMMARY

APLASIA CUTIS CONGENITA

ACC is a clinical finding of scarred or absent skin in the newborn. Associated conditions and presentation are highly variable. Lesions may present with a complete absence of skin structures, with healing erosions, blistering, or well-healed scars. Histologic features depend on the stage and clinical presentation, and may show erosion/ulceration, granulation tissue, and/or epidermal atrophy, and usually lack adnexal structures.

PSEUDOXANTHOMA ELASTICUM

Definition and Epidemiology

PXE is an autosomal recessive disorder featuring calcification and fragmentation of elastic fibers primarily involving the skin, eyes, and vascular system.[38,61] The estimates of

prevalence range from 1 in 25 000 to 1 in 100 000 with a 2:1 female predominance.

Etiology

PXE is primarily a disease of antimineralization factor deficiency.[38] Mutations in *ABCC6* have been found in approximately 80% of cases. To date, there are over 300 loss-of-function mutations in *ABCC6*, which encodes multidrug resistance–associated protein 6 (MRP6). MRP6 is expressed in the liver and kidney and results in the downregulation of systemic antimineralization factors, inorganic pyrophosphate (PPi) and fetuin-A. Dysregulation of PPi can also be caused by homozygous inactivating mutations in the gene product of *ENPP1,* leading to a subset of PXE or generalized arterial calcification of infancy.[62] Finally, compound mutations in γ-glutamyl carboxylase (*GGCX*) and *ABCC6* can also cause PXE.[63] *GGCX* is responsible for the γ-glutamyl carboxylation of the antimineralization factor matrix gla protein and vitamin K–dependent coagulation factors. Double mutations in *GGCX* cause PXE skin lesions with primary coagulopathy.

Clinical Presentation

PXE is clinically heterogeneous due to incomplete expressivity.[38,61,64] Cutaneous findings are typically the first sign of PXE. The eruption of yellow- to skin-colored, nonfollicular papules on the neck and flexural surfaces occurs in the first two decades of life (Figure 9-6). The volar wrist,

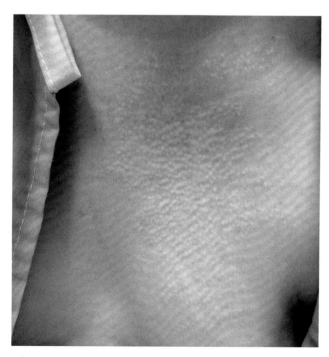

FIGURE 9-6. **Pseudoxanthoma elasticum.** Coalescing skin-colored to yellow papules on the upper chest of an affected teenage girl.

periumbilical, and intertriginous areas can also be affected. Over time, the papules can evolve into firm calcified plaques, and the skin can take on a cobblestoned appearance. Secondary CL due to the loss of normal elastic fibers can manifest as saggy, redundant skin in the axillae, groin, and mental regions. Mucosal involvement appears as yellow papules on the lower lip and the genitals. Perforating PXE can occasionally occur with the transepidermal elimination of dystrophic elastic fibers.[65] Patients with *GGCX* mutations have more extensive PXE-like lesions over the trunk with more severe CL.[66]

Mottling of the retinal pigmented epithelium and angioid streaks, or cracks in the calcified Bruch's membrane, are progressive fundoscopic findings in PXE. These changes eventually lead to neovascularization, retinal hemorrhage, and blindness. Calcified elastic fibers in the walls of the vasculature lead to atherosclerotic changes, eventually resulting in ischemic disease of the gastrointestinal, peripheral arterial, cardiac, and cerebrovascular systems.

Histologic Findings

Clumps of basophilic elastic fiber fragments are most evident in the mid-dermis, with little to mild involvement of the superficial and deeper levels (Figure 9-7).[38,67]

Although the findings are typically evident on standard hematoxylin and eosin-stained sections, calcified deposits along elastic fibers may be best visualized with van Kossa staining. Collagen in the affected regions typically appears normal, although unwinding or fraying of collagen fibers may be seen. The epidermis and dermis are otherwise unremarkable.

Differential Diagnosis

Fundoscopic signs, vascular disease, and ectopic calcification of lesional skin are keys to diagnosing PXE. CL due to other disorders may be considered if PXE-like papules are not present. Fibroelastolytic papulosis is a spectrum of noninflammatory fibroelastolytic disorders (PXE-like papillary dermal elastolysis and white fibrous papulosis of the neck) and can present with similar papules and plaques.[68] They can be differentiated by histologic examination and a lack of calcification of elastic fibers. Late-onset focal dermal elastosis and perforating serpiginous elastosis also lack dermal calcium deposits.[69,70] Perforating calcific elastosis occurs in multiparous women around the periumbilical region and has identical histologic findings to PXE, with the lack of systemic involvement being the only reliable distinction.[71]

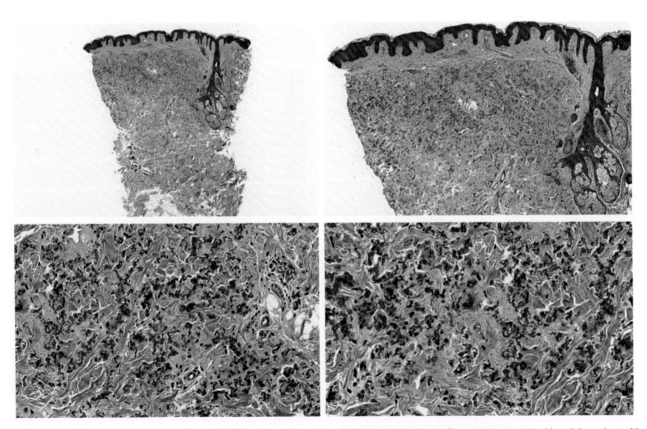

FIGURE 9-7. **Pseudoxanthoma elasticum.** Within the dermis, clumped, basophilic elastic fibers are present with calcium deposition. The latter can be further demonstrated by the use of a Von Kossa stain. Digital slides courtesy of Path Presenter.com.

PSEUDOXANTHOMA ELASTICUM

PXE is an autosomal recessive disorder that causes calcification and fragmentation of elastic fibers in the skin, eyes, and vascular system. Cutaneous findings include yellow- to skin-colored coalescing papules on the neck and flexor surfaces, and the characteristic histologic finding is fragmented, basophilic elastic fibers within the dermis.

ELASTOSIS PERFORANS SERPIGINOSA

Definition and Epidemiology

Elastosis perforans serpiginosa (EPS) is a rare cutaneous disorder characterized by transepidermal elimination of elastin.[72,73] It represents one of the primary perforating dermatoses, which also includes reactive perforating collagenosis (collagen), Kyrle disease (mixed connective tissue), and acquired perforating dermatosis. EPS is often associated with genetic diseases such as EDS, osteogenesis imperfecta, MFS, PXE, and acrogeria. Long-term use of penicillamine and chronic kidney disease are thought to be causes of acquired EPS. Isolated reports show a potential autosomal dominant pattern of inheritance.[74] EPS occurs about three times more frequently in males than in females.

Etiology

The etiology of EPS is unknown.[73,75-77] Possible explanations of the pathogenesis include traumatic erosion of the epidermis, epidermal hyperplasia induced by abnormal connective tissue, and focal inflammation within the dermis. As a cooper chelator, penicillamine is known to inhibit the proper cross-linking of microfibrils. It is also a secondary cause of CL and PXE, and differential factors that determine the clinic manifestation are not clear.

Clinical Presentation

EPS typically presents during childhood or young adulthood. Groups of erythematous or hyperpigmented papules are arranged in annular or serpiginous patterns usually found on the neck, face, and flexural surfaces of the arm. A central keratotic plug in each papule represents the hyperkeratotic epidermis and the transepidermal eruption of elastic fibers (Figure 9-8). Lesions are typically asymptomatic, but may be mildly pruritic. EPS may resolve spontaneously after a chronic course, and is mostly resistant to treatment.[70]

Histologic Findings

An acanthotic epidermis with hyperparakeratosis houses a keratin plug within a central depression.[72,73,78] Transepidermal channels connecting to the plug are filled by eosinophilic aggregates of elastin with basophilic debris of

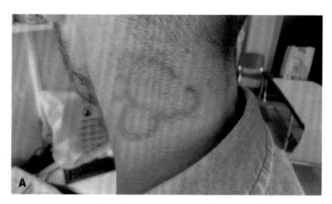
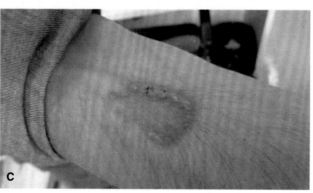
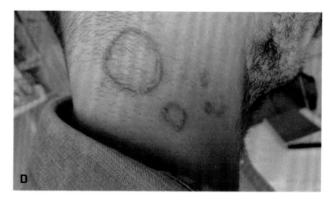

FIGURE 9-8. Elastosis perforans serpiginosa. Annular, hyperkeratotic, slightly erythematous plaques on the neck (**A** and **B**) and forearm of a patient treated with D-penicillamine (**C**). Reprinted with permission from Ranucci G; Di Dato F; Leone F; et al. Penicillamine-induced Elastosis Perforans Serpiginosa in Wilson Disease: Is Useful Switching to Zinc? *Journal of Pediatric Gastroenterology & Nutrition.* 2017; 64(3):e72-e73.

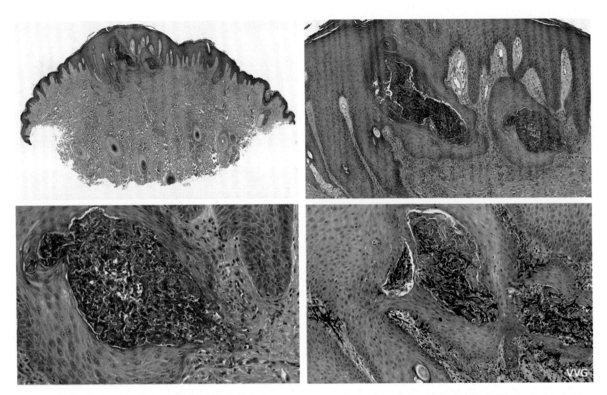

FIGURE 9-9. **Elastosis perforans serpiginosa.** There is transepidermal elimination of elastic fibers. Such finding is best demonstrated with the use of a Verhoeff-Van Gieson stain (bottom right panel). Digital slides courtesy of Path Presenter.com.

inflammatory cells and keratinocytes (Figure 9-9). Channels may be contained within hair follicles. On the papillary dermis side of the channel, elastosis is prominent with twisted and thickened elastic fibers. At the dermal opening of the channel, individual elastic fibers are positioned vertically toward the route of elimination. A mixed dermal infiltrate of lymphocytes, histocytes, and multinucleated giant cells are present. "Lumpy-bumpy"–appearing elastic fibers can be seen in both lesional and nonlesional dermis of penicillamine-induced EPS.[79]

Differential Diagnosis

Elastic stains readily distinguish EPS from the other primary perforating diseases. Perforating PXE can be distinguished by calcification of involved elastic fibers by von Kossa staining.[80] Calcinosis cutis, granuloma annulare, and annular lesions of sarcoidosis can all be easily distinguished with routine histology.

CAPSULE SUMMARY

ELASTOSIS PERFORANS SERPIGINOSA

EPS is a primary perforating dermatosis characterized by annular or serpiginous arrangement of keratotic papules. It can occur as a primary or acquired disorder. Histologically, transepidermal elimination of elastic fibers through a hyperkeratotic core is seen.

FOCAL DERMAL HYPOPLASIA

Definition and Epidemiology

Focal dermal hypoplasia (FDH, Goltz syndrome) is an X-linked dominant disease caused by the dysgenesis of mesoectodermal tissues resulting in a pleiotropic phenotype.[81-83] A total of 90% of all cases are female, 95% of which are from de novo mutations. The range of clinical phenotypes found in heterozygous females is caused by the variable inactivation of the remaining X-chromosome or functional mosaicism.[84] Mosaic males account for 10% of the cases because of the near universal intrauterine demise of hemizygous fetuses.[85]

Etiology

Mutation or deletion of the *PORCN* gene, which encodes the endoplasmic reticulum transmembrane protein Porcupine, results in defective Wnt signaling.[86,87] Wnt signaling is critical in embryonic development and is essential for cell polarization, proliferation, and differentiation.[88] In the skin, Wnt is known to regulate regeneration and hair differentiation from epidermal stem cells. FDH presents a striking illustration of functional mosaicism in ectodermal precursors along Blaschko's lines.

Clinical Presentation

FDH predominantly affects the skin, eyes, and skeleton.[51,82] The range of cutaneous signs represents the degree of skin dysgenesis. Cutaneous findings include red or atrophic cribriform depressions along Blaschko's lines, papules of fat herniation in the popliteal and antecubital fossae, and ACC (Figure 9-10). Dystrophic nails and papillomas at mucocutaneous junctions are also common. Ocular abnormalities include microphthalmia and coloboma of the iris and retina. There are classic skeletal findings of striation of the long bones (osteopathia striata), syndactyly/ectrodactyly of the hands and feet, midline defect associated with aplasia cutis, and dental defects. Characteristic asymmetric facial features are seen, with notched or hypoplastic nasal alae, and small ears.

Histologic Findings

Histopathologic findings correlate with the range of skin lesions.[89,90] Early erythematous Blaschkoid lesions show a thinned epidermis overlying a sclerotic dermis containing variable inflammation. Late dyspigmented and atrophic depressions demonstrate an attenuated dermal layer with perivascular encroachment of adipocytes (Figure 9-11). Finally, protruding fat papules represent the presence of subepithelial fat lobules in place of the dysplastic dermis. Fibrillar components of the connective tissue are markedly

reduced around the encroaching fat papules. Findings in aplasia cutis can range from a complete lack of all layers of the skin to a thinned epidermis over normal dermis and subcutis. The complete absence of appendages is universal. The proliferation of capillaries can be seen in the rete ridges from the lesions of all stages.[91,92]

Differential Diagnosis

Oculocerebrocutaneous syndrome is a rare, sporadic disease featuring the same hypoplastic FDH lesions with severe CNS malformations and orbital cysts.[93] Microphthalmia with linear skin defects is an X-linked dominant disease with similar Blaschkoid lesions of the skin and eye involvement.[94] Familial incontinentia pigmenti also features linear pigmented lesions that progress from vesicles to verrucous plaques that become hyperpigmented and atrophic.[95] Pigmentary mosaicism (Hypomelanosis of Ito) is Blaschkoid hyper- or hypopigmentation that may be focal or widespread, and may be associated with musculoskeletal or neurologic manifestations.[96] *Angioma serpiginosum presents as* red, punctuate ectasias of superficial *dermal vessels* that are not atrophic in appearance.[97] In a single Norwegian family, a distinct deletion of the X-chromosome that

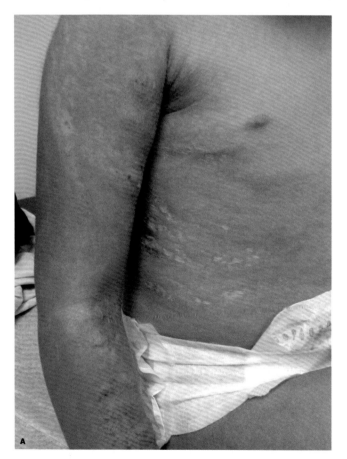
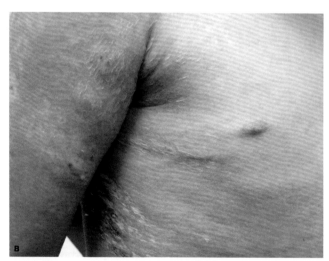
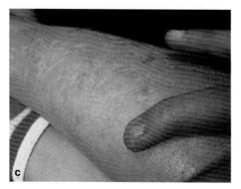

FIGURE 9-10. Focal dermal hypoplasia. A and **B**, Examples of atrophic plaques in a Blaschkoid distribution in an infant. C, Micronychia and Blaschkoid atrophic plaques. Courtesy of Dr. Nnenna Agim, Department of Dermatology, University of Texas Southwestern Medical Center.

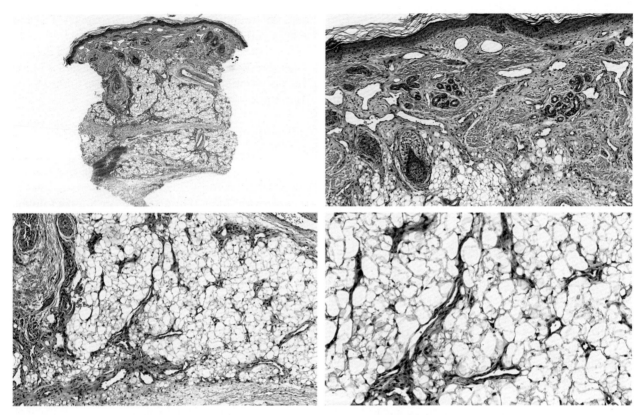

FIGURE 9-11. **Focal dermal hypoplasia.** A slightly acanthotic epidermis overlies a thin dermis. This late lesion demonstrates an attenuated dermal layer with a perivascular encroachment of adipocytes. Digital slides courtesy of Path Presenter.com.

contains the *PORCN* gene was associated with *angioma serpiginosum*.[98] The key skeletal findings of osteopathia striata and digital malformations are specific to FDH and are not seen in related disorders.

CAPSULE SUMMARY

FOCAL DERMAL HYPOPLASIA

FDH or Goltz syndrome is an X-linked dominant disease featuring the atrophy of tissues derived from the ectoderm and mesoderm. The combination of osteopathia striata and syndactyly/ectrodactyly is generally diagnostic. Cutaneous lesions due to skin dysgenesis are found along the Blaschko's lines and present a striking illustration of lyonization. Histopathology is variable, and shows a thinning of the epidermis and/or dermis.

BUSCHKE-OLLENDORFF SYNDROME

Definition and Epidemiology

Buschke-Ollendorff syndrome (BOS) is an autosomal dominant disorder of bone and connective tissue, presenting as a combination of osteosclerotic bone lesions (known as osteopoikilosis) and multiple connective tissue nevi

(dermatofibrosis lenticularis disseminata).[99-101] The prevalence of BOS is estimated at 1:20 000 without known gender predilection.[102]

Etiology

BOS is caused by autosomal dominant, heterozygous, loss-of-function mutations of the *LEMD3* gene.[99,100,103-105] LEMD3, a component of the inner nuclear membrane scaffold, is responsible for the downregulation of TGF-β signaling, which is critical to normal bone and skin morphogenesis.[106] The loss of LEMD3 function results in an enhanced activity of TGF-β and bone morphogenetic protein. Fibroblasts from BOS lesional skin express high levels of elastin mRNA, overproduce the elastin precursor, and have a greater absolute response to TGF-β stimulation.[107] These findings may explain the hyperplastic growths of bone and connective tissue seen in affected patients.

Clinical Presentation

Cutaneous manifestations of BOS begin during early childhood as fleshy or yellow hamartomas of elastin (elastoma), collagen (collagenoma), or mixed connective tissue types.[101,102,108] The skin lesions can be papules, coalescing plaques, or nodules located on the buttocks, trunk, or proximal limbs (Figure 9-12). The characteristic skeletal finding

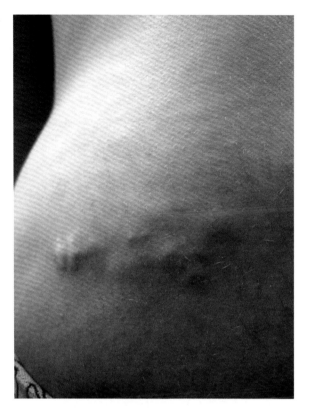

FIGURE 9-12. **Buschke-Ollendorff syndrome.** Dermatofibrosis lenticularis disseminata (collagenomas), appearing as grouped, skin-colored nodules. Courtesy of Dr. Nnenna Agim, Department of Dermatology, University of Texas Southwestern Medical Center.

is osteopoikilosis, which can be detected as symmetric radiopaque foci on the epiphyses and metaphyses of the hands, feet, pelvis, and long bones. Most patients are asymptomatic, although joint pain has been reported. Some affected individuals have isolated skin or bone findings. Melorheostosis, hyperostotic cortical bone that takes on a dripping wax appearance, is also sometimes seen on imaging. The other rare reported findings include short stature, diabetes, craniosynostosis, and otosclerosis.

Histologic Findings

Elastomas are characterized by clumped fragments or a thickened, interlaced meshwork of elastic fibers in the mid- to deep dermis.[109, 111] Collagenomas feature dermal accumulation of hypertrophic collagen bundles with a relative dilution of normal elastic fibers (Figure 9-13).[103,108] Pure collagenous hamartoma is rarely reported in BOS. Mixed connective tissue nevi combine features of both, demonstrating broad elastic fibers enveloping randomly organized, thick collagen bundles in the deeper dermis.[104,112] Dermal edema is present and spaces between fibrillar components may stain positive for mucopolysaccharides.[104] An ultrastructural analysis of elastic fibers variably shows aggregated fragments of the amorphous matrix or massive branching structures that are minimally decorated with microfibrils.[113-115] Cross-sectional contours of collagen fibrils can appear ragged or "flower like".

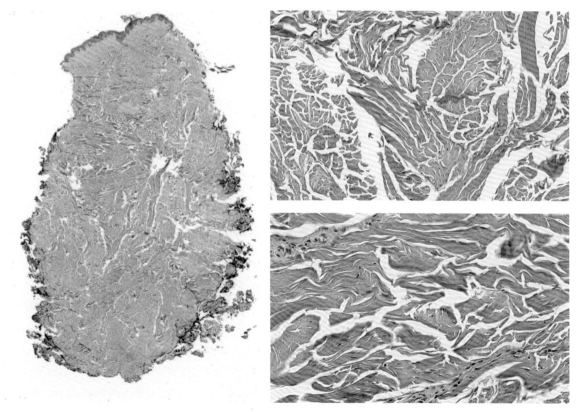

FIGURE 9-13. **Collagenoma.** Collagenomas feature a dermal accumulation of hypertrophic collagen bundles with a relative dilution of normal elastic fibers. Digital slides courtesy of Path Presenter.com.

Differential Diagnosis

The presence of both osteopoikilosis and connective tissue nevi is pathognomonic for BOS. Isolated osteopoikilosis is known to be associated only with *LEMD3* mutations. The other disorders with cutaneous hamartomas include the following: familial collagenoma, eruptive collagenoma, proteus syndrome (cerebriform collagenomas), and tuberous sclerosis.[110] Papular elastorrhexis also presents as white, papular lesions with hypertrophic collagen bundles, but, in contrast to collagenomas, the elastic fibers are fragmented.[116]

STIFF SKIN SYNDROME

Definition and Epidemiology

Stiff skin syndrome (SSS) is a rare autosomal dominant disorder characterized by noninflammatory fibrosis of the skin.[117,118] Only 52 cases have been reported in the literature to date.

Etiology

SSS is caused by mutations in the TGF-β-binding protein-like domain 4 (TB4) of fibrillin-1 *(FBN1)*.[119] MFS is associated with nonoverlapping *FBN1* mutations. Key functional differences exist between the mutated fibrillin-1 found in MFS and SSS. MFS mutations result in the loss of fibrilin-1 expression.[13] In contrast, SSS skin demonstrates large deposits of abnormal fibrilin-1 at the dermal-epidermal junction, and increased expression throughout the dermis, leading to the sequestration of inactive TGF-β at these sites. In these mutations, fibrillin is prevented from binding to integrin, resulting in TGF-β activation and profibrotic signaling. Ongoing studies in the murine models of SSS have yielded an even more complex picture of pathogenesis that could have implications for inflammatory sclerosing disorders.[120]

Clinical Presentation

Often presenting in late infancy and early childhood, typical skin plaques and nodules are woody to palpation with frequent involvement of deep subcutaneous tissue.[117,118] Overlying skin could appear normal or with mild hypertrichosis and hyperpigmentation. Joint immobility favoring the limb girdles and contractures sometimes becomes significant because of the thickened, constricting skin. No other systemic involvement is seen. Both segmental and generalized forms have been described. A slightly more severe phenotype is seen in cases in which the *FBN1* mutations were identified.[119] The clinical assessment of these patients was in late adolescence and adulthood, with other findings including short stature, digital subcutaneous nodules, and neuropathy.

Histologic Findings

Horizontally oriented to the normal epidermis, thickened dermal collagen bundles extend down to a sclerotic fascia with an associated increase in fibroblast

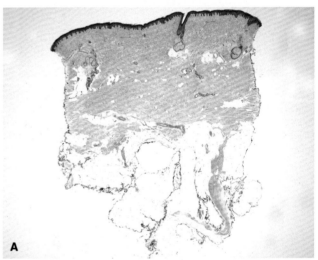

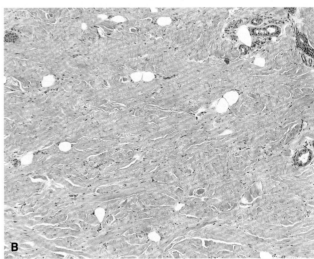

FIGURE 9-14. Stiff skin syndrome. Low (**A**) and high-power (**B**) views show a thickened, sclerotic dermis with the entrapment of adipocytes.

cellularity.[117,118,121,122] There are no inflammatory changes in the dermis, but the accumulation of mucin may be prominent within the collagen clefts, and can be detected by acid Alcian blue or colloidal iron staining. Elastic fibers have normal morphology. In the dermis and subcutis, the entrapment of adipocytes by collagen bundles is a distinctive feature (Figure 9-14).

Differential Diagnosis

Scleredema is typically characterized by uniform edematous changes that start in the neck and face in adults.[123] It can be distinguished from SSS by the increase in mucin deposition that splays apart normal-appearing collagen bundles. In contrast to noninflammatory processes in SSS, localized scleroderma or systemic sclerosis features significant lymphocytic or lymphoplasmacytic infiltration with sclerotic changes.[124,125] Connective tissue nevi are localized hamartomas of collagen and/or elastin without increase in dermal mucin or sclerosis of the reticular dermis and fascia.[126] Nephrogenic systemic fibrosis (NSF) clinically appears as hardened, peau d'orange plaques and is associated with renal insufficiency and exposure to gadolinium.[127] Clinical information is key to making a diagnosis of SSS. Histologically, both feature full thickness sclerosis down to the fascia. Only SSS demonstrates a collagen entrapment of adipocytes, with NSF showing a higher cellularity with more fibroblast proliferation and mild monocytic infiltrates. Scleromyxedema has a striking resemblance to NSF on histology, and the same criteria can help distinguish it from SSS.[128]

CAPSULE SUMMARY

STIFF SKIN SYNDROME

SSS is a rare, autosomal dominant disorder presenting as progressive, noninflammatory fibrosis of the skin. Deep fibrotic plaques or nodules can involve the fascia and cause significant joint immobility. Histopathologic findings include dermal sclerosis, entrapped adipocytes, and an increase in connective tissue mucin.

WINCHESTER SYNDROME AND MULTICENTRIC OSTEOLYSIS, NODULOSIS, AND ARTHROPATHY

Definition and Epidemiology

Winchester syndrome is a heritable disease of connective tissue that has significant clinical overlap with multicentric osteolysis, nodulosis, and arthropathy (MONA).[129,130] Both are rare, autosomal recessive conditions that feature

osteolysis and arthropathy, whereas the presence of subcutaneous skin nodules is unique to MONA.

Etiology

The genetic basis of Winchester syndrome is not firmly established, but it is likely caused by mutation in membrane type-1 metalloproteinase (*MT1-MMP*).[131] The mutation results in a decreased expression of both the zymogen and active MT1-MMP, which leads to a reduced activation of matrix metalloproteinase-2 (*MMP2*). Homozygous mutations in the *MMP2* gene are associated with MONA. MMPs proteolyze and remodel the ECM, which broadly regulates the function of epithelial and mesenchymal tissue.[132] The exact mechanism by which the loss of MT1-MMP and MMP2 function leads to their respective clinical findings is not clear.

Clinical Presentation

Both Winchester syndrome and MONA feature generalized osteoporosis and symmetric osteolysis of the carpal and tarsal bones that lead to joint contractures that begin during the first 6 years of life.[129] Coarse facial features, corneal opacity, EKG changes, and gum hypertrophy are variable findings. Winchester syndrome features more severe, progressive bone disfigurement. Patches of thick, hyperpigmented skin with hypertrichosis can develop over the trunk and limbs, which become softer and paler over time. The presence of subcutaneous nodules favors the diagnosis of MONA.

Histologic Findings

Histopathologic findings in both conditions include deep dermal proliferation of fibroblasts with thickened collagen bundles. The dermis of older lesions evolves to become hypocellular and with homogenized collagen bundles. No accumulation of mucin is seen, and the epidermis appears normal. Ultrastructural studies have demonstrated abnormal fibroblasts with vacuolation of the mitochondria.[133-135]

Differential Diagnosis

The presence of subcutaneous nodules is the most reliable distinguishing feature between Winchester syndrome and MONA. Hyaline fibromatosis syndrome (HFS) is a congenital hyaline deposition disorder caused by recessive mutations in *CMG2*. Multifocal osteolysis, osteoporosis, joint contractures, and a spectrum of other systemic issues can be seen in HFS. Skin lesions range from pearly papules to impressive nodules found on the scalp, ears, neck, face, hands, and perianal region. Histology shows a deposition of hylanized collagen in the dermis with a variable number of fibroblasts. Giant cells, calcospherules, and boney changes can also be seen.[136,137]

CAPSULE SUMMARY

WINCHESTER SYNDROME AND MULTICENTRIC OSTEOLYSIS, NODULOSIS, AND ARTHROPATHY

Winchester syndrome and MONA are primary multicentric osteolytic diseases caused by autosomal recessive defects in ECM remodeling and having significant overlap. In addition to osteolysis, joint contractures, and characteristic facial features, MONA features tender subcutaneous nodules that can differentiate it from Winchester syndrome.

PRIMARY HYPERTROPHIC OSTEOARTHROPATHY

Definition and Epidemiology

Primary hypertrophic osteoarthropathy (PHO), or pachydermoperiostosis, is a rare disease caused by disruptions in prostaglandin metabolism. Patients present with digital clubbing, pachydermia, and periostosis. PHO can be inherited in an autosomal dominant or recessive fashion. There is a male predominance, with a male:female ratio of 7:1.

Etiology

Mutations in the *HPGD* (PHO autosomal recessive, type 1, PHOAR1) and *SLCO2A1* (PHO autosomal recessive, type 2, PHOAR2) genes have been identified as the cause of the recessive PHO, resulting in abnormal prostaglandin metabolism.[138-140] Patients have high levels of serum and urine prostaglandin E2 (PGE2), whose broad, proinflammatory effects lead to the abnormal tissue remodeling seen in PHO.[141] There is no convincing explanation for the difference in prevalence between genders despite some claims of higher PGE2 levels in males.[138,139]

Clinical Presentation

Disease onset typically occurs in infancy (PHOAR1) or adolescence (PHOAR2) with common findings of digital clubbing, pachydermia, and periostitis.[139,140] Progressive skin findings are due to dermal and glandular hypertrophy. Findings include cutis verticis gyrata (CVG), thickened facial skin with the appearance of premature deep furrowing, seborrhea, blepharoptosis, acne, atopic dermatitis, and hyperhidrosis (Figure 9-15). Severe cutis gyrata occurs only with *PHOAR2* mutations. Skeletal involvement results in noninflammatory arthralgia, acroosteolysis, tendon ossification, and radiographic evidence of endosteal and periosteal hyperostosis. Gastrointestinal disease, patent ductus arteriosis (PHOAR1), and myelofibrosis (PHOAR2) have also been documented. On the basis of the clinical severity, PHO is delineated into a complete form (the classical phenotype), an incomplete form (isolated bone involvement with limited skin involvement), and a form fruste (pachydermia and minimal bone disease).[142]

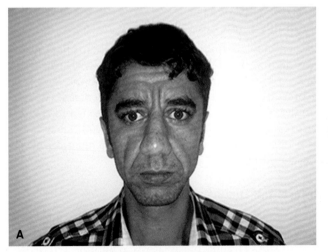

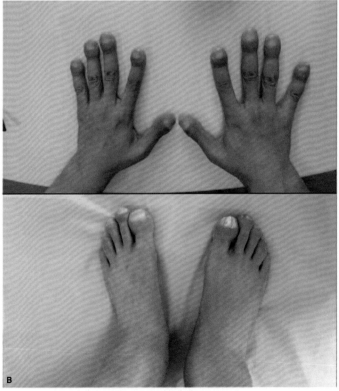

FIGURE 9-15. Primary hypertrophic osteoarthropathy (pachydermoperiostosis). A, Deep furrowing of the face of a 23-year-old man imparting a prematurely aged appearance. **B**, Pachydermodactyly with impressive digital clubbing. **A**, Reprinted with permission from Bingol UA, Cinar C. Pachydermoperiostosis: aesthetic treatment of prematurely aging face with facelift and botulinum toxin a. *J Craniofac Surg*. 2014;25(6):e563-e564. **B**, Reprinted with permission from Zhang H, Yang B. Successful treatment of pachydermoperiostosis patients with etoricoxib, aescin, and arthroscopic synovectomy: two case reports. *Medicine*. 2017;96(47):e8865.

Histologic Findings

A histologic examination of normal-appearing skin may show acanthosis with underlying dermal edema and increased connective tissue mucin.[143] Biopsy samples from the thickened skin show a normal epidermis overlying an edematous dermis, within which there is increased connective tissue mucin. Sebaceous gland hyperplasia, elastin degeneration, and dermal fibrosis are variable, and tend be more marked with increasing clinical severity of pachydermia. Variable lymphohistiocytic and mast cell inflammation of the dermis have been reported.[143-145]

Differential Diagnosis

The secondary causes of hypertrophic osteoarthropathy include intrathoracic tumors, cardiac shunts, and chronic lung disease.[146] Pachydermia has also been reported in secondary disease.[147] CVG can present in an isolated form or can be associated with Turner syndrome, Noonan syndrome, developmental delay, or other conditions.[148-150] Histologically, scleredema and localized myxedema present with dermal edema with a variable separation of collagen bundles by mucin. However, elastic fibers and sebaceous glands are normal, and clinically, furrowing is not present in these conditions.

CAPSULE SUMMARY

PRIMARY HYPERTROPHIC OSTEOARTHROPATHY

PHO is a rare disease caused by defects in prostaglandin metabolism. The congenital elevation of inflammatory prostaglandins leads to pathologic tissue hypertrophy, which manifests as the clinical triad of digital clubbing, pachydermia, and periostosis. Histologic specimens of affected skin show dermal edema, a loss of elastic fibers, increased connective tissue mucin, and enlarged sebaceous glands.

RESTRICTIVE DERMOPATHY

Definition and Epidemiology

Restrictive dermopathy (RD), a rare and lethal progeroid laminopathy, is characterized by pathologically tight skin leading to fetal akinesia and neonatal demise from pulmonary failure.[151-154] RD is the most severe form of the lamin-associated disorder that also includes mandibuloacral dysplasia, *Hutchinson-Gilford progeria syndrome, and others.*[155] Fewer than 100 cases of RD have been reported to date. RD can be inherited in a recessive manner or may result from dominant de novo mutation.

Etiology

RD results from heterozygous or homozygous mutations of the *LMNA* gene or, more commonly, null mutations of the *ZMPSTE24* gene (encoding zinc metalloprotease STE24).[156-159] Lamin A is a structural constituent of the inner nuclear envelope. STE24 is responsible for the processing and maturation of lamin A. There are isolated cases of RD for which causative mutations have not been identified. Mutations in *LMNA* and *ZMPSTE24* result in abnormal nuclear morphology and an accumulation of unprocessed prelamin A. The mechanism that leads to generalized cutaneous deformity is not understood.

Clinical Presentation

Patients are born prematurely with taut, translucent skin with prominent vasculature. Generalized alopecia sparing the head is seen. Characteristic facial features are microstomia fixed in the O position, micrognathia, pinched nose, and wide cranial sutures (Figure 9-16). The features of intrauterine growth restriction can be appreciated with rocker-bottom feet, clavicular dysplasia, and arthrogryposis multiplex congenita.

Histologic Findings

Biopsy specimens show flattened rete overlying a thinned dermis.[152,157,160] There is a scar-like dermal fibrosis, in which collagen bundles are arranged in parallel with the epidermis with sparse elastic fibers. Adnexal structures are uniformly poorly differentiated. The subcutis appears normal. Ultrastructural studies confirm the proliferation of small-caliber

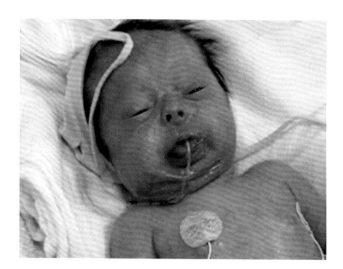

FIGURE 9-16. Restrictive dermopathy. Characteristic facial features of microphthalmia, a pinched nose, and microstomia. Reprinted with permission from Bosque E. Complex case study: nursing care of an infant with restrictive dermopathy. *J Perinat Neonatal Nurs.* 2009;23(2):171-177.

collagen fibrils, the presence of degenerated fibroblasts, and the near absence of elastic fibers.[161]

Differential Diagnosis

A number of lethal congenital syndromes present with fetal akinesia and intrauterine growth restriction. Neu-Laxova features severe CNS malformations with associated tight skin and generalized ichthyosis.[162] Fetal akinesia deformation sequence syndrome, or Pena-Shokeir syndrome, is a clinical sign characterized by dysmorphic facies, pulmonary hypoplasia, and arthrogryposis.[163] It is associated with primary disorders of the neuromuscular junction. Primary cutaneous disorders can also be considered. Autosomal recessive congenital ichthyosis is a heterogeneous group of disorders of keratinization in which hyperkeratosis and scaling are essential features.[164] Histologically, the dermal fibrosis may resemble a scar. Dermatomyofibromas are characterized by a horizontal proliferation of myofibroblasts and collagen, but they are solitary lesions.

CAPSULE SUMMARY

RESTRICTIVE DERMOPATHY

RD is a lethal laminopathy presenting with severe intrauterine growth restriction because of pathologically tight skin. Taut facial skin causes characteristic facies, with the mouth fixed in the O position. The histologic finding of generalized, scar-like dermis is diagnostic for RD.

REFERENCES

1. Malfait F, Francomano C, Byers P, et al. The 2017 international classification of the Ehlers-Danlos syndromes. *Am J Med Genet C Semin Med Genet.* 2017;175(1):8-26.
2. Beighton P, De Paepe A, Steinmann B, Tsipouras P, Wenstrup RJ. Ehlers-Danlos syndromes: revised nosology, Villefranche, 1997. Ehlers-Danlos National Foundation (USA) and Ehlers-Danlos Support Group (UK). *Am J Med Genet.* 1998;77(1):31-77.
3. Shirley ED, DeMaio M, Bodurtha J. Ehlers-Danlos syndrome in orthopaedics: etiology, diagnosis, and treatment implications. *Sports Health.* 2012;4(5):394-403.
4. Germain DP. Ehlers-Danlos syndrome type IV. *Orphanet J Rare Dis.* 2007;2:32.
5. Vanakker O, Callewaert B, Malfait F, Coucke P. The genetics of soft connective tissue disorders. *Annu Rev Genomics Hum Genet.* 2015;16:229-255.
6. Zweers MC, Dean WB, van Kuppevelt TH, Bristow J, Schalkwijk J. Elastic fiber abnormalities in hypermobility type Ehlers-Danlos syndrome patients with tenascin-X mutations. *Clin Genet.* 2005;67(4):330-334.
7. Kapferer-Seebacher I, Pepin M, Werner R, et al. Periodontal Ehlers-Danlos syndrome is caused by mutations in C1R and C1S, which encode subcomponents C1r and C1s of complement. *Am J Hum Genet.* 2016;99(5):1005-1014.
8. Abu A, Frydman M, Marek D, et al. Deleterious mutations in the Zinc-Finger 469 gene cause brittle cornea syndrome. *Am J Hum Genet.* 2008;82(5):1217-1222.
9. Burkitt Wright EMM, Spencer HL, Daly SB, et al. Mutations in PRDM5 in brittle cornea syndrome identify a pathway regulating extracellular matrix development and maintenance. *Am J Hum Genet.* 2011;88(6):767-777.
10. Byers PH, Murray ML. Ehlers-Danlos syndrome: a showcase of conditions that lead to understanding matrix biology. *Matrix Biol.* 2014;33:10-15.
11. Moore MM, Votava JM, Orlow SJ, Schaffer JV. Ehlers-Danlos syndrome type VIII: periodontitis, easy bruising, marfanoid habitus, and distinctive facies. *J Am Acad Dermatol.* 2006;55(2 suppl):S41-S45.
12. Klaassens M, Reinstein E, Hilhorst-Hofstee Y, et al. Ehlers-Danlos Arthrochalasia type (VIIA-B) – expanding the phenotype: from prenatal life through adulthood. *Clin Genet.* 2012;82(2):121-130.
13. Judge DP, Dietz HC. Therapy of Marfan syndrome. *Annu Rev Med.* 2008;59:43-59.
14. Loeys BL, Dietz HC, Braverman AC, et al. The revised Ghent nosology for the Marfan syndrome. *J Med Genet.* 2010;47(7):476-485.
15. Groth KA, Hove H, Kyhl K, et al. Prevalence, incidence, and age at diagnosis in Marfan Syndrome. *Orphanet J Rare Dis.* 2015;10:153.
16. Martinez-Quintana E, Caballero-Sanchez N, Rodriguez-Gonzalez F, Garay-Sanchez P, Tugores A. Novel Marfan syndrome-associated mutation in the FBN1 gene caused by parental mosaicism and leading to abnormal limb patterning. *Mol Syndromol.* 2017;8(3):148-154.
17. Tiecke F, Katzke S, Booms P, et al. Classic, atypically severe and neonatal Marfan syndrome: twelve mutations and genotype-phenotype correlations in FBN1 exons 24-40. *Eur J Hum Genet.* 2001;9(1):13-21.
18. Faivre L, Collod-Beroud G, Child A, et al. Contribution of molecular analyses in diagnosing Marfan syndrome and type I fibrillinopathies: an international study of 1009 probands. *J Med Genet.* 2008;45(6):384-390.
19. Stheneur C, Tubach F, Jouneaux M, et al. Study of phenotype evolution during childhood in Marfan syndrome to improve clinical recognition. *Genet Med.* 2014;16(3):246-250.
20. Grahame R, Pyeritz RE. The Marfan syndrome: joint and skin manifestations are prevalent and correlated. *Br J Rheumatol.* 1995;34(2):126-131.
21. Ledoux M, Beauchet A, Fermanian C, Boileau C, Jondeau G, Saiag P. A case-control study of cutaneous signs in adult patients with Marfan disease: diagnostic value of striae. *J Am Acad Dermatol.* 2011;64(2):290-295.
22. Ghandi Y, K SZ, Mazhari-Mousavi SE, Parvaneh N. Neonatal Marfan syndrome: report of two cases. *Iran J Pediatr.* 2013;23(1):113-117.
23. Tsuji T. Marfan syndrome: demonstration of abnormal elastic fibers in skin. *J Cutan Pathol.* 1986;13(2):144-153.
24. Hollister DW, Godfrey M, Sakai LY, Pyeritz RE. Immunohistologic abnormalities of the microfibrillar-fiber system in the Marfan syndrome. *N Engl J Med.* 1990;323(3):152-159.
25. Pinkus H, Keech MK, Mehregan AH. Histopathology of striae distensae, with special reference to striae and wound healing in the Marfan syndrome. *J Invest Dermatol.* 1966;46(3):283-292.
26. Bergman R, Nevet MJ, Gescheidt-Shoshany H, Pimienta AL, Reinstein E. Atrophic skin patches with abnormal elastic fibers as a presenting sign of the MASS phenotype associated with mutation in the fibrillin 1 gene. *JAMA Dermatol.* 2014;150(8):885-889.
27. Meester JAN, Verstraeten A, Schepers D, Alaerts M, Van Laer L, Loeys BL. Differences in manifestations of Marfan syndrome, Ehlers-Danlos syndrome, and Loeys-Dietz syndrome. *Ann Cardiothorac Surg.* 2017;6(6):582-594.
28. Wang M, Clericuzio CL, Godfrey M. Familial occurrence of typical and severe lethal congenital contractural arachnodactyly caused by missplicing of exon 34 of fibrillin-2. *Am J Hum Genet.* 1996;59(5):1027-1034.
29. Berk DR, Bentley DD, Bayliss SJ, Lind A, Urban Z. Cutis laxa: a review. *J Am Acad Dermatol.* 2012;66(5):842.e1-17.
30. Morava E, Guillard M, Lefeber DJ, Wevers RA. Autosomal recessive cutis laxa syndrome revisited. *Eur J Hum Genet.* 2009;17(9):1099-1110.
31. Lewis PG, Hood AF, Barnett NK, Holbrook KA. Postinflammatory elastolysis and cutis laxa. A case report. *J Am Acad Dermatol.* 1990;22(1):40-48.

32. Na SY, Choi M, Kim MJ, Lee JH, Cho S. Penicillamine-induced elastosis perforans serpiginosa and cutis laxa in a patient with Wilson's disease. *Ann Dermatol.* 2010;22(4):468-471.

33. Isik M, Aydin C. Cutis laxa (elastolysis) in a patient with Sjogren's syndrome. *Eur J Rheumatol.* 2015;2(1):41-42.

34. Tronnier M. Cutaneous disorders characterized by elastolysis or loss of elastic tissue. *J Dtsh Dermatol Ges.* 2018;16(2):183-191.

35. O'Malley JT, D'Agati VD, Sherman WH, Grossman ME. Acquired cutis laxa associated with heavy chain deposition disease involving dermal elastic fibers. *JAMA Dermatol.* 2014;150(11):1192-1196.

36. Garcia-Patos V, Pujol RM, Barnadas MA, et al. Generalized acquired cutis laxa associated with coeliac disease: evidence of immunoglobulin A deposits on the dermal elastic fibres. *Br J Dermatol.* 1996;135(1):130-134.

37. Maruani A, Arbeille B, Machet MC, et al. Ultrastructural demonstration of a relationship between acquired cutis laxa and monoclonal gammopathy. *Acta Derm Venereol.* 2010;90(4):406-408.

38. Marconi B, Bobyr I, Campanati A, et al. Pseudoxanthoma elasticum and skin: clinical manifestations, histopathology, pathomechanism, perspectives of treatment. *Intractable Rare Dis Res.* 2015;4(3):113-122.

39. Patroi I, Annessi G, Girolomoni G. Mid-dermal elastolysis: a clinical, histologic, and immunohistochemical study of 11 patients. *J Am Acad Dermatol.* 2003;48(6):846-851.

40. Graul-Neumann LM, Hausser I, Essayie M, Rauch A, Kraus C. Highly variable cutis laxa resulting from a dominant splicing mutation of the elastin gene. *Am J Med Genet A.* 2008;146a(8):977-983.

41. Van Maldergem L, Yuksel-Apak M, Kayserili H, et al. Cobblestone-like brain dysgenesis and altered glycosylation in congenital cutis laxa, Debre type. *Neurology.* 2008;71(20):1602-1608.

42. Callewaert B, Su CT, Van Damme T, et al. Comprehensive clinical and molecular analysis of 12 families with type 1 recessive cutis laxa. *Hum Mutat.* 2013;34(1):111-121.

43. Fischer-Zirnsak B, Escande-Beillard N, Ganesh J, et al. Recurrent de novo mutations affecting residue arg138 of pyrroline-5-carboxylate synthase cause a progeroid form of autosomal-dominant cutis laxa. *Am J Hum Genet.* 2015;97(3):483-492.

44. Van Damme T, Gardeitchik T, Mohamed M, et al. Mutations in ATP6V1E1 or ATP6V1A cause autosomal-recessive cutis laxa. *Am J Hum Genet.* 2017;100(2):216-227.

45. Syx D, Malfait F, Van Laer L, et al. The RIN2 syndrome: a new autosomal recessive connective tissue disorder caused by deficiency of Ras and Rab interactor 2 (RIN2). *Hum Genet.* 2010;128(1):79-88.

46. Frieden IJ. Aplasia cutis congenita: a clinical review and proposal for classification. *J Am Acad Dermatol.* 1986;14(4):646-660.

47. Demmel U. Clinical aspects of congenital skin defects. I. Congenital skin defects on the head of the newborn. *Eur J Pediatr.* 1975;121(1):21-50.

48. Martinez-Regueira S, Vazquez-Lopez ME, Somoza-Rubio C, Morales-Redondo R, Gonzalez-Gay MA. Aplasia cutis congenita in a defined population from northwest Spain. *Pediatr Dermatol.* 2006;23(6):528-532.

49. Kosnik EJ, Sayers MP. Congenital scalp defects: aplasia cutis congenita. *J Neurosurg.* 1975;42(1):32-36.

50. Hassed S, Li S, Mulvihill J, Aston C, Palmer S. Adams-Oliver syndrome review of the literature: refining the diagnostic phenotype. *Am J Med Genet A.* 2017;173(3):790-800.

51. Mary L, Scheidecker S, Kohler M, et al. Prenatal diagnosis of focal dermal hypoplasia: report of three fetuses and review of the literature. *Am J Med Genet A.* 2017;173(2):479-486.

52. Marneros AG. BMS1 is mutated in aplasia cutis congenita. *PLoS Genet.* 2013;9(6):e1003573.

53. Bessis D, Bigorre M, Malissen N, et al. The scalp hair collar and tuft signs: a retrospective multicenter study of 78 patients with a systematic review of the literature. *J Am Acad Dermatol.* 2017;76(3):478-487.

54. Johnson R, Offiah A, Cohen MC. Fatal superior sagittal sinus hemorrhage as a complication of aplasia cutis congenita: a case report and literature review. *Forensic Sci Med Pathol.* 2015;11(2):243-248.

55. Colon-Fontanez F, Fallon Friedlander S, Newbury R, Eichenfield LF. Bullous aplasia cutis congenita. *J Am Acad Dermatol.* 2003;48(5 suppl):S95-S98.

56. Zhou J, Zheng L, Tao W. Systemic aplasia cutis congenita: a case report and review of the literature. *Pathol Res Pract.* 2010;206(7):504-507.

57. Croce EJ, Purohit RC, Janovski NA. Congenital absence of skin (aplasia cutis congenita). *Arch Surg.* 1973;106(5):732-734.

58. Vijayashankar MR. Aplasia cutis congenita: a case report. *Dermatol Online J.* 2005;11(3):28.

59. Cham PM, Drolet BA, Segura AD, Esterly NB. Congenital Volkmann ischaemic contracture: a case report and review. *Br J Dermatol.* 2004;150(2):357-363.

60. Sauerbrei A, Wutzler P. The congenital varicella syndrome. *J Perinatol.* 2000;20(8 Pt 1):548-554.

61. Uitto J, Jiang Q, Varadi A, Bercovitch LG, Terry SF. Pseudoxanthoma elasticum: diagnostic features, classification, and treatment options. *Expert Opin Orphan Drugs.* 2014;2(6):567-577.

62. Nitschke Y, Baujat G, Botschen U, et al. Generalized arterial calcification of infancy and pseudoxanthoma elasticum can be caused by mutations in either ENPP1 or ABCC6. *Am J Hum Genet.* 2012;90(1):25-39.

63. Li Q, Grange DK, Armstrong NL, et al. Mutations in the GGCX and ABCC6 genes in a family with pseudoxanthoma elasticum-like phenotypes. *J Invest Dermatol.* 2009;129(3):553-563.

64. Chassaing N, Martin L, Calvas P, Le Bert M, Hovnanian A. Pseudoxanthoma elasticum: a clinical, pathophysiological and genetic update including 11 novel ABCC6 mutations. *J Med Genet.* 2005;42(12):881-892.

65. Kocaturk E, Kavala M, Zindanci I, Koc M. Periumbilical perforating pseudoxanthoma elasticum. *Indian J Dermatol Venereol Leprol.* 2009;75(3):329.

66. De Vilder EY, Debacker J, Vanakker OM. GGCX-associated phenotypes: an overview in search of genotype-phenotype correlations. *Int J Mol Sci.* 2017;18(2).

67. Hosen MJ, Lamoen A, De Paepe A, Vanakker OM. Histopathology of pseudoxanthoma elasticum and related disorders: histological hallmarks and diagnostic clues. *Scientifica.* 2012;2012:598262.

68. Patterson AT, Beasley KJ, Kobayashi TT. Fibroelastolytic papulosis: histopathologic confirmation of disease spectrum variants in a single case. *J Cutan Pathol.* 2016;43(2):142-147.

69. Wang AR, Fonder MA, Telang GH, Bercovitch L, Robinson-Bostom L. Late-onset focal dermal elastosis: an uncommon mimicker of pseudoxanthoma elasticum. *J Cutan Pathol.* 2012;39(10):957-961.

70. Lee SH, Choi Y, Kim SC. Elastosis perforans serpiginosa. *Ann Dermatol.* 2014;26(1):103-106.

71. Lopes LC, Lobo L, Bajanca R. Perforating calcific elastosis. *J Eur Acad Dermatol Venereol.* 2003;17(2):206-207.

72. Mehregan AH. Elastosis perforans serpiginosa: a review of the literature and report of 11 cases. *Arch Dermatol.* 1968;97(4):381-393.

73. Lewis KG, Bercovitch L, Dill SW, Robinson-Bostom L. Acquired disorders of elastic tissue: part I. Increased elastic tissue and solar elastotic syndromes. *J Am Acad Dermatol.* 2004;51(1):1-21; quiz 2-4.

74. Langeveld-Wildschut EG, Toonstra J, van Vloten WA, Beemer FA. Familial elastosis perforans serpiginosa. *Arch Dermatol.* 1993;129(2):205-207.

75. Fujimoto N, Tajima S, Ishibashi A. Elastin peptides induce migration and terminal differentiation of cultured keratinocytes via 67 kDa elastin receptor in vitro: 67 kDa elastin receptor is expressed in the keratinocytes eliminating elastic materials in elastosis perforans serpiginosa. *J Invest Dermatol.* 2000;115(4):633-639.

76. Atzori L, Pinna AL, Pau M, Aste N. D-penicillamine elastosis perforans serpiginosa: description of two cases and review of the literature. *Dermatol Online J.* 2011;17(4):3.

77. Thiele-Ochel S, Schneider LA, Reinhold K, Hunzelmann N, Krieg T, Scharffetter-Kochanek K. Acquired perforating collagenosis: is it due to damage by scratching? *Br J Dermatol.* 2001;145(1):173-174.

78. Bergman R, Friedman-Birnbaum R, Ludatscher R, Lichtig C. An ultrastructural study of the reactive type of elastosis perforans serpiginosa. *Arch Dermatol.* 1987;123(9):1127-1129.

79. Bardach H, Gebhart W, Niebauer G. "Lumpy-bumpy" elastic fibers in the skin and lungs of a patient with a penicillamine-induced elastosis perforans serpiginosa. *J Cutan Pathol.* 1979;6(4):243-252.

80. Nasca MR, Lacarrubba F, Caltabiano R, Verzi AE, Micali G. Perforating pseudoxanthoma elasticum with secondary elastosis perforans serpiginosa-like changes: dermoscopy, confocal microscopy and histopathological correlation. *J Cutan Pathol.* 2016;43(11):1021-104.

81. Wang L, Jin X, Zhao X, et al. Focal dermal hypoplasia: updates. *Oral Dis.* 2014;20(1):17-24.

82. Yesodharan D, Buschenfelde UMZ, Kutsche K, Mohandas Nair K, Nampoothiri S. Goltz-Gorlin syndrome: revisiting the clinical spectrum. *Indian J Pediatr.* 2018. Epub 2018/02/01.

83. Goltz RW, Henderson RR, Hitch JM, Ott JE. Focal dermal hypoplasia syndrome. A review of the literature and report of two cases. *Arch Dermatol.* 1970;101(1):1-11.

84. Wechsler MA, Papa CM, Haberman F, Marion RW. Variable expression in focal dermal hypoplasia. An example of differential X-chromosome inactivation. *Am J Dis Child.* 1988;142(3):297-300.

85. Madan S, Liu W, Lu JT, et al. A non-mosaic PORCN mutation in a male with severe congenital anomalies overlapping focal dermal hypoplasia. *Mol Genet Metab Rep.* 2017;12:57-61.

86. Wang X, Reid Sutton V, Omar Peraza-Llanes J, et al. Mutations in X-linked PORCN, a putative regulator of Wnt signaling, cause focal dermal hypoplasia. *Nat Genet.* 2007;39(7):836-838.

87. Grzeschik KH, Bornholdt D, Oeffner F, et al. Deficiency of PORCN, a regulator of Wnt signaling, is associated with focal dermal hypoplasia. *Nat Genet.* 2007;39(7):833-835.

88. Paller AS. Wnt signaling in focal dermal hypoplasia. *Nat Genet.* 2007;39(7):820-821.

89. Ko CJ, Antaya RJ, Zubek A, et al. Revisiting histopathologic findings in Goltz syndrome. *J Cutan Pathol.* 2016;43(5):418-421.

90. Ishii N, Baba N, Kanaizuka I, Nakajima H, Ono S, Amemiya F. Histopathological study of focal dermal hypoplasia (Goltz syndrome). *Clin Exp Dermatol.* 1992;17(1):24-26.

91. del Carmen Boente M, Asial RA, Winik BC. Focal dermal hypoplasia: ultrastructural abnormalities of the connective tissue. *J Cutan Pathol.* 2007;34(2):181-187.

92. Lee IJ, Cha MS, Kim SC, Bang D. Electronmicroscopic observation of the basement membrane zone in focal dermal hypoplasia. *Pediatr Dermatol.* 1996;13(1):5-9.

93. Moog U, Jones MC, Bird LM, Dobyns WB. Oculocerebrocutaneous syndrome: the brain malformation defines a core phenotype. *J Med Genet.* 2005;42(12):913-921.

94. Sharma VM, Ruiz de Luzuriaga AM, Waggoner D, Greenwald M, Stein SL. Microphthalmia with linear skin defects: a case report and review. *Pediatr Dermatol.* 2008;25(5):548-552.

95. O'Doherty M, Mc Creery K, Green AJ, Tuwir I, Brosnahan D. Incontinentia pigmenti: ophthalmological observation of a series of cases and review of the literature. *Br J Ophthalmol.* 2011;95(1):11-16.

96. Happle R. Incontinentia pigmenti versus hypomelanosis of Ito: the whys and wherefores of a confusing issue. *Am J Med Genet.* 1998;79(1):64-65.

97. Chen W, Liu TJ, Yang YC, Happle R. Angioma serpiginosum arranged in a systematized segmental pattern suggesting mosaicism. *Dermatology.* 2006;213(3):236-238.

98. Houge G, Oeffner F, Grzeschik KH. An Xp11.23 deletion containing PORCN may also cause angioma serpiginosum, a cosmetic skin disease associated with extreme skewing of X-inactivation. *Eur J Hum Genet.* 2008;16(9):1027-1028.

99. Hellemans J, Preobrazhenska O, Willaert A, et al. Loss-of-function mutations in LEMD3 result in osteopoikilosis, Buschke-Ollendorff syndrome and melorheostosis. *Nat Genet.* 2004;36(11):1213-1218.

100. Zhang Y, Castori M, Ferranti G, Paradisi M, Wordsworth BP. Novel and recurrent germline LEMD3 mutations causing Buschke-Ollendorff syndrome and osteopoikilosis but not isolated melorheostosis. *Clin Genet.* 2009;75(6):556-561.

101. Ehrig T, Cockerell CJ. Buschke-Ollendorff syndrome: report of a case and interpretation of the clinical phenotype as a type 2 segmental manifestation of an autosomal dominant skin disease. *J Am Acad Dermatol.* 2003;49(6):1163-1166.

102. Pope V, Dupuis L, Kannu P, et al. Buschke-Ollendorff syndrome: a novel case series and systematic review. *Br J Dermatol.* 2016;174(4):723-729.

103. Mumm S, Wenkert D, Zhang X, McAlister WH, Mier RJ, Whyte MP. Deactivating germline mutations in LEMD3 cause osteopoikilosis and Buschke-Ollendorff syndrome, but not sporadic melorheostosis. *J Bone Miner Res.* 2007;22(2):243-250.

104. Yadegari M, Whyte MP, Mumm S, et al. Buschke-Ollendorff syndrome: absence of LEMD3 mutation in an affected family. *Arch Dermatol.* 2010;146(1):63-68.

105. Kratzsch J, Mitter D, Ziemer M, Kohlhase J, Voth H. Identification of a novel point mutation in the LEMD3 gene in an infant with Buschke-Ollendorff syndrome. *JAMA Dermatol.* 2016;152(7):844-845.

106. Bourgeois B, Gilquin B, Tellier-Lebegue C, et al. Inhibition of TGF-beta signaling at the nuclear envelope: characterization of interactions between MAN1, Smad2 and Smad3, and PPM1A. *Sci Signal.* 2013;6(280):ra49.

107. Giro MG, Duvic M, Smith LT, et al. Buschke-Ollendorff syndrome associated with elevated elastin production by affected skin fibroblasts in culture. *J Invest Dermatol.* 1992;99(2):129-137.

108. Schaffenburg WC, Fernelius C, Arora NS. Buschke-Ollendorff syndrome presenting as a painful nodule. *JAAD Case Rep.* 2015;1(2):77-79.

109. Danielsen L, Midtgaard K, Christensen HE. Osteopoikilosis associated with dermatofibrosis lenticularis disseminata. *Arch Dermatol.* 1969;100(4):465-470.

110. McCuaig CC, Vera C, Kokta V, et al. Connective tissue nevi in children: institutional experience and review. *J Am Acad Dermatol.* 2012;67(5):890-897.

111. Maciel MG, Enokihara MM, Seize MB, Marcassi AP, Piazza CA, Cestari SD. Elastoma: clinical and histopathological aspects of a rare disease. *An Bras Dermatol.* 2016;91(5 suppl 1):39-41.

112. Walpole IR, Manners PJ. Clinical considerations in Buschke-Ollendorff syndrome. *Clin Genet.* 1990;37(1):59-63.

113. Uitto J, Santa Cruz DJ, Starcher BC, Whyte MP, Murphy WA. Biochemical and ultrastructural demonstration of elastin accumulation in the skin lesions of the Buschke-Ollendorff syndrome. *J Invest Dermatol.* 1981;76(4):284-287.

114. Trattner A, David M, Rothem A, Ben-David E, Sandbank M. Buschke-Ollendorff syndrome of the scalp: histologic and ultrastructural findings. *J Am Acad Dermatol.* 1991;24(5 Pt 2):822-824.

115. Cole GW, Barr RJ. An elastic tissue defect in dermatofibrosis lenticularis disseminata. Buschke-Ollendorff syndrome. *Arch Dermatol.* 1982;118(1):44-46.

116. Ryder HF, Antaya RJ. Nevus anelasticus, papular elastorrhexis, and eruptive collagenoma: clinically similar entities with focal absence of elastic fibers in childhood. *Pediatric Dermatol.* 2005;22(2):153-157.

117. Myers KL, Mir A, Schaffer JV, Meehan SA, Orlow SJ, Brinster NK. Segmental stiff skin syndrome (SSS): a distinct clinical entity. *J Am Acad Dermatol.* 2016;75(1):163-168.

118. Liu T, McCalmont TH, Frieden IJ, Williams ML, Connolly MK, Gilliam AE. The stiff skin syndrome: case series, differential diagnosis of the stiff skin phenotype, and review of the literature. *Arch Dermatol.* 2008;144(10):1351-1359.

119. Loeys BL, Gerber EE, Riegert-Johnson D, et al. Mutations in fibrillin-1 cause congenital scleroderma: stiff skin syndrome. *Sci Transl Med.* 2010;2(23):23ra0.

120. Gerber EE, Gallo EM, Fontana SC, et al. Integrin-modulating therapy prevents fibrosis and autoimmunity in mouse models of scleroderma. *Nature.* 2013;503(7474):126-130.

121. Jablonska S, Blaszczyk M. Scleroderma-like indurations involving fascias: an abortive form of congenital fascial dystrophy (Stiff skin syndrome). *Pediatr Dermatol.* 2000;17(2):105-110.

122. McCalmont TH, Gilliam AE. A subcutaneous lattice-like array of thick collagen is a clue to the diagnosis of stiff skin syndrome. *J Cutan Pathol.* 2012;39(1):2-4, 1.

123. Cole HG, Winkelmann RK. Acid mucopolysaccharide staining in scleredema. *J Cutan Pathol.* 1990;17(4):211-213.

124. Walker D, Susa JS, Currimbhoy S, Jacobe H. Histopathological changes in morphea and their clinical correlates: results from the Morphea in Adults and Children Cohort V. *J Am Acad Dermatol.* 2017;76(6):1124-1130.

125. Vazquez Botet M, Sanchez JL. The fascia in systemic scleroderma. *J Am Acad Dermatol.* 1980;3(1):36-42.

126. Uitto J, Santa Cruz DJ, Eisen AZ. Connective tissue nevi of the skin. Clinical, genetic, and histopathologic classification of hamartomas of the collagen, elastin, and proteoglycan type. *J Am Acad Dermatol.* 1980;3(5):441-461.

127. Thakral C, Abraham JL. Gadolinium-induced nephrogenic systemic fibrosis is associated with insoluble Gd deposits in tissues: in vivo transmetallation confirmed by microanalysis. *J Cutan Pathol.* 2009;36(12):1244-1254.

128. Kucher C, Xu X, Pasha T, Elenitsas R. Histopathologic comparison of nephrogenic fibrosing dermopathy and scleromyxedema. *J Cutan Pathol.* 2005;32(7):484-490.

129. Bhavani GS, Shah H, Shukla A, et al. Clinical and mutation profile of multicentric osteolysis nodulosis and arthropathy. *Am J Med Genet A.* 2016;170A(2):410-417.

130. Winchester P, Grossman H, Lim WN, Danes BS. A new acid mucopolysaccharidosis with skeletal deformities simulating rheumatoid arthritis. *Am J Roentgenol Radium Ther Nucl Med.* 1969;106(1):121-128.

131. Evans BR, Mosig RA, Lobl M, et al. Mutation of membrane type-1 metalloproteinase, MT1-MMP, causes the multicentric osteolysis and arthritis disease Winchester syndrome. *Am J Hum Genet.* 2012;91(3):572-576.

132. Martins VL, Caley M, O'Toole EA. Matrix metalloproteinases and epidermal wound repair. *Cell Tissue Res.* 2013;351(2):255-268.

133. Cohen AH, Hollister DW, Reed WB. The skin in the Winchester syndrome. *Arch Dermatol.* 1975;111(2):230-236.

134. Sidwell RU, Brueton LA, Grabczynska SA, Francis N, Staughton RC. Progressive multilayered banded skin in Winchester syndrome. *J Am Acad Dermatol.* 2004;50(2 suppl):S53-S56.

135. Nabai H, Mehregan AH, Mortezai A, Alipour P, Karimi FZ. Winchester syndrome: report of a case from Iran. *J Cutan Pathol.* 1977;4(5):281-285.

136. Bernardez C, Martinez Barba E, Kutzner H, Requena L. A mild case of hyaline fibromatosis syndrome, presenting in an adult. *J Eur Acad Dermatol Venereol.* 2016;30(5):902-904.

137. Haleem A, Al-Hindi HN, Juboury MA, Husseini HA, Ajlan AA. Juvenile hyaline fibromatosis: morphologic, immunohistochemical, and ultrastructural study of three siblings. *Am J Dermatopathol.* 2002;24(3):218-224.

138. Uppal S, Diggle CP, Carr IM, et al. Mutations in 15-hydroxyprostaglandin dehydrogenase cause primary hypertrophic osteoarthropathy. *Nat Genet.* 2008;40(6):789-793.

139. Diggle CP, Parry DA, Logan CV, et al. Prostaglandin transporter mutations cause pachydermoperiostosis with myelofibrosis. *Hum Mutat.* 2012;33(8):1175-1181.

140. Seifert W, Kuhnisch J, Tuysuz B, Specker C, Brouwers A, Horn D. Mutations in the prostaglandin transporter encoding gene SLCO2A1 cause primary hypertrophic osteoarthropathy and isolated digital clubbing. *Hum Mutat.* 2012;33(4):660-664.

141. Ricciotti E, FitzGerald GA. Prostaglandins and Inflammation. *Arterioscler Thromb Vasc Biol.* 2011;31(5):986-1000.

142. Rahaman SH, Kandasamy D, Jyotsna VP. Pachydermoperiostosis: incomplete form, mimicking acromegaly. *Indian J Endocrinol Metab.* 2016;20(5):730-731.

143. Oikarinen A, Palatsi R, Kylmaniemi M, Keski-Oja J, Risteli J, Kallioinen M. Pachydermoperiostosis: analysis of the connective tissue abnormality in one family. *J Am Acad Dermatol.* 1994;31(6):947-953.

144. Tanese K, Niizeki H, Seki A, et al. Infiltration of mast cells in pachydermia of pachydermoperiostosis. *J Dermatol.* 2017;44(11):1320-1321.

145. Tanese K, Niizeki H, Seki A, et al. Pathological characterization of pachydermia in pachydermoperiostosis. *J Dermatol.* 2015;42(7):710-714.

146. Fridlington J, Weaver J, Kelly B, Kelly E. Secondary hypertrophic osteoarthropathy associated with solitary fibrous tumor of the lung. *J Am Acad Dermatol.* 2007;57(5 suppl):S106-S110.

147. Cannavo SP, Guarneri C, Borgia F, Vaccaro M. Pierre Marie-Bamberger syndrome (secondary hypertrophic osteoarthropathy). *Int J Dermatol.* 2005;44(1):41-42.

148. Garden JM, Robinson JK. Essential primary cutis verticis gyrata. Treatment with the scalp reduction procedure. *Arch Dermatol.* 1984;120(11):1480-1483.

149. Parolin Marinoni L, Taniguchi K, Giraldi S, Carvalho VO, Furucho M, Bertogna J. Cutis verticis gyrata in a child with Turner syndrome. *Pediatric Dermatol.* 1999;16(3):242-243.

150. Larsen F, Birchall N. Cutis verticis gyrata: three cases with different aetiologies that demonstrate the classification system. *Australas J dermatol.* 2007;48(2):91-94.

151. Nijsten TE, De Moor A, Colpaert CG, Robert K, Mahieu LM, Lambert J. Restrictive dermopathy: a case report and a critical review of all hypotheses of its origin. *Pediatr Dermatol.* 2002;19(1):67-72.

152. Wesche WA, Cutlan RT, Khare V, Chesney T, Shanklin D. Restrictive dermopathy: report of a case and review of the literature. *J Cutan Pathol.* 2001;28(4):211-218.

153. Morais P, Magina S, Ribeiro Mdo C, et al. Restrictive dermopathy: a lethal congenital laminopathy. Case report and review of the literature. *Eur J Pediatr.* 2009;168(8):1007-1012.

154. Verloes A, Mulliez N, Gonzales M, et al. Restrictive dermopathy, a lethal form of arthrogryposis multiplex with skin and bone dysplasias: three new cases and review of the literature. *Am J Med Genet.* 1992;43(3):539-547.

155. Schreiber KH, Kennedy BK. When lamins go bad: nuclear structure and disease. *Cell.* 2013;152(6):1365-1375.

156. Navarro CL, Cadinanos J, De Sandre-Giovannoli A, et al. Loss of ZMPSTE24 (FACE-1) causes autosomal recessive restrictive dermopathy and accumulation of Lamin A precursors. *Hum Mol Genet.* 2005;14(11):1503-1513.

157. Navarro CL, De Sandre-Giovannoli A, Bernard R, et al. Lamin A and ZMPSTE24 (FACE-1) defects cause nuclear disorganization and identify restrictive dermopathy as a lethal neonatal laminopathy. *Hum Mol Genet.* 2004;13(20):2493-2503.

158. Youn GJ, Uzunyan M, Vachon L, Johnson J, Winder TL, Yano S. Autosomal recessive LMNA mutation causing restrictive dermopathy. *Clin Genet.* 2010;78(2):199-200.

159. Moulson CL, Go G, Gardner JM, et al. Homozygous and compound heterozygous mutations in ZMPSTE24 cause the laminopathy restrictive dermopathy. *J Invest Dermatol.* 2005;125(5):913-919.

160. Welsh KM, Smoller BR, Holbrook KA, Johnston K. Restrictive dermopathy. Report of two affected siblings and a review of the literature. *Arch Dermatol.* 1992;128(2):228-231.

161. Paige DG, Lake BD, Bailey AJ, Ramani P, Harper JI. Restrictive dermopathy: a disorder of fibroblasts. *Br J Dermatol.* 1992;127(6):630-634.

162. Manning MA, Cunniff CM, Colby CE, El-Sayed YY, Hoyme HE. Neu-Laxova syndrome: detailed prenatal diagnostic and post-mortem findings and literature review. *Am J Med Genet A.* 2004;125A(3):240-249.

163. Wilbe M, Ekvall S, Eurenius K, et al. MuSK: a new target for lethal fetal akinesia deformation sequence (FADS). *J Med Genet.* 2015;52(3):195-202.

164. Oji V, Tadini G, Akiyama M, et al. Revised nomenclature and classification of inherited ichthyoses: results of the First Ichthyosis Consensus Conference in Soreze 2009. *J Am Acad Dermatol.* 2010;63(4):607-641.

10

Genetic Deposition Disorders

Titilola Sode / Adnan Mir

LIPOID PROTEINOSIS

Definition and Epidemiology

Lipoid proteinosis (LP, hyalinosis cutis et mucosae) is a rare autosomal recessive disease characterized by thickening of the skin and mucosal surfaces. Patients classically present with a hoarse voice early in childhood, variable scarring, and cutaneous yellow beaded papules. It is caused by mutations in extracellular matrix protein 1 (*ECM1*).

The majority of patients are of European ancestry, especially among the Dutch South Afrikaans owing to a founder effect. Fewer than 500 cases have been reported in the literature to date, with more than 50 different reported mutations in *ECM1*.[1,2] Males and females are equally affected. Symptoms typically appear early during childhood.

Etiology

The *ECM1* protein is normally found within the basement membrane zone and acts as a scaffolding molecule, binding to numerous structural proteins, including collagen IV and laminin 332.[3] It also appears to have functions in epidermal differentiation and in angiogenesis. In patients with LP, loss of functional *ECM1* results in hyalinized deposition of protein material at the dermoepidermal junction and within the papillary dermis.

There are several different splice isoforms of *ECM1*, which incorporate different exons. Some mutations cause more severe manifestations of the disease on the basis of which isoform they produce.[3,4] Immune-mediated acquired dysfunction of *ECM1* has been implicated in the pathogenesis of lichen sclerosus et atrophicus.

Clinical Presentation

A hoarse or weak cry is the first identifiable feature of the disease, typically manifesting at birth or within the first few years, and progressively worsening throughout an individual's life. The cutaneous features of the disease vary with age. Infants and young children typically develop vesicles or bullae with hemorrhagic crusting on the face and upper extremities and within the mouth—often secondary to trauma. These lesions heal with varioliform scarring (Figure 10-1A).

Later in childhood, there is an increase in hyaline deposition within the dermis leading to the development of yellow papules and plaques on the face, eyelids, neck, and hands. The scalp can also be affected, resulting in patchy or diffuse hair loss. Thick, waxy yellow plaques favor flexural surfaces, whereas verrucous plaques favor extensor surfaces. In about 50% of individuals, a string of bead-like papules appears on the free eyelid margins, often leading to a loss of lashes (Figure 10-1B and C). Involvement of the eyelid margin may be complicated by corneal ulcers. A cobblestone appearance may appear on mucosal surfaces within the mouth.

Systemic complications of extensive hyaline deposition include movement-limiting woody induration of the tongue, dysphagia, respiratory obstruction, premature tooth loss, parotid pain and swelling, and neurologic complications of grand mal seizures and behavioral changes.

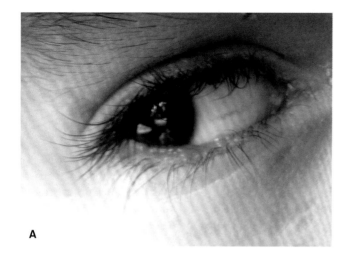

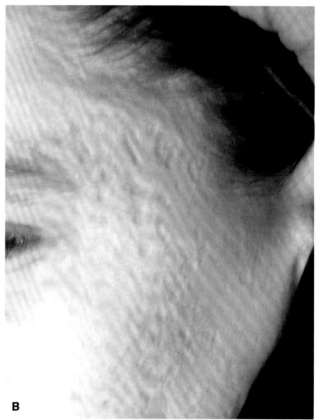

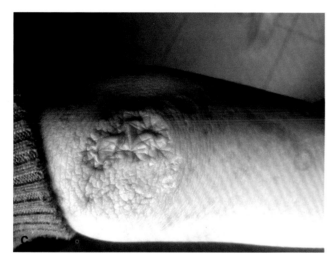

FIGURE 10-1. **Lipoid proteinosis.** A, Beaded, waxy papules along the eyelid margins. B and C, Characteristic, atrophic, varioliform scarring on the face and elbows.

A pathognomonic finding on radiographic examination is bilateral, intracranial, sickle or bean-shaped calcification within the temporal lobes.[5]

Histologic Findings

There is deposition of pale, eosinophilic, amorphous material surrounding small capillaries and eccrine ducts in the superficial dermis. In more developed lesions, deposits undergo hyaline thickening with an "onion-skin" appearance. Sweat glands are damaged with increased hyaline deposition (Figure 10-2). Hyperkeratosis and papillomatous may be seen.[6] The hyaline deposits are periodic acid–Schiff (PAS) positive and diastase resistant, and stain with Alcian blue as well as Sudan black on frozen sections.[7]

Differential Diagnosis

The clinical differential diagnosis of LP includes xanthoma, amyloidosis, colloid milium, leprosy, and scleromyxedema.

Histopathologically, there is significant overlap with erythropoietic protoporphyria (EPP) (Figure 10-3). However, these can be differentiated by the deeper, more extensive involvement of hyalinization in LP, and clinically by the distribution in more sun-exposed areas in EPP. Colloid milium and amyloidosis may be considered, but like EPP, are also typically more superficial.

CAPSULE SUMMARY

LP is a rare genetic condition resulting in hyaline deposition in the skin and mucosae. It causes diffuse waxy papules, nodules, and plaques on the head and upper extremities, as well as mucosal surfaces and in severe cases, internally. Histologically, it is characterized by the deposition of amorphous hyaline material within the dermis surrounding vessels and eccrine glands.

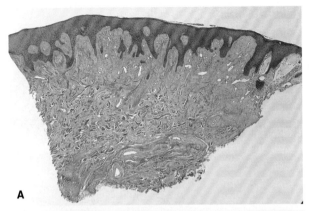

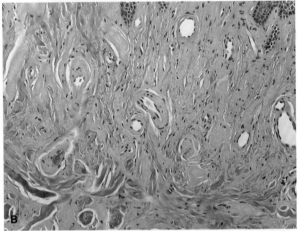

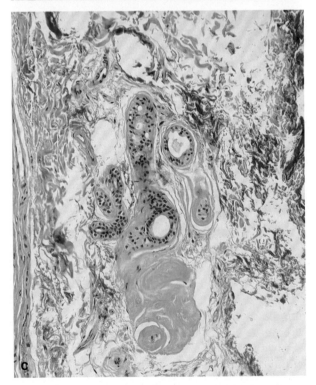

FIGURE 10-2. Lipoid proteinosis. Low- (A) and high-power (B) images showing diffuse deposits of amorphous hyaline material with a thickening of vessel walls. (C) There is involvement of the eccrine coil in this example. Courtesy of Dr. Travis Vandergriff, Department of Dermatology, UT Southwestern Medical Center.

GAUCHER DISEASE

Definition and Epidemiology

Gaucher disease is an autosomal recessive lysosomal storage disease caused by mutation in β-glucosidase. There is resultant accumulation of the glycolipid glucocerebroside, which leads to a variety of complications affecting skin, bones, and liver.

Gaucher disease is a relatively common genetic disease that is classically divided into three clinical subtypes. Type 1, the most common, affects approximately 1/800 births in the Ashkenazi Jewish population, although it is rare in the general population with an incidence of 1 in 40 000 to 60 000.[8,9] Types 2 (which has the most cutaneous findings) and 3 are rare. Males and females are affected equally.

Etiology

Gaucher disease is a sphingolipidosis, a member of the lysosomal storage group of diseases. It is caused by a mutation in β-glucosidase (glucocerebrosidase), which leads to a decrease in the enzyme's ability to break down glucocerebroside. Its accumulation in macrophages results in the formation of Gaucher cells, which in turn accumulate within bone and lead to bone destruction. The pathophysiology of Gaucher disease in the skin is poorly understood, but is likely related to lipid processing and cell membrane formation, much like many of the congenital ichthyoses. Ultrastructural studies of skin from patients with Type 2 Gaucher disease support this explanation.[10]

Clinical Presentation

Type 1 Gaucher disease is categorized as the nonneuronopathic type. The average age of diagnosis ranges from 10 to 20 years. Skin findings are often subtle and include hyperpigmentation and purpura.[11] The hallmarks of this subtype are bone involvement associated with severe pain and progressive splenomegaly. Infiltration of bone marrow by Gaucher cells can lead to pancytopenia, including thrombocytopenia, which may cause widespread purpura.[12] There is an increased risk of multiple myeloma.[13]

Type 2 Gaucher disease is the acute neuronopathic type. It is rapidly progressive and typically lethal by age 2, usually due to aspiration and respiratory complications. It is characterized by the triad of opisthotonus (rigidity/backward arching of the neck and trunk), severe dysphagia, and oculomotor paralysis.[14] A rare subtype of type 2 is fetal Gaucher disease, which presents with a collodion membrane and arthrogryposis (congenital limb contractures). Affected patients tend to die in utero or soon after birth.[15,16]

Type 3 Gaucher disease has no specific cutaneous involvement, but also presents with a heterogeneous range of neurologic abnormalities, typically before the age of 20. Hydrocephaly, cardiac anomalies, and corneal involvement have also been reported.[17]

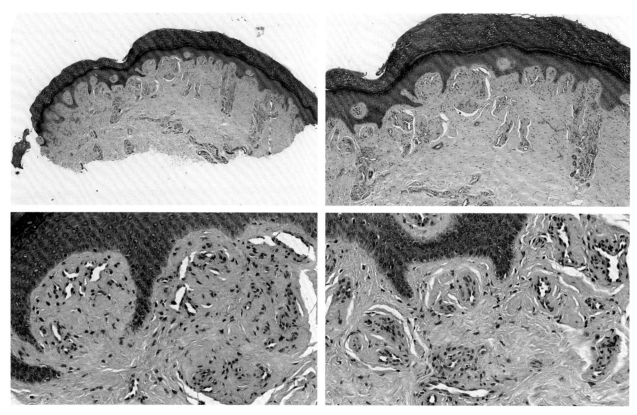

FIGURE 10-3. **Erythropoietic protoporphyria.** In the dermis, eosinophilic hyaline material is deposited in and around blood vessel walls. The deposition is extensive and involves the surrounding dermis to mimic a colloid milium. Impressive thickening of vessels is seen at higher-power examination. Digital slides courtesy of Path Presenter.com.

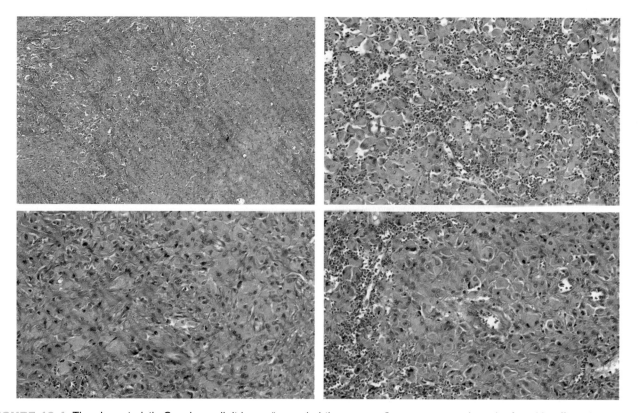

FIGURE 10-4. The characteristic Gaucher cell; it has a "crumpled tissue paper" appearance and can be found in affected bone, liver (current case), and bone marrow, but not in the skin. Digital slides courtesy of Path Presenter.com.

Histologic Findings

There are no specific histologic features in the skin of patients with Gaucher disease. However, low β-glucosidase levels can be detected in fibroblasts cultured from skin biopsies. The characteristic Gaucher cell, which has a "crumpled tissue paper" appearance, can be found in affected bone, liver, and bone marrow, but not in the skin[18] (Figure 10-4).

> ### CAPSULE SUMMARY
>
> Gaucher disease is a member of the lysosomal storage disease group and is caused by mutation in β-glucosidase, resulting in the accumulation of glucocerebroside. Patients with type 1 disease may present with skin hyperpigmentation and purpura, and severe cases of the fatal type 2 disease may present at birth with a collodion membrane and ichthyosis. There are no specific histologic skin findings.

HYALINE FIBROMATOSIS SYNDROME

Definition and Epidemiology

Hyaline fibromatosis syndrome (HFS), which encompasses infantile systemic hyalinosis and juvenile hyaline fibromatosis, is a rare autosomal recessive disorder of the connective tissue characterized by the deposition of hyaline material in the dermis and other organs.[19] Although the two conditions differ in age of onset and severity, both are caused by mutations in anthrax toxin receptor-2 and can be considered on the spectrum of HFS. HFS is rare, but the exact frequency has not been determined. It has been reported worldwide. One retrospective study of 19 Arab patients found that the majority were the result of consanguineous marriage.[20]

Etiology

ANTXR2 encodes a transmembrane receptor that likely plays a role in vasculogenesis and basement membrane matrix integrity. Through an as yet undetermined mechanism, loss or reduction of functional ANTXR2 protein leads to the deposition of hyaline material within the dermis and viscera.

Clinical Presentation

The early-onset form (infantile systemic hyalinosis) typically has a more severe course. Affected patients present at birth with diffusely thickened skin and prominent hyperpigmentation over the joints of the dorsal hands and ankles. There is also malabsorption, protein-losing enteropathy, diarrhea, and recurrent infections, which may cause early mortality in severe cases.[21]

This is in contrast to juvenile hyaline fibromatosis, which typically manifests during early childhood with a

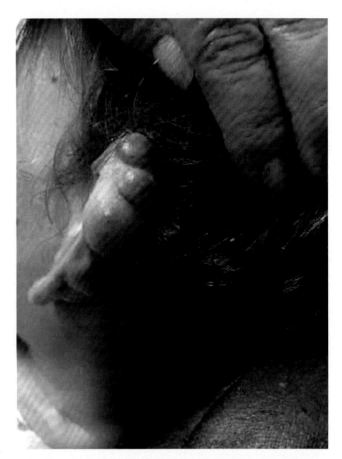

FIGURE 10-5. Hyaline fibromatosis syndrome. A 20-year-old woman with waxy nodules on the helix. Reprinted with permission from Rahvar M, Teng J, Kim J. Systemic hyalinosis with heterozygous CMG2 mutations: a case report and review of literature. *Am J Dermatopathol.* 2016;38(5):e60-e63.

progressive development of disfiguring nodules and papules affecting the perinasal, perioral, and perianal areas; as well as the scalp, face, ears, and hands. They tend to be asymptomatic, and depending on the depth of involvement and level of fibrosis, may be hard or soft, and fixed or mobile (Figure 10-5).[22,23] Large lesions may be prone to ulceration and infection. Oral mucosal involvement has also been described, leading to difficulty feeding and recurrent dental infections.[24] Visceral symptoms of chronic diarrhea and malabsorption are absent in this group.

Other shared manifestations include progressive contractures of hips, elbows, ankles, and wrists that ultimately immobilize the patient; and bone involvement with lytic lesions, osteopenia, and osteoporosis.

Histologic Findings

Histologically, HFS is characterized by ill-defined dermal deposits of brightly eosinophilic hyaline material (Figures 10-6 and 10-7). They are variably sized and contain interspersed plump spindle cells, which may be arranged

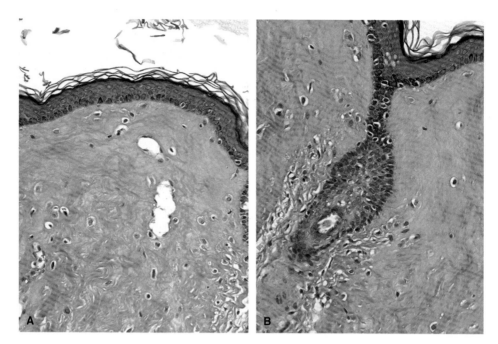

FIGURE 10-6. Hyaline fibromatosis syndrome with amorphous hyaline material within the dermis (A), and interspersed plump spindle cells (B). Reprinted with permission from Antaya RJ, Cajaiba MM, Madri, J, et al. Juvenile hyaline fibromatosis and infantile systemic hyalinosis overlap associated with a novel mutation in capillary morphogenesis protein-2 gene. *Am J Dermatopathol.* 2007;29(1):99-103.

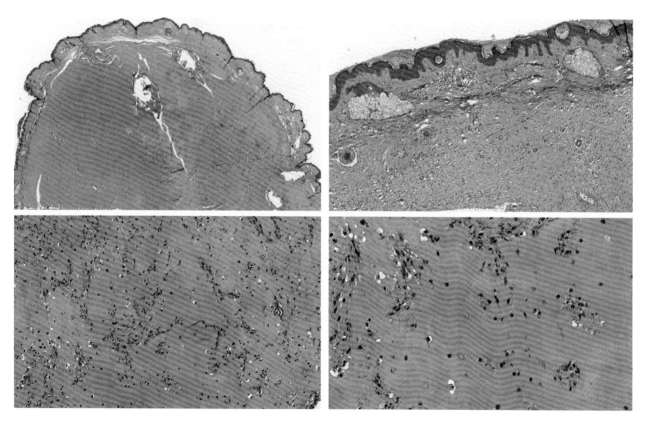

FIGURE 10-7. Juvenile hyaline fibromatosis. There is a characteristic nodular infiltrate in the dermis with sparing of the epidermis. Hyalinized amorphous material is present surrounding curvilinear vessels. Digital slides courtesy of Path Presenter.com.

in pseudovascular-appearing cords. The hyaline material is PAS positive and diastase resistant.[25,26]

Differential Diagnosis

The clinical differential diagnosis includes syndrome and nodulosis–arthropathy–osteolysis syndrome, which are caused by mutations in matrix metalloproteinases.[27,28] Both feature thickening of the skin with joint contractures. Infantile myofibromatosis may present with scattered firm nodules during infancy. Each can be differentiated on a clinical basis from HFS and have distinct histologic findings.

CAPSULE SUMMARY

HFS is a rare, autosomal recessive spectrum of diseases caused by mutations in *ANTXR2*. The early-onset form, infantile systemic hyalinosis, presents with diffusely thickened skin and joint contractures, and early mortality is caused by severe systemic manifestations. The childhood onset form is less severe, presenting with widespread disfiguring nodules and progressive joint contracture. The hallmark pathologic finding is the deposition of dense hyaline material within the dermis.

REFERENCES

1. Kabre V, Rani S, Pai KM, Kamra S. Lipoid proteinosis: A review with two case reports. *Contemp Clin Dent.* 2015;6(2):233-236.
2. Chan I, Liu L, Hamada T, Sethuraman G, McGrath JA. The molecular basis of lipoid proteinosis: mutations in extracellular matrix protein 1. *Exp Dermatol.* 2007;16(11):881-890.
3. Sercu S, Zhang M, Oyama N, et al. Interaction of extracellular matrix protein 1 with extracellular matrix components: ECM1 is a basement membrane protein of the skin. *J Invest Dermatol.* 2008;128(6):1397-1408.
4. Nasir M, Latif A, Ajmal M, Qamar R, Naeem M, Hameed A. Molecular analysis of lipoid proteinosis: identification of a novel nonsense mutation in the ECM1 gene in a Pakistani family. *Diagn Pathol.* 2011;6:69.
5. Touart DM, Sau P. Cutaneous deposition diseases. Part I. *J Am Acad Dermatol.* 1998;39(2, pt 1):149-171; quiz 172-174.
6. Uchida T, Hayashi H, Inaoki M, Miyamoto T, Fujimoto W. A failure of mucocutaneous lymphangiogenesis may underlie the clinical features of lipoid proteinosis. *Br J Dermatol.* 2007;156(1):152-157.
7. Pierard GE, Van Cauwenberge D, Budo J, Lapiere CM. A clinicopathologic study of six cases of lipoid proteinosis. *Am J Dermatopathol.* 1988;10(4):300-305.
8. Grabowski GA. Phenotype, diagnosis, and treatment of Gaucher's disease. *Lancet.* 2008;372(9645):1263-1271.
9. Stirnemann J, Vigan M, Hamroun D, et al. The French Gaucher's disease registry: clinical characteristics, complications and treatment of 562 patients. *Orphanet J Rare Dis.* 2012;7:77.
10. Chan A, Holleran WM, Ferguson T, et al. Skin ultrastructural findings in type 2 Gaucher disease: diagnostic implications. *Mol Genet Metab.* 2011;104(4):631-636.
11. Andersson H, Kaplan P, Kacena K, Yee J. Eight-year clinical outcomes of long-term enzyme replacement therapy for 884 children with Gaucher disease type 1. *Pediatrics.* 2008;122(6):1182-1190.
12. Park JK, Koprivica V, Andrews DQ, et al. Glucocerebrosidase mutations among African-American patients with type 1 Gaucher disease. *Am J Med Genet.* 2001;99(2):147-151.
13. Arends M, van Dussen L, Biegstraaten M, Hollak CE. Malignancies and monoclonal gammopathy in Gaucher disease; a systematic review of the literature. *Br J Haematol.* 2013;161(6):832-842.
14. Mignot C, Doummar D, Maire I, De Villemeur TB; French Type 2 Gaucher Disease Study Group. Type 2 Gaucher disease: 15 new cases and review of the literature. *Brain Dev.* 2006;28(1):39-48.
15. Lui K, Commens C, Choong R, Jaworski R. Collodion babies with Gaucher's disease. *Arch Dis Child.* 1988;63(7):854-856.
16. Mignot C, Gelot A, Bessieres B, et al. Perinatal-lethal Gaucher disease. *Am J Med Genet A.* 2003;120A(3):338-344.
17. Cindik N, Ozcay F, Suren D, et al. Gaucher disease with communicating hydrocephalus and cardiac involvement. *Clin Cardiol.* 2010;33(1):E26-E30.
18. Boven LA, van Meurs M, Boot RG, et al. Gaucher cells demonstrate a distinct macrophage phenotype and resemble alternatively activated macrophages. *Am J Clin Pathol.* 2004;122(3):359-369.
19. Hanks S, Adams S, Douglas J, et al. Mutations in the gene encoding capillary morphogenesis protein 2 cause juvenile hyaline fibromatosis and infantile systemic hyalinosis. *Am J Hum Genet.* 2003;73(4):791-800.
20. Al-Mayouf SM, AlMehaidib A, Bahabri S, Shabib S, Sakati N, Teebi AS. Infantile systemic hyalinosis: a fatal disorder commonly diagnosed among Arabs. *Clin Exp Rheumatol.* 2005;23(5):717-720.
21. Raeeskarami SR, Aghighi Y, Afshin A, Malek A, Zamani A, Ziaee V. Infantile systemic hyalinosis: report of 17-year experience. *Iran J Pediatr.* 2014;24(6):775-778.
22. Muniz ML, Lobo AZ, Machado MC, et al. Exuberant juvenile hyaline fibromatosis in two patients. *Pediatr Dermatol.* 2006;23(5):458-464.
23. Ribeiro SL, Guedes EL, Botan V, Barbosa A, Freitas EJ. Juvenile hyaline fibromatosis: a case report and review of literature. *Acta Reumatol Port.* 2009;34(1):128-133.
24. Lim AA, Kozakewich HP, Feingold M, Padwa BL. Juvenile hyaline fibromatosis: report of a case and comparison with infantile systemic hyalinosis. *J Oral Maxillofac Surg.* 2005;63(2):271-274.
25. Antaya RJ, Cajaiba MM, Madri J, et al. Juvenile hyaline fibromatosis and infantile systemic hyalinosis overlap associated with a novel mutation in capillary morphogenesis protein-2 gene. *Am J Dermatopathol.* 2007;29(1):99-103.
26. Denadai R, Raposo-Amaral CE, Bertola D, et al. Identification of 2 novel ANTXR2 mutations in patients with hyaline fibromatosis syndrome and proposal of a modified grading system. *Am J Med Genet A.* 2012;158A(4):732-742.
27. Bhavani GS, Shah H, Shukla A, et al. Clinical and mutation profile of multicentric osteolysis nodulosis and arthropathy. *Am J Med Genet A.* 2016;170A(2):410-417.
28. Jeong SY, Kim BY, Kim HJ, Yang JA, Kim OH. A novel homozygous MMP2 mutation in a patient with Torg-Winchester syndrome. *J Hum Genet.* 2010;55(11):764-766.

11

Genetic Disorders of DNA Repair Mechanisms

Jennifer A. Day / Adnan Mir

XERODERMA PIGMENTOSUM

Definition and Epidemiology

Xeroderma pigmentosum (XP) is a group of genetically inherited defects caused by mutations in genes responsible for nucleotide excision repair (NER), leading to increased malignancy risk.[1-3] The reported incidence ranges from 1 in 20 000 to 40 000 live births in Japan to 1 in 250 000 to 1 000 000 in the United States and Europe.[4] The prevalence of subtypes varies geographically, with the complementation group XPA being the most common in Japan, and XPC being the most common in the United States and Europe. The Navajo populations in the Southwestern United States manifest an uncommon XPA mutation that has been found in both homozygote and heterozygote states because of a founder effect.[5,6]

Etiology

XP results from mutation of genes in the NER pathway, *XPA-XPG* (Table 11-1). The resultant abnormal repair of ultraviolet (UV) radiation–induced DNA damage is caused by inability to repair pyrimidine dimers, leading to the accumulation of UV signature mutations. XP Variant (XPV) is a related disorder resulting from a defect in a postreplication repair mechanism carried out by a protein encoded by the DNA polymerase η gene.[7]

Clinical Presentation

The clinical manifestations of XP vary by clinical subtype, which are determined by complementation groups (Table 11-1).[8] Generally, complementation groups are divided among those associated with severe photosensitivity and neurologic complications (XPA, XPB, XPD, XPF, and XPG) and those with no neurologic complications (XPC, XPE, and XPV).[9]

Early cutaneous manifestations include photosensitivity, ephelides, lentigines, and poikiloderma (Figure 11-1).[6,7] Photosensitivity manifests as exaggerated sunburn, blisters, and persistent erythema, often after minimal UV exposure.[5] Later findings include premature photoaging and xerosis.[1] The hallmark cutaneous manifestation is the marked predisposition for premature cutaneous malignancy. This increased risk manifests in childhood and adolescence.

TABLE 11-1.	Xeroderma pigmentosum complementation groups
Gene	**Protein**
XPA	DDB1
XPB	ERCC3
XPC	XPC—Endonuclease
XPD	ERCC2
XPE	DDB2
XPF	ERCC4
XPG	ERCC5
XPV	DNA polymerase-η

Abbreviations: DDB, DNA damage binding protein; DNA, deoxyribonucleic acid; ERCC, excision-repair cross-complementing protein.

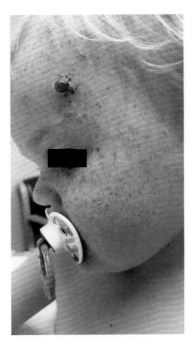

FIGURE 11-1. Early-onset photo damage in a child with xeroderma pigmentosa, with photodistributed actinic damage, solar lentigos, and an early squamous cell cancer (Courtesy Barrett Zlotoff, MD).

The median age for the initial diagnosis of nonmelanoma skin cancer in XP patients is 9 years, with patients under 20 years old having a 10 000-fold increased risk of nonmelanoma skin cancer (typically basal cell carcinoma [BCC] or squamous cell carcinoma [SCC], respectively).[10] The median age for the initial diagnosis of melanoma is 22 years, with a risk 2000 times the typical population.[11,12] There are reports of additional nonmelanoma skin cancers in XP patients, including atypical fibroxanthoma, malignant fibrous histiocytoma, fibrosarcoma, and angiosarcoma.[12]

Ocular manifestations are reported in 40% of XP patients.[2,13] Findings can include photophobia, conjunctivitis, ectropion, and symblepharon (adhesion of the palpebral conjunctiva to the bulbar conjunctiva). Corneal involvement may lead to blindness. Ocular neoplasms occur in about 11% of XP patients, including epithelioma, BCC, SCC, and melanoma.[11] Neurologic findings are highly variable depending on the complementation group, with the highest rate in patients with XPD.[14] Manifestations may include developmental delay, intellectual impairment, sensorineural hearing loss, hyporeflexia, and ataxia.[15] A rare XP phenotype is De Sanctis–Cacchione syndrome, in which patients exhibit severe mental retardation, deafness, ataxia, and paralysis.[16] Notably, neurologic manifestations are absent in XPV.[17] The risk for internal malignancy, most notably brain cancer, is also increased in XP patients.[2,11,18] Mortality typically occurs in the third or fourth decade because of neurologic complications, metastatic SCC, or melanoma.[10,15]

Histologic Findings

Early histologic changes include telangiectasia and pigmentary changes such as prominent epidermal melanin and pigmentary incontinence.[19] Solar elastosis develops within a few years of life. As tumors develop (Figure 11-2A–C), lesional specimens may demonstrate findings of angiomas, actinic keratoses, keratoacanthomas, BCC, SCC, melanoma, and atypical fibroxanthoma.[12]

Differential Diagnosis

The differential diagnosis for photosensitivity seen in XP includes Cockayne syndrome (CS), UV-sensitive syndrome, cerebro-oculo-facio-skeletal syndrome, and erythropoietic protoporphyria. The differential diagnosis for photosensitive disorders with predisposition toward malignancy includes Bloom and Rothmund–Thomson syndromes (RTS).

CAPSULE SUMMARY

XERODERMA PIGMENTOSUM

XP is a rare group of genetic disorders resulting from defective NER, leading to markedly increased risk for cutaneous malignancy at an early age. Specific histologic findings include those related to actinic damage including telangiectasias and pigmentary change. Patients develop actinic keratoses, BCC, SCC, melanoma, and other cutaneous neoplasms.

COCKAYNE SYNDROME

Definition and Epidemiology

CS is a rare group of heritable defects due to mutations in genes involved with NER, leading to photosensitivity.[20] The estimated incidence ranges from 1 in 1.8 to 2.7 million in Europe.[21] It is reportedly more prevalent in Canada, Japan, and Middle Eastern and Western Asian countries.[21]

Etiology

CS results from an autosomal recessive inheritance of genes involved in the transcription-coupled repair arm of NER, proteins CSA and CSB.[22] Mutations result in abnormal RNA synthesis following exposure of DNA to UV radiation.

Clinical Presentation

The clinical findings in CS are related to premature, advanced aging. Major criteria include microcephaly, stunted growth, and progressive neurologic deterioration. Minor criteria include UVB and visible light photosensitivity, dental caries, "salt and pepper" pigmentary retinopathy or cataracts, sensorineural hearing loss, and cachectic dwarfism

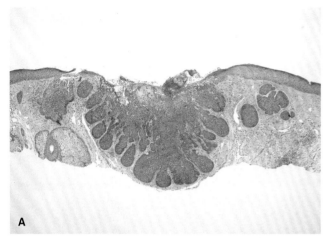

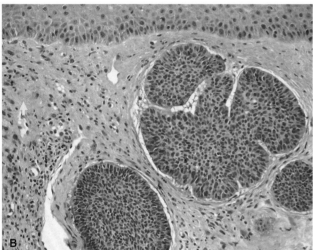

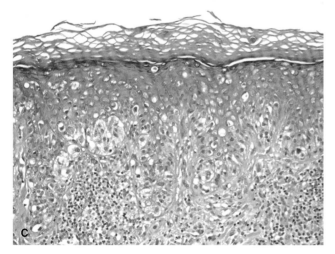

FIGURE 11-2. A, Low-power and B, high-power images of basal cell carcinoma from a 20-year-old patient with Xeroderma Pigmentosum type C. There are typical features of peripheral nuclear palisading, mucinous stroma, and clefting between tumor islands and stroma. Note the presence of background solar elastotic change (arrow), which would not normally be expected at this age. C, Melanoma in situ from the same patient, showing confluent nests and single melanocytes at the dermoepidermal junction, and many atypical melanocytes in the upper layers of the epidermis.

with stooped posture. Cutaneous manifestations include dry, atrophic skin, loss of subcutaneous fat, thinning hair, anhidrosis, and extremity edema. Patients have characteristic facie, which includes microcephaly, a thin nose, and large ears (Figure 11-3A and B). A photosensitive eruption with erythema and scale occurs in the "butterfly" distribution of the face and resolves with hyperpigmentation and mild atrophy.[23]

In contrast to XP, patients with CS do not develop UV-induced pigmentary abnormalities and cancer predisposition.[24,25] Other clinical findings seen in CS include gait abnormalities, contractures, spasticity, and tremors. Comorbidities typically associated with advanced age are noted at much younger ages, including hypertension, atherosclerosis, diabetes, osteoporosis, presbycusis, and cognitive impairment.[22-25]

Histologic Findings and Differential Diagnosis

There are no characteristic histologic findings in CS. Diagnosis is made on the basis of clinical and genetic abnormalities.

The differential diagnosis for photosensitivity seen in CS includes XP, UV-sensitive syndrome, trichothiodystrophy, RTS, and cerebro-oculo-facio-skeletal syndrome.

CAPSULE SUMMARY

COCKAYNE SYNDROME

CS is a rare disorder with a characteristic 'Mickey Mouse' appearance resulting from microcephaly, thin nose, large ears, and disproportionately long limbs. It is caused by genetic defects in transcription-coupled NER, leading to advanced aging and neurologic deterioration without an increased risk of cutaneous malignancy.

ROTHMUND–THOMSON SYNDROME

Definition and Epidemiology

RTS is an autosomal recessive inherited disorder in the DNA helicase gene *RECQL4*, characterized by photosensitivity and an increased risk of malignancy.[25,27] At least 300 patients with RTS have been reported worldwide.[17,28]

Etiology

Most cases of RTS are caused by mutation in *RECQL4*, a DNA helicase, with mutation resulting in abnormal DNA replication and repair, and genomic instability.[25]

Clinical Presentation

Cutaneous findings include photosensitivity in early infancy, manifesting as erythema, edema, and vesiculation starting on the cheeks.[6,27] Eventually, poikiloderma develops on photoexposed areas including the face, dorsal hands,

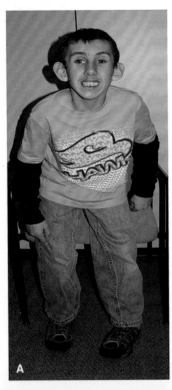

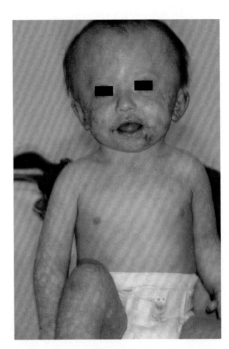

FIGURE 11-4. A child with Rothmund–Thomson Syndrome demonstrating photodistributed and generalized poikiloderma with hypoplastic thumb (Courtesy of Barrett Zlotoff, MD).

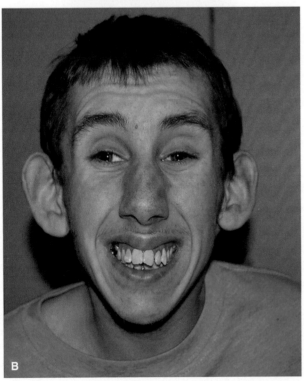

FIGURE 11-3. A child with Cockayne syndrome, and the characteristic features of microcephaly, a thin nose, large ears, dental malocclusion, and prognathism. Reprinted with permission from Trese MGJ, Nudleman ED, Besirli CG. Peripheral retinal vasculopathy in Cockayne Syndrome. *Retin Cases Brief Rep.* 2017;11(3):232-235.

forearms, and sometimes the buttocks (Figure 11-4).[6,28] Affected patients also have sparse hair, hypoplastic nails, and acral verrucous keratoses,[28] which may progress to SCC in less than 5% of patients.[17] Musculoskeletal manifestations include short stature, radial ray defects (hypoplastic or absent thumbs), osteoporosis, dental abnormalities, and midface hypoplasia.[29] Additional associations include juvenile cataracts and pituitary hypogonadism.[6,29] There is an increased risk of osteosarcoma, seen in 10% to 30% of patients.[26,28,30] There are reports of other malignancies including SCC, melanoma, and hematopoietic malignancy.[29-31] Notably, there is normal immune function, intelligence, and life span if unaffected by malignancy.[28]

Histologic Findings

RTS shows typical features of poikiloderma, including hyperkeratosis, epidermal atrophy, and telangiectatic superficial vessels.[32] Additional features include variable dermal inflammation, dermal melanophages, and scattered dyskeratotic keratinocytes.[32] Acral verrucous keratoses display characteristic hyperkeratosis, dyskeratosis, and mild loss of cellular polarity.[33]

Differential Diagnosis

Differential diagnosis includes XP, Bloom syndrome, CS, dyskeratosis congenita, hereditary benign telangiectasia, and Kindler Syndrome. Kindler syndrome presents with congenital or infantile onset trauma-induced bullae, progressive poikiloderma, and photosensitivity that decreases with age. Poikiloderma with neutropenia (HBTPN) is on the differential as well. HBTPN is a rare, autosomal recessive disorder due to mutation in U6 SnRNA biogenesis phosphodiesterase 1 that has been reported mostly in the Navajo population and presents with generalized poikiloderma associated with cyclic neutropenia.[34]

CAPSULE SUMMARY

ROTHMUND–THOMSON SYNDROME

RTS is an autosomal recessive disorder resulting from RECQL4 mutation. It is characterized by photosensitivity, poikiloderma, radial ray defects (presenting as absent or hypoplastic thumbs), and an increased risk of osteosarcoma. Patients should be screened for bone pain, which can be indicative of osteosarcomas.

BLOOM SYNDROME

Definition, Epidemiology, and Etiology

Bloom syndrome (BS) is a rare, autosomal recessive disorder caused by mutations in the DNA helicase *RECQL3*, resulting in an increased rate of sister chromatid exchange.[1,35,36] Fewer than 300 cases have been reported in an international registry.[17,37]

Clinical Presentation

BS is characterized by growth delay and microcephaly. Typical facies feature a narrow face, large ears, malar hypoplasia, and prominent nose (Figure 11-5A and B).[35,38] Cutaneous manifestations of BS include erythema and telangiectasias on malar cheeks, dorsal hands, forearms, and occasionally the lower lip.[35] Additionally, café au lait macules and hypopigmented macules develop in a similar distribution. Systemic manifestations include primary hypogonadism as well as recurrent otic and pulmonary infections.[35] Malignancy predisposition is highest for lymphoma and leukemia, SCC, and adenocarcinoma (particularly of the gastrointestinal tract).[35] Intelligence is normal. Life expectancy is into the third decade, with malignancy being the most common cause of death.[35]

Histologic Findings and Differential Diagnosis

The hallmark diagnostic histologic finding is quadriradial configurations of chromosomes in lymphocytes and fibroblasts.[17,35,38] Telangiectasias are often seen as well. There have been some suggestions that the facial eruption of BS has a lupus-like histology, with hints of vacuolar interface dermatitis, a thickened basement membrane, and follicular plugging (Figure 11-26).[39]

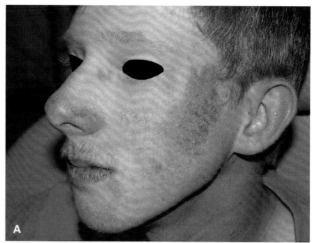
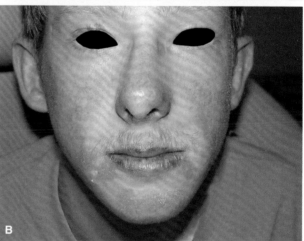

FIGURE 11-5. A and B, A boy with Bloom Syndrome, with characteristic facies featuring a narrow face and prominent ears and nose, as well as telangiectasias and poikiloderma of the malar cheeks. Reprinted with permission from McGowan J, Maize J, Cook J. Lupus-like histopathology in bloom syndrome: reexamining the clinical and histologic implications of photosensitivity. *Am J Dermatopathol.* 2009;31(8):786-791.

The clinical differential diagnosis includes XP, RTS, and dyskeratosis congenita.

CAPSULE SUMMARY

BLOOM SYNDROME

BS is an autosomal recessive disorder due to mutation in *RECQL3*, resulting in photosensitivity, poikiloderma, and an increased risk of leukemia and lymphoma, SCC, gastrointestinal adenocarcinoma, and other malignancies. Lymphocytes and fibroblasts show manifest characteristic quadriradial configurations of chromosomes.

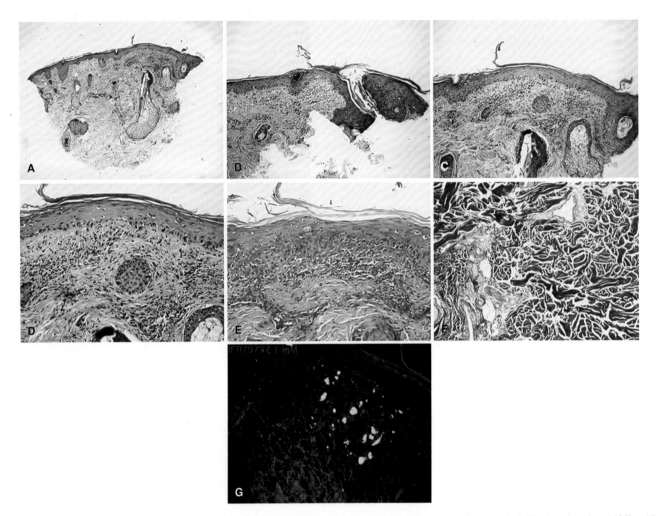

FIGURE 11-6. Histopathology of a case of Bloom syndrome. Effacement of the rete ridges, H&E, ×4. A, follicular plugging, H&E, ×10. B, Squamatization, necrotic keratinocytes, and vacuoles within the basal and parabasal epidermis, H&E, ×40-100. C and D, prominent BM thickening, H&E/PAS, ×100 (E), H&E/colloidal iron, ×200 (F). DIF demonstrated a focal linear presence of shaggy fibrin at the dermoepidermal junction (G). Reprinted with permission from McGowan J, Maize J, Cook J. Lupus-like histopathology in bloom syndrome: reexamining the clinical and histologic implications of photosensitivity. *Am J Dermatopathol.* 2009;31(8):786-91.

REFERENCES

1. Giordano CN, Yew YW, Spivak G, Lim HW. Understanding photodermatoses associated with defective DNA repair: syndromes with cancer predisposition. *J Am Acad Dermatol.* 2016;75(5):855-870.
2. Kraemer KH, Lee MM, Scotto J. Xeroderma pigmentosum: cutaneous ocular, and neurologic abnormalities in 830 published cases. *Arch Dermatol.* 1987;123:241-250.
3. Lambert WC. Genetic diseases associated with DNA and chromosomal instability. *Dermatol Clin.* 1987;5:85-108.
4. Bhutto AM, Kirk SH. Population distribution of xeroderma pigmentosum. *Adv Exp Med Biol.* 2008;637:138-143.
5. Lehmann AR, Norris PG. DNA repair deficient photodermatoses. *Semin Dermatol.* 1990;9:55-62.
6. Chantorn R, Lim HW, Shwayder TA. Photosensitivity disorders in children: part II. *J Am Acad Dermatol.* 2012;67:1113.e1-1113.e15
7. Jung EG: Xeroderma pigmentosum. *Int J Dermatol.* 1986;25:629-633.
8. Fischer E, Jung EG: Photosensitivity and the genodermatoses. *Semin Dermatol.* 1982;1:169-174.
9. Sethi M, Lehmann AR, Fawcett H, et al. Patients with xeroderma pigmentosum complementation groups C, E and V do not have abnormal sunburn reactions. *Br J Dermatol.* 2013;169:1279-1287.
10. DiGiovanna JJ, Kraemer KH. Shining a light on xeroderma pigmentosum. *J Invest Dermatol.* 2012;132:785-796.
11. Halkud R, Shenoy AM, Naik SM, Chavan P, Sidappa KT, Biswas S. Xeroderma pigmentosum: clinicopathological review of the multiple oculocutaneous malignancies and complications. *Indian J Surg Oncol.* 2014;5:120-124.
12. Youssef N, Vabres P, Buisson T, Brousse N, Fraitag S. Two unusual tumors in a patient with xeroderma pigmentosum: atypical fibroxanthoma and basosquamous carcinoma. *J Cutan Pathol.* 1999;26:430-435.
13. Brooks BP, Thompson AH, Bishop RJ, et al. Ocular manifestations of xeroderma pigmentosum: long-term follow-up highlights the role of DNA repair in protection from sun damage. *Ophthalmology.* 2013;120:1324-1336.
14. Taylor EM, Broughton BC, Botta E, et al. Xeroderma pigmentosum and trichothiodystrophy are associated with different mutations in the XPD (ERCC2) repair/transcription gene. *Proc Natl Acad Sci U S A.* 1997;94:8658-8663.
15. Bradford PT, Goldstein AM, Tamura D, et al. Cancer and neurologic degeneration in xeroderma pigmentosum: long term follow-up characterises the role of DNA repair. *J Med Genet.* 2011;48:168-176.
16. Reed WB, Mary SB, Nickel WR. Xeroderma pigmentosum with neurological complications: the De Sanctis-Cacchione syndrome. *Arch Dermatol.* 1965;91:224-226.

17. Lim HW, Hawk JLM, Rosen CF. Photodermatologic disorders. In: Bolognia JL, Jorizzo JL, Rapini RP, eds. *Dermatology.* 4th ed. Philadelphia, PA: Elsevier; 2018:1548-1568.

18. Lai JP, Liu YC, Alimchandani M, et al. The influence of DNA repair on neurological degeneration, cachexia, skin cancer and internal neoplasms: autopsy report of four xeroderma pigmentosum patients (XP-A, XP-C and XP-D). *Acta Neuropathol Commun.* 2013;1:4.

19. Kraemer KH, Slor H: Xeroderma pigmentosum. *Clin Dermatol.* 1985;3:33-69.

20. Yew YW, Giordano CN, Spivak G, Lim HW. Understanding photodermatoses associated with defective DNA repair: photosensitive syndromes without associated cancer predisposition. *J Am Acad Dermatol.* 2016;75(5):873-882.

21. Kleijer WJ, Laugel V, Berneburg M, et al. Incidence of DNA repair deficiency disorders in western Europe: xeroderma pigmentosum, Cockayne syndrome and trichothiodystrophy. *DNA Repair (Amst).* 2008;7:744-750.

22. Laugel V. Cockayne syndrome: the expanding clinical and mutational spectrum. *Mech Ageing Dev.* 2013;134:161-170.

23. Nance MA, Berry SA. Cockayne syndrome: review of 140 cases. *Am J Med Genet.* 1992;42:68-84.

24. Wilson BT, Stark Z, Sutton RE, et al. The Cockayne Syndrome Natural History (CoSyNH) study: clinical findings in 102 individuals and recommendations for care. *Genet Med.* 2016;18:483-493.

25. Frouin E, Laugel V, Durand M, Dollfus H, Lipsker D. Dermatologic findings in 16 patients with Cockayne syndrome and cerebro-oculo-facial-skeletal syndrome. *JAMA Dermatol.* 2013;149:1414-1418.

26. Lu L, Jin W, Liu H, Wang LL. RECQ DNA helicases and osteosarcoma. *Adv Exp Med Biol.* 2014;804:129-145.

27. Oh DH, Spivak G. Hereditary photodermatoses. *Adv Exp Med Biol.* 2010;685:95-105.

28. Wang LL, Levy LL, Lewis RA. Clinical manifestations in a cohort of 41 Rothmund-Thomson syndrome patients. *Am J Med Genet.* 2001;102:11-17.

29. Vennos EM, Collins M, James WD. Rothmund-Thomson syndrome: review of the world literature. *J Am Acad Dermatol.* 1992;27:750-762.

30. Larizza L, Roversi G, Volpi L. Rothmund-Thomson syndrome. *Orphanet J Rare Dis.* 2010;5:2.

31. Stinco G, Governatori G, Mattighello P, Patrone P. Multiple cutaneous neoplasms in a patient with Rothmund-Thomson syndrome: case report and published work review. *J Dermatol.* 2008;35:154-161.

32. Kumar P, Sharma PK, Gautam RK, Jain RK, Kar HK. Late-onset Rothmund–Thomson syndrome. *Int J Dermatol.* 2007;46:492-493.

33. Shuttleworth D, Marks R. Epidermal dysplasia and skeletal deformity in congenital poikiloderma (Rothmund–Thomson syndrome). *Br J Dermatol.* 1987;117:377-384.

34. Arnold AW, Itin PH, Pigors M, et al. Poikiloderma with neutropenia: a novel C16orf57 mutation and clinical diagnostic criteria. *Br J Dermatol.* 2010;163:866-869

35. Arora H, Chacon AH, Choudhary S, et al. Bloom syndrome. *Int J Dermatol.* 2014;53:798-802.

36. Killen MW, Stults DM, Adachi N, Hanakahi L, Pierce AJ. Loss of Bloom syndrome protein destabilizes human gene cluster architecture. *Hum Mol Genet.* 2009;18:3417-3428.

37. Weill Cornell Medical College. Bloom's syndrome registry. 2009. http://www.weill.cornell.edu/bsr/. Accessed April 1, 2017.

38. Gretzula JC, Hevia O, Weber PJ. Bloom's syndrome. *J Am Acad Dermatol.* 1987;17:479-488.

39. McGowan J, Maize J, Cook J. Lupus-like histopathology in bloom syndrome: reexamining the clinical and histologic implications of photosensitivity. *Am J Dermatopathol.* 2009;31(8):786-791.

12

Genetic Mosaic Disorders

Lihi Atzmony / Keith A. Choate

Mosaicism refers to the presence of genetically distinct cells within an organism that result from postzygotic mutation.[1] In contrast to chimerism, in which an individual is comprised of multiple cell lineages derived from distinct fertilized eggs, somatic mosaicism occurs during the development of a single embryo.[2] The timing of postzygotic mutations determines the spectrum of tissues involved, with early mutations affecting pluripotent stem cells, which proliferate and migrate to affect all germ layers and give rise to widespread systemic and cutaneous disease, and with late mutations typically affecting only cutaneous progenitors and giving rise to patterned skin lesions. The patterning and appearance of cutaneous mosaic disorders is largely determined by mutation timing, its pathophysiologic effects, and by the cutaneous progenitor cells it affects.

Historically, mosaicism has been phenotypically recognized in plants, animals, and humans with manifestations including twin stripes in oranges and maze kernel, coat color variegation in animals, and skin lesions that follow the lines of Blaschko and Heterochromia Irides.[2-4]

Prior to the advent of next-generation sequencing technology, there were inadequate tools to determine the genetic basis of a mosaic disorder without prior knowledge of a candidate gene. Initial discoveries were tied to technology employed. For example, chromosomal anomalies in mosaic pigmentary disorders were initially studied via karyotyping,[5,6] and more recently via sequencing and microarray-based approaches to identify chromosomal copy number variations and structural alterations. Rapid advances in understanding the molecular pathogenesis of mosaic disorders have been seen recently with paired whole exome sequencing (WES, high-throughput sequencing, next-generation sequencing) of affected and normal tissue.[7-9]

Cutaneous mosaic disorders provide a unique opportunity to study genetic mosaicism because the affected tissue is easily recognized and affected cells can be easily isolated via skin biopsy. In this chapter, we discuss phenotypic patterns and the classification of cutaneous mosaic disorders, current technologies employed to identify disease-causing mutations in mosaic disorders, and finally exemplary cutaneous mosaic disorders.

PHENOTYPE PATTERNS AND CLASSIFICATIONS

Cutaneous mosaicism can be categorized on the basis of phenotype (patterns of lesion distribution) or genetics.

Phenotype-Based Categorization

Most of the early knowledge of mosaicism was based on clinical recognition of intrapatient phenotypic variation. In 1901, Alfred Blaschko provided the first systematic documentation of cutaneous mosaic disorders. He observed more than 150 cases of various linear skin disorders such as epidermal and sebaceous nevi and carefully transposed the pattern in each patient onto a statue. A composite diagram of these distribution patterns was then published in his atlas of linear skin diseases, and these are now referred to as "Blaschko lines" (Figure 12-1).[10] One hundred years later, Happle used a similar method to define more precisely the

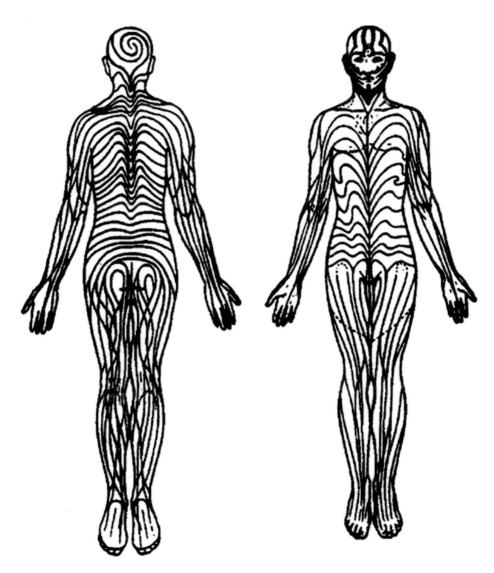

FIGURE 12-1. Lines of Blaschko. From Happle R, Mosaicism in human skin: understanding the Patterns and Mechanisms. *Arch Dermatol.* 1993;129 (11):1460-1470. Reprinted with permission.

Blaschko lines pattern of the head and neck on the basis of more than 180 figures collected from the literature.[3]

More recent classification of other patterns of cutaneous mosaicism was proposed describing five archetypical patterns of cutaneous mosaicism: Blaschko, phylloid, block-like (checkerboard), large patches without midline separation, and lateralization (Figure 12-2).[11] These patterns depend on the type of cell that is affected and the patterns of migration and proliferation of its precursors during embryogenesis. Blaschko's lines represent pathways of ectodermal development, and Blaschko-linear disorders most typically involve keratinocytes and melanocytes. Block-like and phylloid patterns respect the midline; the former is typically found in mosaicism affecting mesodermal derivatives, such as endothelial cells and fibroblasts, or neuroectodermal-derived melanocytes, and the latter is typically found in mosaicism affecting endothelial cells and melanocytes. Large patches without midline separation

(coat-like pattern) are most commonly seen in highly cellular or proliferative lesions such as giant congenital melanocytic nevi or congenital hemangiomas.

More recently, a statement to classify cutaneous mosaic disorders as segmental versus nonsegmental has been proposed.[12] Segmental mosaic disorders encompass the archetypical mosaic patterns that usually respect the midline. Nonsegmental mosaicism demonstrates no predictable pattern and includes single-point mosaicism, disseminated mosaicism, and patchy mosaicism without midline separation. Single-point mosaicism is the commonest type of mosaicism, with almost all solitary tumors belonging to this group. Examples include trichoepitheliomas, seborrheic keratoses, and pyogenic granulomas.[12-14] Disseminated mosaicism encompass autosomal dominant diseases characterized by multiple tumors in which loss of heterozygosity (LOH) occurs. Examples are cylindromatosis, leiomyomatosis, tuberosclerosis, and neurofibromatosis.[12]

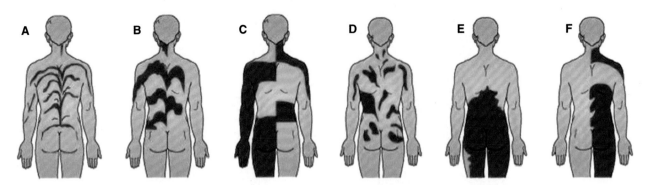

FIGURE 12-2. Patterns observed in cutaneous mosaic disorders. This includes narrow lines of Blaschko (A), broad lines of Blaschko (B), block-like or checkerboard pattern (C), phylloid pattern, (D) and patchy pattern without midline separation (E). Lateralization pattern (F) can be observed in CHILD (congenital hemidysplasia with ichthyosiform erythroderma and limb defects) syndrome, which represents functional mosaicism. Adapted with permission from Molho-Pessach V, Schaffer JV. Blaschko lines and other patterns of cutaneous mosaicism. *Clin Dermatol.* 2011;29(2):205-225.

Genetic Classification of Mosaicism

Postzygotic de novo mutations initiate all forms of genomic mosaicism, which is further classified on the basis of the presence or absence of mutation in gonadal tissue. Germline (gonadal) mosaicism describes genetic heterogeneity within the gametes, permitting mutations to be inherited and expressed constitutionally by subsequent generation. An example is osteogenesis imperfecta type II. Although it was suspected that this disease is autosomal recessive, it was subsequently shown that mosaicism was common in parents of affected siblings.[15] Somatic mosaicism precludes gonadal involvement, restricting mutation to somatic cells, whereas gonosomal mosaicism reflects mosaicism of both germline and somatic tissue and results from mutagenic events occurring early during embryogenesis. Although the same genetic mutation underlying autosomal dominant (AD) disorder can present in a mosaic pattern, other mutations are known to exist only in a mosaic state. As such, genomic mosaic disorders can be subdivided into two subgroups.

Mosaic Manifestation of Mendelian Disorders

These are mosaic patterns of AD disorders. In the constitutional state, AD mutations are present in all cells and are transmitted through the germline to affected offspring. Cutaneous mosaic manifestations of AD Mendelian disorders are segmental and are further subdivided into type I segmental mosaicism in which mutation is confined to the affected segment in an otherwise wild-type individual and type II segmental mosaicism in which a second mutation occurs in the subpopulation of precursor cells in an individual who already carries a germline mutation (Figure 12-3). This leads to segments with more severe phenotypes. An example of type I segmental mosaicism is segmental neurofibromatosis type I where classic skin lesions of cafe-au-lait spots and neurofibromas occur in a confined segment of the body without crossing the midline.[16] Parents with segmental neurofibromatosis (NF) can produce offspring with

a constitutional/generalized form of NF when gonosomal mosaicism underlies their disease.[17] Examples of type II segmental mosaicism are manifestations of Hailey-Hailey and Dariers diseases with stripes of more severe disease.[18-20]

Disorders That Manifest Only as Mosaicism

These mosaic disorders are likely embryonic lethal when constitutionally expressed. Examples are listed in Table 12-1. Revertant mosaicism is a naturally occurring phenomenon involving spontaneous correction of pathogenic mutations in somatic cells. This occurs through second-site mutation that restores completely or partially the normal function of the gene. Although pathogenic somatic mutations give rise to skin lesions in cutaneous mosaic disorders, in revertant mosaicism, an island of healthy skin appears on the background of completely affected skin. Examples are ichthyosis with confetti (*KRT1, KRT10*) and non-Herlitz junctional epidermolysis bullosa (*COL17A1, LAMB3*).[21,22]

Epigenetic modifications are changes in gene function that are mitotically and/or meiotically heritable and that do not entail a change in DNA sequence. These include DNA methylation/demethylation, retrotransposon insertion, and imprinting.[23] In skin disorders that reflect epigenetic mosaicism, a germline mutation is inherited, but its expression is modified within specific skin segments. Random X-linked inactivation (Lyonization) that occurs during early female embryogenesis can generate healthy and diseased skin, often in a Blaschkoid pattern in the setting of X-linked inherited diseases. X-linked epigenetic mosaic skin disorders can be further classified into male-lethal (eg, incontinentia pigmenti and Conradi-Hünermann-Happle syndrome), sublethal (eg, Menkes disease), and nonlethal (eg, hypohidrotic ectodermal dysplasia). In addition to Blaschkoid manifestations, other patterns of X-linked epigenetic mosaic skin disorders are lateralization seen in CHILD syndrome (congenital *h*emidysplasia with *i*chthyosiform nevus and *l*imb *d*efect) and block-like seen in women heterozygous for X-linked congenital hypertrichosis.[24]

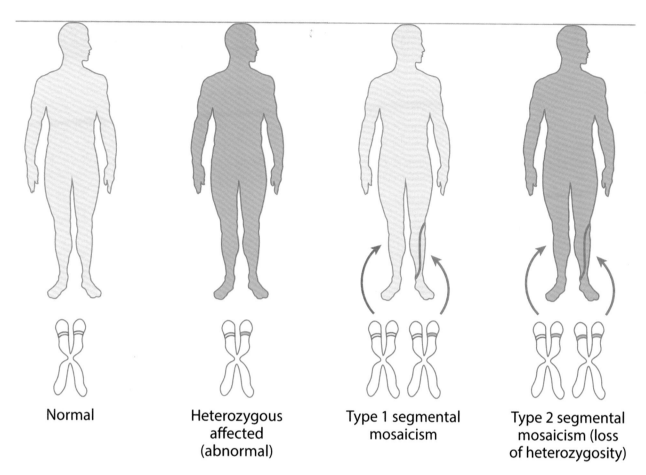

Normal

Heterozygous
affected
(abnormal)

Type 1 segmental
mosaicism

Type 2 segmental
mosaicism (loss
of heterozygosity)

FIGURE 12-3. **Types of segmental mosaicism.** Segmental mosaicism encompasses four phenotypic patterns that respect the midline. In type I segmental mosaicism a postzygotic mutation is limited to the affected segment in an otherwise wild-type individual. In type II mosaicism a second postzygotic mutational event (second-point mutation/ loss of heterozygosity) occurs in an individual already carrying germline (autosomal dominant) mutation, leading to a segment with a more severe phenotype. Adapted with permission from Lim YH, Moscato Z, Choate KA. Mosaicism in cutaneous disorders. *Annu Rev Genet.* 2017;51:123-141.

SAMPLE SELECTION AND IDENTIFICATION OF CAUSAL GENETIC MUTATIONS

Affected tissue in cutaneous mosaic disorders is expected to differ from normal tissue within the same individual only with respect to a single, causal mutation. Thus, a comparison of the genetic composition of affected and unaffected tissue from the same individual is the primary means of analysis. Obtaining a uniformly affected sample of cells, however, can be challenging. Although affected skin may be clearly distinguished from unaffected skin clinically, it often contains an admixture of mutant and wild-type cells, reducing the power to detect causal mutation. For example, a punch biopsy of a linear inflammatory skin disorder contains a variable degree of accompanying immune cell infiltrates, and a biopsy from a keratinocytic lesion contains dermal fibroblasts, endothelial cells, and adipocytes, all of which would be expected to contain DNA, which would dilute a mutant signal. Unaffected control tissues that are usually utilized in cutaneous mosaic disorders are blood (lymphocytes), saliva, and buccal swab (epithelial cells) and

clinically normal skin. It should be kept in mind that in syndromic mosaic disorders a subset of mutant cells may be found in other tissues including blood and saliva, complicating the identification of normal control. In addition, in case of type II segmental mosaicism, especially in the pediatric group, less affected or normal skin will also harbor the germline mutation.[25]

Isolation of Mutant Cells

Pure mutant cell populations can be isolated via laser capture microdissection (LCM) if histologic features or immunostains can delineate affected tissue. The basic principle of LCM is that microscope-controlled laser can be used to dissect specific cells or regions from tissue sections adhered to a thermoplastic membrane (frozen or fixed and paraffin-embedded sections). Cellular components, including RNA, DNA, and protein, can be extracted for analysis.[26] A comparison of sequenced DNA from laser-captured tissue and control DNA can identify mosaic mutations. Alternatively, cell culture can be employed to isolate a specific mutant cell population. For example, in a Blaschko-linear

TABLE 12-1.   Examples of embryonic lethal cutaneous mosaic disorders

Disorder	Syndromic Presentation[a]	Genes
Nevus sabaceus[40]	Schimmelpenning syndrome, phakomatosis pigmentokeratotica (nevus spilus and nevus sebaceous)	*HRAS, KRAS*
Epidermal nevus[8,41,42,43(p3)]	CLOVE **syndrome** (Congenital, Lipomatous, Overgrowth, Vascular Malformations, Epidermal Nevi and Spinal/Skeletal Anomalies and/or Scoliosis)	*PIK3CA*
	Epidermal nevus syndrome, cutaneous-skeletal hypophosphatemia syndrome (*HRAS* and *NRAS* mutations, described with giant congenital melanocytic nevus as well)	*HRAS, KRAS, NRAS,*
	Epidermal nevus syndrome (Garcia-Hafner-Happle syndrome)	*FGFR3*
Proteus syndrome[7]		*AKT1*
Nevus spilus[36]	Papular nevus spilus syndrome, phakomatosis pigmentokeratotica	*HRAS*
Giant congenital melanocytic nevus[37]	Giant congenital melanocytic nevus syndrome, cutaneous skeletal hypophosphatemia syndrome	*RAS*
McCune-Albright syndrome[44]		*GNAS1*
Nevus comedonicus[45]	Nevus comedonicus syndrome	*NEK9*
Port-wine stain[9]	Sturge-Weber syndrome	*GNAQ, GNA11*
Solitary enchondroma[46,b]	Maffucci syndrome	*IDH1*
Becker nevus[47]	Becker nevus syndrome	*ACTB*
Congenital GLUT-negative hemangiomas[13,48] (NICH, RICH)		*GNA11, GNA14, GNAQ, KRAS, NRAS*

[a]If there was no report on nonsyndromic mutation positive skin nevus, then the syndrome is listed under disorder.
[b]Cartilage-forming tumor. Maffucci syndrome is a vascular-skeletal disorder characterized by enchondroma and spindle cell hemangiomas.
Abbreviations: CLOVE, congenital lipomatosus overgrowth, vascular malformation and epidermal nevi; GLUT, glucose transporter; NICH, noninvoluting congenital hemangioma; RICH, rapidly involuting congenital hemangioma

lesion suspected to harbor a mutation in keratinocytes, one can isolate the cells from epidermal sheets of diseased skin and grow them in a culture dish. DNA isolated from cultured keratinocytes can be then compared with DNA from normal tissue.[21]

Detection of Mutation

Karyotype and fluorescence in situ hybridization were successfully employed to study cases of syndromic Blaschkoid and phylloid dyspigmentation, finding distinct karyotypes and aneuploidy within patient cells.[5,27-29] These methods are carried out in a cell-by cell manner and can be challenging in the setting of low-level mosaicism as cells need to be examined individually.[2] Moreover, for some types of mosaicism, the abnormal as well as the normal cells may not divide, so an analysis of metaphases might provide a biased view of the true chromosome constitution of this individual.[30]

Single Nucleotide Polymorphism Array

Beginning in 2005, microarray-based techniques began to replace cytogenetic testing, including array-based comparative genomic hybridization (CGH), which can analyze genomic copy number variants (CNVs), followed by genome-wide single nucleotide polymorphism (SNP) arrays, which provide both genotypes (allele frequency) and CNVs (by calculating the logR ratio for signal intensity). Compared with cytogenetic analyses, these techniques analyze data from many cells simultaneously and permit examination of cells regardless of cell cycle state. SNP arrays are much more sensitive than CGH for detecting mosaicism with a lower level of detection of 5% affected cells. This method was employed to find copy-neutral LOH underlying revertant mosaicism in ichthyosis with confetti.[21]

Next-Generation Sequencing

Next-generation sequencing (NGS) is a high-throughput method, sequencing DNA in a massively parallel fashion. Since 2005, NGS platforms have become widely available, reducing the cost of sequencing of the coding regions of the genome (a.k.a. the "exome") to hundreds of dollars and of whole genome sequencing to thousands.[30] Exons are the protein coding regions within the genome comprising less than 2% of the human genome. However, they are estimated to harbor approximately 85% of disease-causing mutations.[25,30] As such, most studies focus on exome sequencing data in order to identify pathogenic mutations. In WES exons, flanking areas are captured with special probes and separated from noncoding DNA. The separated DNA fragments are amplified and then sequenced in a parallel fashion. Reads are further processed and aligned to a reference genome and single nucleotide variants (deviations from reference sequence) identified and annotated for predicted effect on the encoded protein. In mosaic disorders, paired WES of normal and affected tissue from the same individual are further analyzed to identify only those positions in the genome that differ in affected tissue. Whole genome sequencing provides an unbiased coverage of exons as well as sequencing data of noncoding regions. In cases where causal mutations cannot be identified via WES (eg, a structural rearrangement or mutation in introns or regulatory elements), whole genome sequencing may be necessary.[31]

MOSAIC RASOPATHIES

Ras proteins are small GTPases encoded by three genes *HRAS, KRAS,* and *NRAS* playing a key role in transducing stimuli of extracellular growth factors into the intracellular environment. They function as molecular "switches," switching-on signaling when bound to Guanosine triphosphate (GTP) and off when bound to Guanosine diphosphate (GDP).[32] Following activation, Ras proteins feed two major molecular pathways: Ras-Raf-MEK-ERK and the PI3K-akt signaling pathways. Activation of these pathways influences cell survival, proliferation, and differentiation.

The degree of the pathway activation determines whether mutations are embryonic lethal and can survive only in a mosaic state or are compatible with life and thus can lead to a constitutional disease; critical amino acid residues at codon 12, 13, and 61 mediate the hydrolysis of GTP to GDP that is central to Ras inactivation. Indeed, potent canonical mutations in these three residues lead to constitutively active GTP-bound Ras. These mutations have an incidence of around 20% in cancer and are responsible for mosaic RASopathies that are considered embryonic lethal (Table 12-1).[32,33] Less potent activation of H-Ras caused by recurrent mutation at codon 12 causes germline Costello syndrome as well as Wooly hair nevus, which is caused by somatic mutation.[34]

The timing of mutation during embryogenesis determines the extent of mosaic RASopathies: Keratinocytic epidermal nevus (KEN) and nevus sebaceous (NS) are examples of segmental mosaic RASopathies originating from mutated keratinocytic precursor cells. *RAS* mutations can be restricted to the KEN or NS alone, or if appearing earlier during embryogenesis, can give rise to Schimmelpenning and epidermal nevus syndromes involving tissues derived from additional cell lineages (Table 12-1). Likewise, mutation in a multipotent progenitor cell giving rise to keratinocytic and melanocyte lineages causes phacomatosis pigmentokeratotica, a combination of NS and speckled lentiginous nevi occurring in the Blaschkoid pattern.[35] *RAS* mutations in melanocyte lineage are responsible for spilus nevi and giant congenital melanocytic nevi.[8,36,37] Finally, a

subset of noninvoluting congenital hemangiomas as well as pyogenic granulomas were found to be driven by *RAS* mutations.[13,14] Of note, mutations in non-Ras members of the MAPK pathway are frequently found in cutaneous mosaic RASopathies, and one example is the activating *BRAF* p.V600E mutation that is frequently found, like *RAS* mutations in melanocytic nevi, pyogenic granulomas, and syringocystadenoma papilliferum.[38,39]

SUMMARY

Cutaneous mosaic disorders provide a unique opportunity to study genetic mosaicism because of the accessibility of mosaic tissue and the clinical characteristics that make distinguishing affected and unaffected tissue straightforward and allow the isolation of affected tissue through simple in-office procedures. The discovery of novel mutations underlying cutaneous mosaic disorders is continuing at an unprecedented pace because of technological advances in genetic analysis. Some discoveries made in cutaneous mosaic disorders have revealed novel biologic pathways that are relevant to diseases beyond the skin and may have therapeutic implications for skin and systemic disease.

REFERENCES

1. Strachan T, Read A. *Human Molecular Genetics.* 4th ed. New York, NY: Garland Science; 2010.
2. Biesecker LG, Spinner NB. A genomic view of mosaicism and human disease. *Nat Rev Genet.* 2013;14(5):307-320. doi:10.1038/nrg3424
3. Happle R, Assim A. The lines of Blaschko on the head and neck. *J Am Acad Dermatol.* 2001;44(4):612-615.
4. Happle R. *Mosaicism in Human Skin-Understanding Nevi, Nevoid Skin.* Springer. https://www.springer.com/la/book/9783642387647. Accessed January 1, 2018.
5. Sybert VP. Hypomelanosis of Ito: a description, not a diagnosis. *J Invest Dermatol.* 1994;103(5 suppl):141S-143S.
6. Horn D, Happle R, Neitzel H, Kunze J. Pigmentary mosaicism of the hyperpigmented type in two half-brothers. *Am J Med Genet.* 2002;112(1):65-69. doi:10.1002/ajmg.10600
7. Lindhurst MJ, Sapp JC, Teer JK, et al. A mosaic activating mutation in AKT1 associated with the Proteus syndrome. *N Engl J Med.* 2011;365(7):611-619. doi:10.1056/NEJMoa1104017
8. Lim YH, Ovejero D, Sugarman JS, et al. Multilineage somatic activating mutations in HRAS and NRAS cause mosaic cutaneous and skeletal lesions, elevated FGF23 and hypophosphatemia. *Hum Mol Genet.* 2014;23(2):397-407. doi:10.1093/hmg/ddt429
9. Shirley MD, Tang H, Gallione CJ, et al. Sturge–Weber syndrome and Port-Wine stains caused by somatic mutation in GNAQ. *N Engl J Med.* 2013;368(21):1971-1979. doi:10.1056/NEJMoa1213507
10. Blaschko A. *Die Nervenverteilung in Der Haut in Ihrer Beziehung Zu Den Erkrankungen Der HautDie Nervenverteilung in Der Haut in Ihrer Beziehung Zu Den Erkrankungen Der Haut. Beilage Zu Den Verhandlungen Der Deutschen Dermatologischen Gesellschaft VII Congress Breslau.* Braumuller, Wein; 1901.
11. Happle R. Mosaicism in human skin: understanding the patterns and mechanisms. *Arch Dermatol.* 1993;129(11):1460-1470.
12. Happle R. The categories of cutaneous mosaicism: A proposed classification. *Am J Med Genet A.* 2016;170A(2):452-459. doi:10.1002/ajmg.a.37439
13. Lim YH, Douglas SR, Ko CJ, et al. Somatic activating RAS Mutations cause vascular tumors including pyogenic granuloma. *J Invest Dermatol.* 2015;135(6):1698-1700. doi:10.1038/jid.2015.55

14. Groesser L, Peterhof E, Evert M, Landthaler M, Berneburg M, Hafner C. BRAF and RAS mutations in sporadic and secondary pyogenic granuloma. *J Invest Dermatol.* 2016;136(2):481-486. doi:10.1038/JID.2015.376

15. Byers PH, Tsipouras P, Bonadio JF, Starman BJ, Schwartz RC. Perinatal lethal osteogenesis imperfecta (OI type II): a biochemically heterogeneous disorder usually due to new mutations in the genes for type I collagen. *Am J Hum Genet.* 1988;42(2):237-248.

16. Tinschert S, Naumann I, Stegmann E, et al. Segmental neurofibromatosis is caused by somatic mutation of the neurofibromatosis type 1 (NF1) gene. *Eur J Hum Genet EJHG.* 2000;8(6):455-459. doi:10.1038/sj.ejhg.5200493

17. Callum P, Messiaen LM, Bower PV, et al. Gonosomal mosaicism for an NF1 deletion in a sperm donor: evidence of the need for coordinated, long-term communication of health information among relevant parties. *Hum Reprod Oxf Engl.* 2012;27(4):1223-1226. doi:10.1093/humrep/des014

18. Happle R. [Segmental type 2 manifestation of autosome dominant skin diseases. Development of a new formal genetic concept]. *Hautarzt Z Dermatol Venerol Verwandte Geb.* 2001;52(4):283-287.

19. Boente M del C, Frontini M del V, Primc N-B, Asial R-A. [Linear Darier disease in two siblings. An example of loss of heterozygosity]. *Ann Dermatol Venereol.* 2004;131(8-9):805-809.

20. Itin PH, Büchner SA, Happle R. Segmental manifestation of Darier disease. What is the genetic background in type 1 and type 2 mosaic phenotypes? *Dermatol Basel Switz.* 2000;200(3):254-257. doi:10.1159/000018370

21. Choate KA, Lu Y, Zhou J, et al. Mitotic recombination in patients with ichthyosis causes reversion of dominant mutations in KRT10. *Science.* 2010;330(6000):94-97. doi:10.1126/science.1192280

22. Lai-Cheong JE, McGrath JA, Uitto J. Revertant mosaicism in skin: natural gene therapy. *Trends Mol Med.* 2011;17(3):140-148. doi:10.1016/j.molmed.2010.11.003

23. Dupont C, Armant DR, Brenner CA. Epigenetics: definition, mechanisms and clinical perspective. *Semin Reprod Med.* 2009;27(5):351-357. doi:10.1055/s-0029-1237423

24. X-chromosome inactivation: role in skin disease expression. https://www.ncbi.nlm.nih.gov/pubmed/16720460. Accessed April 10, 2018.

25. Lim YH, Moscato Z, Choate KA. Mosaicism in cutaneous disorders. *Annu Rev Genet.* 2017;51(1):123-141. doi:10.1146/annurev-genet-121415-121955

26. Jensen E. Laser-capture microdissection. *Anat Rec.* 2013;296(11):1683-1687. doi:10.1002/ar.22791

27. Chemke J, Rappaport S, Etrog R. Aberrant melanoblast migration associated with trisomy 18 mosaicism. *J Med Genet.* 1983;20(2):135-137.

28. González-Enseñat MA, Vicente A, Poo P, et al. Phylloid hypomelanosis and mosaic partial trisomy 13: two cases that provide further evidence of a distinct clinicogenetic entity. *Arch Dermatol.* 2009;145(5):576-578. doi:10.1001/archdermatol.2009.37

29. Happle R. Phylloid hypomelanosis is closely related to mosaic trisomy 13. *Eur J Dermatol EJD.* 2000;10(7):511-512.

30. Bamshad MJ, Ng SB, Bigham AW, et al. Exome sequencing as a tool for Mendelian disease gene discovery. *Nat Rev Genet.* 2011;12(11):745. doi:10.1038/nrg3031

31. Weinhold N, Jacobsen A, Schultz N, Sander C, Lee W. Genome-wide analysis of non-coding regulatory mutations in cancer. *Nat Genet.* 2014;46(11):1160-1165. doi:10.1038/ng.3101

32. Prior IA, Lewis PD, Mattos C. A comprehensive survey of Ras mutations in cancer. *Cancer Res.* 2012;72(10):2457-2467. doi:10.1158/0008-5472.CAN-11-2612

33. Hafner C, Groesser L. Mosaic RASopathies. *Cell Cycle.* 2013;12(1):43-50. doi:10.4161/cc.23108

34. Levinsohn JL, Teng J, Craiglow BG, et al. Somatic HRAS p.G12S mutation causes woolly hair and epidermal nevi. *J Invest Dermatol.* 2014;134(4):1149-1152. doi:10.1038/jid.2013.430

35. Groesser L, Herschberger E, Sagrera A, et al. Phacomatosis pigmentokeratotica is caused by a postzygotic HRAS mutation in a multipotent progenitor cell. *J Invest Dermatol.* http://www.jidonline.org/article/S0022-202X(15)36357-0/fulltext. Accessed April 11, 2018.

36. Sarin KY, McNiff JM, Kwok S, Kim J, Khavari PA. Activating HRAS mutation in nevus spilus. *J Invest Dermatol.* 2014;134(6):1766-1768. doi:10.1038/jid.2014.6

37. Kinsler VA, Thomas AC, Ishida M, et al. Multiple congenital melanocytic nevi and neurocutaneous melanosis are caused by postzygotic mutations in codon 61 of NRAS. *J Invest Dermatol.* 2013;133(9):2229-2236. doi:10.1038/jid.2013.70

38. Shen A-S, Peterhof E, Kind P, et al. Activating mutations in the RAS/mitogen-activated protein kinase signaling pathway in sporadic trichoblastoma and syringocystadenoma papilliferum. *Hum Pathol.* 2015;46(2):272-276. doi:10.1016/j.humpath.2014.11.002

39. Levinsohn JL, Sugarman JL, Bilguvar K, et al. Somatic V600E BRAF mutation in linear and sporadic syringocystadenoma papilliferum. *J Invest Dermatol.* http://www.jidonline.org/article/S0022-202X(15)41820-2/fulltext. Accessed April 11, 2018.

40. Levinsohn JL, Tian LC, Boyden LM, et al. Whole-exome sequencing reveals somatic mutations in HRAS and KRAS, which cause nevus sebaceus. *J Invest Dermatol.* 2013;133(3):827-830. doi:10.1038/jid.2012.379

41. Hafner C, Toll A, Real FX. HRAS mutation mosaicism causing urothelial cancer and epidermal nevus. *N Engl J Med.* 2011;365(20):1940-1942. doi:10.1056/NEJMc1109381

42. Hafner C, López-Knowles E, Luis NM, et al. Oncogenic PIK3CA mutations occur in epidermal nevi and seborrheic keratoses with a characteristic mutation pattern. *Proc Natl Acad Sci USA.* 2007;104(33):13450-13454. doi:10.1073/pnas.0705218104

43. García-Vargas A, Hafner C, Pérez-Rodríguez AG, et al. An epidermal nevus syndrome with cerebral involvement caused by a mosaic FGFR3 mutation. *Am J Med Genet A.* 2008;146A(17):2275-2279. doi:10.1002/ajmg.a.32429

44. Weinstein LS, Shenker A, Gejman PV, Merino MJ, Friedman E, Spiegel AM. Activating mutations of the stimulatory G protein in the McCune-Albright syndrome. *N Engl J Med.* 1991;325(24):1688-1695. doi:10.1056/NEJM199112123252403

45. Levinsohn JL, Sugarman JL, McNiff JM, Antaya RJ, Choate KA. Somatic mutations in NEK9 cause nevus comedonicus. *Am J Hum Genet.* 2016;98(5):1030-1037. doi:10.1016/j.ajhg.2016.03.019

46. Pansuriya TC, van Eijk R, Adamo P d', et al. Somatic mosaic IDH1 or IDH2 mutations are associated with enchondroma and spindle cell hemangioma in Ollier disease and Maffucci syndrome. *Nat Genet.* 2011;43(12):1256-1261. doi:10.1038/ng.1004

47. Cai ED, Sun BK, Chiang A, et al. Postzygotic mutations in beta-actin are associated with Becker's nevus and Becker's nevus syndrome. *J Invest Dermatol.* 2017;137(8):1795-1798. doi:10.1016/j.jid.2017.03.017

48. Lim YH, Bacchiocchi A, Qiu J, et al. GNA14 somatic mutation causes congenital and sporadic vascular tumors by MAPK activation. *Am J Hum Genet.* 2016;99(2):443-450. doi:10.1016/j.ajhg.2016.06.010

13

Genetic Autoinflammatory Disorders

Matthew D. Vesely / Chyi-Chia Richard Lee / Edward W. Cowen

The concept of autoimmunity (*horror autotoxicus*) was initially proposed over a century ago by Paul Ehrlich to describe the clinical scenario whereby the components of adaptive immunity damage normal tissue.[1] In contrast, autoinflammation (*horror autoinflammaticus*), a term originally proposed in 1999, describes damage to normal tissue induced by innate immunity.[2,3] Although the immune system is divided into innate and adaptive components, they are intricately linked and function in equilibrium. Perturbations in the adaptive immune system often result in an imbalance among innate immune components; thus, neither autoimmunity nor autoinflammatory disorders have defects isolated to a single branch of the immune system. Nevertheless, a preponderance of innate dysregulation is the characteristic feature of autoinflammation.[4] Defects in the distinct components of innate immunity, in turn, may result in disorders with unique clinicopathologic features. All disorders described herein are rare, monogenic conditions affecting the pediatric population (Table 13-1).

CRYOPYRIN-ASSOCIATED PERIODIC SYNDROME (CAPS)

Definition and Epidemiology

Cryopyrin-associated periodic syndrome (CAPS) is a rare disorder of childhood-onset, characterized by systemic and tissue-specific inflammation of the integumentary, nervous, and musculoskeletal systems.[5] Three related, but distinct, phenotypes encompass the clinical spectrum of CAPS and are referred to as cryopyrinopathies because they have all been linked to mutations in the gene-encoding cryopyrin [*CIAS1* (cold-induced autoinflammatory syndrome 1), also known as *NLRP3* (NACHT domain, leucine-rich repeat, and pyrin-containing protein 3)]. The mildest phenotype is familial cold autoinflammatory syndrome (FCAS), followed by Muckle-Wells syndrome (MWS), which is associated with more systemic inflammation. The most severe phenotype is neonatal-onset multisystem inflammatory disease (NOMID), which is sometimes referred to in Europe as chronic infantile neurological cutaneous and articular (CINCA) syndrome.

MWS was originally described in 1962 in northern European kindreds who suffered recurrent, severe, acute inflammatory episodes.[6] Subsequently, MWS, FCAS, and NOMID/CINCA were all found to be caused by mutations in the *NRLP3* gene.[7-11] It is estimated that CAPS affects 1:1 000 000 people worldwide.[12] However, the true prevalence may be higher, given unfamiliarity among clinicians and the milder phenotype of FCAS that presents in later childhood.[13] In France, the incidence of CAPS has been estimated to be as high as 1:360 000 people.[14] The age of presentation varies with severity, with the most severe phenotype, NOMID, developing within days of birth, whereas the symptoms of FCAS may be delayed for several years.

Etiology

The cryopyrinopathies are associated with autosomal dominant or de novo mutations of *NLRP3/CIAS1*, which encodes the protein cryopyrin. The hallmark of the innate immune dysregulation of CAPS is excessive production of

TABLE 13-1.	Clinical features, histology, and genetics of selected autoinflammatory syndromes with unique histopathologic features			
Disease	**Gene**	**Skin Findings**	**Systemic Manifestations**	**Histology**
CAPS	*NLRP3/CIAS1* Cryopyrin	Urticaria-like eruptions	Fevers arthralgia, eye disease, amyloidosis, neurologic symptoms	Superficial perivascular, and perieccrine infiltrate of mature neutrophils
DIRA	*IL1RN* IL-1 antagonist	Erythematous plaques with follicular pustules	Periostitis, multifocal osteomyelitis, hepalosplenomegaly	Hyperkeratosis, epidermal, and dermal neutrophilic infiltrate with follicular pustules
DADA2	*CERC1* ADA2	Livedo racemosa and painful, pink nodules	Early-onset stroke	Medium-vessel vasculitis
SAVI	*TMEM173* STING	Telangiectatic-purpuric plaques on acral sites, progression to ulcers and eschars, nasal cartilage destruction	Fever, failure to thrive, interstitial lung disease	Vasculopathy with neutrophilic infiltrate, karyorrhexis, intravascular thrombosis,s and fibrinoid necrosis of small vessels
CANDLE Syndrome	*PSMB8* PSMB8	Annular violaceous plaques, periorbital edema, lipodystrophy	Fevers, organomegaly, arthralgia	Perivascular and interstitial atypical mononuclear infiltrate composed of immature neutrophilis and myeloid precursors
Blau Syndrome	*CARD15/NOD2* CARD15/NOD2	Densely populated, small red-brown papules	Fever, granulomatous uveitis, polyarthritis, camptodactyly; granulomatous kidney, liver, lung, and CNS disease	Multicentric, noncaseating, sarcoid-type granulomas, with emperipolesis of lymphocytes in giant cells

Abbreviations: ADA2, adenosine deaminase 2; CANDLE, Chronic Atypical Neutrophilic Dermatosis with Lipodystrophy and Elevated Temperature; CAPS, cryopyrin-associated periodic syndrome; CNS, central nervous system; DADA2, deficiency of adenosine deaminase; DIRA, deficiency of the interleukin-1 receptor antagonist; SAVI, STING-associated vasculopathy with onset in infancy.

interleukin-1β (IL-1β). Cryopyrin is a critical component of the inflammasome, a multiprotein complex responsible for generation IL-1β in response to pathogens or "danger signals" from dead or dying host cells. *NLRP3* mutations in patients with CAPS appear to activate the inflammasome in the absence of pathogenic insults.[3] Nearly all patients with FCAS and MWS have inherited mutations in *NLRP3*, whereas *NLRP3* mutations found in NOMID patients tend to occur de novo.[10] Furthermore, about half of patients with NOMID do not have detectable germline *NLRP3* mutations; however, many somatic mutations have been found in these patients.[15]

Clinical Presentation

CAPS present with urticaria-like papules and plaques, conjunctivitis, fevers, arthralgia, and constitutional symptoms.[5,16] In the case of FCAS, symptoms are triggered within hours of exposure to cold temperatures, resulting in an effervescent urticarial rash followed by scleral injection, fever, and arthralgia, which typically last less than 24 hours. Nonpruritic, erythematous papules, and plaques coalesce to form polycyclic or geographic plaques predominantly on trunk and extremities (Figure 13-1A and B). In patients with MWS, a similar presentation with effervescent urticarial rash, fever, conjunctivitis, and arthralgia occurs in the absence of cold exposure.

Acute inflammatory episodes typically last 24 to 48 hours, and many patients with MWS experience daily symptoms of chronic systemic inflammation including pain (eg, abdominal) and fatigue. Long-standing systemic inflammation results in secondary amyloidosis, and neurologic involvement results in sensorineural hearing loss. The most severe CAPS phenotype, NOMID, is characterized by daily, persistent attacks of fever, urticarial rash, and arthralgia. A defining feature of NOMID is central nervous system (CNS) inflammation, resulting in chronic aseptic meningitis, seizures, cognitive impairment, and hearing and vision loss.[16-18] Extensive bone and joint involvement results in deforming arthropathy with epiphyseal bone formation (Figure 13-1C), joint contractures with limited mobility, and abnormal facial features with frontal bossing and flattening of the nasal dorsum.

Histologic Findings

A skin biopsy of the erythematous and edematous papules and plaques in patients with CAPS shows superficial perivascular and perieccrine infiltrate predominately composed of mature neutrophils and dilated superficial dermal lymphatics (Figure 13-2).[19,20] This is in contrast to the typical superficial perivascular lymphocytic inflammatory infiltrate of classic allergic urticaria. In addition, a helpful identifying

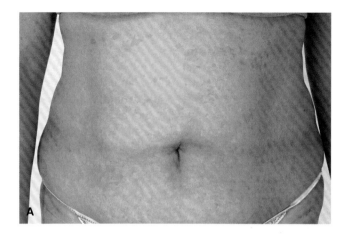

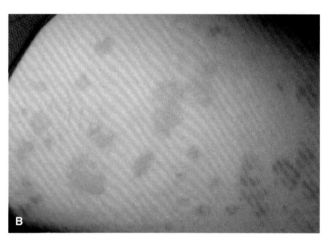

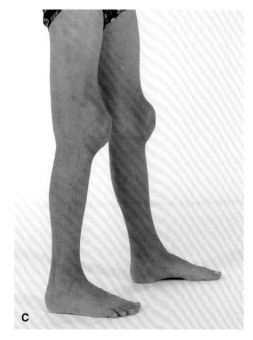

FIGURE 13-1. Cryopyrin-associated periodic syndrome. Urticaria-like papules and plaques in a patient with neonatal-onset multisystem inflammatory disease (NOMID) (A) and Muckle-Wells syndrome (B). C, Extensive bone and joint involvement resulting in deforming arthropathy in a patient with NOMID.

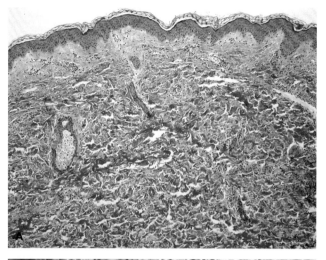

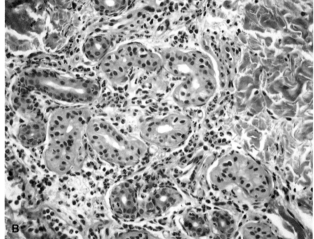

FIGURE 13-2. Histology of neonatal-onset multisystem inflammatory disease. A, The epidermal changes are unremarkable. There is mild papillary dermal edema with superficial perivascular and perieccrine infiltrate of mature neutrophils and dilated superficial dermal lymphatics. There is no histologic evidence of vasculitis. B, Characteristic perieccrine neutrophilic infiltration shows an infiltrate of mature neutrophils between eccrine glands.

feature is characteristic perieccrine neutrophilic infiltration similar to neutrophilic eccrine hidradenitis.[21] There is an absence of karyorrhexis or leukocytoclasis and vasculitis. There are no epidermal changes and no eosinophils.

Differential Diagnosis

Classic urticaria is composed of superficial perivascular infiltrate of lymphocytes and may contain eosinophils. However, a subset of patients with urticaria will present with predominately neutrophil-rich infiltrate, termed neutrophilic urticaria.[22] Since the introduction of the term "neutrophilic urticaria," there have been numerous subtypes described, including autoimmunity-related neutrophilic dermatosis[23], neutrophilic urticaria with systemic inflammation[24], and neutrophilic urticarial dermatoses.[25] These various subtypes are all characterized by superficial perivascular neutrophilic inflammation and leukocytoclasis, but there is an absence of periecrrine involvement, vasculitis, or dermal edema. The histologic pattern found in CAPS characteristically involves periecrrine neutrophilic infiltration but lacks significant leukocytoclasis. Urticarial vasculitis has the presence of both leukocytoclasis and vasculitis. Sweet syndrome is characterized by an intense dermal infiltration of neutrophils with leukocytoclasis and significant dermal edema.

CAPSULE SUMMARY

CRYOPYRIN-ASSOCIATED PERIODIC SYNDROME

CAPS is a group of rare, inherited autoinflammatory disorders that represent a spectrum of disease severity. NOMID/CINCA is the most severe form. Autosomal dominant or de novo gain-of-function mutations in *NLRP3*, a component of the inflammasome, result in an overproduction of IL-1β. The clinical features include acute episodes of fever, arthralgia, and urticaria-like eruptions. CNS inflammation is a hallmark of NOMID/CINCA. The histology of CAPS skin lesions is characterized by superficial perivascular and periecrrine infiltrate of mature neutrophils without eosinophils, leukocytoclasis, or vasculitis. Periecrrine neutrophilic infiltration and an absence of leukocytoclasis may help distinguish CAPS from other neutrophilic urticarial dermatoses.

DEFICIENCY OF THE INTERLEUKIN-1 RECEPTOR ANTAGONIST

Definition and Epidemiology

Deficiency of the interleukin-1 receptor antagonist (DIRA) is a rare autoinflammatory disorder characterized by sterile multifocal osteomyelitis and periostitis, with skin lesions resembling pustular psoriasis in the neonatal period.[26,27] Autosomal recessive mutations in interleukin-1 receptor antagonist (*IL1RN*) result in uncontrolled IL-1α/β signaling.[26,27]

Reports of DIRA to date are predominately described in patients of Puerto Rican, Newfoundland, Lebanese, Dutch, and Brazilian descent.[26-29] The worldwide incidence is unknown given its rarity, but the condition is associated with an estimated 30% mortality during infancy if untreated. It is estimated that 0.2% of the population in Newfoundland are carriers of the mutation with likely similar rates in Lebanon, Brazil, and the Netherlands. The carrier rate in Puerto Rico is approximately 1.3% due to a founder effect, and in the Arecibo region, it is estimated that DIRA may occur in 1:6300 people.[26]

Etiology

DIRA is caused by autosomal recessive mutations in *IL1RN*. The lack of a functional *IL1RN* in DIRA patients results in an unopposed stimulation of the IL-1 receptor by IL-1α and

IL-1β.[30] IL-1β is processed by the myeloid cells of the innate immune system by the inflammasome, whereas IL-1α is preformed and can be released by nonimmune cells such as keratinocytes and endothelial cells.[30] The downstream effects of IL-1α/β result in the production of additional proinflammatory cytokines including tumor necrosis factor (TNF) and IL-17. Although CAPS is the result of the overproduction and secretion of IL-1β, DIRA is the result of an inability to terminate signaling from both IL-1β and IL-1α. In addition, the IL-1 receptor is highly expressed within the epidermis, and unopposed signaling by IL-1α may be responsible for the epidermal changes including hyperkeratosis and subcorneal pustulosis seen in DIRA.

Clinical Presentation

At birth or within a few weeks of age, neonates with DIRA develop a pustular rash, swollen joints, pain with movement, and oral mucosal ulcers.[31] Of note, fever is characteristically absent despite the elevation of inflammatory markers and acute phase reactants. DIRA in utero resulting in fetal demise has also been reported.[32] The rash may consist of discrete erythematous plaques studded with follicular pustules or evolve to generalized pustulosis. Less commonly, ichthyosiform skin changes and nail changes including pitting and onychomadesis are present (Figure 13-3). Superficial trauma of the skin results in pathergy and subsequent pustulosis at the sites of trauma. Although the initial clinical presentation may be confused with pustular psoriasis, the early onset of disease, together with neonatal distress and markers of systemic inflammation, including periostitis, multifocal sterile osteomyelitis, and hepatosplenomegaly, are characteristic of DIRA. The most common radiographic findings include balloon widening of the anterior rib ends, multifocal osteolytic lesions, and periosteal elevation. CNS vasculitis has also been reported.[26] Untreated DIRA results in death during infancy or early childhood from multisystem shock and organ failure secondary to overwhelming systemic inflammation. Treatment with IL-1 blockers is lifesaving.[26]

Histologic Findings

The cutaneous biopsies of the pustular rash show a dense infiltrate of mature neutrophils throughout the dermis with acanthosis, intraepidermal neutrophils, prominent papillary dermal edema, and pustule formation along the hair follicular infundibulum (Figure 13-4).[26,27] Notably, there is a combination of subcorneal pustules as well as dense neutrophilic infiltrate with a destruction of hair follicular infundibula. One patient had histopathologic evidence of vasculitis in the subcutis adjacent to bone inflammation.[26]

Differential Diagnosis

The histopathologic differential diagnosis of DIRA includes other causes of subcorneal pustules. The key distinguishing

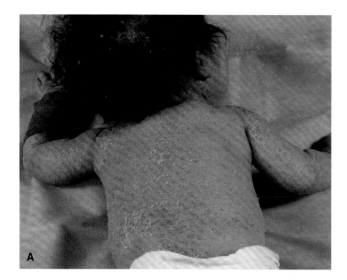

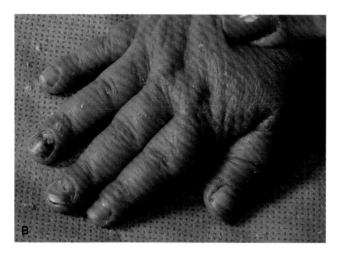

FIGURE 13-3. **Deficiency of the IL-1 receptor antagonist.** A, Erythroderma, pinpoint pustules, and ichthyosiform scale in a neonate. B, Nail changes including pitting and onychomadesis.

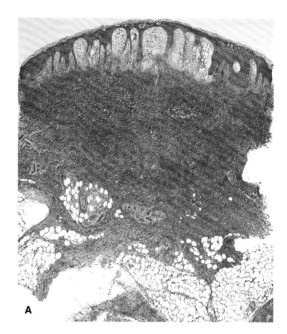

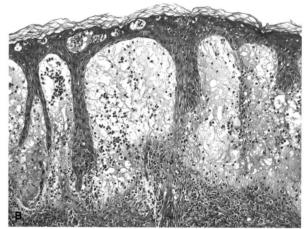

FIGURE 13-4. **Histology of deficiency of the IL-1 receptor antagonist.** A, A dense infiltrate of mature neutrophils throughout the dermis with subcorneal/intraepidermal neutrophilic pustules, prominent papillary dermal edema, and the destruction of hair follicle infundibula. B, There is prominent papillary dermal edema with intraepidermal pustules of mature neutrophils.

feature of DIRA is folliculocentric infiltrate of neutrophils with involvement of the follicular infundibula, as other disorders that present with subcorneal pustules rarely involve the hair follicle. Pustular psoriasis may show features common in more chronic plaque psoriasis such as an elongation of rete ridges, papillary epidermal thinning, and dilated, tortuous papillary vessels. In addition, the lesions of pustular psoriasis are characterized by parakeratosis, spongiosis, and the spongiform pustules of Kogoj. Deficiency of IL-36 receptor antagonist (DITRA) also presents with an erythematous pustular rash mimicking psoriasis but lacks internal organ manifestation.[33-35] The histology of DITRA demonstrates spongiform pustules, acanthosis, and parakeratosis.[34] Subcorneal pustular dermatosis (Sneddon-Wilkinson disease) shows perivascular neutrophilic infiltrate with occasional monocytes and eosinophils. Acute generalized exanthematous pustulosis is nonfollicular and often contains eosinophils.

CAPSULE SUMMARY

DEFICIENCY OF THE INTERLEUKIN-1 RECEPTOR ANTAGONIST

DIRA is a rare, life-threatening inherited autoinflammatory disorder caused by autosomal recessive mutations in *IL1RN*, resulting in an overstimulation by IL-1α/β. The clinical features include neonatal-onset neutrophilic pustules, periostitis, and multifocal sterile osteomyelitis. Estimated mortality in infancy is 30% if untreated. Pustular rash shows a dense infiltrate of mature neutrophils in the epidermis and dermis with acanthosis, hyperkeratosis, and pustule formation along the follicular infundibulum of hair follicles.

DEFICIENCY OF ADENOSINE DEAMINASE 2 (DADA2)

Definition and Epidemiology

Deficiency of adenosine deaminase 2 (DADA2) is a recently identified autoinflammatory syndrome characterized by intermittent fevers, livedo racemosa, and systemic vasculopathy/vasculitis.[36,37] Patients with DADA2 have recurrent lacunar infarcts in early childhood, occurring as early as infancy, as well as cutaneous polyarteritis nodosa (PAN). Loss-of-function, autosomal recessive mutations in cat eye syndrome chromosome region, candidate 1 (*CERC1*), which encodes ADA2, have been identified in patients with DADA2.

Since the initial description of DADA2 in 2014, more than 50 cases have been reported.[38] Given the rarity and very recent description of the disease, the worldwide incidence is unknown. Nevertheless, a significant number of cases of DADA2 have been reported in individuals of Georgian Jewish ancestry. In one study, all 19 Georgian Jewish DADA2 patients shared the same homozygous p.Gly47Arg mutation.[36] Therefore, it has been estimated that the carrier frequency of this mutation in *CERC1* is about 10% of the Georgian Jewish population. The quantity of detectable ADA2 in the serum is lower in DADA2 heterozygote carriers compared with healthy controls, but it is unknown whether this confers a health risk in this carrier population.

Etiology

ADA2 is a secreted protein of the myeloid cell lineage that helps differentiate monocytes into macrophages and dendritic cells. In addition, ADA2 may also play a role in the development and differentiation of endothelial cells. However, very little is known regarding how the loss of ADA2 function results in vasculopathy and vasculitis. An analysis of blood from DADA2 patients reveals an elevated neutrophil and interferon signature, suggesting that there is excessive neutrophil activation in the absence of ADA2.[39]

Clinical Presentation

Livedo racemosa, PAN, and early-onset stroke are the distinguishing early features of DADA2. In addition, intermittent fevers, splenomegaly with consumptive thrombocytopenia, portal hypertension with esophageal varices, hypocellular bone marrow with anemia, and mild immunodeficiency with hypogammaglobulinemia are also commonly present.[40] The most common cutaneous manifestation is livedo racemosa, which is most prominent on the trunk and extremities and is composed of broad, interrupted pink-to-violaceous patches in a branching or net-like configuration (Figure 13-5). Discrete, firm, painful pink nodules on the extremities resembling PAN occur in some patients in early childhood. Recurrent early-onset hemorrhagic and ischemic strokes are a potentially devastating clinical feature and may lead to neurologic deficits in childhood.

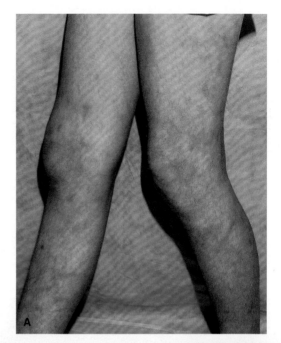

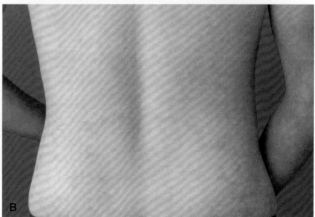

FIGURE 13-5. **Deficiency of adenosine deaminase 2.** Livedo racemosa on the extremities (A) and trunk (B) are composed of broad, interrupted pink-to-violaceous patches in a branching or net-like configuration.

Histologic Findings

A histopathologic examination of the painful, pink subcutaneous nodules demonstrates medium-sized vessel vasculitis at the dermal subcutaneous junction consistent with PAN (Figure 13-6). A dense, transmural neutrophilic and lymphohistiocytic infiltrate with fibrinoid necrosis of the vessel wall is present.[36,37] The cutaneous biopsies of the livedo racemosa rash may show a mild interstitial neutrophilic and mononuclear infiltration with perivascular lymphocytes without vasculitis. However, many biopsies of the livedoid pattern show only dilated superficial small blood vessels with a thickening of the vascular wall.[38]

Differential Diagnosis

A clinicopathologic correlation of early-onset strokes, livedo racemosa, and cutaneous PAN in a child is often needed to

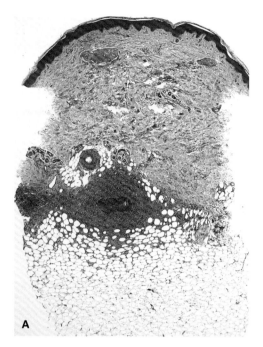
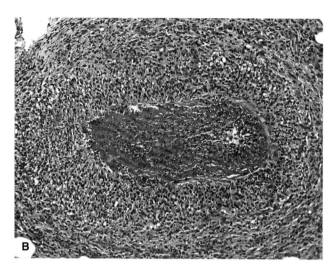

FIGURE 13-6. Histology of deficiency of adenosine deaminase 2. A, There is medium-vessel vasculitis at the dermal subcutaneous junction. B, A dense, transmural neutrophilic and lymphohistiocytic infiltrate with a fibrinoid necrosis of the medium-sized vessel is present, histologically consistent with polyarteritis nodosa.

alert physicians to the potential diagnosis of DADA2. The histologic features of PAN in the setting of DADA2 are indistinguishable from cutaneous PAN occurring in isolation. The same is true for livedo racemosa in the setting of DADA2. Thus, a strong clinical suspicion with characteristic dermatopathology findings is required in the setting of a child with PAN to diagnose DADA2, and further diagnostic confirmation by genome sequencing is required.

CAPSULE SUMMARY

DEFICIENCY OF ADENOSINE DEAMINASE 2

DADA2 is a rare autoinflammatory disorder characterized by early-onset stroke, livedo racemosa, and PAN. Loss-of-function, autosomal recessive mutations in *CERC1*, which encodes ADA2, results in systemic vasculopathy and a vasculitis of unknown mechanism. Painful subcutaneous nodules histologically show medium-sized vessel vasculitis with a dense neutrophilic and lymphohistiocytic infiltrate with fibrinoid necrosis of the vessel wall consistent with PAN. Suspect this disorder with early-onset PAN in a child.

STING-ASSOCIATED VASCULOPATHY WITH ONSET IN INFANCY

Definition and Epidemiology

STING-associated vasculopathy with onset in infancy (SAVI) is characterized by severe cutaneous vasculopathy,

small-vessel vasculitis, interstitial lung disease, and systemic inflammation.[41] Uniquely, cutaneous small-vessel vasculitis and micro-thrombotic vasculopathy are localized to acral sites that worsen in cold temperatures. SAVI is caused by gain-of-function mutations (autosomal dominant) in transmembrane protein 173 (*TMEM173*), which encodes the stimulator of interferon genes (STING), resulting in excessive interferon-β (IFN-β) production and stimulation.

There have been fewer than 30 cases of SAVI reported since its initial description in 2014.[41-44] Cohorts have been identified in European, Turkish, French-Canadian, and Korean ancestry.[45,46] Unlike DADA2, there does not appear to be a population with enriched mutation frequency for SAVI, suggesting that most cases of SAVI are likely due to de novo mutations. However, there is a single report of four affected individuals from a three-generation family of mixed European descent that shared a heterozygous mutation in STING.[42]

Etiology

The interferon pathway is critical for host protection against pathogens, especially viruses. An overproduction of the IFN pathway has been implicated in autoimmunity disorders such as systemic lupus erythematosus and other autoinflammatory disorders such as Aicardi-Goutieres syndrome. STING is downstream of the type 1 IFN receptor, and when activated, STING induces transcription of type I IFNs and IFN-response genes. Thus, gain-of-function mutations in STING, which cause SAVI, results in uncontrolled IFN production, particularly IFN-β.[41,42] STING is expressed in endothelial cells, and in skin biopsies from lesional skin, endothelial cells show an increased expression of certain inflammatory markers, suggesting a possible etiology for the vasculitis and vasculopathy in patients with SAVI.[41] STING is expressed by type II pneumocytes and alveolar macrophages which likely contribute to the pulmonary disease by an unknown mechanism(s).

Clinical Presentation

The earliest clinical manifestations of SAVI occur within the first 6 months of life and include telangiectatic-purpuric patches and plaques on cold-sensitive areas such as cheeks, nose, ears, hands, and feet (Figure 13-7A).[41] Pustular and blistering rashes on acral sites that worsen with cold exposure have also been described. Over time, these lesions progress to painful ulcerations with eschar formation (Figure 13-7B). Cartilage resorption of the ear and nasal septum are common sequelae. In addition, distal digit gangrene may require surgical amputation (Figure 13-7C). Chronic disease is marked by atrophic scars with telangiectasia. The majority of patients develop interstitial lung disease and hilar or paratracheal lymphadenopathy, which often presents as tachypnea. Systemic inflammation associated with intermittent fevers, anemia of chronic disease, and failure to thrive is present in all patients. Some patients succumb to severe pulmonary complications from chronic inflammation and subsequent fibrosis and die in their teenage years.[41]

Histologic Findings

The biopsy of early skin lesions shows an intense inflammation of cutaneous small vessels including a dense neutrophilic and mononuclear inflammatory infiltrate with karyorrhexis and fibrin deposits within the vessel lumen (Figure 13-8A).[41] Chronic cutaneous lesions show variable amounts of intraluminal thrombi within cutaneous small vessels, fibrinoid necrosis of the vessel wall, and a mild dermal neutrophilic infiltrate with sparse leukocytoclasis (Figure 13-8B).[44] In addition, there is a perivascular lymphocytic infiltrate and rare epidermal necrotic keratinocytes. Vasculopathy appears to primarily involve small caliber vessels of the skin, but occasional involvement of medium-sized vessels has been observed. Lung tissue biopsies reveal lymphoid aggregates within lung parenchyma, emphysematous changes in alveolar spaces, and interstitial fibrosis.[41]

Differential Diagnosis

The cutaneous biopsies of SAVI reveal cutaneous small-vessel vasculitis and micro-thrombotic vasculopathy. The combination of both vasculitis and thrombotic vasculopathy is histologically similar to antineutrophil cytoplasmic antibodies–associated small-vessel vasculitis. However, the clinical presentation of early-onset cutaneous vasculitis on acral sites that are cold sensitive is characteristic of SAVI.

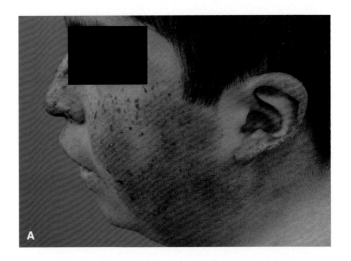

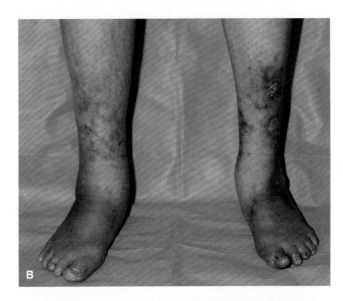

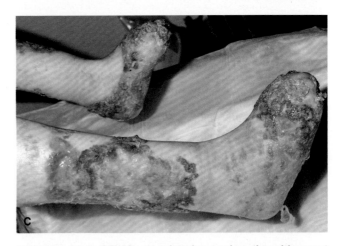

FIGURE 13-7. **STING-associated vasculopathy with onset in infancy.** A, Telangiectatic-purpuric patches and plaques on cold-sensitive areas, including the ears, nose, and cheeks. B, Painful ulcerations with eschar formation. Note the pernio-like lesions of the left toes. C, Cartilage resorption and distal digit gangrene result in tissue loss.

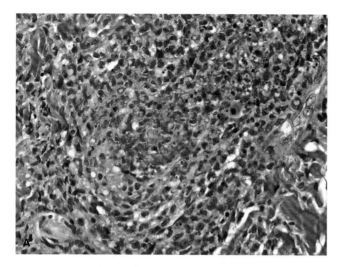

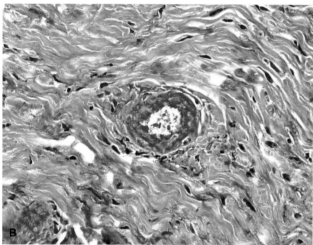

FIGURE 13-8. Histology of STING-associated vasculopathy with onset in infancy. A, The skin biopsies of early lesions reveal cutaneous small-vessel vasculitis, characterized by a dense transmural infiltrate of neutrophils and mononuclear cells with karyorrhexis with the destruction of vessel wall and fibrin thrombi. B, Histologic findings in chronic lesions reveal vasculopathic changes characterized by a fibrinoid necrosis of vascular wall with mild inflammation and karyorrhexis similar to micro-thrombotic vasculopathy.

CAPSULE SUMMARY

STING-ASSOCIATED VASCULOPATHY IN INFANCY

SAVI is a rare, life-threatening inherited autoinflammatory disorder caused by autosomal dominant, gain-of-function mutations in STING, *TMEM173*, resulting in overstimulation by interferon-β. Clinical features include telangiectatic-purpuric patches and plaques on cold-sensitive areas, including the ears, nose, and digits that progress to painful ulcerations with eschar formation. Cartilage resorption and distal digit gangrene are common sequelae. Systemic features include interstitial lung disease. A histology of acute cutaneous lesions shows small-vessel vasculitis with a dense neutrophilic and mononuclear infiltrate, leukocytoclasis, and fibrin deposition. Chronic cutaneous lesions show fibrin thrombi within cutaneous small vessels with fibrinoid necrosis of the vessel wall.

CHRONIC ATYPICAL NEUTROPHILIC DERMATOSIS WITH LIPODYSTROPHY AND ELEVATED TEMPERATURE (CANDLE) SYNDROME

Definition and Epidemiology

Chronic Atypical Neutrophilic Dermatosis with Lipodystrophy and Elevated Temperature (CANDLE) syndrome is characterized by recurrent fevers, periorbital edema with violaceous plaques, and facial lipodystrophy.[47] Systemic features include conjunctivitis, arthralgia, joint contractures, aseptic meningitis, generalized lipodystrophy, and cardiac arrhythmias. Shortly after the initial description of CANDLE, a separate group reported a similar phenotype in a disorder they named joint contractures, muscle atrophy, microcytic anemia, and Panniculitis-induced (JMP) syndrome.[48] Patients with these disorders had a similar constellation of signs previously reported in the Japanese literature, now referred to as Nakajo-Nishimura syndrome.[49]

Subsequent genetic analysis revealed that the majority of patients with all three conditions have heterozygous mutations in proteasome subunit beta type-8 precursor (*PSMB8*). This protein is a key component of the proteasome, an organelle responsible for the degrading and recycling of intracellular protein products. A subset of patients have now been described with mutations in other proteasome components.[50] Given that CANDLE, JMP, and Nakajo-Nishimura syndrome represent the same disorder, some authors have recommended a unifying nomenclature including proteasome-associated autoinflammatory syndrome or autoinflammation, lipodystrophy, and dermatitis syndrome.[51,52]

Approximately 60 cases of CANDLE have been reported since the initial description in 2010.[47] The majority of patients with CANDLE have homozygous or compound heterozygous mutations in proteasome subunits that arise de novo and have been identified in patients belonging to diverse ethnic groups, including mixed European, Hispanic, and Japanese. However, this autosomal recessive disorder has been identified in multiple families, including two siblings from Spain, two siblings from Mexico, and many kindreds of Japanese descent.[47,48,53] Within the Japanese literature, many of the patients described with Nakajo-Nishimura syndrome were from consanguineous parents.[53]

Etiology

CANDLE is caused by homozygous or compound heterozygous mutations in the proteasome or immunoproteasome subunits *PSMB8*, *PSMB3*, *PSMB4*, *PSMB9*, and *PROM* (proteasome maturation protein). Under steady-state conditions, multiple subunits come together within cells to form the proteasome, which degrades and recycles intracellular waste proteins. Under inflammatory conditions, such as a viral infection within a cell, a variant of the proteasome called the immunoproteasome is formed to degrade foreign (ie, viral) proteins for antigen processing and presentation. Proteasome-immunoproteasome dysfunction as seen in CANDLE syndrome results in the accumulation of protein waste, cellular stress, and, ultimately, a hypersecretion of type I interferons.[50,54] Thus, CANDLE represents an inherited interferonopathy that acutely worsens during periods of cellular stress such as viral infections.

Clinical Presentation

CANDLE syndrome manifests within the first 6 months of life with recurrent fever and characteristic intense, red-violaceous edematous plaques on acral sites including nose, ears, fingers, and toes. Later in infancy and early childhood, annular, purpuric, and edematous plaques develop throughout the body and resolve with purpura (Figure 13-9A and B). Overtime, persistent violaceous, periorbital edema develops with occasional perioral involvement. Progressive facial lipodystrophy begins in early childhood with subsequent development of more generalized lipodystrophy (Figure 13-9C), disabling arthritis, and delayed physical development, with systemic inflammation occurring in nearly every organ. A systemic manifestation of inflammation include hepatomegaly, splenomegaly, lymphadenopathy, arthritis, chondritis, aseptic meningitis, myositis, pneumonitis, conjunctivitis, nodular episcleritis, nephritis, and epididymitis.[50]

Histologic Findings

The histology of the cutaneous lesions of CANDLE shows a dense, predominantly interstitial infiltrate composed of atypical mononuclear cells with karyorrhexis throughout the papillary and reticular dermis with extension into the subcutaneous fat with perivascular lymphocytes. Characteristically, this mononuclear cell infiltrate is composed of atypical (immature) myeloid cells with large, vesicular, elongated, or kidney-shaped nuclei, conspicuous nucleoli, mixed with rare mature neutrophils, eosinophils, and scattered mature lymphocytes (Figure 13-10).[47] There is leukocytoclasis in the dermis but an absence of vasculitis. The epidermis is spared, and if subcutaneous tissue is present, then a lobular pattern panniculitis with lipodystrophy is sometimes observed. Histologic studies have confirmed the presence of myeloid lineage cells (positive for Leder stain) and further immunophenotypic analysis has revealed an

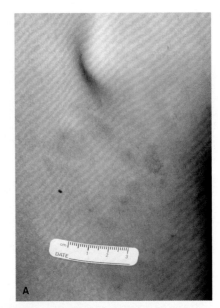

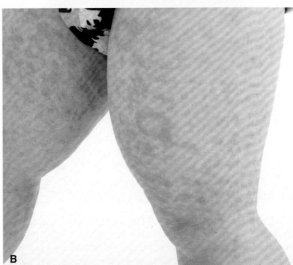

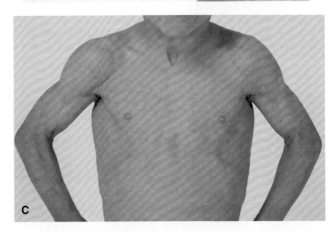

FIGURE 13-9. **Chronic Atypical Neutrophilic Dermatosis with Lipodystrophy and Elevated Temperature syndrome.** A and B, Annular, purpuric, and edematous plaques that resolve with purpura develop in late infancy and early childhood. C, Progressive facial and generalized lipodystrophy are characteristic features.

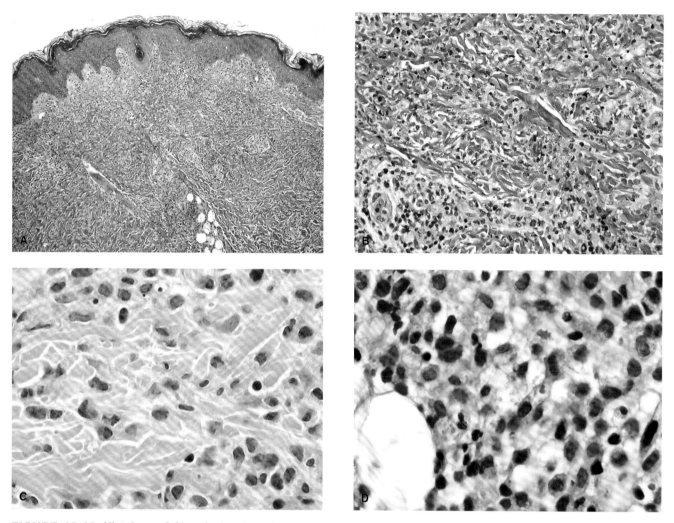

FIGURE 13-10. Histology of Chronic Atypical Neutrophilic Dermatosis with Lipodystrophy and Elevated Temperature syndrome. A, Lower magnification view shows a dense, predominantly interstitial infiltrate of atypical mononuclear cells in the papillary and reticular dermis with perivascular lymphocytes. B, Higher magnification shows large atypical mononuclear cells with leukocytoclasis but without vasculitis. C, The mononuclear cell infiltrate is composed of atypical (immature) myeloid cells with large, vesicular, elongated, or kidney-shaped nuclei, conspicuous nucleoli, mixed with rare mature neutrophils, eosinophils, and scattered mature lymphocytes. D, Lobular pattern panniculitis with lipodystrophy is present in some biopsies.

infiltrate comprised of CD68[+] and CD163[+] macrophages as well as clusters of CD123-positive plasmacytoid dendritic cells, which are the major producers of type I IFN.[55]

Differential Diagnosis

The histopathologic pattern of atypical mononuclear perivascular and interstitial dermal infiltrate seen in CANDLE syndrome resembles leukemia cutis or leukemoid reactions. However, there is no underlying leukemia or bone marrow dysplasia in neonates presenting with CANDLE syndrome or that have been observed after long-term follow-up. In addition, the atypical myeloid infiltrate of CANDLE syndrome may also be confused with the "histiocytoid" variant of Sweet syndrome composed of immature myeloid cells. The immunohistochemistry of cutaneous lesions from CANDLE syndrome patients shows a unique pattern of macrophages (CD68, CD163),

myeloid precursors (Leder) and immature neutrophils (myeloperoxidase), and clusters of CD123-positive plasmacytoid dendritic cells that help establish a diagnosis.[55]

CAPSULE SUMMARY

CHRONIC ATYPICAL NEUTROPHILIC DERMATOSIS WITH LIPODYSTROPHY AND ELEVATED TEMPERATURE

CANDLE syndrome is a rare, autosomal recessive autoinflammatory disorder caused by homozygous or heterozygous, loss-of-function mutations in proteasome subunits (*PSMB8*), resulting in an overproduction of type I interferons. Clinical features include a neonatal onset of acral perniosis-like plaques followed by annular, violaceous-purpuric, edematous plaques, and periorbital edema. Progressive facial and generalized lipodystrophy gives CANDLE patients their unique appearance. The histology of acute cutaneous lesions shows dense perivascular and interstitial dermal infiltrate composed of atypical mononuclear cells with karyorrhexis. Immunohistochemistry shows a unique mix of immature neutrophils, macrophages, and clusters of plasmacytoid dendritic cells. The atypical myeloid infiltrate of CANDLE syndrome can be mistaken for "histiocytoid" Sweet syndrome, but immunohistochemistry is distinctive.

BLAU SYNDROME

Definition and Epidemiology

Blau syndrome is an autosomal dominantly inherited autoinflammatory disorder characterized by granulomatous dermatitis, uveitis, and polyarthritis as independently described in 1985 by Dr. Jabs and Dr. Blau.[56,57] Other names proposed by different groups include juvenile systemic granulomatosis, pediatric granulomatous arthritis, early-onset sarcoidosis, Jabs syndrome, or Jabs-Blau syndrome.[58] Subsequent genetic analysis demonstrated that these disorders are the same disease within a clinical spectrum caused by activating mutations in Caspase recruitment domain-containing protein 15 (CARD15), which is also called nucleotide-binding oligomerization domain protein 2 (NOD2).[59-61] Blau syndrome is a monogenic autoinflammatory disorder characterized by predominantly granulomatous inflammation.

Initial reports of Blau syndrome were restricted to small numbers of families who shared the constellation of granulomatous dermatitis, uveitis, and polyarthritis and were of distinct ethnicities including mixed European and African.[62,63] Sporadic cases of early-onset sarcoidosis have subsequently been shown to have missense mutations in CARD15/NOD2, confirming that Blau syndrome may be inherited (familial) or sporadic.[64] Currently, it is thought that Blau syndrome affects all races, but the exact incidence remains unknown and is considered very rare.

Etiology

CARD15/NOD2 is an intracellular protein that functions as a pathogen recognition receptor within immune cells such as macrophages, monocytes, and dendritic cells. The normal function of CARD15/NOD2 is to recognize pathogens such as viruses and bacteria and activate proinflammatory cytokines (eg, IL-1, IL-6, TNF) through nuclear factor κB (NF-κB).[65] Patients with Blau syndrome have an activating, gain-of-function mutation in CARD15/NOD2 that results in the constitutive activation of NF-κB, resulting in

an overproduction of proinflammatory cytokines.[64] Biopsies from patients with Blau syndrome show a prominent expression of IFN-γ, IL-6, and IL-17.[66] It is not clear exactly how a change in CARD15/NOD2 function results in non-caseating granulomatous inflammation. Polymorphisms in NOD2 and missense mutations in a distinct region of NOD2 are associated with Crohn disease, characterized by a granulomatous inflammation of small bowel.[67] In addition, there was a recent report describing a cohort of patients termed NOD2-associated autoinflammatory disease that develop an overlap of Blau syndrome-like disease after age 40 along with a granulomatous inflammation of the gut similar to Crohn disease.[68]

Clinical Presentation

The earliest clinical presentation of Blau syndrome is the development of slightly scaly, red-brown to dark-red papular, eczematous, or lichenoid rash within the first year of life (Figure 13-11). This densely populated, erythematous papular eruption occurs symmetrically on trunk and extremities and spontaneously resolves. Often, infants are misdiagnosed with atopic dermatitis or ichthyosis vulgaris. Individual lesions can appear similar to lichen nitidus. However, the rash of Blau syndrome tends to be composed of discrete, small, flat-topped papules that are often arranged in clusters or linear arrays and are more widespread than lichen nitidus.[69]

The next classical features of Blau syndrome to develop are granulomatous polyarthritis and intermittent fevers. In the acute arthritis phase, small joints of the hands become hypertrophic and "boggy" because of tenosynovial cysts. Chronic inflammation results in joint deformities including flexion contractures and camptodactyly (fixed flexion deformity of the proximal interphalangeal joints), usually within the first 5 years of age.[70]

Finally, granulomatous eye inflammation, most often chronic, recurrent bilateral uveitis, develops in the first 5 years

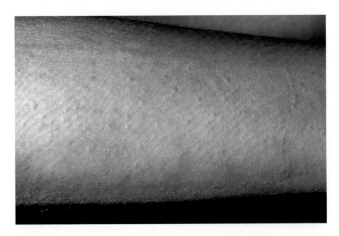

FIGURE 13-11. Blau syndrome. Densely populated, erythematous papular eruption representing miliary granulomas on the forearm. Note the linear array of papules.

of life, resulting in visual impairment and, in some cases, blindness.[71] Other systemic findings include granulomatous inflammation of kidney, liver, lung, and CNS. Additionally, nonspecific cutaneous findings observed in patients with Blau syndrome include erythema nodosum, cutaneous small-vessel vasculitis, and leg ulcers.[70]

Histologic Findings

The skin biopsy of rash during infancy shows noncaseating, sarcoid-type granulomas in a polycyclic configuration (Figure 13-12). Granulomas are a universal feature in all skin biopsies despite an eczematous or lichenoid clinical appearance. Janssen and colleagues characterized the polycyclic granulomas of Blau syndrome with large lymphocytic coronas, extensive emperipolesis of lymphocytes within multinucleated giant cells, multinucleated giant cell death, fibrinoid necrosis, and fibrosis.[66] These unique features are not seen in small bowel granulomas from Crohn

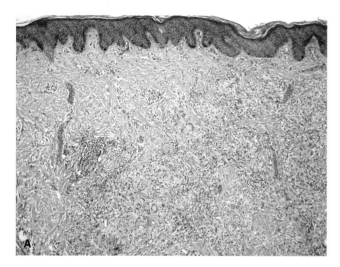

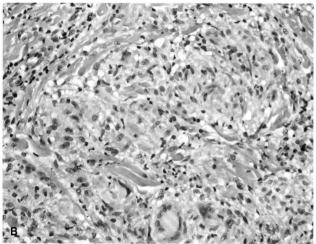

FIGURE 13-12. Histology of Blau syndrome. A, Noncaseating, sarcoid-type granulomas arranged in a polycyclic configuration. B, Granulomas are composed of epithelioid histiocytes, multinucleated giant cells, and scattered lymphocytes.

disease patients. Some reports demonstrate the epithelioid granulomas of Blau syndrome in a periadnexal or perifollicular pattern.[69] The immunohistochemistry of skin lesions shows an expression of IFN-γ, IL-6, IL-17, IL-23 receptor, and transforming growth factor-β (TGF-β).[66]

Differential Diagnosis

The histopathologic differential diagnosis of noncaseating epithelioid granulomas includes sarcoidosis, foreign body granulomatous chronic inflammatory reactions, and infections (mycobacterial and fungal). The perifollicular pattern of granulomas is similar to that observed in lichen scrofulosorum, a tuberculid reaction to tuberculosis. The polarization of specimens with granulomas to rule out foreign body reactions and special stains for a histologic examination of infectious microorganisms is always prudent. However, the neonatal onset of a discrete, erythematous papular rash that shows polycyclic granulomas and emperipolesis strongly suggests Blau syndrome.

CAPSULE SUMMARY

BLAU SYNDROME

Blau syndrome is a rare, autosomal dominant autoinflammatory disorder caused by gain-of-function mutations in *CARD15/NOD2*, resulting in granulomatous inflammation. Clinical features include neonatal-onset red-brown scaly papules and plaques followed by granulomatous polyarthritis with joint deformity (camptodactyly) and granulomatous uveitis. A histology of acute cutaneous lesions shows multifocal sarcoid-type granulomas composed of epithelioid histiocytes with occasional multinucleated giant cells and a few scattered lymphocytes.

REFERENCES

1. Silverstein AM. Autoimmunity versus horror autotoxicus: the struggle for recognition. *Nat Immunol.* 2001;2(4):279-281.
2. McDermott MF, Aksentijevich I, Galon J, et al. Germline mutations in the extracellular domains of the 55 kDa TNF receptor, TNFR1, define a family of dominantly inherited autoinflammatory syndromes. *Cell.* 1999;97(1):133-144.
3. Masters SL, Simon A, Aksentijevich I, Kastner DL. Horror autoinflammaticus: the molecular pathophysiology of autoinflammatory disease (*). *Annu Rev Immunol.* 2009;27:621-668.
4. Nguyen TV, Cowen EW, Leslie KS. Autoinflammation: from monogenic syndromes to common skin diseases. *J Am Acad Dermatol.* 2013;68(5):834-853.
5. Kastner DL. Hereditary periodic fever syndromes. *Hematology Am Soc Hematol Educ Program.* 2005:74-81.
6. Muckle TJ, Wellsm. Urticaria, deafness, and amyloidosis: a new heredo-familial syndrome. *Q J Med.* 1962;31:235-248.
7. Cuisset L, Drenth JP, Berthelot JM, et al. Genetic linkage of the Muckle-Wells syndrome to chromosome 1q44. *Am J Hum Genet.* 1999;65(4):1054-1059.

8. Hoffman HM, Mueller JL, Broide DH, Wanderer AA, Kolodner RD. Mutation of a new gene encoding a putative pyrin-like protein causes familial cold autoinflammatory syndrome and Muckle-Wells syndrome. *Nat Genet.* 2001;29(3):301-305.

9. Hoffman HM, Wanderer AA, Broide DH. Familial cold autoinflammatory syndrome: phenotype and genotype of an autosomal dominant periodic fever. *J Allergy Clin Immunol.* 2001;108(4):615-620.

10. Aksentijevich I, Nowak M, Mallah M, et al. De novo CIAS1 mutations, cytokine activation, and evidence for genetic heterogeneity in patients with neonatal-onset multisystem inflammatory disease (NOMID): a new member of the expanding family of pyrin-associated autoinflammatory diseases. *Arthritis Rheum.* 2002;46(12):3340-3348.

11. Feldmann J, Prieur AM, Quartier P, et al. Chronic infantile neurological cutaneous and articular syndrome is caused by mutations in CIAS1, a gene highly expressed in polymorphonuclear cells and chondrocytes. *Am J Hum Genet.* 2002;71(1):198-203.

12. Farasat S, Aksentijevich I, Toro JR. Autoinflammatory diseases: clinical and genetic advances. *Arch Dermatol.* 2008;144(3):392-402.

13. Stych B, Dobrovolny D. Familial cold auto-inflammatory syndrome (FCAS): characterization of symptomatology and impact on patients' lives. *Curr Med Res Opin.* 2008;24(6):1577-1582.

14. Cuisset L, Jeru I, Dumont B, et al. Mutations in the autoinflammatory cryopyrin-associated periodic syndrome gene: epidemiological study and lessons from eight years of genetic analysis in France. *Ann Rheum Dis.* 2011;70(3):495-499.

15. Tanaka N, Izawa K, Saito MK, et al. High incidence of NLRP3 somatic mosaicism in patients with chronic infantile neurologic, cutaneous, articular syndrome: results of an International Multicenter Collaborative Study. *Arthritis Rheum.* 2011;63(11):3625-3632.

16. Kuemmerle-Deschner JB. CAPS: pathogenesis, presentation and treatment of an autoinflammatory disease. *Semin Immunopathol.* 2015;37(4):377-385.

17. Finetti M, Omenetti A, Federici S, Caorsi R, Gattorno M. Chronic Infantile Neurological Cutaneous and Articular (CINCA) syndrome: a review. *Orphanet J Rare Dis.* 2016;11(1):167.

18. Goldbach-Mansky R, Dailey NJ, Canna SW, et al. Neonatal-onset multisystem inflammatory disease responsive to interleukin-1beta inhibition. *N Engl J Med.* 2006;355(6):581-592.

19. Aubert P, Suarez-Farinas M, Mitsui H, et al. Homeostatic tissue responses in skin biopsies from NOMID patients with constitutive overproduction of IL-1beta. *PLoS One.* 2012;7(11):e49408.

20. Jacob SE, Cowen EW, Goldbach-Mansky R, Kastner D, Turner ML. A recurrent rash with fever and arthropathy. *J Am Acad Dermatol.* 2006;54(2):318-321.

21. Huttenlocher A, Frieden IJ, Emery H. Neonatal onset multisystem inflammatory disease. *J Rheumatol.* 1995;22(6):1171-1173.

22. Peters MS, Winkelmann RK. Neutrophilic urticaria. *Br J Dermatol.* 1985;113(1):25-30.

23. Saeb-Lima M, Charli-Joseph Y, Rodriguez-Acosta ED, Dominguez-Cherit J. Autoimmunity-related neutrophilic dermatosis: a newly described entity that is not exclusive of systemic lupus erythematosus. *Am J Dermatopathol.* 2013;35(6):655-660.

24. Belani H, Gensler L, Bajpai U, et al. Neutrophilic urticaria with systemic inflammation: a case series. *JAMA Dermatol.* 2013;149(4):453-458.

25. Kieffer C, Cribier B, Lipsker D. Neutrophilic urticarial dermatosis: a variant of neutrophilic urticaria strongly associated with systemic disease. Report of 9 new cases and review of the literature. *Medicine (Baltimore).* 2009;88(1):23-31.

26. Aksentijevich I, Masters SL, Ferguson PJ, et al. An autoinflammatory disease with deficiency of the interleukin-1-receptor antagonist. *N Engl J Med.* 2009;360(23):2426-2437.

27. Reddy S, Jia S, Geoffrey R, et al. An autoinflammatory disease due to homozygous deletion of the IL1RN locus. *N Engl J Med.* 2009;360(23):2438-2444.

28. Minkis K, Aksentijevich I, Goldbach-Mansky R, et al. Interleukin 1 receptor antagonist deficiency presenting as infantile

29. Jesus AA, Osman M, Silva CA, et al. A novel mutation of IL1RN in the deficiency of interleukin-1 receptor antagonist syndrome: description of two unrelated cases from Brazil. *Arthritis Rheum.* 2011;63(12):4007-4017.

30. Jesus AA, Goldbach-Mansky R. IL-1 blockade in autoinflammatory syndromes. *Annu Rev Med.* 2014;65:223-244.

31. Naik HB, Cowen EW. Autoinflammatory pustular neutrophilic diseases. *Dermatol Clin.* 2013;31(3):405-425.

32. Altiok E, Aksoy F, Perk Y, et al. A novel mutation in the interleukin-1 receptor antagonist associated with intrauterine disease onset. *Clin Immunol.* 2012;145(1):77-81.

33. Cowen EW, Goldbach-Mansky R. DIRA, DITRA, and new insights into pathways of skin inflammation: what's in a name? *Arch Dermatol.* 2012;148(3):381-384.

34. Marrakchi S, Guigue P, Renshaw BR, et al. Interleukin-36-receptor antagonist deficiency and generalized pustular psoriasis. *N Engl J Med.* 2011;365(7):620-628.

35. Onoufriadis A, Simpson MA, Pink AE, et al. Mutations in IL36RN/IL1F5 are associated with the severe episodic inflammatory skin disease known as generalized pustular psoriasis. *Am J Hum Genet.* 2011;89(3):432-437.

36. Navon Elkan P, Pierce SB, Segel R, et al. Mutant adenosine deaminase 2 in a polyarteritis nodosa vasculopathy. *N Engl J Med.* 2014;370(10):921-931.

37. Zhou Q, Yang D, Ombrello AK, et al. Early-onset stroke and vasculopathy associated with mutations in ADA2. *N Engl J Med.* 2014;370(10):911-920.

38. Pichard DC, Ombrello AK, Hoffmann P, Stone DL, Cowen EW. Early-onset stroke, polyarteritis nodosa (PAN), and livedo racemosa. *J Am Acad Dermatol.* 2016;75(2):449-453.

39. Belot A, Wassmer E, Twilt M, et al. Mutations in CECR1 associated with a neutrophil signature in peripheral blood. *Pediatr Rheumatol Online J.* 2014;12:44.

40. Caorsi R, Penco F, Grossi A, et al. ADA2 deficiency (DADA2) as an unrecognised cause of early onset polyarteritis nodosa and stroke: a multicentre national study. *Ann Rheum Dis.* 2017.

41. Liu Y, Jesus AA, Marrero B, et al. Activated STING in a vascular and pulmonary syndrome. *N Engl J Med.* 2014;371(6):507-518.

42. Jeremiah N, Neven B, Gentili M, et al. Inherited STING-activating mutation underlies a familial inflammatory syndrome with lupus-like manifestations. *J Clin Invest.* 2014;124(12):5516-5520.

43. Melki I, Rose Y, Uggenti C, et al. Disease-associated mutations identify a novel region in human STING necessary for the control of type I interferon signaling. *J Allergy Clin Immunol.* 2017;140(2):543-552 e545.

44. Chia J, Eroglu FK, Ozen S, et al. Failure to thrive, interstitial lung disease, and progressive digital necrosis with onset in infancy. *J Am Acad Dermatol.* 2016;74(1):186-189.

45. Seo J, Kang JA, Suh DI, et al. Tofacitinib relieves symptoms of stimulator of interferon genes (STING)-associated vasculopathy with onset in infancy caused by 2 de novo variants in TMEM173. *J Allergy Clin Immunol.* 2017;139(4):1396-1399 e1312.

46. Jain A, Misra DP, Sharma A, Wakhlu A, Agarwal V, Negi VS. Vasculitis and vasculitis-like manifestations in monogenic autoinflammatory syndromes. *Rheumatol Int.* 2018;38(1):13-24.

47. Torrelo A, Patel S, Colmenero I, et al. Chronic atypical neutrophilic dermatosis with lipodystrophy and elevated temperature (CANDLE) syndrome. *J Am Acad Dermatol.* 2010;62(3):489-495.

48. Garg A, Hernandez MD, Sousa AB, et al. An autosomal recessive syndrome of joint contractures, muscular atrophy, microcytic anemia, and panniculitis-associated lipodystrophy. *J Clin Endocrinol Metab.* 2010;95(9):E58-63.

49. Kanazawa N. Nakajo-Nishimura syndrome: an autoinflammatory disorder showing pernio-like rashes and progressive partial lipodystrophy. *Allergol Int.* 2012;61(2):197-206.

pustulosis mimicking infantile pustular psoriasis. *Arch Dermatol.* 2012;148(6):747-752.

50. Torrelo A. CANDLE syndrome as a paradigm of proteasome-related autoinflammation. *Front Immunol.* 2017;8:927.

51. McDermott A, Jacks J, Kessler M, Emanuel PD, Gao L. Proteasome-associated autoinflammatory syndromes: advances in pathogeneses, clinical presentations, diagnosis, and management. *Int J Dermatol.* 2015;54(2):121-129.

52. Touitou I, Galeotti C, Rossi-Semerano L, et al. The expanding spectrum of rare monogenic autoinflammatory diseases. *Orphanet J Rare Dis.* 2013;8:162.

53. Kitano Y, Matsunaga E, Morimoto T, Okada N, Sano S. A syndrome with nodular erythema, elongated and thickened fingers, and emaciation. *Arch Dermatol.* 1985;121(8):1053-1056.

54. Brehm A, Liu Y, Sheikh A, et al. Additive loss-of-function proteasome subunit mutations in CANDLE/PRAAS patients promote type I IFN production. *J Clin Invest.* 2015;125(11):4196-4211.

55. Torrelo A, Colmenero I, Requena L, et al. Histologic and Immunohistochemical Features of the Skin Lesions in CANDLE Syndrome. *Am J Dermatopathol.* 2015;37(7):517-522.

56. Blau EB. Familial granulomatous arthritis, iritis, and rash. *J Pediatr.* 1985;107(5):689-693.

57. Jabs DA, Houk JL, Bias WB, Arnett FC. Familial granulomatous synovitis, uveitis, and cranial neuropathies. *Am J Med.* 1985;78(5):801-804.

58. Rose CD. Blau syndrome: a systemic granulomatous disease of cutaneous onset and phenotypic complexity. *Pediatr Dermatol.* 2017;34(2):216-218.

59. Miceli-Richard C, Lesage S, Rybojad M, et al. CARD15 mutations in Blau syndrome. *Nat Genet.* 2001;29(1):19-20.

60. Kanazawa N, Matsushima S, Kambe N, Tachibana T, Nagai S, Miyachi Y. Presence of a sporadic case of systemic granulomatosis syndrome with a CARD15 mutation. *J Invest Dermatol.* 2004;122(3):851-852.

61. Rose CD, Doyle TM, McIlvain-Simpson G, et al. Blau syndrome mutation of CARD15/NOD2 in sporadic early onset granulomatous arthritis. *J Rheumatol.* 2005;32(2):373-375.

62. Manouvrier-Hanu S, Puech B, Piette F, et al. Blau syndrome of granulomatous arthritis, iritis, and skin rash: a new family and review of the literature. *Am J Med Genet.* 1998;76(3):217-221.

63. Saini SK, Rose CD. Liver involvement in familial granulomatous arthritis (Blau syndrome). *J Rheumatol.* 1996;23(2):396-399.

64. Kanazawa N, Okafuji I, Kambe N, et al. Early-onset sarcoidosis and CARD15 mutations with constitutive nuclear factor-kappaB activation: common genetic etiology with Blau syndrome. *Blood.* 2005;105(3):1195-1197.

65. Ogura Y, Inohara N, Benito A, Chen FF, Yamaoka S, Nunez G. Nod2, a Nod1/Apaf-1 family member that is restricted to monocytes and activates NF-kappaB. *J Biol Chem.* 2001;276(7):4812-4818.

66. Janssen CE, Rose CD, De Hertogh G, et al. Morphologic and immunohistochemical characterization of granulomas in the nucleotide oligomerization domain 2-related disorders Blau syndrome and Crohn disease. *J Allergy Clin Immunol.* 2012;129(4):1076-1084.

67. Caso F, Galozzi P, Costa L, Sfriso P, Cantarini L, Punzi L. Autoinflammatory granulomatous diseases: from Blau syndrome and early-onset sarcoidosis to NOD2-mediated disease and Crohn's disease. *RMD Open.* 2015;1(1):e000097.

68. Yao Q, Zhou L, Cusumano P, et al. A new category of autoinflammatory disease associated with NOD2 gene mutations. *Arthritis Res Ther.* 2011;13(5):R148.

69. Schaffer JV, Chandra P, Keegan BR, Heller P, Shin HT. Widespread granulomatous dermatitis of infancy: an early sign of Blau syndrome. *Arch Dermatol.* 2007;143(3):386-391.

70. Rose CD, Pans S, Casteels I, et al. Blau syndrome: cross-sectional data from a multicentre study of clinical, radiological and functional outcomes. *Rheumatology (Oxford).* 2015;54(6):1008-1016.

71. Sarens IL, Casteels I, Anton J, et al. Blau syndrome-associated uveitis: preliminary results from an international prospective interventional case series. *Am J Ophthalmol.* 2018;187:158-166.

14

Disorders of Hair, Adnexae, Nails, and Cartilage

Ifeoma U. Perkins / Jarish Cohen / Paradi Mirmirani

TRICHORRHEXIS NODOSA

Definition and Epidemiology

Trichorrhexis nodosa (TN) is an inherited or acquired fragile hair shaft disorder characterized by hair breakage that occurs as a result of damage to hair cuticles.[1] The disease can have a more proximal or distal distribution along the hair shaft. There is a wide age range at presentation. Acquired TN is common in patients of African descent (proximal type) and Caucasian and Asian descent (distal type).

Etiology

Acquired TN can be the result of physical trauma including excessive brushing, heat, pulling, or twisting.[2] It can also be the result of chemical trauma including permanent straightening or waving.

Inherited TN can be caused by arginosuccinic aciduria, a rare metabolic disorder of the urea cycle causing hyperammonemia.[3] If undiagnosed in infancy, neonates can present with failure to feed leading to lethargy and coma in some instances. Congenital TN can also be an incidental finding in patients with other hair shaft disorders including pili torti, monilethrix, and trichothiodystrophy.

Clinical Presentation

TN may present with small, white, or gray flecks on the hair shafts. Hair damage is usually noticed as a change in the quality of the hair or as "dry ends" or "flyaway hair" and may have a "shaggy" or "skimpy" appearance (Figure 14-1).

Hair breakage can result in focal or diffuse alopecia depending on the extent of scalp involvement. A tug test, in which a swatch of hair is held in one hand and the proximal end of the hair is tugged with the other hand, will lead to fragments of shortened hairs that are easily broken off.

Histologic Findings

Each node is formed by cortical fiber separation and fraying of the hair shaft in a manner analogous to the bristles of two paint brushes being pushed together (Figure 14-2).

CAPSULE SUMMARY

TRICHORRHEXIS NODOSA

TN occurs as a result of physical or chemical trauma. The clinical presentation is that of small nodes or white flecks on the affected hair shafts that can result in alopecia of various severity. Light microscopy shows fragile nodes with frayed cortical fibers with a "pushed together" appearance.

MONILETHRIX

Definition and Epidemiology

Monilethrix is a hair shaft disorder characterized by brittle, beaded hairs that emanate from keratotic, follicular papules.[4] The condition usually manifests in the neonatal period or early childhood. In rare instances, babies are born

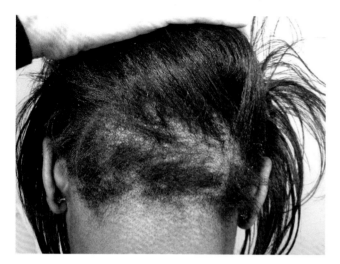

FIGURE 14-1. **Trichorrhexis Nodosa.** Localized area of short hair-blunt ends with positive tug test. From Mirmirani P, Huang KP, Price VH. A practical, algorithmic approach to diagnosing hair shaft disorders. *Int J Dermatol. 2011;50(1):1-12.*

bald with beaded hairs appearing later in life. The course can be seasonal and is variable with some affected patients improving in adulthood, whereas in others it can worsen.

Etiology

Monilethrix is usually inherited in an autosomal dominant fashion with high penetrance and variable expressivity. In the autosomal dominant variant, mutations in 3 type II basic hair keratin genes, *hHb1, hHb3,* and *hHb6* (chromosome 12q13) have been described, with the latter being the most commonly altered.[5-9] An autosomal recessive variant has been reported and is caused by a mutation in desmoglein 4.[10,11] Desmoglein 4 is a transmembrane cell adhesion molecule expressed in the hair cortex and upper cuticle,

which is also associated with localized autosomal recessive hypotrichosis.[8]

Clinical Presentation

Hair shafts rarely grow more than 2 to 3 cm. The hairs break easily, resulting in severe alopecia (Figure 14-3). In severe variants, the affected hair can involve the entire scalp, secondary sexual hair, eyebrows, and eyelashes.[12] Neonates who develop monilethrix initially present with normal lanugo hair and later have characteristic findings when they grow terminal hair. Follicular hyperkeratosis may also be found on the body. Other features may include koilonychia, mental retardation (rare), syndactyly, cataracts, as well as tooth and other nail abnormalities.[13]

Histologic Findings

Hair shafts show regularly spaced, elliptical nodes that are roughly 0.7 to 1.1 mm apart. The nodes are of normal caliber and have a typical air-filled medulla, whereas the areas of constriction show an absence of medulla (Figure 14-4).

CAPSULE SUMMARY

MONILETHRIX

Monilethrix is a hair shaft fragility disorder that typically presents in early childhood and can progress to severe alopecia. The autosomal dominant form is caused by mutations in type II basic keratin genes, and the autosomal recessive variant is caused by mutations in desmoglein 4. Affected hair shafts show elliptical nodes at regular intervals, and internodal regions that are of smaller caliber and lack the hair shaft medulla.

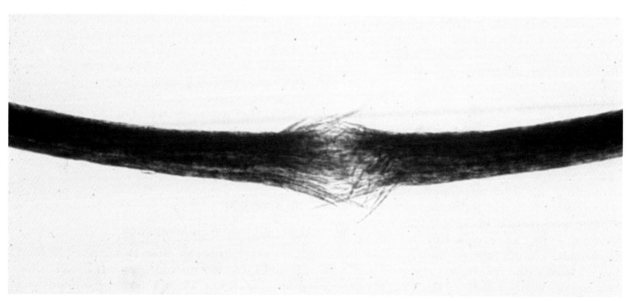

FIGURE 14-2. **Trichorrhexis nodosa.** Hair mount reveals brush-like ends in opposition. From Mirmirani P, Huang KP, Price VH. A practical, algorithmic approach to diagnosing hair shaft disorders. *Int J Dermatol. 2011;50(1):1-12.*

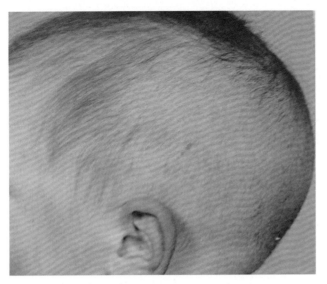

FIGURE 14-3. **Monilethrix.** Short broken hairs noted predominantly in the occipital scalp. Courtesy of Paradi Mirmirani, MD, Kaiser Permanente, Vallejo CA.

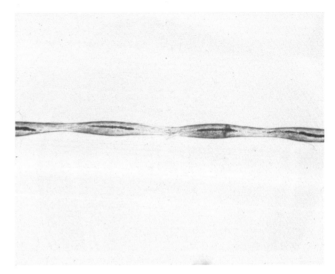

FIGURE 14-4. **Monilethrix.** Hair mount reveals beaded nodes at regular intervals. From Mirmirani P, Huang KP, Price VH. A practical, algorithmic approach to diagnosing hair shaft disorders. *Int J Dermatol.* 2011;50(1):1-12.

TRICHORRHEXIS INVAGINATA

Definition and Epidemiology

Trichorrhexis invaginata is a rare congenital hair shaft abnormality characterized by short, brittle hairs that manifests in patients with Netherton syndrome (NS). NS, and thus trichorrhexis invaginata, affects children. Progressive alopecia and atopic eczema are present at a young age.

Etiology

NS is an autosomal recessive disorder caused by mutations in the *SPINK5* gene, which encodes the serine protease inhibitor LEKTI.[14,15] LEKTI is necessary for proper skin barrier function and desquamation.[16] Although its function in the follicle is not well characterized, LEKTI appears to be highly expressed in sites of keratinization such as the inner root sheath and upper infundibulum.[17]

Clinical Presentation

NS is characterized by the triad of trichorrhexis invaginata, ichthyosis linearis circumflexa, and atopic diathesis.[18] Patients are born with congenital ichthyosiform erythroderma,[19] neonatal dehydration, failure to thrive, and recurrent infections.[20] Ichthyosis linearis circumflexa consists of migratory polycyclic erythematous patches with surrounding serpiginous double-edged scale.[21] An atopic diathesis may include eczema-like eruptions, atopic dermatitis, asthma, pruritus, allergic rhinitis, angioedema, urticaria, elevated serum IgE, and/or hypereosinophilia.[20] The hair findings in NS, including TN, are not present in every hair. Multiple hairs should be tested, and the most high-yield location to pluck and examine is reported to be the lateral eyebrows.[22]

Histologic Findings

In trichorrhexis invaginata, nodes appear at irregular intervals and are composed of a distal portion of the hair shaft that has sunken into the proximal portion creating a "ball-and-socket" appearance[22] (Figure 14-5). Nascent nodes form under torsion, and the distal aspect of the hair shaft undergoes intussusception into the proximal aspect.[23]

CAPSULE SUMMARY

TRICHORRHEXIS INVAGINATA

Trichorrhexis invaginata is one of the triad of signs that define NS, the others being ichthyosis linearis circumflexa, and atopic diathesis. Patients with NS have defects in the *SPINK5* gene, which encodes LEKTI, a serine protease inhibitor integral to normal barrier function. The characteristic light microscopic feature is that of nodes showing the distal portion of the hair shaft herniating into the proximal portion, forming a ball-and-socket joint appearance.

PILI TORTI

Definition and Epidemiology

Pili torti is a hair shaft defect characterized by short, brittle, and spangled hairs and is associated with various syndromes, including Menkes disease, Björnstad syndrome, and p63 mutation–associated ectodermal dysplasia syndromes (referred to in the literature by multiple monikers such as ectrodactyly, ectodermal dysplasia, and cleft lip;

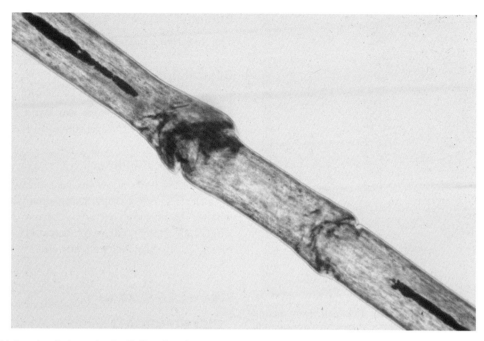

FIGURE 14-5. **Trichorrhexis invaginata.** Ball and socket appearance of hair shaft as it collapses on itself. Courtesy of Paradi Mirmirani, MD, Kaiser Permanente, Valejo CA.

Rapp-Hodgkin syndrome; and ankyloblepharon ectodermal dysplasia cleft lip/palate syndrome/Hay Wells Syndrome). Pili torti usually presents in early childhood, but can sometimes occur at birth or arise after puberty.

Etiology

The twisted appearance may be caused by mitochondrial dysfunction and the buildup of reactive oxygen species particularly in the inner root sheath.[24] Menkes disease is caused by a mutation in the X-linked *ATP7A* gene, which encodes a copper-transporting ATPase.[25-30] Defects in this protein may account for hair twisting by defective incorporation of copper into keratin disulfide bonds and/or by the aforementioned mitochondrial dysfunction mechanism. Mutations in the *BCS1L* gene underlie the phenotype of Björnstad syndrome.[24,31] Hay-Wells and/Rapp Hodgkins syndromes are caused by mutations in the *TP63* gene, which is expressed by many ectodermally derived structures such as the hair follicle.[32]

Clinical Presentation

Variable hair fragility manifests as patchy alopecia, with coarse stubble predominantly seen in the temporal and/or occipital areas presumably due to friction, with areas of hairs of up to 5 cm of length (Figure 14-6). The hairs of the eyelashes and eyebrows can also be involved. In addition to pili torti, patients with Menkes disease have severe developmental and neurologic impairment, connective-tissue abnormalities, and tortuous blood vessels.[25] After lanugo hair is shed, infants develop stubbly, sparse, hypopigmented hair that has been described as "steel wool" in

appearance and texture because it is difficult to comb and fractures with friction.[33] In Björnstad syndrome, pili torti and bilateral sensorineural loss usually manifest before the age of two.[34] The degree of hair shaft fragility correlates to the severity of hearing loss.[34] *TP63* gene mutation–related

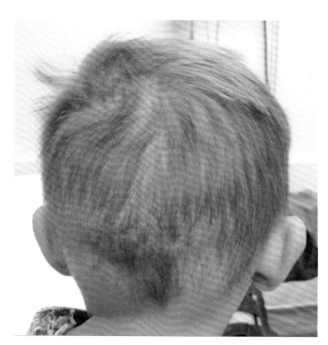

FIGURE 14-6. **Björnstad syndrome; Pili torti.** Short hair in the occipital scalp with spangled appearance. From Mirmirani P, Huang KP, Price VH. A practical, algorithmic approach to diagnosing hair shaft disorders. *Int J Dermatol. 2011;50(1):1-12.*

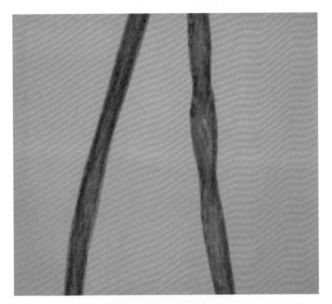

FIGURE 14-7. Björnstad syndrome; Pili torti. Hair mount reveals flattened and twisted hair on the long axis. From Mirmirani P, Huang KP, Price VH. A practical, algorithmic approach to diagnosing hair shaft disorders. *Int J Dermatol. 2011;50(1):1-12.*

ectodermal dysplasias have variable expressivity, but features can include irregular strands of tissue connecting the upper and lower eyelids, termed *ankyloblepharon filiforme adnatum*, hypohidrosis, erythroderma, palmoplantar keratoderma, and cleft lip, cleft palate, or both. There is often also a severe and recalcitrant scalp dermatitis in these patients.[35]

Histologic Findings

Affected hairs are flattened and twisted on the horizontal axis typically by 180° turns. Usually runs of 3 to 10 twists are present at irregular intervals along the hair shaft (Figure 14-7).

CAPSULE SUMMARY

PILI TORTI

Pili torti is a hair fragility condition that can be seen in various syndromes, including Menkes disease, Björnstad syndrome, and p63 mutation–related ectodermal dysplasia syndrome. Pili torti manifests clinically as short, brittle hair that is prone to fracturing, which can eventuate in patchy alopecia accentuated in the temporal and occipital regions. Light microscopy shows abnormal twisting of the hair at irregular intervals.

PILI BIFURCATI

Definition and Epidemiology

Pili bifurcati is a rare hair shaft disorder characterized by thin, short fragile hairs eventuating in diffuse alopecia. Pili bifurcati affects patients in childhood.

Etiology

The underlying pathogenic defect is unknown.

Clinical Presentation

Pili bifurcati usually manifests in children with short fragile hair on the scalp, which can lead to diffuse alopecia.[36] Other sites include the eyelashes and eyebrows.[37]

Histologic Findings

The affected hairs show bifurcated hair shafts. On scanning electron microscopy, a single hair shaft splits into two smaller shafts, which then fuse downstream to again form a single hair shaft.[38] The two bifurcated hair shafts are completely covered by their own cuticles.

CAPSULE SUMMARY

PILI BIFURCATI

Pili bifurcati is a hair shaft fragility disorder characterized by short coarse hair and diffuse alopecia. The hair shafts show nodes of bifurcation with downstream fusion into a single hair shaft.

TRICHOTHIODYSTROPHY

Definition and Epidemiology

Trichothiodystrophy is a hair shaft abnormality characterized by brittle hairs and is associated with neuroectodermal disorders. Trichothiodystrophy presents at birth.

Etiology

Trichothiodystrophy is caused by mutations in xeroderma pigmentosum-B, xeroderma pigmentosum-D, and p8/TTDA helicase/ATPase subunits of the DNA repair/basal transcription factor IIH, which are three genes involved in transcription initiation and nucleotide excision repair.[39] The gene defects result in hair with a significant reduction in sulfur-rich cysteine matrix proteins. Alterations in these genes also give rise to xeroderma pigmentosum and Cockayne syndrome.

Clinical Presentation

Depending on the specific gene mutation, patients with trichothiodystrophy can present with a complex, sometimes referred by the acronym PIBIDS: *p*hotosensitivity, *i*chthyosis, *b*rittle hair, *i*ntellectual impairment, *d*ecreased fertility, *s*hort stature, or IBIDS, when photosensitivity is not present. The hair findings include short, brittle hairs of varying length on the scalp, eyebrows, and eyelashes.[39,40]

Histologic Findings

Affected hairs show a clean transverse break through the hair shaft and an absence of cuticle cells at the fracture site, a defect termed trichoschisis (Figure 14-8). Hairs may be focally flattened or ribbon-like[41] (Figure 14-9). When viewed under polarized light in the dark or "extinguished" position, an alternating light and dark banding pattern (tiger tail banding) can be seen[42,43] (Figure 14-10).

CAPSULE SUMMARY

TRICHOTHIODYSTROPHY

Trichothiodystrophy is a brittle hair disorder caused by a deficiency in sulfur incorporation into the hair shaft due to mutation in genes involved in transcription initiation and DNA repair. Patients typically present in early childhood with ichthyosis and varying degrees of neurologic impairment, as well as short brittle hair.

MARIE-UNNA HEREDITARY HYPOTRICHOSIS

Definition and Epidemiology

Marie-Unna hereditary hypotrichosis (MUHH) is a hair shaft abnormality characterized by coarse, unruly hair, and progressive hair loss. The disorder usually presents in childhood.

Etiology

A subset of patients with MUHH have mutations in the U2HR locus, an upstream regulator of the Hr gene, but the exact mechanism of the disease is not known.[44] Mutations in the epidermal growth factor receptor kinase substrate 8-like protein 3 have also been associated with MUHH.[45]

Clinical Presentation

MUHH can present as an isolated phenomenon or as part of an autosomal dominant inherited syndrome. Typically, patients are born with normal-appearing to slightly coarse hair, although there are cases with sparse to no hair.[46,47] Over time, hair is progressively lost and becomes coarse and wiry. In addition to the scalp, hair can be lost from the eyebrows, eyelashes, and the body. By puberty, a nonscarring alopecia is present, with the vertex and scalp margins being the most affected sites.[48]

Histologic Findings

Affected hairs are deeply pigmented, are of varying caliber, and may be twisted or bent.[49]

CAPSULE SUMMARY

MARIE-UNNA HEREDITARY HYPOTRICHOSIS

MUHH is a hair shaft anomaly that manifests as coarse wiry hair that is gradually lost, resulting in nonscarring alopecia. The hairs in MUHH are twisted and bent and exhibit dark pigmentation.

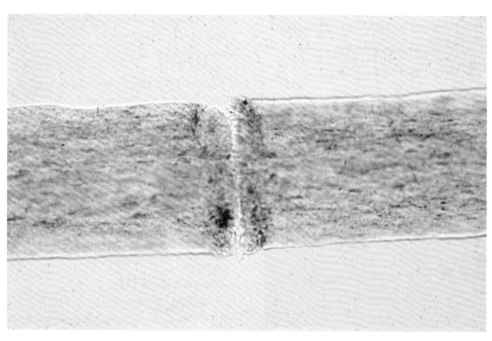

FIGURE 14-8. Trichothiodystrophy: light microscopy reveals trichoschisis. Courtesy of Paradi Mirmirani, MD, Kaiser Permanente, Vallejo CA.

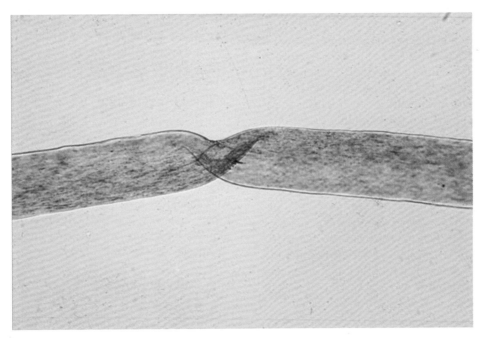

FIGURE 14-9. Trichothiodystrophy: light microscopy reveals ribboning. From Mirmirani P, Huang KP, Price VH. A practical, algorithmic approach to diagnosing hair shaft disorders. *Int J Dermatol. 2011;50(1):1-12.*

PILI ANNULATI

Definition and Epidemiology

Also called "ringed hair," pili annulati is a rare hair shaft disorder characterized by light and dark bands within the hair shaft, leading to a "shiny," "spangled," or "sandy" appearance.

Epidemiology

The disorder is present at birth or arises during infancy.

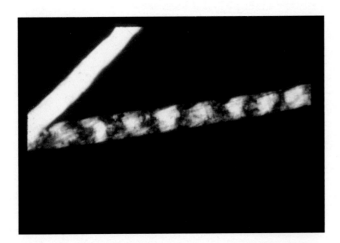

FIGURE 14-10. Trichothiodystrophy: polarizing microscopy reveals tigertail banding. From Mirmirani P, Huang KP, Price VH. A practical, algorithmic approach to diagnosing hair shaft disorders. *Int J Dermatol. 2011;50(1):1-12.*

Etiology

Pili annulati is inherited in an autosomal dominant fashion. The disease-causing locus has been mapped to the telomeric region on chromosome 12q.[50]

Clinical Presentation

The hairs in pili annulati show alternating light and dark banding along the hair shaft with a variable number of hairs affected, often imparting a shiny appearance to the hair (Figure 14-11). It can affect the entire scalp hair or be patchy and can also involve the axillae, beard, and pubic region.[51,52] Hair growth is normal and hairs are typically pliable and strong, but there may be some degree of hair fragility. TN-like fractures may be induced in the dark bands.

Histologic Findings

The clinically apparent light bands appear as dark bands on hair mount because of the inverse effects of reflected and transmitted light (Figures 14-12 and 14-13). The bands correspond to air-filled cavities within the hair shaft that can be appreciated on electron microscopy.[53-55]

CAPSULE SUMMARY

PILI ANNULATI

Pili annulati is characterized by a characteristic banding of hair, resulting in a shiny or sandy appearance. Affected hairs have air-filled cavities in the hair shaft and are typically of normal length and strength, but can have some degree of susceptibility to fracture.

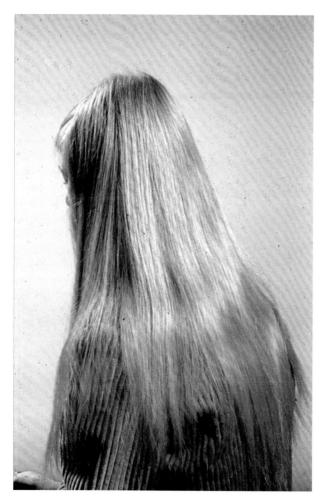

FIGURE 14-11. Pili annulati. Hair has a shiny appearance. From Mirmirani P, Huang KP, Price VH. A practical, algorithmic approach to diagnosing hair shaft disorders. *Int J Dermatol. 2011;50(1):1-12.*

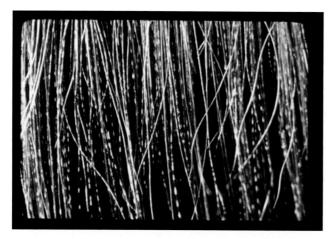

FIGURE 14-12. Pili annulati. Closeup of the hair shafts reveal spangled appearance. From Mirmirani P, Huang KP, Price VH. A practical, algorithmic approach to diagnosing hair shaft disorders. *Int J Dermatol. 2011;50(1):1-12.*

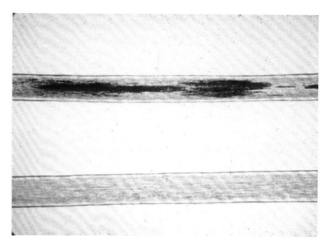

FIGURE 14-13. Pili annulati. Hair mount reveals dark and light bands in comparison with normal hair shaft. From Mirmirani P, Huang KP, Price VH. A practical, algorithmic approach to diagnosing hair shaft disorders. *Int J Dermatol. 2011;50(1):1-12.*

WOOLLY HAIR

Definition and Epidemiology

Woolly hair is a hair shaft disorder characterized by fine, tightly wound hairs that may be associated with other disorders or syndromes. The disorder usually presents in childhood.

Etiology

Mutations that underlie the autosomal recessive presentations of wooly hair affect *P2RY5* gene[56,57] and lipase H gene.[58,59] The *P2RY5* gene encodes a G protein-coupled receptor that is expressed in Henle and Huxley layers of the inner root sheath of the hair follicle. Lipase H gene mutations are also present in isolated hypotrichosis and likely plays a role in hair follicle growth.[58,59] Somatic mosaic *HRAS* mutations can cause the association of woolly hair and epidermal nevi.[60]

Clinical Presentation

Woolly hair can present in isolation on the scalp in a partial or focal manner, such as in the wooly hair nevus, or in a syndromic manner[61,62] (Figure 14-14). Associated findings and syndromes include palmoplantar keratoderma,[63] keratosis pilaris atrophicans fasciei,[64] Noonan syndrome,[65] Carvajal syndrome,[66] cardiofaciocutaneous syndrome,[67] Naxos disease,[68] keratosis follicularis spinulosa decalvans,[69] and epidermal nevi.[60]

Naxos disease is an autosomal recessive disorder characterized by wooly hair from birth, diffuse nonepidermolytic palmoplantar keratoderma, and arrhythmogenic right ventricular dysplasia/cardiomyopathy.[70,71] The latter tends to present in late puberty. In contrast, patients with Carvajal syndrome exhibit epidermolytic palmoplantar keratoderma in addition to wooly hair and cardiac defects.[66,72]

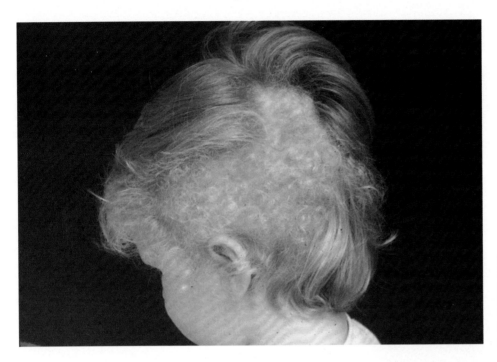

FIGURE 14-14. Woolly hair nevus. Discrete patch of tightly curled hair in an otherwise normal field of scalp. From Mirmirani P, Huang KP, Price VH. A practical, algorithmic approach to diagnosing hair shaft disorders. *Int J Dermatol.* 2011;50(1):1-12.

Histologic Findings

There are no specific pathologic findings on hair mount.

CAPSULE SUMMARY

WOOLLY HAIR

Patients with wooly hair syndrome display fine tightly coiled hairs. The disorder may present in isolation or may be associated with other cutaneous disorders or syndromes.

ACQUIRED PROGRESSIVE KINKING OF THE HAIR

Definition and Epidemiology

Acquired progressive kinking of the hair (APKH) is a rare disorder characterized by a rapid onset of curly, unruly hair. The disorder presents in children and young adults with a peak in adolescence.

Etiology

The underlying pathogenic defect is unknown.

Clinical Presentation

APKH presents as ill-defined patches of frizzy and kinky hairs typically on the frontal, temporal, and vertex of the scalp.[73,74] Hairs can be hypopigmented, hyperpigmented, or of normal color compared with the surrounding unaffected hairs.[75]

Histologic Findings

Hairs are apparently normal on light microscopy, but partial twisting along the long axis of the hair shaft and shallow canalicular grooves can be seen on scanning electron microscopy.[76,77]

CAPSULE SUMMARY

ACQUIRED PROGRESSIVE KINKING OF THE HAIR

APKH is a rare acquired hair shaft disorder that manifests with patches of unruly, frizzy hair typically in adolescence. Electron microscopy shows irregular twisting of the hair and grooves along the long axis.

UNCOMBABLE HAIR SYNDROME

Definition and Epidemiology

Uncombable hair syndrome is a hair shaft disorder characterized by unruly hair that is difficult to style. The condition is also known as pili trianguli et canaliculi, and spun glass hair. The disorder usually manifests in childhood, but acquired cases that present later in life have been reported.

Etiology

Uncombable hair syndrome is caused by mutations in peptidylarginine deiminase 3 (*PADI3*), transglutaminase 3 (*TGM3*), and trichohyalin (*TCHH*). PADI3 and TGM3 mediate posttranslational modification of TCHH, and all three

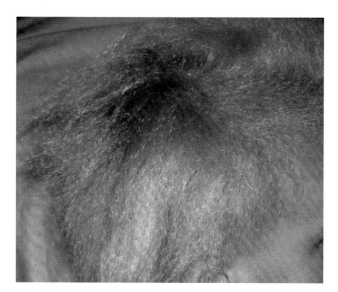

FIGURE 14-15. Uncombable hair syndrome: hair has an unruly, spangled appearance and is difficult to comb. Courtesy of Ken Greer, MD, University of Virginia Health Sciences Center, Charlottesville, VA.

genes are involved in the formation of the hair shaft.[78] An autosomal recessive inheritance pattern is implicated in the majority of cases.

Clinical Presentation

The hair is usually blonde to light brown with a frizzy, spangled texture, and projects outward from the scalp[79,80] (Figure 14-15).

Histologic Findings

The hair shaft is triangular or bean-shaped on cross-section. Hairs may have longitudinal grooves along one or two facets[81] (Figure 14-16A and B).

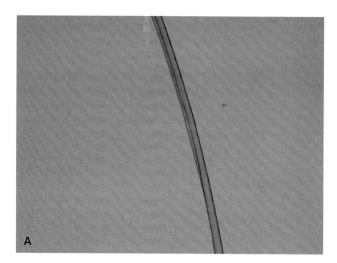

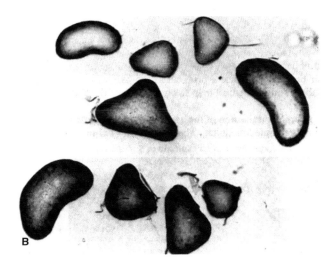

FIGURE 14-16. A, Uncombable hair syndrome: hair mount reveals longitudinal groove along hair shaft. B, Uncombable hair syndrome: hair mount cross-section of hair shaft reveals triangular or kidney bean–shaped formation. From Mirmirani P, Huang KP, Price VH. A practical, algorithmic approach to diagnosing hair shaft disorders. *Int J Dermatol. 2011;50(1):1-12.*

CAPSULE SUMMARY

UNCOMBABLE HAIR SYNDROME

Uncombable hair syndrome typically manifests in infancy or childhood and patients show disorderly hairs that stand out from the scalp and are difficult to style. Hairs may show a triangular or reniform configuration on cross-section and may exhibit longitudinal ridging.

LOOSE ANAGEN SYNDROME

Definition and Epidemiology

Loose anagen syndrome (LAS) is a disorder of abnormal anchorage of the hair to the follicles in the scalp and is a potential cause of noncicatricial alopecia in the pediatric population. True incidence of LAS is not well known.

However, it is believed to be common and underrecognized. LAS most commonly presents in children with low density or thin hair.[82] It is thought to affect Caucasian females, often after the age of 2. More recently, however, it has been described in all skin types and all hair types.[83]

Etiology

The true etiology of this disease is still not clear; however, studies of hair follicles from patients with LAS have shown structural abnormalities of the inner root sheath complex of the anagen follicle. This perturbation of the normal supportive and anchoring function of the inner root sheath likely results in a loose attachment of the hair shaft to the anagen follicle.[84]

Clinical Presentation

Younger pediatric patients may be brought in by family members and caregivers with complaints of an inability to grow hair long and hair that pulls out easily from the scalp usually without evidence of breakage.

On physical exam, patients are often Fitzpatrick skin type 2, although it has been reported in all skin types. On scalp exam, there are often no findings of scalp inflammation such as erythema or perifollicular scale. The scalp hair may be any color or texture. It is often appreciably thin, wispy, and short in length, seldom longer than the nape of the neck in pediatric patients.[82] A minority of patients may also have "bed head," or hair that is heavily knotted, particularly in the occipital scalp (Figure 14-17).

Histologic Findings

Diagnosis of LAS can be made by performing a hair pull test or trichogram analysis showing the classic findings in at least 50% of examined hairs. Light microscopic evaluation shows a predominance of anagen hairs characterized by abnormally keratinized inner root sheaths, pigmented and bent or squared-off hair bulbs (so-called hockey stick-shaped hair bulbs), lack of external root sheaths, and proximal ruffling of the cuticle of the hair shaft (Figure 14-18).[82,84]

Scalp biopsy is rarely performed for the diagnosis of LAS. However, limited small cases series report a variety of histologic findings from scalp exam. Few report normal hair follicular histology; others report abnormal histopathology of the inner root sheath including fracturing and fragmentation and clefting within the inner root sheath and between

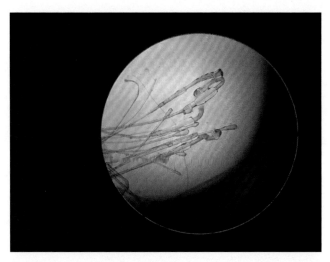

FIGURE 14-18. Loose anagen syndrome: hair mount reveals bent or squared-off hair bulbs (so-called hockey stick-shaped), abnormally keratinized inner root sheath, and proximal ruffling of the cuticle of the hair shaft. Courtesy of Barrett Zlotoff MD, University of Virginia Health Science Center.

the inner and outer root sheaths.[82] The keratinized Henle cell layer may also show a tortuous and irregular swelling. Irregular keratinization of the cuticle cells of the inner root sheath and a swollen appearance of Huxley cells. Absent hair shafts and collapsed root sheaths and abnormal hair shaft shapes have been reported in a minority of cases.

Differential Diagnosis

The clinical differential diagnosis includes telogen effluvium (TE) and diffuse alopecia areata. However, the histologic findings on scalp biopsy can resolve this. Histologically, diagnostic considerations include TE and trichotillomania. TE, unlike LAS, frequently lacks hair shaft abnormalities. Although trichotillomania may show loss of hair shafts like LAS histologically, the former often has loss of the inner root sheath as well as prominent trichomalacia, pigmented hair casts, and follicular hemorrhage, features notably absent in LAS.

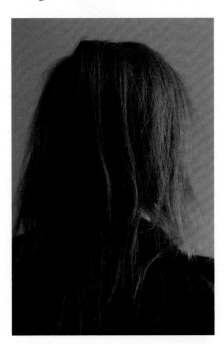

FIGURE 14-17. Loose anagen syndrome: hairs of various lengths. Courtesy of Barrett Zlotoff, MD, University of Virginia Health Sciences Center, Charlottesville, VA.

CAPSULE SUMMARY

LOOSE ANAGEN SYNDROME

LAS is a potential cause of noncicatricial alopecia caused by an abnormal lack of anchorage of anagen hairs to the scalp hair follicles. It commonly presents in young children as hair that pulls out painlessly and easily, is easily tangled, and cannot be grown long. It is diagnosed with a hair pull test or trichogram analysis showing abnormal anagen hairs. The condition is often self-limited and improves with age in most patients.

CONGENITAL TRIANGULAR ALOPECIA (TEMPORAL TRIANGULAR ALOPECIA)

Definition and Epidemiology

Congenital triangular alopecia (CTA), also known as temporal triangular alopecia, is a localized form of noncicatricial alopecia characterized by the absence of terminal hairs in the affected scalp region.[85] Characteristically, this condition presents in infancy or early childhood. Not infrequently however, the lesions may not be noticed until later in childhood within the first decade of life. Rare cases of acquired disease in adulthood have been described. Its true incidence is unknown. Rarely has it been described in coexistence with a variety of disorders, including aplasia cutis congenita, Trisomy 21 (Down syndrome), mental retardation, epilepsy, phakomatosis pigmentovascularis, and congenital heart disease.[85]

Etiology

The exact cause of CTA is largely unknown. The prevailing hypothesis is that this disease arises in utero as a failure of the formation of terminal hairs within the affected segment of the scalp skin. Alternatively, others believe that the disease represents abnormal miniaturization of preexistent terminal hairs. This latter hypothesis may in part explain the rare cases of presentation in adults.[85]

Clinical Presentation

Clinically, patients with CTA present with a triangular or round patch of alopecia typically along the frontotemporal hairline (Figure 14-19). The hair loss can be unilateral or bilateral. Although there is a loss of terminal hairs, vellus hairs at this site are unaffected.[85] There is neither scarring nor inflammation present. The remainder of the scalp is often clinically normal.

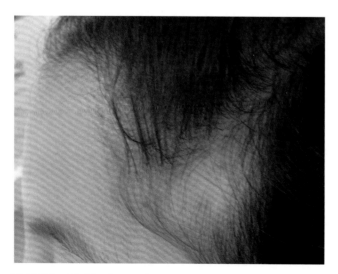

FIGURE 14-19. Congenital triangular alopecia. Courtesy of Paradi Mirmirani, MD, Kaiser Permanente, Vallejo CA.

Histologic Findings

On light microscopy, there is a preservation of the normal number of hair follicles. However, almost all of these follicle are vellus hairs; terminal hairs are few or absent entirely.[85] Inflammation and scarring are absent, and sebaceous lobules remain intact. Fibrous streamers or follicular stelae are notably absent.

Differential Diagnosis

Clinically, these lesions may be mistaken for alopecia areata. However, a detailed clinical history and careful physical examination often readily point to the more correct diagnosis. When in doubt, a scalp biopsy may be performed. In alopecia areata, the biopsy shows a lymphocyte-mediated process, distinguishing this entity quite clearly from CTA. Histologically, other diagnostic considerations include end-stage traction alopecia and androgenetic alopecia. In the latter entity, numerous follicular stelae are often present, distinguishing it from CTA. Although androgenetic alopecia with marked follicular miniaturization may mimic CTA, the finding of follicular stelae lends support to the former as the correct diagnosis.[85]

CAPSULE SUMMARY

CONGENITAL TRIANGULAR ALOPECIA

CTA, also known as temporal triangular alopecia, is a noncicatricial alopecia characterized by an asymptomatic triangular or round patch of hair loss on the frontotemporal hairline that presents in infancy or childhood.

Histologically, a transversely sectioned scalp biopsy reveals the preservation of follicular quantity, and a marked increased proportion of vellus hairs with a concurrent decrease or near absence of terminal hairs.

KERATOSIS PILARIS

Definition and Epidemiology

Keratosis pilaris (KP) is an autosomal dominant disorder of keratinization with variable penetrance. It is characterized by the presence of small pruritic follicular based papules.[86] Up to 40% of adults are estimated to be affected, with the condition presenting in young women more commonly. It is often noted in the first two decades of life.[86] Notably, this population of patients has an increased incidence of atopy as well.

Etiology

Although the exact cause of the disorder unknown, it is thought to represent the follicular variant of ichthyosis vulgaris in some cases. KP is thought to be caused by abnormal keratinization around the follicular orifice that results in plugging.[86]

Clinical Presentation

Clinically, patients present with small 2 to 6 mm pink to hyperpigmented (in darker skin) pruritic follicularly based papules most commonly on the lateral segments of the arms and thighs (Figures 14-20 and 14-21). Other areas frequently involved include the face, buttocks, and trunk.[86] These papules on occasion are associated with distorted and dystrophic hair shafts clinically.

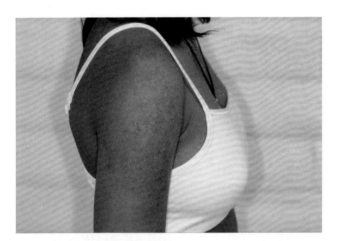

FIGURE 14-20. **Keratosis pilaris.** Multiple follicularly based hyperpigmented papules on the arm of darker-skinned patient. Courtesy of Barrett Zlotoff, MD, University of Virginia Health Sciences Center, Charlottesville, VA.

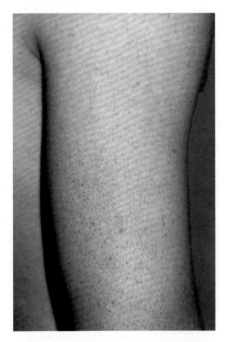

FIGURE 14-21. **Keratosis pilaris.** Multiple follicularly based pink papules on the arm. Courtesy of Barrett Zlotoff, MD, University of Virginia Health Sciences Center, Charlottesville, VA.

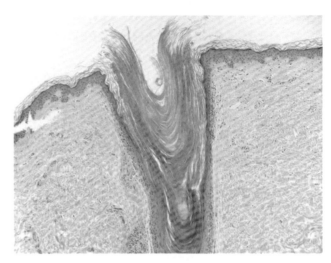

FIGURE 14-22. **Keratosis pilaris.** Histopathology: there is prominent follicular plugging, perifolliculitis, and perifollicular fibrosis (×100).

Histologic Findings

Histologically, biopsy of the papules reveals papillated epidermal hyperplasia with basket-weave orthokeratosis and follicular plugging. There is almost always accompanying follicular dilatation with thinning and atrophy of the follicular infundibulum (Figure 14-22).[86] Rarely, intact hair shafts captured in the planes of sectioning may appear bent or distorted.

Differential Diagnosis

Clinical differential diagnosis for these lesions include lichen spinulosus and the follicular lesions of pityriasis rubra pilaris. Biopsy findings can often distinguish these entities as lichen spinulosus and pityriasis rubra pilaris show epidermal spongiosis as the dominant inflammatory pattern. Although spongiosis may be a secondary finding histologically in KP from the frequent excoriation, it is not the dominant finding. Histologically, inflamed excoriated lesions of KP can mimic acneiform disorders such as suppurative folliculitis.[5] However, the physical examination and a detailed history should help sort between these two entities because acne will have actual comedones.

CAPSULE SUMMARY

KERATOSIS PILARIS

KP is a common disorder of keratinization thought to represent the follicular variant of ichthyosis vulgaris. Many patients suffering from this disorder also have atopy. It often presents as pruritic tiny follicular based papules along the arms and thighs. Histologically, these papules represent foci of perifollicular epidermal hyperplasia, marked follicular dilatation, and follicular plugging.

DISORDERS OF THE NAILS IN CHILDREN

Definition and Epidemiology

Disorders of the nail unit in children are rare, but increasing in prevalence worldwide. Nail changes can be categorized as congenital or acquired. Congenital nail disorders may provide clues in the diagnosis of hereditary diseases; however, because these disorders are rare, the focus of this section will be on acquired nail disorders. The most common acquired nail disorders include onychomycosis, melanonychia, trachyonychia, onychomadesis, and nail pitting. As such, the discussion herein will focus on these five disorders.[87]

Onychomycosis is defined as a fungal infection of the nail plate. Melanonychia is brownish or black discoloration of the nail attributed to increased melanin pigment deposition. Trachyonychia is defined as roughness of the nails. Onychomadesis is the abnormal separation of the proximal nail plate from the nail bed, frequently resulting in loss of the entire nail. Lastly, nail pitting is defined as the presence of punctate and superficial depressions in the nail.

Disorders of the nail are present among all age groups and thus may be found at any point during childhood. Onychomycosis is rare in the pediatric population, estimated to affect 0.3% of children below the age of 18 worldwide.[87] The incidence of trachyonychia, melanonychia, onychomadesis, and nail pitting is largely unknown.

Etiology

Onychomycosis is most often caused by a dermatophytic infection of the nail plate, the most common species identified being *Trichophyton*, *Epidermophyton*, and *Microsporum*. Of these, *Trichophyton rubrum* is the most common offender.[87] Less often, onychomycosis may be caused by nondermatophytes, molds, and Candida species. Infection of the nail plate is thought to occur by secondary spread or rather direct extension from primary infection of the adjacent acral skin.

With respect to melanonychia, the mechanisms through which increased melanin is deposited in the nail unit are variable and include a spectrum of pigmented disorders from functional melanonychia (also known as lentigo or benign melanocytic hyperplasia) to melanocytic nevi and melanoma in situ. Functional melanonychia, attributed to melanocytic activation or hypermelanosis, is the most common overall cause of melanonychia. However, within the pediatric population, nail matrix melanocytic nevi are the primary cause of melanonychia. A small series of 40 cases of longitudinal melanonychia by Goettmann-Bonvallo and colleagues identified benign melanocytic proliferations (nevi and melanocytic hyperplasia) in 77% of all patients evaluated.[88] Of note, primary invasive melanoma of the nail unit has not been reported in a pediatric patient in the literature and is consequently thought to be exceedingly rare. When melanonychia is noted to involve more than one nail, a genetic syndrome such as Peutz Jeghers and Laugier-Hunziker syndrome or a medication reaction may be implicated.[89]

Trachonychia often occurs idiopathically; however, it has also been described in children as part of a constellation of other skin disorders, including alopecia areata, lichen planus, and psoriasis.[87]

Onychomadesis is thought to occur secondary to disruption and arrest of nail matrix production, often secondary to an acute systemic event such as high fever, infection, acute exacerbation of a chronic systemic disorder, medications including chemotherapeutic agents, nail trauma, periungual inflammation of any etiology, and a nutritional deficiency.[87] However, onychomadesis has also been reported as part of a constellation of findings in a host of chronic disorders as well, such as Kawasaki syndrome, Stevens-Johnson syndrome, systemic lupus erythematosus, alopecia areata, pemphigus vulgaris, and epidermolysis bullosa.[87] A minority of cases have also been reported in the setting of a varicella zoster virus infection as well as hand, foot, and mouth disease.

Nail pitting is thought to arise from a disruption of the nail matrix in the proximal nail fold. These most often occur idiopathically in children, but a minority of cases are associated with pediatric psoriasis or alopecia areata.

Clinical Presentation

Onychomycosis often presents with a yellow discoloration of the affected nail, most commonly the distal and lateral segments of the nail plate (Figure 14-23). This is not infrequently associated with a thickening of the nail, subungual debris, and onycholysis. Importantly, because this hyperkeratotic subungual debris often carries a high organismal burden, it is important to scrape and submit this material

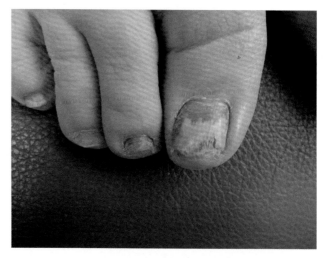

FIGURE 14-23. Onychomycosis. Hyperkeratotic toenail with discoloration, onychodystrophy, and fissuring. Courtesy of Barrett Zlotoff, MD, University of Virginia Health Sciences Center, Charlottesville, VA.

when submitting nail clippings for histologic evaluation. A minority of cases may present with leukonychia (white discoloration of the nail).

Clinically, melanonychia presents as a black or brown longitudinal band of varied thickness spanning the length of the entire nail. Usually, the streak extends from the proximal nail fold to the hyponychium; however, a few cases of transverse melanonychia with horizontal pigmented bands have also been described.[88] Rarely, the entire nail unit may be involved (total melanonychia). In neoplastic etiologies, the presentation is often limited to the involvement of one nail; the involvement of multiple or all nails is unusual and should prompt a consideration of a potential underlying genetic syndrome. Contrary to in the adult population, the findings of periungual pigmentation, variegation in the coloration of the streak, and a thick band on exam are not uncommon in the pediatric melanonychia of benign etiologies.[87]

Trachyonychia may present clinically as "shiny trachyonychia" or "opaque trachyonychia," referring to the severity of the thickening and coarseness of the affected nail(s).[87] This likely represents a spectrum of disease manifestation based on the severity of disease.

Onychomadesis presents with lifting of the nail plate from the proximal nail fold (Figure 14-24). Often times, this partially detached nail will eventually fall off.[87]

In superficial nail pitting, the longitudinal length of segment of the nail plate involved (from proximal nail fold to hyponychium) is related to the length of time of disease.[87] Fingernails are more often affected than toe nails, and multiple digits are often involved (Figure 14-25). In patients

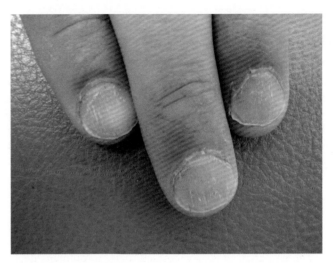

FIGURE 14-25. Nail pitting. Courtesy of Paradi Mirmirani, MD, Kaiser Permanente, Vallejo CA.

with psoriasis, the classic dermatologic findings of psoriasis may concurrently be present, and other nail changes such as oil spotting and thickening are often present. Of note, studies show that the presence of less than 20 pits overall suggests an idiopathic or nonpsoriatic etiology to the disorder. However, patients with more than 20 pits are at an increased likelihood of having psoriasis.[87,89] Along similar lines, children with more than 60 pits almost always have psoriasis. The pitting associated with alopecia areata is often in a more regular, evenly spaced grid-like pattern. A complete history and physical exam must be performed for these children in search of not only features suggestive of psoriasis, alopecia areata, atopy, or other papulosquamous skin diseases with nail findings.

Histologic Findings

On light microscopy, the presence of multiple fungal organisms makes the diagnosis of onychomycosis (Figure 14-26). Dermatophytic and mold-mediated infections exhibit hyphal structures, whereas infections mediated by candida species have yeasts and pseudohyphae. If the diagnosis is in question, a periodic acid–Schiff (PAS) or silver stain may be performed to highlight the organisms. Tissue culture and polymerase chain reaction evaluation serve increasingly as great ancillary tests to corroborate biopsy findings.

Rarely, melanonychia are biopsied for histologic evaluation in children.[88] Partial biopsies are strongly discouraged in this setting because they frequently lead to inconclusive diagnoses. Nail biopsy findings for the lesions of melanonychia vary depending on the etiology of the pigment deposition. In the case of a functional melanonychia, there is increased melanin pigment within the nail matrix epithelium appreciable increase in the number of melanocytes (Figure 14-27). This increase in pigment may not be readily appreciable on hematoxylin- and eosin-stained sections;

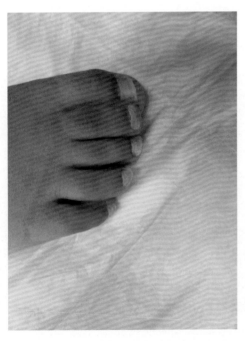

FIGURE 14-24. Onychomadesis lifting of nail fold. Courtesy of Barrett Zlotoff, MD, University of Virginia Health Sciences Center, Charlottesville, VA.

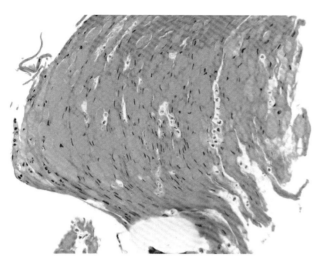

FIGURE 14-26. **Onychomycosis.** Histopathology: hyperkeratotic and parakeratotic nail plate with many fungal hyphae and spores (×400).

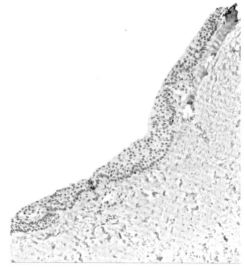

FIGURE 14-28. **Lentigo (functional melanonychia).** Histopathology: SOX-10 (red chromogen) immunostain showing no increase in melanocytes (×200).

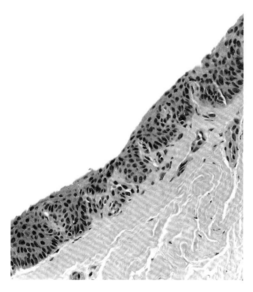

FIGURE 14-27. **Lentigo (functional melanonychia).** Histopathology: focal pigment within the basilar layer of ungula matrical epithelium (×400).

special stains for the melanin pigment, such as a Fontana argentaffin reaction, show strong pigmentation in both the overlying nail plate and the nail matrix. Melanocytic immunohistochemical stains such as S100 protein or SOX-10 show no increase in intraepithelial melanocytes (Figure 14-28). In the case of nail unit melanocytic nevi, a moderate increase in heavily pigmented, and often dendritic, melanocytes is identified within the nail matrix epithelium, which is often arranged in a combination of single cells (lentiginous) and small nests.[90] The overlying nail plate often shows "pigment columns," foci of melanin pigment in linear array oriented perpendicular to the long axis of the nail plate within cells corresponding clinically to anatomic.[90] As

a well-described "special site," nail matrix nevi are known for occasionally exhibiting some features often deemed as atypical in the melanocytic proliferations of nonacral sites, including suprabasilar scatter and poor nesting pattern (lentiginous predominant architecture). In the nail unit, such features are still within the spectrum of that observed in benign acral nevi. Most nail unit nevi are of the conventional type; rarely, Spitz and blue nevi have also been reported.[90] The features of melanoma and melanoma in situ include cytologic atypia of the nail matrix melanocytes, predominantly lentiginous melanocytes in confluence, irregular distribution of these melanocytes in the matrix epithelium, prominent and marked pagetoid spread of the melanocytes, multinucleation, and the presence of mitotic figures within melanocytes in the underlying subepithelial connective tissue.[90]

The findings of a nail plate biopsy of trachyonychia often show thickened and fissuring of the nail plate or onychodystrophy.[87] This finding is not specific to the etiology. The additional presence of hypergranulosis, a lichenoid interface dermatitis at the junction of the nail matrix epithelium and the subjacent connective tissue, dyskeratotic keratinocytes within the epithelium, and irregular epithelial hyperplasia may point to the diagnosis of lichen planus as the cause for trachyonychia in some cases. Similarly, accompanying acanthosis of the nail matrix epithelium with elongated rete ridges, overlying parakeratosis, and neutrophilic epithelial collections suggest trachyonychia due to psoriasis.

As onychomadesis is often a clinical diagnosis and is self-limited, nail plate biopsy is often not necessary for diagnosis or management. Similarly, nail biopsy is seldom performed for nail pits.

Differential Diagnosis

Clinically, it is important to note that the lesions of onychomycosis, particularly pigmented lesions, may be confused for subungual hematoma or a melanocytic lesion. On the other hand, less pigmented lesions of onychomycosis may be overlooked on clinical exam and are consequently underdiagnosed. Histologically, several factors contribute to false-negative results in onychomycosis, including suboptimal biopsy (minimal nail clippings and/or failure to submit subungual hyperkeratotic debris), low organismal burden, and sampling error.

The differential diagnosis for melanonychia includes onychomycosis, trauma and subungual hematoma, and exogenous pigment deposition. Histologically, the diagnostic distinction between a nail matrix nevus and melanocyte hyperplasia is often based on the number and distribution of the dendritic melanocytes. In melanocytic hyperplasia, there are less melanocytes, and melanocytes are confined to the nail matrix epithelium. Abnormal cytology and architecture distinguishes melanoma in situ and invasive melanoma from more benign entities.

With all findings of trachyonychia, a careful skin and mucous membrane exam should be performed for findings suggestive of onychomycosis, lichen planus, psoriasis, alopecia areata, and eczema at minimum. Histologically, the finding of onychodystrophy is nonspecific and may also be observed in onychomycosis. PAS or silver stain may help identify fungal organisms in the latter.

The findings of onychomadesis clinically should prompt an evaluation for the inciting cause so as to prevent persistence and recurrence in other intact nails.

CAPSULE SUMMARY

DISORDERS OF THE NAILS IN CHILDREN

Disorders of the nail unit are rare in the pediatric population. The most common include onychomycosis, melanonychia, trachyonychia, onychomadesis, and nail pitting. However, some cases manifest as a part of constellation of findings in patients with chronic disorders such as alopecia areata, lichen planus, psoriasis, eczema, and systemic lupus erythematosus.

The most common cause of onychomycosis is a dermatophytic fungal infection. When obtaining nail clippings, submission of subungual hyperkeratotic debris is important for improving the diagnostic yield of the specimen. The most common cause of melanonychia is a nail matrix melanocytic nevus. Melanoma of the nail unit is exceedingly rare in the pediatric population. In a minority of cases, onychodystrophy may be associated with an underlying genetic syndrome.

ACNE VULGARIS

Definition and Epidemiology

Acne vulgaris is a common chronic inflammatory disorder affecting the pilosebaceous unit in the skin and is often characterized by variable degrees of follicular occlusion and inflammation.

The prevalence of acne is thought to reach as much as 95% during adolescent years.[91,92] However, it can also present in younger children. Neonatal acne is reported to affect up to 20% of neonates; similarly, two additional studies identified acne in up to 78% of girls between 8 and 12 years of age, with the presence of more than ten comedones in up to half of boys 10 and 11 years of age.[92]

Etiology

The lesions of acne vulgaris are thought to be initiated by follicular occlusion, often secondary to debris, sebum, and desquamated follicular keratinocytes. Entrapped microorganisms, including *Propionibacterium acnes*, subsequently proliferate.[93] This process, often eventuating in follicular rupture, incites an inflammatory response within the dermis of the skin, resulting in the characteristic inflammatory dermatologic lesions. Sebum overproduction in the prepubescent and adolescent population is frequently touted as a reason for the well-documented increase of disease prevalence during teenage years.[93]

Clinical Presentation

Patients present with a variable combination of comedones, inflammatory papules, pustules, nodules, and cysts often located on sebum-rich skin sites (i.e., face, neck, chest, and back) (Figures 14-29 and 14-30).

Histologic Findings

Histologically, acne vulgaris is characterized by a dilation of hair follicles, follicular plugging, and perifollicular

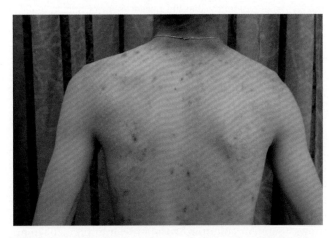

FIGURE 14-29. Acne vulgaris. Cystic and scarring pattern. Courtesy of Barrett Zlotoff, MD, University of Virginia Health Sciences Center, Charlottesville, VA.

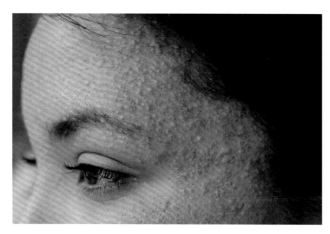

FIGURE 14-30. **Acne vulgaris.** Comedonal pattern. Courtesy of Barrett Zlotoff, MD, University of Virginia Health Sciences Center, Charlottesville, VA.

inflammation, typically consisting of neutrophils, lymphocytes, and plasma cells (suppurative folliculitis and perifolliculitis) (Figure 14-31).[93] Plugged follicles are often filled with neutrophils, keratin debris, and bacteria. Follicular rupture along with a concurrent granulomatous reaction may also be observed. In more exuberant inflammatory lesions, the inflammatory infiltrate may also involve other adnexal structures such as the arrector pili muscles and sebaceous glands.[93]

Differential Diagnosis

Clinical differential diagnosis for acne lesions in the pediatric population varies considerably by the age of the patient (Table 14-1). Histologically, all variants of acne can appear morphologically similar, including acne rosacea, steroid acne, perioral dermatitis, and steroid rosacea. Clinical correlation is essential in making the correct diagnosis. Notably,

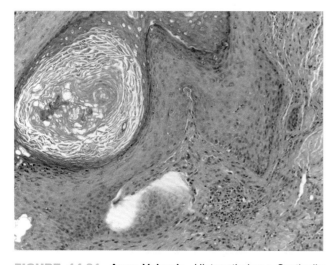

FIGURE 14-31. **Acne Vulgaris.** Histopathology: Cystically dilated follicle (comedone), folliculitis (neutrophils, lymphocytes, and rare eosinophils within the follicular epithelium), and perifolliculitis (inflammatory cells around the follicle) (×200).

TABLE 14-1.	Clinical differential diagnosis for acne vulgaris
Patient Age of Onset	**Clinical Differential Diagnosis for Acne Vulgaris**
Neonate (up to 6 wk)	Neonatal cephalic pustulosis
	Infectious agents
	Transient neonatal pustular melanosis
	Nevus comedonicus
	Erythema toxicum neonatorum
	Sebaceous gland hyperplasia
	Milia
	Miliaria
	Maternal medications (eg, lithium, phenytoin, corticosteroids)
	Congenital adrenal hyperplasia
	Virilizing tumor
	Underlying endocrinopathy
Infant (6 wk to 1 y)	Infectious agents (eg, molluscum contagiosum)
	Periorificial dermatitis
	Keratosis pilaris
	Exogenous causes (eg, acne pomade, chloracne, steroid acne)
Mid-childhood (1-7 y)	Underlying hyperandrogenic state
	Flat warts
	Demodicosis
	Molluscum contagiosum
	Periorificial dermatitis
	Pityrosporum folliculitis
	Pseudoacne of the nasal crease
	Idiopathic facial aseptic granuloma
	Keratosis pilaris
Preadolescent (7-12 y)	Flat warts
	Demodicosis
	Molluscum contagiosum
	Periorificial dermatitis
	Pityrosporum folliculitis
	Pseudoacne of the nasal crease
	Idiopathic facial aseptic granuloma
	Keratosis pilaris
Adolescent (12-18 y)	Steroid acne
	Acne rosacea
	Perioral dermatitis

acneiform drug eruptions may also be seen in association with epidermal growth factor receptor inhibitors.

CAPSULE SUMMARY

ACNE VULGARIS

Acne vulgaris is a common chronic inflammatory disorder that may present at any age during childhood. The prevalence of this disease is highest in the adolescent population where up to 95% are reported to have some degree of acne. Histologically, these lesions represent inflammation of the components of the pilosebaceous units often with some degree of follicular plugging and bacterial overgrowth.

PERIORAL DERMATITIS

Definition and Epidemiology

Perioral dermatitis (POD) is a chronic inflammatory skin disorder characterized by erythema, papules, and pustules around the mouth, eyes, and nose. The variants of this condition include childhood granulomatous periorificial dermatitis, facial Afro-Caribbean eruption, and lupus miliaris disseminatus faciei.[94,95] Ninety percent of cases of POD have been described in young adult women.[94,95] However, an increasing number of cases are being described in children under the age of 5.

Etiology

Most cases of POD are idiopathic, and the exact mechanism of disease is not well understood. However, many cases have been reported shortly after the use of a potent topical steroid; a few have been reported after the use of systemic corticosteroids or in children with the use of inhaled corticosteroids with poor technique and resultant facial exposure to those steroids.[94]

Clinical Presentation

Clinically, patients present with a rosacea-like eruption consisting of erythema and small pink or skin-colored papules and pustules in the perioral, perinasal, and periocular distribution, most often with a rim of sparing just around the vermillion border (Figure 14-32).[94,95] The rash is usually asymptomatic, often present for weeks, months, or years. A minority of patients endorse pruritis, burning, and tenderness.

Histologic Findings

The histologic findings of POD are essentially identical to that of rosacea: perifollicular telangiectasia with a variable lymphocytic infiltrate consisting predominantly of lymphocytes and histiocytes with rare plasma cells (Figure 14-33).[94,95] Papules may occasionally histologically exhibit acanthosis or epidermal spongiosis. The lesions of childhood granulomatous periorificial dermatitis show caseating granulomas additionally.[94,95]

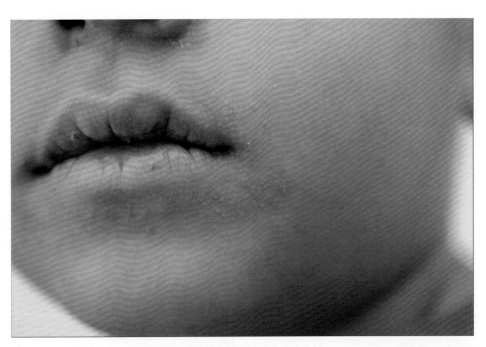

FIGURE 14-32. **Perioral dermatitis.** Small pink perioral papules and pustules. Courtesy of Barrett Zlotoff, MD, University of Virginia Health Sciences Center, Charlottesville, VA.

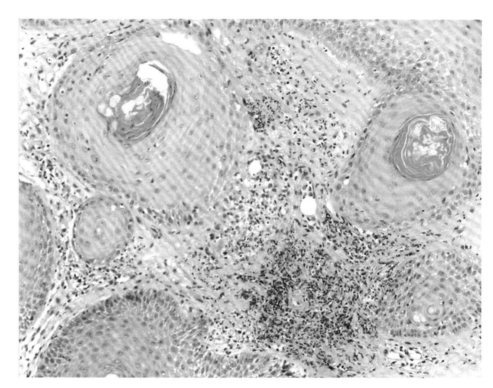

FIGURE 14-33. **Perioral dermatitis.** Histopathology: perifolliculitis, follicular spongiosis, epidermal spongiosis, and focal perifollicular telangiectatic vessels (×200).

Differential Diagnosis

Clinically, the differential diagnosis includes rosacea, allergic contact dermatitis, irritant contact dermatitis, seborrheic dermatitis, impetigo, dermatophytosis, and multiple angiofibromas. Histologic findings from a skin biopsy should clarify the diagnosis amid these entities. Histologic considerations are the same for rosacea, given the identical features in both entities.

CAPSULE SUMMARY

PERIORAL DERMATITIS

Periorificial dermatitis is an underdiagnosed chronic inflammatory disorder that often mimics rosacea in the pediatric population. Characteristically, it presents with papules, pustules, and erythema in perioral, perinasal, and periocular skin. Histologically, periorificial dermatitis resembles rosacea.

FOX-FORDYCE DISEASE

Definition and Epidemiology

Fox-Fordyce disease (FF), also known as apocrine miliaria, is a chronic rare dermatologic disorder characterized by inflammation of the apocrine duct and subsequent development of papules in apocrine gland–bearing skin sites.[96] The

frequency of FF in the pediatric population is unknown. This disorder is thought to occur very rarely in children.[96]

Etiology

The cause of this FF is still unknown. However, it is postulated that follicular occlusion of unclear etiology leads to the accumulation of apocrine gland secretion within the duct and gland, with subsequent secretion extravasation into the surrounding dermis.[96] This generates an inflammatory response within the dermis that is thought to cause the patient intense pruritus. Several isolated case reports and small case series report the occurrence of FF after laser hair removal and a variety of hormonal therapies.[97]

Clinical Presentation

Clinically, these patients present with firm painless follicularly based papules, often described as pruritic in the axillae, periareolar region, and anogenital region (Figure 14-34).[96] Less-described sites include lips, proximal thighs, umbilicus, perineum, and sternum.

Histologic Findings

Histologically, FF exhibits dilation of hair follicular infundibulum overlying the affected apocrine gland. There is spongiosis and hyperkeratosis of the follicular epithelium (Figure 14-35). Deeper in the biopsy, within the reticular dermis, there are often dilated apocrine glands and ducts

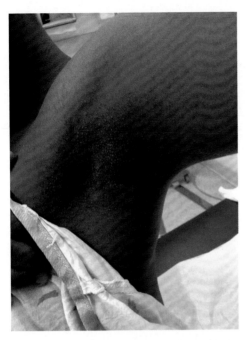

FIGURE 14-34. **Fox-Fordyce disease.** Follicularly based papules in the axillae. Clinical image (A) courtesy of Barrett Zlotoff, MD, University of Virginia Health Sciences Center, Charlottesville, VA.

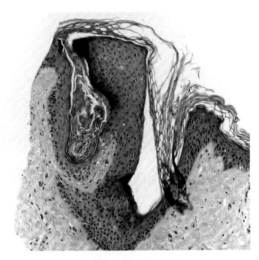

FIGURE 14-35. **Fox-Fordyce disease.** Histopathology: dilated infundibulum with follicular spongiosis and parakeratosis arranged in a column.

with associated periductular lymphohistiocytic inflammation and fibrosis.[96]

Differential Diagnosis

The clinical differential diagnosis for FF includes Graham-Little-Piccardi-Lasseur syndrome and trichostasis spinulosa.[96] Histologically, the differential diagnosis for FF includes other spongiotic dermatitides such as follicular atopic dermatitis, seborrheic dermatitis, and miliaria rubra.

CAPSULE SUMMARY

FOX-FORDYCE DISEASE

FF disease is a rare dermatologic disorder characterized by the presence of small firm pruritic follicularly based papules in the axillae, groin, and periareolar region. It is very rarely observed in the pediatric population. Histologically, there is spongiosis and hyperkeratosis of follicular epithelium with dilation and inflammation of apocrine glands and ducts.

HIDRADENITIS SUPPURATIVA

Definition and Epidemiology

Hidradenitis suppurativa (HS), also known as acne inversa, is a scarring chronic painful inflammatory skin disorder characterized by episodic inflammation of the sweat glands and associated structures in the skin. HS is less commonly

recognized in the pediatric population. Although it is estimated to affect up to 2% of children under the age of 18, studies show that many patients diagnosed in adulthood report the first onset of symptoms before the age of 13.[98] Consequently, it is suspected to be underdiagnosed in the pediatric population much like in the adult population.[99] Of the cases of childhood HS reported, approximately 30% present during adolescence and 7% before adolescence.[98] Notably, few cases report a link between the prepubertal onset of HS and premature adrenarche, adrenal hyperplasia, or metabolic syndrome.[98]

Etiology

Abnormalities in the pilosebaceous-apocrine unit could lead to follicular occlusion, which is considered an early pathogenic subclinical event. The abnormalities could include loss-of-function mutations in gamma-secretase genes, altered apocrine gland receptor sensitivity, variations in apocrine gland composition due to *ABCC11* polymorphisms, missing sweat gland proteins, and changes in the anatomy of the hair follicle infundibular region.

Although the true cause of HS is still not clearly understood, a well-supported hypothesis suggests follicular occlusion of a variety of proposed causes as a key inciting event to the pathogenesis of the disorder. As HS frequently manifests with cutaneous lesions affecting apocrine gland-rich skin, many experts hold the theory that this follicular occlusion results in the accumulation of apocrine secretions and the proliferation of entrapped microorganisms within the pilosebaceous unit.[98,100,101] These dilated follicles are thought to eventually rupture, spilling a slew of antigenic material (e.g, hair shaft, keratin, bacteria) into the dermis and inciting a dense inflammatory response that is difficult to contain. Multiple episodes are thought to lead

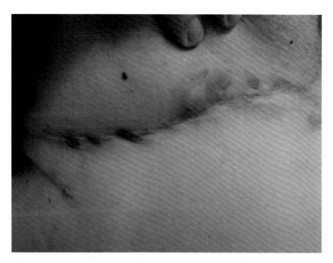

FIGURE 14-36. Hidradenitis suppurativa. Courtesy of Barrett Zlotoff, MD, University of Virginia Health Sciences Center, Charlottesville, VA.

to scarring of the affected skin, entrapment of lesional microorganisms, and subsequent impaired wound healing, thus perpetuating the cycle. Increasingly, alterations of the skin microbiota and biofilms are being implicated in disease pathogenesis and propagation. Obesity and metabolic syndrome have also been identified as risk factors for HS in the pediatric population.[100]

Clinical Presentation

Patients most often present with exquisitely painful comedones, cysts, inflammatory papules, pustules, nodules, plaques, abscesses, and draining sinus tracts and fistulas preferentially in intertriginous areas (Figure 14-36). Quality of life is often profoundly impaired in the pediatric population, as has been reported in the adult HS literature as well.[99] One recent study reported the presence of a psychiatric disorder in up to 23% of patients with childhood-onset HS by the age of 23.[99]

Histologic Findings

The histologic features of HS are comparable to those of acne. These include follicular hyperkeratosis, follicular hyperplasia, and follicular occlusion or plugging (Figure 14-37). There is almost always spongiosis of the follicular infundibulum as well as suppurative folliculitis and perifolliculitis. Keratin-filled cysts, either intact, or ruptured with concomitant granulomatous reaction and perifollicular fibrosis, are often present. Rarely, the presence of abnormal sinus tracts may be captured histologically: full thickness defects or channels within the dermis with a moderately dense mixed inflammatory cell infiltrate and dermal fibrosis. Sebaceous gland involution and apocrine gland hyperplasia may also be present. Of note, the components of the inflammatory infiltrate varies largely by the age and stage of the lesion sampled.

Differential Diagnosis

Appropriate/accurate diagnosis of HS may not occur for 7 to 14 years after the onset of symptoms.[98,99] Cases of childhood onset are thought to be particularly underdiagnosed. The clinical differential diagnosis includes acne vulgaris,

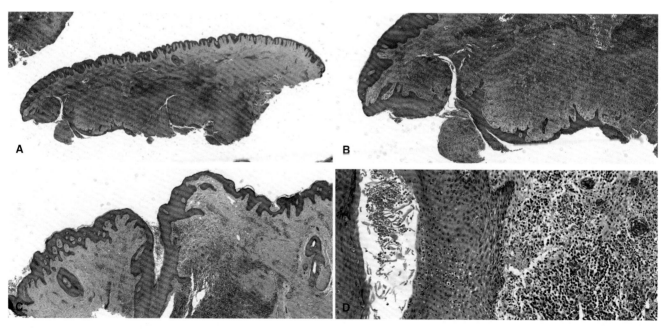

FIGURE 14-37. A skin biopsy shows marked dermal inflammation and a sinus tract (A and B). A closer inspection shows areas of folliculitis, follicular hyperkeratosism and a brisk perifollicular lymphoplasmacytic infiltrate (C and D).

CAPSULE SUMMARY

HIDRADENITIS SUPPURATIVA

HS is a chronic inflammatory disorder of the sweat glands characterized by painful nodules, inflammatory papules, and plaques in intertriginous areas. It is thought to be underdiagnosed in children, much like in adults. Of the children with childhood-onset HS, 30% presented during their teenage years. Biopsy often demonstrates dense perifollicular and periadnexal inflammation consisting of varying proportions of neutrophil, lymphocytes, histiocytes, multinucleated giant cells, and plasma cells based on the age and stage of the lesion sampled.

folliculitis, carbuncles, furuncles, granuloma inguinale, and lymphogranuloma venereum. The histologic differential diagnosis involves acneiform lesions that histologically can look identical to HS.

MILIARIA

Definition and Epidemiology

Miliaria is a common skin disorder in children caused by an obstruction of the eccrine duct. It exists on clinical spectrum that is largely based on the site of obstruction within the eccrine sweat apparatus within the skin (eg, miliaria crystallina, miliaria rubra, and miliaria pustulosa).[102,103]

Miliaria is common in children. It is estimated to affect up to 40% of infants and often presents within the first month of life.[103]

Etiology

Miliaria crystallina is thought to result from premature superficial eccrine acrosyringial blockage within the level of the epidermis.[102,103] Miliaria rubra is caused by blockage of the eccrine duct within the level of the mid-epidermis. Miliaria pustulosis is caused by an obstruction of the apparatus within the level of the dermis.

Clinical Presentation

Clinically, the physical exam findings of miliaria are dependent on the level of obstruction of the duct within the skin. In miliaria crystallina, as the obstruction is superficial, small, clear thin-walled vesicles are present on the head and neck as well as trunk (Figure 14-38). These vesicles frequently rupture, leaving a collarette of scale but no erythema.[103] Miliaria rubra, also known as "heat rash," presents with small erythematous papules, some of which harbor intact microvesicles.[103] Lastly, miliaria pustulosis presents with pustules present on covered portions of skin.

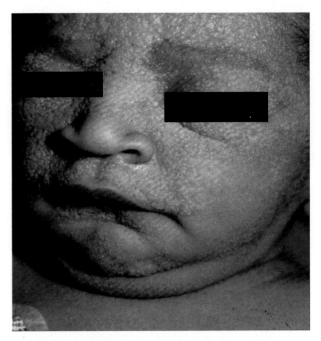

FIGURE 14-38. **Miliaria crystallina.** Numerous small clear thin-walled fluid-filled vesicles. Courtesy of Barrett Zlotoff, MD, University of Virginia Health Sciences Center, Charlottesville, VA.

Histologic Findings

Histologically, skin biopsies of the lesions in miliaria crystallina show a pauciinflammatory subcorneal vesicle overlying the acrosyringium of the blocked eccrine duct (Figure 14-39).[102,103] In miliaria rubra, there is often the additional finding of spongiosis of the affected acrosyringium. Subcorneal neutrophils and lymphocytes may also be present. Lastly, miliaria pustulosis may show more prominent features of the latter two, with several intraepidermal microabscesses all overlying the affected eccrine duct acrosyringium.

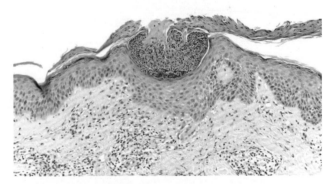

FIGURE 14-39. **Miliaria pustulosis.** Histopathology: intraepidermal pustule present above the eccrine duct (×100).

Differential Diagnosis

The clinical differential diagnosis for miliaria includes milia, acne neonatorum, and transient neonatal pustular melanosis.[103] Histologically, lesions of miliaria should be distinguished from other follicular-occlusive inflammatory disorders such as acne neonatorum, HS, and suppurative folliculitis. Rarely, in miliaria crystallina, a primary immunobullous disorder may be considered; however, the latter are exceedingly rare in very young children.

CAPSULE SUMMARY

MILIARIA

Miliaria is a very common disorder of occlusion of the eccrine duct acrosyringium. It affects up to 40% of infants and may be confused with milia, acne neonatorum, and folliculitis both clinically and histologically.

RELAPSING POLYCHONDRITIS

Definition and Epidemiology

Relapsing polychondritis is a rare autoimmune connective tissue disorder characterized by an inflammation of hyaline, elastic, and fibrous cartilaginous tissue; it is frequently associated with multiorgan dysfunction, including dermatologic manifestations.[104] Although more common in adults aged 30 to 50 years old, relapsing polychondritis has been described in a limited number of small case series in the pediatric population.[105,106] In children, it is believed to affect females more than males and present over a wide range of ages, from age 1 to 17.

Etiology

The exact cause of relapsing polychondritis is unknown. It is, however, postulated that this disorder arises as a result of CD4+ T-cell and collagen II antibody–mediated destruction of proteoglycan-rich tissue located not only in cartilage but also in the inner and outer ear, eyes, heart, and blood vessels. Pediatric cases are reported to have an increased incidence of having a personal (concurrent) or a family history of autoimmune disease. Reported associated syndromes include retroperitoneal fibrosis, Goodpasture syndrome, Henoch-Schönlein purpura, psoriasis, Takayasu arteritis, common variable immunodeficiency, and Sjögren syndrome.[104-107]

Clinical Presentation

One-third of adult patients with relapsing polychondritis present with chondritis as the sentinel symptom. However, children usually present with arthritis (36%), auricular chondritis (27%), respiratory tract chondritis (25%), and ocular inflammation (50%).[105,106] Pediatric patients are also reported to have a higher incidence of laryngotracheal involvement. This differs from the adult patients who have been reported to have ear involvement in 78% of cases, nasal chondritis in 39%, airway in 50%, eye in 46%, ear in 27%, and cardiac in 7%.

The arthritis of relapsing polychondritis is often episodic, asymmetric, peripheral, and nonerosive. The segments of skin overlying the affected sites are often tender, swollen, and erythematous. Notably, the ear lobe, containing no cartilage, is often spared in the inflammatory process.

Histologic Findings

Histologically, sampled cartilaginous tissue shows a loss of basophilic staining of cartilaginous matrix with vacuolated chondrocytes with pyknotic nuclei, perichondrial inflammation consisting of lymphocytes, histiocytes, and plasma cells, and replacement of cartilaginous tissue by fibrous tissue.[105,106] Although these findings are nonspecific per se, they appear to be fairly reproducible in this patient population. Some biopsies yield only granulation tissue.

Differential Diagnosis

Clinical differential diagnosis for relapsing polychondritis includes inflammatory arthritis and autoimmune disorders affecting the joints such as rheumatoid arthritis. Histologically, the findings are somewhat nonspecific and may be seen in the clinical setting of localized trauma of a variety of etiologies.

CAPSULE SUMMARY

RELAPSING POLYCHONDRITIS

Relapsing polychondritis is a rare autoimmune disorder characterized by asymmetric arthritis and ear chondritis in the pediatric population. There is a higher incidence of respiratory tract chondritis in cases of childhood onset. Unlike adults, children less often have other associated autoimmune diseases. The histologic features include altered cartilage, perichondral inflammation, granulation tissue, and fibrosis.

REFERENCES

Trichorrhexis nodosa

1. Rogers M. Hair shaft abnormalities: Part I. *Australas J Dermatol.* 1995;36:179-184; quiz 185-176.
2. Mirmirani P. Ceramic flat irons: improper use leading to acquired trichorrhexis nodosa. *J Am Acad Dermatol.* 2010;62:145-147.
3. Fichtel JC, Richards JA, Davis LS. Trichorrhexis nodosa secondary to argininosuccinicaciduria. *Pediatr Dermatol.* 2007;24:25-27.

Monilethrix

1. Bentley-Phillips B, Bayles MA. A previously undescribed hereditary hair anomaly (pseudo-monilethrix). *Br J Dermatol.* 1973;89:159-167.
2. Winter H, Clark RD, Tarras-Wahlberg C, Rogers MA, Schweizer J. Monilethrix: a novel mutation (Glu402Lys) in the helix termination motif and the first causative mutation (Asn114Asp) in the helix initiation motif of the type II hair keratin hHb6. *J Invest Dermatol.* 1999;113:263-266.
3. Healy E, Holmes SC, Belgaid CE, et al. A gene for monilethrix is closely linked to the type II keratin gene cluster at 12q13. *Hum Mol Genet.* 1995;4:2399-2402.
4. Birch-Machin MA, Healy E, Turner R, et al. Mapping of monilethrix to the type II keratin gene cluster at chromosome 12q13 in three new families, including one with variable expressivity. *Br J Dermatol.* 1997;137:339-343.
5. Schweizer J, Langbein L, Rogers MA, Winter H. Hair follicle-specific keratins and their diseases. *Exp Cell Res.* 2007;313:2010-2020.
6. Winter H, Labreze C, Chapalain V, et al. A variable monilethrix phenotype associated with a novel mutation, Glu402Lys, in the helix termination motif of the type II hair keratin hHb1. *J Invest Dermatol.* 1998;111:169-172.
7. Schaffer JV, Bazzi H, Vitebsky A, et al. Mutations in the desmoglein 4 gene underlie localized autosomal recessive hypotrichosis with monilethrix hairs and congenital scalp erosions. *J Invest Dermatol.* 2006;126:1286-1291.
8. Zlotogorski A, Marek D, Horev L, et al. An autosomal recessive form of monilethrix is caused by mutations in DSG4: clinical overlap with localized autosomal recessive hypotrichosis. *J Invest Dermatol.* 2006;126:1292-1296.
9. Summerly R, Donaldson EM. Monilethrix. A family study. *Br J Dermatol.* 1962;74:387-391.
10. Karincaoglu Y, Coskun BK, Seyhan ME, Bayram N. Monilethrix: improvement with acitretin. *Am J Clin Dermatol.* 2005;6:407-410.

Trichorrhexis Invaginata

1. Chavanas S, Bodemer C, Rochat A, et al. Mutations in SPINK5, encoding a serine protease inhibitor, cause Netherton syndrome. *Nat Genet.* 2000;25:141-142.
2. Chavanas S, Garner C, Bodemer C, et al. Localization of the Netherton syndrome gene to chromosome 5q32, by linkage analysis and homozygosity mapping. *Am J Hum Genet.* 2000;66:914-921.
3. Ong C, O'Toole EA, Ghali L, et al. LEKTI demonstrable by immunohistochemistry of the skin: a potential diagnostic skin test for Netherton syndrome. *Br J Dermatol.* 2004;151:1253-1257.
4. Bitoun E, Micheloni A, Lamant L, et al. LEKTI proteolytic processing in human primary keratinocytes, tissue distribution and defective expression in Netherton syndrome. *Hum Mol Genet.* 2003;12:2417-2430.
5. Greene SL, Muller SA. Netherton's syndrome. Report of a case and review of the literature. *J Am Acad Dermatol.* 1985;13:329-337.
6. Pruszkowski A, Bodemer C, Fraitag S, Teillac-Hamel D, Amoric JC, de Prost Y. Neonatal and infantile erythrodermas: a retrospective study of 51 patients. *Arch Dermatol.* 2000;136:875-880.
7. Sun JD, Linden KG. Netherton syndrome: a case report and review of the literature. *Int J Dermatol.* 2006;45:693-697.
8. Altman J, Stroud J. Netherton's disease and ichthyosis linearis circumflexa. *Arch Dermatol.* 1969;100:248-249.
9. Powell J, Dawber RP, Ferguson DJ, Griffiths WA. Netherton's syndrome: increased likelihood of diagnosis by examining eyebrow hairs. *Br J Dermatol.* 1999;141:544-546.
10. Netherton EW. A unique case of trichorrhexis nodosa;bamboo hairs. *AMA Arch Derm.* 1958;78:483-487.

Pili Torti

1. Hinson JT, Fantin VR, Schonberger J, et al. Missense mutations in the BCS1L gene as a cause of the Bjornstad syndrome. *N Engl J Med.* 2007;356:809-819.
2. Moller LB, Mogensen M, Horn N. Molecular diagnosis of Menkes disease: genotype-phenotype correlation. *Biochimie.* 2009;91:1273-1277.
3. Tang J, Donsante A, Desai V, Patronas N, Kaler SG. Clinical outcomes in Menkes disease patients with a copper-responsive ATP7A mutation, G727R. *Mol Genet Metab.* 2008;95:174-181.
4. Park HD, Moon HK, Lee J, et al. A novel ATP7A gross deletion mutation in a Korean patient with Menkes disease. *Ann Clin Lab Sci.* 2009;39:188 191.
5. Bertini I, Rosato A. Menkes disease. *Cell Mol Life Sci.* 2008;65:89-91.
6. de Bie P, Muller P, Wijmenga C, Klomp LW. Molecular pathogenesis of Wilson and Menkes disease: correlation of mutations with molecular defects and disease phenotypes. *J Med Genet.* 2007;44:673-688.
7. Ambrosini L, Mercer JF. Defective copper-induced trafficking and localization of the Menkes protein in patients with mild and copper-treated classical Menkes disease. *Hum Mol Genet.* 1999;8:1547-1555.
8. Lubianca Neto JF, Lu L, Eavey RD, et al. The Bjornstad syndrome (sensorineural hearing loss and pili torti) disease gene maps to chromosome 2q34-36. *Am J Hum Genet.* 1998;62:1107-1112.
9. Koster MI. p63 in skin development and ectodermal dysplasias. *J Invest Dermatol.* 2010;130(10):2352-2358.
10. Hart DB. Menkes' syndrome: an updated review. *J Am Acad Dermatol.* 1983;9:145-152.
11. Robinson GC, Johnston MM. Pili torti and sensory neural hearing loss. *J Pediatr.* 1967;70:621-623.
12. Knaudt B, Volz T, Krug M, et al. Skin symptoms in four ectodermal dysplasia syndromes including two case reports of Rapp-Hodgkin-Syndrome. *Eur J Dermatol.* 2012;22(5):605-613.

Pili Bifurcati

1. Weary PE, Hendricks AA, Wawner F, Ajgaonkar G. Pili bifurcati: a new anomaly of hair growth. *Arch Dermatol.* 1973;108:403-407.
2. Camacho FM, Happle R, Tosti A, Whiting D. The different faces of pili bifurcati. A review. *Eur J Dermatol.* 2000;10(5):337-340.
3. Echeverría XP, Romero WA, Carreño NR, Zegpi MS, González SJ. Hair shaft abnormalities. Pili bifurcati: a scanning electron microscopy analysis. *Pediatr Dermatol.* 2009;26(2):169-170.

Trichothiodystrophy

1. Itin PH, Sarasin A, Pittelkow MR. Trichothiodystrophy: update on the sulfur-deficient brittle hair syndromes. *J Am Acad Dermatol.* 2001;44:891-920;quiz 921-894.
2. Price VH, Odom RB, Ward WH, Jones FT. Trichothiodystrophy: sulfur-deficient brittle hair as a marker for a neuroectodermal symptom complex. *Arch Dermatol.* 1980;116:1375-1384.
3. Liang C, Morris A, Schlucker S, et al. Structural and molecular hair abnormalities in trichothiodystrophy. *J Invest Dermatol.* 2006;126:2210-2216.
4. Dawber RP. An update of hair shaft disorders. *Dermatol Clin.* 1996;14:753-772.
5. Sperling LC, DiGiovanna JJ. "Curly" wood and tiger tails: an explanation for light and dark banding with polarization in trichothiodystrophy. *Arch Dermatol.* 2003;139:1189-1192.

Marie-Unna Hereditary Hypotrichosis

1. Wen Y, Liu Y, Xu Y, et al. Loss-of-function mutations of an inhibitory upstream ORF in the human hairless transcript cause Marie Unna hereditary hypotrichosis. *Nat Genet.* 2009;41(2):228-233.

2. Zhang X, Guo BR, Cai LQ, et al. Exome sequencing identified a missense mutation of EPS8L3 in Marie Unna hereditary hypotrichosis. *J Med Genet.* 2012;49(12):727-730.

3. Unna M. Uber hypotrichosis congenita. *Derm Wochenschr.* 1925;81:1167-1178.

4. Argenziano G, Sammarco E, Rossi A, Delfino M, Calvieri S. Marie Unna hereditary hypotrichosis. *Eur J Dermatol.* 1999;9(4):278-280.

5. Podjasek JO, Hand JL. Marie-Unna hereditary hypotrichosis: case report and review of the literature. *Pediatr Dermatol.* 2011;28(2):202-204.

6. Roberts JL, Whiting DA, Henry D, Basler G, Woolf L. Marie Unna congenital hypotrichosis: clinical description, histopathology, scanning electron microscopy of a previously unreported large pedigree. *J Investig Dermatol Symp Proc.* 1999;4(3):261-267.

Pili Annulati

1. Green J, Fitzpatrick E, de Berker D, Forrest SM, Sinclair RD. A gene for pili annulati maps to the telomeric region of chromosome 12q. *J Invest Dermatol.* 2004;123:1070-1072.

2. Giehl KA, Ferguson DJ, Dean D, et al. Alterations in the basement membrane zone in pili annulati hair follicles as demonstrated by electron microscopy and immunohistochemistry. *Br J Dermatol.* 2004;150:722-727.

3. Cady L, Trotter, M. A study of ringed hair. *Arch of Derm Syph.* 1922;6:301-317.

4. Giehl KA, Ferguson DJ, Dawber RP, Pittelkow MR, Foehles J, de Berker DA. Update on detection, morphology and fragility in pili annulati in three kindreds. *J Eur Acad Dermatol Venereol.* 2004;18:654-658.

5. Price VH, Thomas RS, Jones FT. Pili annulati. Optical and electron microscopic studies. *Arch Dermatol.* 1968;98:640-647.

6. Gummer CL, Dawber RP. Pili annulati: electron histochemical studies on affected hairs. *Br J Dermatol.* 1981;105:303-309.

Wooly Hair

1. Shimomura Y, Garzon MC, Kristal L, Shapiro L, Christiano AM. Autosomal recessive woolly hair with hypotrichosis caused by a novel homozygous mutation in the P2RY5 gene. *Exp Dermatol.* 2009;18:218-221.

2. Pasternack SM, Murugusundram S, Eigelshoven S, et al. Novel mutations in the P2RY5 gene in one Turkish and two Indian patients presenting with hypotrichosis and woolly hair. *Arch Dermatol Res.* 2009;301:621-624.

3. Shimomura Y, Wajid M, Zlotogorski A, Lee YJ, Rice RH, Christiano AM. Founder mutations in the lipase h gene in families with autosomal recessive woolly hair/hypotrichosis. *J Invest Dermatol.* 2009;129:1927-1934.

4. Shimomura Y, Wajid M, Ishii Y, et al. Disruption of P2RY5, an orphan G protein-coupled receptor, underlies autosomal recessive woolly hair. *Nat Genet.* 2008;40:335-339.

5. Levinsohn JL, Teng J, Craiglow BG, et al. Somatic HRAS p. G12S mutation causes woolly hair and epidermal nevi. *J Invest Dermatol.* 2014;134(4):1149-1152.

6. Lantis SD, Pepper MC. Woolly hair nevus. Two case reports and a discussion of unruly hair forms. *Arch Dermatol.* 1978;114:233-238.

7. Ormerod AD, Main RA, Ryder ML, Gregory DW. A family with diffuse partial woolly hair. *Br J Dermatol.* 1987;116:401-405.

8. Tosti A, Misciali C, Piraccini BA, Fanti PA, Barbareschi M, Ferretti RM. Woolly hair, palmoplantar keratoderma, and cardiac abnormalities: report of a family. *Arch Dermatol.* 1994;130:522-524.

9. McHenry PM, Nevin NC, Bingham EA. The association of keratosis pilaris atrophicans with hereditary woolly hair. *Pediatr Dermatol.* 1990;7:202-204.

10. Neild VS, Pegum JS, Wells RS. The association of keratosis pilaris atrophicans and woolly hair, with and without Noonan's syndrome. *Br J Dermatol.* 1984;110:357-362.

11. Carvajal-Huerta L. Epidermolytic palmoplantar keratoderma with woolly hair and dilated cardiomyopathy. *J Am Acad Dermatol.* 1998;39:418-421.

12. Roberts A, Allanson J, Jadico SK, et al. The cardiofaciocutaneous syndrome. *J Med Genet.* 2006;43:833-842.

13. Chien AJ, Valentine MC, Sybert VP. Hereditary woolly hair and keratosis pilaris. *J Am Acad Dermatol.* 2006;54:S35-39.

14. Lacarrubba F, Dall'Oglio F, Rossi A, Schwartz RA, Micali G. Familial keratosis follicularis spinulosa decalvans associated with woolly hair. *Int J Dermatol.* 2007;46:840-843.

15. Djabali K, Martinez-Mir A, Horev L, Christiano AM, Zlotogorski A. Evidence for extensive locus heterogeneity in Naxos disease. *J Invest Dermatol.* 2002;118:557-560.

16. Gregoriou S, Kontochristopoulos G, Chatziolou E, Rigopoulos D. Palmoplantar keratoderma, woolly hair and arrhythmogenic right ventricular cardiomyopathy. *Clin Exp Dermatol.* 2006;31:315-316.

17. Protonotarios N, Tsatsopoulou A. Naxos disease and Carvajal syndrome: cardiocutaneous disorders that highlight the pathogenesis and broaden the spectrum of arrhythmogenic right ventricular cardiomyopathy. *Cardiovasc Pathol.* 2004;13:185-194.

Acquired Progressive Kinking of the Hair

1. Wise F, Sulzberger MB. Acquired progressive kinking of the scalp hair accompanied by changes in its pigmentation: correlation of an unidentified group of cases presenting circumscribed areas of kinky hair. *Arch Dermatol.* 1932;25:99.

2. Rebora A, Guarrera M. Acquired progressive kinking of the hair. *J Am Acad Dermatol.* 1985;12(5 Pt 2):933-936.

3. Mortimer PS, Gummer C, English J, Dawber RP. Acquired progressive kinking of hair. Report of six cases and review of literature. *Arch Dermatol.* 1985;121(8):1031-1033.

4. Tosti A, Piraccini BM, Pazzaglia M, Misciali C. Acquired progressive kinking of the hair: clinical features, pathological study, and follow-up of 7 patients. *Arch Dermatol.* 1999;135(10):1223-1226.

5. Tran JT, Lucky AW, Subramaniam S. What syndrome is this? Acquired progressive kinking of the hair. *Pediatr Dermatol.* 2004;21(3):265-268.

Uncombable Hair Syndrome

1. Ü Basmanav FB, Cau L, Tafazolli A, Mechin MC, et al. Mutations in three genes encoding proteins involved in hair shaft formation causes uncombable hair syndrome. *Am J Hum Genet.* 2016;99(6):1292-1304.

2. Kuhn CA, Helm TN, Bergfeld WF, McMahon JT. Acquired uncombable hair. *Arch Dermatol.* 1993;129:1061-1062.

3. Shelley WB, Shelley ED. Uncombable hair syndrome: observations on response to biotin and occurrence in siblings with ectodermal dysplasia. *J Am Acad Dermatol.* 1985;13:97-102.

4. Jarell AD, Hall MA, Sperling LC. Uncombable hair syndrome. *Pediatr Dermatol.* 2007;24:436-438.

Loose Anagen Syndrome

1. Swink SM, Castelo-Soccio L. Loose anagen syndrome: a retrospective chart review of 37 cases. *Pediatr Dermatol.* 2016;33(5):507-510. doi:10.1111/pde.12912

2. Agi C, Cohen B. A case of loose anagen syndrome in an African American girl. *Pediatr Dermatol.* 2015;32(3):e128-e129. doi:10.1111/pde.12554

3. Mirmirani P, Uno H, Price VH. Abnormal inner root sheath of the hair follicle in the loose anagen hair syndrome: an ultrastructural study. *J Am Acad Dermatol.* 2011;64(1):129-134.

Congenital Temporal Alopecia

1. Sperling L. Chapter 14, Temporal triangular alopecia. In: *An Atlas of Hair Pathology With Clinical Correlations*. 2nd ed. London, UK: Informa Healthcare; 2012:75-78.

Keratosis Pilaris

1. Metze D. Chapter 3, Disorders of keratinization. In: *McKee's Pathology of the Skin*. 4th ed. Philadelphia, PA: Elsevier Saunders; 2012:46-96.

Disorders of the nail

1. Chu DH, Rubin AI. Diagnosis and management of nail disorders in children. *Pediatr Clin North Am*. 2014;61(2):293-308. doi:10.1016/j.pcl.2013.11.005
2. Goettmann-Bonvallot S, André J, Belaich S. Longitudinal melanonychia in children: a clinical and histopathologic study of 40 cases. *J Am Acad Dermatol*. 1999;41(1):17-22.
3. Rubin B. Chapter18, Neoplastic and non-neoplastic disorders of the nail apparatus. In: *Dermatopathology*. 2nd ed. Philadelphia, PA: Elsevier Saunders; 2016:691-718.
4. Haneke E. Chapter 15, Melanocytic lesions. In: *Histopathology of the nail: onychopathology*. 1st ed. Boca Raton, FL: CRC Press; Taylor & Francis Group; 2017:263-273.

Acne Vulgaris

1. Maroñas-Jiménez L, Krakowski AC. Pediatric acne: clinical patterns and pearls. *Dermatol Clin*. 2016;34(2):195-202. doi:10.1016/j.det.2015.11.006.
2. Bhate K, Williams HC. Epidemiology of acne vulgaris. *Br J Dermatol*. 2013;168(3):474-485. doi:10.1111/bjd.12149.
3. Fung M. Chapter1, Inflammatory diseases of the dermis and epidermis. In: *Dermatopathology*. 2nd ed. Philadelphia, PA: Elsevier Saunders; 2016:11-78.

Perioral Dermatitis

1. Goel NS, Burkhart CN, Morrell DS. Pediatric periorificial dermatitis: clinical course and treatment outcomes in 222 patients. *Pediatr Dermatol*. 2015;32(3):333-336. doi:10.1111/pde.12534.
2. Kellen R, Silverberg NB. Pediatric periorificial dermatitis. *Cutis*. 2017;100(6):385-388.

Fox-Fordyce Disease

1. Blasco-Morente G, Naranjo-Díaz MJ, Pérez-López I, Martínez-López A, Ruiz-Villaverde R, Aneiros-Fernández J. Fox-fordyce disease. *Sultan Qaboos Univ Med J*. 2016;16(1):e119-e1120. doi:10.18295/squmj.2016.16.01.025.

2. Tetzlaff MT, Evans K, DeHoratius DM, Weiss R, Cotsarelis G, Elenitsas R. Fox-fordyce disease following axillary laser hair removal. *Arch Dermatol*. 2011;147(5):573-576. doi:10.1001/archdermatol.2011.103.

Hidradenitis Suppurativa

1. Mehdizadeh A, Alavi A, Alhusayen R, et al. Proceeding report of the Symposium on Hidradenitis Suppurativa Advances (SHSA). *Exp Dermatol*. 2018;27(1):104-112. doi:10.1111/exd.13445.
2. Tiri H, Jokelainen J, Timonen M, Tasanen K, Huilaja L. Somatic and psychiatric comorbidities of hidradenitis suppurativa in children and adolescents. *J Am Acad Dermatol*. 2018; pii: S0190-9622(18)30353-0. doi:10.1016/j.jaad.2018.02.067.
3. Pink A, Anzengruber F, Navarini AA. Acne and hidradenitis suppurativa. *Br J Dermatol*. 2018;178(3):619-631. doi:10.1111/bjd.16231.
4. Shah N. Hidradenitis suppurativa: a treatment challenge. *Am Fam Physician*. 2005;72(8):1547-1552.

Miliaria

1. Junkins-Hopkins J, Busam K. Chapter 5, Blistering skin diseases. In: *Dermatopathology*. 2nd ed. Philadelphia, PA: Elsevier Saunders; 2016:207-248.
2. O'Connor NR, McLaughlin MR, Ham P. Newborn skin: Part I. Common rashes. *Am Fam Physician*. 2008;77(1):47-52.

Relapsing polychondritis

1. Matsuo H, Asahina A, Fukuda T, Umezawa Y, Nakagawa H. Relapsing polychondritis associated with psoriasis vulgaris successfully treated with adalimumab: a case report with published work review. *J Dermatol*. 2017;44(7):826-829. doi:10.1111/1346-8138.13796.
2. Fonseca AR, de Oliveira SK, Rodrigues MC, Aymoré IL, Domingues RC, Sztajnbok FR. Relapsing polychondritis in childhood: three case reports, comparison with adulthood disease and literature review. *Rheumatol Int*. 2013;33(7):1873-8. doi:10.1007/s00296-011-2336-6.
3. Xiao J, Liu WJ, Song HM, Wei M, You X, Jiang Y. Relapsing polychondritis in childhood: report of three cases and review of the literature. *Zhonghua Er Ke Za Zhi*. 2009;47(11):814-819.
4. Karaca NE, Aksu G, Yildiz B, et al. Relapsing polychondritis in a child with common variable immunodeficiency. *Int J Dermatol*. 2009;48(5):525-528. doi:10.1111/j.1365-4632.2009.03809.x.

Cutaneous Mucinosis, Deposits, and Cysts

15

Shivani S. Patel / Anna L. Grossberg / Mark R. Wick

Deposition Disorders of the Skin

Several cutaneous deposition disorders may affect children. These can be grouped into conditions that feature excess stromal mucin or mucopolysaccharide in the corium, forms of amyloidosis, and deposits of minerals or mineral salts.

Mucin Deposition Disorders and Mucopolysaccharidoses

MYXEDEMA AND PRETIBIAL MYXEDEMA

Etiology, Definition and Epidemiology

Myxedema and pretibial myxedema are both rare in children. The former is associated with congenital hypothyroidism, which has largely been eliminated as a medical problem in the modern world because of common screening studies for thyroid function in newborns. Pretibial myxedema is a thyroid dermopathy characteristic of Graves' disease.

The incidence is 1 per 100 000 and occurs in approximately 4% of patients with Graves' disease.[1] There is a female predominance. Pretibial myxedema is rare in children but has been reported in adolescents.

Clinical Presentation and Pathogenesis

Myxedema classically presents on the shins, but has also been reported on the arms, shoulders, and upper back at the sites of trauma.[1,2] There is usually symmetric, nonpitting edema resembling an orange peel both in appearance and texture because of hair follicle accentuation (Figures 15-1 and 15-2).

Up to 40% of patients will also develop overlying erythematous or skin-colored plaques and nodules. There is usually no associated pain or pruritus.[1] This manifestation usually appears 1 to 2 years after a diagnosis of Graves' disease and is more common in patients with associated ophthalmopathy.

Pathophysiology is poorly understood but may involve an overexpression of the thyrotropin receptor serving as a nonspecific antigen on fibroblasts, leading to Interleukin-1 and transforming growth factor-beta release. Cytokine production then stimulates a synthesis of glycosaminoglycans by dermal fibroblasts.[1-3] The skin becomes thickened and "doughy" because of this excess production of stromal mucin by dermal fibroblasts. Studies also demonstrate an

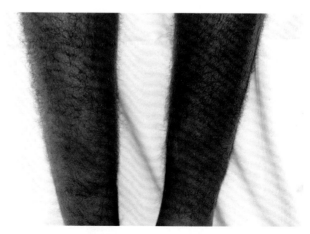

FIGURE 15-1. Pretibial myxedema of the shins in a young boy with thyroid disease.

357

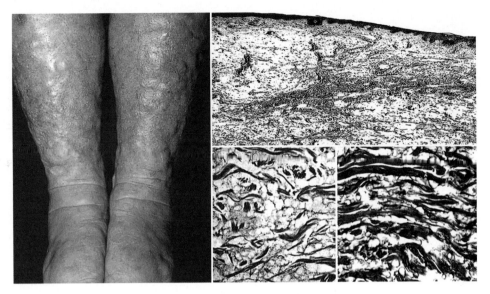

FIGURE 15-2. This adolescent girl with thyroid disease has irregular thickening of the pretibial skin (left panel). A skin biopsy shows a diffuse deposition of stromal mucin in the dermal interstitium (top right and first bottom right panels). It labels with the colloidal iron stain (second bottom right panel).

upregulation of insulin-like growth factor (IGF-1), leading to fibroblast activation and T-cell response in the dermis. Pretibial myxedema has been reported in skin harvested from other sites and grafted to the legs, suggesting a role for dependent position and mechanical stress.[3]

With treatment of thyroid disease, pretibial myxedema has the potential to self-involute, with 70% of mild cases resolving after 25 years.[3]

Histologic Findings and Differential Diagnosis

One sees spaces between dermal collagen bundles, containing the mucinous deposits in the interstitium of the corium. This change may be subtle, especially in myxedema. The mucin is labeled with the colloidal iron or alcian blue techniques (Figure 15-3), and a diminution in the number of dermal elastic fibers may also be apparent with the Verhoeff-Van Gieson stain. There is no cellular proliferation in either myxedema or pretibial myxedema.

Diagnosis is usually made with an evidence of characteristic skin lesions, a history of Graves' disease, and the presence of Graves' ophthalmopathy. Serological testing and skin biopsy can aid in diagnosis.

CAPSULE SUMMARY

MYXEDEMA AND PRETIBIAL MYXEDEMA

Myxedema and pretibial myxedema are both rare in children. The former is associated with congenital hypothyroidism. Pretibial myxedema is a thyroid dermopathy characteristic of Graves' disease. Histologically, one sees spaces between dermal collagen bundles, containing the mucinous deposits in the interstitium of the corium. This change may be subtle, especially in myxedema. The mucin is labeled with the colloidal iron or alcian blue techniques.

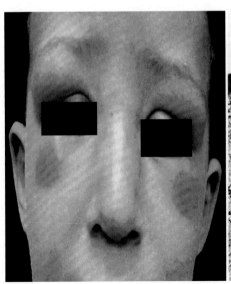

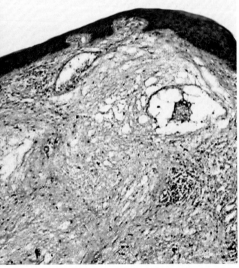

FIGURE 15-3. Self-healing mucinosis of the face in a young body, represented by periorbital swelling and erythema. Histologically, this process features a diffuse deposition of stromal mucin in the dermis, with the formation of mucin "pools."

CUTANEOUS MUCINOSIS OF INFANCY

Definition, Epidemiology, and Etiology

Cutaneous mucinosis of infancy (CMI) is a rare localized variant of cutaneous mucinoses with less than 10 reported cases. It was initially recognized in 1980 and often considered a variant of papular mucinosis.[4,5] Etiology is unknown with pathogenesis likely involving fibroblast overstimulation.[4]

Clinical Presentation and Pathogenesis

CMI is characterized by firm, skin-colored to opalescent papules in a grouped, linear, or generalized distribution. The most commonly affected sites are the upper extremities, thighs, and trunk. The disorder usually presents at birth or shortly after and there is a slight female predominance.[4,6] There is no systemic involvement with localized forms unlike other variants that may have associated thyroid abnormalities or paraproteinemias.[7] The disease often has a persistent and gradual progression without tendency for self-involution. The distribution and the young age of affected individuals may raise the possibility that such lesions are connective tissue nevi of the proteoglycan type (nevus mucinosus).

Histologic Findings

One typically sees mucin in the papillary dermis with no fibroblastic proliferation and scant dermal perivascular chronic inflammatory cells. However, rare cases have histologic features that are reminiscent of adult scleromyxedema of the lichen myxedematosus type.

CAPSULE SUMMARY

CUTANEOUS MUCINOSIS OF INFANCY

CMI is a rare localized variant of cutaneous mucinoses with less than 10 reported cases. CMI is characterized by firm, skin-colored to opalescent papules in a grouped, linear, or generalized distribution. Histologically, there is mucin in the papillary dermis with no fibroblastic proliferation, and scant dermal perivascular chronic inflammatory cells.

SELF-HEALING JUVENILE CUTANEOUS MUCINOSIS

Definition, Epidemiology, and Etiology

Self-healing juvenile cutaneous mucinosis (SHJCM) is a form of localized primary cutaneous mucinosis.[8] SHJCM is a rare disorder with less than 10 reported cases in the literature.[9] The most common age of onset is between 5 and 15, although one reported case occurred in an infant less than

14 months of age.[8] The etiology is unclear, but the proposed mechanism involves fibroblast stimulation by nonspecific antigens, including reports of SHJCM developing after viral illness, Bartonella exposure, and chemotherapy use in a nephroblastoma patient.[9-11]. There is no proven link between SHJCM and autoimmune disease. However, there are two reported cases of high-serum aldolase levels, suggesting a potential association with juvenile dermatomyositis.[12]

Clinical Presentation and Pathogenesis

The disease is characterized by three cutaneous findings: periorbital edema, deep-seated nodules, and ivory white papules. They are located most commonly on the face and periarticular regions.[10,13] The distinguishing features reported by Bonerandi include young age at onset, the distribution of cutaneous findings on the face, scalp, neck, and joints; the absence of systemic symptoms including thyroid disease and paraproteinemia; acute onset; and spontaneous resolution.[8] There are often associated arthralgias, fevers, and leukocytosis during the rapid proliferation phase. In most patients, the disease will clear within 7 months, but some reports have persisted for greater than 2.5 years.[10]

Histologic Findings

Microscopically, it features interstitial deposits of dermal stromal mucin, as described earlier in connection with myxedema. Fibroblastic proliferation has been reported only rarely. Scant perivascular chronic inflammation may again be apparent (Figure 15-4). Self-healing mucinosis may also manifest with subcutaneous nodules of mucin that are separated by fibrous septae, with limited chronic inflammation. In some instances, the nodules contain stellate, rhabdoid, or ganglion-like mesenchymal cells as well, yielding a superficial morphologic resemblance to proliferative fasciitis.

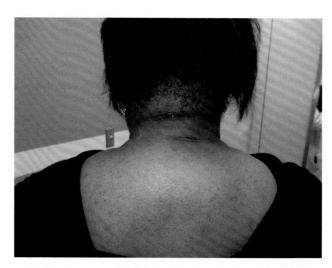

FIGURE 15-4. Scleredema of the mid upper back in a young African-American female.

SELF-HEALING JUVENILE CUTANEOUS MUCINOSIS

SHJCM is a rare disorder with less than 10 reported cases in the literature. The disease is characterized by three cutaneous findings: periorbital edema, deep-seated nodules, and ivory white papules. Microscopically, it features interstitial deposits of dermal stromal mucin, as described earlier in connection with myxedema.

SCLEREDEMA

Definition, Epidemiology, and Etiology

Scleredema, or Scleredema of Buschke, is a rare disorder characterized by progressive symmetric skin induration and thickening around the trunk, shoulders, and neck with associated woody nonpitting edema (Figure 15-5). There is often an association with Type I diabetes. There is no racial or ethnic predilection for any of the types, although there is a moderately increased propensity in females.[14] Distal extremity involvement is very rare. Most cases occur before the age of 20.[14-17]

Clinical Presentation and Pathogenesis

There are three distinct entities. Type I is the most common occurring in the pediatric population, accounting for 55% of total cases. Type I usually has a preceding febrile illness, such as streptococcal pharyngitis, influenza, scarlet fever, or mumps and carries a good prognosis.[17] The disease starts with an active inflammatory state with increased induration and skin thickening over 6 to 8 weeks followed by complete resolution and return to normal state by 6 months to 2 years.[16] There are rare reports of progressively fatal disease.[18] Type II accounts for 25% of cases and usually has an associated monoclonal gammopathy. Type III is slowly progressive and accounts for 20% of cases.

The pathogenesis is poorly understood. One proposed mechanism involves potential allergic sensitization by pathogens to collagen, leading to a disruptive antigen-antibody reaction. Diabetes-associated cases may involve glucose-mediated fibroblast stimulation, leading to increased collagen production.[15]

Histologic Findings

The epidermis in scleredema may show partial effacement of the rete ridges and slight basilar hyperpigmentation. One regularly sees a thickened reticular dermis, with partial collagenization of the superficial subcutis. The collagen fibers are separated by variably dense deposits of interstitial mucopolysaccharide, and these tend to diminish as the duration of the disease increases. The mucin can be labeled with alcian blue or colloidal iron stains (Figure 15-4).

SCLEREDEMA

Scleredema, or Scleredema of Buschke, is a rare disorder characterized by progressive symmetric skin induration and thickening around the trunk, shoulders, and neck with associated woody nonpitting edema. There is often an association with Type I diabetes. The epidermis in scleredema may show partial effacement of the rete ridges and slight basilar hyperpigmentation. The collagen fibers are separated by variably dense deposits of interstitial dermal mucin.

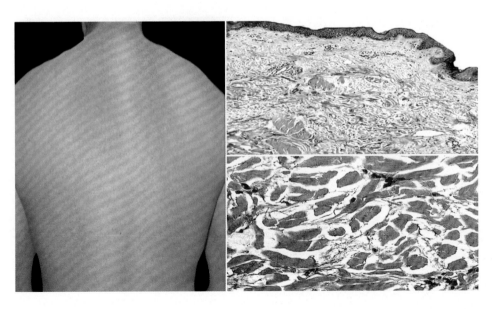

FIGURE 15-5. Scleredema in the skin of the back in an adolescent boy (left panel). Microscopically, this process is typified by a deposition of dermal interstitial stromal mucin, together with fibrosis (right panels).

MUCOPOLYSACCHARIDE STORAGE DISEASES

Mucopolysaccharidoses (MPS) are a rare group of inherited lysosomal enzyme and storage deficiencies characterized by an aberrant catabolism of glycosaminoglycans. These fragments, including dermatan sulfate, heparin sulfate, and chondroitin sulfate, subsequently accumulate in various tissues. Affected children are often normal at birth and present with symptoms during infancy with a wide variation in phenotype.

Clinical Presentation and Pathogenesis

MPS can be classified into eight disorders, and the most common types will be discussed in the following paragraphs. All types of MPS can have many nonspecific cutaneous features, including prominent forehead, macroglossia, flat nasal bridge, and stubby hands.[19-21]

MPS I, or Hurler syndrome, is the most common type occurring in 1 of 100 000 births. Hurler syndrome is autosomal recessive with a deficiency in α-L-iduronidase, leading to the accumulation of heparin sulfate and dermatan sulfate. Infants present with widened nasal bridge and macroglossia by the first year of life, followed by progressive decline in cognition and motor skills with death from cardiorespiratory failure by age 10. They can also have generalized Mongolian spots, which can persist and progress into adulthood.[20]. Mongolian spots may be secondary to the association of heparin sulfate with high-affinity tyrosine kinase receptor and nerve growth factor, which are chemotropic for melanocytes.[19]

MPS II, or Hunter syndrome, is an X-linked recessive disorder with a deficiency in iduronate-2-sulfatase. The disease is rare with incidence 0.3 to 1.3 per 100 000 infants with male predominance. Children are often diagnosed later in childhood, around age 4 to 8. They can present with umbilical hernias and cardiomyopathy. They can also develop ivory papules in a reticular pattern over the scapula and lateral arms before age 10. These cutaneous findings are seen in 13% of patients and often have spontaneous regression.[21] Death from systemic complications usually occurs around the third to fourth decade. Skin tightening and thickening is a feature of both MPS I and MPS II. This occurs most commonly on the hands and can lead to contractures, often mistaken for scleroderma.

Histologic Findings

Hurler and Hunter syndromes are typified pathologically by the presence of metachromatic granules in dermal fibroblasts, and occasionally in eccrine sweat glands as well. Interstitial mucin is also seen diffusely in the corium, and it can be highlighted with the Giemsa, alcian blue, and colloidal iron methods (Figure 15-6).

CAPSULE SUMMARY

MUCOPOLYSACCHARIDE STORAGE DISEASES

MPS are a rare group of inherited lysosomal enzyme and storage deficiencies characterized by an aberrant catabolism of glycosaminoglycans. All types of MPS can have many nonspecific cutaneous features, including prominent forehead, macroglossia, flat nasal bridge, and stubby hands. Hurler and Hunter syndromes are typified pathologically by the presence of metachromatic granules in dermal fibroblasts, and occasionally in eccrine sweat glands as well.

AMYLOIDOSES

Definition, Epidemiology, and Etiology

Amyloidosis can be characterized as localized, systemic, or familial. Primary localized cutaneous amyloidosis is a rare condition characterized by the deposition of extracellular

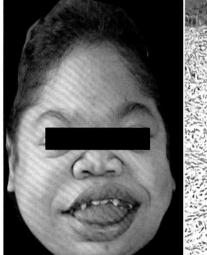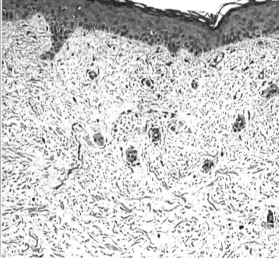

FIGURE 15-6. This female child has gargoylism, with distortion of the facial features caused by dermal deposition of mucopolysaccharide (left panel). Histologically, the dermis is largely effaced by mucoid material (right panel).

amyloid fibril deposition in the dermis without any systemic involvement. There are several different subtypes, including lichen amyloidosis, macular amyloidosis, and nodular amyloidosis.[22-31] Lichen and macular amyloidosis consist of keratin deposition, whereas nodular amyloidosis involves AL-type light chain deposition. Macular amyloidosis is characterized by aggregated brown papules with a rippled appearance, most commonly on the upper back. There is a strong female predominance, and it occurs most commonly in middle age.[23] Nodular amyloidosis affects equal sexes and consists of waxy translucent nodules on acral sites, the face, and mucocutaneous junctions.[23,24] There is a 9% risk of recurrence with nodular amyloidosis with a possible association with Sjogren syndrome.[22,24]

Lichen amyloidosis is a form of localized cutaneous amyloidosis characterized by intensely pruritic, hyperpigmented, discrete papules and plaques without any evidence of systemic involvement. This form of amyloidosis makes up 10% of all cutaneous amyloidoses.[26] The disease occurs more commonly on the shins but has also been reported in the interscapular region and upper back.[27] Although the disease is more common in the 5th and 6th decades of life, lichen amyloidosis has been reported infrequently in adolescents.[28] There is a slight male predominance in the South American, Chinese, and Southeast Asian populations.[29] Lichen amyloidosis has been associated with atopic dermatitis, mycosis fungoides, systemic lupus erythematous, and multiple endocrine neoplasia (MEN) 2A or Sipple syndrome.[30] Up to 36% of MEN 2A patients have this form of localized cutaneous amyloidosis.[27] Etiology is unknown but may be related to viral and genetic factors, atopy, and localized friction.[26] Pathogenesis is poorly understood but involves faulty neurotransmitter release in localized areas with resultant chronic rubbing and trauma. Repeated friction progresses to keratinocyte apoptosis and peptide degeneration. Dermal fibroblasts and macrophages convert these peptides into amyloid fibrils.[29] The intense pruritus characteristically improves with sun exposure and worsens with stress.[27] This process dictates clinical morphology with transition from intense pruritus to subtle hyperpigmentation to the formation of aggregated papules.[31] Familial variants with autosomal dominant transmission have also been reported.[31]

Familial amyloid deposition disorders include Muckle-Wells (urticarial–deafness–amyloidosis) syndrome, Familial Mediterranean Fever, and Schnitzler syndrome.[23] Secondary cutaneous amyloidosis is usually the result of an underlying inflammatory process. Secondary forms can be seen in conditions such as basal cell carcinoma, porokeratoses, and adnexal tumors.[25] The etiology involves aberrant keratinocyte apoptosis with filamentous degradation and deposition of amyloid.[23] All forms of amyloidosis are extremely rare in the pediatric population.

Histologic Findings and Differential Diagnosis

Both macular and lichen amyloidosis show amorphous eosinophilic deposits of amyloid in the dermal papillae (Figure 15-7). Apoptotic keratinocytes are present in the epidermis over the amyloid, often with pigment incontinence as well. The lesions of lichen amyloidosis may also include hyperkeratosis and acanthosis, as seen in lichen simplex chronicus. Cutaneous abnormalities in systemic amyloidosis likewise include dermal amyloid deposition, with virtually no inflammation. Amyloid is particularly seen in blood vessel walls, the basement membrane of sweat gland units, and adipocytes (Figure 15-8). In our experience, skin biopsies are as effective as fat-pad aspiration for the diagnosis of systemic amyloidosis.

Histochemical stains for amyloid include the Congo red, pagoda red, crystal violet, and thioflavine-T methods. It should be noted that affinity for Congo red is usually, but not always, absent in secondary systemic amyloidosis.

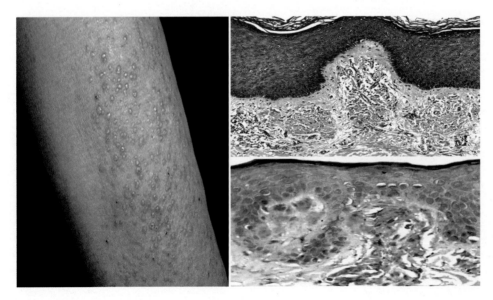

FIGURE 15-7. Lichen amyloidosis on the forearm of an adolescent boy, represented by small papulonodular lesions that were intensely pruritic (left panel). Microscopically, amorphous eosinophilic deposits are present in the upper dermis (top right panel), which label with the Congo red stain (bottom right panel).

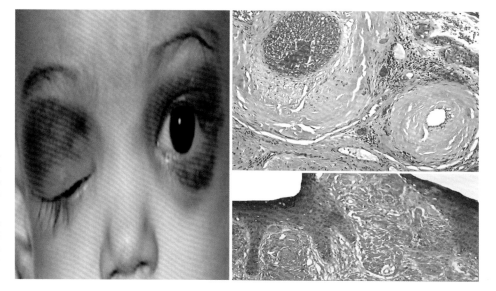

FIGURE 15-8. A child with systemic amyloidosis has "raccoon eyes," which are the result of vascular fragility in periorbital blood vessels (left panel). Microscopically, amorphous eosinophilic deposits are present in the walls of deep dermal blood vessels (top right panel), and these label with the Congo red stain (bottom right panel).

Immunohistochemical reagents are available for putatively specific staining of amyloid types AA and AL, but our experience with them has been disappointing diagnostically.

Cutaneous amyloid deposits may resemble the material seen in juvenile colloid milia. However, the latter do not label with Congo red and instead are immunoreactive for keratin. Other histologic differential diagnostic considerations include erythropoietic protoporphyria and lipoid proteinosis, in which acellular eosinophilic intradermal material may also be present. The eosinophilic material does not label with histochemical stains for amyloid in either of those conditions.

CAPSULE SUMMARY

AMYLOIDOSES

Amyloidosis can be characterized as localized, systemic, or familial. Primary localized cutaneous amyloidosis is a rare condition characterized by the deposition of extracellular amyloid fibril deposition in the dermis without any systemic involvement. There are several different subtypes, including lichen amyloidosis, macular amyloidosis, and nodular amyloidosis. Familial amyloid deposition disorders include Muckle-Wells (urticarial deafness–amyloidosis) syndrome, Familial Mediterranean Fever, and Schnitzler syndrome. Both macular and lichen amyloidosis show amorphous eosinophilic deposits of amyloid in the dermal papillae.

CALCINOSIS CUTIS

Definition, Epidemiology, and Etiology

Calcinosis cutis is a rare disorder characterized by the deposition of calcium phosphate or hydroxyapatite in areas of microtrauma. Most cases are diagnosed before the age of 10, approximately 2 to 3 years after diagnosis. A possible etiology involves the release of calcium from muscle cells affected by myopathy.[32,33]

Clinical Presentation and Pathogenesis

The deposition of calcium phosphate or hydroxyapatite leads to the formation of palpable yellow to white nodules with or without associated contractures (Figure 15-9). Local inflammation can subsequently lead to ulceration or the discharge of milky white substrate. There is predilection for the forearms, elbows, and fingers.[32-36]

Calcinosis cutis can be classified into four subtypes: metastatic, dystrophic, idiopathic, and iatrogenic.[34,35] Metastatic calcinosis cutis occurs with elevated serum calcium and or phosphate levels and can be seen in conditions such as sarcoidosis, chronic renal failure, or hyperparathyroidism.

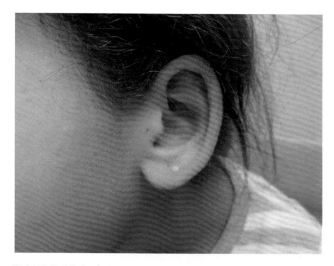

FIGURE 15-9. Calcinosis cutis of the lobule in a young healthy girl without any underlying systemic illness.

Dystrophic calcinosis is the most common subtype. It occurs in previously inflamed tissues in the setting of normal serum calcium and phosphate levels. Dystrophic calcinosis can be seen with CREST syndrome, system lupus erythematosus, and approximately 30% to 70% of juvenile dermatomyositis. This form is also seen in inherited syndromes such as Ehler-Danlos, Werner, and pseudoxanthoma elasticum.[32,33,36] Ulceration and infection are common in juvenile dermatomyositis, and calcinosis can be superficial or extend to the underlying fascia and muscle with limitations in movement.[32]

Idiopathic calcinosis is a diagnosis of exclusion that also occurs in the setting of normal serum calcium and phosphate levels. It can often be seen with Down syndrome and scrotal calcinosis (Figure 15-10). Iatrogenic calcinosis cutis is often seen after the placement of calcium electrodes for electrocardiograms or repeated heel pricks in neonatal infants in the intensive care unit. Heel stick calcinosis appears usually by 4 months of age with spontaneous resolution by 18 to 30 months of age. The etiology of this condition involves repeated phlebitis with the release of alkaline phosphatase and increased pH, leading to calcium salt deposition.[35] A second pathogenesis has been described, which involves tissue damage with denatured proteins that preferentially bind phosphate. Calcium then binds phosphate ions, leading to precipitation.[34]

Histologic Findings

All forms of calcinosis cutis feature the histologic presence of calcium phosphate deposits in the dermis or subcutis, unassociated with inflammation or foreign body reaction (Figure 15-10). The lesions can be labeled with histochemical stains for calcium, such as the von Kossa or alizarin-red methods.

CAPSULE SUMMARY
CALCINOSIS CUTIS
Calcinosis cutis is a rare disorder characterized by the deposition of calcium phosphate or hydroxyapatite in areas of microtrauma. The deposition of calcium phosphate or hydroxyapatite leads to the formation of palpable yellow to white nodules with or without associated contractures. All forms of calcinosis cutis feature the histologic presence of calcium phosphate deposits in the dermis or subcutis.

OSTEOMA CUTIS
Definition, Epidemiology, and Etiology

Osteoma cutis is characterized by heterotopic bone formation in the skin and consists of firm, nontender subcutaneous papules and nodules. It is further classified as primary or secondary, with the latter applying if the process arises in a preexisting skin lesion.[37] Primary osteoma cutis is associated mostly with inherited syndromes with inactivating mutations in *GNAS* including Albright's Hereditary Osteodystrophy (AHO), progressive osseous heteroplasia, fibrodysplasia ossificans progressiva, or plate-like osteoma cutis.[38-40] Osteoma cutis is seen in 25% to 50% of patients with AHO and presents in early infancy.[41]

Clinical Presentation and Pathogenesis

Plate-like osteoma cutis presents in newborns and young children with large skin-colored plaques ranging from 1 to 15 cm on the scalp[38] (Figure 15-11). Progressive osseous heteroplasia is the most severe form, presenting with dermal ossification in infancy with extension to skeletal

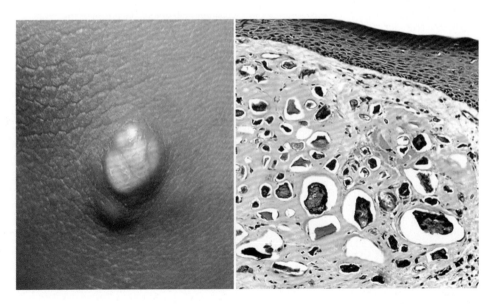

FIGURE 15-10. Calcinosis cutis on the buttock in a child, taking the form of hard white nodular lesions (left panel). Histologically, basophilic calcium salts are distributed throughout a fibrotic dermis (right panel).

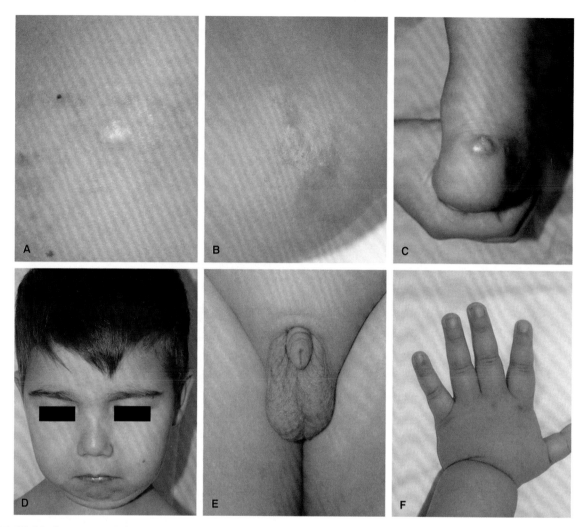

FIGURE 15-11. Osteoma cutis in the setting of Albright hereditary osteodystrophy. Osteoma cutis: a bluish or erythematous, indurated plaque on the back (A) and the lower limb (B), or a reddish, stone-hard, dome-shaped nodule located on the heel (C). D, A characteristic round face with flattened nasal bridge and short neck. E, Micropenis. F, A typical short, stubby hand with brachydactyly. Reprinted with permission from Kacerovska D, Nemcova J, Pomahacova R, Michal M, Kazakov D. Cutaneous and superficial soft tissue lesions associated with albright hereditary osteodystrophy: clinicopathological and molecular genetic study of 4 cases, including a novel mutation of the *GNAS* gene. *Am J Dermatopathol.* 2008;30(5):417-424.

muscle.[37] Secondary osteoma cutis accounts for 85% of total cases. This subtype arises from preexisting skin lesions, the sites of prior trauma, or surgical procedures including scars, acne, and basal cell carcinoma. Miliary osteoma cutis usually occurs in females at the sites of prior acne scars.[38,42]

Pathogenesis is unknown, but it is speculated to involve differentiation of mesenchymal cells, such as fibroblasts, into osteoblasts.[43] Prognosis is good, with most cases remaining stable. However, patients should be monitored for associated conditions and progression to cosmetic defects.[37]

The mechanism of heterotopic bone formation in the skin is not altogether clear, but, as stated earlier, one theory suggests that fibroblasts in the dermis undergo metaplasia to osteoblasts, as a result of abnormalities in the genes that

govern bone formation.[44] A skin biopsy is necessary for a definitive diagnosis of osteoma cutis, in which mature cortical bone is present in the dermis or subcutis (Figures 15-12 and 15-13). Conventional nevus with secondary ossification (osteonevus of Nanta) is seldom encountered in routine dermatopathologic practice. This type of nevus is usually located in the upper part of the body, with the predilection in females.

Histologic Findings

The ossification is usually in the form of the small islands of compact lamellar or structureless bone at the base of the lesion (Figure 15-14). In some cases, trabecular bone with bone marrow and adipocytes may also be present.

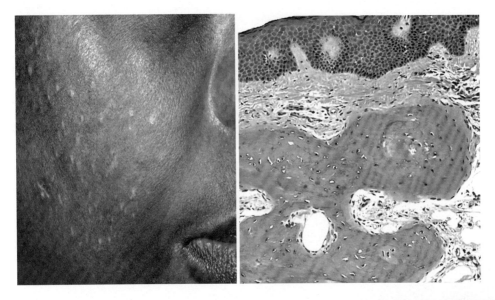

FIGURE 15-12. An adolescent girl had scarring acne vulgaris and has now developed firm white papules in the facial skin (left panel). Microscopically, they represent osteomas that are centered on the former foci of acne (right panel).

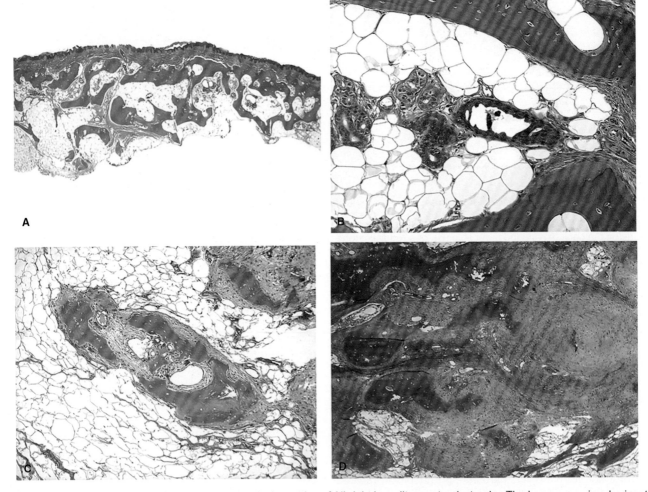

FIGURE 15-13. The so-called plaque-like osteoma in the setting of Albright hereditary osteodystrophy. The bone grows in a horizontal plaque-like fashion (A), often wrapping around eccrine or apocrine ducts, some of which manifested dilatation and hyperplasia with intraluminal bridges (B). Although the bone lamellae are sharply segregated from the surrounding fat (C), another lesion from this patient showed curved bone in the background of immature mesenchymal cell proliferation, occasioning resemblance to fibrous dysplasia (D). Reprinted with permission from Kacerovska D, Nemcova J, Pomahacova R, Michal M, Kazakov DV. Cutaneous and superficial soft tissue lesions associated with albright hereditary osteodystrophy: clinicopathological and molecular genetic study of 4 cases, including a novel mutation of the *GNAS* gene. *Am J Dermatopathol.* 2008;30(5):417-424.

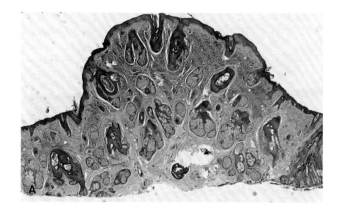

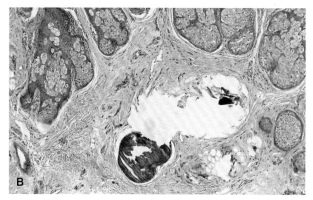

FIGURE 15-14. Osteonevus of Nanta. A, There is an intradermal melanocytic nevus with a congenital pattern (nested melanocytes are tracking down adnexal structures). B, At the base of the lesion, a focus of metaplastic bone formation is present. Digital slides courtesy of Path Presenter.com.

ARGYRIA

Definition, Epidemiology, and Etiology

Argyria is a rare condition characterized by the development of slate gray to blue mucocutaneous discoloration following chronic exposure to silver-containing products. The discoloration is likely secondary to melanocyte stimulation and degradation of elemental silver.[45] Argyria is worsened by sunlight, which can act as a catalyst for the reduction of silver. The dyspigmentation can take several months to appear after the chronic use of silver-containing products.[31] Several culprits have been reported in the literature, including the use of colloidal silver supplements in cystic fibrosis patients for mucous clearance and topical silvadene cream

in a young adult with dystrophic epidermolysis bullosa.[46,47] Despite the discontinuation of silver-containing products, the discoloration can persist lifelong.

Histologic Findings

Microscopically, silver granules in argyria are found along the basement membranes of sweat glands, hair follicles, and the epidermis. They are most easily seen as refractile granules with darkfield microscopy (Figures 15-15 and 15-16). Slight melanosis of the epidermis or dermal melanin incontinence may accompany the silver deposition.

Cutaneous Cysts

Cutaneous cysts are among the most commonly seen lesions in dermatopathology, and they are seen in patients of all ages. Simply defined, a "cyst" is an enclosed space in a tissue compartment that is lined by epithelium and that contains fluid or semisolid material. Most cysts in the skin are thought to derive from the dermal appendages, as "retention" phenomena. Developmental cysts are less common, having their origins in the vestigial remnants of embryonic tissue.

As one might expect, the epithelial lining of cutaneous cysts is potentially variable in nature morphologically, reflecting the spectrum of differentiation that is seen in the normal epidermis and its appendages. Salient pathologic features of the lesions discussed in this chapter are presented in Table 15-1. Additional types of cysts exist in the skin, but they are seen in adults and therefore have been omitted from consideration here.

TRUE CUTANEOUS CYSTS

Epithelial Cysts Lacking Ciliated Cells

EPIDERMAL (EPIDERMOID) CYST, MILIA, AND COMEDONAL CYST

Definition, Epidemiology, Clinical Presentation, and Pathogenesis

Epidermal, or infundibular cysts are flesh-colored firm mobile papules and nodules, often with central puncta (Figure 15-17). Rupture may occur either spontaneously or

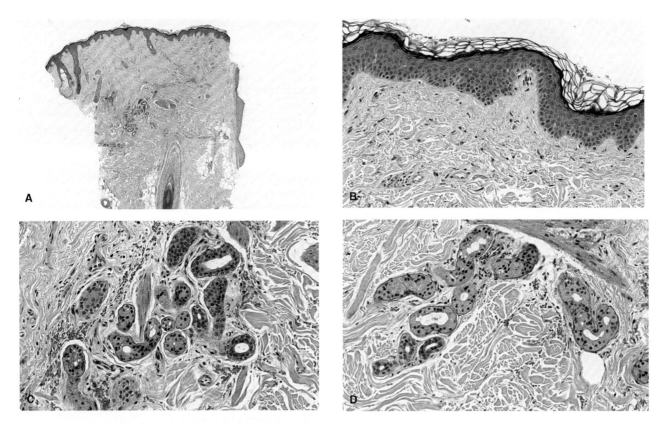

FIGURE 15-15. **Argyria**. The routine hematoxylin and eosin (H and E) examination shows a "normal" skin biopsy (A). There is a slight increased melanin pigmentation of the basal keratinocytes (B). Refractile particles are present along the basement membrane of the sweat ducts (C and D). Digital slides courtesy of Path Presenter.com.

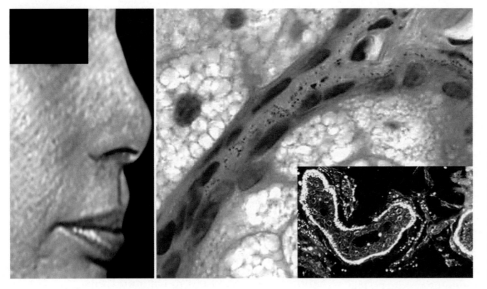

FIGURE 15-16. This teenage girl took colloidal silver for a prolonged period as a dietary supplement. She now has gray-blue discoloration of the facial skin (left panel), representing argyria. Histologically, silver particles can be seen in the dermal appendages by conventional microscopy (right panel) as well as darkfield microscopy (right panel inset).

as a result of trauma, with the extrusion of foul-smelling contents and secondary inflammation. This incites an inflammatory foreign body-type reaction to keratinous cyst contents in the surrounding tissue. They are twice as common in males as in females and usually appear in the third to fourth decade of life but can arise during childhood or puberty.[48] In the pediatric population, approximately 13%

of all head cysts are characterized as epidermoid cysts and favor the eyebrows and postauricular region. Epidermoid cysts are also associated with several genetic syndromes, including Gardner syndrome, occurring in 36% to 50% of these patients.[49] Gardner syndrome is an autosomal dominant disease complex caused by mutations in the *APC* gene. Affected individuals may have multiple adenomatous

TABLE 15-1.	Microscopic characteristics of selected cutaneous cysts
Type of Cyst	**Salient Pathologic Attributes**
Epidermal (epidermoid) [includes milia as well]	Lining epithelium is squamous with keratohyaline granules; keratinization simulates that of normal epidermis
Trichilemmal (pilar)	"Abrupt" trichilemmal keratinization; absence of keratohyaline granules in epithelial lining; contents often include cholesterol clefts and calcifications
Keratocyst	Corrugated configuration to squamous lining epithelium; lack of a granular layer; contents may include vellus hairs
Gardner syndrome	Columns of shadow cells projecting into cyst lumen and attached to groups of basaloid hair matrix-like cells in cyst lining; pilar-type keratinization may also be present
Vellus hair	Multiple cysts with epidermis-like squamous lining epithelium; multiple luminal vellus hairs
Steatocystoma	Epidermis-like epithelial lining with attached sebaceous glands; contents may include vellus hairs
Hidrocystoma	Lining cells may be cuboidal with a luminal cuticle (eccrine hidrocystoma) or low-columnar with decapitation secretion (apocrine hidrocystoma); micropapillary epithelial hyperplasia sometimes present
Comedonal	Epidermis-like epithelial lining with lamellated luminal keratin; may connect to skin surface (open comedone) or not (closed comedone)
Bronchogenic	Principally midline in anatomic location with pseudostratified ciliated columnar epithelial lining; cyst wall may contain small muscle, cartilage, and mucous glands
Branchial cleft	Lateral cervical location; squamous and/or ciliated columnar epithelial lining; lymphoid tissue may be present in wall
Thyroglossal	Midline cervical location; associated cutaneous sinus may be present; respiratory and/or squamous epithelial lining; thyroid parenchymal tissue in wall in a majority of cases
Cervical thymic	Squamous epithelial cyst lining; cholesterol clefts in cyst lumen; thymic tissue including Hassall corpuscles may be seen
Cutaneous ciliated	Seen on legs in female patients; ciliated cuboidal or columnar epithelial lining
Median raphe	Ventral penile location; pseudostratified columnar epithelial lining ± squamous epithelium
True dermoid	Periorbital or midline location; epidermis-like epithelial lining with attached pilosebaceous units; smooth muscle may also be present
Omphalomesenteric	Associated with persistent primitive yolk stalk; lining tissue resembles normal bowel and may also contain heterotopic pancreas; associated omphalocele or umbilical hernia may be present
Digital mucous	Most common between distal interphalangeal joint and cuticle; actually a "pseudocyst" because no epithelial lining is present; mucinous contents stain with alcian blue and colloidal iron methods
Cystic hygroma	Another "pseudocyst" with no epithelial components; interanastomosing vascular channels containing lymph fluid; lymphoid tissue common in lesional stroma

intestinal polyps, soft tissue fibromas and desmoid tumors, osteomas, and cutaneous cysts beginning in childhood. The risk for the eventual development of colorectal adenocarcinoma is high.

Milia, a subtype of epidermoid cysts, are small 1 to 3 mm superficial epidermoid cysts without an associated hair follicle. Congenital milia occur in 40% to 50% of newborns and favor the face and nose. They usually resolve within weeks.[50] Primary milia can occur in children and favor the eyelids; they are believed to occur in the setting of skin trauma and have a predilection for scars and conditions that predispose to skin trauma and healing, such as epidermolysis bullosa.[50] To prevent recurrence, epidermoid cysts need surgical excision with complete removal of the cyst wall.[48]

A comedonal cyst, or closed comedone, is a 1 to 2 mm white papule without a visual orifice found most commonly on the face. They usually appear around age 8 to 10 and can be the earliest sign of acne vulgaris. The cyst is usually filled with lipids, keratinous debris, and bacteria. They result from an abnormal proliferation of ductal keratinocytes because of increased sebum production, local cytokine release, bacteria, and androgen stimulation. They usually resolve within 2 weeks.

Histologic Findings

Epidermal inclusion cysts (EICs) are lined by stratified squamous epithelium, mirroring the structure of the normal epidermis. Importantly, a granular layer is included in the lining. Cyst contents are represented by anucleate and lamellated keratin, as well as keratin "flakes." The epithelium in ruptured EICs may be effaced by a granulomatous foreign body reaction, and the accompanying inflammation comprises neutrophils, lymphocytes, and histiocytes (Figure 15-18).

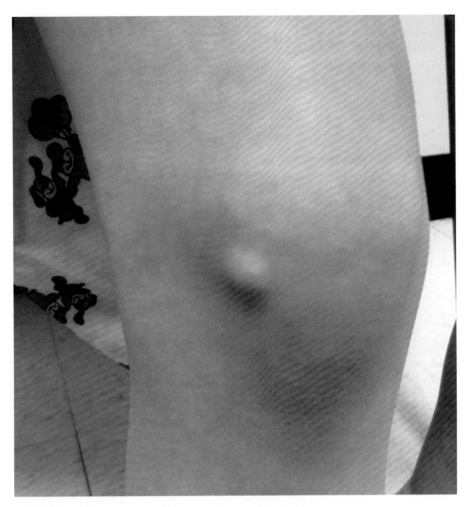

FIGURE 15-17. Epidermal inclusion cyst on the knee of an adolescent female.

Multinucleated giant cells in the infiltrate may contain intra-cytoplasmic keratinous debris.

Most cysts in persons with Gardner syndrome have the microscopic attributes of banal EIC. However, a minority contain peculiar intracystic columns of "shadow" keratinocytes, like those seen in pilomatrixomas. Indeed, such columns appear to be attached to groups of basaloid, hair matrix-like cells in the cyst lining (Figure 15-19), simulating those of pilomatrical tumors. The other descriptions of cysts in Gardner syndrome have included some with

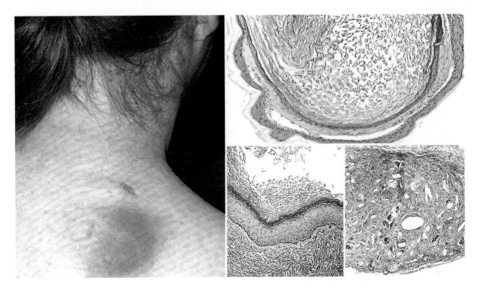

FIGURE 15-18. This adolescent girl has a fluctuant, tender, reddish nodule on the back (left panel). Microscopically, an epidermoid inclusion cyst is seen (top right panel), containing lamellated keratinous material (first bottom right panel). The cyst has ruptured and incited the formation of foreign body granulomas (second bottom right panel).

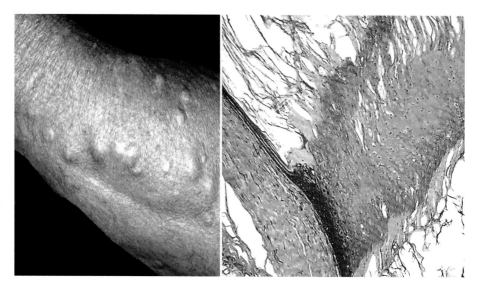

FIGURE 15-19. A teenage boy with Gardner syndrome has several inclusions cysts in the skin of the arms (left panel). Histologically, these resemble epidermoid inclusion cysts, except that they also contain foci of pilomatrical-type tissue associated with parakeratotic columns (right panel).

internal trichilemmal keratinization, and lesions with sebaceous glands attached to their walls.[50]

In some instances, the squamous lining of EICs becomes proliferative ("pseudoepitheliomatous"), producing irregular epithelial nests that project into the cyst lumen or the surrounding dermis (Figure 15-20). One must avoid interpreting such findings as evidence for malignant change in such lesions in children.

Milia histologically resemble the closed comedones that are seen in acne vulgaris, except that the dense intracystic accumulations of cornified cells observed in comedones are lacking in milia (Figure 15-21). In our opinion, large cystic lesions that otherwise have the appearance of open or closed comedones (Figure 15-22) should be designated as such, instead of using the ambiguous term of "comedonal cysts."

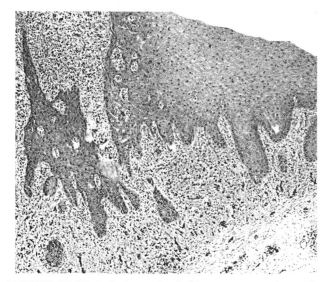

FIGURE 15-20. Inclusion cysts of all types may contain proliferative epithelium that protrudes into the cyst cavity or the pericystic soft tissue. This finding should not be misinterpreted as malignant change.

CAPSULE SUMMARY

EPIDERMAL (EPIDERMOID) CYST, MILIA, AND COMEDONAL CYST

Epidermal or infundibular cysts are flesh-colored firm mobile papules and nodules, often with central puncta. Rupture may occur either spontaneously or as a result of trauma, with the extrusion of foul-smelling contents and secondary inflammation. Epidermoid cysts are also associated with several genetic syndromes, including Gardner syndrome, occurring in 36% to 50% of these patients. EICs are lined by stratified squamous epithelium, mirroring the structure of the normal epidermis. Importantly, a granular layer is included in the lining.

TRICHILEMMAL (PILAR OR ISTHMUS-CATAGEN) CYST

Definition, Epidemiology, and Etiology

Trichilemmal cysts (TLCs) are solitary, smooth, firm nodules with overlying alopecia. Up to 90% of TLCs are found on the scalp with a female predominance. They usually occur after the age of 60. TLCs account for 20% of all cutaneous cysts and are derived from the isthmus of the hair follicle.[51] Rupture is possible and can result in a similar inflammatory reaction as described in EICs. An autosomal dominant variant of familial TLCs has been described, usually in patients with larger cysts (>5 cm), and multiple cysts may occur in this setting.[52] TLCs have been described rarely in the pediatric population, arising on the genitalia and within a nevus sebaceus.[52,53] Complete excision usually prevents further recurrence.

Histologic Findings

Several histologic differences exist between TLC and EIC. The former lacks keratohyaline granules in its epithelial

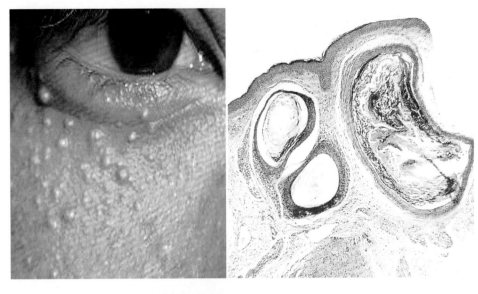

FIGURE 15-21. Numerous milia are seen in the periocular skin in this teenage boy (left panel). Histologically, they resemble miniature epidermoid inclusion cysts (right panel).

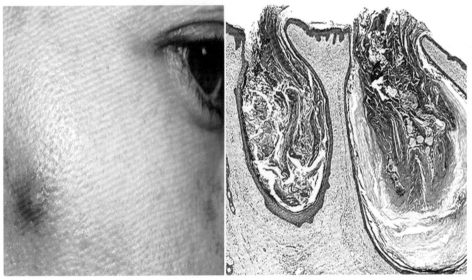

FIGURE 15-22. Acne vulgaris may assume a cystic form, as shown in this clinical photograph of an adolescent boy (left panel). Microscopically, large comedones that may be either open or closed are present (right panel). These should not be called "comedonal cysts."

lining and shows "abrupt" (pilar) keratinization in the cyst contents, with homogeneity of the keratin rather than lamellation (Figure 15-23). Dystrophic calcification and formation of cholesterol clefts are also common in TLC, but not in EIC.

Occasional cysts have microscopic features of both EIC and TLC in the same lesion, and these may also show connection to the skin surface. The terms "hybrid inclusion cyst" or "infundibular inclusion cyst" have been used to describe them. TLC shows a greater tendency for intracystic epithelial proliferation ("proliferating TLC/tumor") (Figure 15-24) than EIC does. However, if that process is confined by the cyst wall, it should not be construed as malignant change. Ruptured and inflamed TLCs also differ from ruptured EICs. In trichilemmal cysts, breaks in the cyst wall allow for the entry of inflammatory cells and fibroblasts into the cyst contents, with subsequent organization.

CAPSULE SUMMARY

TRICHILEMMAL (PILAR OR ISTHMUS-CATAGEN) CYST

TLCs are solitary, smooth, firm nodules with overlying alopecia. TLCs account for 20% of all cutaneous cysts and are derived from the isthmus of the hair follicle. TLCs lack keratohyaline granules in its epithelial lining and shows "abrupt" (pilar) keratinization in the cyst contents, with homogeneity of the keratin rather than lamellation.

CUTANEOUS KERATOCYST

Definition, Epidemiology, and Etiology

Cutaneous keratocysts often present as skin-colored mobile subcutaneous nodules.[54] They can occur as a solitary lesion

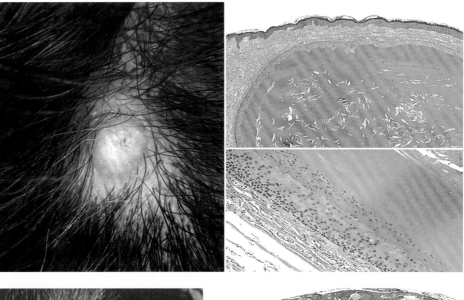

FIGURE 15-23. A pilar inclusion cyst ("wen") is seen in the scalp of this adolescent girl (left panel). Microscopically, it contains brightly eosinophilic ("bubble gum") trichilemmal-type keratin (top right panel). The cyst lining does not contain granulated keratinocytes (bottom right panel).

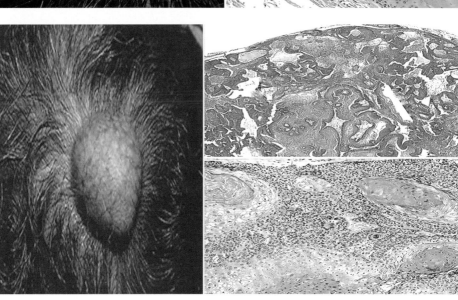

FIGURE 15-24. Another pilar cyst is seen in the scalp of an adolescent boy (left panel). Like the lesion depicted in Figure 15-16, it shows the presence of proliferating epithelium which fills the cyst lumen (top right panel). The lesional cells produce trichilemmal keratin (bottom right panel).

in otherwise healthy individuals but are characteristically associated with nevoid basal cell syndrome when they are multiple.[54] Also known as Gorlin syndrome, nevoid basal cell syndrome is an autosomal dominant disorder with variable penetrance, caused by mutations in the *PTCH1* gene.

Clinical Presentation

Its major features include multiple basal cell carcinomas, odontogenic keratocysts, palmoplantar pits, and calcification of the falx cerebri. Multiple EICs are also a common feature, but are not specific for the condition. Unlike other cutaneous cysts, keratocysts have a tendency to recur after surgery.[54]

Histologic Findings

In 1986, Barr et al described lesions in the skin in adult patients with Gorlin syndrome that had comparable histologic appearances to those in the jaws.[55] They had a squamous lining that lacked a granular layer and an eosinophilic cuticle

that was corrugated or festooned. Parakeratosis and orthokeratosis were apparent in the cyst cavity, and no sebaceous glands were seen (Figure 15-25). Baselga and coworkers[54] subsequently documented a similar case in a 15-year-old girl. Occasional cutaneous keratocysts have also been described in adult patients who did not have Gorlin syndrome.[56-58]

CAPSULE SUMMARY

CUTANEOUS KERATOCYST

Cutaneous keratocysts often present as skin-colored mobile subcutaneous nodules. They can occur as a solitary lesion in otherwise healthy individuals but are characteristically associated with nevoid basal cell syndrome when they are multiple. They have a squamous lining that lacks a granular layer and an eosinophilic cuticle that is corrugated or festooned. No sebaceous glands attached to the wall are seen.

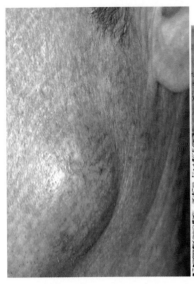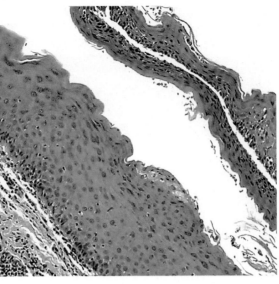

FIGURE 15-25. A teenage boy with the Gorlin-Goltz syndrome has a large inclusion cyst in the skin of the face (left panel). Microscopically, it has a squamous lining with a prominent luminal eosinophilic cuticle, representing a keratocyst (right panel).

STEATOCYSTOMA

Definition, Epidemiology, and Etiology

A steatocystoma is a slow-growing skin-to-yellow-colored cyst derived from sebaceous glands. The overlying epidermis is usually smooth without a central punctum.[58-62] When found in multiple, they are called steatocystoma multiplex. They are found most commonly on the chest, arms, and axilla and will often contain oily yellow discharge. An autosomal dominant variant has been described with mutations in keratin 17 and has also been associated with eruptive vellus hair cysts and pachyonychia congenita type 2.[62] They tend to occur during adolescence or young adulthood and rarely present at birth.[59,61,62] There is no sex predilection.[63] The etiology is unknown but is speculated to involve hamartoma malformation of the pilosebaceous junction.[64,65] The cysts will persist indefinitely unless treated.

Histologic Findings

Steatocystomas have eosinophilic luminal cuticles that are corrugated or undulating. Beneath the eosinophilic cuticle, several layers of attenuated squamous epithelium are present, and the outer layer of the cyst has several attached sebaceous lobules (Figure 15-26). Amorphous material and vellus hairs may be seen in the cyst cavity; indeed, some steatocystomas appear to be hybrid lesions, with concurrent microscopic features of vellus hair cysts, and it is likely that the two exist in a continuum.

CAPSULE SUMMARY

STEATOCYSTOMA

A steatocystoma is a slow-growing skin-to-yellow-colored cyst derived from sebaceous glands. When found in multiple, they are called steatocystoma multiplex. Steatocystomas have eosinophilic luminal cuticles that are corrugated or undulating. Beneath the eosinophilic cuticle, several layers of attenuated squamous epithelium are present, and the outer layer of the cyst has several attached sebaceous lobules.

VELLUS HAIR CYST

Definition and Epidemiology

A vellus hair cyst (VHC) is characterized by the presence of an asymptomatic, smooth, flesh-colored papule approximately 1 to 7 mm in diameter, often with white greasy discharge. More than 85% of cases occur before the age of 25, with diagnosis usually around age 16. There is a slight female predominance.[66-69]

Clinical Presentation and Pathogenesis

The most common location is the parasternal and inframammary region followed by the forehead. The volar forearms are another typical area of involvement. Eruptive VHCs consist of multiple papules, most commonly on the chest[66] (Figure 15-27). They are usually sporadic but rarely transmitted in an autosomal dominant pattern. They can be associated with steatocystoma multiplex and pachyonychia congenita.[66-69] Pathogenesis is unknown, but it is postulated to be a hamartoma of the pilosebaceous unit.[66] Another theory involves an aberrant development of the infundibulum, resulting in the retention of keratin and vellus hairs.[68] Up to 25% of patients will have spontaneous resolution.

Histologic Findings

Microscopically, VHC comprises a cystic collection of squamoid cells that may also contain parts of a telogen follicle and attached slips of the arrector pilorum muscle. The cyst

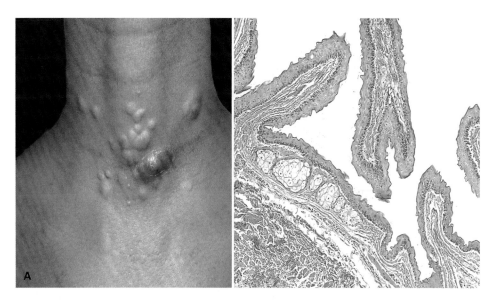

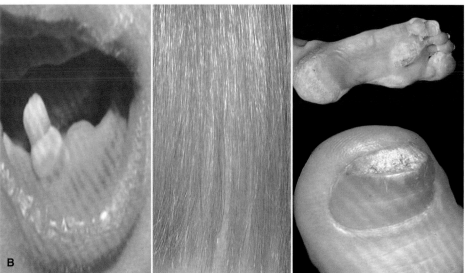

FIGURE 15-26. A, A teenage boy has several cutaneous nodules in the skin of the anterior neck (left panel). Microscopically, they are lined by squamous epithelium with an eosinophilic luminal cuticle, and sebaceous glands that are incorporated into the cyst wall (right panel). These lesions represent steatocystoma multiplex. B, An infant with a related syndrome—pachyonychia congenita (PC)—has a natal tooth (left panel), and an adolescent boy with PC has alopecia (middle panel) with plantar keratoderma, and thickened nails (right panel).

lumen contains keratinous debris and portions of vellus hairs (Figure 15-28). Communication between the cyst lumen and the skin surface may be present, and granulomatous inflammation may surround VHCs.

CAPSULE SUMMARY

VELLUS HAIR CYST

A VHC is characterized by the presence of an asymptomatic, smooth, flesh-colored papule, often with white greasy discharge. Eruptive VHCs consist of multiple papules, most commonly on the chest. Microscopically, VHC comprises a cystic collection of squamoid cells that contains keratinous debris and portions of vellus hairs.

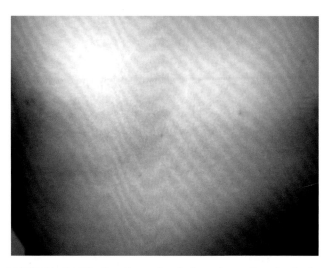

FIGURE 15-27. Eruptive vellus hair cysts on the chest of a young adolescent male.

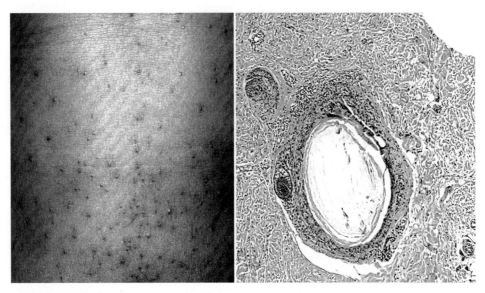

FIGURE 15-28. Multiple cystic lesions are seen in the skin of the chest in this young boy (left panel). Microscopically, they represent cysts that contain vellus hairs (right panel).

HIDROCYSTOMAS

Definition, Epidemiology, and Etiology

Hidrocystomas (Figure 15-29) are benign translucent nodules with a bluish hue found on the head and neck region. They are further classified as eccrine or apocrine. Eccrine hidrocystomas are small, thin-walled, unilocular cysts found predominantly in females in the periorbital region. They usually occur between age 30 and 70.[63-65,70,71] Apocrine hidrocystomas are usually solitary multilocular cysts on the inner canthus. They occur most commonly in adulthood.[64,70,71] They can be associated with Goltz-Gorlin Syndrome, a sporadic disorder with malformed ears,

oral papillomas, and skeletal abnormalities and Schopf–Schultz–Passage Syndrome, an autosomal recessive disorder with multiple eyelid hidrocystomas, hypotrichosis, and palmoplantar hyperkeratosis.[70,72]

Clinical Presentation and Pathogenesis

There is a rare congenital variant located on the anterior orbit with associated eyelid swelling.[73] Pathogenesis is unknown, but some reports suggest occlusion of the eccrine and apocrine ducts as a possible cause.[71] They will usually persist without excision. However, some rare reports demonstrate enlargement during the summer months with

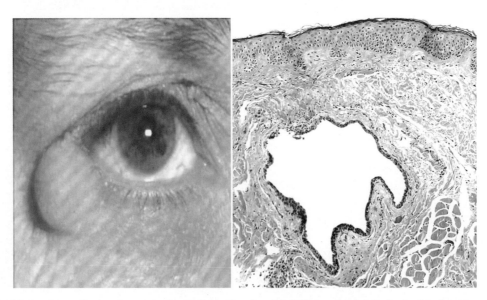

FIGURE 15-29. This boy has a fluctuant cystic lesion in the periocular skin (left panel). Histologically, it is lined by cuboidal epithelium with a thin eosinophilic luminal cuticle, representing an eccrine hidrocystoma (right panel).

spontaneous resolution in cooler weather. Incomplete excision can lead to recurrence in less than 6 weeks.[70]

Histologic Findings

Hidrocystomas are characterized by dilatation of the sweat ducts and potential secondary proliferation of cytologically bland ductal epithelium. The latter phenomenon may produce micropapillary intraluminal cell profiles, resulting in an alternate designation of "cystadenoma." Apocrine hidrocystomas of the eyelids have also been described as "Moll's gland cysts" in the ophthalmologic literature.[74] Lesions in this general category are pseudoneoplastic in nature, and they represent reactions to terminal sweat duct obstruction with an inspissation of secretions.

CAPSULE SUMMARY

HIDROCYSTOMAS

Hidrocystomas are benign translucent nodules with a bluish hue found on the head and neck region. They can be associated with Goltz-Gorlin Syndrome and Schopf–Schultz–Passage Syndrome. Hidrocystomas are characterized by dilatation of the sweat ducts and potential secondary proliferation of cytologically bland ductal epithelium.

CERVICAL THYMIC CYST

Abnormalities in the migration and development of the thymopharyngeal duct may cause thymic cysts to form in the neck. They can be unilocular or multilocular, with a squamous epithelial lining and keratinous debris in the lumen of the cyst.[75-77] Thymic parenchyma is often seen in the cyst wall, including Hassall corpuscles and lymphoid tissue (Figure 15-30). Lesional lymphocytes have the immunophenotype of thymocytes; they are reactive for CD1a, CD2, CD3, and terminal deoxynucleotidyl transferase.

Epithelial Cysts That Contain Ciliated Cells
BRONCHOGENIC CYST

Definition, Epidemiology, and Etiology

Bronchogenic cysts (Figure 15-31) are congenital anomalies of the primitive foregut that occur around the 6th week of gestation. These cysts are found in approximately 1 out of every 42 000 to 68 000 patients with a 4:1 male to female ratio.[78,79] They have a varied age at presentation from 4 days after birth to 13 years of age.[80]

Clinical Presentation and Pathogenesis

The cyst forms after the separation of respiratory tissue from the tracheobronchial tree.[73,78,79,81-83] They are usually unilocular and contain clear fluid. They most commonly present as superficial presternal or suprasternal masses of the lower midline neck, and they comprise approximately 7% of all mediastinal masses in pediatric patients.[78] Approximately 15% to 20% of bronchogenic cysts will originate in the lung parenchyma.[79] Rarely, they can be found in the subcutaneous tissue or abdomen. They are usually asymptomatic but can be associated with chronic cough, wheezing, secondary infection, and rarely cardiac arrest.[79,83] Removal of the cyst is recommended given the possibility of rupture and airway obstruction. They do not regress spontaneously and can often fluctuate in size.[78,79]

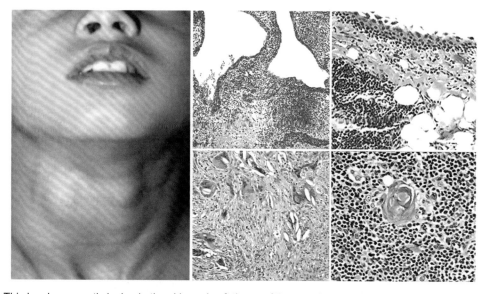

FIGURE 15-30. This boy has a cystic lesion in the skin and soft tissue of the anterior neck (left panel). It contains cystic locules lined by epithelium and invested by lymphoid cells (top right panels). Cholesterol granulomas (first bottom right panel) and Hassall's corpuscles (second bottom right panel) are also seen, establishing the diagnosis of cervical thymic cyst.

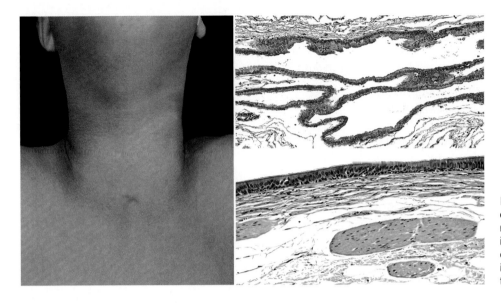

FIGURE 15-31. This boy has a cyst at the base of the neck in the midline (left panel). Histologically, it is lined by ciliated respiratory-type epithelium and has smooth muscle in its walls (right panels), establishing the diagnosis of bronchogenic cyst.

Histologic Findings

The bronchogenic cyst is lined by flat or pseudostratified columnar epithelium that is ciliated. Micropapillary intraluminal projections may also be present. The other cellular components of bronchogenic cysts may include goblet cells, smooth muscle, and cartilage.

CAPSULE SUMMARY

BRONCHOGENIC CYST

Bronchogenic cysts are congenital anomalies of the primitive foregut that occur around the 6th week of gestation. The cyst forms after the separation of respiratory tissue from the tracheobronchial tree. The bronchogenic cyst is lined by flat or pseudostratified columnar epithelium that is ciliated. Micropapillary intraluminal projections may also be present.

THYROGLOSSAL DUCT CYST

Definition, Epidemiology, and Etiology

Thyroglossal duct cysts account for more than 75% of congenital midline neck masses. They present as soft mobile nodules, usually 2 to 4 cm in size that move with tongue protrusion. They occur in 7% of the population.[84-88] More than 50% of cases are diagnosed in childhood with a peak around age 6.[87,88] There is no gender predilection.

Clinical Presentation and Pathogenesis

They originate from persistent epithelial remnants of the thyroglossal duct after descent of the thyroid gland to the anterior neck from the foramen cecum.[85] They most likely occur in the midline neck, and 90% of cases are located

inferior to the hyoid bone. Some cases have also been reported at the base of the tongue causing airway obstruction.[87,88] They are usually asymptomatic but can cause infection and abscess formation with rare reports of ectopic thyroid tissue and papillary thyroid carcinoma.[87,88] Adults are more likely to present with fistulas, dysphagia, and dysphonia. The cyst will often persist without removal. The standard of care involves the Sistrunk procedure, which entails removal of the cyst with the mid portion of the hyoid bone, with recurrence rates of 3% to 6%. Young children have a higher risk of recurrence, with reported recurrences up to 50% in children less than 1 year of age.[87]

Histologic Findings

The cyst lining is cuboidal or columnar, and cilia can be seen in the lesional cells. Benign thyroid tissue is often incorporated into the wall of the cyst (Figure 15-32).

CAPSULE SUMMARY

THYROGLOSSAL DUCT CYST

Thyroglossal duct cysts account for more than 75% of congenital midline neck masses. They present as soft mobile nodules of usually 2 to 4 cm in size that move with tongue protrusion. More than 50% of cases are diagnosed in childhood. The cyst lining is cuboidal or columnar, and cilia can be seen in the lesional cells. Benign thyroid tissue is often incorporated into the wall of the cyst.

BRANCHIAL CLEFT CYST

Definition, Epidemiology, and Etiology

Branchial cleft cysts are developmental anomalies of the lateral neck. They are one of the most common congenital

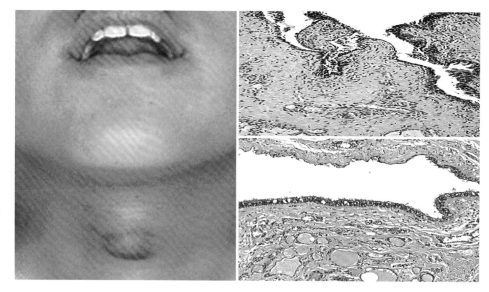

FIGURE 15-32. Another boy with a midline cyst of the anterior neck (left panel). Microscopically, it is lined by respiratory-type epithelium, with thyroid follicles in the adjacent tissue (right panels). The lesion is a thyroglossal duct cyst.

neck masses, accounting for more than 80% of all branchial anomalies.[80,89-91] Up to 95% of these cysts arise from the second branchial arch and occur in the upper lateral neck along the anterior border of the sternocleidomastoid muscle.[80,89] Although they are congenital, they do not clinically appear until adolescence and young adulthood, with the average age of onset 19 years old.

They are more common in males. There are four theories of etiology. First, the congenital theory states that the cyst develops from embryonic gill remnants. The lymph node theory postulates that the cyst arises from trapped parotid epithelium in the upper cervical nodes. The branchial theory states that the cyst develops from the pharyngeal cleft, whereas the precervical sinus theory postulates development of the cyst from the cervical sinus.[80,89-91]

Clinical Presentation and Pathogenesis

They present as soft fluctuant masses. Most patients identify a preceding trigger such as a tooth infection, upper respiratory infection, or pregnancy. They are usually asymptomatic, but some cases have reported tenderness and dysphagia depending on the location.[90] Up to two-third occur on the left side of the neck. Complete surgical excision is the treatment of choice, although 5% of cases will recur following complete removal.[90]

Histologic Findings

The lining is represented by a combination of squamous and columnar-ciliated epithelium, with goblet cells. Abundant lymphoid tissue is present in the walls of many branchial cleft cysts (Figure 15-33). Thyroid tissue is absent.

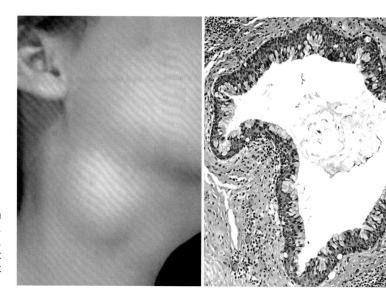

FIGURE 15-33. This girl has a cyst in the lateral neck (left panel). It is lined with respiratory epithelium, admixed with lymphoid stroma (right panel), representing a branchial cleft cyst.

BRANCHIAL CLEFT CYST

Branchial cleft cysts are developmental anomalies of the lateral neck. They are one of the most common congenital neck masses, accounting for more than 80% of all branchial anomalies. Up to 95% of these cysts arise from the second branchial arch and occur in the upper lateral neck along the anterior border of the sternocleidomastoid muscle. The lining is represented by a combination of squamous and columnar-ciliated epithelium, with goblet cells. Abundant lymphoid tissue is present.

CUTANEOUS CILIATED CYST

Definition, Epidemiology, and Etiology

Cutaneous ciliated cysts are soft, painless subcutaneous nodules most commonly found on the lower legs of young girls. They usually arise during puberty and other high estrogen states, including pregnancy. Most reported cases are diagnosed between age 15 and 30.[92-96] There are less than 50 reported cases worldwide.

Clinical Presentation and Pathogenesis

There are two main theories regarding pathogenesis. Some reports favor the migration of heterotopic-ciliated epithelium from Mullerian tissue during embryonic development. With hormonal stimulation at puberty, the cyst becomes functional.[92] However, rare cases have been reported in males and unusual locations such as the scalp and upper extremities.[92,94] Therefore, some reports favor a ciliated metaplasia of eccrine glands.[92] There are no reports of spontaneous regression. Surgical excision is curative.

Histologic Findings

The cyst lining comprises ciliated cuboidal or columnar epithelium, with a micropapillary configuration. The overall image resembles that of normal fallopian tube, supporting a Mullerian origin for this subtype of ciliated cyst. That premise is further supported by immunoreactivity for estrogen and progesterone receptor proteins (Figure 15-34).

CUTANEOUS CILIATED CYST

Cutaneous ciliated cysts are soft, painless subcutaneous nodules most commonly found on the lower legs of young girls. The cyst lining comprises ciliated cuboidal or columnar epithelium, with a micropapillary configuration.

MEDIAN RAPHE CYST

Definition, Epidemiology, and Etiology

Median raphe cysts are benign, translucent congenital cysts that occur anywhere along the midline external urethral meatus to the anal orifice[97-101] (Figure 15-35). They are usually located along the ventral portions of the shaft and glans penis without underlying urethral communication, although rare reports of perineal extension have been observed.[98] The cysts usually grow gradually and often cause discomfort with sexual intercourse, secondary infection, or disfigurement.[100] Although congenital, they often go unnoticed until early adulthood.[97] They are thought to arise from an abnormal closure of the urethral folds.[97] Excision is typically curative.

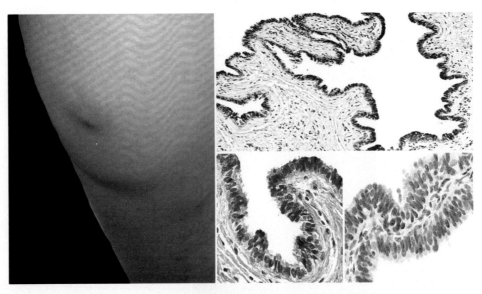

FIGURE 15-34. An adolescent girl has a cyst in the skin of the thigh (left panel). It is lined by ciliated epithelium, which resembles that of the fallopian tube (top right panel and first bottom right panel). That similarity is furthered by immunoreactivity for estrogen receptor protein (second bottom right panel) in this ciliated cutaneous cyst.

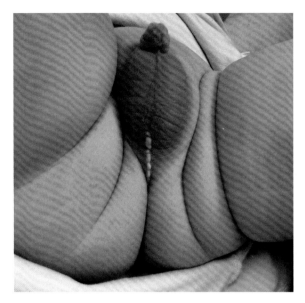

FIGURE 15-35. Multiple median raphe cysts in an infant.

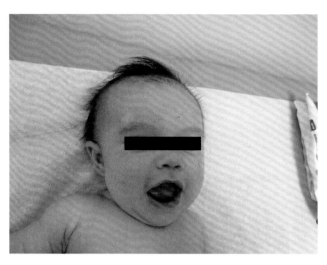

FIGURE 15-37. Dermoid cyst of the lateral eyebrow in an infant.

Histologic Findings

Median raphe cysts contain pseudostratified columnar epithelium that is potentially ciliated (Figure 15-36). Mucous-containing cells may be present as well. Current thought favors the idea that these cysts are caused by a sequestration of ectopic urethral mucosa during embryogenesis.

CAPSULE SUMMARY

MEDIAN RAPHE CYST

Median raphe cyst is a congenital cyst on the ventral surface of the penis, probably caused by abnormal closure of the urethral folds. Histologically, its lining contains ciliated epithelium, with squamoid and cuboidal elements potentially being present as well. Simple excision is curative.

TRUE DERMOID CYST (TERATOMA)

Definition, Epidemiology, and Etiology

Dermoid cysts, or true dermoid cysts (TDCs), are congenital, firm, slightly compressible, skin-colored nodules containing mature skin appendages including keratin, hair, and adnexal structures. More than 50% of cases are diagnosed and treated before 1 year of age.[102] There is no racial or gender predilection.

Clinical Presentation and Pathogenesis

A central punctum with protrusion of hairs is often diagnostic.[102-105] Dermoid cysts favor craniofacial sites, with more than 65% located at the outer third of the eyebrow (Figure 15-37). They can rarely occur on the chest. They often grow slowly for the first few years of life and then stabilize. There are rare reports of swelling, osteomyelitis, sinus tract formation, and extrusion of yellow sebaceous discharge.[103,104] Pathogenesis involves entrapment

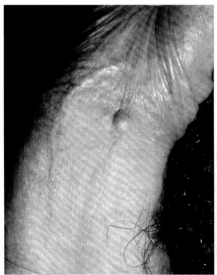

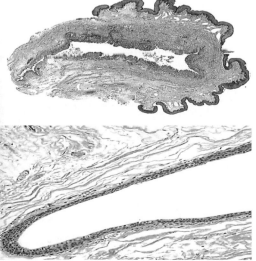

FIGURE 15-36. Another median raphe cyst is seen on the ventral surface of the penile shaft in an adolescent boy. This cyst type may be lined by cuboidal, ciliated, or squamous epithelium, sometimes with interspersed mucin-containing cells (right panels).

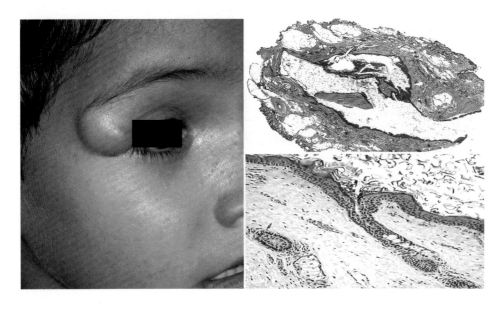

FIGURE 15-38. This cystic lesion of the periorbital skin in a young girl (left panel) contains a squamous epithelial lining with attached dermal appendages (right panels). It is a true dermoid cyst.

of ectodermal tissue at embryonic fusion plates.[102,103] They have also been called "cutaneous teratomas," but they lack the necessary tissue elements for that designation because all of their components are ectodermal in origin. Midline dermoid cysts, particularly nasal dermoid cysts, may require imaging to rule out underlying dysraphism. Complete excision without cyst wall disruption is the treatment of choice because spontaneous regression is uncommon.[102]

Histologic Findings

Microscopically, TDCs have a stratified squamous epithelial lining, with luminal keratinous debris. Pilosebaceous units are attached to the squamous epithelium (Figure 15-38), and sweat gland units or smooth muscle may also be present.

CAPSULE SUMMARY

TRUE DERMOID CYST (TERATOMA)

Dermoid cysts, or TDCs, are congenital, firm, slightly compressible, skin-colored nodules containing mature skin appendages including keratin, hair, and adnexal structures. Microscopically, TDCs have a stratified squamous epithelial lining, with luminal keratinous debris. Pilosebaceous units are attached to the squamous epithelium.

OMPHALOMESENTERIC DUCT CYST

Omphalomesenteric duct (OMD) cysts are rare congenital, red, shiny nodules that occur on the umbilicus after failure of obliteration of the OMD in which the intermediate portion remains patent, whereas the ends are sealed[106-111] (Figure 15-39). The duct is a connection between the yolk sac and foregut and starts to regress around the 8th week of gestation. Failure to obliterate the duct can lead to polyps, cysts,

or diverticula[106] These anomalies can occur in up to 2% of the population, and the cyst is the rarest type.[110] The OMD cyst is more common in males with 4:1 predominance. They can often contain remnants of gastrointestinal tract tissues and can lead to small bowel obstruction. Prior to surgical excision, ultrasound is recommended to evaluate for any secondary abnormalities including sinus tract formation and rarely omphalocele.

Histologic Findings

OMD cysts contain enteric epithelium, which resembles that of the normal intestine or stomach (Figure 15-40). Ectopic pancreatic tissue, smooth muscle, lymphoid tissue, and proliferating blood vessels may also be seen in the cyst wall. OMD cysts may induce marked acanthosis in the overlying or adjacent epidermis.

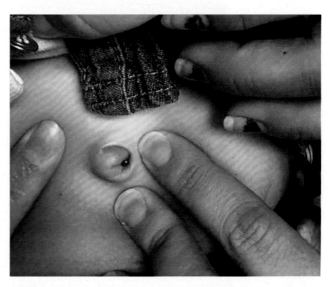

FIGURE 15-39. Omphalomesenteric duct cyst in a young male.

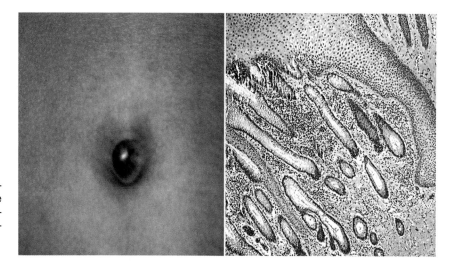

FIGURE 15-40. This umbilical cyst in an adolescent boy (left panel) contains enteric-type glandular epithelium in apposition to the epidermis (right panel), representing an omphalomesenteric duct cyst.

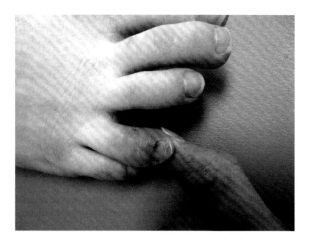

FIGURE 15-41. Digital mucous cyst in a teenage boy.

CAPSULE SUMMARY

OMPHALOMESENTERIC DUCT CYST

Omphalomesenteric duct cysts are developmental in nature, caused by abnormal closure of the Omphalomesenteric duct. They present as paraumbilical masses that contain enteric epithelium microscopically. Ectopic pancreatic, mascular, lymphoid, and vascular tissue may also be part of such lesions.

CUTANEOUS PSEUDOCYSTS

Three lesions are correctly categorized as "pseudocysts" of the skin, because they lack an epithelial lining. These include digital mucous cyst, cystic hygroma, and mucocele.

DIGITAL MUCOUS CYST

Definition, Epidemiology, Clinical Presentation, and Pathogenesis

Digital mucous cysts are asymptomatic, translucent, blue dome-shaped nodules presenting most commonly on the dominant hand along the dorsal aspect of the proximal interphalangeal joint and distal interphalangeal joint[112-114] (Figure 15-41). In 25% of patients, there is associated nail dystrophy in the form of longitudinal depression of the nail plate or onycholysis.[113] Nail dystrophy is more common if the cyst involves the proximal nail fold. Digital mucous cysts usually occur in women around age 50 to 70 and are associated with underlying osteophyte formation and osteoarthritis.[112-114] In childhood, they are often multiple and can be associated with underlying juvenile rheumatoid arthritis or trauma.[113] They are usually asymptomatic, with some reports of pain, swelling, and decreased range of motion. Pathogenesis involves herniation and degeneration of the joint capsule, leading to fibroblast disarray and increased hyaluronic acid production.[113] Spontaneous regression is rare, and surgical excision leads to a 90% cure rate.[114]

Histologic Findings

Puncture or biopsy of the papule yields a gelatinous clear liquid, principally comprising hyaluronic acid, which is seen histologically as a subepidermal collection of amorphous basophilic material (Figure 15-42). No epithelium is present. Digital mucous "cyst" is felt to represent a singular form of dermal mucinosis.

CAPSULE SUMMARY

DIGITAL MUCOUS CYST

Digital mucous cysts are asymptomatic, translucent, blue dome-shaped nodules presenting most commonly on the dominant hand along the dorsal aspect of the proximal interphalangeal joint and distal interphalangeal joint. Histologically, they are pseudocysts with a subepidermal collection of amorphous basophilic material without a true lining.

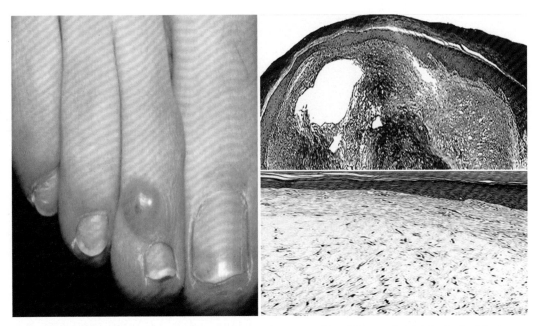

FIGURE 15-42. Another adolescent boy has a digital cyst on the right second toe (left panel). Histologically, it lacks an epithelial lining and contains only mucinous stroma (right panels), establishing the diagnosis of digital mucous (pseudo-) cyst.

CYSTIC HYGROMA (MACROCYSTIC LYMPHATIC MALFORMATIONS)

Definition, Etiology, and Clinical Presentation

Cystic hygromas are congenital macrocystic lymphatic malformations that present as large (often several centimeters) translucent masses with overlying normal appearing skin along the posterior triangle of the right side of the neck (75%) or axillae[76,115-117] (Figure 15-43). The malformation will enhance with transillumination and are often diagnosed on antenatal ultrasound studies.[115] They can be incidental findings, but more than 60% of cases are associated with chromosome abnormalities, most commonly Turner Syndrome (33%) but also Noonan Syndrome, and Trisomy 13, 18, and 21.[116] They occur in 1:6000 to 16 000 births.[117] More than 50% of cases are present at birth and 90% will present by age 2. Complications can arise, including lymphedema, heart failure, intrauterine demise, and facial deformities.

Pathogenesis

Pathogenesis involves failure of the primitive lymph sac connecting to the venous system or improper sequestration of lymph tissue during embryogenesis. Sclerosing agents followed by surgical excision are the treatments of choice with moderate recurrence rates of 10% to 15%.[117] Most recurrences will occur within 1 year of treatment.

Histologic Findings

A profusion of thin-walled vessels throughout the dermis and superficial subcutis is observed (Figure 15-44). The endothelial lining cells are attenuated, with flattened nuclei, amphophilic cytoplasm, and a lack of mitoses. The vascular channels comprising macrocystic lymphatic malformations are variable in diameter, but some may attain large, cystic proportions. Mature lymphocytes are often admixed throughout these tumors, and small collections of such cells may be observed within the vascular lumina along with serum. Intravascular erythrocytes are typically scant or absent.

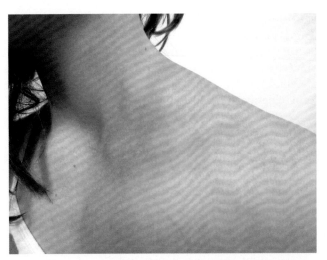

FIGURE 15-43. Cystic hygroma of the left lateral neck in a young adolescent female.

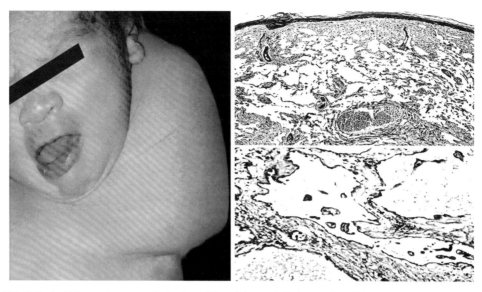

FIGURE 15-44. This infant girl has a large cystic lesion of the right neck (left panel), which comprises numerous lymphatic vascular channels of various sizes (right panels). Although the term "cystic hygroma" is used for such masses, they are actually lymphangiomas.

CAPSULE SUMMARY

CYSTIC HYGROMA (MACROCYSTIC LYMPHATIC MALFORMATIONS)

Cystic hygromas are congenital macrocystic lymphatic malformations that present as large (often several centimeters) translucent masses with overlying normal appearing skin along the posterior triangle of the right side of the neck (75%) or axillae. Histologically, the vascular channels comprising macrocystic lymphatic malformations are variable in diameter, but some may attain large, cystic proportions. Mature lymphocytes are often admixed throughout these tumors.

MUCOCELE

Definition, Etiology, and Clinical Presentation

Mucoceles are benign soft tissue masses with an elastic consistency that present as translucent blue nodules on the lower labial mucosa (Figure 15-45). They can rarely occur on the floor of the mouth or the hard palate.[118-123] They are the second most common oral cavity lesion and account for 10% to 20% of all oral biopsies in pediatric patients.[122,123] Up to 85% of pediatric cases involve the lower labial mucosa. Mucoceles have an equal predominance in both sexes and affects all races. The incidence is highest in the second decade of life, and 35% of patients usually present before age 15.[123] Mucoceles are associated with trauma and lower lip biting.[16,18]

Clinical Presentation and Pathogenesis

Although mucoceles usually have a rapid growth phase, they are usually asymptomatic. Rarely, they can cause swelling or pain with swallowing and mastication.[19] Without treatment, they can persist unchanged for years. There may be periods of episodic improvement with resorption of mucus followed by eventual reaccumulation.[122,123]

Histologic Findings

Mucoceles are subdivided into two microscopic types: mucous retention cysts and mucous extravasation pseudocysts. The former represents a distended salivary duct that retains

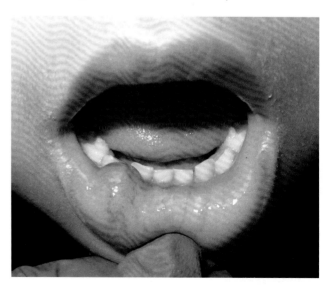

FIGURE 15-45. A mucocele on the lower vermillion lip of a young girl.

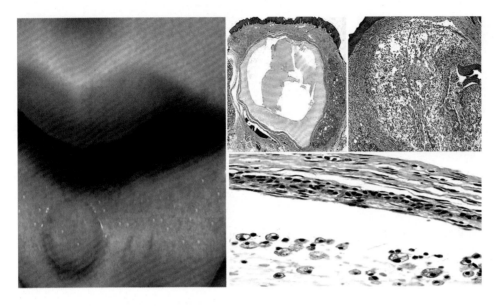

FIGURE 15-46. A cystic lesion of the lip in a young boy (left panel) is represented by a spherical accumulation of mucus that is only partially mantled by flattened epithelial cells (right panels). It is a mucocele.

its epithelial lining. The latter results from rupture of an obstructed or damaged duct, with extravasation of mucus into the surrounding tissue. No epithelium is present within extravasation mucoceles (Figure 15-46). Extravasation mucoceles undergo three phases of development. In the first phase, mucus is spilled from a damaged salivary duct into the surrounding tissues. In the second phase, a foreign body reaction is engendered by the mucus. Finally, a pseudocapsule—without an epithelial lining—surrounds the extravasated mucus and the granulomatous reaction to it.

CAPSULE SUMMARY

MUCOCELE

Mucoceles are benign soft tissue masses with an elastic consistency that present as translucent blue nodules on the lower labial mucosa. Mucoceles are subdivided into two microscopic types: mucous retention cysts and mucous extravasation pseudocysts. The former represents a distended salivary duct that retains its epithelial lining. The latter results from rupture of an obstructed or damaged duct, with extravasation of mucus into the surrounding tissue.

REFERENCES

1. Kim WB, Mistry N, Alavi A, Sibbald C, Sibbald RG. Pretibial myxedema: case presentation and review of treatment options. *Int J Low Extrem Wounds.* 2014;13(2):152-154.
2. Shroff A, Simpson G. Cutaneous manifestations of thyroid disease: a case of thyroid-induced myxedema. *Case Rep Dermatol Med.* 2011;2011:386081.
3. Fatourechi V. Pretibial myxedema: pathophysiology and treatment options. *Am J Clin Dermatol.* 2005;6(5):295-309.
4. Reddy SC, Baman JR, Morrison CS, Scott GA. Cutaneous mucinosis of infancy. *JAAD Case Rep.* 2016;2(3):250-252.
5. Lum D. Cutaneous mucinosis of infancy. *Arch Dermatol.* 1980;116(2):198-200.
6. Stokes KS, Rabinowitz LG, Segura AD, Esterly NB. Cutaneous mucinosis of infancy. *Pediatr Dermatol.* 1994;11(3):246-251.
7. Eichenfield L, Frieden I, Zaenglein A, Mathes E. *Neonatal and Infant Dermatology.* 1st ed. Elsevier Health Sciences; 2014; New York, NY.
8. Carder KR, Fitzpatrick JE, Weston WL, Morelli JG. Self-healing juvenile cutaneous mucinosis. *Pediatr Dermatol.* 2003;20(1):35-39.
9. Cowen EW, Scott GA, Mercurio MG. Self-healing juvenile cutaneous mucinosis. *J Am Acad Dermatol.* 2004;50(5 suppl):S97-S100.
10. Nagaraj LV, Fangman W, White WL, et al. Self-healing juvenile cutaneous mucinosis: cases highlighting subcutaneous/fascial involvement. *J Am Acad Dermatol.* 2006;55(6):1036-1043.
11. Luchsinger I, Coulombe J, Rongioletti F, et al. Self-healing juvenile cutaneous mucinosis: Clinical and histopathologic findings of nine cases: the relevance of long-term follow-up. *J Am Acad Dermatol.* 2018;78(6):1164-1170
12. Steffes WE, Bezalel SA, Church AA, Vincek V, Wesson SK. A case of self-healing juvenile cutaneous mucinosis. *Dermatol Online J.* 2015;21(6).
13. Kofler H, Lipsker D, Maurer H, et al. Self-healing juvenile cutaneous mucinosis: challenging diagnosis and management. *J Dtsch Dermatol Ges.* 2014;12(9):815-817.
14. Beers WH, Ince A, Moore TL. Scleredema adultorum of Buschke: a case report and review of the literature. *Semin Arthritis Rheum.* 2006;35(6):355-359.
15. Lewis CM, Sanchez AT, Davis LS. Atypical scleredema involving the hands in an adolescent. *Pediatr Dermatol.* 2016;33(6):e342-e343.
16. Shrestha B, Neopane AK, Panth R. Scleredema: an uncommon cause of swelling in a child: case report and review of the literature. *BMC Res Notes.* 2014;7:571.
17. Rani JD, Patil SG, Murthy STS, Koshy AV, Nagpal D, Gupta S. Juvenile scleredema of Buschke. *J Contemp Dent Pract.* 2012;13(1):111-114.
18. Sansom JE, Sheehan AL, Kennedy CT, Delaney TJ. A fatal case of scleredema of Buschke. *Br J Dermatol.* 1994;130(5):669-670.
19. Tran MC, Lam JM. Cutaneous manifestations of mucopolysaccharidoses. *Pediatr Dermatol.* 2016;33(6):594-601.
20. Ashrafi MR, Tavasoli A, Shiva S, Parvaneh N, Tamizifar B. Diffuse dermal melanocytosis in two patients with Sandhoff disease and mucopolysaccharidosis VI. *Int J Dermatol.* 2014;53(6):736-738.
21. Marín LL, Gutiérrez-Solana LG, Fernβndez AT. Hunter syndrome: resolution of extensive typical skin lesions after 9 months of enzyme replacement therapy with idursulfase. *Pediatr Dermatol.* 2012;29(3):369-370.

22. Kaltoft B, Schmidt G, Lauritzen AF, Gimsing P. Primary localised cutaneous amyloidosis: a systematic review. *Dan Med J*. 2013;60(11):A4727.

23. Fernandez-Flores A. Cutaneous amyloidosis: a concept review. *Am J Dermatopathol*. 2012;34(1):1-14; quiz 15-17.

24. Moon AO, Calamia KT, Walsh JS. Nodular amyloidosis: review and long-term follow-up of 16 cases. *Arch Dermatol*. 2003;139(9):1157-1159.

25. Vijaya B, Dalal BS, Sunila, Manjunath GV. Primary cutaneous amyloidosis: a clinico-pathological study with emphasis on polarized microscopy. *Indian J Pathol Microbiol*. 2012;55(2):170-174.

26. Andrese E, Vâță D, Ciobanu D, Stătescu L, Solovăstru LG. The autoimmune constellation in lichen amyloidosis. *Rev Med Chir Soc Med Nat Iasi*. 2015;119(4):1045-1050.

27. Verga U, Fugazzola L, Cambiaghi S, et al. Frequent association between MEN 2A and cutaneous lichen amyloidosis. *Clin Endocrinol (Oxf)*. 2003;59(2):156-161.

28. Ladizinski B, Lee KC. Lichen amyloidosis. *CMAJ*. 2014;186(7):532.

29. Behr FD, Levine N, Bangert J. Lichen amyloidosis associated with atopic dermatitis: clinical resolution with cyclosporine. *Arch Dermatol*. 2001;137(5):553-555.

30. Verga U, Beck-Peccoz P, Cambiaghi S. Cutaneous lichen amyloidosis in multiple endocrine neoplasia type 2A. *Thyroid*. 2002;12(12):1149.

31. Schachner L, Hansen R. *Pediatric Dermatology*. 4th ed. Philadelphia, PA: Elsevier Health Sciences; 2011:1912.

32. Reiter N, El-Shabrawi L, Leinweber B, Berghold A, Aberer E. Calcinosis cutis: part I. Diagnostic pathway. *J Am Acad Dermatol*. 2011;65(1):1-12; quiz 13-14.

33. Reiter N, El-Shabrawi L, Leinweber B, Berghold A, Aberer E. Calcinosis cutis: part II. Treatment options. *J Am Acad Dermatol*. 2011;65(1):15-22; quiz 23-24.

34. Gupta V, Balaga R, Banik S. Idiopathic calcinosis cutis over elbow in a 12-year old child. *Case Rep Orthop*. 2013;2013:241891.

35. Rodríguez-Cano L, García-Patos V, Creus M, Bastida P, Ortega JJ, Castells A. Childhood calcinosis cutis. *Pediatr Dermatol*. 1996;13(2):114-117.

36. Welborn MC, Gottschalk H, Bindra R. Juvenile dermatomyositis: a case of calcinosis cutis of the elbow and review of the literature. *J Pediatr Orthop*. 2015;35(5):e43-e46.

37. Ward S, Sugo E, Verge CF, Wargon O. Three cases of osteoma cutis occurring in infancy. A brief overview of osteoma cutis and its association with pseudo-pseudohypoparathyroidism. *Australas J Dermatol*. 2011;52(2):127-131.

38. Caravaglio JV, Gupta R, Weinstein D. Multiple miliary osteoma cutis of the face associated with Albright hereditary osteodystrophy in the setting of acne vulgaris: a case report. *Dermatol Online J*. 2017;23(3).

39. Martin J, Tucker M, Browning JC. Infantile osteoma cutis as a presentation of a GNAS mutation. *Pediatr Dermatol*. 2012;29(4):483-484.

40. Mariani M, Rigante D, Guerriero C, Ricci F, Sani I, Rossodivita A. Progressive osseous heteroplasia in a 7-year-old girl with osteoma cutis and autoimmune thyroiditis: the importance of investigating GNAS mutations. *J Eur Acad Dermatol Venereol*. 2016;30(5):905-907.

41. Kucukemre Aydin B, Yazganoglu KD, Baykal C, et al. Osteoma cutis, *Pediatr*. 2013;55(2):257-258.

42. Chabra IS, Obagi S. Evaluation and management of multiple miliary osteoma cutis: case series of 11 patients and literature review. *Dermatol Surg*. 2014;40(1):66-68.

43. Bouraoui S, Mlika M, Kort R, Cherif F, Lahmar A, Sabeh M. Miliary osteoma cutis of the face. *J Dermatol Case Rep*. 2011;5(4):77-81.

44. Happle R. Progressive osseous heteroplasia is not a Mendelian trait but a type 2 segmental manifestation of GNAS inactivation disorders: a hypothesis. *Eur J Med Genet*. 2016;59(5):290-294.

45. Gulbranson SH, Hud JA, Hansen RC. Argyria following the use of dietary supplements containing colloidal silver protein. *Cutis*. 2000;66(5):373-374.

46. Baker CD, Federico MJ, Accurso FJ. Case report: skin discoloration following administration of colloidal silver in cystic fibrosis. *Curr Opin Pediatr*. 2007;19(6):733-735.

47. Browning JC, Levy ML. Argyria attributed to silvadene application in a patient with dystrophic epidermolysis bullosa. *Dermatol Online J*. 2008;14(4):9.

48. Fogelson S, Dohil M. Papular and nodular skin lesions in children. *Semin Plast Surg*. 2006;20(3):180-191.

49. Armon N, Shamay S, Maly A, Margulis A. Occurrence and characteristics of head cysts in children. *Eplasty*. 2010;10:e37.

50. Berk DR, Bayliss SJ. Milia: a review and classification. *J Am Acad Dermatol*. 2008;59(6):1050-1063.

51. Satyaprakash AK, Sheehan DJ, Sangüeza OP. Proliferating trichilemmal tumors: a review of the literature. *Dermatol Surg*. 2007;33(9):1102-1108.

52. Madan S, Joshi R. Trichilemmal cyst of the penis in a paediatric patient. *Sultan Qaboos Univ Med J*. 2015;15(1):e129-e132.

53. Pelivani N, Houriet C, Haneke E. Trichilemmal cyst nevus with a sebaceous nevus component. *Dermatol Basel Switz*. 2010;221(4):289-291.

54. Baselga E, Dzwierzynski WW, Neuburg M, Troy JL, Esterly NB. Cutaneous keratocyst in naevoid basal cell carcinoma syndrome. *Br J Dermatol*. 1996;135(5):810-812.

55. Barr RJ, Headley JL, Jensen JL, Howell JB. Cutaneous keratocysts of nevoid basal cell carcinoma syndrome. *J Am Acad Dermatol*. 1986;14(4):572-576.

56. Cassarino DS, Linden KG, Barr RJ. Cutaneous keratocyst arising independently of the nevoid basal cell carcinoma syndrome. *Am J Dermatopathol*. 2005;27(2):177-178.

57. Peñaranda JM, Aliste C, Forteza J. Cutaneous keratocyst not associated to gorlin syndrome: an incidental finding in a healthy male. *Am J Dermatopathol*. 2007;29(6):584-585.

58. Mortazavi H, Taheri A, Mansoori P, Kani ZA. Localized forms of steatocystoma multiplex: case report and review of the literature. *Dermatol Online J*. 2005;11(1):22.

59. Teng J, Marqueling A, Benjamin L. *Therapy in Pediatric Dermatology*. Vol. 1. Springer International Publishing; 2017; Geneva, Switzerland.

60. Araujo KM, Denadai R. Clinical misdiagnosis of steatocystoma simplex of eyebrow in a pediatric patient. *Chin Med J (Engl)*. 2016;129(3):377-378.

61. Park YM, Cho SH, Kang H. Congenital linear steatocystoma multiplex of the nose. *Pediatr Dermatol*. 2000;17(2):136-138.

62. Kamra HT, Gadgil PA, Ovhal AG, Narkhede RR. Steatocystoma multiplex-a rare genetic disorder: a case report and review of the literature. *J Clin Diagn Res*. 2013;7(1):166-168.

63. Nam J-H, Lee G-Y, Kim W-S, Kim KJ. Eccrine hidrocystoma in a child: an atypical presentation. *Ann Dermatol*. 2010;22(1):69-72.

64. Samplaski MK, Somani N, Palmer JS. Apocrine hidrocystoma on glans penis of a child. *Urology*. 2009;73(4):800-801.

65. Malihi M, Turbin RE, Mirani N, Langer PD. Giant orbital hydrocystoma in children: case series and review of the literature. *Orbit Amst Neth*. 2015;34(5):292-296.

66. Torchia D, Vega J, Schachner LA. Eruptive vellus hair cysts: a systematic review. *Am J Clin Dermatol*. 2012;13(1):19-28.

67. Erltek E, Kurtipek GS, Duman D, Sanli C, Erdoğan S. Eruptive vellus hair cysts: report of a pediatric case with partial response to calcipotriene therapy. *Cutis*. 2009;84(6):295-298.

68. Zaharia D, Kanitakis J. Eruptive vellus hair cysts: report of a new case with immunohistochemical study and literature review. *Dermatol Basel Switz*. 2012;224(1):15-19.

69. Khatu S, Vasani R, Amin S. Eruptive vellus hair cyst presenting as asymptomatic follicular papules on extremities. *Indian Dermatol Online J*. 2013;4(3):213-215.

70. Sarabi K, Khachemoune A. Hidrocystomas: a brief review. *MedGenMed*. 2006;8(3):57.

71. Kikuchi K, Fukunaga S, Inoue H, Miyazaki Y, Ide F, Kusama K. Apocrine hidrocystoma of the lower lip: a case report and literature review. *Head Neck Pathol*. 2014;8(1):117-121.

72. Weston W, Lane A, Morelli JG. *Color Textbook of Pediatric Dermatology*. 4th ed. Mosby Elsevier; 2007; New York, NY.

73. Sarper A, Ayten A, Golbasi I, Demircan A, Isin E. Bronchogenic cyst. *Tex Heart Inst J.* 2003;30(2):105-108.

74. Sacks E, Jakobiec FA, McMillan R, Fraunfelder F, Iwamoto T. Multiple bilateral apocrine cystadenomas of the lower eyelids. Light and electron microscopic studies. *Ophthalmology.* 1987;94(1):65-71.

75. Prosser JD, Myer CM III. Branchial cleft anomalies and thymic cysts. *Otolaryngol Clin North Am.* 2015;48(1):1-14.

76. Gaddikeri S, Vattoth S, Gaddikeri RS, et al. Congenital cystic neck masses: embryology and imaging appearances, with clinicopathological correlation. *Curr Probl Diagn Radiol.* 2014;43(2):55-67.

77. Petropoulos I, Konstantinidis I, Noussios G, Karagiannidis K, Kontzoglou G. Thymic cyst in the differential diagnosis of paediatric cervical masses. *B-ENT.* 2006;2(1):35-37. PubMed PMID: 16676846.

78. Moz U, Gamba P, Pignatelli U, et al. Bronchogenic cysts of the neck: a rare localization and review of the literature. *Acta Otorhinolaryngol Ital.* 2009;29(1):36-40.

79. Ahrens B, Wit J, Schmitt M, Wahn U, Niggemann B, Paul K. Symptomatic bronchogenic cyst in a six-month-old infant: case report and review of the literature. *J Thorac Cardiovasc Surg.* 2001;122(5):1021-1023.

80. Valentino M, Quiligotti C, Carone L. Branchial cleft cyst. *J Ultrasound.* 2013;16(1):17-20.

81. Manchanda V, Mohta A, Khurana N, Das S. Subcutaneous bronchogenic cyst. *J Cutan Aesthetic Surg.* 2010;3(3):181-183.

82. Harle CC, Dearlove O, Walker RW, Wright N. A bronchogenic cyst in an infant causing tracheal occlusion and cardiac arrest. *Anaesthesia.* 1999;54(3):262-265.

83. Frye SA, Decou JM. Pediatric bronchogenic cyst complicated by atypical mycobacterium infection: a case report. *Cases J.* 2009;2:8070.

84. Thabet H, Gaafar A, Nour Y. Thyroglossal duct cyst: variable presentations. *Egypt J Ear Nose Throat Allied Sci.* 2011;12:13-20.

85. Moorthy S, Arcot R. Thyroglossal duct cyst—more than just an embryological remnant. *Indian J Surg.* 2011;73(1):28-31.

86. Bai W, Ji W, Wang L, Song Y. Diagnosis and treatment of lingual thyroglossal duct cyst in newborns. *Pediatr Int.* 2009;51(4):552-554.

87. Ren W, Zhi K, Zhao L, Gao L. Presentations and management of thyroglossal duct cyst in children versus adults: a review of 106 cases. *Oral Surg Oral Med Oral Pathol Oral Radiol Endod.* 2011;111(2):e1-e6.

88. Mondin V, Ferlito A, Muzzi E, et al. Thyroglossal duct cyst: personal experience and literature review. *Auris Nasus Larynx.* 2008;35(1):11-25.

89. Nahata V. Branchial cleft cyst. *Indian J Dermatol.* 2016;61(6):701.

90. Chavan S, Deshmukh R, Karande P, Ingale Y. Branchial cleft cyst: a case report and review of literature. *J Oral Maxillofac Pathol.* 2014;18(1):150.

91. Panchbhai AS, Choudhary MS. Branchial cleft cyst at an unusual location: a rare case with a brief review. *Dento Maxillo Facial Radiol.* 2012;41(8):696-702.

92. Fontaine DG, Lau H, Murray SK, Fraser RB, Wright JR Jr. Cutaneous ciliated cyst of the abdominal wall: a case report with a review of the literature and discussion of pathogenesis. *Am J Dermatopathol.* 2002;24(1):63-66.

93. Reserva JL, Carrigg AB, Schnebelen AM, Hiatt KM, Cheung WL. Cutaneous ciliated cyst of the scalp: a case report of a cutaneous ciliated eccrine cyst and a brief review of the literature. *Am J Dermatopathol.* 2014;36(8):679-682.

94. Swarbrick N, Harvey NT, Wood BA. Cutaneous ciliated cyst of the scrotum. *Pathology (Phila).* 2015;47(6):593-595.

95. Chong S-J, Kim S-Y, Kim H-S, Kim GM, Kim SY, Jung J-H. Cutaneous ciliated cyst in a 15-year-old girl. *J Am Acad Dermatol.* 2007;56(1):159-160.

96. Kavishwar VS, Waghmare RS, Puranik GV, Chadha K. Cutaneous ciliated cyst of right popliteal fossa. *J Assoc Physicians India.* 2014;62(10):85-87.

97. Sagar J, Sagar B, Patel AF, Shak DK. Ciliated median raphe cyst of perineum presenting as perianal polyp: a case report with immunohistochemical study, review of literature, and pathogenesis. *ScientificWorld Journal.* 2006;6:2339-2344.

98. Arer IM, Yilmaz D, Ozek OC, Yabanoglu H, Caliskan K. Unusual location of median raphe cyst presenting as perianal polyp: a case report. *Dermatol Online J.* 2016;22(6).

99. Yu A, Capolicchio J-P. A case of epidermoid median raphe cyst traversing the corpora cavernosa. *Can Urol Assoc J.* 2017;11(3-4):E119-E121.

100. Navarro HP, Lopez PC, Ruiz JM, et al. Median raphe cyst. Report of two cases and literature review. *Arch Esp Urol.* 2009;62(7):585-589.

101. Kumar P, Das A, Savant SS, Barkat R. Median raphe cyst: report of two cases. *Dermatol Online J.* 2017;23(2).

102. Paradis J, Koltai PJ. Pediatric teratoma and dermoid cysts. *Otolaryngol Clin North Am.* 2015;48(1):121-136.

103. Orozco-Covarrubias L, Lara-Carpio R, Saez-De-Ocariz M, Duran-McKinster C, Palacios-Lopez C, Ruiz-Maldonado R. Dermoid cysts: a report of 75 pediatric patients. *Pediatr Dermatol.* 2013;30(6):706-711.

104. Yan C, Low DW. A rare presentation of a dermoid cyst with draining sinus in a child: case report and literature review. *Pediatr Dermatol.* 2016;33(4):e244-e248.

105. Hills SE, Maddalozzo J. Congenital lesions of epithelial origin. *Otolaryngol Clin North Am.* 2015;48(1):209-223.

106. Bagade S, Khanna G. Imaging of omphalomesenteric duct remnants and related pathologies in children. *Curr Probl Diagn Radiol.* 2015;44(3):246-255.

107. Ballester I, Betlloch I, Pérez-Crespo M, Toledo F, Cuesta L. Atypical presentation of an omphalomesenteric duct cyst. *Dermatol Online J.* 2009;15(6):13.

108. Iwasaki M, Taira K, Kobayashi H, Saiga T. Umbilical cyst containing ectopic gastric mucosa originating from an omphalomesenteric duct remnant. *J Pediatr Surg.* 2009;44(12):2399-2401.

109. Hsu JW, Tom WL. Omphalomesenteric duct remnants: umbilical versus umbilical cord lesions. *Pediatr Dermatol.* 2011;28(4):404-407.

110. Annaberdyev S, Capizzani T, Plesec T, Moorman M. A rare case presentation of a symptomatic omphalomesenteric cyst in an adult, 24-year-old patient, treated with laparoscopic resection. *J Gastrointest Surg.* 2013;17(8):1503-1506.

111. Ratan SK, Rattan KN, Kalra R, Maheshwari J, Parihar D, Ratan J. Omphalomesenteric duct cyst as a content of omphalocele. *Indian J Pediatr.* 2007;74(5):500-502.

112. Paller A, Mancini A. *Hurwitz Clinical Pediatric Dermatology.* 5th ed. Elsevier Health Sciences; 2015:640; New York, NY.

113. Li K, Barankin B. Digital mucous cysts. *J Cutan Med Surg.* 2010;14(5):199-206.

114. Jabbour S, Kechichian E, Haber R, Tomb R, Nasr M. Management of digital mucous cysts: a systematic review and treatment algorithm. *Int J Dermatol.* 2017;56(7):701-708.

115. Brown RE, Harave S. Diagnostic imaging of benign and malignant neck masses in children-a pictorial review. *Quant Imaging Med Surg.* 2016;6(5):591-604.

116. Mehta MR. Cystic hygroma: presentation of two cases with a review of the literature. *Indian J Otolaryngol Head Neck Surg.* 2000;52(3):319-322.

117. Singh Bakshi S. Cystic hygroma. *Acta Clin Belg.* 2017;72(2):146.

118. Nico MMS, Park JH, Lourenço SV. Mucocele in pediatric patients: analysis of 36 children. *Pediatr Dermatol.* 2008;25(3):308-311.

119. Shapira M, Akrish S. Mucoceles of the oral cavity in neonates and infants: report of a case and literature review. *Pediatr Dermatol.* 2014;31(2):e55-e58.

120. Abdel-Aziz M, Khalifa B, Nassar A, Kamel A, Naguib N, El-Tahan A-R. Mucocele of the hard palate in children. *Int J Pediatr Otorhinolaryngol.* 2016;85:46-49.

121. Bhargava N, Agarwal P, Sharma N, Agrawal M, Sidiq M, Narain P. An unusual presentation of oral mucocele in infant and its review. *Case Rep Dent.* 2014;2014:723130.

122. More CB, Bhavsar K, Varma S, Tailor M. Oral mucocele: a clinical and histopathological study. *J Oral Maxillofac Pathol.* 2014;18(suppl 1):S72-S77.

123. Nallasivam KU, Sudha BR. Oral mucocele: review of literature and a case report. *J Pharm Bioallied Sci.* 2015;7 (suppl 2):S731-S733.

16

Alopecia

Scott Walter / Mary Barrett / Lynne J. Goldberg

Nonscarring Alopecia

ANDROGENETIC ALOPECIA

Definition and Epidemiology

Androgenetic alopecia (AGA), which is the most common alopecia in adults, can occur in children and adolescents. It is characterized not by a true loss of hair, but by a slow and progressive miniaturization of the hair follicle, with an increase in the telogen to anagen hair ratio.[1] This leads to an apparent thinning of the hair in characteristic patterns on the scalp. Both a genetic predisposition and androgen hormones play a role in the pathogenesis of AGA.[1,2]

The exact incidence and prevalence of AGA in children is not well established. One study of nearly 500 15- to 17-year-old males found that 15.5% had some degree of AGA.[3] For most children, onset is typically after puberty, but can occur in prepubertal children as young as 6.[4] The average age of onset in children ranges from 13.5 to 15 years old.[4,5] Two larger studies in adolescents showed a male predominance, with male to female ratio ranging from 2:1 to 4.3:1, which is similar to the adult population.[5,6] Other studies have shown a slight female predominance in children.[4,7] A strong family history of alopecia is common in children with AGA, present in 72.1% to 83% of affected patients, which is greater than that reported for adults (30% to 64.5%).[5,6] In a series of 20 prepubertal children with AGA, all had a strong family history—with 9 patients having one parent affected and 11 having both parents affected.[4] Some other dermatologic disorders have been associated with

AGA, including seborrheic dermatitis, acne vulgaris, and atopic dermatitis.[6] Severe acne and hirsutism in females is associated with a more severe AGA presentation.[1]

Etiology

As the name suggests, AGA is both androgen-dependent and genetically inherited. Males castrated before puberty do not develop AGA, which supports the role of androgens.[8] However, the exact mechanism of pathogenesis is not well understood—especially in the pediatric population.

Miniaturization occurs when androgen hormones act directly upon terminal follicles, converting them to vellus-like follicles. As they miniaturize, the hair cycle shortens, leading to increasingly smaller and more superficial follicles with shorter, thinner, and paler hair shafts. Shortening of the anagen phase results in a greater number of overall hairs in the telogen phase.[1] Certain follicles on the scalp have been found to be more susceptible to the effects of excess androgens, which leads to the characteristic male and female patterns of hair loss—in males on the vertex and frontotemporal scalp and on the crown in females.[1] Androgen receptors and type II 5-α reductase, the enzyme that converts testosterone to the active metabolite dihydrotestosterone, are found in higher levels in the outer root sheath and dermal papillae of follicles in these areas.[9,10] The relationship between blood levels of androgen hormones in the development of AGA is controversial, with studies in children and adolescents yielding conflicting results. Nevertheless, hyperandrogenemia has been detected in association with some cases of pediatric AGA, including in patients with polycystic ovarian syndrome and late-onset congenital adrenal hyperplasia.[4,5,6,11,12]

Studies in children with AGA consistently show a family history of patterned hair loss, and concordance rates in monozygotic twins range from 80% to 90%, suggesting a strong genetic predisposition.[2,4,6] Although the exact genetic inheritance is not known, it is most likely polygenic.[13-15] In adults, polymorphisms in the 5-alpha-reductase enzyme and androgen receptor have been found to be associated with AGA, and mutations in 17-α-hydroxylase are associated with premature AGA.[14-16]

Clinical Presentation

AGA presents with gradual onset hair thinning localized to the androgen-dependent parts of the scalp. Hair in affected areas is thinner, shorter, and finer, leading to classic patterns of loss as described originally by Hamilton and Ludwig.[17,18] The majority of adult men have loss localized to the vertex and recession in the frontotemporal region, whereas adult females typically preserve their frontal hairline with loss more prominent on the crown of the scalp. The patterns of hair loss in children with AGA vary, and usually present more mildly compared with adults.[19] Prepubertal males may present with classically female pattern, and sometimes show frontal prominence.[4,5] This is characterized by a widened central part (Figure 16-1). Onset in adolescents usually presents in classic gender-specific patterns.[6] The occiput is usually spared in all patients. Diagnosis in children is supported by trichoscopy showing greater than 20% hair diameter diversity (miniaturization).[4]

Histologic Findings

The major histopathologic finding in AGA is miniaturization of hair follicles with a subsequent decrease in the terminal:vellus (T:V) size ratio (Figure 16-2). The normal T:V ratio is approximately 6-8:1,[20] but a ratio of 4:1 or less is considered compatible with AGA,[21] and a ratio of 2:1 or less is common. Additional findings include a normal overall number of follicles, a slight increase in the percentage of follicles in catagen or telogen phase (up to 20%), and the presence of follicular stelae (fibrous tracts or streamers) underlying the miniaturized hairs.[22] In a small study of biopsies of pediatric AGA, 57% showed varying degrees of a lymphocytic perifollicular inflammation and accompanying fibrosis.[5] However, inflammation is not a consistent feature, and peribulbar inflammation or associated follicular destruction should be absent. Scarring may occur in long-standing AGA,[22] but is unlikely in the pediatric population.

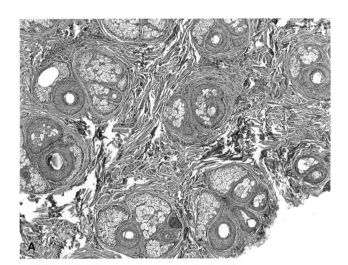

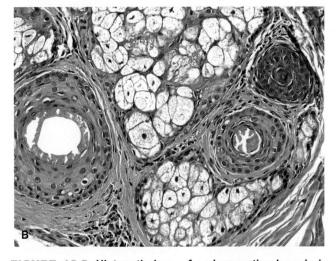

FIGURE 16-2. **Histopathology of androgenetic alopecia in a 16-year-old girl.** A, Low-power view of the isthmus reveals a mixture of terminal and vellus hair follicles with a terminal to vellus ratio of approximately 1:1 (H&E, ×4). B, Higher power of a follicular unit with one terminal and two vellus hair follicles (H&E, ×20).

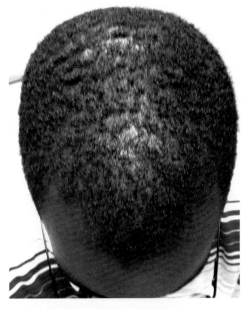

FIGURE 16-1. **Male pattern hair loss in a 17-year-old boy.** Note the bitemporal recession of the hair line and the thinning of hair on the crown.

Differential Diagnosis

The clinical differential diagnosis of AGA includes alopecia areata (AA) and telogen effluvium (TE). In most cases, these can be distinguished by the pattern of hair loss, with AA typically leading to patchy hair loss in well-demarcated areas, and TE causing more global hair thinning. Diffuse AA lacks the typical patchy distribution of the classic type and may pose a diagnostic challenge.

Histologically, AA shares some common features with AGA, but typically shows a much more marked shift away from anagen, with catagen/telogen counts from 50% to 100%. Additionally, peribulbar lymphocytic inflammation is often present,[23] along with dilated follicular infundibula, trichomalacia, and small follicles with abnormal morphology lacking a central hair shaft.

TE in its acute form displays a normal total number of follicles with an increased proportion in catagen and telogen phases (not exceeding 50%), and fibrous stelae underlying these follicles. Chronic TE can have a variable percentage of catagen/telogen follicles and may closely mimic a normal scalp biopsy. Neither acute nor chronic TE displays the miniaturization of follicles characteristic of AGA.

CAPSULE SUMMARY

ANDROGENETIC ALOPECIA

AGA is an uncommon cause of alopecia in children. It is caused by the action of androgen hormones on scalp hair follicles, leading to miniaturization and the appearance of hair loss. It is polygenic in inheritance, and presents as a gradual thinning of hair at the vertex and frontotemporal regions of the scalp in males or on the crown of the scalp in females and prepubertal children. Histopathologic findings include miniaturization of hair follicles with an associated decrease in the T:V size ratio and a mild increase in the number of catagen/telogen follicles.

TELOGEN EFFLUVIUM

Definition and Epidemiology

TE is a nonscarring, diffuse alopecia characterized by a disproportionate loss of telogen hairs after a trigger that disrupts the normal hair cycle.[24,25]

The exact prevalence and incidence of TE is not known in adults or children, but is likely similar in the two groups.[26] It is one of the most common causes of nonscarring hair loss in children, accounting for 10% to 17.6% all forms of alopecia in one case series.[5,27,28] The mean age at presentation has been reported as 8 years, with females being more commonly affected.[28]

Etiology

Normally, hair follicles cycle asynchronously, with about 10% in telogen phase at any given time.[29] This leads to a normal daily physiologic hair shedding of 100 to 200 hairs. In TE, a trigger causes a synchrony of the hair cycle, such that a large number of follicles shift together from anagen to telogen phase, resulting in marked hair shedding 2 to 3 months after the trigger.[26]

Potential triggers include psychologic or physiologic stress, or hormonal changes. The most common causes in children are high-grade fever, frequent illness, and iron deficiency anemia.[28] Other causes may include surgery, medications, other nutritional deficiency (zinc, protein, essential fatty acids), endocrine disorders, and immunizations.[30-33] No trigger is identified in about one-third of cases. Commonly used medications in the pediatric population that may trigger TE include psychotropics (lithium and antidepressants), systemic retinoids, anticonvulsants, and oral contraceptives.[24,34] The exact mechanism behind how these triggers lead to TE is not well understood.

Clinical Presentation

Patients with TE present with an acute and diffuse decrease in density of hair, typically with a loss of less than 50% of the hair.[35] Onset occurs approximately 2 to 3 months after the triggering event, is reversible, and lasts a total of 6 months.[24] Shedding that persists longer than 6 months is classified as chronic TE,[35] which is typically seen in middle-aged women, but has been reported in children experiencing chronic starvation.[36] Distribution of hair loss is usually diffuse, but may be more noticeable in the bitemporal area in some patients.[35] Although trichoscopic findings are nonspecific, they may provide clues to the diagnosis and include empty follicles, lack of variability in diameter, brown perifollicular discoloration, and short, upright regrowing hairs during the regrowth phase.[37-39]

Histologic Findings

A biopsy of TE may show very subtle findings, as the total number of hair follicles is normal. Acute cases often show a shift toward catagen and telogen phases (generally greater than 20%), although a lower percentage does not exclude the diagnosis.[31] Chronic TE may have a normal percentage of follicles in catagen/telogen phases because of the waxing and waning nature of the disease.[40] Biopsies with an increase in catagen/telogen follicles show normal counts superficially at the level of the isthmus, with decreased numbers of follicles and fibrous stelae at deeper levels. Importantly, neither acute nor chronic TE features loss or miniaturization of follicles or significant inflammation.[41]

Differential Diagnosis

The clinical differential diagnosis of TE includes AGA and AA. AGA tends to follow a slower course without regrowth. AA has a similarly abrupt onset, but tends to lead to patchy hair loss. Diffuse AA may be difficult to differentiate from TE on a clinical basis.

The histopathologic differential diagnosis of TE is quite broad, as a variety of etiologies can result in an increased percentage of catagen/telogen-phase follicles. These include AGA, AA, traction alopecia, trichotillomania, and psoriatic alopecia. Accurate diagnosis often depends on the presence of a characteristic clinical history.

AGA may show an increase in catagen/telogen follicles, but a more conspicuous finding is miniaturization of follicles. Similarly, AA displays prominent miniaturization, as well as findings such as peribulbar lymphocytic inflammation, trichomalacia, a lack of hair shaft production in miniaturized follicles, and dilation and keratotic plugging of follicular infundibula. Traction alopecia may show normal follicular size and number in addition to a mildly elevated catagen/telogen count, but there is often follicular dropout, and the presence of trichomalacia, pigment casts within follicles, and sebaceous glands that lack associated follicles may help distinguish it from TE. Trichotillomania shows features similar to those of traction alopecia, with the addition of disrupted and deformed follicles. Finally, psoriatic alopecia often has a markedly increased catagen/telogen count, but overlying changes of psoriasis are also seen.

CAPSULE SUMMARY

TELOGEN EFFLUVIUM

TE is a diffuse, nonscarring alopecia that is relatively common in children. It is often triggered by an illness or a medication and presents with acute diffuse hair loss. It begins 2 to 3 months after the trigger and lasts approximately 6 months. The pathophysiology involves a large number of follicles simultaneously undergoing premature or prolonged shift from the anagen growth phase to catagen and telogen phases. Histologically, it displays a normal number of follicles with a shift from anagen to catagen and telogen phases, but findings may be subtle or absent. It is a histopathologic diagnosis of exclusion, best made when there is a characteristic clinical history combined with a lack of additional findings such as miniaturization, trichomalacia, or inflammation.

ALOPECIA AREATA

Definition and Epidemiology

AA is the most common type of alopecia seen in children and is characterized by an acute onset, nonscarring alopecia of the scalp or any hair-bearing area.[5,42] It is classified as a polygenic, lymphocyte-mediated autoimmune disease specific to the hair follicle.

The estimated prevalence is 0.1% to 0.2% in the general population, with 20% of cases occurring in the pediatric population.[43,44] Although there is no gender ratio difference in adults, studies in children favor a slight female predominance, with a female to male ratio ranging from 1.6 to 2.5:1.[43,45,46] There is no racial predilection.[46] The mean age of onset in children ranges from 4.2 to 5.7, with onset peaking between ages 2 and 6.[43,45] AA is rare in infancy, but has been reported.[45] A total of 10% to 19% of patients have a positive family history of AA.[45,47-49]

Etiology

AA is a lymphocyte-mediated, genetically influenced autoimmune disease restricted to the hair follicle.[50,51] It is likely polygenic in nature, with numerous genes identified that are involved with both the innate and acquired immune system. Genes encoding cytotoxic T-lymphocyte-associated antigen 4, regulatory T cells, interleukin-2, and human leukocyte antigen class II have all been implicated.[52] There is a positive family history in 4% to 28% of patients with AA, and 55% concordance in monozygotic twins.[53,54]

Hair loss in AA is mediated by CD8+ T-lymphocytes activated by disruption of the immune privilege inherent to the hair follicle.[55,56] T cells found in the peribulbar infiltrate induce keratinocyte apoptosis, leading to aberration in the follicle growth cycle.[51,57] The degree of inflammation determines whether the hair follicle remains in anagen or converts to telogen phase, with more inflammation leading to the latter.[50,51]

AA is commonly seen in association with other inflammatory and autoimmune disorders. Atopic dermatitis is the most commonly associated disorder in children, with prevalence ranging from 28% to 61% among children with AA. It is associated with more severe alopecia.[45,58] Other associated disorders include thyroid disease, Down syndrome, vitiligo, juvenile idiopathic arthritis, psoriasis, and other autoimmune diseases.[45,58] A recent study in children found that an increased incidence of thyroid disease was seen in AA patients with concomitant atopy, Down syndrome, or a family history of thyroid disease.[58]

Environmental factors such as stress, hormones, and infectious agents have been linked to the development of AA, although clear etiologic evidence is lacking.[50]

Clinical Presentation

AA presents acutely with asymptomatic patches of hair loss on any hair-bearing area. It affects the scalp in the majority of patients and typically appears as well-defined, focal patches of alopecia without epidermal change (Figure 16-3).[46] AA can be classified either on the basis of pattern of hair loss or severity. Patterns include patchy alopecia with partial loss, typically on the scalp; alopecia totalis (AT) defined by a complete loss of scalp hair; and alopecia universalis (AU)

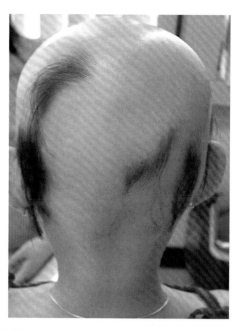

FIGURE 16-3. Alopecia areata in a 6-year-old girl. Extensive, patchy, nonscarring hair loss.

with complete loss of scalp and body hair. The ophiasis pattern presents with band-like, circumferential loss of hair across the temporal, parietal, and occipital scalp. Severity is classified by an overall percentage of hair loss: mild (<25%), moderate (26% to 50%), or extensive (>50%).[59] The reported prevalence of severe disease in affected children of different populations ranges from 13% to 66%.[43,47-49,58,60,61] Early age of onset is associated with more severe disease,[60,62] and 5% of all AA cases may progress to AT/AU.[63]

The characteristic lesions of AA are well-defined, round, or oval patches of complete hair loss with underlying normal skin tone. Patches occasionally have a slight red or orange-pink hue.[50] Closer examination often reveals "exclamation point" hairs, which represent short, proximally tapered hairs most often seen at the border or within the patch.[46] The other trichoscopic features of AA include black dots (44%-70% of patients), yellow dots (63%-94%), broken hairs (45%-58%), and vellus hairs (33%-72%).[37] Black dots represent fractured hair shafts in active disease, whereas yellow dots are enlarged follicular infundibula containing keratinous and sebaceous material, indicating inactive, late-stage, or severe disease.[37,51,64] Early regrowth of hair is often non- or hypopigmented.[65] Hairs at the periphery of active disease patches may be extracted with minimal force and no pain, indicating a positive hair-pull test.[66]

Nail changes are seen in AA in 26.5% to 40% of children, with pitting being the most common change observed.[43,48,49,51,67,68] Others include onychorrhexis (longitudinal splitting of the plate), Beau lines (horizontal grooves), onychomadesis (shedding at the proximal end), trachyonychia (rough, longitudinally ridged nails), koilonychia (spoon-shaped nails), leukonychia (white macules),

and red-spotted lunulae.[66] Nail disease is associated with a more severe disease in children.[43,48,49]

Histologic Findings

The pathologic changes in AA depend on the stage of disease. In early (acute or subacute) disease, hair counts are normal, but there is a shift to catagen and telogen phases.[41,69] Over time, there is a marked decrease in follicular size (Figure 16-4). An infiltrate of lymphocytes around follicular bulbs is a classic, albeit inconsistent finding (Figure 16-4).[23] Other diagnostic features are the presence of follicles that either produce minute or no hair shafts, deformed or distorted hair shafts (trichomalacia), lymphocytic exocytosis into follicular epithelium, pigment casts (fragments of displaced pigmented matrix or cortical cells),[41] and dilated follicular infundibula plugged with keratin.[23]

Chronic AA also typically has a normal or near-normal number of follicles,[69] with most or all follicles being miniaturized, and a marked shift approaching 100% to catagen and telogen phases. Peribulbar inflammation may be sparse or absent in chronic disease.[41] If AA persists for many years, permanent follicular loss may occur.[70]

Differential Diagnosis

AGA also features follicle miniaturization, but has a more modest shift to catagen and telogen phases, and does not feature peribulbar inflammation, trichomalacia, or dilated follicular infundibula. Psoriatic alopecia typically has accompanying changes of psoriasis and sebaceous gland atrophy.[69] Trichotillomania can also have a shift into catagen/telogen phases, trichomalacia, and pigment casts, but these may be less pronounced, and miniaturization is absent. Syphilitic alopecia can closely mimic AA, featuring extensive miniaturization of follicles, a marked shift to catagen/telogen counts approaching 100%, and a peribulbar infiltrate of lymphocytes with an occasional extension of the inflammation up the follicle to the isthmus. However, syphilis is more likely to have plasma cells in the inflammatory infiltrate than AA.[71-73]

CAPSULE SUMMARY

ALOPECIA AREATA

AA is the most common cause of hair loss in children. It is acute in onset and may present with discrete round patches of hair loss, band-like loss, diffuse loss, or a total loss of all scalp or body hair. Histologically, AA features miniaturization of follicles and an increase in catagen/telogen hairs, with both changes becoming more marked as the disease progresses. Peribulbar lymphocytic inflammation is a characteristic finding, but is not always present. Although AA does not cause scarring, longstanding disease may progress to follicular dropout and permanent hair loss.

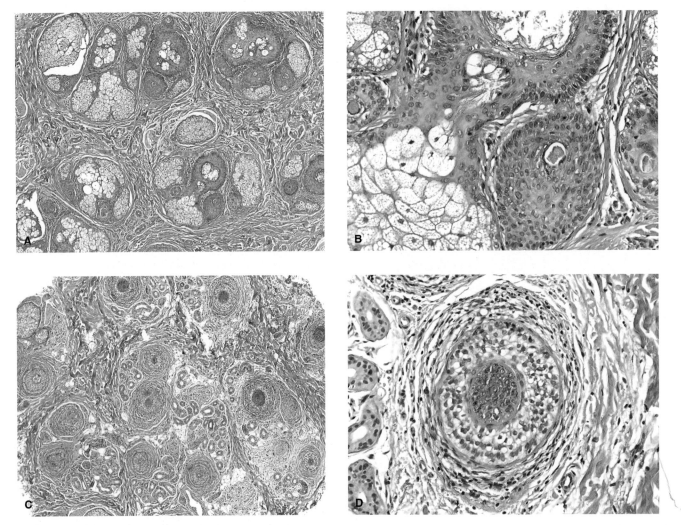

FIGURE 16-4. Histopathology of alopecia areata in an 18-year-old boy. A, Low-power view of the isthmus showing the absence of terminal hair shafts (H&E, ×4). B, High-power view of follicles with absent hair shafts typical of alopecia areata (H&E, ×20). (C) Low- and (D) high-power view at the suprabulbar level showing marked perifollicular inflammation (H&E, ×4; H&E, ×20).

TRICHOTILLOMANIA

Definition and Epidemiology

Trichotillomania (TTM) is a self-induced form of traction alopecia caused by habitual plucking, pulling, or twisting of hairs, that is classified as an obsessive compulsive disorder.

The prevalence of TTM in children with alopecia ranges from 2% to 9.8%,[5,28,74] with an estimated lifetime prevalence of 0.6% to 4.0%.[75] In young children, males and females tend to be effected equally, with female predominance increasing with age.[76-78] Peak onset occurs between 9 and 13 years, but has been reported in children as young as 1.[78-81] Later age of onset is associated with increased severity, less responsiveness to treatment, and a higher likelihood of psychiatric comorbidities.[76,80] About 5% to 8% of patients endorse a family history of TTM.[82]

Etiology

The exact etiology of TTM is not well understood. Concordance in monozygotic twins ranges from 38.1% to 58.3%, suggesting a genetic component.[83] Mutations in serotonin 2A receptor and *SLITRK1* (a tyrosine kinase receptor) have been identified at higher rates in TTM patients.[84,85] The serotonin, glutamate, and dopamine pathways may play a pathogenic role.[76]

Behavioral and psychosocial factors may also play a role in TTM. It is often seen in association with other habitual behaviors such as nail biting and skin picking. The onset of TTM often coincides with periods of psychosocial stress at home or school.[76,80,86] Adolescents with TTM have a higher incidence of comorbid psychiatric disorders such as depression, obsessive compulsive disorder, and phobias.[87,88]

Clinical Presentation

TTM presents with irregularly shaped patches of non-scarring alopecia, most commonly on the scalp. Any hair-bearing area may be affected, including the eyebrows, eyelashes, and pubic hair.[30,86] Patches of alopecia have broken hairs of varying lengths and lack scale.[86,89] Younger children are more likely to be limited to one site, whereas the majority of adolescents and adults have multiple foci of involvement.[75,90,91] Two types of hair pulling have been described in TTM—automatic and focused.[92] In focused pulling, patients are aware that they are pulling and devote their attention to it.[92,93] In the automatic type, patients are unaware and often pull hair while performing other daily activities.[92,93] Younger children tend to exhibit automatic pulling, but a combination can exist.[92,93]

TTM has a variety of trichoscopic findings, most commonly multiple broken hairs varying in shape and length.[37] Exclamation point hairs, black dots, split ends, and coiled hairs are also characteristic, but not specific.[37] Flame hairs, a recently described trichoscopic finding described as semitransparent, cone shaped, wavy hair residue stuck to the scalp, are seen in 25% of patients and are highly specific.[94] Other characteristic findings include the V-sign (greater than two hairs arising from one follicular unit and broken at same level) and tulip hairs (tulip-shaped ends on short hairs).[94]

Histologic Findings

TTM retains a normal number of terminal and vellus hairs. The trauma of hair plucking results in incomplete, distorted follicles. Other findings include trichomalacia (Figure 16-5), fractured hair shafts, collapsed inner root sheaths, pigment casts in follicular lumina, intrafollicular hemorrhage,[41,95] and distorted sebaceous lobules.[96] There is often a shift to catagen/telogen phases.[41,95] Inflammation is typically mild and is not peribulbar in location.[95] Importantly, the changes described earlier are predominantly seen in terminal hairs—vellus hairs are usually normal in morphology, as they escape plucking.[96]

Differential Diagnosis

The clinical and histopathologic differential diagnosis for TTM includes traction alopecia, AA, and TE. Traction alopecia has overlapping features with TTM, but a distortion of follicular epithelium and/or hair shafts is rare to absent. AA may feature trichomalacia and pigment casts, but the proportion of follicles in catagen/telogen is typically much higher in AA, which also lacks follicular epithelium and shaft distortion. TE may have increased catagen/telogen follicles and a lack of inflammation, but it also lacks signs of traumatic changes to the follicles.

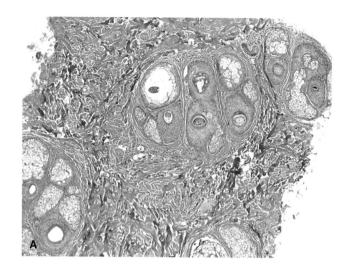

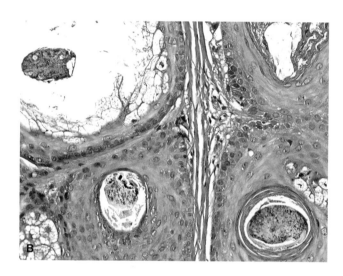

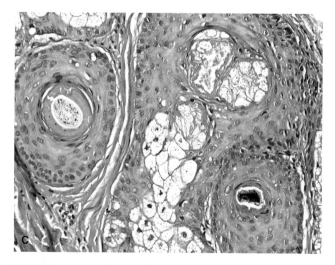

FIGURE 16-5. Histopathology of trichotillomania in a 15-year-old girl. A, Low-power view of the isthmus showing normal follicular size and trichomalacia (H&E, ×4). B and C, Higher-power view of trichomalacia in trichotillomania (H&E, ×20).

CAPSULE SUMMARY

TRICHOTILLOMANIA

TTM is a poorly understood form of self-induced, non-scarring hair loss that is thought to have both genetic and psychosocial contributing factors. It presents most often as an irregular patch of hair loss on the scalp, but may be seen on any hair-bearing region, and patients may or may not be aware of their hair-pulling behavior. Histologically, TTM has a variety of findings, including distortion of follicles and hair shafts, trichomalacia, pigment casts, and an increase in catagen/telogen follicles. These findings preferentially affect terminal hairs.

TINEA CAPITIS

Definition and Epidemiology

Tinea capitis (TC) is a superficial dermatophyte fungal infection of the scalp that is often associated with hair loss.[97] Its prevalence ranges from 4% to 15% in the United States, and its incidence has varied with time across geographic and demographic populations.[98-103] Prepubertal children are most highly affected, with the peak age of diagnosis ranging from 5 to 10 years.[98] Many studies have shown higher incidence in male children than in females, although some show equal gender predilection.[99,100,102,104,105] It is most common in African-American children for reasons that are unknown.[98,99] In one large cross-sectional study, the rate of infection in African-American children was 12.9% compared with 1.6% and 1.1% in Hispanic and Caucasian children, respectively.[99] The most common coexisting conditions are atopic dermatitis and asthma.[98]

Etiology

Dermatophytes are the filamentous fungi that cause tinea. *Trichophyton tonsurans*, an anthropophilic (human source) dermatophyte, is the most common cause of TC in the United States, Canada, and United Kingdom.[98,106] The second most common is *Microsporum canis*, a zoophilic (animal source) dermatophyte, which accounts for less than 10% of cases in the United States.[98,107]

Infection is caused by a direct inoculation of the scalp with the causative dermatophyte from an infected individual, animal, or contaminated object, and can be transmitted by asymptomatic carriers.[108] Dermatophytes specifically target the stratum corneum using cell wall glycoproteins for adherence and proteolytic keratinase enzymes to invade the skin and hair shafts.[109,110] Although the prepubertal predilection has not been fully explained, it may be due to the inhibitory properties of fatty acids found in postpubertal sebum.[111]

Infection occurs in three patterns on the scalp: ectothrix, endothrix, and favus. The ectothrix pattern results from infection by arthroconidia (fungal spores) outside the hair shaft and is most commonly seen in the *Microsporum* genus.[112] The endothrix pattern is characterized by arthroconidia within the hair shaft and is seen in *T. tonsurans* and *T. violaceum* species.[112] Favus is a rare and severe form most commonly caused by *T. schoenleinii*, in which hyphae and air spaces are found within the hair shaft.[112,113]

Clinical Presentation

The clinical presentation and severity of TC varies both by causative organism and by host immune response, and can be both noninflammatory and inflammatory in nature. The most common presentation is single or multiple patches of alopecia with or without scale, ranging in size from very small to several centimeters in diameter (Figure 16-6).[112] Scaly gray patches are common in ectothrix infections,[112] and patches that contain "black dots", which represent broken hair shafts at the follicle orifice, can be seen in endothrix infections.[110] A subtle seborrheic dermatitis-like presentation can also be seen in infection with *T. tonsurans,* in which there is diffuse scaling and little hair loss.[112] Comma hairs and corkscrew hairs are characteristic trichoscopic findings for tinea capitis.[114,115]

As inflammation and host response increases, TC can present on a spectrum from scaly pustules and suppurative folliculitis to a large inflammatory pustular plaque known as a kerion.[116] Kerions are usually boggy and have pustules, thick crust, drainage, and associated tenderness/pain.[116] Favus presents with thick yellow crusts composed of keratin debris and hyphae known as scutula, which adhere to the scalp and are associated with severe alopecia.[113,117] Scarring can occur if left untreated.[117]

Children often have associated cervical lymphadenopathy (Figure 16-6) in all forms of TC.[117] Associated "id" or

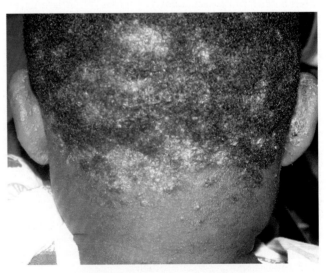

FIGURE 16-6. Tinea capitis in a young boy. Patchy hair loss with crusting. Note the fullness in his neck due to lymphadenopathy.

autoeczematization reactions can be seen in children after antifungal therapy is initiated, but may precede treatment.[117,118] This is characterized by a pruritic, eczematous, or pustular eruption typically starting on the face and spreading to the trunk, often in a perifollicular pattern.

Histologic Findings

The presence of spores (sometimes with hyphae) in or on hair shafts is pathognomonic of TC. Spores are found surrounding the outside of the hair shaft in ectothrix infections, and within the shaft itself in endothrix infections (Figure 16-7).[119] In any given biopsy for TC, only a few follicles may contain infected shafts (Figure 16-7).[120] Both endothrix and ectothrix organisms may be highlighted by special stains for fungi, such as periodic acid-Schiff (PAS) and silver-based stains.[119]

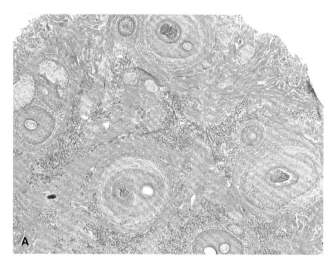

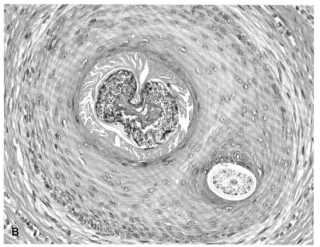

FIGURE 16-7. Histopathology of tinea capitis in a 19-year-old woman. A, Low-power view of the isthmus revealing three enlarged hair shafts filled with fungal spores. Note the presence of perivascular inflammation, mild perifollicular fibrosis, and uninvolved hair shafts (H&E, ×4). B, High-power view of an endothrix dermatophyte infection of the hair shaft (H&E, ×40).

Inflammation is present in variable degrees and usually consists of a mixed infiltrate of neutrophils, lymphocytes, and eosinophils. It may be present superficially, in both the superficial and deep dermis, or only in the deep dermis. Granulomatous inflammation is sometimes present, particularly in older lesions.[119,121] If longstanding and untreated, TC can result in scarring and permanent follicular loss.[119,122]

Differential Diagnosis

The main clinical differential diagnosis for TC is AA. The histopathologic diagnosis of TC is straightforward when fungal organisms are seen within hair follicles. In their absence, the differential diagnosis is quite broad, and can include several entities that share findings with TC. In a new lesion with active inflammation, an early neutrophilic scarring alopecia could be considered. Folliculitis decalvans displays a dense mixed inflammatory infiltrate with neutrophils around follicles in the superficial and mid dermis, and dissecting cellulitis has a similar infiltrate that is centered on the deep dermis and subcutis.[119,123] Untreated or longstanding lesions of TC that show scarring may resemble the end-stage cicatricial alopecias. Bacterial or *Pityrosporum* folliculitis may show a superficial (and sometimes deep) mixed inflammatory infiltrate with neutrophils, but the changes are usually confined to one or two discrete follicles, and organisms are often seen within the follicular lumen. If the clinical presentation is suspicious for TC but the biopsy does not show fungus, a fungal culture may be helpful.

CAPSULE SUMMARY

TINEA CAPITIS

TC is a relatively common cause of hair loss in children, caused by a variety of dermatophyte fungal infections of the hair shaft. *Trichophyton tonsurans* and *microsporum canis* are the two most common causative agents. Clinically, it typically presents with patchy alopecia, often with scale, and may progress to pustules or boggy plaques. The histologic sine qua non of TC is the presence of fungal elements within or on the surface of hair shafts. TC responds to antifungal treatment, but untreated or longstanding infections can lead to permanent hair loss.

TEMPORAL TRIANGULAR ALOPECIA

Definition and Epidemiology

Temporal triangular alopecia (TTA) is a nonscarring alopecia that most commonly presents from birth to age 9 with an oval or triangular-shaped patch of alopecia on one or both temples.[124] The peak age of onset is between 3 and 6 years.[125] Males and females are equally affected.[126] A family history is occasionally noted.[126]

Etiology

The etiology of TTA is not known. In the majority of patients, the scalp is normal prior to presentation, suggesting that terminal hairs undergo miniaturization to vellus hairs.[127]

Clinical Presentation

TTA presents as a noninflammatory, nonscarring, somewhat ill-defined patch of hair loss, usually unilaterally on the temporal scalp (Figure 16-8). The patch is often triangular, oval or lancet-shaped.[125,127] The left side is favored over the right (55.8 vs. 30.8%),[126] although it can present bilaterally in 7.5% to 20% of cases.[126,128] The patch may be completely bald, but is often composed of vellus hairs with sparse terminal hairs near the borders. It typically remains unchanged throughout life.[127] Trichoscopic features include white hairs, diversity in diameter, terminal hair surrounding vellus hairs, white dots, and empty follicles.[128] TTA can be associated with congenital conditions including phakomatosis pigmentovascularis and Down syndrome.[126]

Histologic Findings

TTA displays a normal number of hair follicles, but most or all of the follicles are vellus in size.[125-127] Underlying fibrous stelae, which indicate miniaturization in diseases such as AGA and AA, are absent in TTA.[127,129] Thus, there are a lack of follicles when sampled in the subcutis and deep dermis, with an increase to a normal total through the isthmus and infundibular levels. The vellus hairs are morphologically normal, with intact sebaceous glands, and sparse or absent

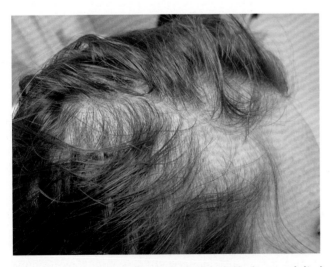

FIGURE 16-8. Temporal triangular alopecia in an adult. A characteristic noninflammatory patch of alopecia at the right temple, present unchanged since childhood.

inflammation.[125,127,129] In rare cases, the overall number of follicles may be reduced.[129]

Differential Diagnosis

The clinical and histologic differential diagnosis of TTA includes AGA, AA, and end-stage traction alopecia. The clinical setting can be very helpful. Miniaturized or vellus hairs in AGA and AA have underlying fibrous stelae to mark their former positions in the subcutaneous fat. Additionally, AA typically shows a marked shift to catagen/telogen phase, and may have peribulbar inflammation, trichomalacia, and dilated follicular infundibula. End-stage traction alopecia has a reduced total number of follicles, with some being replaced by fibrous stellae, leaving only vellus hairs and intact sebaceous glands in the biopsy.[41]

CAPSULE SUMMARY

TEMPORAL TRIANGULAR ALOPECIA

TTA is a nonscarring alopecia that presents in infants or young children as an ill-defined oval or triangular-shaped patch of hair loss on one or both temples, remaining unchanged as the patient ages. Histopathology demonstrates a predominance of vellus-sized hairs, possibly with rare terminal hairs, in an otherwise normal epidermis and dermis. Fibrous stelae underlying the vellus follicles are not seen.

Cicatricial (Scarring) Alopecia

Scarring alopecias are a group of diseases in which the hair follicle is destroyed by an inflammatory process, leading to permanent hair loss. The causative entities are classified according to the type of inflammation present.[130] The common lymphocytic scarring alopecias consist of lichen planopilaris (LPP), discoid lupus erythematosus (DLE), and central centrifugal cicatricial alopecia (CCCA). The neutrophilic alopecias include folliculitis decalvans and dissecting cellulitis of the scalp. All of these disorders are relatively rare in children and will be discussed briefly.

LYMPHOCYTIC SCARRING ALOPECIAS
Epidemiology, Etiology, and Clinical Presentation

LPP is an uncommon cause of scarring alopecia in children that typically causes small areas of hair loss, often on the crown, with a smooth scalp surface and perifollicular erythema and scale. In the limited reported cases of LPP in children, there is a male predominance, which differs from the female predominance seen in adults.[131,132] The age at presentation ranges from 8 to 16.[131]

The etiology of LPP is not well understood. Patients often report scalp pruritus, burning, and pain.[133] Like adults, about half of children show extracutaneous signs of lichen planus. However, unlike adults, children tend to be asymptomatic.[131]

Frontal fibrosing alopecia (FFA), thought to be a form of LPP, is typically seen in postmenopausal women, but three cases have been reported in the pediatric population. Onset ranged from age 5 to 7.[134]FFA presents with a band-like patch of scarring alopecia across the frontal scalp and often has associated eyebrow alopecia.

DLE is an autoimmune disease of the skin that results in scarring alopecia when present on the scalp. It is uncommon in children, with approximately 2% of all patients with DLE presenting before the age of 10.[135,136] There is no racial predilection. One cases series in children found a mean age of onset of 10.3 with a range of 6 months to 16 years.[135] A female predominance has been observed, as in the adult population.[135-137] Children are more likely to present with or progress to systemic lupus erythematosus (38% in children compared with 5% to 10% in adults).[136,138] The majority of children have lesions limited to the head/neck (63% in one series), but it can present in a generalized fashion.[137] On the scalp, lesions are typically hyperkeratotic, inflammatory, erythematous patches and plaques that evolve with central depigmentation, atrophy, and peripheral hyperpigmentation.[137]

CCCA is a scarring alopecia most often seen in middle-aged African or African-American women and rarely in children.[139] A case series of six children showed a mean age of onset of 14 years, with the majority (83%) being of African American descent and having a family history of CCCA.[140] Children are unlikely to have undergone chemical treatments to the hair.[140] The exact etiology of CCCA is not well understood. Hair care practices are suspected, but a genetic component is likely based upon a pedigree analysis in a South African family showing autosomal dominant inheritance.[141] CCCA classically presents on the vertex of the scalp with a centrifugally expanding patch of scarring alopecia, or rarely with diffuse thinning.[142] Associated symptoms include tender papules, pruritus, and scaling.[140]

Histologic Findings

The entities LPP and FFA are histologically indistinguishable and share multiple histologic features with CCCA.[143] Common findings among the three include a perifollicular lymphocytic infiltrate at the level of the isthmus (often with extension up and down the follicle), lymphocytic exocytosis into follicular epithelium, perifollicular fibrosis, follicular epithelial thinning with the development of follicular asymmetry, a loss of sebaceous glands, and a fusion of follicles into compound structures containing 2 to 4 hair shafts (polytrichia).[119,143,144] In follicles that have been

completely destroyed, a fibrous tract or scar may remain in the subcutis and dermis, indicating the follicle's former position. LPP and FFA can show focal basal layer vacuolization and necrotic epithelial cells in the follicle, as well as focal interface changes in the overlying interfollicular epidermis.[145,146] A premature desquamation of the inner root sheath of the follicle (desquamation below the level of the isthmus) can occur in all scarring alopecias, but is an early finding in CCCA that can be seen in otherwise unaffected follicles.[147] It is typically seen only in affected follicles in LPP and FFA.[143,147]

DLE has findings that can significantly overlap with those in the other lymphocytic scarring alopecias. There is a typically moderate-to-dense lymphoplasmacytic infiltrate that often extends the entire length of the follicle and affects the superficial and deep vascular plexus, a distinguishing feature from LPP and CCCA (Figure 16-9).[148] Rarely, the deep portion of the inflammatory infiltrate can form lymphoid follicles.[123] There can be associated vacuolization of the follicular epithelial basal layer, apoptotic epithelial cells, and lymphocytic infiltration into the follicular epithelium.[143,145,149] A perieccrine infiltrate of lymphocytes and plasma cells is usually present (Figure 16-9),[143] and sebaceous glands may be involved by the infiltrate, reduced in size or completely destroyed.[123,150] The epidermis frequently shows classic changes of DLE, including epidermal atrophy, follicular plugging, interface changes of the dermoepidermal junction (Figure 16-9), basement membrane thickening along the epidermis and adnexae,[149]papillary dermal edema and hyalinization, and increased dermal mucin.[143,145] A recent study outlined the histopathologic features of DLE in transverse section, describing patterns that resemble AA and LPP.[151] Direct immunofluorescence studies of DLE may be helpful and are characterized by a deposition of IgG and C3 in a granular pattern along the dermoepidermal and dermofollicular junctions.[152,153]

CAPSULE SUMMARY

LYMPHOCYTIC SCARRING ALOPECIAS

The lymphocytic scarring alopecias are a group of entities that are rare in the pediatric population. Clinically, FFA presents as a band of hair loss along the frontal hairline, CCCA starts as a patch of loss on the vertex that expands outward, and LPP and DLE present with variably patchy alopecia (with plaques in the case of DLE). Histologically common findings include lymphocytic infiltrates around hair follicles with associated perifollicular fibrosis and destruction of follicular epithelium and sebaceous glands. The lymphocytic scarring alopecias progress to a final end stage where most or all follicles, along with their sebaceous glands, are replaced by fibrosis in the dermis and subcutis.

The lymphocytic scarring alopecias can be difficult to distinguish histologically. LPP and FFA are best distinguished by clinical presentation and can sometimes coexist. CCCA differs in clinical presentation from LPP and FFA, may display a premature desquamation of the inner root sheath in otherwise unaffected follicles, and lacks an interfollicular epidermal evidence of interface changes. DLE usually has more prominent epidermal changes of interface dermatitis, particularly a thickened basement membrane zone, increased interstitial dermal mucin, and a dense superficial and deep infiltrate that involves blood vessels, eccrine coils, and ducts.

NEUTROPHILIC SCARRING ALOPECIA

Epidemiology, Etiology, and Clinical Presentation

Folliculitis decalvans (FD) is a neutrophilic scarring alopecia primarily seen in young to middle-aged adults.[119,154] It is more common in males and African-American patients.[119,154] It has rarely been reported in the pediatric population.[28] The etiology is not well understood, but *S. aureus* is thought to play a role, as it can be isolated from most patients.[155,156] Reported familial cases suggest a genetic component.[155,157] Dissecting cellulitis of the scalp (DCS) aka "perifolliculitis capitis abscedens et suffodiens" is a chronic neutrophilic inflammatory disease of the scalp most commonly seen in young African-American adults aged 20 to 40, although it can be seen in other ethnicities.[158,159] It has rarely been reported in the pediatric population.[160-162] The exact etiology of DCS is unknown. Disruption in follicular

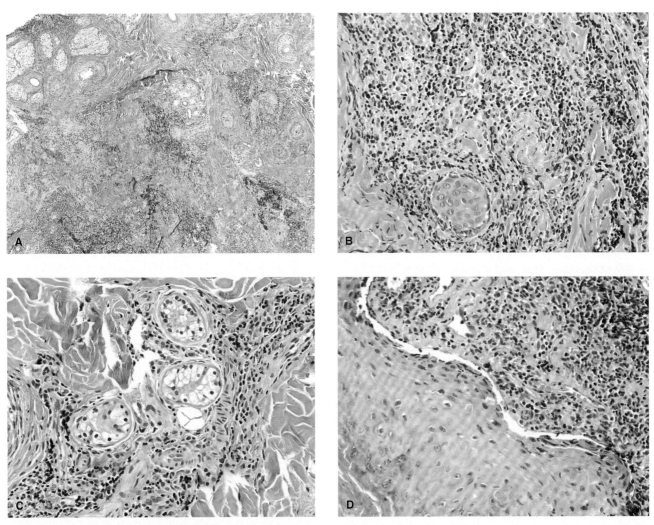

FIGURE 16-9. Histopathology of discoid lupus erythematosus in a 16-year-old boy. A, Low-power view of the isthmus revealing a decreased number of hair follicles and marked perivascular inflammation (H&E, ×4). B, Higher power of the isthmus shows a heavy lymphocytic infiltrate that is not particularly centered on the remnant of follicular epithelium present (H&E, ×20). C, Perieccrine inflammation (H&E, ×20). D, The dermoepidermal junction in transverse section exhibits interface dermatitis with individually necrotic keratinocytes and subepidermal clefting, a heavy lymphocytic infiltrate and melanophages (H&E, ×20).

keratinization is thought to play a role, leading to the accumulation of keratin and sebaceous material in the follicle. The follicle then dilates and ruptures, stimulating a neutrophilic and granulomatous response that may become secondarily infected, creating abscesses and sinus tracts.[145,159] Familial cases have been reported, suggesting a genetic component to the pathophysiology.[163] DCS is a component of the follicular occlusion tetrad, which also includes hidradenitis suppurativa, acne conglobate, and pilonidal sinus.[164] Other systemic associations include musculoskeletal problems and arthropathy.[159]

FD presents first with erythematous follicular papules and pustules most commonly on the vertex and occipital scalp.[165] Patients often have associated erythema, perifollicular scale, hemorrhagic crust, and erosions.[165] Over time, without treatment, this can lead to focal or widespread scarring.[166] Tufting is a common trichoscopic feature—typically with at least six hairs per follicle.[167] Other trichoscopic clues include perifollicular pustules and inter- and perifollicular white scale.[167] DCS presents with boggy and suppurative nodules and favors the vertex and occipital scalp. The nodules can be interconnected via sinus tracts and often drain blood and pus spontaneously and with pressure.[159,161] Alopecia typically occurs overlying the nodules and is reversible early in the course of the disease, but scarring can occur in persistent cases.[168] Scarring can be both hypertrophic and keloidal.[159] Patients often experience associated pain and pruritus.[161] Yellow and black dots can be seen on trichoscopy.[167]

Histologic Findings

The neutrophilic scarring alopecias are characterized by a perifollicular and intrafollicular infiltrate that contains neutrophils and, especially in later stages, plasma cells, mixed with lymphocytes, eosinophils, and histiocytes. In later lesions, granulomata and foreign body-type multinucleated giant cells may be seen, often in association with hair shafts that are displaced into the dermis. A mild increase in the percentage of catagen/telogen follicles is often seen. In FD, the inflammation targets the superior portion of the follicle, the isthmus and infundibulum, whereas in DCS, it is predominantly located in the deep dermis and subcutaneous tissue (Figure 16-10). Both entities display dilated infundibula, follicular epithelial infiltration by neutrophils, dilation of the follicular lumen with intraluminal neutrophils and keratin debris, destruction of follicular epithelium with fibrous tract formation, and involvement of the interfollicular dermis by the inflammation.[70,123,165,169] Follicles disrupted by inflammation may merge into compound structures containing five or more hair shafts.[165] Neutrophilic abscesses, usually sterile, form in the dermis or subcutis in DCS, and in some cases, squamous epithelium-lined sinus tracts associated with granulation tissue may be appreciated (Figure 16-10).[70,119] Sebaceous

glands are destroyed in both FD and DCS, but this is a late finding in DCS, where the inflammation is mostly lower in the dermis than the level of the sebaceous glands (Figure 16-10). As with lymphocytic scarring alopecia, end-stage neutrophilic scarring alopecia will be devoid of follicles and sebaceous glands. However, neutrophilic scarring alopecias usually have interfollicular scarring (fibrosis of dermis between follicles) owing to an extensive inflammation of the interfollicular dermis.[70,119,146]

Differential Diagnosis

In an active neutrophilic scarring alopecia, the dilated follicles and neutrophilic infiltrate may mimic an acute bacterial or fungal folliculitis, including TC. Gram stain and PAS stain for organisms may be useful in distinguishing these entities. Late-stage neutrophilic scarring alopecia can look very similar to late-stage lymphocytic scarring alopecia. Changes such as perifollicular fibrosis and a predominantly lymphocytic infiltrate around remaining follicles may mark a late-stage lymphocytic scarring alopecia, whereas the presence of interfollicular fibrosis and plasma cells in the infiltrate may suggest burned-out neutrophilic scarring alopecia.

CAPSULE SUMMARY

NEUTROPHILIC SCARRING ALOPECIA

The neutrophilic scarring alopecias, comprising FD and DCS, are usually seen in young to middle-aged adults and are relatively rare in the pediatric population. Although both entities are typically seen on the vertex and occipital scalp, FD usually presents with erythematous, crusted follicular papules and pustules, whereas DCS displays boggy papules and plaques that drain pus and blood and can form sinus tracts. Histologically, both FD and DCS display a neutrophil-heavy peri- and intrafollicular infiltrate, with inflammation in FD concentrated at the isthmus and inflammation in DCS around the deep follicle and into the subcutaneous tissue. Both processes can result in scarring and permanent hair loss. Late-stage neutrophilic scarring alopecias show interfollicular fibrosis and inflammation containing plasma cells.

ACNE KELOIDALIS

Definition and Epidemiology

Acne keloidalis (AK) is a primary scarring alopecia that occurs primarily on the occipital scalp and the nape of the neck, often leading to the formation of keloidal scarring. It is a distinct inflammatory disorder with little pathophysiologic resemblance to acne.

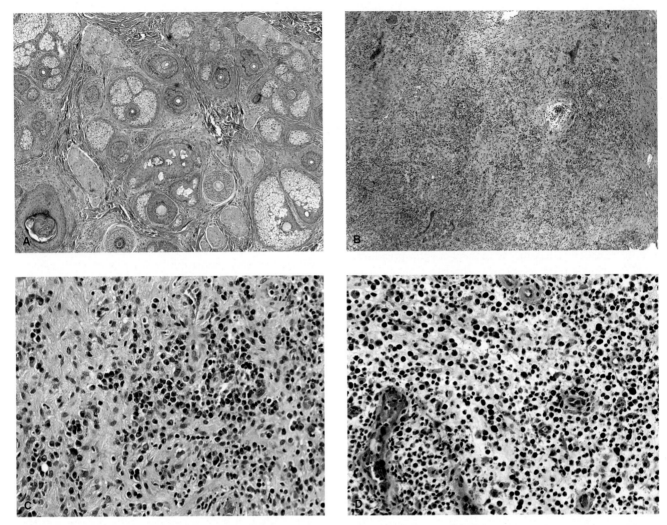

FIGURE 16-10. **Histopathology of dissecting cellulitis in an 18-year-old man.** A, Low-power view of the isthmus reveals a decrease in follicular size and could be read as nonscarring (H&E, ×2). B, Low-power view of the deep dermis shows diffuse inflammation and absent hair follicles (H&E, ×20). C, Higher-power view of the inflammation in the deep dermis revealing a predominance of plasma cells (H&E, ×20). D, Higher-power view of the bottom of the specimen reveals replacement of the subcutis by granulation tissue with plasma cells and neutrophils (H&E, ×4).

AK primarily affects men of African descent starting during adolescence, although it has been described in uncommonly in patients of other ethnicities, as well as in women.[170-174] The male to female ratio is approximately 20:1.[175]

Etiology

Although AK was previously thought to be simply a response to ingrown hairs, studies of the histopathology have suggested that it is actually a primary scarring alopecia.[176] The pathogenic mechanism, however, is not well understood. The primary inflammation leads to weakening and degeneration of the follicle and hair shaft, with secondary inflammation caused by free hair shafts and subsequent keloidal scarring.

A mechanical component is also likely, as frequent haircuts, shaving, and trauma often lead to exacerbations.[177] Additionally, a number of medications have been implicated

in causing or exacerbating AK, including cyclosporine and carbamazepine.[170,178]

Clinical Presentation

AK typically presents in adolescents and young men as firm, asymptomatic, small papules and occasional pustules on the occipital scalp and posterior neck (Figure 16-11). Pruritus is occasional, and pain is infrequent. These papules may resolve with a resultant alopecic patch or coalesce and form larger keloidal plaques. Polytrichia can be seen, and bacterial infections and draining sinuses may complicate severe cases.

Histologic Findings

The biopsy specimens of AK show perifollicular lympho-plasmacytic inflammation at the level of the isthmus and

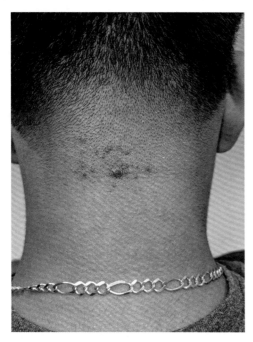

FIGURE 16-11. Acne keloidalis on the posterior neck of a teenager. Hyperpigmented, folliculocentric papules that are asymptomatic.

lower infundibulum, with associated thinning of the epithelium, and concentric fibroplasia. The sebaceous glands are lost in affected follicles, and advanced cases show complete destruction of the follicle with associated neutrophilic inflammation (Figure 16-12). Affected follicles can be seen even in clinically unaffected areas.[176]

Differential Diagnosis

The clinical differential diagnosis includes dissecting cellulitis, acne conglobate, and hidradenitis suppurativa. Histopathologically, AK must be differentiated from CCCA and other scarring alopecias.

CAPSULE SUMMARY

ACNE KELOIDALIS

AK is a primary scarring alopecia affecting primarily the posterior neck of young men of African descent. It is characterized by the development of firm, inflammatory papules that either resolve with alopecia or coalesce to form larger keloidal papules and plaques. Histopathologically, a lymphoplasmacytic inflammatory infiltrate is seen at the level of the isthmus in early lesions, with a thinning of the follicular epithelium, fibroplasia, and the loss of sebaceous glands. Later lesions show a destruction of the follicle with massive neutrophilic inflammation around free hair shafts and other follicular components.

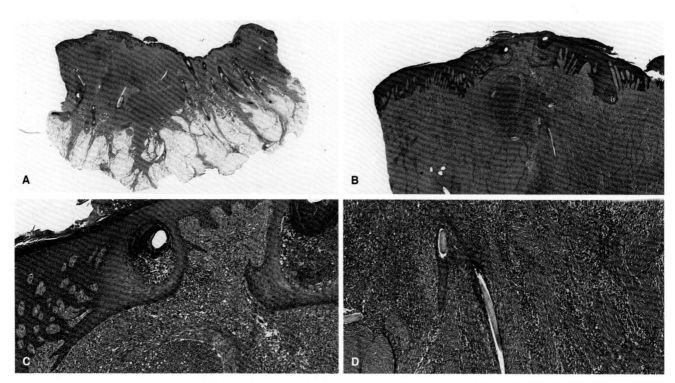

FIGURE 16-12. There is a localized area of fibrosis and acute folliculitis with loss of sebaceous glands (A and B). A closer view highlights a focus of marked acute pustular folliculitis (C). The adjacent dermis shows marked chronic lymphoplasmacytic inflammation and extruded hair shafts (D). Digital slides courtesy of Path Presenter.com.

REFERENCES

1. Tosti A, Piraccini BM. Androgenetic alopecia. *Int J Dermatol.* 1999;38(S1):1-7. doi:10.1046/j.1365-4362.1999.00002.x
2. Chumlea WC, Rhodes T, Girman CJ, et al. Family history and risk of hair loss. *Dermatology.* 2004;209(1):33-39. doi:10.1159/000078584
3. Setty LR. A Comparative study of the distribution of hair of the hand and the foot of white and negro males. *Am J Phys Anthropol.* 1970;33(1):131-137. doi:10.1002/ajpa.1330330108
4. Tosti A, Iorizzo M, Piraccini BM. Androgenetic alopecia in children: report of 20 cases. *Br J Dermatol.* 2005;152(3):556-559. doi:10.1111/j.1365-2133.2004.06279.x
5. Gonzalez ME, Cantatore-Francis J, Orlow SJ. Androgenetic alopecia in the paediatric population: A retrospective review of 57 patients. *Br J Dermatol.* 2010;163(2):378-385. doi:10.1111/j.1365-2133.2010.09777.x
6. Kim BJ, Kim JY, Eun HC, Kwon OS, Kim MN, Ro BI. Androgenetic alopecia in adolescents: a report of 43 cases. *J Dermatol.* 2006;33(10):696-699. doi:10.1111/j.1346-8138.2006.00161.x
7. Paik JH, Yoon JB, Sim WY, Kim BS, Kim NI. The prevalence and types of androgenetic alopecia in Korean men and women. *Br J Dermatol.* 2001;145(1):95-99. doi:10.1046/j.1365-2133.2001.04289.x
8. Hamilton JB. Effect of castration in adolescent and young adult males upon further changes in the proportions of bare and hairy scalp. *J Clin Endocrinol Metab.* 1960;20(10):1309-1318. doi:10.1210/jcem-20-10-1309
9. Sawaya ME, Price VH. Different levels of 5alpha-reductase type I and II, aromatase, and androgen receptor in hair follicles of women and men with androgenetic alopecia. *J Invest Dermatol.* 1997;109(3):296-300. doi:10.1111/1523-1747.ep12335779
10. Randall VA, Thornton MJ, Messenger AG. Cultured dermal papilla cells from androgen-dependent human hair follicles (e.g. beard) contain more androgen receptors than those from non-balding areas of scalp. *J Endocrinol.* 1992;133(1):141-147. doi:10.1677/joe.0.1330141
11. Pitts RL. Serum elevation of dehydroepiandrosterone sulfate associated with male pattern baldness in young men. *J Am Acad Dermatol.* 1987;16(3):571-573. doi:10.1016/S0190-9622(87)70075-9
12. Orme S, Cullen DR, Messenger AG. Diffuse female hair loss: are androgens necessary? *Br J Dermatol.* 1999;141(3):521-523. doi:10.1046/j.1365-2133.1999.03049.x
13. Küster W, Happle R. The inheritance of common baldness: two B or not two B? *J Am Acad Dermatol.* 1984;11(5):921-926. doi:10.1016/S0190-9622(84)80498-3
14. Ellis J A, Stebbing M, Harrap SB. Genetic analysis of male pattern baldness and the 5alpha-reductase genes. *J Invest Dermatol.* 1998;110(6):849-853. doi:10.1046/j.1523-1747.1998.00224.x
15. Ellis JA, Stebbing M, Harrap SB. Polymorphism of the androgen receptor gene is associated with male pattern baldness. *J Invest Dermatol.* 2001;116(3):452-455. doi:10.1046/j.1523-1747.2001.01261.x
16. Carey AH, Waterworth D, Patel K, et al. Polycystic ovaries and premature male pattern baldness are associated with one allele of the steroid metabolism gene CYP17. *Hum Mol Genet.* 1994;3(10):1873-1876. doi:10.1093/hmg/3.10.1873
17. Hamilton JB. Patterned loss of hair in man; types and incidence. *Ann N Y Acad Sci.* 1951;53(3):708-728.
18. Ludwig E. Classification of the types of androgenetic alopecia (common baldness) occurring in the female sex. *Br J Dermatol.* 1977;97(3):247-254.
19. Price VH. Androgenetic alopecia in adolescents. *Cutis.* 2003;71(2):115-121.
20. Whiting DA. Diagnostic and predictive value of horizontal sections of scalp biopsy specimens in male pattern androgenetic alopecia. *J Am Acad Dermatol.* 1993;28(5):755-763. doi:10.1016/0190-9622(93)70106-4
21. Sundberg JP, Beamer WG, Uno H, Van Neste D, King LE. Androgenetic alopecia: in vivo models. *Exp Mol Pathol.* 1999;67(2):118-130. doi:10.1006/exmp.1999.2276

22. Olsen EA, Messenger AG, Shapiro J, et al. Evaluation and treatment of male and female pattern hair loss. *J Am Acad Dermatol.* 2005;52(2):301-311. doi:10.1016/j.jaad.2004.04.008
23. Müller CSL, El Shabrawi-Caelen L. "Follicular Swiss cheese" pattern: another histopathologic clue to alopecia areata. *J Cutan Pathol.* 2011;38(2):185-189. doi:10.1111/j.1600-0560.2010.01640.x
24. Malkud S. Telogen effluvium: a review. *J Clin Diagnostic Res.* 2015;9(9):WE01-WE03. doi:10.7860/JCDR/2015/15219.6492
25. Harrison S, Sinclair R. Telogen effluvium. *Clin Exp Dermatol.* 2002;27(5):389-395.
26. Bedocs L, Bruckner A. Adolescent hair loss. *Curr Opin Pediatr.* 2008;20(4):431-435. doi:10.1097/MOP.0b013e328305e285
27. Atton AV, Tunnessen WW, Afton V. Alopecia common in children: causes. 2013;12(1). doi:10.1542/pir.12-1-25
28. Al-Refu K. Hair loss in children: common and uncommon causes; clinical and epidemiological study in Jordan. *Int J Trichology.* 2013;5(4):185-189. doi:10.4103/0974-7753.130393
29. Price VH. Treatment of hair loss. *N Engl J Med.* 1999;341(13):964-973. doi:10.1056/NEJM199909233411307
30. Castelo-Soccio L. Diagnosis and management of alopecia in children. *Pediatr Clin North Am.* 2014;61(2):427-442. doi:10.1016/j.pcl.2013.12.002
31. Kligman AM. Pathologic dynamics of human hair loss. *Arch Dermatol.* 1961;83(2):175. doi:10.1001/archderm.1961.01580080005001
32. Headington JT. Telogen effluvium. New concepts and review. *Arch Dermatol.* 1993;129(3):356-363. doi:10.1001/archderm.1993.01680240096017
33. Harrison S, Sinclair R. Optimal management of hair loss (alopecia) in children. *Am J Clin Dermatol.* 2003;4(11):757-770. doi:10.2165/00128071-200304110-00004
34. Patel M, Harrison S, Sinclair R. Drugs and hair loss. *Dermatol Clin.* 2013;31(1):67-73. doi:10.1016/j.det.2012.08.002
35. Trüeb RM. Systematic approach to hair loss in women. *JDDG Dtsch Dermatol Ges.* 2010;8(4):284-297. doi:10.1111/j.1610-0387.2010.07261.x
36. Kaufman JP. Telogen effluvium secondary to starvation diet. *Arch Dermatol.* 1976;112(5):731. doi:10.1001/archderm.1976.01630290073022
37. Mubki T, Rudnicka L, Olszewska M, Shapiro J. Evaluation and diagnosis of the hair loss patient: part II. Trichoscopic and laboratory evaluations. *J Am Acad Dermatol.* 2014;71(3):431.e1-431.e11. doi:10.1016/j.jaad.2014.05.008
38. Olszewska M, Warszawik O, Rakowska A, Słowinska M, Rudnicka L. [Methods of hair loss evaluation in patients with endocrine disorders]. *Endokrynol Pol.* 2011;6(suppl 1):29-34.
39. Rakowska A, Slowinska M, Kowalska-Oledzka E, Olszewska M, Rudnicka L. Dermoscopy in female androgenic alopecia: method standardization and diagnostic criteria. *Int J Trichology.* 2009;1(2):123-130. doi:10.4103/0974-7753.58555
40. Whiting DA. Chronic telogen effluvium: increased scalp hair shedding in middle-aged women. *J Am Acad Dermatol.* 1996;35(6):899-906.
41. Sperling LC, Lupton GP. Histopathology of non-scarring alopecia. *J Cutan Pathol.* 1995;22(2):97-114. doi:10.1111/j.1600-0560.1995.tb01391.x
42. Kyriakis KP, Paltatzidou K, Kosma E, Sofouri E, Tadros A, Rachioti E. Alopecia areata prevalence by gender and age. *J Eur Acad Dermatology Venereol.* 2009;23(5):572-573. doi:10.1111/j.1468-3083.2008.02956.x
43. Nanda A, Al-Fouzan AS, Al-Hasawi F. Alopecia areata in children: a clinical profile. *Pediatr Dermatol.* 2002;19(6):482-485. doi:10.1046/j.1525-1470.2002.00215.x
44. Safavi K. Prevalence of alopecia areata in the first national health and nutrition examination survey. *Arch Dermatol.* 1992;128(5):702. doi:10.1001/archderm.1992.01680150136027
45. Sorrell J, Petukhova L, Reingold R, Christiano A, Garzon M. Shedding light on alopecia areata in pediatrics: a retrospective analysis of comorbidities in children in the national alopecia areata registry. *Pediatr Dermatol.* 2017;34(5):e271-e272. doi:10.1111/pde.13238

46. Wasserman D, Guzman-Sanchez DA, Scott K, McMichael A. Alopecia areata. *Int J Dermatol.* 2007;46(2):121-131. doi:10.1111/j.1365-4632.2007.03193.x

47. Muller SA, Winkelmann RK. Alopecia areata. *Arch Dermatol.* 1963;88(3):290. doi:10.1001/archderm.1963.01590210048007

48. Sharma VK, Kumar B, Dawn G. A clinical study of childhood alopecia areata in Chandigarh, India. *Pediatr Dermatol.* 1996;13(5):372-377. doi:10.1111/j.1525-1470.1996.tb00703.x

49. De Waard-Van der Spek FB, Oranje AP, De Raeymaecker DM, Peereboom-Wynia JD. Juvenile versus maturity-onset alopecia areata. A comparative retrospective clinical study. *Clin Exp Dermatol.* 1989;14(6):429-433. doi:10.1111/j.1365-2230.1989.tb02604.x

50. Alkhalifah A, Alsantali A, Wang E, McElwee KJ, Shapiro J. Alopecia areata update. Part I. Clinical picture, histopathology, and pathogenesis. *J Am Acad Dermatol.* 2010;62(2):177-188. doi:10.1016/j.jaad.2009.10.032

51. Trüeb RM, Dias MFRG. Alopecia areata: a comprehensive review of pathogenesis and management. *Clin Rev Allergy Immunol.* 2018;54(1):68-87. doi:10.1007/s12016-017-8620-9

52. Petukhova L, Duvic M, Hordinsky M, et al. Genome-wide association study in alopecia areata implicates both innate and adaptive immunity. *Nature.* 2010;466(7302):113-117. doi:10.1038/nature09114

53. McDonagh AJG, Tazi-Ahnini R. Epidemiology and genetics of alopecia areata. *Clin Exp Dermatol.* 2002;27(5):405-409. doi:10.1046/j.1365-2230.2002.01077.x

54. Jackow C, Puffer N, Hordinsky M, Nelson J, Tarrand J, Duvic M. Alopecia areata and cytomegalovirus infection in twins: genes versus environment? *J Am Acad Dermatol.* 1998;38(3):418-425. doi:10.1016/S0190-9622(98)70499-2

55. Paus R, Ito N, Takigawa M, Ito T. The hair follicle and immune privilege. *J Investig Dermatology Symp Proc.* 2003;8(2):188-194. doi:10.1046/j.1087-0024.2003.00807.x

56. Paus R, Bertolini M. The role of hair follicle immune privilege collapse in alopecia areata: status and perspectives. *J Investig Dermatology Symp Proc.* 2013;16(1):S25-S27. doi:10.1038/jidsymp.2013.7

57. Dressel D, Brütt CH, Manfras B, et al. Alopecia areata but not androgenetic alopecia is characterized by a restricted and oligoclonal T-cell receptor-repertoire among infiltrating lymphocytes. *J Cutan Pathol.* 1997;24(3):164-168.

58. Patel D, Li P, Bauer AJ, Castelo-Soccio L. Screening guidelines for thyroid function in children with alopecia areata. *JAMA Dermatology.* 2017;19104:1-4. doi:10.1001/jamadermatol.2017.3694

59. Olsen E, Hordinsky M, McDonald-Hull S, et al. Alopecia areata investigational assessment guidelines. National Alopecia Areata Foundation. *J Am Acad Dermatol.* 1999;40(2 Pt 1):242-246.

60. Xiao FL, Yang S, Liu JB, et al. The epidemiology of childhood alopecia areata in China: a study of 226 patients. *Pediatr Dermatol.* 2006;23(1):13-18. doi:10.1111/j.1525-1470.2006.00161.x

61. Ikeda T. A new classification of alopecia areata. *Dermatology.* 1965;131(6):421-445. doi:10.1159/000254503

62. Kakourou T, Karachristou K, Chrousos G. A case series of alopecia areata in children: Impact of personal and family history of stress and autoimmunity. *J Eur Acad Dermatology Venereol.* 2007;21(3):356-359. doi:10.1111/j.1468-3083.2006.01931.x

63. Price VH. Therapy of alopecia areata: on the cusp and in the future. *J Investig Dermatol Symp Proc.* 2003;8(2):207-211. doi:10.1046/j.1087-0024.2003.00811.x

64. Inui S, Nakajima T, Nakagawa K, Itami S. Clinical significance of dermoscopy in alopecia areata: analysis of 300 cases. *Int J Dermatol.* 2008;47(7):688-693. doi:10.1111/j.1365-4632.2008.03692.x

65. Messenger AG, de Berker DAR, Sinclair RD. Disorders of hair. In: *Rook's Textbook of Dermatology.* Oxford: Wiley-Blackwell; 2010:1-100. doi:10.1002/9781444317633.ch66

66. Madani S, Shapiro J. Alopecia areata update. *J Am Acad Dermatol.* 2000;42(4):549-566; quiz 567-570.

67. Gandhi V, Baruah MC, Bhattacharaya SN. Nail changes in alopecia areata: incidence and pattern. *Indian J Dermatol Venereol Leprol.* 69(2):114-115.

68. Kasumagic-Halilovic E, Prohic A. Nail changes in alopecia areata: frequency and clinical presentation. *J Eur Acad Dermatology Venereol.* 2009;23(2):240-241. doi:10.1111/j.1468-3083.2008.02830.x

69. Messenger AG, Slater DN, Bleehen SS. Alopecia areata: alterations in the hair growth cycle and correlation with the follicular pathology. *Br J Dermatol.* 1986;114(3):337-347.

70. Sperling LC, Solomon AR, Whiting DA. A new look at scarring alopecia. *Arch Dermatol.* 2000;136(2):235-242.

71. Lee JY, Hsu ML. Alopecia syphilitica, a simulator of alopecia areata: histopathology and differential diagnosis. *J Cutan Pathol.* 1991;18(2):87-92.

72. Cuozzo DW, Benson PM, Sperling LC, Skelton HG. Essential syphilitic alopecia revisited. *J Am Acad Dermatol.* 1995;32(5 PART 2):840-843. doi:10.1016/0190-9622(95)91543-5

73. Jordaan HF, Louw M. The moth-eaten alopecia of secondary syphilis. A histopathological study of 12 patients. *Am J Dermatopathol.* 1995;17(2):158-162.

74. Stroud JD. Hair loss in children. *Pediatr Clin North Am.* 1983;30(4):641-657.

75. Panza KE, Pittenger C, Bloch MH. Age and gender correlates of pulling in pediatric trichotillomania. *J Am Acad Child Adolesc Psychiatry.* 2013;52(3):241-249. doi:10.1016/j.jaac.2012.12.019

76. Duke DC, Keeley ML, Geffken GR, Storch EA. Trichotillomania: a current review. *Clin Psychol Rev.* 2010;30(2):181-193. doi:10.1016/j.cpr.2009.10.008

77. Cohen LJ, Stein DJ, Simeon D, et al. Clinical profile, comorbidity, and treatment history in 123 hair pullers: a survey study. *J Clin Psychiatry.* 1995;56(7):319-326.

78. Sah DE, Koo J, Price VH. Trichotillomania. *Dermatol Ther.* 2008;21(1):13-21. doi:10.1111/j.1529-8019.2008.00165.x

79. Tay Y-K, Levy ML, Metry DW. Trichotillomania in childhood: case series and review. *Pediatrics.* 2004;113(5):e494-e498. doi:10.1542/peds.113.5.e494

80. Chandran NS, Novak J, Iorizzo M, Grimalt R, Oranje AP. Childhood trichotillomania: diagnostic algorithm and systematic problem-solving management using the 5W1H (Kipling's principle). In: Oranje AP, Al-Mutairi N, Shwayder T, eds. *Practical Pediatric Dermatology.* Cham: Springer International Publishing; 2016:143-154. doi:10.1007/978-3-319-32159-2_15

81. Walsh KH, McDougle CJ. Trichotillomania. Presentation, etiology, diagnosis and therapy. *Am J Clin Dermatol.* 2001;2(5):327-333. doi:10.2165/00128071-200102050-00007

82. Christenson GA, Mackenzie TB, Reeve EA. Familial trichotillomania. *Am J Psychiatry.* 1992;149(2):283. doi:10.1176/ajp.149.2.aj1492283

83. Novak CE, Keuthen NJ, Stewart SE, Pauls DL. A twin concordance study of trichotillomania. *Am J Med Genet B Neuropsychiatr Genet.* 2009;150B(7):944-949. doi:10.1002/ajmg.b.30922

84. Hemmings SMJ, Kinnear CJ, Lochner C, et al. Genetic correlates in trichotillomania: a case-control association study in the South African Caucasian population. *Isr J Psychiatry Relat Sci.* 2006;43(2):93-101.

85. Züchner S, Wendland JR, Ashley-Koch AE, et al. Multiple rare SAPAP3 missense variants in trichotillomania and OCD. *Mol Psychiatry.* 2009;14(1):6-9. doi:10.1038/mp.2008.83

86. Papadopoulos AJ, Janniger CK, Chodynicki MP, Schwartz RA. Trichotillomania. *Int J Dermatol.* 2003;42(5):330-334. doi:10.1046/j.1365-4362.2003.01147.x

87. O'Sullivan RL, Keuthen NJ, Christenson GA, Mansueto CS, Stein DJ, Swedo SE. Trichotillomania: behavioral symptom or clinical syndrome? *Am J Psychiatry.* 1997;154(10):1442-1449. doi:10.1176/ajp.154.10.1442

88. Oranje AP, Peereboom-Wynia JD, De Raeymaecker DM. Trichotillomania in childhood. *J Am Acad Dermatol.* 1986;15(4 Pt 1):614-619.

89. Xu L, Liu KX, Senna MM. A practical approach to the diagnosis and management of hair loss in children and adolescents. *Front Med.* 2017;4:1-13. doi:10.3389/fmed.2017.00112

90. Wright HH, Holmes GR. Trichotillomania (hair pulling) in toddlers. *Psychol Rep.* 2003;92(1):228-230. doi:10.2466/pr0.2003.92.1.228

91. Woods DW, Flessner C, Franklin ME, et al. Understanding and treating trichotillomania: what we know and what we don't know. *Psychiatr Clin North Am.* 2006;29(2):487-501, ix. doi:10.1016/j.psc.2006.02.009

92. Christenson GA, Crow SJ. The characterization and treatment of trichotillomania. *J Clin Psychiatry.* 1996;57(suppl 8):42-47; discussion 48-49.

93. Harrison JP, Franklin ME. Pediatric trichotillomania. *Curr Psychiatry Rep.* 2012;14(3):188-196. doi:10.1007/s11920-012-0269-8

94. Rakowska A, Slowinska M, Olszewska M, Rudnicka L. New trichoscopy findings in trichotillomania: flame hairs, V-sign, hook hairs, hair powder, tulip hairs. *Acta Derm Venereol.* 2014;94(3):303-306. doi:10.2340/00015555-1674

95. Muller SA. Trichotillomania: A histopathologic study in sixty-six patients. *J Am Acad Dermatol.* 1990;23(1):56-62. doi:10.1016/0190-9622(90)70186-L

96. Lachapelle JM, Pierard GE. Traumatic alopecia in trichotillomania: a pathogenic interpretation of histologic lesions in the pilosebaceous unit. *J Cutan Pathol.* 1977;4(2):51-67.

97. Pomeranz A, Sabnis S. Tinea capitis epidemiology, diagnosis and management strategies. *Pediatr Drugs.* 2002;4(12):779-783. doi:10.1016/j.medcli.2013.04.021

98. Mirmirani P, Tucker LY. Epidemiologic trends in pediatric tinea capitis: a population-based study from Kaiser Permanente Northern California. *J Am Acad Dermatol.* 2013;69(6):916-921. doi:10.1016/j.jaad.2013.08.031

99. Abdel-Rahman SM, Farrand N, Schuenemann E, et al. The prevalence of infections with trichophyton tonsurans in schoolchildren: the CAPITIS Study. *Pediatrics.* 2010;125(5):966-973. doi:10.1542/peds.2009-2522

100. Panackal AA, Halpern EF, Watson AJ. Cutaneous fungal infections in the United States: Analysis of the national ambulatory medical care survey (NAMCS) and national hospital ambulatory medical care survey (NHAMCS), 1995-2004. *Int J Dermatol.* 2009;48(7):704-712. doi:10.1111/j.1365-4632.2009.04025.x

101. Ghannoum MA, Isham N, Hajjeh R, et al. Tinea capitis in Cleveland: survey of elementary school students. *J Am Acad Dermatol.* 2003;48(2 SUPPL.):189-193. doi:10.1067/mjd.2003.109

102. Lobato MN, Vugia DJ, Frieden IJ. Tinea capitis in California children: a population-based study of a growing epidemic. *Pediatrics.* 1997;99:551-554.

103. Cantrell WC, Jacobs MK, Sobera JO, Parrish CA, Warner J, Elewski BE. Tinea capitis in Birmingham: Survey of elementary school students. *Pediatr Dermatol.* 2011;28(4):476-477. doi:10.1111/j.1525-1470.2010.01166.x

104. Laude TA, Shah BR, Lynfield Y. Tinea capitis in Brooklyn. *Am J Dis Child.* 1982;136(12):1047-1050. doi:10.1001/archpedi.1982.03970480013002

105. Gupta AK, Summerbell RC. Increased incidence of Trichophyton tonsurans tinea capitis in Ontario, Canada between 1985 and 1996. *Med Mycol.* 1998;36(2):55-60. doi:10.1046/j.1365-280X.1998.00129.x

106. Fuller LC, Child FC, Midgley G, Higgins EM. Scalp ringworm in south-east London and an analysis of a cohort of patients from a paediatric dermatology department. *Br J Dermatol.* 2003;148(5):985-988. doi:10.1046/j.1365-2133.2003.05022.x

107. Higgins EM, Fuller LC, Smith CH. Guidelines for the management of tinea capitis. *Br J Dermatol.* 2000;143(1):53-58. doi:10.1046/j.1365-2133.2000.03530.x

108. Kawachi Y, Ikegami M, Takase T, Otsuka F. Chronically recurrent and disseminated tinea faciei/corporis: autoinoculation from asymptomatic tinea capitis carriage. *Pediatr Dermatol.* 2010;27(5):527-528. doi:10.1111/j.1525-1470.2010.01270.x

109. Nenoff P, Krüger C, Ginter-Hanselmayer G, Tietz HJ. Mykologie - ein update. Teil 1: Dermatomykosen: Erreger, epidemiologie und pathogenese. *JDDG - J Ger Soc Dermatol.* 2014;12(3):188-212. doi:10.1111/ddg.12245

110. Hay RJ. Tinea capitis: current status. *Mycopathologia.* 2017;182(1-2):87-93. doi:10.1007/s11046-016-0058-8

111. Shy R. Tinea corporis and tinea capitis. *Pediatr Rev.* 2007;28(5):164-174. doi:10.1542/pir.28-5-164

112. Bolognia J, Jorizzo J, Schaffer J. *Dermatology.* Philadelphia, PA: Elsevier; 2012. doi:10.1017/CBO9781107415324.004

113. Ilkit M. Favus of the scalp: an overview and update. *Mycopathologia.* 2010;170(3):143-154. doi:10.1007/s11046-010-9312-7

114. Slowinska M, Rudnicka L, Schwartz RA, et al. Comma hairs: a dermatoscopic marker for tinea capitis. A rapid diagnostic method. *J Am Acad Dermatol.* 2008;59(5 suppl). doi:10.1016/j.jaad.2008.07.009

115. Hughes R, Chiaverini C, Bahadoran P, Lacour JP. Cockscrew hair: a new dermoscopic for diagnosis of tinea capitis in black children. *Arch Dermatol.* 2011;147(3):355-356. doi:10.1007/s13398-014-0173-7.2.

116. Isa-Isa R, Arenas R, Isa M. Inflammatory tinea capitis: kerion, dermatophytic granuloma, and mycetoma. *Clin Dermatol.* 2010;28(2):133-136. doi:10.1016/j.clindermatol.2009.12.013

117. Elewski BE. Tinea capitis: a current perspective. *J Am Acad Dermatol.* 2000;42(1 Pt 1):1-20-24. doi:10.1016/S0190-9622(00)90001-X

118. Cheng N, Rucker Wright D, Cohen BA. Dermatophytid in tinea capitis: rarely reported common phenomenon with clinical implications. *Pediatrics.* 2011;128(2):e453-e457. doi:10.1542/peds.2010-2757

119. Whiting DA. Cicatricial alopecia: clinico-pathological findings and treatment. *Clin Dermatol.* 2001;19(2):211-225. doi:10.1016/S0738-081X(00)00132-2

120. Graham JH, Johnson WC, Helwig EB. Tinea capitis. *Arch Dermatol.* 1964;89(4):528. doi:10.1001/archderm.1964.01590280028004

121. Arenas R, Toussaint S, Isa-Isa R. Kerion and dermatophytic granuloma. Mycological and histopathological findings in 19 children with inflammatory tinea capitis of the scalp. *Int J Dermatol.* 2006;45(3):215-219. doi:10.1111/j.1365-4632.2004.02449.x

122. Strober BE. Tinea capitis. *Dermatol Online J.* 2001;7(1):12.

123. Sellheyer K, Bergfeld WF. Histopathologic evaluation of alopecias. *Am J Dermatopathol.* 2006;28(3):236-259.

124. Kubba R, Rook A. Congenital triangular alopecia. *Br J Dermatol.* 1976;95(6):657-659.

125. Tosti A. Congenital triangular alopecia: report of fourteen cases. *J Am Acad Dermatol.* 1987;16(5):991-993. doi:10.1016/S0190-9622(87)70127-3

126. Yamazaki M, Irisawa R, Tsuboi R. Temporal triangular alopecia and a review of 52 past cases. *J Dermatol.* 2010;37(4):360-362. doi:10.1111/j.1346-8138.2010.00817.x

127. Trakimas C, Sperling LC, Skelton HG, Smith KJ, Buker JL, Sperling LC. Clinical and histologic findings in temporal triangular alopecia. *J Am Acad Dermatol.* 1994;31(2):205-209. doi:10.1016/S0190-9622(94)70147-4

128. Fernández-Crehuet P, Vaño-Galván S, Martorell-Calatayud A, Arias-Santiago S, Grimalt R, Camacho-Martínez FM. Clinical and trichoscopic characteristics of temporal triangular alopecia: a multicenter study. *J Am Acad Dermatol.* 2016;75(3):634-637. doi:10.1016/j.jaad.2016.04.053

129. Silva CY, Lenzy YM, Goldberg LJ. Temporal triangular alopecia with decreased follicular density. *J Cutan Pathol.* 2010;37(5):597-599. doi:10.1111/j.1600-0560.2009.01388.x

130. Olsen EA, Bergfeld WF, Cotsarelis G, et al. Summary of North American Hair Research Society (NAHRS)-sponsored workshop on cicatricial alopecia, Duke University Medical Center, February 10 and 11, 2001. *J Am Acad Dermatol.* 2003;48(1):103-110. doi:10.1067/mjd.2003.68

131. Christensen KN, Lehman JS, Tollefson MM. Pediatric lichen planopilaris: clinicopathologic study of four new cases and a review of the literature. *Pediatr Dermatol.* 2015;32(5):621-627. doi:10.1111/pde.12624

132. Assouly P, Reygagne P. Lichen planopilaris: update on diagnosis and treatment. *Semin Cutan Med Surg.* 2009;28(1):3-10. doi:10.1016/j.sder.2008.12.006

133. Cevasco NC, Bergfeld WF, Remzi BK, de Knott HR. A case-series of 29 patients with lichen planopilaris: The Cleveland Clinic Foundation experience on evaluation, diagnosis, and treatment. *J Am Acad Dermatol.* 2007;57(1):47-53. doi:10.1016/j.jaad.2007.01.011

134. Atarguine H, Hocar O, Hamdaoui A, Akhdari N, Amal S. Alopécie frontale fibrosante: à propos de trois cas pédiatriques. *Arch Pediatr.* 2016;23(8):832-835. doi:10.1016/j.arcped.2016.05.006

135. Sampaio MC, De Oliveira ZN, Machado MC, Dos Reis VM, Vilela MA. Discoid lupus erythematosus in children: a retrospective study of 34 patients. *Pediatr Dermatol.* 2008;25(2):163-167. doi:10.1111/j.1525-1470.2008.00625.x

136. Arkin LM, Ansell L, Rademaker A, et al. The natural history of pediatric-onset discoid lupus erythematosus. *J Am Acad Dermatol.* 2015;72(4):628-633. doi:10.1016/j.jaad.2014.12.028

137. Moises-Alfaro C, Berro-Peez R, Carrasco-Daza D, Gutierez-Castrello P, Ruiz-Maldonado R. Discoid lupus erythematosus in children: clinical, histopathologic, and follow-up features in 27 cases. *Pediatr Dermatol.* 2003;20(2):103-107.

138. Hymes SR, Jordon RE. Chronic cutaneous lupus erythematosus. *Med Clin North Am.* 1989;73(5):1055-1071.

139. Gathers RC, Lim HW. Central centrifugal cicatricial alopecia: past, present, and future. *J Am Acad Dermatol.* 2009;60(4):660-668. doi:10.1016/j.jaad.2008.09.066

140. Eginli A, Dlova NC, McMichael A. Central centrifugal cicatricial alopecia in the pediatric population: a case series and review of the literature. *Pediatr Dermatol.* 2015;34(2):1-5. doi:10.1111/pde.13046

141. Dlova NC, Jordaan FH, Sarig O, Sprecher E. Autosomal dominant inheritance of central centrifugal cicatricial alopecia in black South Africans. *J Am Acad Dermatol.* 2014;70(4):679-682. doi:10.1016/j.jaad.2013.11.035

142. de Oliveira Góes HF, Reis Gavazzoni Dias MF, de Abreu Neves Salles S, dos Santos Lima C, da Silva Vieira M, Pantaleão L. Lichen planopilaris developed during childhood*. 2017;92(4):543-545. doi:10.1590/abd1806-4841.20174890

143. Stefanato CM. Histopathology of alopecia: a clinicopathological approach to diagnosis. *Histopathology.* 2010;56(1):24-38. doi:10.1111/j.1365-2559.2009.03439.x

144. Headington JT. Cicatricial alopecia. *Dermatol Clin.* 1996;14(4):773-782. doi:10.1016/S0733-8635(05)70403-4

145. Sperling LC. Scarring alopecia and the dermatopathologist. *J Cutan Pathol.* 2001;28(7):333-342. doi:http://dx.doi.org/10.1034/j.1600-0560.2001.280701.x

146. Bernárdez C, Molina-Ruiz AM, Requena L. Histopatología de las alopecias. Parte II: alopecias cicatriciales. *Actas Dermosifiliogr.* 2015;106(4):260-270. doi:10.1016/j.ad.2014.06.016

147. Sperling LC. Premature desquamation of the inner root sheath is still a useful concept! [4]. *J Cutan Pathol.* 2007;34(10):809-810. doi:10.1111/j.1600-0560.2006.00707.x

148. Nambudiri VE, Vleugels RA, Laga AC, Goldberg LJ. Clinicopathologic lessons in distinguishing cicatricial alopecia: 7 Cases of lichen planopilaris misdiagnosed as discoid lupus. *J Am Acad Dermatol.* 2014;71(4):e135-e138. doi:10.1016/j.jaad.2014.04.052

149. Fabbri P, Amato L, Chiarini C, Moretti S, Massi D. Scarring alopecia in discoid lupus erythematosus: a clinical, histopathologic and immunopathologic study. *Lupus.* 2004;13(6):455-462. doi:10.1191/0961203304lu1041oa

150. Wilson CL, Burge SM, Dean D, Dawber RP. Scarring alopecia in discoid lupus erythematosus. *Br J Dermatol.* 1992;126(4):307-314.

151. Chung HJ, Goldberg LJ. Histologic features of chronic cutaneous lupus erythematosus of the scalp using horizontal sectioning: emphasis on follicular findings. *J Am Acad Dermatol.* 2017;77(2):349-355. doi:10.1016/j.jaad.2017.02.039

152. Trachsler S, Trueb RM. Value of direct immunofluorescence for differential diagnosis of cicatricial alopecia. *Dermatology.* 2005;211(2):98-102. doi:10.1159/000086436

153. Ohyama M. Primary cicatricial alopecia: recent advances in understanding and management. *J Dermatol.* 2012;39(1):18-26. doi:10.1111/j.1346-8138.2011.01416.x

154. Tan E, Martinka M, Ball N, Shapiro J. Primary cicatricial alopecias: clinicopathology of 112 cases. *J Am Acad Dermatol.* 2004;50(1):25-32. doi:10.1016/j.jaad.2003.04.001

155. Annessi G. Tufted folliculitis of the scalp: a distinctive clinicohistological variant of folliculitis decalvans. *Br J Dermatol.* 1998;138(5):799-805.

156. Powell JJ, Dawber RP, Gatter K. Folliculitis decalvans including tufted folliculitis: clinical, histological and therapeutic findings. *Br J Dermatol.* 1999;140(2):328-333.

157. Douwes KE, Landthaler M, Szeimies RM. Simultaneous occurrence of folliculitis decalvans capillitii in identical twins. *Br J Dermatol.* 2000;143(1):195-197.

158. Ramesh V. Dissecting cellulitis of the scalp in 2 girls. *Dermatologica.* 1990;180(1):48-50.

159. Scheinfeld NS. A case of dissecting cellulitis and a review of the literature. *Dermatol Online J.* 2003;9(1):87-93. doi:10.1007/s11845-008-0177-4

160. Halder RM. Hair and scalp disorders in blacks. *Cutis.* 1983;32(4):378-380.

161. Badaoui A, Reygagne P, Cavelier-Balloy B, et al. Dissecting cellulitis of the scalp: a retrospective study of 51 patients and review of literature. *Br J Dermatol.* 2016;174(2):421-423. doi:10.1111/bjd.13999

162. Arneja JS, Frcsc M, Vashi CN, et al. Management of fulminant dissecting cellulitis of the scalp in the pediatric population: case report and literature review. *Can J Plast Surg.* 2007;1515(44):211-214.

163. Bjellerup M, Wallengren J. Familial perifolliculitis capitis abscedens et suffodiens in two brothers successfully treated with isotretinoin. *J Am Acad Dermatol.* 1990;23(4):752-753. doi:10.1016/S0190-9622(08)81076-6

164. Chicarilli ZN. Follicular occlusion triad: hidradenitis suppurativa, acne conglobata, and dissecting cellulitis of the scalp. *Ann Plast Surg.* 1987;18(3):230-237. doi:10.1097/00000637-198703000-00009

165. Otberg N, Kang H, Alzolibani AA, Shapiro J. Folliculitis decalvans. *Dermatol Ther.* 2008;21(4):238-244. doi:10.1111/j.1529-8019.2008.00204.x

166. Ross EK, Tan E, Shapiro J. Update on primary cicatricial alopecias. *J Am Acad Dermatol.* 2005;53(1):1-37. doi:10.1016/j.jaad.2004.06.015

167. Miteva M, Tosti A. Hair and scalp dermatoscopy. *J Am Acad Dermatol.* 2012;67(5):1040-1048. doi:10.1016/j.jaad.2012.02.013

168. Mundi JP, Marmon S, Fischer M, Kamino H, Patel R, Shapiro J. Dissecting cellulitis of the scalp. *Dermatol Online J.* 2012;18(12):8.

169. Vañó-Galván S, Molina-Ruiz AM, Fernández-Crehuet P, et al. Folliculitis decalvans: a multicentre review of 82 patients. *J Eur Acad Dermatology Venereol.* 2015;29(9):1750-1757. doi:10.1111/jdv.12993

170. Azurdia RM, Graham RM, Weismann K, Guerin DM, Parslew R. Acne keloidalis in caucasian patients on cyclosporin following organ transplantation. *Br J Dermatol.* 2000;143(2):465-467.

171. Dinehart SM, Tanner L, Mallory SB, Herzberg AJ. Acne keloidalis in women. *Cutis.* 1989;44(3):250-252.

172. Loayza E, Cazar T, Uraga V, Lubkov A, Garces JC. Acne keloidalis nuchae in Latin American women. *Int J Dermatol.* 2015;54(5):e183-e185.

173. Knable AL, Jr., Hanke CW, Gonin R. Prevalence of acne keloidalis nuchae in football players. *J Am Acad Dermatol.* 1997;37(4):570-574.

174. Su HJ, Cheng AY, Liu CH, et al. Primary scarring alopecia: a retrospective study of 89 patients in Taiwan. *J Dermatol.* 2018;45(4):450-455.

175. Alexis A, Heath CR, Halder RM. Folliculitis keloidalis nuchae and pseudofolliculitis barbae: are prevention and effective treatment within reach? *Dermatol Clin.* 2014;32(2):183-191.

176. Sperling LC, Homoky C, Pratt L, Sau P. Acne keloidalis is a form of primary scarring alopecia. *Arch Dermatol.* 2000;136(4):479-484.

177. Shapero J, Shapero H. Acne keloidalis nuchae is scar and keloid formation secondary to mechanically induced folliculitis. *J Cutan Med Surg.* 2011;15(4):238-240.

178. Grunwald MH, Ben-Dor D, Livni E, Halevy S. Acne keloidalis-like lesions on the scalp associated with antiepileptic drugs. *Int J Dermatol.* 1990;29(8):559-561.

17

Cutaneous Bacterial Infections

Francisco G. Bravo

The skin is the immediate interface between humans and their environment and serves as an effective barrier to a host of microorganisms that are present ambiently throughout the world. Some are normal cutaneous flora, whereas others are potential pathogens. This chapter summarizes the cutaneous bacterial infections that children may develop with emphasis on a synthesis of the clinical and histologic features.

IMPETIGO

Definition and Epidemiology

Impetigo is one of the most common bacterial infections in dermatology and general medicine. It is caused by Group A beta-hemolytic *Streptococcus pyogenes*, *Staphylococcus aureus*, or a combination of both.

Impetigo is the most common infection between the ages of 2 and 5 years, but can be seen at any age. It is highly transmissible.

Etiology

Impetigo has two clinical forms, represented by "honey-crusted," nonbullous impetigo, caused by *S. pyogenes* and *S. aureus*, and a bullous form, caused exclusively by the specific phage types of *S. aureus*.

Group A streptococci are highly pathogenic in comparison with other groups of streptococci. They can be isolated from the skin up to 10 days before the disease manifests clinically, and they can be isolated from the oropharynx 14 to 20 days after appearing on the skin.[1,2]

Bullous impetigo is mostly produced by *S. aureus* group II, phage type 71, and also phage types 3A, 3C, and 55. Two toxins, with desmoglein 1 as their target, have been described. The exfoliative toxins produced by Staphylococcus can produce impetigo and staphylococcal scalded skin syndrome by cleaving a peptide bound in desmoglein 1, imitating the mechanisms seen in pemphigus foliaceus.[3]

Clinical Presentation

Nonbullous impetigo (crusted impetigo, impetigo contagiosa) is the most common form seen in children over 2 years of age, as well as in adults. It represents 70% of all impetigo cases. *S. aureus*, either alone or in combination with Group A beta-hemolytic streptococci, is responsible for 80% of cases.[1] The infection may arise in normal skin or in already damaged skin, including atopic dermatitis, insect bites, scabies, or pediculosis. The lesions are round, with a very fragile central vesicle that breaks easily and becomes a honey crust (Figure 17-1). They measure 2 to 4 cm, grow centrifugally, and develop satellite lesions. They are preferably located on exposed areas, such as the face and extremities. The patient may develop regional lymphadenopathy and fever. The skin lesions can self-resolve in 2 to 3 weeks without therapy.

Bullous impetigo starts with smaller blisters that are initially tense, with clear contents. These later become flaccid and contain pus (Figure 17-2). The lesions are usually multiple, with satellites; they can reach up to 2 cm in diameter, and when the blister breaks, the center looks erythematous and the roof remnants give the lesion an

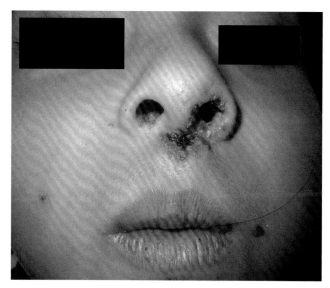

FIGURE 17-1. Clinical image of honey-crusted impetigo. Courtesy of Dr Karina Feria.

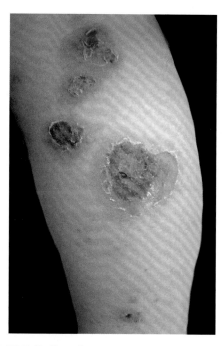

FIGURE 17-3. Bullous impetigo: remnants of the roof of the blisters are seen at the lesional edges, giving the lesions an annular appearance. Courtesy of Dr Rosa Ines Castro.

represented by a histologic crust, containing a mixture of serum with parakeratotic and neutrophilic debris.

Classical bullous impetigo shows a subcorneal epidermal blister containing neutrophils (Figure 17-4).[4] Spongiosis and focal acantholysis may also be seen (Figure 17-5).[5] The underlying dermis contains variable inflammation, commonly featuring neutrophils, which may also invade the epidermis. Tissue Gram stains may show cocciform bacteria, representing either *S. aureus* or *S. pyogenes*.

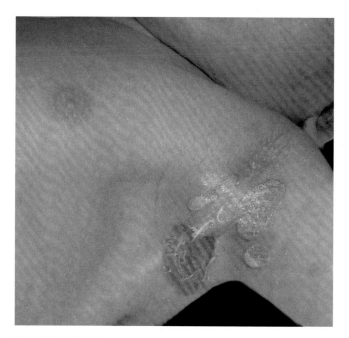

FIGURE 17-2. Clinical image of bullous impetigo in a neonate. Courtesy of Dr Karina Feria.

annular morphology. They may occasionally be polycyclic (Figure 17-3). The lesions are mostly located on intertriginous areas such as diaper zone, axillae and neck, but they can also be acral in location. Regional lymphadenopathy is rare.

Histologic Findings

Nonbullous impetigo (which is only rarely biopsied) may initially show a few neutrophils at the subcorneal level and in the underlying epidermis. Crusted impetigo is

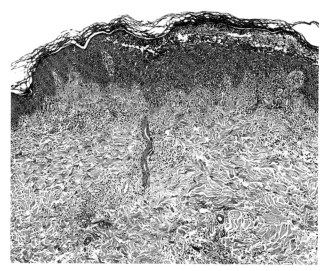

FIGURE 17-4. Bullous impetigo: subcorneal blister with acantholysis. Hematoxylin and eosin (H&E) stain. ×200. Courtesy of Dr Luis Requena.

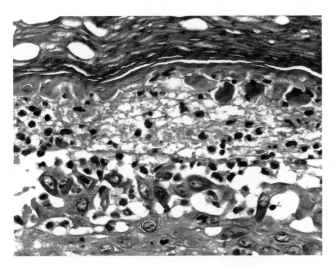

FIGURE 17-5. Bullous impetigo: high power of the case in Figure 17-3. H/E ×400. Courtesy of Dr Luis Requena.

Differential Diagnosis

Commonly, in the first hours of its evolution, tinea corporis may be associated with a honey crust, and it can be confused with crusted nonbullous impetigo. In *Herpes simplex* infection, cutaneous vesicles are smaller and have a more grayish color than those of impetigo. Histologically, herpetic lesions show nuclear molding and multinucleated giant cells. Subcorneal blisters with neutrophils can be seen in acute generalized eruptive pustulosis, early psoriasis, candidiasis, tinea, and acropustulosis of infancy. The clinical context and periodic acid–Schiff (PAS) staining will help in establishing the correct diagnosis.

CAPSULE SUMMARY

IMPETIGO

Impetigo is caused by beta-hemolytic *S. pyogenes* and *S. aureus*. Nonbullous impetigo is most commonly associated with *S. aureus* and *S. pyogenes*. It is usually located on exposed areas such as face and extremities, and honey-crusted lesions predominate. Bullous impetigo is most commonly associated with *S. aureus* group II, phage type 71. On intertriginous areas, lesions are flaccid and vesicular. They later break, leaving annular lesions with a collarette. Histologic findings include either a subcorneal blister containing neutrophils or a crust over the epidermis with spongiosis.

Infections With Methicillin-Resistant *S. Aureus*

The first strain of *S. aureus* that was resistant to methicillin was described in 1961. In the general population, one in three people carries *S. aureus* in the nose, without

any manifestations, whereas 2 out of 100 people harbor methicillin-resistant *S. aureus* (MRSA). MRSA was initially seen in hospitalized patients who required invasive interventions, such as placement of intravenous lines, bladder catheters, and mechanical ventilation. By the end of the 1990s, another variant of MRSA was described in the mid-western United States, which was associated with skin and soft tissue infection in persons in the general populace. It was named "community-acquired" MRSA (CA-MRSA).

MRSA bacteria are different from staphylococci that produce exfoliative toxins and those associated with bullous impetigo. They carry the gene that allows the production of the Panton-Valentine Leucocidin exotocin.[1] In the community, MRSA is considered to be a rare cause of impetigo. CA-MRSA infections are more likely to present with the formation of furuncles and abscesses than with impetigo. MRSA is now the most common cause of purulent skin and soft tissue infections in many regions of the United States.[6]

ECTHYMA

Definition and Epidemiology

Ecthyma is a bacterial infection that is deeply seated in the skin and has a tendency to affect the lower dermis, producing ulceration with crusting. Ecthyma gangrenosum (EG) is the term used for a similar, ulcerated lesion caused by a hematogenous spread of infections with *Pseudomonas aeruginosa* or other causes of bacterial septicemia.

Ecthyma is commonly seen on the legs in children and elderly persons, and it is a frequent complication of papular urticaria. EG is more commonly encountered in immunocompromised patients with Gram-negative sepsis, most often but not exclusively caused by *P. aeruginosa*.

Etiology

Most ecthymas are produced by Group A streptococci, either as a primary infection or as a complication of preexisting conditions such as an insect bite or excoriation. Coagulase-positive staphylococci have also been isolated as coinfectants from the lesions of streptococcal ecthyma. EG is mostly seen in immunocompromised patients, particularly those with underlying malignancies. Once considered a clinical entity that was pathognomonic of *P. aeruginosa* infection, it is now known to be potentially associated with additional microorganisms, including other *Pseudomonas* species, *Escherichia coli*, *Citrobacter*, *Klebsiella*, *Morganella*, *Candida*, and *Fusarium*.[7]

Clinical Presentation

Classical ecthyma begins as a vesicle or a pustule, surrounded by a zone of erythema. As it enlarges, it will develop a central yellow-green crust, with a "punched-out" appearance (Figure 17-6).[8] If the overlying scab is removed,

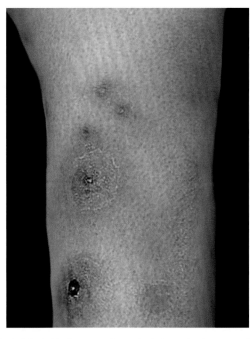

FIGURE 17-6. **Ecthyma: ulcerated deep lesions on the pretibial areas.**

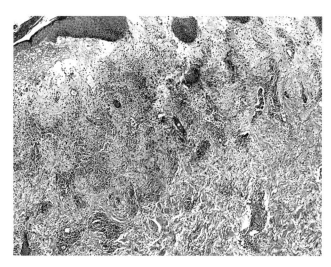

FIGURE 17-7. **Ecthyma, histologic findings include edema in the papillary dermis and neutrophils in the mid-dermis.** H/E ×100. Courtesy of Dr Luis Requena.

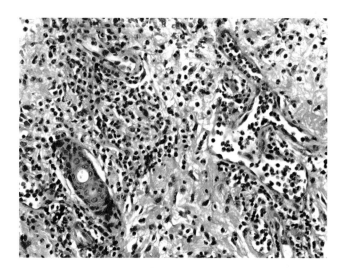

FIGURE 17-8. **Ecthyma, histologic findings include a large number of neutrophils in the mid-dermis.** H/E ×400. Courtesy of Dr Luis Requena.

a saucer-shaped ulcer will be revealed with elevated borders and a grainy base. Typical locations are the shins and the dorsa of the feet. Lesions can be multiple. In addition to children, ecthyma also occurs in intravenous drug users, patients infected with HIV, and individuals with poor hygiene, malnutrition, or previous trauma.[9]

EG starts as a hemorrhagic pustule that evolves into a necrotic ulcer; rather than a crust, it is covered by a black scab and surrounded by a red halo. EG is predominantly located on the gluteal and perineal skin, but up to 30% of cases may be seen on the extremities or the face.[8] Lesions are larger than those of classical ecthyma. EG has also been reported in other circumstances besides malignancy, and even in immunocompetent persons.[8] Healthy infants may develop EG in the diaper area after receiving antibiotics, in conjunction with maceration of the skin.

Histologic Findings

The histologic appearance of classical ecthyma shows ulceration, with superficial crusting and many neutrophils in the underlying dermis (Figures 17-7 and 17-8). Accumulations of cocci can be seen inside the crust.

In EG, necrosis is present in the epidermis and dermis, along with hemorrhage and a mixed inflammatory cell infiltrate around an area of infarction, caused by vascular thrombosis. Vasculitis can be seen at the edges of the ulcer. Sometimes, the inflammatory infiltrate is sparse. Gram-negative bacteria can be detected in the vessel walls.[10]

Differential Diagnosis

Ecthyma can be confused clinically with excoriated papules of prurigo nodularis. Well-developed lesions can be mistaken for leishmaniasis. The histologic findings in EG can also be seen in cutaneous infections with *Vibrio vulnificus*.

CAPSULE SUMMARY

ECTHYMA

Classical ecthyma is streptococcal in nature, located on the pretibial areas with crusted and punched-out lesions. Affected patients are usually children. Biopsies show ulceration and neutrophilia, and bacteria can be seen in the crust.

EG is associated with sick, immunocompromised patients. *P. aeruginosa* is the predominant, but not the only, etiologic agent. The lesions are more necrotic than crusted. Histologically, necrosis is evident, and the inflammatory infiltrate is mixed and sometimes sparse. There may be evidence of vasculitis, with bacteria in the vessel walls.

BACTERIAL FOLLICULITIS

Definition and Epidemiology

Bacterial folliculitis is the infection of hair follicles and perifollicular areas by bacteria, presenting with multiple dome-shaped pustules that are centered on the follicular ostia. The most common causative organism is *S. aureus*.

Folliculitis in children most commonly affects the scalp, whereas in adults it has a predilection for the bearded portion of the face, the axillae, the gluteal area, and the extremities. Excessive sweating, a humid environment, poor hygiene, the use of occlusive preparations and dressings, and maceration of the skin are predisposing factors, as is continuity with draining abscesses. Repeated bathing in poorly chlorinated swimming pools, hot tubs, and whirlpools is associated with *Pseudomonas* folliculitis. Gram-negative bacterial folliculitis may be seen in patients who have had a prolonged treatment of acne with oral antibiotics.

Etiology

The most common causative agent for bacterial folliculitis is *S. aureus*, but occasionally coagulase-negative *Staphylococcus* species can cause the condition. "Hot tub folliculitis" is classically associated with infections by *P. aeruginosa*. Bacteria seen in posttreatment folliculitis in acne patients are usually *Enterobacteriaceae* and *Proteus* species.

Clinical Presentation

Bacterial folliculitis can be divided into superficial and deep forms. The superficial variant, known as impetigo of Bockhart, comprises tiny, fragile pustules, centered on the follicular ostia. In children, it usually affects the scalp. Hair shafts can be seen piercing the pustules. Preexisting conditions such as living in hot humid climates, obesity, the use of occlusive dressings, and diabetes mellitus all favor the appearance of folliculitis. Deep forms of folliculitis include furuncles—most commonly caused by *S. aureus* infection—and folliculitis barbae or sycosis barbae.[8] Patients with hot tub folliculitis caused by *P. aeruginosa* develop lesions on the buttocks, hips, and axillae.[11] Otitis and mastitis are possible, as well as systemic symptoms such as fever and malaise. Children and adolescents may have a singular presentation of folliculitis, with the development of red papules and nodules on the hands and feet.[12,13]

Histologic Findings

In the superficial form of bacterial folliculitis, a subcorneal neutrophilic pustule is seen that is centered on the follicular infundibulum and the surrounding dermis. Lymphocytes and macrophages may be present as well. The inflammatory infiltrate may involve the entirety of the follicle.

In the deeper variants of folliculitis such as the furuncle, one sees dermal abscesses that are centered on the mid or lower portions of the follicle; the follicular epithelium may be destroyed, but a remnant of hair shafts can be seen. The epidermis is only secondarily involved and is replaced by a crust, and the process may extend into the subcutis.

Pseudomonas folliculitis presents histologically with a combination of superficial and deep folliculitis. There is a predominance of neutrophils in the infiltrate with the destruction of follicular walls. Gram-negative folliculitis in acne patients is also superficial and deep.

Differential Diagnosis

Tinea on the face may have a follicular component that remains when pediatric patients are treated only with topical antimycotic therapy. The associated lesions may histologically show either suppurative or lymphocytic inflammation, sometimes with giant cells. An important clue is the presence of spores or hyphae in the follicular lumina. *Pityrosporum* folliculitis can cause a rupture of the follicles, and yeast forms are seen inside of them, sometimes spilling into the surrounding dermis. Eosinophilic pustular folliculitis of infancy occurs during the first 14 months of life, presenting as crops of papules and pustules on the scalp with possible extension to other sites. Many eosinophils are seen microscopically, and the infiltrate may be interfollicular rather than follicle centered.[14]

CAPSULE SUMMARY

FOLLICULITIS

Superficial folliculitis is most commonly associated with infection by *S. aureus* (impetigo of Bockhart). Clinically, it comprises tiny pustules on the scalp with hair shafts in the center of them. Histologically, one sees a neutrophilic infundibulitis and peri-infundibulitis. Chronic folliculitis is a deep process, either a follicle-centered abscess (furuncles caused by *Staphylococcus*) or a superficial and deep suppurative infection as in *P.* folliculitis.

ERYSIPELAS

Definition and Epidemiology

Erysipelas is an acute infection of the skin that involves the superficial dermal lymphatics, with well-demarcated borders and the presence of systemic symptoms. Erysipelas is most commonly seen in newborn infants and children, or in adults between the ages of 40 and 60.

Etiology

The vast majority of erysipelas cases are caused by infection with Group A beta-hemolytic *S. pyogenes*. Group B *S. pyogenes* may also produce disease in newborns. Other potentially causative microbes include *S. pyogenes* of Group G, C, and D, as well as *S. aureus, Streptococcus pneumoniae, Klebsiella pneumoniae,* and *Yersinia enterocolitica.*

Clinical Presentation

Currently, the most common location for erysipelas is the legs (Figure 17-9), with the face being next in frequency. This infection is commonly associated with a break in the skin, such as a fissure, an insect bite, or superficial dermatophytosis. In infants, the disease may disseminate from the umbilical stump to the skin of the abdomen or from a circumcision site to the genitoperineum. Predisposing conditions include venous or lymphatic obstruction, diabetes mellitus, and nephrotic syndrome. Erysipelas commonly debuts with the sudden onset of fever, chills, and malaise.

Clinical findings include a rapidly developing red plaque that is warm, tender, shiny, elevated, sharply demarcated, and confluent, occasionally with a "peau d´orange" appearance. Vesicles, bullae, and ecchymotic lesions may develop as the infection progresses. When erysipelas subsides, mild hyperpigmentation and fine scaling may be the residua. Complications include bacteremia, local abscess formation, thrombophlebitis, gangrene, and glomerulonephritis.

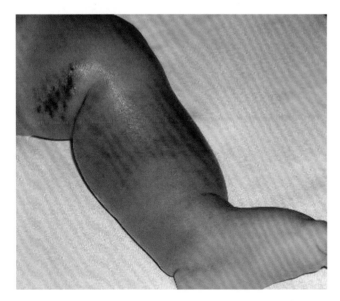

FIGURE 17-9. Erysipelas on the lower extremity. Courtesy Dra. Rosa Ines Castro.

Histologic Findings

Histologically, erysipelas is characterized by marked subepidermal edema, and a diffuse, variably dense interstitial infiltrate of neutrophils in the underlying dermis, without abscess formation.[10] The infiltrate is accentuated around blood vessels, and nuclear dust may be present. Capillary and lymphatic vessels may be dilated, and granulation tissue may be located beneath the zone of papillary edema as the disease subsides.

Differential Diagnosis

The principal histologic differential diagnoses for erysipelas are Sweet syndrome, which usually has a denser mid-dermal infiltrate of neutrophils, and leukocytoclastic vasculitis. Rheumatoid dermatitis-panniculitis and erythema marginatum may also be neutrophilic, but they have different clinical manifestations.

CAPSULE SUMMARY

ERYSIPELAS

Clinically, presentation is an acute onset of fever, chills, and malaise and the subsequent appearance of a red, shiny, warm, tender plaque on a leg or the face. Histologically, one sees edema of the papillary dermis and a diffuse interstitial dermal infiltrate of neutrophils.

ERYSIPELOID

Definition and Epidemiology

This uncommon cutaneous infection, also known as "erysipeloid of Rosenbach," is caused by *Erysipelothrix rhusiopathiae*, a Gram-positive pleomorphic bacillus. The distribution of the causative microorganism is worldwide. Domestic swine, rodents, and birds are the most common reservoirs. Fish flesh is usually not infected, but the bacteria commonly contaminates the slimy coating over fish scales. Erysipeloid is typically occupationally acquired, and it is seen in butchers, fishermen, fish handlers, slaughterhouse workers, veterinarians, and other persons having contact with the animal vectors. The infection is rare in children.

Etiology

E. rhusiopathiae is a linear or slightly curved thin bacillus, measuring 0.8 to 2.5 in length. Sometimes, the organisms are arranged in single, short chains, or they may occur in groups with a "v" configuration. They are Gram-positive bacteria, but may look Gram-negative because the organisms decolorize easily. *Erysipelothrix* is not acid-fast. Isolation from the skin requires taking a sample from the edges of cutaneous lesions, keeping in mind that the bacteria typically are most numerous in the deep tissues. Isolation in culture is difficult. Biochemically, the bacteria produce neuraminidase and hyaluronidase.[15]

Clinical Presentation

Erysipeloid is a form of bacterial cellulitis. The lesions are commonly located on the hands. Edema, erythema, and throbbing pain are part of the classical presentation. A history of a cut or a puncture while handling contaminated material can often be obtained. Systemic symptoms are uncommon. The cutaneous lesions are well-demarcated violaceous plaques, with a clear center and a diamond shape. Suppuration is rare, and lesional pain is often severe. The latter two findings separate erysipeloid from erysipelas and other types of bacterial cellulitis.

Pediatric cases are uncommon and are usually seen in immunocompromised patients. Their lesions may also be located on the feet, evolving from hemorrhagic blisters to eschars, and a discrete history of environmental exposure to the organism may be absent.[16]

Histologic Findings

The epidermis in erysipeloid is spongiotic or necrotic, and subepidermal bulla formation has also been described. Massive edema of the papillary dermis is common, and the subjacent corium contains neutrophils, eosinophils, lymphocytes, plasma cells, and histiocytes. Blood vessels may be dilated, with enlarged endothelial cells.[17] The classical description of erysipeloid states that bacteria cannot be seen histologically in the lesions. However, a recently reported case in a child did feature visible bacteria in a tissue Gram stain.[16]

Differential Diagnosis

The main differential diagnoses for erysipeloid are other infections that can involve the hands and feet, such as erysipelas, other forms of bacterial cellulitis, cutaneous anthrax, and blistering distal dactylitis (BDD). Viral infections, including herpetic whitlow and orf, may be considered, as well as "fish tank granuloma," caused by *Mycobacterium marinum* infection. The dense neutrophilic infiltrate is an important clue to the presence of a bacterial infection.

CAPSULE SUMMARY

ERYSIPELOID

Erysipeloid of Rosenbach is a rare cutaneous infection of the hands and feet that is caused by *E. rhusiopathia*. Butchers, fish handlers, veterinarians, and other persons who have contact with animal vectors are predisposed to this disease, but a clear environmental exposure history may be lacking in children with erysipeloid.

BLISTERING DISTAL DACTYLITIS

Definition and Epidemiology

Blistering distal dactylitis (BDD) is a bacterial infection that affects the volar images of the distal fingers or toes. It is caused in the majority of cases by Group A *S. pyogenes*.

The disease was initially described as one that was mainly seen in children between the ages of 2 and 16 years. Recently, adult cases have also been reported in immunocompromised and diabetic patients[18,19] as well as in infants who are less than 9 months of age.[20] So far, no examples have been described in elderly persons.

Etiology

The microorganism considered as the most common cause of BDD is Group A, beta-hemolytic *S. pyogenes*. In a minority of cases, *S. aureus* and Group B streptococci have been implicated as well.

Clinical Presentation

Blisters develop on the distal volar fat pad of a finger or occasionally on a toe. The proximal phalanges and palms are more rarely involved. The lesions may evolve into erosion, which may be variably painful or asymptomatic. More than one digit can be affected, and more than 1 lesion can be seen (Figure 17-10); cutaneous bullae are oval, measuring 1 to 3 cm. Many patients have associated oropharyngitis, conjunctivitis, and perianal cellulitis, but systemic symptoms are usually absent.

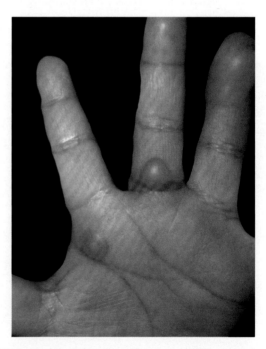

FIGURE 17-10. **Blistering distal dactylitis.** Courtesy Dra. Rosa Ines Castro.

Findings

The only reference regarding histologic findings in BD is a description of blistering due to massive subepidermal edema.[21]

Differential Diagnosis

The most common differential diagnosis is that of herpetic whitlow; indeed, cases of combined streptococcal dactylitis and herpetic infection have been described. Trauma, burns, dyshidrosis, contact eczema, psoriasis, and insect bites can also be considered as clinical possibilities.

CAPSULE SUMMARY

BLISTERING DISTAL DACTYLITIS

This presents as a distal blister on a finger pad of a child or teenager that is caused by Group A Streptococcus. Massive subepidermal edema may be present histologically.

BACTERIAL CELLULITIS

Definition and Epidemiology

Cellulitis is an infection of the dermis and subcutaneous tissue by *Staphylococcus* or *Streptococcus* sp. or Gram-negative bacteria. The main difference between this condition and erysipelas is that the infection is more deeply seated.

Cellulitis can occur at any age, especially when there is a break in the skin. Special types worth mentioning include newborn cellulitis caused by Group B streptococci and *Haemophilus influenzae* type b cellulitis. The latter is still prevalent in developing countries where *Haemophilus* vaccines are not routinely used.

Etiology

Common pathogens that cause cellulitis in children include *S. pyogenes* and *S. aureus*, followed by *S. pneumoniae*; Groups B, G, or C streptococci, *E. coli,* and *H. influenzae* type b.

Clinical Presentation

Redness, swelling, tenderness, increased local temperature, and poor demarcation of the cutaneous lesions are classically seen in the presentation of cellulitis. Most patients have fever, chills, and malaise, and some may develop sepsis. Periorbital cellulitis can be associated with MRSA (Figure.17-11).

Perianal cellulitis affects young children. It manifests with striking erythema of the anus (Figure 17-12), painful defecation, and bloody stools. The etiology is almost always *S. pyogenes,*[22] and affected individuals may also have simultaneous streptococcal pharyngitis. *Haemophilus* cellulitis

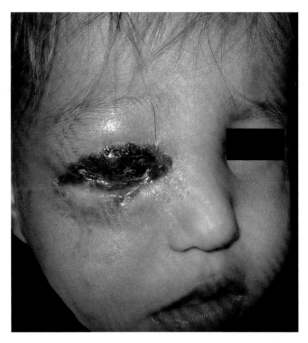

FIGURE 17-11. **Cellulitis of the periorbital area.** The patient subsequently developed osteitis. Courtesy of Dra. Rosa Ines Castro.

has special characteristics in pediatric patients. It is usually facial, with either a perioral or periorbital plaque, and a reddish-blue to purple color. This condition occurs in children who are less than 2 years old, following a respiratory or sinus infection, and it has the potential to involve the central nervous system.

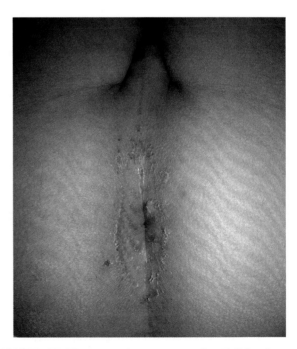

FIGURE 17-12. **Perianal streptococcal cellulitis.** Courtesy Dra. Rosa Ines Castro.

Histologic Findings

Bacterial cellulitis is characterized by a deep dermal and subcutaneous infiltrate of neutrophils. When suppurative ulceration is seen clinically, necrotizing vasculitis and thrombosis are common histologically. In necrotizing forms of cellulitis, bacteria are usually visible microscopically, but they may be absent otherwise.

Differential Diagnosis

The main clinical differential diagnosis includes various infections with organisms that are capable of producing cellulitis, including fungi, *Vibrio vulnificus*, and other bacteria.[23] As true of erysipelas, Sweet syndrome and rheumatoid dermatosis can also be considered.

CAPSULE SUMMARY

BACTERIAL CELLULITIS

Bacterial cellulitis is a deeply seated bacterial infection. Diffuse neutrophilic infiltrates are present in the deep dermis and subcutaneous tissue.

NECROTIZING FASCIITIS

Definition and Epidemiology

Necrotizing fasciitis (NF) is a rare but aggressive infection of the skin and soft tissue that involves subcutaneous tissue and fascia. It has the potential for widespread tissue destruction and carries a high mortality rate.

The estimated prevalence of NF in pediatric patients is 0.08 per 100 000 children per year,[24] and overall mortality is around 15%. The incidence of this condition in children is bimodal, with 2 peaks—less than 2 years and around 10 years of age. Mortality in adults can be as high as 30%, even with appropriate therapy.[25]

Etiology

Group A streptococci and *S. aureus* are the main isolates in reported pediatric cases of NF. Superantigens of streptococci, such as SpeG and the streptococcal mitogen exotoxin Z (SmeZ), bind to CD4+ T cells, B cells, monocytes, and dendritic cells, overstimulating the local immune response and causing tissue necrosis.[24]

Many instances of staphylococcal NF are caused by community-acquired MRSA. *P. aeruginosa* is the third most common bacterial cause and is always associated with some sort of immunodeficiency.[26] Polymicrobial infections are less common in children with NF when compared with adults.

Clinical Presentation

Although preceding trauma is a common inciting factor for NF, children may develop the condition without it. In adults, symptoms and signs that raise the suspicion of NF include pain out of proportion to the clinical lesions, rapidly enlarging, bullae, ecchymoses, anesthesia, crepitation on palpation, and accompanying sepsis. In children, tenderness may be more common than pain. Fever is common in neonates, and also in teenagers. The anatomic location for the lesions varies depending on patient age; under 1 year, truncal disease predominates, whereas the extremities or head and neck are the most common locations in older children. Fournier gangrene can occur in children under 3 years of age; it is related to unsanitary diaper use (Figure 17-13).

Histologic Findings

Microscopic findings include dense neutrophilic infiltrates in the deep dermis, subcutaneous tissue, and underlying fascia (Figures 17-14 and 17-15). Tissue necrosis and vascular thrombosis are commonly seen, and Weedon defines NF as a form of septic vasculitis.[21] Bacteria can be present in sheets, and they may be seen with Hematoxylin and eosin (H&E) stain.

Differential Diagnosis

NF is distinguished from erysipelas and cellulitis by a greater intensity of necrosis and vascular abnormalities. Ischemic conditions, such as calciphylaxis and the bullae of barbiturate intoxication, may also feature wholesale necrosis, but they lack the intense neutrophilic reaction of NF. Pyoderma gangrenosum can also imitate NF, but the former of those

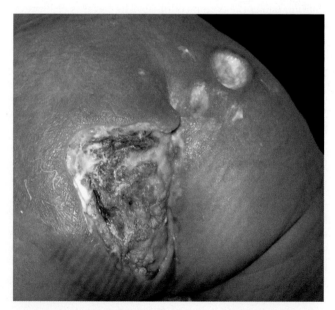

FIGURE 17-13. Necrotizing fasciitis in the gluteal area. In this case, the disease was related to improper diaper use. Courtesy Dra. Rosa Ines Castro.

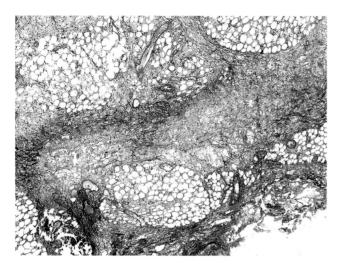

FIGURE 17-14. **Necrotizing fasciitis—histologic examination shows a clear necrosis of the subcutaneous fat.** H/E ×100.

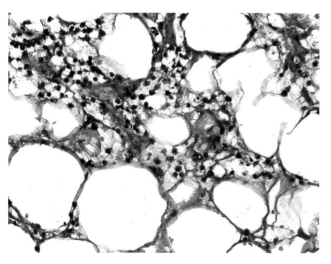

FIGURE 17-15. **Necrotizing fasciitis, showing neutrophils in the necrotic fat.** H/E ×400.

conditions has sharper demarcation and more subepidermal edema, with no deep vessel thrombosis. A distinction should be made between NF and the necrotizing form of Sweet syndrome, which is usually associated with a hematologic malignancy. Myonecrosis is seen only in late-stage NF.

CAPSULE SUMMARY

NECROTIZING FASCIITIS

It is clinically characterized by necrosis, bullae formation, ecchymosis, crepitation, as well as pain and tenderness that are disproportionate to other cutaneous abnormalities. Early diagnosis is crucial, and proper medical and surgical therapy is mandatory. Microscopically, deep dermal, subcutaneous, and fascial infiltrates of neutrophils are present, with necrosis and vascular thrombosis.

STAPHYLOCOCCAL SCALDED SKIN SYNDROME (SSSS)

Definition and Epidemiology

Staphylococcal scalded skin syndrome (SSSS) is a life-threatening, diffuse, blistering disorder produced by infection with phage group II *S. aureus*. It affects children under the age of 5 and adults with various predisposing disorders.

SSSS is a rare disorder. The disease can occur at any age but most commonly affects newborns and children under the age of 5. Why pediatric patients are more susceptible to the disease can be explained by their poor production of antibodies against staphylococcal toxins and suboptimal renal clearance of the toxins themselves.

Etiology

Only certain strains (5%)[27] of *S. aureus* can produce the exfoliative toxin that causes SSSS. Phage group II staphylococci, particularly strains 71 and 55/71, are recognized as the classical pathogens in SSSS. The onset of the disease in nurseries may be explained by the existence of asymptomatic carriage of such bacteria in healthy caregivers, with involuntary transmission to infants. The responsible toxins—exfoliative toxin A, exfoliative toxin B, and exfoliative toxin D—are atypical glutamate-specific trypsin-like serine proteases that accumulate in the skin. They mediate a digestion of the desmoglein-1 cadherin, functionally altering keratinocyte desmosomes and resulting in intraepidermal separation. The lesions of SSSS imitate those of pemphigus foliaceus; most of them are linked to exfoliative toxin B.

Clinical Presentation

Children affected by SSSS present with systemic symptoms such as fever, malaise, and irritability. Early cutaneous denudation, with a Nikolsky sign, may be induced by lateral friction over the skin surface. The child may complain of abdominal pain and manifest exquisite truncal skin tenderness. Patches of redness may appear abruptly, which become well demarcated and confluent, later evolving into a scarlatiniform eruption. The next phase is the formation of large blisters around the central face, axillae, and groin, which break easily and leave a moist surface that looks scalded. The denuded skin facilitates the loss of fluid, with dehydration and thermal dysregulation. After 24 hours, the "scalded" areas become covered by a thin crust, resulting in fissuring in the perioral and periorbital areas (Figure 17-16). In a few days, the skin heals without scarring.

Histologic Findings

The typical microscopic findings in SSSS include an intraepidermal cleft at the subcorneal level in the absence of significant inflammation except for a few neutrophils

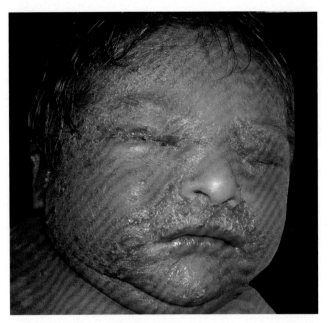

FIGURE 17-16. Staphylococcal scalded skin syndrome, featuring erythema, crusting, and early perioral fissuring in a newborn. Courtesy of Dra. Rosa Ines Castro.

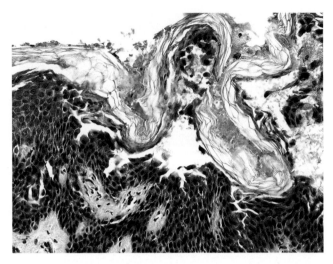

FIGURE 17-18. Staphylococcal scalded skin syndrome, demonstrating subcorneal separation and acantholytic cells. H/E ×400. Courtesy of Dr Luis Requena.

(Figures 17-17 and 17-18). As opposed to the image of toxic epidermal necrolysis (TEN), no necrotic keratinocytes are seen. Sparse mixed inflammation may be seen in the dermis.

Differential Diagnosis

Important clinical differential diagnoses in SSSS cases include TEN (erythema multiforme major), bullous impetigo, and pemphigus foliaceus. In TEN, mucosal involvement is common, but SSSS spares the mucous membranes. Histologically, necrotic keratinocytes are widespread in TEN but is absent in SSSS. Bullous impetigo always features an abundance of neutrophils; pemphigus foliaceus also shows more inflammation than expected in SSSS, potentially including eosinophils.

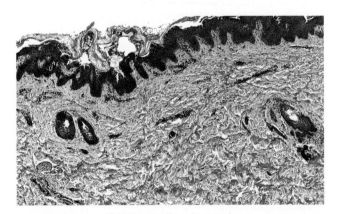

FIGURE 17-17. Histopathologically, Staphylococcal scalded skin syndrome shows a subcorneal separation. H/E ×100. Courtesy of Dr Luis Requena.

CAPSULE SUMMARY

STAPHYLOCOCCAL SCALDED SKIN SYNDROME

SSSS is a blistering disease of children caused by the specific strains of *S. aureus*. The blistering effect is caused by exfoliative toxins that are produced by the microorganisms. Clinically, children with SSSS have fever, red patches in the skin that are exquisitely tender. The lesions evolve into a scarlatiniform eruption with later formation of large, fragile blisters. Once they break, "scalded" areas predominate, and fine fissuring with crusting appears around the mouth and eyes. Histologically, the characteristic intraepidermal cleft in SSSS is subcorneal, in the absence of necrotic keratinocytes, and with insignificant inflammatory infiltrates.

ERYTHRASMA

Definition and Epidemiology

Erythrasma is a cutaneous infection caused by *Corynebacterium minutissimum*, a lipophilic and filamentous Gram-positive bacillus. Its clinical presentation is identical to that of intertriginous tinea, except for the production of red fluorescence under the Wood's light in erythrasma.

Erythrasma is seen mainly in people who are exposed to a warm, damp environment. It is seen at all ages, but with the incidence being higher in adults; children are rarely affected.

Etiology

Erythrasma is classically associated with infection by *C. minutissimum*, although that name may in fact represent up to eight different bacterial species that are able to produce porphyrin.[28] They are part of the normal flora of intertriginous areas of the body surface.

Clinical Presentation

Typical erythrasma manifests with tan to brown patches in the toe webs, axillae, groin, intergluteal crease, and inframammary skin. It can be associated with variable degrees of scaling, odor, and maceration. Erythrasma is particularly symptomatic in obese patients and those with diabetes mellitus. In the toe webs, it may coexist with classical tinea dermatophytosis. Erythrasma produces coral-red or orange fluorescence with Wood's lamp. Disseminated forms may occur uncommonly.

Histologic Findings

Small coccobacilli may be seen in the stratum corneum histologically. Filamentous forms are arranged as "Chinese letters" and are surrounded by the cocciform organisms.[29] These microorganisms may be difficult to see in H/E-stained slides, but they are visible with Gram, PAS, and methenamine silver stains.[10] Inflammatory response to the infection is usually minimal or absent.

Differential Diagnosis

The main differential diagnosis of erythrasma is with candidiasis and the tineas. Extensive cases may be confused with pityriasis rotunda and pityriasis versicolor.

CAPSULE SUMMARY

ERYTHRASMA

Clinical presentation is tan to brown patches in the toe webs, axillae, groin, intergluteal crease, and inframammary skin, particularly in obese patients and those with diabetes mellitus. Lesions show coral-red or orange fluorescence with Wood's lamp. Histologic findings are minimal—numerous bacteria in the stratum corneum, with only modest dermal perivascular chronic inflammation or none at all.

TRICHOMYCOSIS

Definition and Epidemiology

Trichomycosis (TM) is a bacterial infection of the hair follicles, appearing as nodular concretions along hair shafts. It is caused by infection with *C. flavescens*, also called *C. tenuis*. Because it is commonly located in the axillae, the disease is also known as trichomycosis axillaris. Bonifaz proposed the name trichobacteriosis as a more appropriate designation because of the bacterial etiology.[30]

Affected patients are otherwise healthy. Although the infection has been described as "cosmopolitan," it is seen most commonly in adolescents and young adults who live in hot climates.

Etiology

As stated earlier, the causative agent is *Corynebacterium flavescens*. This bacterium was previously called *C. tenuis*, but most recent studies place it in the 2(LD2) group of corynebacterial microorganisms.[30] Currently, they are simply reported as *Corynebacterium* "species."

It is likely that the intrafollicular concretions are caused by the deposition of a cement-like substance that is produced by the bacteria, mixed with the components of apocrine sweat. That premise would explain the predilection for axillary skin.

Clinical Presentation

Clinically, TM manifests as tiny nodular concretions along hair shafts, in the axillae, the pubic area, the intergluteal cleft, or, rarely, the scalp. Concretions may be yellow or *flava* (98% of cases), red (*rubra*), or black (*nigra*); the postulated causative agents for the last two versions are *Micrococcus* species, but that supposition requires further confirmation. TM is seen more frequently in males, perhaps because of common depilatory practices in women. Male–male transmission has been reported in situations where persons live in close contact with one another, as true of military personnel and athletes. Patients may have more than one site of disease. An unpleasant odor and a strange texture of the hair are common complaints. Wood's lamp examination is positive, and it helps delineate the extent of the lesions.

Histologic Findings

Direct examination of hair under the microscope reveals the aforementioned concretions that are adherent to the hair cortex (Figure 17-19). The microorganisms are masses of coccoid or rod-shaped bacteria, each measuring 0.5 to 1 μm. Lesional concretions surround the hair shafts.

Differential Diagnosis

The principal differential diagnoses for TM are ectothrix and endothrix tinea, and Piedra. Direct examination of the hair helps distinguish TM from pediculosis corporis.

CAPSULE SUMMARY

TRICHOMYCOSIS

The etiological agent is *Corynebacterium sp*. Clinical presentation includes odor and abnormal hair texture in body areas where apocrine glands are numerous. On examination, one can see the presence of hard bacterial concretions along the hair shafts.

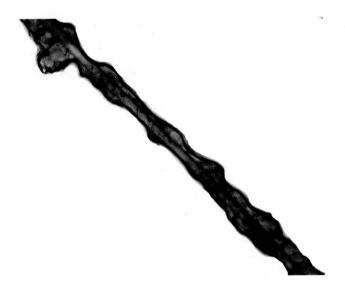

FIGURE 17-19. **Trichomycosis in a child.** The hair is from the scalp. *Corynebacterium* sp. were isolated in culture. Courtesy of Karina Feria, MD. KOH preparation. ×100.

PITTED KERATOLYSIS

Definition and Epidemiology

Also known also as "keratolysis punctata," pitted keratolysis (PK) is an infection that may be caused by infection with several bacteria, including *Corynebacterium* spp. along with other synergistic microbes. The clinical presentation is that of macerated pitting of the stratum corneum on the soles and palms, accompanied by an unpleasant odor.

PK occurs worldwide, but it predominates in the tropics. Affected persons often like to walk barefoot, or they commonly immerse their feet in water repeatedly or have hyperhidrosis. PK is common in adolescents and young adults, and it appears to favor males.[31] It has been said that young children are less often affected,[32] but in rural areas, the percentage of children with the disease may be as high as 8%.[33]

Etiology

The disease is the result of a synergistic infection with *Corynebacterium* spp., *Micrococcus sedentarius*, and *Dermatophilus congolensis*. All of those microbes have the potential to dissolve the stratum corneum, leaving holes or pits on its surface.

Clinical Presentation

Patients with PK usually complain of an unpleasant odor on their hands and feet. Frequent contact with water is a common risk factor; manual workers and students are often affected. The disease is principally localized to the feet, followed by the hands. On the soles, the pedal balls, ventral toes, and heels are especially affected. One sees a whitish macerated surface with abundant, asymmetrically distributed pits, which may coalesce to form large depressed areas

(Figure 17-20). These are associated with a pungent smell and often with hyperhidrosis.

Histologic Findings

A microscopic examination of skin scrapings or a shave biopsy will show two groups of histologic findings. In the superficial form of PK, coccoid bacteria are seen on the skin surface, associated with punctate lysis of the stratum corneum. In the deep form, the organisms are dimorphic; in addition to cocciform bacteria, filamentous ones are also seen in twisted arrangements inside keratolytic holes, deep in the stratum corneum (Figure 17-21).[32]

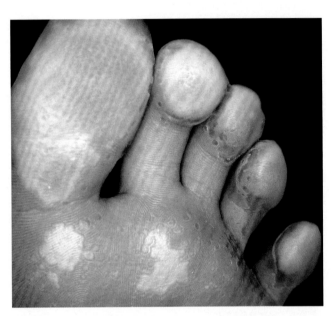

FIGURE 17-20. **Pitted keratolysis, showing lesions ranging from small pits to large depressed areas.**

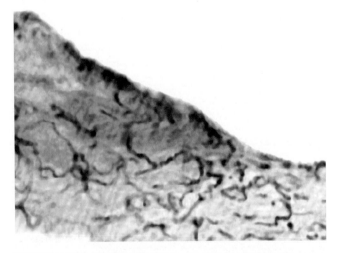

FIGURE 17-21. **Pitted keratolysis, demonstrating the presence of filamentous bacteria at the bottom of a pit.** PAS ×100. Courtesy of Dr Roberto Arenas.

Differential Diagnosis

The clinical differential diagnosis for PK centers on tinea pedis and circumscribed plantar hypokeratosis. The latter condition is seen in older patients, in whom the skin looks dry rather than macerated. The foul odor of PK is not shared by either of the other two conditions.

CAPSULE SUMMARY

PITTED KERATOLYSIS

Seen in persons with hyperhidrosis or exposed to a repeated immersion of the hands and feet in water, the clinical presentation is whitish, macerated palms or soles with surface pits and foul odor. Histologically, cocciform and/or filamentous bacteria are seen in the stratum corneum with a multifocal lysis of the stratum corneum.

PEDIATRIC CUTANEOUS TUBERCULOSIS

Definition and Epidemiology

Tuberculosis (TB) is one of the most important chronic bacterial infections internationally. The causative organism is *Mycobacterium tuberculosis*. Most patients with TB have pulmonary lesions, but up to 25% of them also have extrathoracic disease. From 1% to 4% of those lesions involve the skin.[34] Cutaneous TB is characterized by substantial clinical heterogeneity, and it is always difficult to isolate *M. tuberculosis* from the infected tissues in such cases.

In 2016, the estimated number of persons with active TB was 10.4 million; 6.3 million of those had new infections and 1.7 million died of the disease. Approximately 95% of all cases occurred in developing nations, often affecting people with low incomes. Patients in India, Indonesia, China, the Philippines, and Pakistan accounted for 56% of all cases, followed by others in Nigeria and South Africa. Around 1 million children were reported to have active TB in 2016.[35]

It commonly affects those people who are infected by HIV. Particular forms of cutaneous TB, such as scrofuloderma and lichen scrofulosorum, seem to occur more commonly in children than in adults.

Etiology

Examples of cutaneous TB can be caused not only by *M. tuberculosis*, but also by *M. bovis* and the *Bacillus Calmette–Guerin* (BCG). The disease may be acquired as a result of primary external inoculation (primary inoculation TB or chancre), external inoculation in an already-sensitized individual (tuberculosis verrucosa cutis and lupus vulgaris on the extremities), propagation by continuity from infection in underlying structures (tuberculosis periorificialis and scrofuloderma), and hematogenous or lymphatic spread (tuberculous gummas and facial lupus vulgaris). Cutaneous TB cases represent a spectrum, depending on the mycobacterium load. Some examples have a negligible number of cutaneous organisms (the "tuberculids"), whereas others are paucibacillary (lupus vulgaris) or multibacillary (primary inoculation TB). Active pulmonary TB can also spread to the mouth, the perioral skin, and the dorsa of the hands and the forearms, caused by coughing up infected sputum while covering the mouth ("snuffbox tuberculosis").

Clinical Presentation

Pediatric patients may be more prone to develop certain clinical forms of cutaneous TB. Adults tend to have lesions of lupus vulgaris on the face, whereas children, especially those between 10 and 14 years old, more often develop them on the buttocks and the legs.[36,37] One report of Indian children with cutaneous TB described a high number of scrofuloderma cases, possibly explained in part by the consumption of milk contaminated with *M. bovis*.[36] Lichen scrofulosorum is also mainly reported in children in that country. Children appear to have systemic TB more often than adults do[37]

Primary inoculation TB, or tuberculous chancre, is an uncommon form of cutaneous TB. In young infants, it presents with ulcerations on the cheek or in the mouth, associated with an enlarged cervical lymph node. That association is analogous to a pulmonary Ghon complex (Figure 17-22), and it is related to the inoculation of mycobacteria in the skin through close contact with another infected individual. Other clinical variants of cutaneous TB

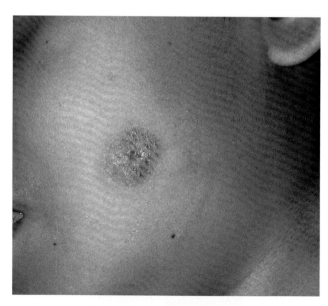

FIGURE 17-22. Primary inoculation tuberculosis in the cheek of a child. Upper cervical lymphadenopathy is also seen.

include scrofuloderma, tuberculosis periorificialis, tuberculous gumma, miliary cutaneous TB, and lupus vulgaris. The last of those forms can be located on the face (as classically described in the past in European adults) or on the extremities and buttocks of young patients.[37,38] Lupus vulgaris may also develop secondarily in patients with scrofula (Figure 17-23) or at a BCG vaccination site, especially in immunocompromised individuals.

Tuberculosis verrucosa cutis is principally seen on the legs, and it is a common form of cutaneous TB in Indian children. "Tuberculids" (paucibacillary cutaneous TB) includes erythema induratum of Bazin (nodular vasculitis), papulonecrotic tuberculid, and lichen scrofulosorum. Molecular techniques in such cases have demonstrated the presence of the antigens of *M. tuberculosis* in the skin lesions, but direct tissue examination and cultures are always negative for that organism.[37]

Lichen scrofulosorum is a generalized, papular, and lichenoid eruption, initially described in association with scrofuloderma in adults. Currently, it is a common tuberculid in Indian children, and is usually associated with active pulmonary TB. Cutaneous lesions range from pinhead-sized to larger lichenoid papules, organized in a discoid pattern, with spared areas and a spiny surface. They have a follicular or perifollicular distribution.

Papulonecrotic tuberculid is a symmetrical eruption that favors the extensor surfaces of the extremities. The earlobes and acral loci are classical locations as well. Individual lesions are umbilicated, and they heal with a varioliform scar. Many patients have simultaneous phlyctenular keratoconjunctivitis. Erythema induratum of Bazin is a form

of panniculitis in which ulcerated nodules appear on the posterior images of the legs, usually in adult women. It is rare in children.

Histologic Findings

The histologic appearance of TB varies, depending on the particular clinical form of the disease that is being studied. Well-organized tuberculous granulomas with necrosis are seen in scrofuloderma, usually in the deep corium (Figure 17-24). In conventional punch biopsies, the roof of an underlying abscess is often represented. Granulomas are also present in primary inoculation TB (superficial granulomas with necrosis beneath an ulcerated epidermis), gummas (tuberculoid [TT] granulomas surrounded by granulation tissue), tuberculosis periorificialis, and miliary forms (necrotizing granulomas). Mycobacteria can be identified using Ziehl-Neelsen (ZN) or Fite-Faraco stains (FFS), but it is rare to see numerous organisms.

Lupus vulgaris on the face comprises large, epithelioid, almost sarcoidal granulomas with lymphocytic cuffs and no necrosis. On the extremities, that form of cutaneous TB and tuberculosis verrucosa cutis induce pseudocarcinomatous epidermal hyperplasia, with small TT granulomas touching the surface epithelium (Figure 17-25). The inflammatory infiltrate may also extend into the deep reticular dermis. Mycobacteria are not visible in most cases, even with histochemical or immunohistochemical stains.

In lichen scrofulosorum, cutaneous granulomas are very superficial, located around the follicular infundibula and the eccrine ducts. Constituent histiocytes are epithelioid, and a lymphocytic cuff is either patchy or completely absent, again simulating the microscopic image of sarcoidosis.

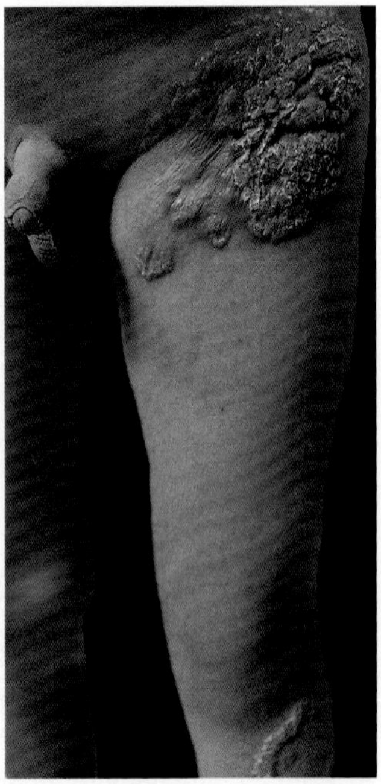

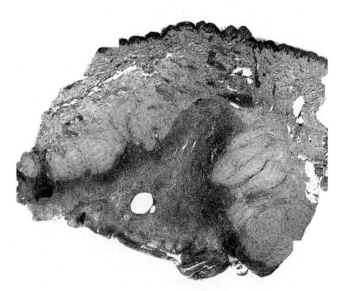

FIGURE 17-23. Lupus vulgaris after inguinal scrofula. Notice the satellite lesion near the knee.

FIGURE 17-24. Scrofula—the granulomatous process is reaching the skin surface from below. H/E ×20.

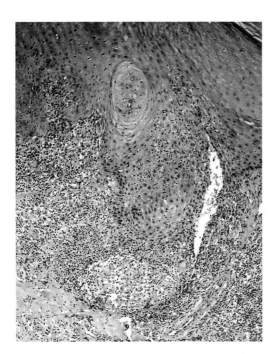

FIGURE 17-25. Lupus vulgaris on an extremity. Small tuberculous granulomas are in contact with a hyperplastic epidermis. H/E ×20.

The lesions of papulonecrotic tuberculid exhibit wedge-shaped areas of necrosis surrounded by TT granulomas. Associated foci of vasculitis may be seen.

Erythema induratum of Bazin is a lobular panniculitis, with zones of necrosis, granulomatous inflammation, and vasculitis affecting small-to-medium-sized blood vessels in the subcutis. Affected vessels can be located in either the fat lobules or the interlobular septa.

If cutaneous TB is suspected, it is mandatory to order special stains for mycobacteria. However, in most instances, the number of bacteria seen in tissue is extremely limited or nil. Thus, it is improper to exclude TB diagnostically simply on the basis of negative staining results.

Differential Diagnosis

When TT granulomas are seen microscopically, the differential diagnosis concerns sarcoidosis and several infectious processes. Those include leishmaniasis, sporotrichosis, and others. Nontuberculous mycobacteria, such as *M. marinum*, *M. chelonae, M. abscessus*, and *M. fortuitum*, may produce a histologic pattern similar to that of cutaneous infection with *M. tuberculosis*, or they may simulate the image of a syphilitic gumma. The identification of *M. tuberculosis* in culture establishes a definitive diagnosis. Nevertheless, in cases of tuberculosis verrucosa, lupus vulgaris, or the tuberculids, negative culture results are not uncommon. Presently, molecular studies for mycobacteria in tissue are highly sensitive but unstandardized.

CAPSULE SUMMARY

CUTANEOUS TUBERCULOSIS

Cutaneous TB has several clinical forms in children, including scrofuloderma, lupus vulgaris, and tuberculids such as lichen scrofulosorum. A common denominator in cutaneous TB is the histologic presence of granulomas. Each form of the disease has a characteristic pathologic appearance. In scrofuloderma, well-formed TT granulomas are seen with necrosis; lupus vulgaris shows epidermal hyperplasia and "hanging" granulomas; and lichen scrofulosorum manifests sarcoidal, nonnecrotizing granulomas around follicular infundibula and sweat ducts.

CUTANEOUS LEPROSY (HANSEN'S DISEASE)

Definition and Epidemiology

Leprosy is a chronic infection caused by *Mycobacterium leprae*, with a special predilection for the peripheral nerves and the skin. Around 220 000 new cases of leprosy are seen every year, with three countries accounting for 81% of that number: India, Brazil, and Indonesia.[39] Although the main population that is affected is young adults, children under 15 years of age comprise about 9% of the total. The incidence of leprosy in that patient group is considered to be an indicator of increasing new cases, active transmission in the community, and inefficiency of local control programs.

Etiology

The causative agent of leprosy is *M. leprae*, a fuchsin-positive, acid-fast, non-toxin-producing bacillus, with an extremely slow replication rate (12-30 days). It cannot be isolated in vitro. In infected animals and persons, the organism shows a special tropism for Schwann cells in cutaneous nerves. The main mode of transmission is by direct contact with secretions from the upper airway of infected patients. Around 90% of people will then be able to clear the infection spontaneously because of genetically determined resistance. The latter appears to be linked to several genes, including *PRAK2, PARCRG, CCDC122, C13orf31, NOD2, TNFSF15, HLADR, RIPK2*, and *LRRK2*.[39] Only a small number of patients develop the indeterminate form of leprosy, with later progression into an spectrum extending from the tuberculoid to lepromatous poles.

Clinical Presentation

Leprosy mainly affects the skin and peripheral nerves. It can produce purely neurologic symptoms and signs, or neurologic and cutaneous findings together. Although the Ridley and Jopling classification system (RJCS) helps understand the disease, it is a bit complex. Hence, the World Health

Organization has divided cases simply into paucibacillary and multibacillary types. In contrast, the RJCS includes several categories. The indeterminate form of leprosy is represented by one or a few macular lesions. They may be located on the face or elsewhere. Four A words typify their clinical features: achromic, anesthetic, anhidrotic, and alopecic.

Indeterminate leprosy is the earliest cutaneous manifestation of the condition; it is commonly seen in children and may easily be confused with pityriasis alba, vitiligo, nevus anemicus, and pityriasis versicolor. The lesions are transient, but they have the potential either to resolve or to progress to a spectrum between two poles, the tuberculoid (TT) and the lepromatous (LL), with three additional intermediate states. Intermediate leprosy is further subdivided into borderline-tuberculoid (BT), the borderline-borderline (BB), and the borderline-lepromatous variants (BL). The "polar" forms of the disease (TT and LL) tend to be stable, but BT, BB, and BL variants can go up or down the immune scale, by presenting with type I reaction.

The TT pole of leprosy is characterized by one to three lesions, localized to one body site, as anesthetic macules or plaques. They have smooth surfaces and well-defined borders, can be erythematous or hypochromic, and may be associated with thickened peripheral nerves. At the LL pole, the lesions are multiple and bilateral, potentially having a macular, papular, or nodular appearance (lepromas). Anesthetic areas may be extensive and numerous; they can have a "gloves and socks" distribution. Neurologic involvement can evolve to cause permanent functional disabilities. Other cutaneous findings include localized alopecia (except on the scalp) with a characteristic loss of the eyebrows (madarosis), a leonine facies, enlarged ear lobes, a destruction of nasal cartilage, and a shortening of fingers and toes with a reabsorption of the distal phalanxes, keratitis, iritis, and pressure ulcers. As patients go from BT to BL disease, one sees a greater number of lesions, a tendency for bilaterality, potential satellite lesions (in BT), "punched-out" lesions (in BB and BL) (Figure 17-26), and disseminated papules (in BL).

"Type I" systemic reactions in leprosy manifest with fever, malaise, arthralgias, and myalgias in patients with BT, BB, or BL forms of the disease. "Type II" reactions or "erythema nodosum lepromatosum" (ENL) are almost exclusively seen with BL or LL variants, and are typified by fever, malaise, and "hot" erythematous skin lesions, caused by a neutrophilic Sweet syndrome-like reaction. That process is thought to derive from a deposition of immune complexes. Both reactions produce progressive nerve and skin damage with pain and destruction of joints and bones, causing substantial morbidity. Most children manifest leprosy in its indeterminate, TT, or BT forms. Hence, one tends to see localized, unilateral, paucibacillary, single lesions.[39] Only a few published series have contained a predominance of LL cases, with disseminated multibacillary eruptions. One must bear in mind that it is difficult to assess neurologic function and neural thickening in children.[38] Musculoskeletal manifestations such as arthralgia, arthritis, and

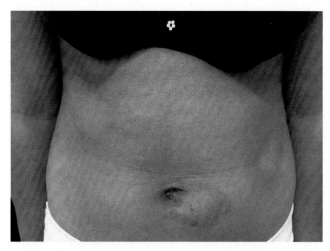

FIGURE 17-26. Leprosy in an adolescent—multiple "punched-out" plaques are seen in this patient with borderline leprosy. Courtesy of Dr Karina Feria.

myalgia may be present in up to 14% of pediatric leprosy cases.[39]

A particular type of TT leprosy in children, called "nodular leprosy of childhood," presents with a single nodule on the face or arm. It is seen most commonly when the child's mother has multibacillary leprosy.[40]

Histologic Findings

The principal histologic finding in leprosy is an inflammation of peripheral nerves in the skin. To evaluate the number of bacilli that are present in a microscopic section, histochemical staining is required. The most sensitive method is the Fite-Faraco stain (FFS), which is a modification of the Ziehl-Neelsen (ZN) technique. The FFS incorporates peanut oil as a reagent, to avoid washing lipids out of bacterial cell walls when exposed to organic solvents. Leprosy bacilli can indeed be seen sometimes with the ZN, but the FFS is more sensitive. Immunostains against lipoarabinomannan and phenolic-glycolipid PGL-1 (constituents of *M. leprae*) have been developed but are not widely available.

In histologic analysis, it is useful to divide lesions into two groups—paucibacillary (corresponding to the TT pole), and multibacillary (the LL pole). Indeterminate leprosy is characterized microscopically by modest perivascular, periadnexal, perineural, superficial, and deep lymphohistiocytic infiltrates. A few foamy histiocytes around nerve fibers can be a clue to the diagnosis.

TT leprosy can be suspected when linear, elongated, perivascular, periadnexal, and perineural granulomatous infiltrates are present in the dermis (Figure 17-27). True TT granulomas are seen, containing histiocytes and multinucleated giant cells with a cuff of lymphocytes, but necrosis is rare. Bacilli are usually absent in TT (paucibacillary lesions). Nerve fibers may be necrotic, but vasculitis is absent. The infiltrates in TT usually spare the papillary dermis, a criterion that can be used when to distinguish that disease from sarcoidosis histologically. The latter condition also

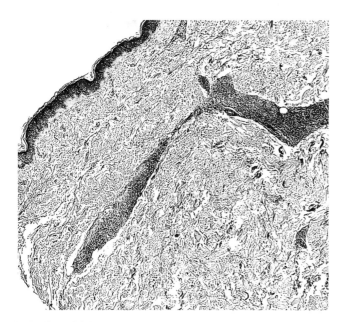

FIGURE 17-27. Tuberculoid leprosy histology—a linear granulomatous infiltrate is present along a nerve fiber. H/E ×100. Courtesy of Dr Cesar Salinas.

tends to feature "naked" granulomas with no lymphocytic cuffs.

Lepromatous leprosy produces a diffuse, dense, cellular dermal infiltrate, mainly represented by histiocytes. The cells have "foamy" cytoplasm and are called "lepra" or "Virchow" histiocytes; they contain "globi," which are intracellular accumulations of bacilli. A Grenz zone is commonly present (Figure 17-28), and the FFS demonstrates lesional bacilli in great numbers.

Borderline leprosy lesions are histologically represented by a mixed image, with both epithelioid granulomas and

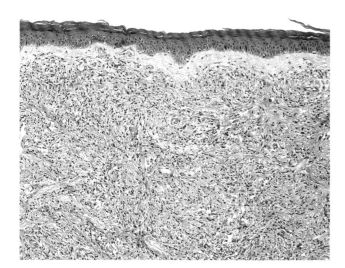

FIGURE 17-28. Lepromatous leprosy—a Grenz zone separates the epidermis from a diffuse foamy infiltrate that fills the entire dermis. H/E ×200.

foamy histiocytes. They may resemble either TT or LL, at least focally.

Histioid leprosy is a variant of LL disease that clinically resembles a neoplasm and histologically may simulate the appearance of dermatofibroma or another form of fibrous histiocytoma. The principal lesional cell form is epithelioid, with foamy cytoplasm that contains many bacilli.

Type I leprosy reactions are easily identified clinically, but not histologically. The only clue may be a greater number of lymphocytes in the lesional granulomas. Type II reactions (ENL) are characterized by dense dermal neutrophilic infiltrates and marked edema of the papillary dermis. The inflammation may extend into the subcutis in some cases, and superficial or deep leukocytoclastic vasculitis can also be seen.

The Lucio phenomenon is characterized microscopically by a dense lymphohistiocytic infiltrate around cutaneous blood vessels, with foamy endothelial cells that are loaded with intracellular bacilli. Thrombosis and vascular necrosis in medium-sized vessels can also be seen.

Differential Diagnosis

Indeterminate and TT leprosy has a substantial clinical differential diagnosis, but the main histologic considerations are sarcoid and facial lupus vulgaris. Lupus vulgaris on the extremities shows epidermal hyperplasia, and that finding is shared by the lesions of deep mycosis. Surface epithelial changes are typically absent in leprosy.

Lepromatous leprosy is microscopically singular. A perineural distribution has been described in cutaneous sarcoidosis, but the presence of mycobacteria in TT allows for its identification as such. If LL leprosy has been treated before a biopsy is done, the bacterial load may be nil. ENL can be confused with Sweet syndrome if foam cells are overlooked, or if the neutrophilic infiltrate is so dense that it obscures the histiocytic component.

CAPSULE SUMMARY

LEPROSY

Clinical manifestation is one or several anesthetic macules, plaques, or nodules, and in advanced cases, there is a destruction of skin and soft tissue. Histologic findings are elongated linear dermal granulomas or diffuse histiocytic infiltration by foamy cells containing many bacteria. Granulomas are centered on cutaneous nerves. FF staining is mandatory for diagnosis.

CAT-SCRATCH DISEASE

Definition and Epidemiology

Cat-scratch disease (CSD) is an infection of the skin and lymphoid tissues, caused by *Bartonella henselae*. The main reservoirs for that organism in nature are the cat and the cat flea. The disease is acquired from bacteremic cats that transmit the microorganism through the saliva while biting and clawing humans.

CSD has a worldwide distribution. Children and adolescents are most often affected, but adults can also get the disease. Approximately 50% of all cats harbor *B. henselae* in an asymptomatic fashion.[41] A history of personal contact with a cat is not always remembered, and it may indeed be absent because the cat flea can also transmit the infection.

Etiology

Bartonella henselae is a small Gram-negative rod that is very difficult to isolate in cultures. The genus to which it belongs also includes *Bartonella bacilliformis* (the agent of Carrion disease and verruga peruana) and *Bartonella quintana* (the cause of trench fever and bacillary angiomatosis). In immunocompromised patients, especially those infected with HIV, *B. henselae* can also cause bacillary angiomatosis.

Clinical Presentation

CSD manifests itself with the development of a papule at the site of a cat scratch or flea bite.[42] If the history includes known contact with felines, the diagnosis is straightforward. The lesions evolve from flat erythematous macules to either papules or vesicles, and they become crusted after 3 to 10 days.

Regional lymphadenopathy appears 1 to 3 weeks after the skin lesions, and it may resolve spontaneously or persist for months. Many patients do not recall being scratched by a cat, and they may not even remember having any skin lesions. A single enlarged lymph node is present in 85% of cases. Most commonly, affected nodes are axillary, epitrochlear, cervical, or inguinal. They are painful, mobile, and solid on palpation. Purulent discharge from the node may be seen in 30% of cases. About one-half of patients with CSD develop systemic symptoms, such as malaise, myalgias, and abdominal pain. Roughly 10% will have visceral complications including endocarditis, encephalitis, uveitis, conjunctivitis, or hepatitis.

Histologic Findings

The skin papules in CSD show areas of acellular dermal necrosis, with various forms and shapes—round, triangular, or stellate. Groups of epithelioid histiocytes surround the necrosis, and they often manifest a palisaded arrangement. A few multinucleated giant cells and a small cuff of lymphocytes may also be present. Plasma cells and eosinophils can be a part of the infiltrate as well.

Histologic findings in lymph nodes are similar, except for the additional presence of neutrophilic abscesses inside the zones of stellate necrosis. Clumped bacilli can be seen with Warthin-Starry stains, both in the skin and in the lymph nodes. Indirect immunofluorescence assays are also useful.[43]

Differential Diagnosis

The clinical differential diagnosis for CSD includes viral lymphadenopathies such as mononucleosis, as well as staphylococcal and streptococcal lymphadenitis, toxoplasmosis, tularemia, TB, and atypical mycobacterial infections. Viral lymphadenitis tends to be bilateral, in contrast to that seen with CSD.

Histologically, other considerations can include Kikuchi disease, Kawasaki disease, and infections such as tularemia, atypical mycobacteriosis, TB, brucellosis, deep mycoses, lymphogranuloma venereum, and lymphadenopathy accompanying idiopathic granulomatous mastitis. A histochemical or immunohistochemical demonstration of the causative bacilli in CSD is definitive diagnostically.

CAPSULE SUMMARY

CAT-SCRATCH DISEASE

CSD is caused by infection with Bartonella henselae, acquired through a cat-scratch or a flea bite. Crusted skin lesions and/or lymphadenopathy are seen. Microscopically, dermal necrosis with surrounding palisaded histiocytes is present. In lymph nodes, neutrophilic microabscesses are associated with the zones of necrosis.

CUTANEOUS ACTINOMYCOSIS AND NOCARDIOSIS

Definition and Epidemiology

Cutaneous actinomycosis (CA) is the involvement of skin and soft tissue by a spreading infection originating in underlying structures. It results in swelling, sinus formation, and the draining of tissue "grains." This condition is caused by actinomyces species, including *A. israelii.*

Nocardiosis of the skin (NOS) is an unusual disease that is caused by microorganisms in the genus *Nocardia*. The typical clinical picture associated with this entity includes superficial abscesses, cellulitis, and "sporotrichoid" lesions.

Actinomycosis is now considered to be rare in industrialized countries and is principally seen in the developing world. The disease is related to poor oral hygiene, especially in its orocervicofacial form. Male predominance is the rule, except in the pelvic form, which is associated with the use of intrauterine contraceptive devices.

Most pulmonary nocardiosis cases occur in the context of immunosuppression, but primary NOS can be seen in immunocompetent patients.

Etiology

Actinomyces sp. are Gram-positive, non-acid-fast anaerobic to microaerophilic bacteria that are part of the usual flora of the oropharynx, gastrointestinal tract, and urinary system. As opposed to the *Actinomyces* sp. that cause myce-toma, which are environmental, those that are associated with CA are endogenous; the infection develops when a mucosal surface is broken. The most common pathogen in human cases is *A. israelii*. This species, along with *A. gerencseriae*, is responsible for almost 70% of cases of orocervicofacial actinomycosis.[44] Actinomycosis is frequently a part of a polymicrobial infection.

Nocardiosis was originally felt to be caused by a single species, *Nocardia asteroides*. However, current canon states that it instead represents an etiologic complex, including *N. abscessus*, *N. brevicatena-paucivorans*, *N. nova complex*, *N. transvalensis complex*, *N. farcinica*, and *N. asteroides*.[45] Nocardia is a Gram-positive, aerobic bacterium that adopts a filamentous configuration, with hypha-like branching on direct microscopy. That microorganism shows a variable degree of acid-fastness with the ZN stain.

In cases of primary NOS, *N. brasiliensis* is the most commonly isolated agent. Unlike other forms of nocardiosis, NOS usually develops in immunocompetent patients.[45]

Clinical Presentation

CA has several potential variants—orocervicofacial (the most common), thoracic, abdominal, and pelvic. The usual clinical presentation is that of an indurated mass located along the mandible ("lumpy jaw") or in the neck. The swelling is only variably painful, and it is so hard on palpation that the examiner often considers it to represent a malignant tumor. Eventually, CA progresses to form draining sinuses. Similar lesions can occur in the thoracic or abdominal walls or in the pelvic area.

Primary NOS may be associated with a prior history of local trauma. The disease manifests itself with the formation of skin abscesses or localized cellulitis. Lesions can infect lymphatic vessels, inducing a linear pattern known as "sporotrichoid" nocardiosis. The latter condition has been described on the face in children.

Histologic Findings

Microscopically, CA resembles an ordinary subcutaneous abscess. The general appearance features central, loculated spaces, separated by granulation tissue and associated with the infiltrates of foamy macrophages. The adjacent tissue is fibrotic with a lymphoplasmocytic infiltrate. The presence of "grains" is a clue to the diagnosis. These are roughly spherical structures comprising bluish material, surrounded by an eosinophilic amorphous ring (the "Splendore-Hoeppli" phenomenon) and abundant neutrophils. Constituent filamentous bacteria may have club-shaped ends at the periphery of the grains.

In NOS, histologic findings are nonspecific. One may see ulceration and abscesses containing many neutrophils, hemorrhage, and necrosis, with contiguous fibrosis. Grains are rarely seen in NOS. The filamentous bacteria are difficult to see in H- and E-stained sections, but they are visible with both the Gram and ZN methods.

Differential Diagnosis

The clinical differential diagnosis of orocervicofacial actinomycosis includes TB and other mycobacterioses. Histologically, one should distinguish actinomycosis from actinomycetoma, eumycetoma, and botryomycosis. If grains are not seen histologically, it is not possible to identify actinomycosis with certainty, and microbiologic studies will be required to do so.

Other diagnostic considerations in cases of NOS include infections capable of causing sporotrichoid lesions, such as sporotrichosis, leishmaniasis, and atypical mycobacterioses. Tissue Gram, PAS, and ZN stains help distinguish nocardiosis from the other conditions.

CAPSULE SUMMARY

CUTANEOUS ACTINOMYCOSIS AND NOCARDIOSIS

Actinomycosis is a lumpy mass in specific sites, with draining sinuses and the presence of microscopic "grains." Primary cutaneous nocardiosis is characterized by clinical abscess formation, localized cellulitis, or sporotrichoid lesions. Histologic findings are suppurative acute inflammation with a low likelihood of identifying the microorganisms in H- and E-stained sections.

NEISSERIAL INFECTIONS

Definition and Epidemiology

The two main human pathogens in the genus *Neisseria* are *N. meningitidis* and *N. gonorrhoeae*, the respective causes of meningococcal meningitis and gonorrhea. Both diseases have septicemic forms that may yield cutaneous lesions, which feature the presence of infectious vasculitis.

Historically, meningococcal disease was cyclical over spans of several years, and its incidence was declining even before the introduction of effective vaccines. The disease typically occurs in outbreaks, affecting young adults preferentially. The risk of developing it is higher in college attendees or military recruits who live in close quarters with one another.

The incidence of disseminated gonococcal infection parallels that of gonorrhea in general. Gonococcal septicemia is seen classically in adolescents and young adults.

Etiology

N. meningitidis is a Gram-negative diplococcus that grows easily in solid media. Through agglutination testing with immune sera, 13 serogroups have been identified. Groups A, B, C, X, Y, and W-135 are responsible for 98% of cases.[46]

N. gonorrhoeae is a Gram-negative, intracellular anaerobic diplococcus. It is transmitted by sexual contact or vertically during childbirth. Porin channels, known as Porin A and Porin B, play an important role in the virulence of this organism. Strains with Porin A have the potential to invade epithelial cells and to cause bacteremia.[47]

Clinical Presentation

Up to 20% of patients with meningococcal infections present with sepsis. Affected patients have fever, hypotension, multiorgan failure, and disseminated intravascular coagulation . Cutaneous petechiae, purpura, or a maculopapular rash are often part of the clinical picture. The skin eruption is most pronounced on the extremities. An unusual clinical variant is known as chronic meningococcemia, defined by bacteremia that lasts at least 1 week and is associated with intermittent fever, migratory arthralgias, and a rash comprising macules, papules, nodules, petechiae, or polymorphous lesions.[48] It is seen in immunocompetent patients.

Disseminated gonococcal infection is a rare complication of mucosal gonorrhea; it typically presents 1 to 3 weeks after initial infection. Symptoms and signs include fever, malaise, rigors, migratory arthralgias, myalgias, tenosynovitis, and skin lesions. The latter are represented by macules, papules, or pustules, on an erythematous or hemorrhagic base. Abscess formation, cellulitis, NF, and vasculitis have also been described.[47] Skin lesions are usually located on the extremities.

Histologic Findings

The histologic appearance of cutaneous lesions in acute meningococcal disease reflects what is seen clinically—a dominant component of vascular involvement, including fibrin thrombi in small vessels and a neutrophilic infiltrate with little, if any, leukocytoclasia. Diplococci may be seen with the tissue Gram stain, and the polymerase chain reaction (PCR) has also been used with skin biopsies to confirm the diagnosis.[49] Skin findings in chronic meningococcemia feature a perivascular lymphocytic infiltrate, few neutrophils, and no vascular thrombi.[48]

In disseminated gonococcal infections, one sees septic vasculitis, with thrombi occluding small vessels containing swollen endothelial cells, surrounded by many neutrophils. Epidermal necrosis and bulla formation may occur in the context of leukocytoclastic vasculitis.[47] Tissue Gram staining and PCR are again useful diagnostically.

Differential Diagnosis

Fever and a rash comprising papules or pustules can also be seen in staphylococcal septicemia. A distinction must also be made between neisserial infections and cases of bacterial endocarditis with cutaneous manifestations.

CAPSULE SUMMARY

NEISSERIAL INFECTIONS

Sepsis with either *N. meningitides* or *N. gonorrhoeae* can produce skin lesions that are macular, papular, petechial, and pustular. Histologically, variably dense dermal infiltrates of neutrophils, often associated with vasculitis and vascular thrombosis, are present.

LYME DISEASE

Definition and Epidemiology

Lyme disease is a systemic infection that is caused by spirochetes, including *Borrelia burgdorferi* and related species. The disease is transmitted through tick bites. Lyme disease is characterized by a specific dermatologic condition called "erythema migrans (EM)," which may be accompanied by arthritis, neurologic deficits, cardiac dysfunction, and ophthalmologic disorders.

Lyme disease occurs mainly in the northern hemisphere, principally the United States, European countries including part of Russia, and some countries in Asia and northern Africa. The true incidence of the disease is uncertain, because of differing criteria for reporting it. In the United States, primary endemic areas are the Northeast and mid-Atlantic regions as well as in the upper Midwest. People living in rural areas, who spend substantial time outdoors, and those who live in or visit areas with a high concentration of tick vectors have the highest risk. The more tick bites one has, or the longer a tick remains attached to a bite, the greater the chance of infection. The age distribution for Lyme disease is bimodal, with the greatest incidence in children between 5 and 9 years of age and also in adults above 50 years.[50]

Etiology

B. burgdorferi belongs to the phylum *Spirochetes*, organisms that have an outer membrane surrounding a protoplasmic cylinder. They are long (10-30 µm) and thin (0.18-0.25 µm in diameter), irregularly coiled, and highly mobile, possessing 7 to 11 polar flagella. The chromosome for such microbes is linear, and it includes variable numbers of circular plasmids.

In Europe, Lyme disease can also be caused by *B. afzelli* and *B. garinii*. Currently, *Borrelia* is considered to represent a complex of organisms, including at least 20 species. Major tick vectors in North America include *Ixodes scapularis* in the East and Midwest, and *Ixodes pacificus* in the Western states. In Europe, the main vector is *Ixodes ricinus*.

Clinical Presentation

The clinical evolution of Lyme disease occurs in three stages. The primary lesion or stage produces the lesions of

EM, also known as erythema chronicum migrans. It comprises erythematous papules that enlarge at their peripheries, becoming a coalescent plaque measuring 5 to 70 cm in diameter, with central clearing and an erythematous center. The lesions have a targetoid, "bulls-eye" appearance (Figure 17-29); they may be pruritic or painful, potentially accompanied by fever, malaise, and headache. Some patients develop regional lymphadenopathy, which, in 20% of cases, is the only disease manifestation. Spontaneous regression is not uncommon. Secondarily, multiple EM-like lesions develop that are smaller than those in stage 1 of the illness. They may be accompanied by early neurologic manifestations and endocarditis. European patients may develop lymphocytoma cutis (lymphadenoma benigna cutis) at this stage as well. Tertiary lesions have the appearance of acrodermatitis chronica atrophicans (ACA). They are mainly seen in Europe, usually accompanied by neurologic deficits. Arthritis is likewise seen in late-stage disease.

EM is seen in 70% of reported cases, constituted by more than 90% of pediatric cases and 75% to 90% of all European cases. In children, tick bites are most common in the head and neck; adults tend to get them on the extremities.

The disease is more common in the summer months. Borrelia lymphocytomas are commonly seen in European patients and especially in children. They are usually solitary and located on the earlobes, the scrotum, and the axillary folds. In adults, the areola of the breast is a common site. ACA is more seen in middle-aged to elderly women; it has an insidious progression, being unilateral at the outset but then involving greater portions of the skin surface. Initially, ACA is an inflammatory lesion, but it becomes atrophic

with time. About 20% of patients develop fibrous nodules around the elbows; others have band-like fibrous lesions over the ulna and tibia. About 30% to 40% of ACA patients have a concomitant sensorimotor polyneuropathy. Other neuropathic manifestations include lymphocytic meningitis, cranial neuritis, and radiculoneuritis. Children tend not to have radicular pain, but they develop frequent headaches, clinical signs of meningitis, and facial palsy.

Arthritis is more likely if the diagnosis and treatment are delayed; it is seen in up to 60% of untreated patients. If Lyme disease is correctly identified in its early stage, only 6% of cases show the presence of arthritis. Cardiac involvement is most commonly represented by conduction defects.

Histologic Findings

EM is characterized by a patchy superficial perivascular lymphohistiocytic infiltrate, with a variable number of plasma cells. In early lesions, a few eosinophils may also be part of the infiltrate.[51] Neutrophils and eosinophils may be seen at the borders of annular lesions. Boer described the histologic patterns in cutaneous Lyme disease as a spectrum. They can include superficial and deep, predominantly perivascular lymphoid inflammation, preferentially interstitial histiocytic infiltrates, variable numbers of plasma cells—which may sometimes be absent—and a variable density of the inflammation (Figures 17-30 and 17-31).[52] The more prominent the lymphoid infiltrate, the more likely it will involve the subcutis and manifest the presence of germinal centers.[52] In one series, a relatively high frequency of subtle

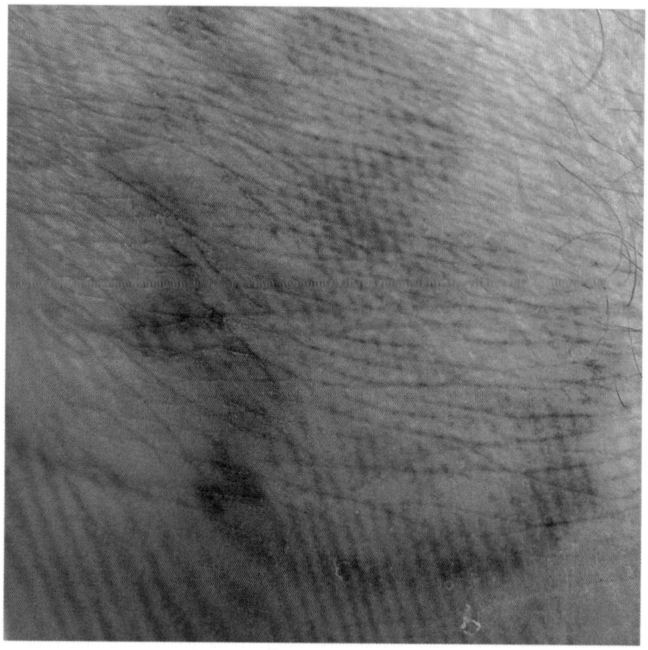

FIGURE 17-29. Erythema migrans—a classical lesion is seen on the wrist. Courtesy of Dr Heinz Kutzner.

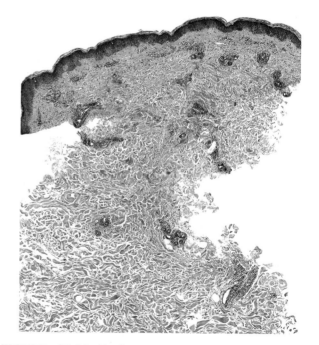

FIGURE 17-30. Erythema migrans—histopathologic features include a superficial and deep perivascular inflammatory infiltrate. In this particular case, no epidermal changes are seen. H/E. ×2.5. Courtesy of Dr Heinz Kutzner.

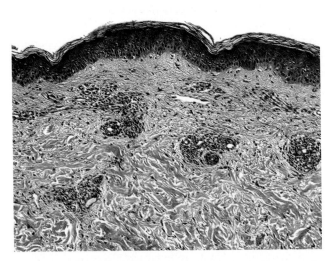

FIGURE 17-31. **This high-power view is from the case depicted in Figures 17-18 and 17-19. The infiltrate comprises lymphocytes, plasma cells, and eosinophils. H/E ×200.** Courtesy of Dr Heinz Kutzner.

epidermal changes was seen, including spongiosis, exocytosis, scattered necrotic keratinocytes, and basal vacuolar changes.

Warthin–Starry stains may allow for the visualization of an occasional spirochete in the papillary dermis. PCR studies for Borrelia-specific DNA have variable sensitivity and specificity in paraffin-embedded tissues, ranging from 30% to 90%, depending on the details of the cases that are studied and the method that is used. Floating microscopy may facilitate the visualization of Borrelia in EM.[53]

In Borrelia lymphocytomas, the dermal lymphoid infiltrate is more diffuse. It characteristically includes germinal centers (seen in 80% of cases) that are rich in centroblasts, immunoblasts, and tingible body macrophages. The interfollicular infiltrate includes lymphocytes, histiocytes, eosinophils, and plasma cells. In some instances, large follicles may become confluent and produce an image that resembles that of a B-cell lymphoma.

The inflammatory infiltrate in ACA is superficial, patchy, or band like, and disposed around dilated dermal blood vessels. It contains many plasma cells. Later lesions manifest a lesser inflammatory density; the epidermis flattens and becomes more atrophic. Collagen and elastic fibers in the corium diminish in number, and the skin generally becomes thinner and atrophic.

Differential Diagnosis

The diagnosis of EM is based on its typical macroscopic appearance and the clinical context. Differential diagnosis includes other gyrate and annular lesions, but a large size and solitary nature favor EM.

Borrelial lymphocytomas likewise has a broad differential diagnosis. Vaccination site pseudolymphomas and

Kimura disease may be considered in the histologic differential diagnosis.

The clinical appearance of ACA can be confused with that of venous insufficiency, perniosis, aged skin, and morphea. The inflammatory infiltrate in ACA, which is rich in plasma cells, must be separated from that seen in syphilis, morphea, and atrophoderma.

CAPSULE SUMMARY

CUTANEOUS LYME DISEASE

Erythema migrans—large clinical solitary annular lesions— are seen in those having been in an endemic area or bitten by a tick. Histologically, numerous plasma cells favor this diagnosis. Borrelial lymphocytoma cutis is rich in plasma cells and eosinophils, and may contain germinal centers. ACA usually presents as single or multiple atrophic plaques on the extremities. Histologically, the epidermis is flattened and atrophic, with a dermal lichenoid infiltrate of plasma cells.

RICKETTSIAL INFECTIONS

Definition and Epidemiology

Rickettsial infections (Rickettsioses) constitute a large group of vector-borne, zoonotic diseases, caused by several species of small bacterial organisms belonging to the genera *Rickettsia* and *Ehrlichia*. These microorganisms are defined as alpha-proteobacteria, that is, organisms that require the parasitization of eukaryotic cells to survive and proliferate.

Different species cause specific diseases in particular endemic areas of the world. Some have high mortality rates, such as endemic and epidemic typhus and Rocky Mountain Spotted Fever (RMSF). On the other hand, Mediterranean Spotted Fever (MSF) is uncommonly fatal. Males around 40 years of age are at particular risk if they live in rural areas and have contact with arthropod or insect vectors (eg, ticks, fleas, body lice) and host animals. However, vector bites are reported by patients in only 5% of cases. In cases of RMSF, children between 5 and 9 years of age, immunosuppressed individuals, and persons over 70 years of age have a higher risk of mortality.[54]

Etiology

Each disease is linked to a specific pathogen. *R. rickettsia* causes RMSF, *R. conorii* causes MSF in Europe and Africa, *R. sibirica* causes North Asian tick typhus, *R. japonica* causes oriental (Japanese) spotted fever, and *R. akari* causes rickettsialpox. The typhus group is represented by *R. typhi* in endemic typhus and *R. prowazekii* in epidemic typhus. Vectors are also specific. In RMSF, they include several species of ticks, including *Dermacentor variabilis*, *D. andersoni*, *Rhipicephalus sanguineus*, and *Amblyomma cajennense*. The microorganisms are present in the feces of the vector organisms, and they gain access to the human body through erosions caused by scratching bites. They then enter human cells, live in the cytosol, and finally kill the hosting cell, passing into intercellular spaces to continue spreading. The organisms have a special predilection for growth in endothelial cells.

Clinical Presentation

All rickettsioses cause similar systemic symptoms, manifesting as acute febrile illnesses in persons who have traveled or lived in endemic areas. Associated cutaneous rashes appear 3 to 7 days after a vector bite, and they evolve from a purely macular rash to a maculopapular eruption with central petechiae. The lesions first appear on the extremities (especially the ankles and wrists) and involve the truncal skin. Later, they become hemorrhagic or necrotic, potentially causing gangrene. Occasionally, a black, eschar-like lesion, known as the "tache noir," develops at the site of initial inoculation.[55] In rickettsialpox, lesions are papulovesicular, resembling those of chickenpox. Infection of the lungs, central nervous system, and kidneys may appear subsequently.

Histologic Findings

Most rickettsial infections show a superficial and deep dermal perivascular infiltrate of lymphocytes and macrophages, accompanied by edema and endothelial swelling. Perivascular and periadnexal cuffing by inflammation, especially around eccrine glands and ducts, may be noticed.[55] Extravasated red blood cells appear as the rash progresses. Fibrin may be present in vessel walls, and thrombosis and necrosis of vessels can be seen in late-stage lesions. These diseases are primarily lymphocytic small vessel vasculitides, although neutrophilic vasculitis is occasionally seen. Plasma cells and eosinophils are part of the infiltrate in 20% to 40% of cases.[56] Epidermal necrosis can be observed at the inoculation site.[55] Several immunofluorescence and immunohistochemical techniques are available to allow visualization of the microorganisms in the endothelial cells of the skin.

Differential Diagnosis

A maculopapular erythematous eruption with central petechiae, located on the wrists and ankles in the context of a febrile illness and a suitable geographic history, is helpful in raising the diagnostic possibility of a rickettsiosis. Other diseases to be considered include the gloves and socks eruption of Parvovirus B19 infection, as well as secondary syphilis. However, the overall clinical contexts of those conditions differ from those of rickettsial infections.

Microscopically, superficial and deep dermal perivascular lymphocytic infiltrates are associated with a sizable differential diagnosis, but clinical information in the rickettsioses should prompt the observer to evaluate the cutaneous

endothelial cells for swelling and necrosis. Dengue fever is an alternate consideration, but it produces a more superficial perivascular infiltrate with less endothelial swelling. The other causes of lymphocytic vasculitis, such as pityriasis lichenoides and perniosis, should also be remembered.

CAPSULE SUMMARY

RICKETTSIAL INFECTIONS OF THE SKIN

Fever and an epidemiologic history consistent with rickettsial exposure are present. A maculopapular rash is seen with central petechiae, beginning on the distal extremities with progression centripetally to involve the trunk. Histologically, a superficial and deep perivascular dermal lymphocytic infiltrate is present, with an evidence of endothelial damage or overt vasculitis.

REFERENCES

1. Pereira LB. Impetigo: review. *An Bras Dermatol*. 2014;89:293-299.
2. Hartman-Adams H, Banvard C, Juckett G. Impetigo: diagnosis and treatment. *Am Fam Physician*. 2014;90:229-235.
3. Amagai M, Stanley JR. Desmoglein as a target in skin disease and beyond. *J Invest Dermatol*. 2012;132(3 Pt 2):776-784.
4. Wick MR. Bullous, pseudobullous, & pustular dermatoses. *Semin Diagn Pathol*. 2017;34:250-260.
5. Phung TL, Wrigth TS, Pourciau CY, Smoller BR, eds. *Pediatric Dermatopathology*. New York, NY: Springer; 2017.
6. Calfee DP. Trends in community versus health care-acquired methicillin-resistant *Staphylococcus aureus* infections. *Curr Infect Dis Rep*. 2017;19:48.
7. Vaiman M, Lazarovitch T, Heller L, Lotan G. Ecthyma gangrenosum and ecthyma-like lesions: review article. *Eur J Clin Microbiol Infect Dis*. 2015;34:633-639.
8. Carroll JA. Common bacterial pyodermas: taking aim against the most likely pathogens. *Postgrad Med*. 1996;100:311-322.
9. Matz H, Orion E, Wolf R. Bacterial infections: uncommon presentations. *Clin Dermatol*. 2005;23:503-508.
10. Patterson JW. *Weedon´s Skin Pathology*. 5th ed. New York, NY: Churchill-Elsevier; 2016.
11. Segna KG, Koch LH, Williams JV. "Hot tub" Folliculitis from a nonchlorinated children's pool. *Pediatr Dermatol*. 2011;28:590-591.
12. Dietrich KA, Ruzicka T, Herzinger T. Whirlpool-dermatitis with "hot hands." *Dtsch Med Wochenschr*. 2014;139:1459-1461.
13. Yu Y, Cheng AS, Wang L, Dunne WM, Bayliss SJ. Hot tub folliculitis or hot hand-foot syndrome caused by *Pseudomonas aeruginosa*. *J Am Acad Dermatol*. 2007;57:596-600.
14. Hernández-Martín Á, Nuño-González A, Colmenero I, Torrelo A. Eosinophilic pustular folliculitis of infancy: a series of 15 cases and review of the literature. *J Am Acad Dermatol*. 2013;68:150-155.
15. Reboli AC, Farrar WE. *Erysipelothrix rhusiopathiae*: an occupational pathogen. *Clin Microbiol Rev*. 1989;2:354-359.
16. Boyd AS, Ritchie C, Fenton JS. Cutaneous *Erysipelothrix rhusiopathiae* (erysipeloid) infection in an immunocompromised child. *Pediatr Dermatol*. 2014;31:232-235.
17. Barnett JH, Estes SA, Wirman JA, Morris RE, Staneck JL. Erysipeloid. *J Am Acad Dermatol*. 1983;9:116-123.
18. Scheinfeld N. A review and report of blistering distal dactylitis due to *Staphylococcus aureus* in two HIV-positive men. *Dermatol Online J*. 2007;13:8.

19. Scheinfeld NS. Is blistering distal dactylitis a variant of bullous impetigo? *Clin Exp Dermatol.* 2007;32(3):314-316

20. Lyon M, Doehring MC. Blistering distal dactylitis: a case series in children under nine months of age. *J Emerg Med.* 2004;26:421-423.

21. Weedon D. *Skin Pathology.* 4th ed. London: Elsevier; 2010.

22. Šterbenc A, Seme K, Lah LL, Točkova O, et al. Microbiological characteristics of perianal streptococcal dermatitis: a retrospective study of 105 patients in a 10-year period. *Acta Dermatovenerol Alp Pannonica Adriat.* 2016;25:73-76.

23. Poblete R, Andresen M, Perez C, Dougnac A, Díaz O, Tomicic V. *Vibrio vulnificus*: una causa infrecuente de shock séptico. *Rev Méd Chil.* 2002;130:787-791.

24. Walker MJ, Barnett TC, McArthur JD, et al. Disease manifestations and pathogenic mechanisms of Group A streptococci. *Clin Microbiol Rev.* 2014;27:264-301.

25. Chen KJ, Klingel M, McLeod S, Mindra S, Ng VK. Presentation and outcomes of necrotizing soft tissue infections. *Int J Gen Med.* 2017;10:215-220.

26. Zundel S, Lemaréchal A, Kaiser P, Szavay P. Diagnosis and treatment of pediatric necrotizing fasciitis: a systematic review of the literature. *Eur J Pediatr Surg.* 2017;27:127-137.

27. Handler MZ, Schwartz RA. Staphylococcal scalded skin syndrome: diagnosis and management in children and adults. *J Eur Acad Dermatol Venereol.* 2014;28:1418-1423.

28. Roth RR, James WD. Microbiology of the skin: resident flora, ecology, and infection. *J Am Acad Dermatol.* 1989;20:367-390.

29. Morales-Trujillo ML, Arenas R, Arroyo S. Eritrasma interdigital; datos clínicos, epidemiológicos y microbiológicos. *Actas Dermosifiliogr.* 2008;99:469-473.

30. Bonifaz A, Váquez-González D, Fierro L, Araiza J, Ponce RM. Trichomycosis (trichobacteriosis): clinical and microbiological experience with 56 cases. *Int J Trichology.* 2013;5:12-16.

31. Pinto M, Hundi GK, Bhat RM, et al. Clinical and epidemiological features of coryneform skin infections at a tertiary hospital. *Indian Dermatol Online J.* 2016;7:168-173.

32. Prado N, Vera-Izaguirre V, Arenas R, Toussaint S, Castillo M , Ruiz-Esmenjaud J. Queratolisis plantar en pediatría. Informe clínico e histopatológico de 13 casos. *Dermatol Pediatr Lat.* 2004;2:117-122.

33. García-Romero MT, Lara-Corrales I, Kovarik CL, Pope E, Arenas R. Tropical skin diseases in children: a review- part I. *Pediatr Dermatol.* 2016;33:253-263.

34. Ramírez-Lapausa M, Menéndez-Saldaña A, Noguerado-Asensio A. Extrapulmonary tuberculosis. *Rev Esp Sanid Penit.* 2015;17:3-11.

35. World Health Organization. *Global Tuberculosis Report 2017.* Geneva: World Health Organization; 2017.

36. Gupta V, Ramesh V. Understanding cutaneous tuberculosis in children. *Int J Dermatol.* 2017;56:242-244.

37. Singal A, Sonthalia S. Cutaneous tuberculosis in children: the Indian perspective. *Indian J Dermatol Venereol Leprol.* 2010;76:494-503.

38. Bravo FG, Gotuzzo E. Cutaneous tuberculosis. *Clin Dermatol.* 2007;25:173-180.

39. Barreto JG, Frade MAC, Bernardes Filho F, da Silva MB, Spencer JS, Salgado CG. Leprosy in children. *Curr Infect Dis Rep.* 2017;19:23.

40. Butlin CR, Saunderson P. Children with leprosy. *Lepr Rev.* 2014; 85:69-73.

41. Klotz SA, Ianas V, Elliott SP. Cat-scratch disease. *Am Fam Physician.* 2011;83:152-155.

42. Mazur-Melewska K, Mania A, Kemnitz P, Figlerowicz M, Służewski W. Cat-scratch disease: a wide spectrum of clinical pictures. *Postepy Dermatol Alergol.* 2015;32:216-220.

43. Shin OR, Kim YR, Ban TH, et al. A case report of seronegative cat scratch disease, emphasizing the histopathologic point of view. *Diagn Pathol.* 2014;19:62.

44. Wong VK, Turmezei TD, Weston VC. Actinomycosis. *BMJ.* 2011;343: d6099.

45. Wilson JW. Nocardiosis: update and clinical overview. *Mayo Clin Proc.* 2012;87:403-407.

46. Horino T, Kato T, Sato F, et al. Meningococcemia without meningitis in Japan. *Intern Med.* 2008;47:-1543-1547.

47. Beatrous SV, Grisoli SB, Riahi RR, Matherne RJ, Matherne RJ. Cutaneous manifestations of disseminated gonococcemia. *Dermatol Online J.* 2017;15:23.

48. Bonville CA, Suryadevara M, Ajagbe O, Domachowske JB. Chronic meningococcemia presenting as a recurrent painful rash without fever in a teenage girl. *Pediatr Infect Dis J.* 2015;34:670-672.

49. Parmentier L, Garzoni C, Antille C, Kaiser L, Ninet B, Borradori L. Value of a novel *Neisseria meningitidis*-specific polymerase chain reaction assay in skin biopsy specimens as a diagnostic tool in chronic meningococcemia. *Arch Dermatol.* 2008;144:770-773.

50. Borchers AT, Keen CL, Huntley AC, Gershwin ME. Lyme disease: a rigorous review of diagnostic criteria and treatment. *J Autoimmun.* 2015;57:82-115.

51. Müllegger RR, Glatz M. Skin manifestations of Lyme borreliosis: diagnosis and management. *Am J Clin Dermatol.* 2008;9:355-368.

52. Böer A, Bresch M, Dayrit J, Falk TM. Erythema migrans: a reassessment of diagnostic criteria for early cutaneous manifestations of borreliosis with particular emphasis on clonality investigations. *Br J Dermatol.* 2007;156:1263-1271.

53. Eisendle K, Grabner T, Zelger B. Focus floating microscopy: "gold standard" for cutaneous borreliosis? *Am J Clin Pathol.* 2007;127:213-222.

54. Kollypara R. Rikettsial infections. In: Tyring S, Lupi O, eds. *Tropical Dermatology.* 2nd ed. Edinburgh: Elsevier; 2017.

55. Sangueza O, Bravo Puccio F, Sangueza M. *Dermatopathology of Tropical Diseases.* London: JP Medical Ltd; 2017.

56. Kao GF, Evancho CD, Ioffe O, Lowitt MH, Dumler JS. Cutaneous histopathology of rocky mountain spotted fever. *J Cutan Pathol.* 1997;24:604-610.

18

Cutaneous Protozoal Infections

Francisco G. Bravo

LEISHMANIASIS

Definition and Epidemiology

Leishmaniasis is defined as a cutaneous, mucocutaneous, or visceral anthropozoonotic disease, resulting from the inoculation of protozoa belonging to the genus *Leishmania*.

The World Health Organization classifies leishmaniasis as one of the most important neglected tropical diseases. It is considered endemic in at least 97 countries, with 1 000 000 cases reported in the last 5 years.[1]

Regarding "old world" cutaneous leishmaniasis (OWCL), the disease has classically been seen most often in children. In contrast, "new world" leishmaniasis of the skin typically affects adult patients who live in rural areas, usually doing agricultural work. Over time, however, an increased number of pediatric cases have been reported in Latin America, which would be considered the "new world." Affected countries include Brazil, Colombia, Argentina, and Venezuela, where the number of cases in children ranges from 6% to 35% of all patients with leishmaniasis.[2,3] The important population at risk in developed countries include adventurous tourists, migratory workforce, and military personnel. They are exposed to the disease when visiting or inhabiting endemic areas around the world. The vectors for leishmaniasis are sandflies, either *Phlebotomus* (in old world disease) or *Lutzomyia* (for new world leishmaniasis). Other humans, dogs, and rodents represent the main reservoirs for the microorganisms in nature.

Etiology

More than 20 species of *Leishmania* may cause disease in humans. Each one is associated with a particular clinical presentation (Table 18-1). Sandflies acquire the microorganisms when they bite infected animals or people. The flies then transmit flagellated promastigotes from their probascises, by biting other hosts. Once inside macrophages, dermal dendrocytes, or Langerhans cells, the promastigotes lose their flagella and become amastigotes. In that form, they multiply and infect neighboring cells and live in the cytoplasm. If a Th1 response is activated, the production of IL-2 and interferon-γ can eradicate the organisms. However, if the response is inadequate or is instead the Th2 form—with the production of IL-4, IL-5, and IL-10—the disease process continues and becomes chronic.[4]

Clinical Presentation

Children have been always an important population affected by OWCL, either in wet, rural, areas where *Leishmania major* is the dominant pathogen or in dry, urban regions in which *Leishmania tropica* is preponderant. Although the classical form of new world cutaneous leishmaniasis (NWCL) was associated with young males working in rural areas, an increasing number of children have recently been affected. They may live in rural locales that are affected by deforestation or in crowded periurban areas.

The usual presentation of cutaneous leishmaniasis (CL) is in its ulcerated form, beginning either as a papule or as a nodule (Figures 18-1 and 18-2). The lesional ulcer is shallow with elevated borders, and it is either covered by a crust or open with a red, granulomatous bottom. OWCL tends to resolve spontaneously in a matter of months, although *Leishmania aethiopica* may be associated with a more protracted course. In NWCL, cases caused by *Leishmania mexicana* often

433

TABLE 18-1.	Leishmania species and the diseases associated with them

Cutaneous leishmaniasis
  Old world leishmaniasis
    Leishmania major
    Leishmania tropica
    Leishmania aethiopica (causes diffuse cutaneous leishmaniasis)
    Leishmania pifanoi
  New world leishmaniasis
    Leishmania mexicana complex
    Leishmania mexicana
    Leishmania amazonensis (causes diffuse cutaneous leishmaniasis)
    Leishmania pifanoi
    Leishmania venezuelensis
    Leishmania viannia complex
    Leishmania braziliensis
    Leishmania peruviana
    Leishmania panamensis
    Leishmania guyanensis
Mucocutaneous leishmaniasis
  Old world leishmaniasis
    Leishmania aethiopica
  New world leishmaniasis
    Leishmania braziliensis
Visceral leishmaniasis
  Old world leishmaniasis
    Leishmania donovani
    Leishmania infantum (can cause pure cutaneous leishmaniasis)
  New world leishmaniasis
    Leishmania chagasi

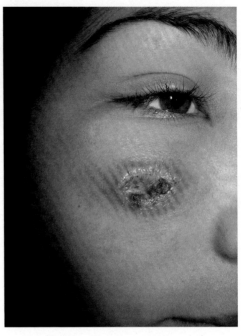

FIGURE 18-2. Cutaneous leishmaniasis: ulcerated lesion in a child. A facial location is common in children.

remit spontaneously as well, but those caused by *Leishmania braziliensis* are usually chronic. They carry a risk for evolution to mucocutaneous leishmaniasis. Lesions are solitary or few in number; common locations include exposed areas of the face, upper extremities, hands, ears, and legs.

CL may be clinically polymorphic, rather than being represented by a single ulcer. Other variants include impetigo-like, lupoid, plaque-like (Figure 18-3), sporotrichoid, agminate, zosteriform, verruciform, or pustular, imitating acute folliculitis or a furuncle. Multiple papular lesions in several sites typify the disseminated form of CL. A particular variant seen in the pediatric population is leishmaniasis recidiva cutis (Figure 18-4); in such cases, a few papular lesions manifest as recurrent disease around a scar caused by a previous, ulcerated lesion. They may subsequently become annular and tend to be chronic.[5-7]

Mucocutaneous lesions are associated with infections by *L. braziliensis* or *L. aethiopica*. The ulcers in this condition usually begin in the nasal septum and progress to involve

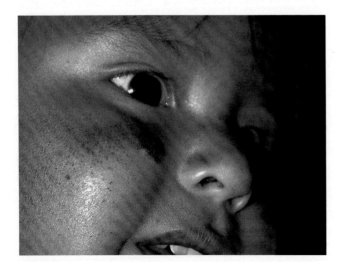

FIGURE 18-1. Cutaneous leishmaniasis: nonulcerated lesion in a child.

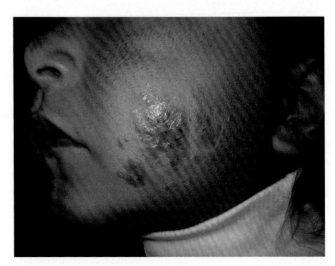

FIGURE 18-3. Cutaneous leishmaniasis: multiple lesions, with a tendency to form a plaque.

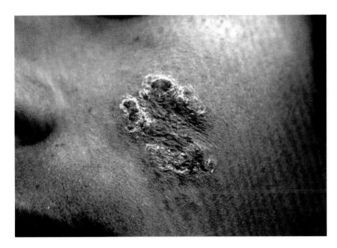

FIGURE 18-4. Cutaneous leishmaniasis recidivans cutis. Courtesy of Braulio Valencia, MD.

the perinasal skin, nasopharynx, or larynx. Children can also have labial and oral involvement. Mucocutaneous lesions usually follow cutaneous disease by months to a few years.

Diffuse CL is the anergic form of leishmaniasis, very similar pathophysiologically to the lepromatous form of leprosy. It is caused in Central and South America by *Leishmania amazonensis*, and in Africa by *L. aethiopica*. The clinical presentation features multiple papules, nodules, and plaques located in any skin area, but they are usually situated on the face and extremities. A response to treatment may be seen initially, but it is usually followed by persistent recurrences and then unremitting lesions.[8]

Histologic Findings

The skin biopsy is one of the most useful tools for the diagnosis of CL. Appropriate samples are either punch or incisional biopsies from the edge of an ulcer or the center of a solid lesion, and they should include the deep dermis.

Pathologic findings are similar in OWCL and NWCL. The most common observation is a diffuse inflammatory affecting both the papillary and reticular dermis. In some instances, the pattern is more focal and band-like, or perivascular and interstitial throughout the corium. Less commonly, one can see well-formed granulomas of the tuberculous type, which are sometimes necrotizing. They are surrounded by a diffuse lymphoplasmacytic and histiocytic infiltrate. Overt granulomas tend to be observed most often in chronic lesions, such as those of recidivans cutis and lupoid forms of CL.

The usual components of the inflammatory infiltrate include lymphocytes, plasma cells, and histiocytes with clear cytoplasm, as well as isolated giant cells. The epidermis may be normal in appearance, hyperplastic, or ulcerated. The papillary dermis usually contains a histiocytic infiltrate, but it may be completely spared, with a Grenz zone. Because of the abundance of plasma cells, Russell bodies are not uncommon. Other occasional constituents of the infiltrate include neutrophils and eosinophils.

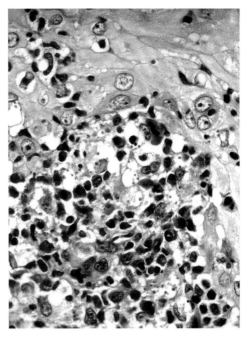

FIGURE 18-5. Cutaneous leishmaniasis: multiple amastigotes in the papillary dermis. H/E, ×1000.

The diagnosis of CL can be made if one sees amastigotes, the nonflagellated forms of the causative microorganisms. They have an oval to round shape and measure 2 to 4 μm in diameter, and are seen inside the histiocytes. The nucleus of amastigotes tends to be located at one pole of the organism, and a smaller structure, the kinetoplast, is present at the other pole. The best place to look for amastigotes is the papillary dermis (Figure 18-5), where the infiltrate is mostly histiocytic and less lymphoplasmacytic. However, they can also be located more deeply. The diagnosis is definitive when multiple microorganisms are seen in each histiocyte; they tend to be located at the periphery of the cells (the "marquee sign") (Figure 18-6).[9] Calcifications are rarely

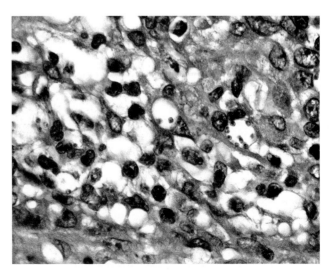

FIGURE 18-6. Cutaneous leishmaniasis: amastigotes organized as the "marquee sign." H/E ×1000.

present,[10] as occasionally seen in tuberculosis and paracoccidioidomycosis. The infiltrates are histologically similar in mucocutaneous leishmaniasis.

Hematoxylin and eosin-stained sections usually allow the amastigotes to be visualized as pale blue-gray intracellular inclusions. Other histochemical methods such as Giemsa, Wright, Feulgen, or Romanowsky stains also give the leishmanial organisms a pale blue color.[11] The number of amastigotes tends to be higher in new lesions and those with a diffuse lymphoplasmacytic and histiocytic infiltrate. They are scarce or completely absent in well-defined granulomas. As a rule, amastigotes are seen in only 50% to 60% of skin biopsies from CL patients. Various immunohistochemical methods have been devised for the direct recognition of leishmanial protozoa, but the only commercially available stain is for CD1a, which is serendipitously present in the infected histiocytes of OWCL. It has yet to be proven useful in the diagnosis of NWCL.[9]

Differential Diagnosis

Important histologic differential diagnoses for CL include sporotrichosis and tuberculosis. Other deep fungal infections may present with pseudoepitheliomatous hyperplasia and granulomas, but the responsible etiologic agents are easily seen, as in chromoblastomycosis or paracoccidioidomycosis. Regarding other microorganisms that may simulate the microscopic appearance of CL, most of them are seen principally in the context of HIV infection. They include *Histoplasma capsulatum*, *Talaromyces marneffei* (formerly *Penicillium marneffei*)[12], and *Emergomyces africanus* (formerly *Emmonsia pasteurina*).[13,14] All of those agents are roughly the size of *Leishmania*, at 2 to 4 μm. Although histoplasmosis is seen all around the world, *Talaromyces* infections occur mostly in South East Asia. *Emergomyces* is seen mainly in HIV+ patients in Africa. Those microorganisms will label with histochemical techniques used for fungi, such as Periodic acid–Schiff (PAS) and Gomori methenamine silver, whereas *Leishmania* sp. do not.

CAPSULE SUMMARY

LEISHMANIASIS

Leishmaniasis is one of the most important tropical diseases, and it is endemic in many countries around the world. Many species of Leishmania are potentially responsible for the disease. CL is the most common, with children usually being affected. Common locations include the head, arms, and legs. The lesions are usually chronic shallow ulcers with elevated borders; however, CL shows a considerable clinical variability in appearances. Skin biopsy is a useful tool for diagnosis, both because of the pattern of infiltration and the presence of intracellular microorganisms.

AMOEBIASIS CUTIS WITH *ENTAMOEBA HISTOLYTICA*

Definition and Epidemiology

Amoebiasis cutis is caused by infestation with *Entamoeba histolytica*. It occurs by fecal–oral transmission, with primary intestinal disease and secondary involvement of the skin, or by the direct intracutaneous inoculation of material that is contaminated with feces.

Cases of amoebiasis cutis are seen frequently in tropical areas of the world, such as Central and South America, Africa, and Asia. Yearly, around 50 million cases of invasive amoebiasis are reported worldwide, causing 100 000 deaths.[15] Adults and children can both be affected. Although it is rare, amoebiasis cutis is still seen in places like Mexico City.[15] When children develop that condition, they are usually baby boys wearing diapers.[4]

Etiology

The amoeba life cycle includes cystic and trophozoitic stages; the latter form is the one seen in tissue. The cystic form is responsible for transmission, via contaminated food or water. When a lectin protein in the surface of trophozoites comes into contact with the epithelial lining cells of the intestine, active infection begins. The infection may remain intraluminal, but if the lectin interacts with N-acetyl-D-galactosamine residues on the epithelium, invasion is enabled.[16] Contaminated diapers and poor hygiene represent the underpinnings of most amoebiasis cutis cases.[17]

Clinical Presentation

Clinical lesions comprise one or several painful ulcers, located on the perianal area, perineum, groin, scrotum, penis, vulva, vagina, and cervix, or near intestinal fistulae, colostomy stomas, and laparotomy incision sites. In children less than 2 years old, the diaper area is the most common location, but such distant sites as the periorbital area and inner ocular canthus have also been reported.[17,18] Amoebiasis cutis may be the first sign of an otherwise-undetected colonic infestation.[19] In children, the disease is associated with active dysentery, fever, irritability, weight loss, anemia, and leukocytosis.[17] Although the disease has a high mortality in adults, especially in patients with HIV, pediatric cases respond better to therapy. Sometimes, however, significant scarring remains.[17,19]

Histologic Findings

The main microscopic characteristic of cutaneous amoebiasis is necrosis en masse. The epidermis may be modestly acanthotic or it may show marked pseudoepitheliomatous hyperplasia. The centers of the lesions are necrotic with abundant nuclear debris, surrounded by an inflammatory infiltrate of neutrophils, lymphocytes, and eosinophils with many extravasated red blood cells. Trophozoites are regularly present in large numbers in the necrotic areas and in the overlying epidermis. The size of the microorganism is 20 to 50 μm; they are surrounded many times by a clear halo. The nuclei measure 4 to 7 μm and have central small karyosomes. Phagocytized erythrocytes may be present in the cytoplasm of the organisms, and an invasion of capillary walls is possible.[17,19] The PAS stain often labels viable microorganisms.

Differential Diagnosis

The histologic differential diagnosis centers on abscess-forming bacterial infections, including mycobacterioses. The absence of granulomas in amoebiasis separates it from tuberculosis cutis. Recognition of the trophozoites is critical for the definitive diagnosis of amoebiasis cutis.

CAPSULE SUMMARY

AMOEBIASIS CUTIS

Classical lesions are painful ulcers in the diaper area in young children, and symptoms include fever and dysentery. The most important findings in the skin biopsy are en masse tissue necrosis, acute inflammation, and the presence of amoebic trophozoites. One must be careful not to confuse the organisms with degenerated histiocytes or cellular debris.

INFECTIONS WITH FREE-LIVING AMOEBAE, WITH EMPHASIS ON *BALAMUTHIA MANDRILLARIS*

Definition and Epidemiology

Free-living amoebae are represented by a group of rare organisms that have a tendency to involve the central nervous system (CNS), causing acute and subacute meningoencephalitis. The more insidious forms associated with granulomatous amoebic meningoencephalitis are caused by several *Acanthamoeba* species and *Balamuthia mandrillaris* (BM). They may also produce characteristic skin lesions, even before CNS lesions appear.

Acanthamoeba is most commonly associated with disease in immunosuppressed patients. On the contrary, the majority of infections with BM occur in immunocompetent individuals, and more than 200 cases have been described worldwide.[20] Countries with the highest incidence include Peru and the United States. California, Texas, and other southwestern states account for the majority of American cases, and pediatric patients with BM infection have particularly been reported in California. Around 50% of Peruvian BM infestations are seen in patients less than 15 years of age,[21] many of whom have cutaneous involvement. That feature is less common in the rest of the world.

Etiology

Both *Acanthamoeba* and BM are environmental amoebae. They live freely in stagnant water and soil. A history of swimming in brackish water is not as often reported as it is in cases of infestation with *Naegleriasis*. The organisms typically enter the body through the skin.

Clinical Presentation

The most common presentation in infestations with BM and *Acanthamoeba* is the presence of an asymptomatic plaque with slightly elevated borders. Ulceration is more common with *Acanthamoeba* than with BM. The typical location for the lesions is the central face, either with symmetric involvement of both cheeks or an asymmetric distribution on one side of the face (Figure 18-7). If untreated, the entire face may become involved. Other common lesional sites are the knees and upper legs (Figure 18-8), and satellitosis may be seen. If the disease is detected only in skin initially, it may take up to a year for CNS involvement to become manifest.

Histologic Findings

Skin biopsies usually show an inflammatory infiltrate throughout the entire dermis. It comprises lymphocytes, plasma cells, histiocytes, and many giant cells, with the possible formation of ill-defined granulomas (Figure 18-9). Neutrophils, eosinophils, and nuclear dust are seen as well. Trophozoites are scarce, with not as many being seen as in amoebiasis cutis. They measure 15 to 30 μm with a central nucleus and a distinct nucleolus. The cytoplasm of the organisms may have an irregular outline (Figure 18-10), or the

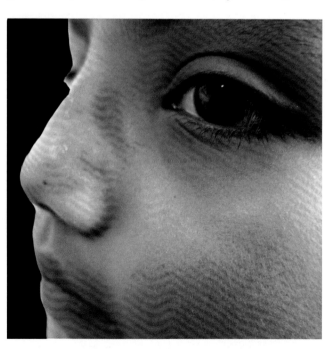

FIGURE 18-7. *Balamuthia mandrillaris* **infection: a plaque on the central face.**

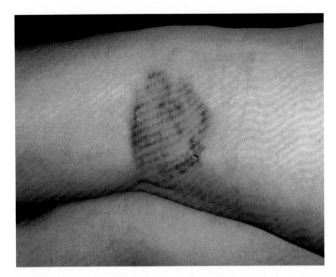

FIGURE 18-8. *Balamuthia mandrillaris* infection: a plaque behind the knee.

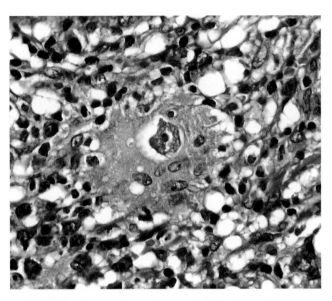

FIGURE 18-10. *Balamuthia mandrillaris*: high-power image of trophozoite, as seen in Figure 18-9. H/E ×400.

whole trophozoite may adopt an oval shape inside a vacuole (Figure 18-11). On high-power microscopy, the cytoplasm may look bubbly. If organismal nuclei are not apparent, trophozoites may be easily confused with histiocytes. Occasionally, the microorganisms are located in giant cells (Figure 18-10). No hemophagocytosis is seen, allowing a distinction from *E. histolytica*.

Differential Diagnosis

Similar central facial lesions can be seen in tuberculosis, leishmaniasis, sarcoidosis, conidiobolomycosis, and

nasal-type NK-T cell lymphomas. Histologically, the appearance of infestations with BM or *Acanthamoeba* similarly imitates that of tuberculosis, other mycobacteriosis, leishmaniasis, sporotrichosis, and other deep mycoses. The Center for Disease Control (Atlanta, Georgia, US) has developed reliable methods for identifying amoebic trophozoites, including direct immunofluorescence and immunoperoxidase stains. These are species specific. The polymerase chain reaction and other molecular techniques for the identification of the organisms are available at research centers.

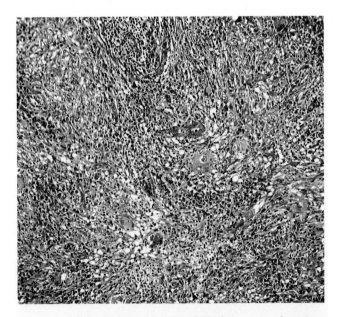

FIGURE 18-9. *Balamuthia mandrillaris*: a granulomatous pattern is present, with multiple giant cells. At the center, a trophozoite is present inside a giant cell. H/E, ×200.

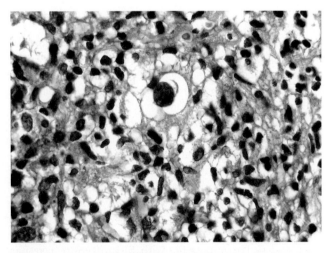

FIGURE 18-11. *Balamuthia mandrillaris*: another high-power picture of a round trophozoite with bubbly cytoplasm, inside a vacuole H/E ×400.

CAPSULE SUMMARY

INFESTATIONS WITH FREE-LIVING AMOEBAE

BM, and, less commonly, *Acanthamoeba* infestations may present with asymptomatic cutaneous plaques on the central face, the knees, or elsewhere, without any other symptoms. If the histologic image is that of a granulomatous process with many multinucleated giant cells, either isolated or forming ill-defined granulomas, infestation with a free-living amoeba is a possibility. One must look actively for trophozoites amidst the inflammatory infiltrate in the dermis. They have bubbly cytoplasm, and a nucleus and nucleolus.

REFERENCES

1. World Health Organization. Leishmaniasis. http://www.who.int/leishmaniasis/en/. Accessed December 19, 2017.
2. Paniz-Mondolfi AE, Talhari C, García Bustos MF, et al. American cutaneous leishmaniasis in infancy and childhood. *Int J Dermatol*. 2017; 56(12):1326-1341.
3. Blanco VM, Cossio A, Martinez JD, Saravia NG. Clinical and epidemiologic profile of cutaneous leishmaniasis in Colombian children: considerations for local treatment. *Am J Trop Med Hyg*. 2013;89(2):359-364.
4. Sangueza O, Bravo Puccio F, Sangueza M. *Dermatopathology of Tropical Diseases*. London: JP Medical Ltd; 2017.
5. Dassoni F, Daba F, Naafs B, Morrone A. Leishmaniasis recidivans in Ethiopia: cutaneous and mucocutaneous features. *J Infect Dev Ctries*. 2017 30;11(1):106-110.
6. Ardic N, Yesilova Y, Gunel IE, Ardic IN. Leishmaniasis recidivans in pediatric patients. *Pediatr Infect Dis J*. 2017; 36(5):534-540.
7. Sharifi I, Fekri AR, Aflatoonian MR, Khamesipour A, et al. Leishmaniasis recidivans among school children in Bam, Southeast Iran, 1994-2006. *Int J Dermatol*. 2010;49(5):557-561.
8. Barral A, Costa JM, Bittencourt AL, Barral-Netto M, Carvalho EM. Polar and subpolar diffuse cutaneous leishmaniasis in Brazil: clinical and immunopathologic aspects. *Int J Dermatol*. 1995;34(7):474-479.
9. Sundharkrishnan L, North JP. Histopathologic features of cutaneous leishmaniasis and use of CD1a staining for amastigotes in Old World and New World leishmaniasis. *J Cutan Pathol*. 2017;44(12): 1005-1011.
10. Alvarez P, Salinas C, Bravo F. Calcified bodies in New World cutaneous leishmaniasis. *Am J Dermatopathol*. 2011;33(8):827-830.
11. Mehregan DR, Mehregan AH, Mehregan DA. Histologic diagnosis of cutaneous leishmaniasis. *Clin Dermatol*. 1999;17(3):297-304.
12. Nguyen K, Taylor S, Wanger A, Ali A, Rapini RP. A case of *Penicillium marneffei* in a US hospital. *J Am Acad Dermatol*. 2006;54(4):730-732.
13. Kenyon C, Bonorchis K, Corcoran C, et al. A dimorphic fungus causing disseminated infection in South Africa. *N Engl J Med*. 2013; 10;369(15):1416-1424.
14. Dukik K, Muñoz JF, Jiang Y, et al. Novel taxa of thermally dimorphic systemic pathogens in the *Ajellomycetaceae (Onygenales)*. *Mycoses*. 2017;60(5):296-230.
15. Magaña M, Magaña ML, Alcántara A, Pérez-Martín MA. Histopathology of cutaneous amebiasis. *Am J Dermatopathol*. 2004;26(4):280-284.
16. Stauffer W, Ravdin JI. *Entamoeba histolytica*: an update. *Curr Opin Infect Dis*. 2003;16(5):479-485.
17. Magaña ML, Fernández-Díez J, Magaña M. Cutaneous amebiasis in pediatrics. *Arch Dermatol*. 2008;144(10):1369-1372.
18. Parshad S, Grover PS, Sharma A, Verma DK, Sharma A. Primary cutaneous amebiasis: case report with review of the literature. *Int J Dermatol*. 2002;41(10):676-680.
19. Ramdial PK, Calonje E, Singh B, Bagratee JS, Singh SM, Sydney C. Amebiasis cutis revisited. *J Cutan Pathol*. 2007;34(8):620-628.
20. Diaz JH. The public health threat from *Balamuthia mandrillaris* in the southern United States. *J La State Med Soc*. 2011;163(4):197-204.
21. Bravo FG, Seas C. *Balamuthia mandrillaris* amoebic encephalitis: an emerging parasitic infection. *Curr Infect Dis Rep*. 2012;14(4):391-396.

19

Cutaneous Viral Infections

Jessica Kaffenberger / Richard H. Flowers / Barrett J. Zlotoff / Mark R. Wlck

Viral diseases of the skin are relatively common in children and are more varied in nature than that seen in adults. The current widespread practice of early vaccination in pediatrics has markedly decreased the number of active viral infections, when compared with historical data. However, many children are still affected by them yearly on an international scale. This chapter outlines the spectrum of cutaneous viral infections in early life, along with possible associated complications.

HERPES SIMPLEX VIRUS

Definition and Epidemiology

Herpes simplex virus (HSV) is a part of the herpesvirus family that includes herpes simplex virus-1 (HSV-1), herpes simplex virus-2 (HSV-2), varicella-zoster virus, cytomegalovirus, Epstein-Barr virus, and human herpesviruses and 6-8.[1] HSV causes a vesicular rash that periodically flares throughout the patient's life.

HSV-1, a ubiquitous virus, is typically transmitted during childhood via nonsexual contact. It predominantly affects the oral mucosa, pharynx, and lips. HSV-2 is primarily linked with sexual transmission and affects the genital tract; however, in the United States, HSV-1 is becoming an increasingly prevalent cause of genital herpes.[2] In neonates, HSV-2 can be acquired via vertical transmission from the mother to child during passage through the birth canal.[3]

Between 2005 and 2010, HSV-1 seroprevalence was 30% between ages 14 and 19, 50% by age 20 to 29, and 62% by ages 30 and 39. (4) Between the same years, HSV-2 had a seroprevalence of 1.2% between the ages of 14 and 19, 10% by age 20 to 29, and 19% by ages 30 to 39.[4]

Etiology

Herpesvirus family consists of large, enveloped, double-stranded DNA viruses. HSV-1 and 2 serotypes have a similar DNA sequence but carry different envelope proteins.[1]

HSV-1 and 2 proliferate intracellularly after entering the skin or the mucous membranes, resulting in a vesicular eruption. The primary episode in most immunocompetent hosts will clear after a few weeks; however, the virus will travel in a retrograde manner along axons to neuronal cell bodies. Here, the virus will establish a life-long latent infection. The trigeminal and sacral ganglia are the primary sites of HSV1 and HSV2 latency.[1,5] At periodic times, the virus reenters the lytic phase, travels back to the skin or mucous membranes, and creates another vesicular outbreak.[6] The recurrences may be spontaneous or a result of numerous triggers, including stress, sunlight, heat, cold, menstruation, fevers, trauma, or immunosuppression.[7]

Clinical Presentation

The classic lesions of HSV-1 and 2 are grouped vesicles on an erythematous base (Figure 19-1). The sensations of burning, numbness, or pain often precede the vesicular outbreak. Although often asymptomatic, initial exposure to HSV-1 can result in primary gingivostomatitis and most commonly occurs in young children between 1 and 5 years old.[1] This primary infection can be widespread, with lesions occurring both intraorally and periorally on the lips, cheeks, and chin (Figure 19-2).[1,3,8] Children are often unable to swallow because of the pain and are at risk of dehydration.

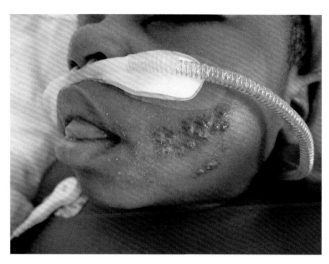

FIGURE 19-1. Grouped vesicles and vesiculopustules on an erythematous base in neonatal herpes simplex virus infection.

Associated fevers and lymphadenopathy may also be present. Severe cases of herpetic gingivostomatitis often warrant hospitalization where hydration and pain control can be provided. Recurrences of HSV-1 are generally less severe than the primary infection and present as the classic "cold sore" (Figure 19-3).[3]

Primary HSV-1 can also affect the eye and is a leading cause of corneal blindness in the United States.[9] Patients often have concurrent primary oral HSV infection or a prior history of oral HSV.[1] Clinical signs include conjunctivitis, edema, erythema, and erosions of the cornea. Patients often experience severe pain, photophobia, and eye watering. Urgent ophthalmologic evaluation is essential.[1]

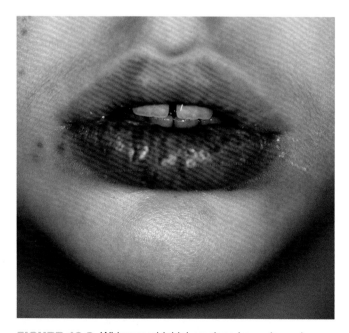

FIGURE 19-2. Widespread labial erosions in a primary herpes simplex virus-1 infection.

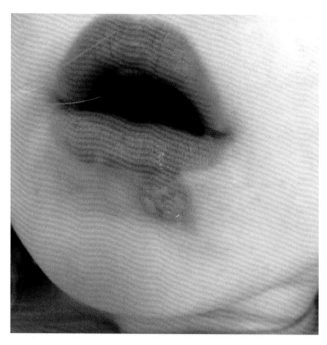

FIGURE 19-3. The classic "cold sore" of recurrent labial herpes simplex virus-1 infection.

Neonates are also susceptible to HSV, and the virus can be transmitted in utero, peripartum, or postpartum. Around 95% of neonatal HSV infections are acquired during the peri- or postpartum periods with the greatest risk of transmission from a mother with a primary genital HSV infection at or near the time of delivery. Neonatal HSV most commonly affects the mouth, skin, or eyes, yet rarely can lead to central nervous system (CNS) or disseminated disease.[10]

HSV-2 is primarily responsible for genital tract disease. Like HSV-1, most primary HSV-2 infections are subclinical and are, therefore, unnoticed.[11] However, if symptomatic, primary HSV-2 typically affects the vulva, labia, vagina, perineum, penis, or urethra. Cervical lesions in females are also common in primary infections. Widespread vesicles rupture, leaving painful erosions and ulcers.[1]

Children are more prone to cutaneous HSV than adults, with one study citing that 60% of children who visited an academic dermatology center for HSV had no labial or mucosal involvement.[8] Cutaneous HSV can occur in any location, but there are several distinct subtypes that are often seen in children. In neonates, HSV can infect traumatic wound from scalp electrodes and prevent healing of scalp erosions.[12] Herpetic whitlow is a distinct form of HSV involving the distal phalanx (Figure 19-4). Herpes gladiatorum refers to widespread HSV1 inoculation through abraded skin from sports such as wrestling or rugby. Finally, eczema herpeticum, also known as Kaposi's varicelliform eruption, is a widespread HSV infection of the impaired skin of patients with atopic dermatitis (Figure 19-5) or other condition causing an impaired skin barrier.[1]

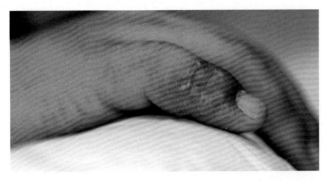

FIGURE 19-4. Vesiculobullous eruption on distal finger in herpetic whitlow.

Histologic Findings & Differential Diagnosis

HSV dermatitis begins as an intraepidermal process, proceeding to the formation of subepidermal blisters. Infected keratinocytes in the epidermis and hair follicles undergo "ballooning" degeneration and acantholysis, and they may form multinucleated cells. Nuclei often have a "gun-metal gray" color, with margination and homogenization of chromatin (Figure 19-6). At least some contain eosinophilic viral inclusions, surrounded by clear halos. As the lesions age, the keratinocytes become intensely eosinophilic and the cited nuclear changes tend to disappear. Dermal inflammation is variable in quantity and constituency; it may include a mixture of mononuclear cells and neutrophils, and, in rare cases, lymphoid cells in the infiltrate are numerous and cytologically atypical (Figure 19-7). Indeed, on many occasions, a rich CD30-positive infiltrate is seen. Vasculitic changes are also

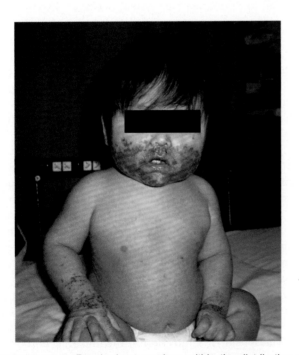

FIGURE 19-5. Punched-out erosions within the distribution of eczema in eczema herpeticum.

very frequent in the biopsies. The presence of inflammation of the sebaceous glands attached to the hair follicles can also point toward the diagnosis of HSV infection.[13-19] Immunostains for HSV-1 or HSV-2 are positive in active skin lesions. As mentioned earlier, the microscopic changes of erythema multiforme may develop subsequently.[16]

CAPSULE SUMMARY

HERPES SIMPLEX VIRUS INFECTION

Up to 62% of people are infected by HSV by age 40. The DNA virus remains latent in neural ganglia. HSV infection causes a vesicular painful eruption on an erythematous base and may cause "eczema herpeticum" in atopic patients. The histopathology of the infection shows intraepidermal vesicles and subepidermal blisters, with "ballooning" degeneration and acantholysis of keratinocytes. The nuclei of infected cells show margination and homogenization of chromatin, and intranuclear viral inclusions are surrounded by a halo. Inflammation is variable, but may simulate lymphoma in some cases.

VARICELLA-ZOSTER VIRUS

Definition and Epidemiology

Varicella-zoster virus (VZV) is a part of the herpesvirus family that includes HSV-1, HSV-2, VZV, cytomegalovirus, Epstein-Barr virus, and human herpesviruses 6 and 8.[1] Acute infection with VZV causes a widespread vesicular eruption called varicella, also frequently known as chickenpox. The reactivation of VZV that is latent in the sensory nerve ganglia causes herpes zoster (HZ), often known as shingles. The terms "shingles" and "zoster" derive from the Latin and Greek words for "girdle", referring to the girdle-like dermatomal distribution of recurrent VZV infections.

VZV is predominately transmitted via air droplets, but can also be spread by direct contact with lesions. VZV is extremely contagious when spread in an airborne fashion. Prior to vaccine development, studies report that 60% to 100% of susceptible household contacts would develop a clinically evident infection.[20] VZV's incidence has dramatically decreased after the development of a varicella vaccine that has been available in the United States since 1995.[21,22] One dose of varicella vaccine was reported to be 80% to 85% effective in preventing varicella.[23] Although excellent, this was not sufficient to prevent community outbreak, and a two-dose varicella vaccine was approved for children in June 2006.[21] A 2017 meta-analysis found the incidence of breakthrough varicella to be 2.2 cases per 1,000 person years in healthy children after two doses of the vaccine, as against 8.5 cases per 1,000 person years for those who received one dose.[22]

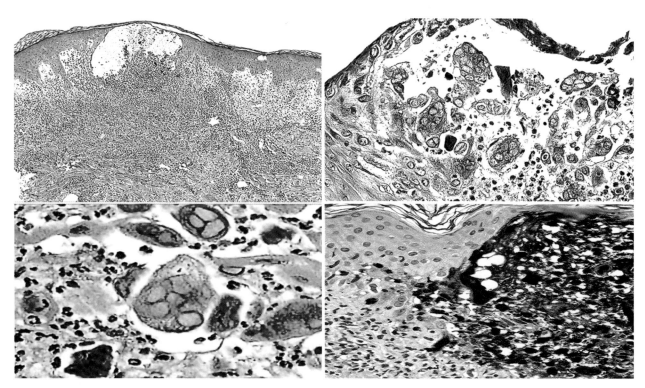

FIGURE 19-6. Microscopic images of cutaneous infection with herpes simplex virus-1. (Top left)—An intraepidermal vesicle is present, with underlying acute and chronic inflammation. (Top right)—The vesicle contains multinucleated cells with marginated chromatin and intranuclear inclusions. (Bottom left)—Nuclear details of the infected keratinocytes are seen well in this image. (Bottom, right)—An immunostain for herpes simplex virus-1 is diffusely positive in the lesional cells.

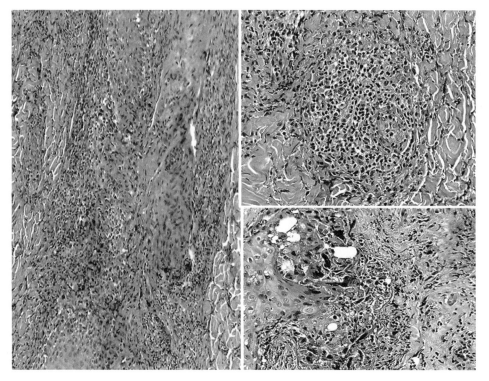

FIGURE 19-7. A marked lymphoid infiltrate is centered on hair follicles in this case of herpes simplex virus (HSV-1) infection (left panel). It comprises lymphoid cells with cytologic atypia, potentially causing confusion over a possible lymphoreticular neoplasm (top right). In other areas, the cytopathic cells of HSV-1 can be seen in the infiltrate (bottom right).

Herpes zoster, which is caused by the reactivation of VZV, has also seen a decline after the institution of the varicella vaccine, and its prevalence has been reported to be 79% lower among vaccinated than among unvaccinated children. Wild-type virus causes over half of HZ cases in children who have been vaccinated. Skin-to-skin contact with fluid from HZ vesicles can transmit VZV to susceptible individuals.[24]

Etiology

Herpes virus family consists of large, enveloped, double-stranded DNA viruses. When transmitted via respiratory droplets, the virus disseminates hematogenously, causing a systemic infection. The virus then invades the capillary endothelial cells in order to invade the epidermis and cause cutaneous lesions. Once the primary infection resolves, VZV travels in a retrograde fashion back to the dorsal root ganglia where it establishes latency. The reactivation of VZV can occur years after primary infection, and usually presents in a dermatomal distribution as HZ. Like HSV, reactivation can be spontaneous or occur because of stress, sunlight, heat, cold, menstruation, fevers, trauma, or immunosuppression.[25]

Clinical Presentation

VZV is usually preceded by a prodrome of fever, malaise, and myalgia. Following this prodrome, vesicles surrounded by a rim of erythema, colloquially described as "dewdrops on a rose petal", erupt on the scalp and face and then spread to the trunk and extremities (Figure 19-8). Vesicles quickly form pustules or crusts and then heal within 7 to 10 days. The presence of lesions in numerous stages of development is a hallmark of varicella in contrast to smallpox, which presents with all lesions in the same stage of development.[25]

Maternal VZV during the first 20 weeks of pregnancy can put the fetus at risk for developing congenital varicella syndrome, which is characterized by multisystem abnormalities, including ocular abnormalities, low birth weight, brain abnormalities, cutaneous scarring, and hypoplastic limbs.[26] Transplacental transmission can also cause outbreaks within the first 10 to 12 days of life.[27]

Like VZV and HSV, HZ is characterized by vesicles on an erythematous base. HZ is classically confined to a dermatomal distribution (Figure 19-9), with more than 50% of cases exhibiting a thoracic distribution. Vesicles usually appear proximally and then spread distally along the affected dermatome.[28] HZ is often preceded by and then accompanied by severe hyperesthesia, pain, and tenderness. After the cutaneous lesions resolve, some patients develop postherpetic neuralgia, which manifests as recurrent sharp, "lightening-like" pain, and paresthesia in the previously affected areas. Fortunately, in otherwise healthy children, postherpetic neuralgia is very rare.[29]

Histologic Findings

The microscopic features of skin lesions in shingles and PV are largely superimposable on those of HSV. All of those disorders feature the presence of distinctive multinucleated cells in cytologic scrape preparations of unroofed blisters (Tzanck smears) (Figure 19-10). Inflammation is least prominent in the early lesions of primary varicella, compared with those of HSV and shingles. Immunostains for VZV are positive in the infected keratinocytes of both primary varicella and shingles.

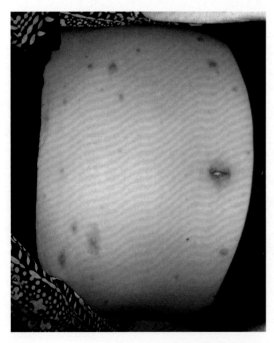

FIGURE 19-8. Vesicles on an erythematous base in the "dew drops on a rose petal" pattern found in primary varicella-zoster virus infection, commonly known as "chicken pox."

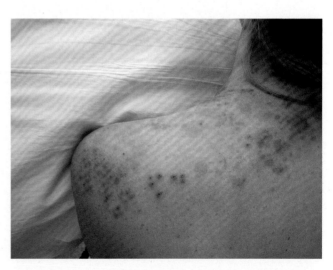

FIGURE 19-9. Punched-out erosions, vesicles, and erythematous-eroded plaques in a dermatomal distribution in recurrent varicella-zoster infection, commonly known as "shingles."

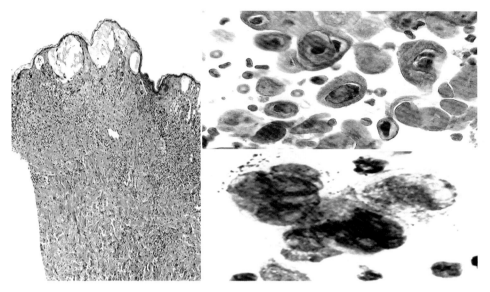

FIGURE 19-10. This example of varicella-zoster virus dermatitis shows findings that are comparable to those seen in Figure 19-6, including intraepidermal vesicles with reticular degeneration (left panel), marginated nuclear chromatin, and intranuclear inclusions (top right). A Tzanck smear from one of the vesicles demonstrates the multinucleated lesional cells, as seen with a Papanicolaou stain.

CAPSULE SUMMARY

VARICELLA-ZOSTER VIRUS INFECTION

Infection by VZV occurs by airborne spread as well as by contact with lesions from infected individuals. Maternal transmission can result in dermatomal scar-type presentation with systemic sequela. There has been a decreased incidence since the development of an effective vaccine, but the infection can still occur in vaccinated children. VZV is a DNA virus that remains latent in neural ganglia; chickenpox in children can be followed by "shingles" in adolescence or adulthood, sometimes with multiple episodes. Postinfectious neuralgia may follow shingles, but this is rare in children. The clinical and histologic features of VZV lesions are superimposable to those of HSV.

WARTS

Definition and Epidemiology

Warts (verrucae) are caused by human papillomaviruses (HPV) that infect the epithelial tissues of the skin and mucous membranes. HPV is a ubiquitous virus with over 200 distinct HPV genotypes currently characterized.[30,31] Some subtypes of HPV, especially HPV-16 and 18, are classified as high risk and can incite changes leading to numerous malignancies; to cite an example, cervical cancer.[31]

Verruca vulgaris, also known as common warts, are most commonly associated with HPV types 1, 2, 27, 57, with type 1 most commonly occurring in children under 12 years old.[32] Verruca plana (flat warts) are primarily associated with HPV types 3, 10.[33] Palmar-plantar (myrmecial) verruca are most commonly associated with HPV type 1, but types 2, 27, and 57 are also seen.[32-34] Condyloma (genital warts) are associated

predominately with HPV subtypes 6 and 11.[35] Verruca are transmitted via skin-to-skin contact or from fomites on warm, wet areas such as public pools or showers.[33] Common warts have a prevalence of up to 25% in schoolchildren and often go untreated.[36] However, even without treatment, most common warts will spontaneously regress.[31]

Condyloma acuminata (CA) is one of the most common sexually transmitted diseases in adolescents and adults. The prevalence of this condition in infants and children remains poorly studied. A female predominance has been reported.[37] Condyloma in children should always warrant at least a consideration of sexual abuse. However, autoinoculation or heteroinoculation from mothers, siblings, or caretakers are frequently responsible for transmission.[34,38] After a thorough investigation, one study indicated that only 3 of 131 patients were ruled suspicious for sexual abuse.[38] The older the child the more likely sexual abuse is a cause. Vertical transmission from maternal birth canal is most likely for those under 2 years. Abuse is rare for those under 4 years; for 4 to 8-year-olds, it is still rare but more of a consideration, and in the 8 or older age group, abuse is 12 times more likely than in the 4 and under age group.[39]

Etiology

HPVs are small, nonenveloped, circular, double-stranded DNA viruses. The virus infects the basal cells of the stratified epithelium.[31] In order for the HPV to reach the basal layer, it is likely that microabrasions in the skin serve as a portal of entry for the virus. HPV utilizes numerous mechanisms to avoid inciting an immune response. The virus does not cause cell death, which would trigger inflammation and a subsequent immune response. Instead, the infected cell is shed during the natural turnover of keratinocytes. Additionally, HPV downregulates interferon gene expression, thereby preventing a robust immune response.[40]

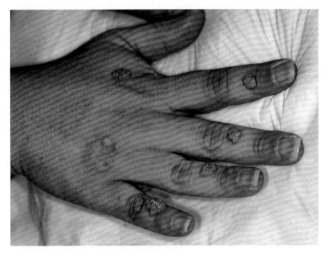

FIGURE 19-11. Hyperkeratotic papules with a "verrucous" surface in verrucous vulgaris.

Clinical Presentation

Verruca Vulgaris

Verruca vulgaris are most commonly flesh-colored, pink, or light brown papules with a verrucal (rough) surface. They may be dome-shaped, hyperkeratotic, exophytic, or filiform and often affect the dorsal hands (Figure 19-11) or periungal areas, but can also be seen on the face and extremities.[33,34] Upon close examination, verruca vulgara often have black puncta that reflect thrombosed capillaries. A linear formation created by autoinoculation secondary to scratching or a ringed appearance (Figure 19-12) following aggressive topical therapies are examples of koebnerization of the disease.

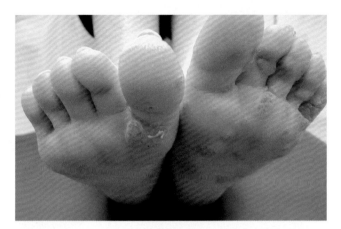

FIGURE 19-13. Plantar warts demonstrating thrombosed capillaries, which are visualized as black dots within the "mosaic" coalescing hyperkeratotic plaques.

Verruca Plana

Verruca plana are flesh-colored, pink, or light brown flat-topped papules. Unlike verruca vulgaris, verruca plana are smooth and are usually small with a diameter under 5 mm.[33] Verruca plana koebnerize easily and are commonly found on the dorsal hands, arms, face, or legs.

Palmoplantar Verrucae

Palmar and plantar verrucae are thick, hyperkeratotic papules or plaques found on the palms or soles. These warts are often on pressure points of the foot and therefore can cause significant discomfort (Figure 19-13).[33] The thick keratotic plug is often surrounded by a hyperkeratotic rim, and removal of the plug leaves a central depression behind.[33] The presence of thrombosed capillaries is helpful to distinguish these warts from corns or calluses (Figure 19-14).[34]

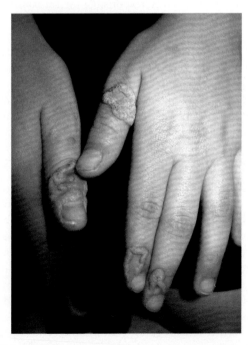

FIGURE 19-12. "Donut" or ringed warts occurring post cryotherapy.

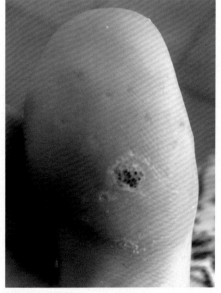

FIGURE 19-14. A plantar wart on the great toe displaying a hyperkeratotic rim with a central depression and thrombosed capillaries.

Condyloma Acuminata

These are pink, soft, exophytic papules most commonly found perianally in children.[38] Lesions can also occur on the penis, scrotum, and vulva. Multiple lesions are usually present, and these lesions can coalesce into large, exophytic plaques. Small lesions are frequently asymptomatic; however, these large plaques are easily irritated, resulting in pain and bleeding.[33]

Histologic Findings

Histologically, verruca vulgaris (VV) shows epidermal hyperkeratosis and parakeratosis. The second of those changes often assumes the appearance of peaked columns ("peaking parakeratosis"). Other typical changes include hypergranulosis with a clumping of cytoplasmic keratohyaline; papillomatosis with lengthening of the rete ridges; hypervascularity of the upper dermis; and bowing of the peripheral rete in the lesion, toward its center. The last of those changes may ultimately cause fusion of the rete ridges, producing a flat lesional base. Evidence of intranuclear viral replication includes perinuclear halos in infected keratinocytes ("koilocytes"), with possible binucleation, as well as crenation and hyperchromasia of the nuclei or homogenization of chromatin (Figure 19-15).

Ordinary and myrmecial plantar warts have different appearances. The first of those lesional groups shows exophytic, papillomatous epidermal growth with koilocyte formation and prominent cytoplasmic keratohyaline granules. In myrmecial verrucae, one sees endophytic epidermal growth, with large eosinophilic granules in the cytoplasm and nuclei of infected keratinocytes. Cellular vacuolization is also common (Figure 19-16).[41-44]

Microscopically, CA show epidermal papillomatosis, often yielding frond-like profiles or a more blunted "roller-coaster" surface configuration (Figure 19-17).

Variable parakeratosis is apparent, along with possible epidermal koilocytosis and nuclear crenation. Another peculiarity of CA is that they may virtually perfectly imitate the histologic appearance of extragenital seborrheic keratoses, with interlocking bars of bland epidermal epithelium that are punctuated by keratinous "horn cysts."[45]

CAPSULE SUMMARY

HUMAN PAPILLOMAVIRUS INFECTION

Over 200 DNA viral HPV genotypes belong to this category. They are transmitted by skin to skin or fomite to skin transfer. HPV does not cause cell death; virus is shed during keratinocyte turnover. Multiple clinical forms like verruca vulgaris, verruca plana, palmoplantar verruca, and condyloma acuminatum exist. The histologic features of HPV infection include epidermal papillomatosis, clumping of keratinocyte keratohyaline, bowing of peripheral rete to a central focal point, and koilocytosis.

EPIDERMODYSPLASIA VERRUCIFORMIS

Definition and Epidemiology

Epidermodysplasia verruciformis (EV) is a rare autosomal recessive genodermatosis that predisposes patients to widespread infections with specific HPV subtypes, most commonly HPV 5 and 8.

EV was first described by Lewandowsky and Lutz in 1922.[46] Reports first mapped the disease to several consanguineous EV families.[47] However, since this time, genetic cases of EV have been documented worldwide. The disease likely carries genetic heterogeneity, with only 75% of the affected individuals carrying the known inactivating mutations of *EVER1/ TMC6 (transmembrane channel-like)* and *EVER2/TMC8*.[48-50]

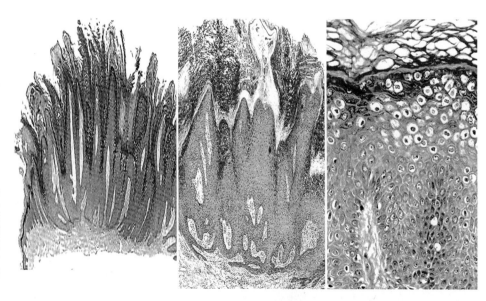

FIGURE 19-15. Verrucae show marked papillomatosis of the epidermis, with overlying parakeratosis (left panel), inward bowing and fusion of rete ridges (middle panel), and viral cytologic changes including nuclear crenation and cytoplasmic clearing (koilocytosis) (right panel).

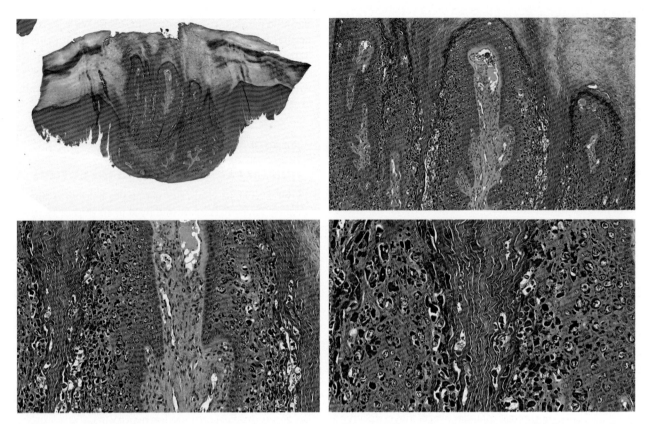

FIGURE 19-16. Myrmecial verrucae. Viral replication is high, producing marked cytologic changes in the infected keratinocytes (right panels). As opposed to molluscum viral cytopathic changes, the viral inclusions do not displace the nuclei of the infected cells. Digital slides courtesy of Path Presenter.com.

In 2009, the term "acquired EV" (AEV) was adopted to describe an EV-like syndrome that developed in immunosuppressed patients.[51]

Etiology

EV is a genodermatosis caused by mutations in two adjacent genes, *EVER1/TMC6* and *EVER2/TMC8*.[47] *EVER* genes encode endoplasmic reticulum transmembrane proteins that are important in ion transport and signal transduction.[47,48]

It is proposed that TMC6 and TMC8 provide resistance to HPV by regulating intracellular zinc and by increasing tumor necrosis factor-alpha.[50]

At least 20 HPV subtypes have been found in EV patients. The most common subtypes are HPV 5 and 8, both of which are associated with malignant transformation.[48]

AEV has been described in patients with defective cell-mediated immunity such as infection (HIV), non-Hodgkin lymphoma, leprosy, or medications. This entity is very

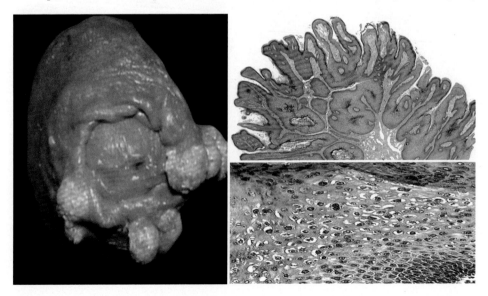

FIGURE 19-17. Condyloma acuminata (CA) are represented by nodular excrescences in modified mucosal skin, as shown here on the penis (left panel). They manifest similar microscopic changes to those of verrucae, except that epithelial papillomatosis in CA is more blunted (top right). Koilocytosis is again a feature (bottom right).

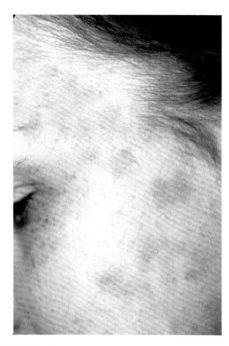

FIGURE 19-18. Slightly scaly, reddish thin plaques with a "tinea versicolor-like" morphology occurring in epidermodysplasia verruciformis. Courtesy of Kenneth Greer MD, University of Virginia.

rare, with several scientists suggesting that affected patients have an unknown genetic susceptibility to EV infections.[50]

Clinical Presentation

EV skin lesions begin in early childhood and are often characterized by slightly scaly, reddish-brown papules and patches that resemble pityriasis versicolor (Figure 19-18). Lesions can also resemble flat warts and usually start on the dorsal hands (Figure 19-19) and forehead and then spread to the arms, legs, neck, and trunk, with particular involvement of the gluteal cleft area (Figure 19-20). The buttocks and other non-sun-exposed skin are an unusual site for flat

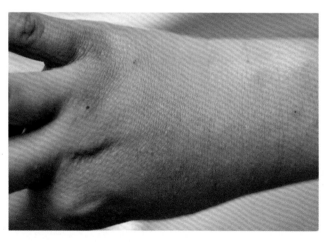

FIGURE 19-19. Thin, flat wart-like papules dorsum of hands in epidermodysplasia verruciformis.

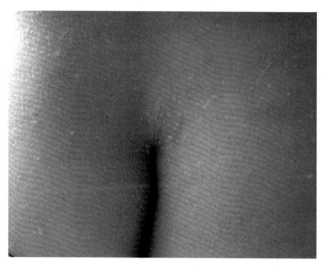

FIGURE 19-20. Thin, flat wart-like papules in gluteal cleft, an unusual site for flat warts but common in epidermodysplasia verruciformis.

warts outside of EDV. Mucosal membranes are spared. Lesions are refractory to treatment.[50] Malignant transformation, most commonly to squamous cell carcinoma, occurs in 30% to 70% of patients by early adulthood. Carcinomas are predominantly found in sun-exposed areas, suggesting a role of UV irradiation in malignant transformation.[48,50,52]

Clinically, AEV resembles EV. It has been reported in patients of all ages and in both sexes equally.[51]

Histologic Findings

Histologic findings in EV differ somewhat from those associated with ordinary VV or CA. The biopsies of EV show viral changes over a relatively broad expanse of epidermis, or multiple "islands" thereof in the surface epithelium. One sees enlarged keratinocytes in the upper epidermis; these often have blue-gray cytoplasm and may also demonstrate koilocytosis. Hypergranulosis is commonly present, but, in some cases, it affects only small islands of keratinocytes that are scattered throughout the upper epidermis (Figures 19-21 and 19-22).[53-57]

CAPSULE SUMMARY

EPIDERMODYSPLASIA VERRUCIFORMIS

EV is an autosomal recessive genodermatosis that predisposes to infection with specific HPV types—usually 5 and 8. Mutations in 2 adjacent genes—*EVER1/TMC6* and *EVER2/TMC8* on chromosome 17 can be seen. "Acquired" EV is associated with defective cellular immunity, as seen in infection with human immunodeficiency virus, non-Hodgkin lymphoma, and patients undergoing intense chemotherapy. Clinically, the lesions appear in early childhood as scaly red-brown papules

and patches, which multiply in number and involve the neck, extremities, and trunk, mimicking tinea versicolor in some cases. There is no mucosal involvement. Squamous cell carcinoma complicates EV in 3% to 70% of cases, usually on sun-exposed skin. The biopsies of EV show changes associated with HPV infection over a broad expanse of epidermis or multiple islands of infected cells in the surface epithelium.

CYTOMEGALOVIRUS

Definition and Epidemiology

Cytomegalovirus (CMV) or human herpes virus-5 is a ubiquitous double-stranded DNA virus. It is an opportunist infection in the setting of immunosuppression especially in transplant and AIDS patients. CMV is a very common infection, with 70% to 90% of individuals being infected worldwide. CMV is the most common congenital infection, affecting up

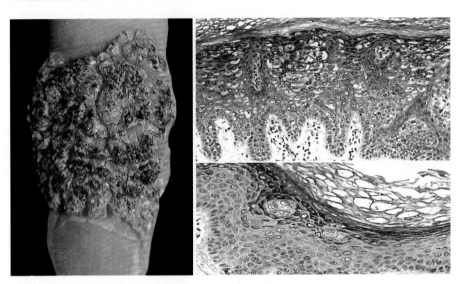

FIGURE 19-21. Epidermodysplasia verruciformis may occupy significant portions of the skin surface, as shown on the finger in the left panel. Keratinocytes infected with human papillomavirus are larger than those seen in ordinary warts, with lavender cytoplasm (top right). In some cases, small islands of such cells are scattered throughout the epidermis (bottom right).

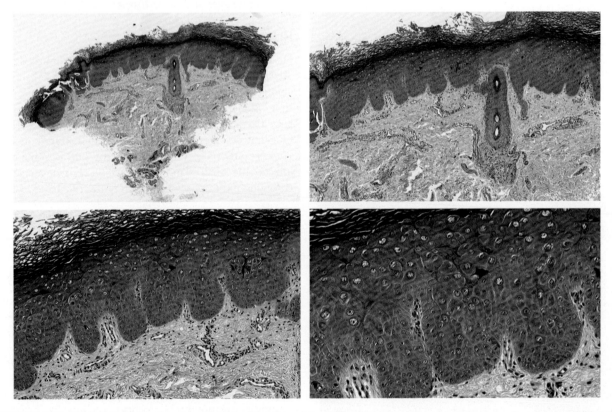

FIGURE 19-22. Epidermodysplasia verruciformis. Alteration of the maturation of individual keratinocytes is seen, in addition to numerous cells containing a bluish cytoplasm with vacuolation. Digital slides courtesy of Path Presenter.com.

to 2% of newborns[58] and 0.7% of newborns in the United States.[59] Infection is asymptomatic in up to 90% of neonates.[60]

Etiology

CMV is transmitted via urine, saliva, sexual fluids, and breast milk. Blood transfusions may also transmit CMV. Transmission from mother to fetus/infant may occur via the placenta, during delivery via cervical secretions and postnatally via breast milk or saliva. Transmission rates are higher in women with primary CMV infection versus women with reactivation.[60] Following primary infection, CMV establishes life-long latency within the host. Periodic reactivation may result in viral shedding; reinfection is not uncommon with other viral strains. Systemic infection may occur in neonates and in immunosuppressed populations.[58]

Clinical Presentation

Symptomatic manifestations in neonates are similar to other TORCH infections (toxoplasmosis, syphilis, rubella, CMV, herpes simplex). The liver, spleen, gastrointestinal tract, and CNS are prominently affected, with the later classically resulting in deafness, encephalitis, and intracranial calcifications. Severe neurologic damage, sensorineural hearing loss, and permanent developmental delay may occur, even in asymptomatic individuals. Cutaneous manifestations include jaundice, purpura, and a "blueberry muffin" appearance.[61] The latter describes dark blue-red papules and nodules representing extramedullary erythropoiesis. Cutaneous vesicles may rarely occur.[62]

Aside from congenital infection, CMV-associated disease occurs most commonly in adults and children with immunodeficiency where it may manifest infection of the retina, CNS, lungs, and gastrointestinal tract. This occurs characteristically in the setting of HIV/AIDS but also in immunocompromised patients with hematologic malignancy or postorgan transplantation. The most common cutaneous manifestation in this setting is sharply demarcated anogenital ulcerations, but lesions may be extragenital in children. These ulcers are often coinfected with HSV in patients with AIDS, but not in patients who are immunocompromised from other etiologies.[63,64] A diaper dermatitis-like presentation in a child with disseminated CMV has been described.[65] Gianotti-Crosti syndrome in children may result from CMV.[66] CMV can cause a heterophil-antibody-negative mononucleosis-like syndrome (fevers, myalgias, abnormal liver function tests, atypical lymphocytosis) with a "rubelliform" rash in adolescents/young women.[61,67] A small-vessel vasculitis with livedo-like changes was reported in this setting.[68] Scleredema-like changes in an infant with CMV pneumonia has been reported as well.[69] A variety of other nonspecific lesions, including purpuric papules and plaques, exanthems, crusted papules, vesiculobullae and prurigo nodularis-like lesions, have been reported, although predominantly in adults.[70]

Histologic Findings

In the skin, CMV can actively proliferate in vascular endothelium, the epidermis, or dermal appendages. Cutaneous biopsies show possible ulceration and mixed acute and chronic inflammation in the corium. CMV-infected cells often contain characteristic large, eosinophilic nuclear inclusions surrounded by a halo (Figure 19-23). They are easily visible by routine microscopy, but may be accentuated with immunostains for CMV-early antigen or in situ hybridization for CMV DNA.[71-74]

CAPSULE SUMMARY

CYTOMEGALOVIRUS INFECTION

CMV is synonymous with human herpesvirus-5. Congenital CMV infection can cause purpura and "blueberry muffin" lesions in the skin of babies. CMV causes an opportunistic infection in immunocompromised hosts. Clinically, there are sharply demarcated cutaneous ulcers in diaper area, and other locations may be CMV-infected in immunodeficient individuals. The virus is transmitted by contact with bodily secretions. Adolescents may develop CMV-related illness resembling infectious mononucleosis. Histologically, CMV infects vascular endothelium, epidermal keratinocytes, and dermal appendageal epithelium, with possible ulceration. Infected cells contain large intranuclear eosinophilic viral inclusions, surrounded by halos.

EPSTEIN-BARR VIRUS

Definition and Epidemiology

Epstein-Barr virus (EBV) or human herpes virus-4 is a double-stranded DNA virus. It is a very common human pathogen resulting in a wide range of clinical manifestations particularly in the pediatric population.

EBV infection is ubiquitous, with prevalence reaching 95% in adults worldwide.[75] The incidence by age varies in different countries; in the United States for example, approximately 50% of the population have seroconverted by age 5. In developing countries, children acquire the infection earlier, with universal seroconversion occurring by age 3 to 4. By adulthood, the vast majority of individuals regardless of socioeconomic status or nationality would have seroconverted.[76]

Etiology

EBV infection is transmitted through bodily fluids, primarily oral secretions but also blood transfusions, genital secretions, and breast milk.[77] The virus infects the oropharynx and then targets circulating B-lymphocytes via the binding of CD21. Following acute infection, EBV establishes latency

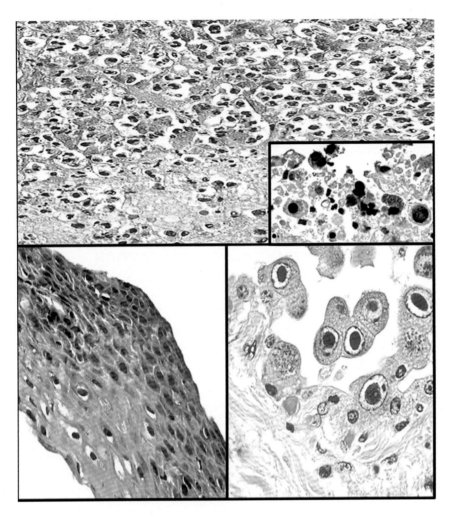

FIGURE 19-23. Cytomegalovirus (CMV) infection of the skin can produce ulceration, with a fibrinoinflammatory exudate (top panel); an immunostain for CMV-early antigen is intensely positive in the infected keratinocytes (top panel inset). In some instances, nuclear viral inclusions in keratinocytes are subtle in appearance (bottom left panel), whereas other examples of the disease manifest obvious inclusion bodies (bottom right panel).

within the B-cells. It escapes immune recognition by limiting viral gene expression. In the presence of compromised cell-mediated immunity, B-cells become immortalized and may lead to EBV-induced malignancy. Cell-mediated immunity is protective against primary infection, but an internal reactivation of the virus leads to periodic viral shedding.[78]

Clinical Presentation

EBV is associated with a variety of mucocutaneous manifestations in children, including nonspecific exanthem, infectious mononucleosis, Gianotti-Crosti syndrome, non-sexually-related acute genital ulcers, oral hairy leukoplakia, and hydroa vacciniforme (HV), in addition to a host of neoplastic and lymphoproliferative diseases. Nonspecific manifestations including erythema multiforme, acute urticarial, and leukocytoclastic vasculitis, have also been described.

Infants and young children infected with EBV will develop a mild nonspecific febrile illness, if symptoms occur at all. Adolescents and young adults generally develop infectious mononucleosis. The classic triad of fever, lymphadenopathy, and pharyngitis occur in approximately half of patients.[78] Fatigue and malaise linger. Patients may also

have splenomegaly (leading to feared splenic rupture), hepatomegaly, hemolytic anemia, myocarditis, or CNS disease. The cutaneous manifestations of infectious mononucleosis include palatal petechiae, genital ulcers, jaundice, and a transient pink exanthematous rash. Bilateral upper eyelid edema (Hoagland sign) is an early manifestation.[79] Up to 90% to 100% of patients with infectious mononucleosis who are given ampicillin will develop a diffuse morbilliform eruption (Figure 19-24),[80,81] but a recent study suggested that the number may be closer to 30%. This rash has been described in the setting of EBV to a variety of antibiotics, including amoxicillin, penicillin, tetracycline, and macrolides.[82]

Gianotti-Crosti syndrome or papular acrodermatitis of childhood is a distinct eruption of monomorphic edematous papules or papulovesicles (Figure 19-25) on the extensor extremities, cheeks, and buttocks, most often occurring in children younger than 4 years old. Although originally described secondary to hepatitis B infection and also linked to a variety of viral and bacterial infections, the majority of cases are linked to primary EBV infection. The rash generally resolves within 2 to 4 weeks.[83]

Non-sexually-related acute genital ulcers, or Lipschütz ulcers, are painful genital ulcers often occurring on the labia

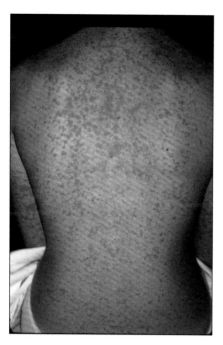

FIGURE 19-24. Classic morbilliform rash of mononucleosis after ampicillin exposure.

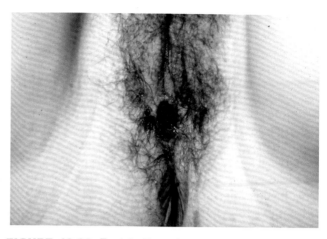

FIGURE 19-26. **Epstein-Barr virus is a common cause of Lipschütz ulcers.** These are punched-out genital ulcers that are not sexually transmitted and occur in children and adolescent girls. Photo courtesy of Kenneth Greer MD, University of Virginia.

minora of adolescent females. They are described as purple-red ulcers with ragged edges (Figure 19-26).[77] They are not sexually transmitted and are often associated with systemic symptoms and a history of aphthosis.[84] EBV is the most commonly associated infection, although often no etiology is found.[85]

Oral hairy leukoplakia (OHL) is a benign EBV-associated mucosal disease. It is most commonly associated with HIV, but is seen in a variety of immunosuppressive states as well. OHL often presents as white plaques on the lateral tongue with a corrugated surface. The plaques cannot be scraped off, unlike oral candidiasis. OHL is generally asymptomatic but can cause burning, soreness, or taste changes. The appearance of OHL is similar in adults and children, but the incidence of clinical disease may be much less frequent in children.[86] Unlike in adults, OHL in children with HIV has not been shown to have predictive value for progression to AIDS.[87]

Typical HV is a rare generally self-limited photosensitizing disorder of childhood, associated with EBV infection. HV features painful recurrent papulovesicles on the sun-exposed areas of the cheeks, nose, ears, and dorsal hands/arms that heal with pox-like scars (Figure 19-27). Severe ulcerating lesions are seen in atypical HV, which features less

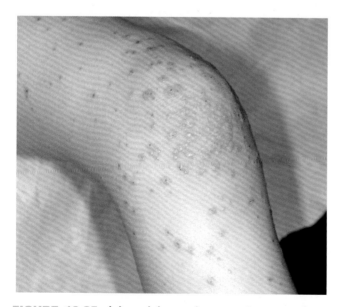

FIGURE 19-25. **Juicy, pink papules on extensor surfaces with concentration over elbows in Gianotti-Crosti syndrome.** Similar papules occur in high number over knees, buttocks, and cheeks.

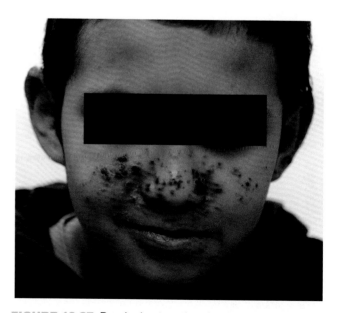

FIGURE 19-27. Punched-out erosions in sun-exposed areas including the bridge of nose, cheeks, and rims of ears typical of hydroa vacciniforme in a patient of South American ethnicity. Photo courtesy of Aimee Smidt MD, University of New Mexico.

photosensitivity. This disease could sometimes progress to an HV-like lymphoma, a cutaneous T- or NK-cell lymphoma. The most recent update in the WHO classification has changed the terminology of HV to HV-lymphoproliferative disorder. These children and adolescents may develop fever, lymphadenopathy, and hepatosplenomegaly. Children may develop hypersensitivity to mosquito bites (Figure 19-28), with erythema, bullae, and ulceration as well as systemic symptoms. Underlying chronic active EBV infection as well as NK/T-cell leukemia and lymphoma are associated.[77]

EBV was the first virus to be associated with oncogenesis in humans. A host of neoplasms are associated, including a variety of B-cell lymphomas, extranodal NK/T-cell lymphoma, HV-like lymphoma, Hodgkin lymphoma, and hemophagocytic syndrome. Malignancies that are more commonly seen in children include endemic Burkitt lymphoma, HV-like lymphoma, and hemophagocytic syndrome.[77]

Burkitt lymphoma is a poorly differentiated, aggressive non-Hodgkin B-cell lymphoma. Endemic disease (eBL) is most common in equatorial Africa, Brazil, and Papua New Guinea and is associated with EBV infection as well as *Plasmodium falciparum* infection.[88] The average age of eBL in endemic areas is around 5 to 8 years old.[89,90] eBL often arises in the head and neck and presents as an enlarging jaw mass.

Cutaneous disease is uncommon but is generally erythematous nodules or plaques.[77]

Hemophagocytic syndrome or macrophage activation syndrome is a rare progressive histiocytosis that is often fatal. A variety of infectious triggers are cited as causing secondary/reactive hemophagocytic syndrome, with EBV being the most common.[91] Fever, hepatosplenomegaly, liver disease, and pancytopenia are characteristic. Cutaneous involvement may occur in up to 65% of patients and features nonspecific purpuric macules, papules, or subcutaneous nodules.[92,93]

Histologic Findings

In the exanthem of acute mononucleosis, skin lesions demonstrate rather nonspecific histologic findings. They include a superficial and deep perivascular lymphoid infiltrate with a potential extravasation of erythrocytes (Figure 19-29), lichenoid, and spongiotic inflammation, a vacuolation of basal epidermal keratinocytes, and keratinocyte apoptosis. The lesional lymphocytes include both CD4+ and CD8+ cells.[94,95]

The lesions of Gianotti-Crosti syndrome histologically show modest epidermal spongiosis with marked papillary dermal edema (Figure 19-30). The latter finding is particularly present in cases caused by EBV infection. The dermis

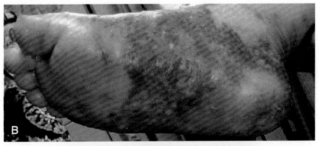

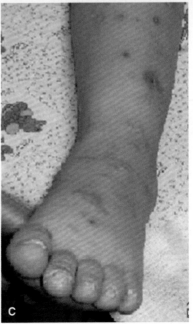

FIGURE 19-28. Severe mosquito bite allergy. There are clear and hemorrhagic bulla with intense erythematous swelling at mosquito-bitten sites on the (A) right leg dorsum and (B) palm. Necrosis and ulcers clustered on the base of the toes and turned into escar formation after recovery. C, Previous escar scar remitted and centrally dipped like a volcano on the left. Lee W-I, Lin J-J, Hsieh M-Y, Lin S-J, Jaing T-H, Chen S-H, et al. (2013) Immunologic Difference between Hypersensitivity to Mosquito Bite and Hemophagocytic Lymphohistiocytosis Associated with Epstein-Barr Virus Infection. *PLoS ONE* 8(10): e76711.

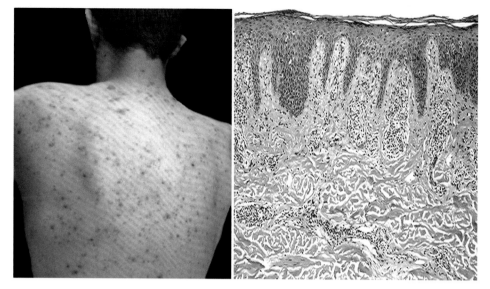

FIGURE 19-29. A morbilliform rash may be seen in infectious mononucleosis, caused by acute infection with Epstein-Barr virus (left panel). Histologic findings in such cases are nondescript, represented by slight papillary dermal edema and perivascular dermal lymphoid infiltrates (right panel).

contains a perivascular and interstitial inflammatory infiltrate, dominated by mononuclear cells but with scattered eosinophils. Immunohistologic and in situ hybridization studies are negative for EBV-related markers, and an etiologic association with that virus is usually established using serologic findings instead. Among the lesional inflammatory cells, cytotoxic T-cells are overrepresented.[96-98]

Mucosal epithelial ulceration of the genital skin is seen microscopically in some patients who are infected with EBV, with an overlying fibrinoinflammatory exudate ("Lipschütz ulcers"). The underlying tissue contains a dense and deep infiltrate of lymphocytes (Figures 19-31 and 19-32), most of which are CD4+ T-cells. Other findings in that study included venulitis, endarteritis obliterans, neutrophilic sebaceous adenitis, and mucosal lymphoid hyperplasia. Endothelial and vascular smooth muscle cells were seen to express cytoplasmic EBV latent membrane protein-1, and

lesional lymphocytes were positive in over one-third of cases for early EBV mRNA (EBER) by in situ hybridization.[99-101]

In OHL, mild papillary mucosal acanthosis is evident, along with hyperkeratosis and parakeratosis. Epithelial cells in this disorder demonstrate cytoplasmic lucency and may resemble the koilocytes of HPV infection. Their nuclei have a homogenous ground-glass appearance, and intranuclear inclusions may be seen. A definitive pathologic diagnosis of OHL requires a demonstration of EBV-DNA, RNA, or latent membrane protein in the lesional epithelial cells. That can be accomplished by in situ hybridization and immunohistochemistry (Figure 19-33).[102-104]

Histologically, the skin lesions in severe mosquito bite allergy exhibit epidermal necrosis and ulceration. Pronounced dermal edema can be present, with interstitial and perivascular infiltrates of neutrophils and lymphocytes. Vasculitis is usually present, with karyorrhectic cell debris and extravasated

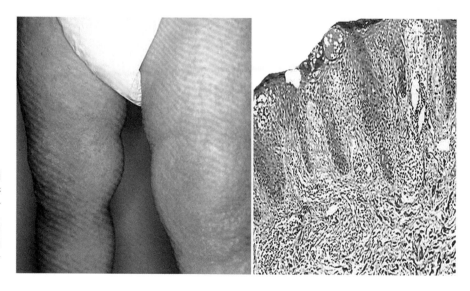

FIGURE 19-30. The Gianotti-Crosti syndrome presents with monomorphic edematous papules, as seen on the anterior thighs of this young child (left panel). Histologic findings include epidermal spongiosis, papillary dermal edema, and a mixed dermal perivascular and interstitial inflammatory infiltrate (right panel).

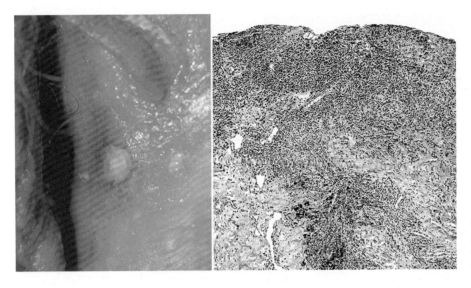

FIGURE 19-31. Lipschütz ulcers of the vulva (left panel) show a dense and deep infiltrate of lymphocytes, and vasculitis or endarteritis obliterans may also be present (right panel).

erythrocytes in the corium (Figure 19-34). The lesional lymphocytes in severe mosquito bite allergy comprise a mixture of CD4 and CD8-positive T-cells and NK-cells. Approximately 10% are positive for EBER by in situ hybridization.[105-107]

Another allied disorder is that of vasculitic purpura (VP) in children with chronic active EBV infection. It is predominantly seen in patients between the ages of 5 and 11 years, with a clinical constellation of findings that closely simulates those of Henoch-Schonlein purpura (Figure 19-35). However, immunohistologic studies in VP have failed to demonstrate the presence of IgA deposits.[108]

In HV-like lymphoproliferative disease, the lymphoid infiltrate comprises small-to-medium-sized cells with hyperchromatic nuclei, which are centered in the dermis with

a perivascular and periadnexal distribution. Epidermal necrosis is also common, together with spongiosis, intraepidermal and subepidermal vesicle formation, and exocytosis of the atypical lymphocytes. Biologically aggressive lesions—with markedly increased levels of EBV-DNA in the peripheral blood—demonstrate a higher level of cytologic atypia (Figure 19-36), and deep extension into the subcutis is possible. Angiotropism of the lymphoid infiltrate may be seen as well, with fibrinoid changes in affected vessels.[109-112]

The EBV-infected cells are a mixture of cytotoxic T-cells (CD3+, CD8+, TIA-1+, granzyme B+, perforin+) and NK-cells (CD56+). The number of EBER-positive cells is variable. T-cells can express either T-cell receptor (TCR)-$\alpha\beta$ or TCR-$\gamma\delta$. Clonal rearrangements of the T-cell receptor can be demonstrated.[107,113]

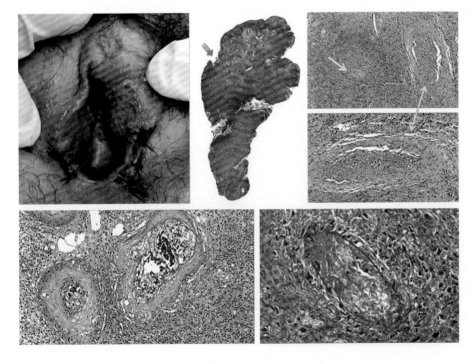

FIGURE 19-32. **Arteritis and venulitis associated with thrombosis.** A 15-year-old girl with infectious mononucleosis (fever, malaise, lymphadenopathy, lymphocytosis with atypical lymphocytes) developed painful, deep vulvar ulcers (top left panel, sutures mark biopsy sites). Arrow points to ulcer bed (top middle panel) where foci of venulitis with thrombosis (double-sided arrow) and arteritis (blue arrow) are admixed with diffuse mixed inflammatory infiltrates (top right and right mid-panels). Elastic tissue stain highlights loss and disruption of elastic lamina (bottom right panel). In this patient, sebaceous lobules exhibited coagulative necrosis and degeneration of sebocytes, but no herpetic nuclear viropathic changes (bottom left panel). Obtained with permission from Barrett MM, Sangüeza M, Werner B, Kutzner H, Carlson JA. Lymphocytic arteritis in Epstein-Barr virus vulvar ulceration (Lipschütz Disease): a report of 7 cases. *Am J Dermatopathol.* 2015;37(9):691-698.

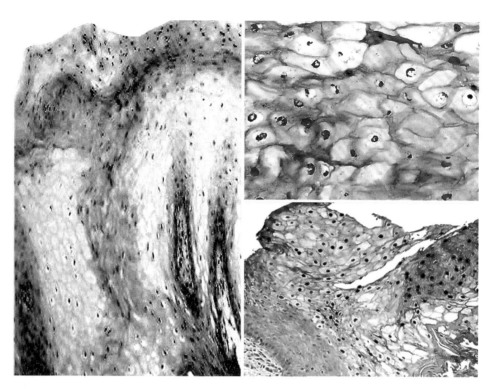

FIGURE 19-33. Oral hairy leuko-plakia is typified microscopically by mucosal acanthosis, hyperkeratosis, and parakeratosis (left panel). Infected cells resemble those seen in human papillomavirus infection, except that the degree of cytoplasmic lucency is greater (top right panel). In situ hybridization for Epstein-Barr virus-related nucleic acid is positive in such lesions (bottom right panel).

Histologic findings in drug-induced hypersensitivity and drug-related eruption with systemic symptoms can include a nondescript spongiotic dermatitis, with possible vesiculation and dermal eosinophilia (Figure 19-37), or a lymphocytic interface dermatitis with basal epidermal vacuolar degeneration and wholesale epidermal apoptosis. The latter picture is usually associated with prominent visceral organ dysfunction.[114,115]

CAPSULE SUMMARY

EPSTEIN-BARR VIRUS INFECTION

EBV is synonymous with human herpesvirus-4. Approximately 95% of children are infected in the United States by age 5. It is transmitted by contact with bodily secretions. EBV targets circulating B-lymphocytes, in which latent infection follows. The infection is associated with several potential clinical presentations, including a nonspecific exanthema, bilateral upper eyelid edema, Gianotti-Crosti syndrome, acute ulcers of the genital skin, HV, severe mosquito bite allergy, drug hypersensitivity syndromes, and lymphoproliferative disorders including Burkitt lymphoma. The histologic features are variable, potentially including nonspecific dermatitis, skin ulceration, mucosal papillomatosis with koilocytosis, prominent dermal edema, subepidermal vesicles, vasculitis, and cytologically atypical lymphoid proliferations.

HUMAN HERPESVIRUS 6

Definition and Epidemiology

Human herpesvirus 6 (HHV6) is a part of the herpesvirus family that includes HSV-1, HSV-2, VZV, CMV, EBV, and human herpesviruses 6-8. HHV-6 is most commonly associated with a rash called roseola, also known as erythema subitum. This virus has also been cited as a trigger for pityriasis rosea.[1]

HHV 6 is a ubiquitous virus that infects 75% to 90% of children by 2 years of age. HHV-6 is predominantly spread via saliva, but can also be acquired in utero. The virus is spread year-round without a season preference, and infected individuals can continue to shed the virus for years after the acute primary infection.[116] Pityriasis rosea (PR) is more commonly seen between 10 and 35 years of age, but is also often attributed to HHV 7.[117,118]

Etiology

Herpesvirus family consists of large, enveloped, double-stranded DNA viruses. Like other herpesviruses, HHV6 establishes latency following the primary infection and can reactivate during times of immunosuppression.[119] HHV-6 has two variants: HHV-6A and HHV-6B. HHV-6B is the primary agent responsible for childhood illness.[121,122]

Clinical Presentation

Nearly all children who acquire HHV-6 have symptoms of infection, with the most common symptoms being

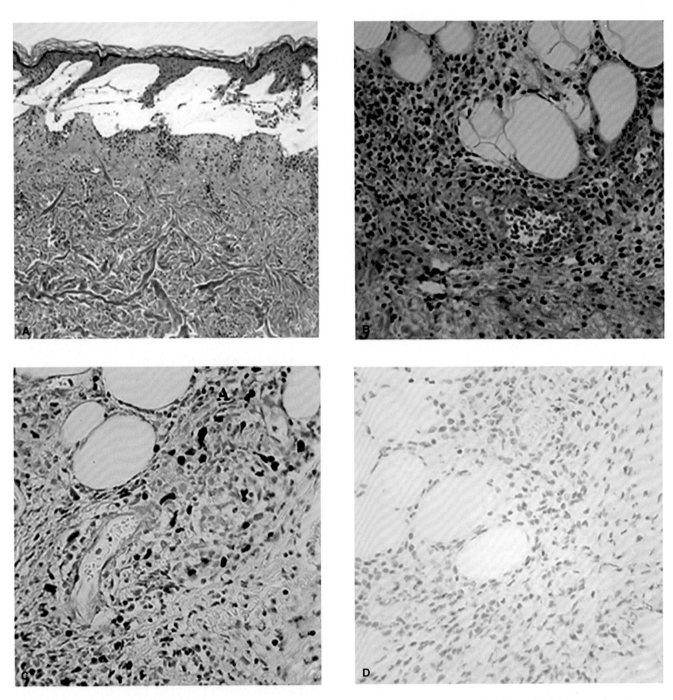

FIGURE 19-34. **Pathologic findings in severe mosquito bite allergy.** (A: H&E, ×100, B: ×400) Histopathologic examination of the skin biopsy specimen showed intraepidermal vesicles with interstitial and perivascular infiltration of lymphocytes, neutrophils, eosinophils, and histiocytes. C, In situ hybridization analysis for Epstein-Barr-related ribonucleic acid (EBER) was positive (dark brown color, ×400). D, Immunohistochemical staining with CD56 was negative (×400). Seon HS, Roh JH, Lee SH, Kang EK. A Case of Hypersensitivity to Mosquito Bites without Peripheral Natural Killer Cell Lymphocytosis in a 6-Year-Old Korean Boy. *J Korean Med Sci*. 2013 Jan;28(1):164-166. https://doi.org/10.3346/jkms.2013.28.1.164.

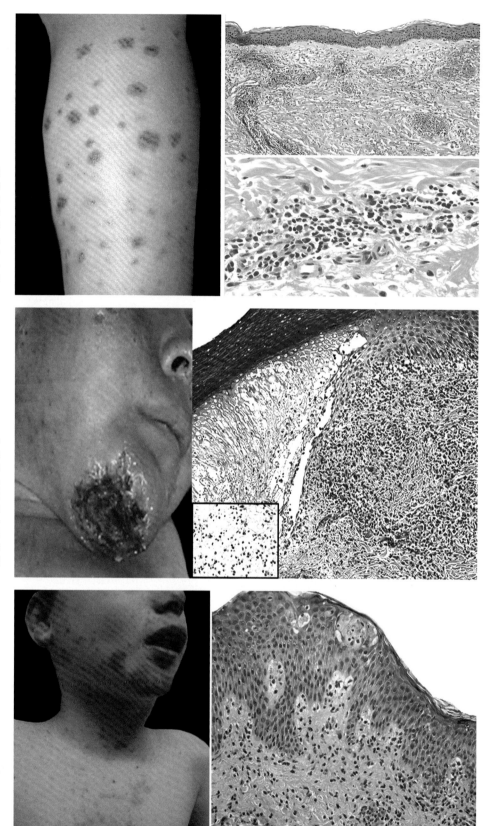

FIGURE 19-35. Vasculitic purpura may be seen in children with chronic Epstein-Barr virus infection, with palpable purpuric lesions like those seen in Henoch-Schonlein purpura (left panel). A small-vessel vasculitis, mediated by neutrophils, lymphocytes, and eosinophils, is also apparent (right panel), but affected vessels do not contain IgA deposits.

FIGURE 19-36. **Hydroa vacciniforme-like lymphoproliferative disease is also associated with Epstein-Barr virus (EBV) infection.** This child has a large ulcerated lesion on the face (left panel), with a bulky dermal infiltrate of atypical lymphoid cells (right panel). The lesional cells contain EBV-related nucleic acid by in situ hybridization (right panel inset).

FIGURE 19-37. Children infected with Epstein-Barr virus are susceptible to drug-induced hypersensitivity dermatitides, as seen in this boy who was given an antibiotic before developing this eruption (left panel). Histologically, most examples of this phenomenon are nondescript spongiotic dermatitides with variable numbers of dermal eosinophils (right panel). However, occasional reactions have the clinicopathologic features of erythema multiforme.

fever, fussiness, and rhinorrhea.[116,122] Cough, diarrhea, and seizures have also been linked to HHV-6, with approximately 20% of childhood seizures attributed to HHV-6.[122]

Roseola

Approximately a third of patients with primary HHV-6 infection develop a characteristic rash called roseola, also called sixth disease or exanthema subitum. Classically, patients experience a high fever, often over 103 F for 3 to 5 days. As the fever subsides and the patient begins to feel well, the child develops a rapid-onset (subitum is Latin for sudden) erythematous, blanchable macules and papules over the trunk which then spreads to the extremities and face (Figure 19-38).[116,119] Reddish-pink papules on the soft palate and uvula, called Nagayama spots, can also be present. The rash is asymptomatic and lasts 1 to 3 days before fading.[119]

Pityriasis Rosea

PR is characterized by pink, oval patches with fine scale. The disease usually starts with a single "herald patch" on the trunk. After about 2 weeks, a generalized eruption of smaller patches develops. The smaller patches favor the trunk and limbs and are often oriented with their long axis on cleavage lines, earning the description of a "Christmas tree" distribution (Figure 19-39).[118] Lesions usually spare the face, scalp, palms, and soles. Oral lesions, almost always asymptomatic, have been reported in up to 28% of cases. Oral lesions manifest most commonly as petechial and

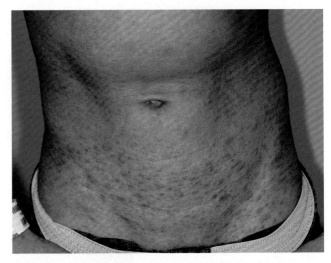

FIGURE 19-39. "Christmas tree pattern" of ovoid, thin, scaly, erythematous plaques lining up on skin lines with a larger "herald patch" on the patients left hip in pityriasis rosea

macular-papular patterns, but can also present with erythematovesicular and erythematomacular patterns.[123,124] The rash, including oral lesions, typically lasts about 1 to 2 months.[118]

Histologic Findings

To date, no systematic histologic evaluations of roseola have been conducted. That is probably because the diagnosis is obvious on clinical grounds and biopsies are not usually obtained. However, anecdotal cases seen by the authors have shown nonspecific dermal perivascular lymphocytic infiltrates that are modest in density (Figure 19-40). PR typically manifests itself as a mild subacute spongiotic dermatitis, sometimes with extravasated erythrocytes in the papillary dermis.[125]

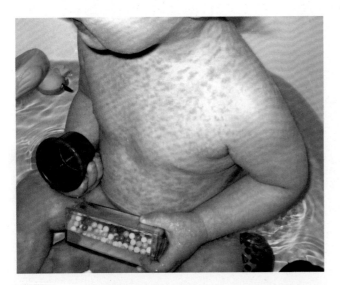

FIGURE 19-38. Erythematous macules and papules over the trunk which then spread to the extremities and face in roseola. Photo courtesy of Kenneth Greer MD, University of Virginia.

CAPSULE SUMMARY

HUMAN HERPESVIRUS-6 INFECTION

Seventy percent to ninety percent of children are infected by HHV-6 by age 2. The virus is primarily spread via saliva. The infection is associated with fever and possible childhood seizures. Clinically, cutaneous lesions show the features of roseola with multiple erythematous macules, potentially involving oral mucosa, or PR with pink oval patches on the trunk having a "Christmas tree" distribution. Histologically, roseola and PR show nonspecific perivascular chronic inflammation, sometimes with erythrocyte extravasation, and variable epidermal spongiosis.

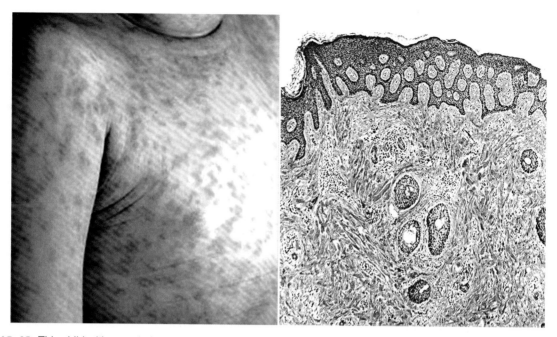

FIGURE 19-40. This child with roseola has an eruption comparable to that shown in Figure 19-39 (left panel). Microscopically, only an unremarkable dermal perivascular infiltrate of lymphocytes is present (right panel).

HAND-FOOT-AND-MOUTH DISEASE

Definition and Epidemiology

Hand-foot-and-mouth disease (HFMD) is caused by enteroviruses and is characterized by fever, oral vesicles, and papules and vesicles predominately affecting the palms and soles classically. A more widespread, atypical form is increasing in prevalence in many geographic areas.

HFMD predominately affects children between 1 and 4 years of age, but older children and adults can also contract the disease. It is spread most commonly via the fecal-oral method, although oral-oral transmission is possible.[126] HFMD is most prevalent in the summer and fall[127] and is very contagious, with reports of large-scale outbreaks. Numerous enteroviruses can cause HFMD; so although the patient acquires immunity after infection, HFMD can reoccur with a different enterovirus.[128]

Etiology

Enteroviruses are small, single-stranded RNA viruses that include echovirus, coxsackie viruses (A and B subtypes), enterovirus, and poliovirus.[129] Coxsackie A16 (CV-A16) is the leading cause of HFMD, with enterovirus 71 as the second most common cause.[130] Coxsackie A6 (CV-A6) has been emerging as an increasingly common cause of a more severe atypical HFMD.[131] Several other serotypes of enteroviruses, such as Coxsackie A10, have also been linked to HFMD.[132]

Clinical Presentation

Patients initially often suffer from fever and malaise 1 to 2 days prior to the vesicular eruption. The oral-cutaneous eruption is characterized by oval-shaped vesicles with a rim of erythema that favor the palms, soles, oral mucosa, and buttocks.[126] On the hands and feet, the football-shaped vesicles are often parallel to skin lines (Figure 19-41). Vesicles can also be present on the thighs and external genitalia, and may spread to more diffuse involvement. Vesicles may be asymptomatic, but are often very painful.[133]

Although it has been the causative agent in the epidemics of HFMD, CV-A16 is usually characterized by mild infection where lesions usually crust and resolve within 10 days.[128,133] Enterovirus 71, with predominance in Asia, has

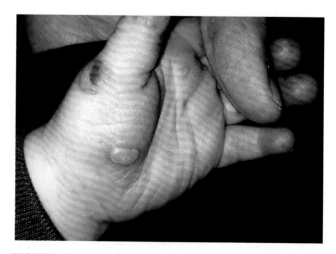

FIGURE 19-41. Football-shaped vesicles on the palm parallel to skin lines on palmar surface in classic coxsackievirus A16-related hand, foot, and mouth disease.

been associated with more critical disease, causing some patients to develop encephalitis, aseptic meningitis, and flaccid paralysis.[134]

CV-A6 has been reported to cause an "atypical HFMD" characterized by a more severe, widespread eruption, with numerous lesions spreading to the trunk and extremities (Figure 19-42A and B). The distribution of papulovesicles and even bullae is more often on extensor extremities, buttocks, dorsal hands and feet, and periorally, along with palmar and sole lesions (Figure 19-43). It can also have an

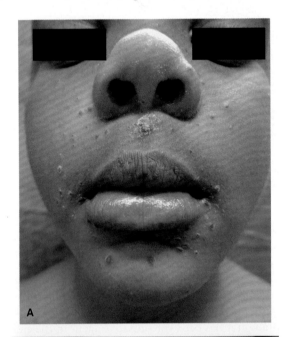

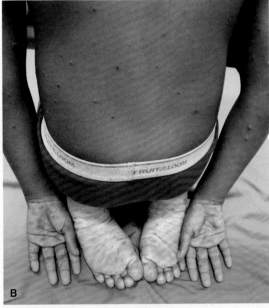

FIGURE 19-42. A and B, Widespread vesicles around the mouth, scattered over extensor arms and legs and over the trunk along with erythematous macules on palms and soles seen in the more dramatic eruption of "atypical hand-foot-and-mouth disease" associated with coxsackievirus A6.

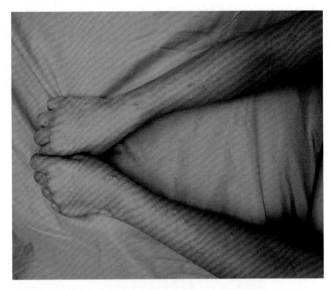

FIGURE 19-43. **Vesicles are present on the distal extremities.**

"eczema coxsackium"-type presentation, with lesions occurring within a background of eczematous dermatitis.[135] Unlike the other strains, CV-A6 is prevalent in the late fall to winter and also affects adults more often.[131] Nail involvement, mainly presenting as onychomadesis, is often present with CV-A6.[136,137]

Histologic Findings

Cutaneous and mucosal lesions show intraepithelial vesicles of variable size, associated with reticular degeneration. No multinucleated keratinocytes or viral inclusions are apparent. The papillary dermis or upper submucosa is often edematous, and a superficial perivascular infiltrate of lymphocytes is evident (Figures 19-44 and 19-45). These histologic changes are surprisingly unremarkable, when compared with the level of clinical illness that is associated with HFMD lesions.[138-140]

CAPSULE SUMMARY

HAND-FOOT-MOUTH DISEASE

This disease is caused by an infection by enteroviruses (especially coxsackievirus). Classical presentation includes fever, oral vesicles, and papules and football-shaped vesicles on palms and soles with a rim of erythema. Recently, outbreaks of coxsackie virus A6 have manifested as atypical presentations with an increased number of lesions, increased severity of lesions, and a more extensor, perioral and buttock concentration and lesions. It is spread via fecal-oral transmission and is extremely contagious. Histologic findings include intraepithelial vesicles with reticular degeneration, a lack of viral inclusions, dermal or submucosal edema, and superficial perivascular infiltrates of lymphocytes.

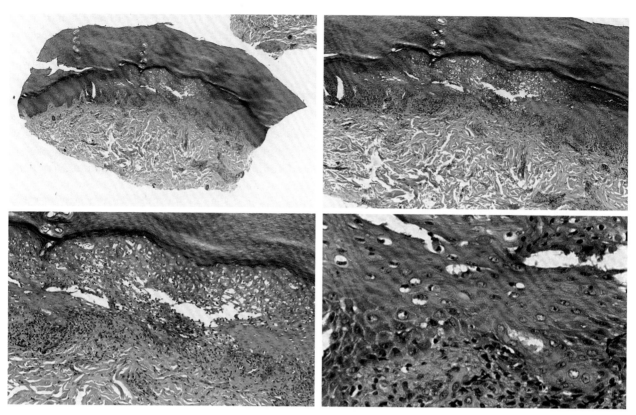

FIGURE 19-44. Hand-foot-mouth disease. Histologic changes in this disorder include epidermal necrosis, frequent apoptotic keratinocytes, and a perivascular lymphocytic infiltrate. Digital slides courtesy of Path Presenter.com.

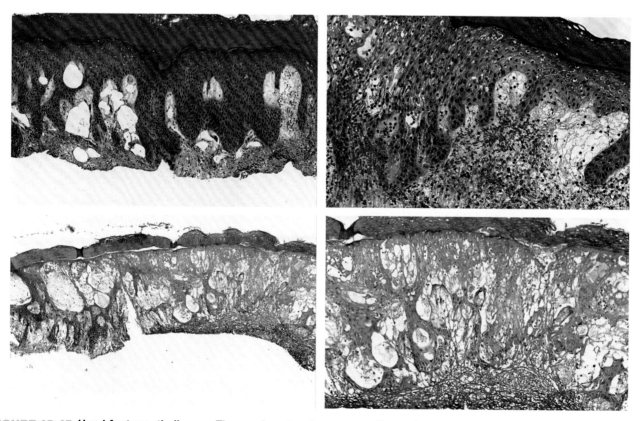

FIGURE 19-45. Hand-foot-mouth disease. The panels on top show a case with prominent edema and superficial dermal hemorrhage. The panels down show numerous intraepidermal vesicles. Digital slides courtesy of Path Presenter.com.

PARVOVIRUS B19

Definition and Epidemiology

Parvovirus B19 is a virus that can cause numerous clinical manifestations, including erythema infectiosum (fifth disease), papular-purpuric gloves and socks syndrome, oligoarthritis, aplastic anemia, hydrops fetalis, and fetal demise.[141]

Parvovirus B19 predominantly affects school-age children with half of 15-year-old children having B19 antibodies.[142] Transmission predominantly occurs via the respiratory tract, however, transmission can also occur via blood, and in utero. Peak incidence occurs during the late winter and spring.[141-143]

Etiology

Parvovirus B19 (B19), the only parvovirus that is pathologic in humans, is a single-stranded DNA virus.[142] B19 targets erythroid progenitor cells by binding to the P antigen. A small proportion of patients lack the P antigen and are thus resistant to B19 infection.[144] Following transmission from the respiratory tract, the virus multiples in the throat and causes viremia by day 6. B19 infection of erythroblasts causes apoptosis of infected cells and arrest of reticulocytes, thereby resulting in a transient aplastic crisis in healthy individuals. However, in patients with chronic blood disorders such as sickle cell anemia, spherocytosis, and thalassemia, this may result in a life-threatening aplastic crisis.[142]

Clinical Presentation

Parvovirus B19 can manifest with hematologic, rheumatologic, and dermatologic manifestations. The primary two dermatologic manifestations are erythema infectiosum and papular-purpuric gloves and socks syndrome (PPGSS).[142,145]

Erythema Infectiosum

Erythema infectiosum (EI), or fifth disease, generally begins with prodromal symptoms including headaches, fevers and chills, which coincide with the viremic phase. As anti-B-19 antibodies develop, patients erupt with the characteristic bright red, symmetric erythema of bilateral cheeks, sparing the nasal bridge.[142,143] This eruption is often described as "slapped cheek" (Figure 19-46). One or two days later,

the second stage of EI manifests with erythematous macular eruption on the extremities and trunk in a reticulated, "lacy" pattern (Figure 19-47). Palms and soles are usually unaffected. In the final recrudescence stage, the exanthem starts to fade, but reappears or flares with heat, sunlight, or emotional upset.[143]

Papular-purpuric Gloves and Socks Syndrome

PPGSS classically affects young adults during the spring and summer.[146] It presents with edema and erythema of the hands and feet.[147] The diffuse erythema is often associated with petechiae and purpura, with a sharp cut-off at the wrists and ankles (Figure 19-48).[148] Extreme pruritus can be present.[146] Petechiae and erythema are also often seen on the oral mucosa. Patients with PPGSS can have associated fevers, malaise, and arthralgias, suggesting that the cutaneous eruptions coincide with the viremic phase. Thus, unlike EI, patients with PPGSS are considered contagious when their rash erupts.[147,148]

A juvenile version of PPGSS, most commonly affecting children 1 to 3 years old, has also been described. Juvenile PPGSS mimics that of classic PPGSS; however, petechiae are much less pronounced, and fever, lymphadenopathy, and mucosal involvement are rare.[146]

Although the majority of PPGSS is associated with B19, PPGSS has also been reported to be caused by several other viruses, including VZV, EBV, CMV, herpesviruses 6 and 7, coxsackie, and rubella.[147,148]

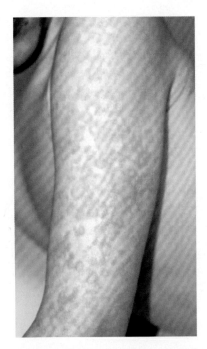

FIGURE 19-47. Erythematous macules in a "lacy" pattern on the arm, the extremities, and trunk in a reticulated, "lacy" pattern appearing after the "slapped cheeks" in erythema infectiosum.

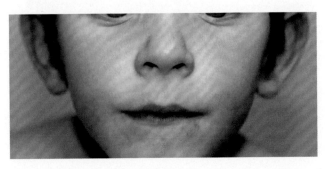

FIGURE 19-46. "Slapped cheek" with a symmetric erythema of bilateral cheeks in erythema infectiosum.

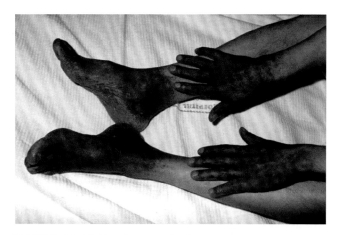

FIGURE 19-48. Papular-purpuric gloves and socks syndrome exhibiting diffuse petechial patches with erythema with a sharp cut-off at the wrists and ankles. Photo compliments of Margarita Larralde, MD, Hospital Aleman, Buenos Aires Argentina.

Histologic Findings

Regardless of the clinical cutaneous manifestations of parvovirus infection (erythema infectiosum [fifth disease], purpura, or the petechial "socks and gloves" syndrome), histologic findings in skin biopsies are comparable. They can be remarkably modest and nonspecific, principally represented by dermal vascular dilatation with slight endothelial swelling and a moderate perivascular lymphocytic infiltrate. Interstitial erythrocyte extravasation may be seen in the corium as well. The virus can be demonstrated in endothelial cells using immunohistochemistry (Figure 19-49). In other cases, one may see interstitial histiocytic infiltrates with piecemeal fragmentation of collagen and a vascular injury pattern, or interface dermatitis, eczematous alterations, intraepidermal pustule formation, and papillary dermal edema. Overall, the pathologic features of B19 infection suggest a delayed-type hypersensitivity reaction via antibody-dependent cellular immunity.[149-152]

CAPSULE SUMMARY

PARVOVIRUS B19 INFECTION

This is an infection predominantly seen in school-age children, and transmission is primarily respiratory. Parvovirus B19 is the only pathogenic parvovirus in humans. The infection may have rheumatologic, hematologic, and cutaneous manifestations, with the latter being represented by "fifth disease" (erythema infectiosum) and PPGSS. Histologic findings are typically modest and nonspecific, usually represented by dermal vascular dilatation, endothelial swelling, and perivascular lymphocytic infiltrates, with or without erythrocyte extravasation. Some cases may feature dermal necrobiosis, interface dermatitis, or intraepidermal pustule formation.

MOLLUSCUM CONTAGIOSUM

Definition and Epidemiology

Molluscum contagiosum (MC) is an infection of the skin and, rarely the mucous membranes, caused by the molluscipox virus (MCV), a double-stranded DNA virus belonging to the Poxviridae family. MCV is common in young children, immunocompromised children and adults, and HIV-infected persons and often presents as a sexually transmitted disease in adolescents and young adults.[153]

The prevalence of MC varies greatly depending on what population is studied, but as any pediatrician will attest to, it is not uncommon. Best estimates are that the prevalence ranges from 2% to 5% in children. Infection is more common in those with atopic dermatitis, and there seems to be an association with recent swimming by the affected children.[154] One study indicates that sharing of fomites such as bath sponges or towels is more predictive of infection than just being in the same pool.[155] Importantly, although

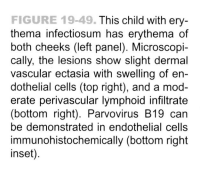

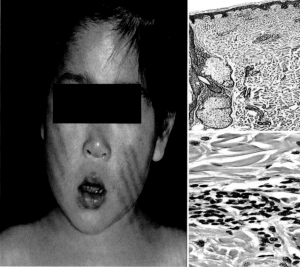

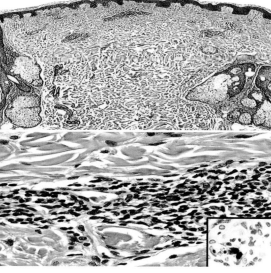

FIGURE 19-49. This child with erythema infectiosum has erythema of both cheeks (left panel). Microscopically, the lesions show slight dermal vascular ectasia with swelling of endothelial cells (top right), and a moderate perivascular lymphoid infiltrate (bottom right). Parvovirus B19 can be demonstrated in endothelial cells immunohistochemically (bottom right inset).

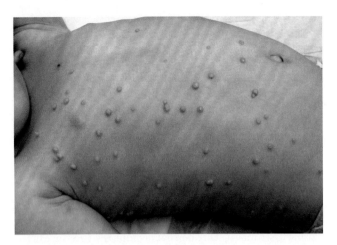

FIGURE 19-50. Numerous "pearly" white- or flesh-colored papules that are smooth surfaced and dome shaped with central umbilication consistent with molluscum infection in an immunosuppressed patient.

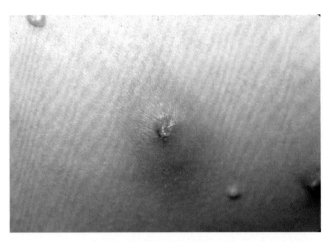

FIGURE 19-51. Inflammation occurring from follicular involvement of molluscum that is often mistaken for bacterial superinfection.

molluscum is often sexually transmitted in adults and adolescents, genital and perianal molluscum in children is most often thought to be related to autoinoculation.[156]

Etiology

MC is usually spread by skin to skin and fomite to skin contact. Rare cases of vertical transmission to neonates have been reported.[157] The virus replicates only within the human epidermis, enhancing cell mitosis and disrupting epidermal cell differentiation, leading to the characteristic papules. The virus replicates in the cytoplasm and viral cores mature into Henderson-Paterson bodies as they move from the basal layer upward in the epidermis. The stratum corneum ultimately disintegrates as the inclusions enlarge and release mature virions from the umbilicated center of the lesion.[158]

Clinical Presentation

MC usually initially presents as small 1 to 3 mm "pearly" white-or flesh-colored papules that are smooth surfaced and dome shaped with central umbilication. The papules grow to around 3 to 5 mm in diameter and in an average infection number 11 to 20. However, some children, particularly those that are immunocompromised, can develop innumerable lesions (Figure 19-50). Dermoscopy can help identify molluscum lesions, demonstrating a multilobulated, white-to-yellow, amorphous central structure surrounded by a "crown" of blood vessels. Once the immune system recognizes and attacks the virus, the surrounding erythema often develops, sometimes progressing to an intense inflammatory reaction that can even result in large inflammatory papules or pustules (Figure 19-51) that are often mistaken for *Staphylococcal* abscesses. The formation of abscess-like lesions occurs in follicular-centered lesions. A pox-like scar can occur in lesions, with and without this follicular inflammation, upon resolution of the papule.[159]

The time to resolution of individual lesions is thought to be around 2 months and is usually much shorter than the overall resolution of the eruption in the affected patient due to autoinoculation from scratching and other trauma. The spread and formation of new lesions lasts for an average of about 1 year but can last for 2 to 4 years, with an average of 13% of patients still manifesting lesions after 24 months in one study.[160]

In addition to eczematous reactions surrounding molluscum papules, a number of interesting "id reactions" (hypersensitivity reactions distant from the site of infection) are known to occur to this viral infection. Eczematous eruptions at distant sites and/or a Gianotti-Crosti syndrome (papular acrodermatitis of childhood) like the eruption of juicy papules on extensor surfaces, elbows, and knees are not uncommon. More rarely, an erythema multiforme-like eruption (Figure 19-52) or erythema annulare centrifugum and even pseudolymphomas[161] can occur in association with molluscum.[162,163]

Eruptive MC with innumerable lesions can occur in immunocompromised individuals or atopics and may be worsened by corticosteroid or calcineurin usage.[164,165] Other unusual forme fruste of this disorder include giant molluscum lesions that usually occur in immunocompromised patients.[166]

Clinically, molluscum can have multiple mimics. Histoplasmosis, cryptococcosis, coccidiomycosis, and other infections such as *Penicillium marneffei, Blastomyces dermatitidis, Paracoccidioides brasiliensis, Sporothrix schenckii, or atypical and typical mycobacteria; leishmaniasis; bacterial infections caused by Bartonella quintana and B. henselae; human papillomavirus infections; and Kaposi's sarcoma* have been known to mimic molluscum.[167,168] Preputial ectopic sebaceous glands,[169] lymphangioma circumscriptum,[170] Langerhans cell histiocytosis,[171] subepidermal calcified nodules,[171] leprosy,[173] squamous cell cancers,[174] and a variety of other entities have all been reported to present with molluscum-like

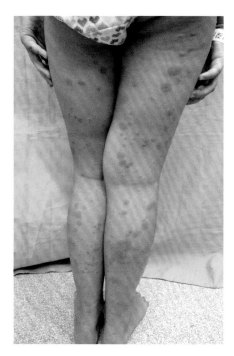

FIGURE 19-52. Targetoid plaques of an erythema multiforme type "id" reaction associated with the scattered molluscum seen in the background.

umbilicated papules. This author has biopsied skin-colored papules with a molluscum-like appearance that were found to be multiple juvenile xanthogranuloma.

Histologic Findings

MC shows an endophytic proliferation of squamous lobules with variable connection to the skin surface. They are separated from one another by delicate fibrous septa. The most striking histologic feature of MC lesions is the formation of large eosinophilic inclusions in the cytoplasm of infected keratinocytes; they are relatively small in the inferior aspects of the lesional lobules, but occupy virtually the entire cell volume more superficially (Figure 19-53). The inclusions are extruded into ectatic ostia that lead to the skin surface. As true of other intradermal proliferations such as dermatofibromas, MC lesions may induce basal epidermal hyperplasia which resembles the image of superficial basal cell carcinoma.[175]

In the early stages of MC, virtually no inflammation is apparent. However, as the lesions enlarge and potentially ulcerate, a lymphoid infiltrate may appear. This is particularly true in regressing foci. The infiltrate may uncommonly be so dense that a lymphoproliferative lesion could be considered microscopically.[176]

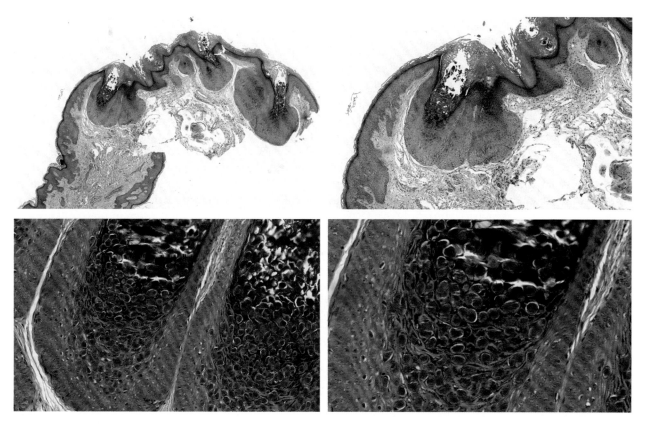

FIGURE 19-53. Histologically, molluscum contagiosum manifests with endophytic lobules of squamous epithelium, with large, brightly eosinophilic intracellular inclusions of viral particles. The viral inclusions displaced the nuclei to the side of the cell. Digital slides courtesy of Path Presenter.com.

Conventional H&E staining is sufficient to establish the diagnosis of MC. However, because the eosinophilic inclusions represent agglomerations of this DNA virus, they will label brightly with the Feulgen histochemical stain as well.[177]

CAPSULE SUMMARY

MOLLUSCUM CONTAGIOSUM

MC is caused by cutaneous infection by molluscipox DNA virus and is common in young children and immunocompromised individuals. The infection is probably transmitted via skin-skin or skin-fomite contact. Clinical presentation includes small pearly white- or flesh-colored, dome-shaped papules with central umbilication and may be innumerable in immunodeficient patients. It may be associated with "id" reactions. Histologic findings are singular with an endophytic proliferation of squamous lobules, the cells of which contain large eosinophilic inclusions. Large lesions may be associated with a lymphocytic inflammatory reaction that may be florid in some instances.

COWPOX/"CATPOX"

Definition and Epidemiology

Cowpox is an orthopoxvirus that presents similarly to orf, but is transmitted to humans by cattle, cats, and possibly rodents. This is thought to be the virus that Edward Jenner utilized in his original 18th-century experiments with prevention of smallpox (also an orthopoxvirus) by vaccination. Pseudocowpox (also referred to as milker's nodules, milker's node, or paravaccinia), on the other hand, was referred to by Jenner as "spurious cowpox", as exposure to this parapoxvirus did not confer any immunity to the smallpox virus.[178]

Cowpox is probably limited to Europe, Eastern Europe, and some areas in Russia. One review found that there is a high proportion of girls aged 12 or younger who have been infected. This has been ascribed to their habit of cat cuddling.[179]

Etiology

Despite the moniker, the cowpox virus in recent times is usually acquired from cats, which are likely infected by rodents. Affected cats usually have a history of a single primary lesion with a scabbed wound or large abscess most often involving the head, neck, or forelimb.[180]

Clinical Presentation

The incubation period for this virus is about 1 week. Painful papules then develop, which can quickly become vesicles. Classically, in about 5 to 7 days, an umbilicated pustule then forms with surrounding edema and erythema, and this lesion then develops into a crust, eschar, or ulcer. The lesion (most patients only have one) takes about 6 to 8 weeks to resolve, and often does scar. The patient may have single or multiple lesions, usually on the hands or face. Draining lymph nodes often become enlarged, swollen, and painful. There have been atopic patients who develop an "eczema vaccinatum"-type reaction with lesions that resemble smallpox.[178]

CAPSULE SUMMARY

COWPOX-CATPOX

Cowpox is caused by an orthopoxvirus that is carried by cattle, cats, and rodents, with the most recent cases spread by cats. The disease is generally restricted to Europe and parts of Asia. Clinical presentation includes painful papules that become vesicular and pustular with surrounding erythema. The lesions then develop into ulcers or eschars. Regional lymphadenitis may be present. Histologic findings are similar to those of HSV infection and pseudopox (Milker's Nodule; see the next section).

PSEUDOPOX (MILKER'S NODULE)

Definition and Epidemiology

Milker's nodules are caused by a parapoxvirus that infects the teats of cattle. There is controversy about whether orf, milker's nodules, and the bovine papular stomatitis virus are actually distinct viral strains. However, multiple investigators have looked at their DNA and found distinctions.[181] The parapoxvirus that causes milker's nodules has also been referred to as paravaccinia or pseudocowpox. This comes from the historical distinction that Jenner made regarding this strain as "spurious cowpox" to indicate that inoculation did not confer immunity against smallpox.[178]

Pseudocowpox has a worldwide distribution and usually occurs in those with occupational or other exposure to cow teats. It seems to occur more often in "new milkers"—those who have not had long-time experience with milking, such as young people—perhaps because chronic exposure confers some immunologic protection.[182]

Etiology

The pseudocowpox virus is transmitted by infected lesions on cows by direct contact and often occurs in previously traumatized skin. Bovine papular stomatitis can occur with exposure to the mouth of infected animals.[178,182]

Clinical Presentation

Lesions are morphologically similar to orf (see figures). They start as a tiny red macule or papule that enlarges at the periphery and elevates centrally to form a targetoid round, oval, or dome-shaped, well-demarcated nodule that is usually 1 to 2 cm in diameter. The papular stage is about a week and it is another week to develop into the tartoid nodule with a red center and surrounding white ring and red halo. Resolution into a firm-crusted nodules occurs over the next week and then regression with crusting in the final weeks. Lesions are usually painless, with occasional mild swelling of draining lymph nodes. The lesions are often solitary but can be multiple. It is unusual to have more than six lesions in a patient.[182]

There have been rare reports of erythema nodosum, erythema multiform, or other exanthems distant from the primary lesions of milker's nodules.[183] In immunocompromised hosts, there have been reports of erythema multiforme the triggering of graft versus host disease.[183]

Histologic Findings

The lesions of cutaneous cowpox and pseudopox exhibit histologic changes that are similar to those seen in infections with *Herpes simplex* or *Varicella-zoster*. They feature cytoplasmic vacuolization, ballooning, and reticular degeneration of keratinocytes, prominent epidermal acantholysis, vesicle formation, and eventual ulceration (Figure 19-54). Viral inclusions in cowpox are cytoplasmic rather than intranuclear, and they have a brightly eosinophilic appearance. Multinucleation of the infected cells is uncommon. Inflammation is mononuclear and relatively scanty in evolving lesions, but ulcerated ones are associated with neutrophilic infiltrates as well.

Viral antigens can be demonstrated immunohistochemically in the intracytoplasmic inclusions of cowpox. Ultrastructural features of poxviruses in general include a nucleocapsid core, an intermediate coat, and a lipoprotein envelope.[185-189]

CAPSULE SUMMARY

MILKER'S NODULE (PSEUDOPOX)

The disease is caused by a DNA parapoxvirus that is present in the teats of cattle. It has a worldwide distribution, is transmitted by direct contact with bovine teats, and tends to develop in previously damaged skin. Clinical presentation includes a small red maculopapule on a hand that becomes targetoid, round, and dome-shaped, attaining a size of 1 to 2 cm. It is self-regressing and crusted, and multiple lesions are unusual. Pathologic findings include cytoplasmic vacuolization of infected keratinocytes with ballooning or reticular degeneration, epidermal acantholysis, vesicle formation, and ulceration. Inflammatory response may be absent, lymphocytic, or neutrophilic.

ORF

Definition and Epidemiology

Orf is a zoonotic parapoxvirus infection that infects sheep, goats, and the humans who work with those animals. It has alternatively been referred to as scabby mouth or sore mouth in animals because of the orofacial vesicles and scabs. In humans, it is also known as ecthyma contagiosum, contagious pustular dermatosis, and infectious pustular dermatitis. The name "orf" is derived from the Anglo Saxon name for cattle.[190]

Young animals are more susceptible to orf virus, and many cases occur in the spring and early summer; these are related to bottle-feeding and close contact with lambs. The incidence of orf virus infection in children is not totally clear, but multiple case reports indicate that some of their

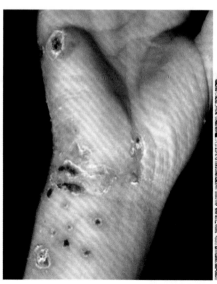 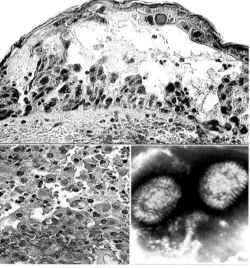

FIGURE 19-54. **Crusted lesions of cow-catpox are seen on the hand and wrist of this adolescent girl.** Microscopically, marked epidermal acantholysis is apparent, with reticular degeneration (top right panel) and eosinophilic, cytoplasmic viral inclusions (first bottom right panel). Parapox virions are seen in the cytoplasm of infected cells using transmission electron microscopy (second bottom right panel).

behaviors—nuzzling animals, sustaining animal bites, practicing poor hand hygiene, and general willingness to come into close contact with sick animals—make zoonoses more common than in adults.[191] Farmers and their children, wool shearers, veterinarians, and other individuals with close contact with animals are most commonly infected, with rare cases associated with religious feasts involving sacrificial goats or sheep. There have been reported outbreaks involving multiple children and adults on a particular farm.[192]

Etiology

Orf is caused by the double-stranded DNA parapoxvirus shed from the scab of the animal host lesions entering through traumatized skin and then replicating in epidermal cells. The infection is associated with an increase in epidermal keratinocyte replication and viral angiogenic factors. This hyperproliferation, angiogenesis, and accompanying influx of neutrophils followed by the accumulation of T-cells, B-cells, and MHC Class II dendritic cells lead to the evolution of the clinical presentation, as described in the next section. Viruses with features similar to those of the orf parapoxvirus are also found in camels, red squirrels, seals, musk ox, cats, and reindeer.[193-195]

Clinical Presentation

Orf lesions develop in six sequential stages on the skin, each stage lasting about 6 days. The initial stage is an erythematous macule with central papule (Figure 19-55). This progresses to a target lesion with a red center surrounded by a

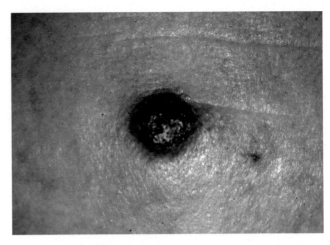

FIGURE 19-56. **Orf lesion in red papule stage of development, beginning to become weepy.** Photo courtesy of Kenneth Greer MD, University of Virginia.

white middle ring, with a peripheral red halo. A nodule arises from the center of the target lesion (Figure 19-56) and begins a weeping phase, which then forms a dry crust with black dots at its apex (Figure 19-57). Finally, there is a papillomatous stage that looks verrucous in morphology and then a regressive stage with dry crust and eventual shedding of the scab. Systemic symptoms may include localized lymphadenopathy and lymphangitis. Fever, rigors, drenching sweats, malaise, and urticaria are rare.[196] The most variable clinical feature seems to be pain, with some patients reporting painless lesions and others complaining of severe pain.[191]

Unusual presentations of orf include giant lesions and the development of satellite lesions around the primary lesion; large progressive lesions may be more common in immunosuppressed patients.[197,198] Rarely, the orf virus can cause cutaneous manifestations remote from primary lesion or lesions at the sites of inoculation. An Orf-induced

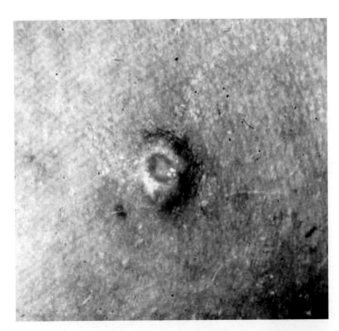

FIGURE 19-55. Early developing lesion of orf with erythematous background and central ring of pallor that is rising up into a papule. Photo courtesy of Kenneth Greer MD, University of Virginia.

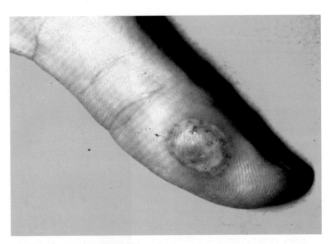

FIGURE 19-57. Maturing orf lesion with black dots and vesiculation of surface. Photo courtesy of Kenneth Greer MD, University of Virginia.

immunobullous disease with tense bullae clinically similar to bullous pemphigoid has been reported to manifest subepidermal blisters with a mixed inflammatory cell infiltrate containing neutrophils and eosinophils at the base. The direct immunofluorescence in these cases demonstrates IgG and C3 at the dermoepidermal junction, with indirect immunofluorescence demonstrating circulating antibasement membrane IgG binding to the dermal side of salt-split skin. The antigen for this immunobullous reaction is unknown at this time.[199] Multiple cases of erythema multiforme, as well as cases described as Stevens-Johnsons syndrome and papulovesicular eruptions, have been reported in association with primary Orf infections as well.[200]

Histologic Findings

The microscopic features of skin lesions in milker's nodule and orf are virtually identical. Both diseases are caused by *Paravaccinia* viruses. Histologically, one sees loculated intraepidermal blisters that are caused by a massive ballooning degeneration of infected keratocytes. They may subsequently rupture and ulcerate. Intracytoplasmic or, rarely, intranuclear inclusions may be present in the infected epithelial cells; they are eosinophilic but can be difficult to see. Papillary dermal edema is common, with inflammatory infiltrates of lymphocytes, histiocytes, plasma cells, and eosinophils throughout the corium. Mature lesions also exhibit marked epidermal acanthosis (Figures 19-58 and 19-59). The reaction pattern that has just been described is common to all of the diseases caused by poxviruses. Thus, the clinical history is important in deciding whether milker's nodule or orf is the proper final diagnosis. Both disorders manifest immunoreactivity for *Paravaccinia* virus in the epidermis, and Lendrum's phloxine-tartrazine histochemical stain will also label the cytoplasmic viral inclusions.[201-204]

CAPSULE SUMMARY

ORF (ECTHYMA CONTAGIOSUM)

Orf is caused by a parapoxvirus carried in the mouths of sheep and goats. Transmission is by direct skin contact with infected animal mucosa and is seen primarily in farmers, wool shearers, and veterinarians.

Several clinical stages are recognized, beginning with an erythematous, variably painful maculopapule on a hand, followed by targetoid, nodular, verrucoid, and crusted stages. Lymphadenitis, fever, and rigors are rarely present. Microscopic findings are essentially identical to those of Milker's Nodule, except that orf may show epidermal acanthosis and a more intense inflammatory reaction.

CUTANEOUS MANIFESTATIONS OF HIV IN CHILDREN

Definition and Epidemiology

Human immunodeficiency virus is a retrovirus infecting cells of the human immune system, resulting in acquired immunodeficiency syndrome and ultimately death without treatment. Pediatric infection results in a variety of infectious, inflammatory, and neoplastic cutaneous manifestations.

Pediatric HIV is acquired vertically in approximately 90% of cases. Historic transmission from infection mother to child was around 30%, but rates have dropped considerably with the advent of highly active retroviral therapy.[205,206] Transfusion of blood products may also result in pediatric infection. Most studies show that around half of children with HIV will have cutaneous manifestations, but some studies show rates of over 80%.[207,208]

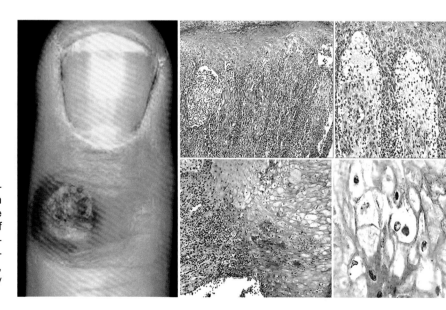

FIGURE 19-58. Pseudopox (milker's nodule) is seen on the finger of an adolescent boy, in its crusting phase (left panel). Microscopic features of pseudopox include ballooning degeneration of infected keratinocytes, dermal edema, cytoplasmic inclusions, and a dense dermal inflammatory infiltrate (right panels).

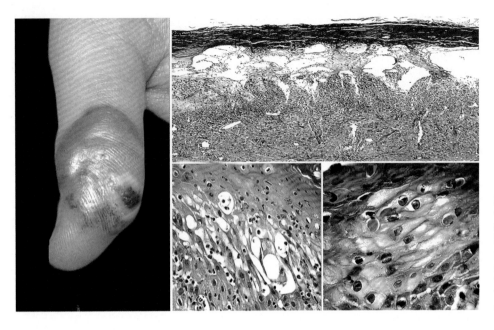

FIGURE 19-59. A nodular lesion with an erythematous periphery is seen in this case of orf, in an adolescent girl (left panel). As seen in pseudopox, dermal edema (top right panel), reticular epidermal degeneration (first bottom right panel), and cytoplasmic inclusions (second bottom right panel) are evident.

Etiology

As a retrovirus, HIV is a single-stranded DNA virus that uses reverse transcriptase, ribonuclease, and integrase to transcribe double-strand DNA and integrate it into host chromosome. HIV preferentially targets CD4+ helper T-cells, leading to selective depletion via apoptosis and other mechanisms.[209] Immunodeficiency, especially of the cellular immune system, in turn, predisposes to infections as well as malignancies; alterations in immune response may result in the exaggeration of common inflammatory dermatoses as well.

Clinical Presentation

In general, infectious and inflammatory conditions in the setting of HIV, while clinically similar to those that are common in the general population, are more severe and less responsive to therapy.[210] The incidence and the severity of dermatologic findings in pediatric HIV are correlated with the degree of immunosuppression, specifically CD4 count.[211,212] Although acute primary infection is infrequently seen in children, older individuals often develop a maculopapular exanthem on the face and upper trunk (Figure 19-60).[213]

Cutaneous candidiasis is the most common infectious manifestation and may occur as erythematous plaques, papules, and pustules in the neck folds, diaper area, or axillae. Pseudomembranous plaques on the oral mucosa can be scraped off with a tongue depressor in thrush. Chronic candida paronychia affects slightly older children. Unusual or severe dermatophytosis is common as well.[210]

Varicella (chickenpox) infection may be severe with internal complications.[208,214] Children with HIV have increased incidence of zoster (shingles), which can be chronic, widespread, nodular, and ulcerative.[210,215] Herpes simplex infection in HIV children most commonly presents as an acute

gingivostomatitis with painful ulcers on the lips, tongue, palate, and buccal mucosa. Severe, current, and chronic disease may occur.[216] MC infection can feature numerous, large, atypical, and verrucous lesions of uncommon locations, like the head and neck.[208] These may mimic cryptococcosis and histoplasmosis and are refractory to conventional therapy.[216]

Human papillomavirus infections, especially plane warts, are common in children with HIV and are often difficult to treat.[208] CMV manifests as perianal ulcerations and may also cause diaper dermatitis.[65] EBV is associated with corrugated adherent white plaques on the lateral tongue (OHL).

Bacterial infections including impetigo, ecthyma, and cellulitis are increased in children with HIV, and *Staphylococcus aureus* is a common culprit. Internal and systemic infections are common as well.[214] Scabies may be severe, and

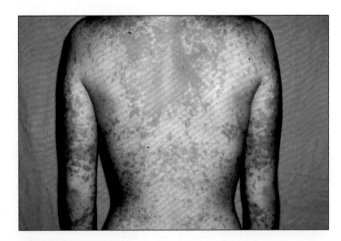

FIGURE 19-60. Nonspecific morbilliform, maculopapular erythematous eruption of primary HIV. Photo courtesy of Kenneth Greer MD, University of Virginia.

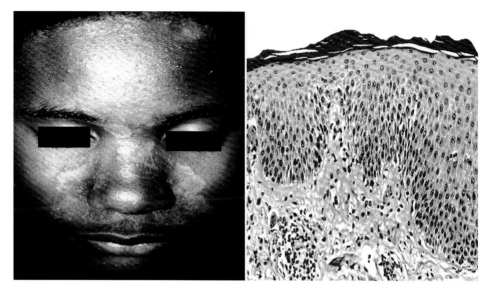

FIGURE 19-61. This adolescent boy who is infected with HIV has the typical scaly facial eruption of seborrheic dermatitis (left panel). Microscopically, one sees a subacute spongiotic dermatitis with intermittent parakeratosis (right panel).

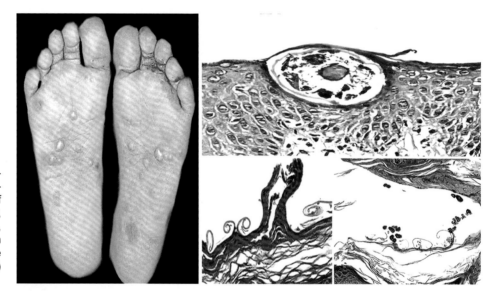

FIGURE 19-62. Another HIV-infected child shows the lesions of scabies mite infestation on the soles of the feet (left panel). Microscopically, complete mites (top right panel), "pigtails" in the stratum corneum (first bottom right panel), and mite scybala (second bottom right panel) are present.

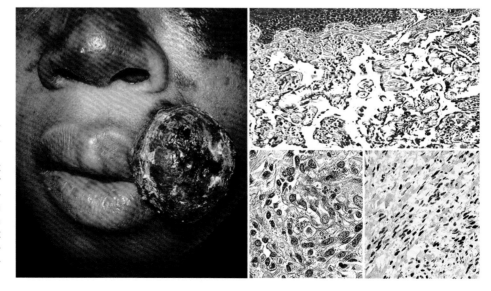

FIGURE 19-63. This African boy with HIV infection has a large, ulcerated nodular lesion of the face, representing Kaposi's sarcoma (left panel). Histologically, that tumor demonstrates random dermal neovascularization (top right panel), with eosinophilic cytoplasmic inclusions in some lesional cells (first bottom right panel). The tumor cells are immunoreactive for HHV8-latent nuclear antigen-1 (second bottom right panel).

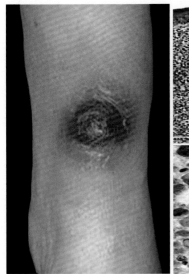

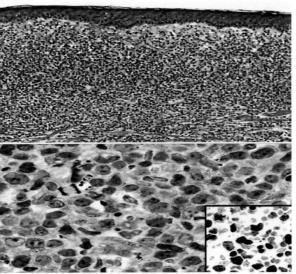

FIGURE 19-64. Another HIV-infected child has a nodular, violaceous, ulcerated lesion of the lower leg (left panel). It comprises a dense infiltrate of large, atypical lymphoid cells, representing large-cell lymphoma (right panels). The lesional cells are immunoreactive for HHV8-latent nuclear antigen-1 (bottom right panel inset).

TABLE 19-1.	**Cutaneous disorders in patients with HIV infection.**
Infections	**Viral**—molluscum contagiosum; herpes simplex; varicella-zoster; verruca vulgaris and condyloma acuminata; cytomegalovirus
	Bacterial—mycobacteria; bacillary angiomatosis
	Spirochetal—syphilis
	Fungal—candidiasis; superficial dermatophytoses; histoplasmosis; cryptococcosis; phaeohyphomycosis; nocardiosis; zygomycosis; pneumocystosis
Parasitoses	Amebiasis; acanthamebiasis; Leishmaniasis; scabies
Dermatoses	psoriasis; seborrheic dermatitis; pityriasis rubra pilaris; acquired ichthyosis; asteatosis; porokeratosis; leukocytoclastic vasculitis; eosinophilic folliculitis; papular pruritic eruption; palmoplantar keratoderma; acrodermatitis enteropathica; neutrophilic eccrine hidradenitis
Neoplasms	Kaposi's sarcoma; cutaneous lymphomas; squamous and basal cell carcinomas; Merkel cell carcinoma; malignant melanoma

crusted (Norwegian) scabies may occur in the setting of severely depressed CD4 count.[216]

Seborrheic dermatitis is the most common inflammatory dermatosis in HIV-positive children.[208] Infants may have erythema and scale of the face, scalp, and diaper area, whereas older children have a distribution more similar to that of adults.[216] Drug reactions are particularly common in HIV patients; up to 16% of children in one study developed a hypersensitivity reaction to trimethoprim-sulfamethoxazole.[217] Severe generalized atopic dermatitis occurs in these children.[210] Papular pruritic eruptions of the extremities may represent exaggerated arthropod bite reactions.[218]

A variety of nonspecific cutaneous manifestations, including vasculitis, aphthous ulcers, and sequelae of nutritional deficiencies (xerosis, alopecia, acrodermatitis enteropathica-like changes), may be observed in children with HIV.[217] Noncutaneous manifestations that may be evident of skin examination include generalized lymphadenopathy and chronic parotitis with parotid swelling. In contrast to adults with HIV, children are unlikely to develop Kaposi's sarcoma.[210]

Histologic Findings

HIV may directly cause a transient viral exanthem in patients who have been only recently infected. It clinically and pathologically resembles roseola (see previous paragraphs). In addition, the compromise in systemic immunity that HIV produces is associated with a host of secondary conditions that may affect the skin. These include various dermatoses, infections, infestations, and neoplastic proliferations, as summarized in Table 19-1 and discussed in detail elsewhere in this book. Selected examples are also illustrated in Figures 19-56 through 19-64.

REFERENCES

1. Fatahzadeh M, Schwartz RA. Human herpes simplex virus infections: Epidemiology, pathogenesis, symptomatology, diagnosis, and management. *J Am Acad Dermatol.* 2007;57(5):737-763.
2. Roberts CM, Pfister JR, Spear SJ. Increasing proportion of herpes simplex virus type 1 as a cause of genital herpes infection in college students. *Sex Trans Dis.* 2003;30(10): 797-800.
3. Simmons A. Clinical manifestations and treatment considerations of herpes simplex virus infection. *J Infect Dis.* 2002;186(suppl 1): S71-77.
4. Bradley H, Markowitz LE, Gibson T, McQuillan GM. Seroprevalence of Herpes simplex virus types 1 and 2—United States, 1999–2010. *J Infect Dis.* 2014;209(3):325-333.

5. Miller CS, Danaher RJ, Jacob RJ. Molecular aspects of herpes simplex virus I latency, reactivation, and recurrence. *Crit Rev Oral Biol Med.* 1998;9(4):541-562.

6. McAdam AJ, Milner DA, Sharpe AH. Infectious diseases. In: Kumar V, Abbas AK, Aster JC, eds. *Robbins & Cotran Pathologic Basis of Disease.* Philadelphia, PA: Elsevier; 2015:341-402.

7. Ichihashi M, Nagai H, Matsunaga K. Sunlight is an important causative factor of recurrent herpes simplex. *Cutis.* 74(5, Suppl): 14-18.

8. Gittler JK, Mu EW, Orlow SJ. Characterization of herpes simplex virus infections seen in the pediatric dermatology office. *Pediatr Dermatol.* 2017;34(4):446-449.

9. Al-Dujaili LJ, Clerkin PP, Clement C, et al. Ocular herpes simplex virus: how are latency, reactivation, recurrent disease and therapy interrelated? *Future Microbiol.* 2011;6(8):877-907.

10. Harris JB, Holmes AP. Neonatal herpes simplex viral infections and acyclovir: an update. *J Pediatr Pharmacol Therap.* 2017;22(2):88-93.

11. Xu F, Sternberg MR, Kottiri BJ, et al. Trends in herpes simplex virus type 1 and type 2 seroprevalence in the United States. *JAMA.* 2006;296(8): 964-973.

12. Goldkrand JW. Intrapartum inoculation of herpes simplex virus by fetal scalp electrode. *Obstet Gynecol.* 1982;59(2):263-265.

13. Friedrich ER, Cole W, Middelkamp JN. Herpes simplex. Clinical aspects and electron microscopic findings. *Am J Obstet Gynecol.* 1969;104(5): 758-779.

14. Singer DB. Pathology of neonatal Herpes simplex virus infection. *Perspect Pediatr Pathol.* 1981;6:243-278.

15. Nikkels AF, Hermanns-Lê T, Nikkels-Tassoudji N, Piérard GE. [Diagnosis of skin infections caused by simplex-type herpes virus and by varicella zona]. *Rev Med Liege.* 1993;48(7):401-405.

16. Spijkervet FK, Vissink A, Raghoebar GM, van der Waal I. [Vesiculobullous lesions of the oral mucosa]. *Ned Tijdschr Tandheelkd.* 2001;108(6): 223-228.

17. Yirrell DL, Norval M, Reid HW. Local epidermal viral infections: comparative aspects of vaccinia virus, herpes simplex virus and human papillomavirus in man and orf virus in sheep. *FEMS Immunol Med Microbiol.* 1994;8(1):1-12.

18. Schneider LC, Schneider AE. Diagnosis of oral ulcers. *Mt Sinai J Med.* 1998;65(5-6): 383-387.

19. Requena L, Requena C. [Histopathology of the more common viral skin infections]. *Actas Dermosifiliogr.* 2010;101(3): 201-216.

20. Seward JF, Zhang JX, Maupin TJ, Mascola L, Jumaan AO. Contagiousness of varicella a household contact study. *JAMA.* 2004;292(6):704-708.

21. Seward JF, Marin M, Vázquez M. Varicella vaccine effectiveness in the US vaccination program: a review. *J Infect Dis.* 2008;197(Suppl 2):S82-89

22. Zhu S, Zeng F, Xia L, He H, Zhang J. Incidence rate of breakthrough varicella observed in healthy children after 1 or 2 doses of varicella vaccine: results from a meta-analysis. *Am J Infect Control.* 2017;S0196-6553(17):30945-30948.

23. Edmunds WJ, Brisson, M. The effect of vaccination on the epidemiology of varicella zoster virus. *J Infect.* 2002;44(4):211-219.

24. Weinmann S, Chun C, Schmid DS, et al. Incidence and clinical characteristics of herpes zoster among children in the varicella vaccine era, 2005–2009. *J Invest Dermatol.* 2013;208(11):1859-1868.

25. Kawaguchi Y, Mori Y, Kimura H (Editors): *Human Herpesviruses.* New York, NY: Springer; 2018.

26. Ahn KH, Park YJ, Hong SC1, et al. Congenital varicella syndrome: a systematic review. *J Obstet Gynecol.* 2016;36(5):563-566.

27. Sauerbrei A, Wutzler P. Neonatal varicella. *J Perinatol.* 2001;21(8):5450549-5450549.

28. Weinberg JM. Herpes zoster: epidemiology, natural history, and common complications. *J Am Acad Dermatol.* 2007;57(6):S130-135.

29. Paller A, Mancini AJ. *Viral Diseases of the Skin.* Philadelphia, PA: Elsevier; 2011: 348-369.

30. Bernard HU, Burk RD, Chen Z, van Doorslaer K, zur Hausen H, de Villiers EM. Classification of papillomaviruses (PVs) based on 189 PV types and proposal of taxonomic amendments. *Virology.* 2010;401(1):70-79.

31. Egawa N, Doorbar J. The low-risk papillomaviruses. *Virus Res.* 2017;231:119-127.

32. Bruggink SC, de Koning MN, Gussekloo J, et al. Cutaneous wart-associated HPV types: Prevalence and relation with patient characteristics. *J Clin Virol.* 2012;55(3):250-255.

33. Jabłonska S, Majewski S, Obalek S, Orth G. Cutaneous warts. *Clin Dermatol.* 1997;15(3):309-319.

34. Cardoso JC, Calonje E. Cutaneous manifestations of human papillomaviruses: a review. *Acta Dermatovenerol APA.* 2011;20(3):145-154.

35. Monk BJ, Tewari KS. The spectrum and clinical sequelae of human papillomavirus infection. *Gynecol Oncol.* 2007;107(2):S6-S13.

36. Kilkenny M, Merlin K, Young R, Marks R. The prevalence of common skin conditions in Australian school students: 1. Common, plane and plantar viral warts. *Br J Dermatol.* 1998;138(5):840-845.

37. Stefanaki C, Barkas G, Valari M, et al. Condylomata acuminata in children. *Pediatr Infect Dis.* 2012;31(4): 440-442.

38. Jones V, Smith SJ, Omar HA. Nonsexual transmission of anogenital warts in children: a retrospective analysis. *Sci World J.* 2007;(7):1896-1899.

39. Sinclair KA, Woods CR, Sinal SH. Venereal warts in children. *Pediatr Rev.* 2011;32(3):115-121; quiz 121.

40. Stanley M. Immune responses to human papillomavirus. *Vaccine.* 2006;24(suppl 1):S16-S22.

41. Orth G, Jablonska S, Breitburd F, Favre M, Croissant O. The human papillomaviruses. *Bull Cancer.* 1978;65(2): 151-164.

42. Prasad CJ. Pathobiology of human papillomavirus. *Clin Lab Med.* 1995;15(3): 685-704.

43. Cheah PL, Looi LM. Biology and pathological associations of the human papillomaviruses: a review. *Malays J Pathol* 1998;20(1):1-10.

44. Fazel N, Wilczynski S, Lowe L, Su LD. Clinical, histopathologic, and molecular aspects of cutaneous human papillomavirus infections. *Dermatol Clin.* 1999;17(3):521-536, viii.

45. Ahmed AM, Madkan V, Tyring SK. Human papillomaviruses and genital disease. *Dermatol Clin.* 2006;24(2):157-165, vi.

46. Lewandowsky F, Lutz W. Ein Fall einer bisher nicht beschrie- benen Hauterkrankung. *Arch Dermatol Syph.* 1992;141:193-203.

47. Ramoz N, Rueda LA, Bouadjar B, Montoya LS, Orth G, Favre M. Mutations in two adjacent novel genes are associated with epidermodysplasia verruciformis. *Nat Genet.* 2002;32(4):579-581.

48. Orth G. Genetics of epidermodysplasia verruciformis: insights into host defense against papillomaviruses. *Semin Immunol.* 2006;18(6): 362-374.

49. Hampras SS, Rollison DE, Tommasino M, et al. Genetic variations in the epidermodysplasia verruciformis (EVER/TMC) genes, cutaneous human papillomavirus infection and squamous cell carcinoma of the skin. *Br J Dermatol.* 2015;173(6):1532-1535.

50. Przybyszewska J, Zlotogorski A, Ramot Y. Re-evaluation of epidermodysplasia verruciformis: Reconciling more than 90 years of debate. *J Am Acad Dermatol.* 2017,76(6): 1161-1175.

51. Rogers HD, MacGregor JL, Nord KM, et al. Acquired epidermodysplasia verruciformis. *J Am Acad Dermatol.* 2009;60(2): 315-320.

52. Soyer HP, Rigel D, Wurm EMT. *Actinic Keratosis, Basal Cell Carcinoma, and Squamous Cell Carcinoma.* Philadelphia, PA: Elsevier; 2017.

53. Lutzner MA, Blanchet-Bardon C. Epidermodysplasia verruciformis. *Curr Probl Dermatol.* 1985;13:164-185.

54. Dubina M, Goldenberg G. Viral-associated nonmelanoma skin cancers: a review. *Am J Dermatopathol.* 2009;31(6):561-573.

55. Burger B, Itin PH. Epidermodysplasia verruciformis. *Curr Probl Dermatol.* 2014;45:123-131.

56. Smola S. Human papillomaviruses and skin cancer. *Adv Exp Med Biol.* 2014;810:192-207.

57. Fernandez-Flores A. Lesions With an Epidermal Hyperplastic Pattern: Morphologic Clues in the Differential Diagnosis. *Am J Dermatopathol.* 2016;38(1): 1-16; quiz 17-19.

58. Drago F, Aragone MG, Lugani C, Rebora A. Cytomegalovirus infection in normal and immunocompromised humans: a review. *Dermatology.* 2000;200(3):189-195.

59. Kenneson A, Cannon MJ. Review and meta-analysis of the epidemiology of congenital cytomegalovirus (CMV) infection. *Rev Med Virol.* 2007;17(4): 253-276.

60. Malm G, Engman ML. Congenital cytomegalovirus infections. *Semin Fetal Neonatal Med.* 2007;12(3):154-159.

61. Lesher JL Jr. Cytomegalovirus infections and the skin. *J Am Acad Dermatol.* 1988;18(6):1333-1338.

62. Blatt J, Kastner O, Hodes DS. Cutaneous vesicles in congenital cytomegalovirus infection. *J Pediatr.* 1978;92(3):509.

63. Dauden E, Fernández-Buezo G, Fraga J, Cardeñoso L, García-Díez A. Mucocutaneous presence of cytomegalovirus associated with human immunodeficiency virus infection: discussion regarding its pathogenetic role. *Arch Dermatol.* 2001;137(4):443-448.

64. Choi YL, Kim JA, Jang KT, et al. Characteristics of cutaneous cytomegalovirus infection in non-acquired immune deficiency syndrome, immunocompromised patients. *Br J Dermatol.* 2006;155(5):977-982.

65. Thiboutot DM, Beckford A, Mart CR, Sexton M, Maloney ME. Cytomegalovirus diaper dermatitis. *Arch Dermatol.* 1991;127(3):396-398.

66. Caputo R, Gelmetti C, Ermacora E, Gianni E, Silvestri A. Gianotti-Crosti syndrome: a retrospective analysis of 308 cases. *J Am Acad Dermatol.* 1992;26(2, Pt 1):207-210.

67. Jordan MC, Rousseau W, Stewart JA, Noble GR, Chin TD. Spontaneous cytomegalovirus mononucleosis. Clinical and laboratory observations in nine cases. *Ann Intern Med.* 1973;79(2):153-160.

68. Weigand DA, Burgdorf WH, Tarpay MM. Vasculitis in cytomegalovirus infection. *Arch Dermatol.* 1980;116(10):1174-1176.

69. Heilbron B, Saxe N. Scleredema in an infant. *Arch Dermatol.* 1986;122(12):1417-1419.

70. Chiewchanvit S, Thamprasert K, Siriunkgul S. Disseminated cutaneous cytomegalic inclusion disease resembling prurigo nodularis in a HIV-infected patient: a case report and literature review. *J Med Assoc Thai* 1993;76(10):581-584.

71. Swanson S, Feldman PS. Cytomegalovirus infection initially diagnosed by skin biopsy. *Am J Clin Pathol.* 1987;87(1):113-116.

72. Toome BK, Bowers KE, Scott GA. Diagnosis of cutaneous cytomegalovirus infection: a review and report of a case. *J Am Acad Dermatol.* 1991;24(5 Pt 2):860-867.

73. Chisholm C, Lopez L. Cutaneous infections caused by Herpesviridae: a review. *Arch Pathol Lab Med.* 2011;135(10):1357-1362.

74. Garib G, Hughey LC, Elmets CA, Cafardi JA, Andea AA. Atypical presentation of exophytic herpes simplex virus type 2 with concurrent cytomegalovirus infection: a significant pitfall in diagnosis. *Am J Dermatopathol.* 2013;35(3):371-376.

75. Thompson MP, Kurzrock R. Epstein-Barr virus and cancer. *Clin Cancer Res.* 2004;10(3): 803-821.

76. Hjalgrim H, Friborg J, Melbye M. The epidemiology of EBV and its association with malignant disease. In: Arvin A, Campadelli-Fiume G, Mocarski E, et al, eds. *Human Herpesviruses: Biology, Therapy, and Immunoprophylaxis.* Cambridge: Cambridge University Press; 2007.

77. Eminger LA, Hall LD, Hesterman KS, Heymann WR. Epstein-Barr virus: dermatologic associations and implications: part II. Associated lymphoproliferative disorders and solid tumors. *J Am Acad Dermatol.* 2015;72(1):21-34; quiz 35-26.

78. Cohen JI. Epstein-Barr virus infection. *N Engl J Med.* 2000;343(7):481-492.

79. Bass MH. Periorbital edema as the initial sign of infectious mononucleosis. *J Pediatr.* 1954;45(2): 204-205.

80. Patel BM. Skin rash with infectious mononucleosis and ampicillin. *Pediatrics.* 1967;40(5): 910-911.

81. Pullen H, Wright N, Murdoch JM. Hypersensitivity reactions to antibacterial drugs in infectious mononucleosis. *Lancet.* 1967;2(7527): 1176-1178.

82. Chovel-Sella A, Tov AB, Lahav E, et al. Incidence of rash after amoxicillin treatment in children with infectious mononucleosis. *Pediatrics.* 2013;131(5):e1424-1427.

83. Hofmann B, Schuppe HC, Adams O, Lenard HG, Lehmann P, Ruzicka T. Gianotti-Crosti syndrome associated with Epstein-Barr virus infection. *Pediatr Dermatol.* 1997;14(4): 273-277.

84. Lehman JS, Bruce AJ, Wetter DA, Ferguson SB, Rogers RS 3rd. Reactive nonsexually related acute genital ulcers: review of cases evaluated at Mayo Clinic. *J Am Acad Dermatol.* 2010;63(1):44-51.

85. Rosman IS, Berk DR, Bayliss SJ, White AJ, Merritt DF. Acute genital ulcers in nonsexually active young girls: case series, review of the literature, and evaluation and management recommendations. *Pediatr Dermatol.* 2012;29(2): 147-153.

86. Ketchem L, Berkowitz RJ, McIlveen L, Forrester D, Rakusan T. Oral findings in HIV-seropositive children. *Pediatr Dent.* 1990;12(3):143-146.

87. Dias EP, Israel MS, Silva Junior A, Maciel VA, Gagliardi JP, Oliveira RH. Prevalence of oral hairy leukoplakia in 120 pediatric patients infected with HIV-1. *Braz Oral Res.* 2006;20(2):103-107.

88. Moormann AM, Snider CJ, Chelimo K. The company malaria keeps: how co-infection with Epstein-Barr virus leads to endemic Burkitt lymphoma. *Curr Opin Infect Dis.* 2011;24(5):435-441.

89. Burkitt, D, Wright D. Geographical and tribal distribution of the African lymphoma in Uganda. *Br Med J.* 1966;1(5487):569-573.

90. Ogwang MD, Bhatia K, Biggar RJ, Mbulaiteye SM. Incidence and geographic distribution of endemic Burkitt lymphoma in northern Uganda revisited. *Int J Cancer.* 2008;123(11):2658-2663.

91. Rouphael NG, Talati NJ, Vaughan C, Cunningham K, Moreira R, Gould C. Infections associated with haemophagocytic syndrome. *Lancet Infect Dis.* 2007;7(12): 814-822.

92. Fisman DN. Hemophagocytic syndromes and infection. *Emerg Infect Dis.* 2000;6(6):601-608.

93. Di Lernia V, Mansouri Y. Epstein-Barr virus and skin manifestations in childhood. *Int J Dermatol.* 2013;52(10):1177-1184.

94. Wenner HA. Virus diseases associated with cutaneous eruptions. *Prog Med Virol.* 1973;16:269-336.

95. Bodemer, C. [Febrile eruptions and herpesviruses]. *Rev Prat.* 1997;47(13):1422-1427.

96. Baleviciene G, Maciuleviciené R, Schwartz RA. Papular acrodermatitis of childhood: the Gianotti-Crosti syndrome. *Cutis.* 2001;67(4):291-294.

97. Brandt O, Abeck D, Gianotti R, Burgdorf W. Gianotti-Crosti syndrome. *J Am Acad Dermatol.* 2006;54(1):136-145.

98. Chuh A, Zawar V, Sciallis GF, Lee A. The diagnostic criteria of pityriasis rosea and Gianotti-Crosti syndrome—a protocol to establish diagnostic criteria of skin diseases. *J R Coll Physicians Edinb.* 2015;45(3):218-225.

99. Ales-Fernandez M, Rodríguez-Pichardo A, García-Bravo B, Ferrándiz-Pulido L, Camacho-Martínez FM. Three cases of Lipschutz vulval ulceration. *Int J STD AIDS.* 2010;21(5):375-376.

100. Haidari G, MacMahon E, Tong CY, White JA. Genital ulcers: it is not always simplex. *Int J STD AIDS.* 2015;26(1):72-73.

101. Stojanov IJ, Woo SB. Human papillomavirus and Epstein-Barr virus associated conditions of the oral mucosa. *Semin Diagn Pathol.* 2015;32(1):3-11.

102. Reichart PA, Langford A, Gelderblom HR, Pohle HD, Becker J, Wolf H. Oral hairy leukoplakia: observations in 95 cases and review of the literature. *J Oral Pathol Med.* 18(7):410-415.

103. Zunt SL, Tomich CE. Oral hairy leukoplakia. *J Dermatol Surg Oncol.* 1990;16(9): 812-816.

104. Cruchley AT, Williams DM, Niedobitek G, Young LS. Epstein-Barr virus: biology and disease. *Oral Dis.* 1997;3(Suppl 1):S156-163.

105. Tokura Y, Tamura Y, Takigawa M, et al. Severe hypersensitivity to mosquito bites associated with natural killer cell lymphocytosis. *Arch Dermatol.* 1990;126(3):362-368.

106. Satoh M, Oyama N, Akiba H, Ohtsuka M, Iwatsuki K, Kaneko F. Hypersensitivity to mosquito bites with natural-killer cell lymphocytosis: the possible implication of Epstein-Barr virus reactivation. *Eur J Dermatol.* 2002;12(4): 381-384.

107. Kimura H, Kawada J, Ito Y. Epstein-Barr virus-associated lymphoid malignancies: the expanding spectrum of hematopoietic neoplasms. *Nagoya J Med Sci.* 2013;75(3/4):169-179.

108. Gru AA, Jaffe ES. Cutaneous EBV-related lymphoproliferative disorders. *Semin Diagn Pathol.* 2017;34(1):60-75.

109. Kim TH, Lee JH, Kim YC, Lee SE. Hydroa vacciniforme-like lymphoma misdiagnosed as cutaneous lupus erythematosus. *J Cutan Pathol.* 2015;42(3):229-231.

110. Chen CC, Chang KC, Medeiros LJ, Lee JY. Hydroa vacciniforme and hydroa vacciniforme-like T-cell lymphoma: an uncommon event for transformation. *J Cutan Pathol.* 2016;43(12):1102-1111.

111. Paik JH, Choe JY, Kim H, et al. Clinicopathological categorization of Epstein-Barr virus-positive T/NK-cell lymphoproliferative disease: an analysis of 42 cases with an emphasis on prognostic implications. *Leuk Lymphoma.* 2017;58(1): 53-63.

112. Toksoy A, Strifler S, Benoit S, et al. Hydroa vacciniforme-like skin lesions in Epstein-Barr-virus-associated T-cell lymphoproliferation with subsequent development of aggressive NK/T-cell lymphoma. *Acta Derm Venereol.* 2017;97(3): 379-380.

113. Wang RC, Chang ST, Hsieh YC, et al. Spectrum of Epstein-Barr virus-associated T-cell lymphoproliferative disorder in adolescents and young adults in Taiwan. *Int J Clin Exp Pathol.* 2014;7(5):2430-2437.

114. Tohyama M, Hashimoto K. New aspects of drug-induced hypersensitivity syndrome. *J Dermatol.* 2011;38(3):222-228.

115. Stander S, Metze D, Luger T, Schwarz T. [Drug Reaction with Eosinophilia and Systemic Symptoms (DRESS): a review]. *Hautarzt.* 2013;64(8):611-622; quiz 623-614.

116. Zerr D, Meier AS, Selke SS, et al. A population-based study of primary human herpesvirus 6 infection. *N Engl J Med.* 2005;352(8):768-776.

117. Broccolo F, Drago F, Careddu AM, et al. Additional evidence that pityriasis rosea is associated with reactivation of human herpesvirus-6 and -7. *J Invest Dermatol.* 2005;124(6):1234-1240.

118. Drago F, Broccolo F, Rebora A. Pityriasis rosea: An update with a critical appraisal of its possible herpesviral etiology. *J Am Acad Dermatol.* 2009;61(2):303-318.

119. Stone RC, Micali GA, Schwartz RA. Roseola infantum and its causal human herpesviruses. *Int J Dermatol.* 2014;53(4):397-403.

120. Leach CT, Sumaya CV, Brown NA. Human herpesvirus-6: Clinical implications of a recently discovered, ubiquitous agent. *J Pediatr.* 1992;121(2):173-181.

121. Ablashi D, Agut H, Alvarez-Lafuente R, et al. Classification of HHV-6A and HHV-6 B as distinct viruses. *Arch Virol.* 2014;159:863-870.

122. Mohammadpour Touserkani F, Gaínza-Lein M, Jafarpour S, Brinegar K, Kapur K, Loddenkemper T. HHV-6 and seizure: A systematic review and meta-analysis. *J Med Virol.* 2017;89(1):161-169.

123. Vidimos AT, Camisa C. Tongue and cheek: oral lesions in pityriasis rosea. *Cutis.* 1992;50(4):276-280.

124. Ciccarese, G., Broccolo F, Rebora A, Parodi A, Drago F. Oropharyngeal lesions in pityriasis rosea. *J Am Acad Dermatol.* 2017;77(5):833-837.e834.

125. Panizzon R, Bloch PH. Histopathology of pityriasis rosea Gibert. Qualitative and quantitative light-microscopic study of 62 biopsies of 40 patients. *Dermatologica.* 1982;165(6): 551-558.

126. Ventarola D, Bordone L, Silverberg N. Update on hand-foot-and-mouth disease. *Clin Dermatol.* 2015;33(3):340-346.

127. Harvell JD, Selig DJ. Seasonal variations in dermatologic and dermatopathologic diagnoses: a retrospective 15-year analysis of dermatopathologic data. *Int J Dermatol.* 2016;55(10):1115-1118.

128. Rao DC, Naidu JR, Maiya PP, Babu A, Bailly JL. Large-scale HFMD epidemics caused by Coxsackievirus A16 in Bangalore, India during 2013 and 2015. *Infect Genet Evol.* 2017;(55):228-235.

129. Aswathyraj S, Arunkumar G, Alidjinou EK, Hober D. Hand, foot and mouth disease (HFMD): emerging epidemiology and the need for a vaccine strategy. *Med Microbiol Immunol.* 2016;205(5):397-407.

130. Mao Q, Wang Y, Yao X, et al. Coxsackievirus A16: epidemiology, diagnosis, and vaccine. *Hum Vaccin Immunother.* 2014;10(2):360-367.

131. Lott JP, Liu K, Landry ML. Atypical hand-foot-and-mouth disease associated with coxsackievirus A6 infection. *J Am Dermatol.* 2013;69(5): 736-741.

132. Guan H, Wang J, Wang C, et al. Etiology of multiple Non-EV71 and Non-CVA16 enteroviruses associated with hand, foot and mouth disease in Jinan, China, 2009-June 2013. *PLOS One.* 2015;10(11): e0142733-e0142733.

133. Scott LA, Stone MS. Viral exanthems. *Dermatol Online J.* 2003;9(3):4-4.

134. Ooi MH, Wong SC, Lewthwaite P, Cardosa MJ, Solomon T. Clinical features, diagnosis, and management of enterovirus 71. *Lancet Neurol.* 2010;9(11): 1097-1105.

135. Mathes EF, Oza V, Frieden IJ, et al. "Eczema coxsackium" and unusual cutaneous findings in an enterovirus outbreak. *Pediatrics.* 2013; 132(1):e149-157.

136. Shin JY, Cho BK, Park HJ. A clinical study of nail changes occurring secondary to hand-foot-mouth disease: onychomadesis and Beau's lines. *Ann Dermatol.* 2014;26(2):280-283.

137. Long D-l, Zhu SY, Li CZ, Chen CY, Du WT, Wang X. Late-onset nail changes associated with hand, foot, and mouth disease: a clinical analysis of 56 cases. *Pediatr Dermatol.* 2016;33(4):424-428.

138. Parra CA. Hand, foot and mouth disease. Light and electron microscopic observations. *Arch Dermatol Forsch.* 1972;245(2): 147-153.

139. Barriere H, Berger M, Billaudel S. [Hand, foot and mouth disease]. *Sem Hop.* 1976;52(39):2215-2220.

140. Buchner A. Hand, foot, and mouth disease. *Oral Surg Oral Med Oral Pathol.* 1976;41(3):333-337.

141. Servant-Delmas A, Morinet F. Update of the human parvovirus B19 biology. *Transfusion clinique et biologique.* 2016;23(1):5-12.

142. Young NS, Brown KE. Parvovirus B19. *N Engl J Med.* 2004;350(6): 586-597.

143. Vafaie J, Schwartz RA. Parvovirus B19 infections. *Int J Dermatol.* 2004;43(10):747-749.

144. Brown KE, Anderson SM, Young NS. Erythrocyte P antigen: cellular receptor for B19 parvovirus. *Science.* 1993;262(5130):114-117.

145. Kerr JR. The role of parvovirus B19 in the pathogenesis of autoimmunity and autoimmune disease. *J Clin Pathol.* 2016;69(4):279-291.

146. Hsieh MY, Huang PH. The juvenile variant of papular–purpuric gloves and socks syndrome and its association with viral infections. *Br J Dermatol.* 2004;151:201-206.

147. Gutermuth J, Nadas K, Zirbs M, et al. Papular-purpuric gloves and socks syndrome. *Lancet.* 2011;378(9786):198-198.

148. Fretzayas A, Douros K, Moustaki M, Nicolaidou P. Papular-purpuric gloves and socks syndrome in children and adolescents. *Pediatr Infect Dis.* 2009;28(3):250-252.

149. Magro CM, Dawood MR, Crowson AN. The cutaneous manifestations of human parvovirus B19 infection. *Hum Pathol.* 2000;31(4):488-497.

150. McNeely M, Friedman J, Pope E. Generalized petechial eruption induced by parvovirus B19 infection. *J Am Acad Dermatol.* 2005;52(5, Suppl 1):S109-S113.

151. Ofuji S, Yamamoto O. Acute generalized exanthematous pustulosis associated with a human parvovirus B19 infection. *J Dermatol.* 2007;34(2):121-123.

152. Parez N, Dehée A, Michel Y, Veinberg F, Garbarg-Chenon A. Papular-purpuric gloves and socks syndrome associated with B19V infection in a 6-year-old child. *J Clin Virol.* 2009;44(2):167-169.

153. Dohil MA, Lin P, Lee J, Lucky AW, Paller AS, Eichenfield LF. The epidemiology of molluscum contagiosum in children. *J Am Acad Dermatol.* 2006;54(1):47-54.

154. Olsen JR, Gallacher J, Piguet V, Francis NA. Epidemiology of molluscum contagiosum in children: a systematic review. *Fam Pract.* 2014;31(2):130-136.

155. Choong KY, Roberts LJ. Molluscum contagiosum, swimming and bathing: a clinical analysis. *Australas J Dermatol.* 1999;40(2):89-92.

156. Bargman, H. Is genital molluscum contagiosum a cutaneous manifestation of sexual abuse in children? *J Am Acad Dermatol.* 1986;14(5 Pt 1):847-849.

157. Luke JD, Silverberg NB. Vertically transmitted molluscum contagiosum infection. *Pediatrics.* 2010;125(2):e423-e425.

158. Chen X, Anstey AV, Bugert JJ. Molluscum contagiosum virus infection. *Lancet Infect Dis.* 2013;13(10): 877-888.

159. Brown J, Janniger CK, Schwartz RA, Silverberg NB. Childhood molluscum contagiosum. *Int J Dermatol.* 2006;45(2):93-99.

160. Olsen JR, Gallacher J, Finlay AY, Piguet V, Francis NA. Time to resolution and effect on quality of life of molluscum contagiosum in children in the UK: a prospective community cohort study. *Lancet Infect Dis.* 2015;15(2):190-195.

161. de Diego J, Berridi D, Saracibar N, Requena L. Cutaneous pseudolymphoma in association with molluscum contagiosum. *Am J Dermatopathol.* 1998;20(5):518-521.

162. Vasily DB, Bhatia SG. Erythema annulare centrifugum and molluscum contagiosum. *Arch Dermatol.* 1978;114(12): 1853.

163. Lee HJ, Kwon JA, Kim JW. Erythema multiforme-like molluscum dermatitis. *Acta Derm Venereol.* 2002;82(3):217-218.

164. Solomon LM, Telner P. Eruptive molluscum contagiosum in atopic dermatitis. *Can Med Assoc J.* 1966;95(19): 978-979.

165. Goksugur N, Ozbostanci B, Goksugur SB. Molluscum contagiosum infection associated with pimecrolimus use in pityriasis alba. *Pediatr Dermatol.* 2007;24(5):E63-E65.

166. Lew W, Lee SH. Scalp mass. Giant molluscum contagiosum. *Arch Dermatol.* 1995;131(6):719, 722.

167. de Souza JA. Molluscum or a mimic? *Am J Med.* 2006;119(11): 927-929.

168. Antinori S. Molluscum or a mimic? Add Penicillium marneffei! *Am J Med.* 2007;120(11):e19-20; author reply e21.

169. Piccinno R, Carrel CF, Menni S, Brancaleon W. Preputial ectopic sebaceous glands mimicking molluscum contagiosum. *Acta Derm Venereol.* 1990;70(4): 344-345.

170. Gupta S, Radotra BD, Javaheri SM, Kumar B. Lymphangioma circumscriptum of the penis mimicking venereal lesions. *J Eur Acad Dermatol Venereol.* 2003;17(5):598-600.

171. Huang JT, Mantagos J, Kapoor R, Schmidt B, Maguiness S. Langerhans cell histiocytosis mimicking molluscum contagiosum. *J Am Acad Dermatol.* 2012;67(3):e117-118.

172. Kim HS, Kim MJ, Lee JY, Kim HO, Park YM. Multiple subepidermal calcified nodules on the thigh mimicking molluscum contagiosum. *Pediatr Dermatol.* 2011;28(2):191-192.

173. Chander R, Jabeen M, Malik M. Molluscum contagiosum-like lesions in histoid leprosy in a 10-year-old Indian boy. *Pediatr Dermatol.* 2013;30(6):e261-262.

174. Binitha MP, Sarita SP, Manju M. Photoletter to the editor: Squamous cell carcinoma associated with and masquerading as molluscum contagiosum. *J Dermatol Case Rep.* 2013;7(3):103-105.

175. Requena L, Requena C. [Histopathology of the more common viral skin infections]. *Actas Dermosifiliogr.* 2010;101(3): 201-216.

176. Kazakov DV, Burg G, Dummer R, Kempf W. Cutaneous lymphomas and pseudolymphomas: newly described entities. *Recent Results Cancer Res.* 2002;160:283-293.

177. Smith KJ, Yeager J, Skelton H. Molluscum contagiosum: its clinical, histopathologic, and immunohistochemical spectrum. *Int J Dermatol.* 1999;38(9): 664-672.

178. Diven DG. An overview of poxviruses. *J Am Acad Dermatol.* 2001;44(1): 1-16.

179. Wienecke R, Wolff H, Schaller M, Meyer H, Plewig G. Cowpox virus infection in an 11-year-old girl. *J Am Acad Dermatol.* 2000;42(5, Pt 2):892-894.

180. Haenssle HA, Kiessling J, Kempf VA, Fuchs T, Neumann C, Emmert S. Papular-purpuric gloves and socks syndrome. *J Am Acad Dermatol.* 2006;54(2, Suppl):S1-S4.

181. Gassmann U, Wyler R, Wittek R. Analysis of parapoxvirus genomes. *Arch Virol.* 1985;83(1/2):17-31.

182. Cawley EP, Wheeler CE. The etiology of Milker's nodules. *AMA Arch Derm.* 1957;75(2):249-259.

183. Kuokkanen K, Launis J, Mörttinen A. Erythema nodosum and erythema multiforme associated with milker's nodules. *Acta Derm Venereol.* 1976;56(1):69-72.

184. Handler NS, Handler MZ, Rubins A. Milker's nodule: an occupational infection and threat to the immunocompromised. *J Eur Acad Dermatol Venereol.* 2018;32(4):537-541.

185. Vestey JP, Yirrell DL, Aldridge RD. Cowpox/catpox infection. *Br J Dermatol.* 1991;124(1):74-78.

186. Vestey JP, Yirrell DL, Norval M. What is human catpox/cowpox infection? *Int J Dermatol.* 1991;30(10):696-698.

187. Baxby D, Bennett M, Getty B. Human cowpox 1969-93: a review based on 54 cases. *Br J Dermatol.* 1994;131(5): 598-607.

188. Bennett M, Baxby D. Cowpox in cats and man. *Vet Q.* 1995;17(suppl 1):16.

189. Drago F, Rampini P, Rampini E, Rebora A. Atypical exanthems: morphology and laboratory investigations may lead to an aetiological diagnosis in about 70% of cases. *Br J Dermatol.* 2002;147(2): 255-260.

190. Johannessen JV, Krogh HK, Kjeldsberg E. Orf. *Contact Dermatitis.* 1980;6(1):36-39.

191. Lederman ER, Austin C, Trevino I, et al. ORF virus infection in children: clinical characteristics, transmission, diagnostic methods, and future therapeutics. *Pediatr Infect Dis J.* 2007;26(8):740-744.

192. Bayindir Y, Bayraktar M, Karadag N. Investigation and analysis of a human orf outbreak among people living on the same farm. *New Microbiol.* 2011;34(1): 37-43.

193. Falk ES. Parapoxvirus infections of reindeer and musk ox associated with unusual human infections. *Br J Dermatol.* 1978;99(6):647-654.

194. Haig DM. Orf virus infection and host immunity. *Curr Opin Infect Dis.* 2006;19(2):127-131.

195. Fairley RA, Whelan EM, Pesavento PA, Mercer AA. Recurrent localised cutaneous parapoxvirus infection in three cats. *N Z Vet J.* 2008;56(4):196-201.

196. Tyring S. *Mucocutaneous Manifestations of Viral Diseases: an Illustrated Guide to Diagnosis and Management.* 2nd ed. Informa Healthcare: 1 online resource (544); 2010.

197. Key SJ, Catania J, Mustafa SF, et al. Unusual presentation of human giant orf (ecthyma contagiosum). *J Craniofac Surg.* 2007;18(5): 1076-1078.

198. Lederman ER, Green GM, DeGroot HE. Progressive ORF virus infection in a patient with lymphoma: successful treatment using imiquimod. *Clin Infect Dis.* 2007;44(11):e100-e103.

199. White KP, Zedek DC, White WL, et al. Orf-induced immunobullous disease: a distinct autoimmune blistering disorder. *J Am Acad Dermatol.* 2008;58(1):49-55.

200. Joseph RH, Haddad FA, Matthews AL, Maroufi A, Monroe B, Reynolds M. Erythema multiforme after orf virus infection: a report of two cases and literature review. *Epidemiol Infect.* 2015;143(2):385-390.

201. Huerter CJ, Alvarez L, Stinson R. Orf: case report and literature review. *Cleve Clin J Med.* 1991;58(6):531-534.

202. Haig DM, McInnes C, Deane D, Reid H, Mercer A. The immune and inflammatory response to orf virus. *Comp Immunol Microbiol Infect Dis.* 1997;20(3):197-204.

203. Haig DM, Mercer AA. Ovine diseases. Orf. *Vet Res.* 1998;29(3/4):311-326.

204. Al-Salam S, Nowotny N, Sohail MR, Kolodziejek J, Berger TG. Ecthyma contagiosum (orf)--report of a human case from the United Arab Emirates and review of the literature. *J Cutan Pathol.* 2008;35(6): 603-607.

205. Blanche S, Rouzioux C, Moscato ML, et al. A prospective study of infants born to women seropositive for human immunodeficiency virus type 1. HIV Infection in Newborns French Collaborative Study Group. *N Engl J Med.* 1989;320(25):1643-1648.

206. De Cock KM, Fowler MG, Mercier E, et al. Prevention of mother-to-child HIV transmission in resource-poor countries: translating research into policy and practice. *JAMA.* 2000;283(9):1175-1182.

207. El Hachem M, Bernardi S, Pianosi G, Krzysztofiak A, Livadiotti S, Gattinara GC. Mucocutaneous manifestations in children with HIV infection and AIDS. *Pediatr Dermatol.* 1998;15(6):429-434.

208. Mankahla A, Mosam A. Common skin conditions in children with HIV/AIDS. *Am J Clin Dermatol.* 2012;13(3):153-166.

209. Douek DC, Roederer M, Koup RA. Emerging concepts in the immunopathogenesis of AIDS. *Annu Rev Med.* 2009;60: 471-484.

210. Prose NS. HIV infection in children. *J Am Acad Dermatol.* 1990;22(6, Pt 2): 1223-1231.

211. Lim W, Sadick N, Gupta A, Kaplan M, Pahwa S. Skin diseases in children with HIV infection and their association with degree of immunosuppression. *Int J Dermatol.* 1990;29(1):24-30.

212. Lowe S, Liu K, Landry ML, et al. Skin disease among human immunodeficiency virus-infected adolescents in Zimbabwe: a strong indicator of underlying HIV infection. *Pediatr Infect Dis J.* 2010;29(4): 346-351.

213. Lapins J, Gaines H, Lindbäck S, Lidbrink P, Emtestam L. Skin and mucosal characteristics of symptomatic primary HIV-1 infection. *AIDS Patient Care STDS.* 1997;11(2):67-70.

214. Domachowske JB. Pediatric human immunodeficiency virus infection. *Clin Microbiol Rev.* 1996;9(4):448-468.

215. Gershon AA, Mervish N, LaRussa P, et al. Varicella-zoster virus infection in children with underlying human immunodeficiency virus infection. *J Infect Dis.* 1997;176(6):1496-1500.

216. Stefanaki C, Stratigos AJ, Stratigos JD. Skin manifestations of HIV-1 infection in children. *Clin Dermatol.* 2002;20(1):74-86.

217. Straka BF, Whitaker DL, Morrison SH, Oleske JM, Grant-Kels JM. Cutaneous manifestations of the acquired immunodeficiency syndrome in children. *J Am Acad Dermatol.* 1988;18(5 Pt 1):1089-1102.

218. Resneck JS Jr, Van Beek M, Furmanski L, et al. Etiology of pruritic papular eruption with HIV infection in Uganda. *JAMA.* 2004;292(21): 2614-2621.

219. Ramoz N, Favre M, Orth G, Rueda LA, Bouadjar B. A susceptibility locus for epidermodysplasia verruciformis, an abnormal predisposition to infection with the oncogenic human papillomavirus type 5, maps to chromosome 17qter in a region containing a psoriasis locus. *J Invest Dermatol.* 1999;112(3):259-263.fv

220. Tyring SK. *Mucocutaneous Manifestations of Viral Diseases.* Abingdon: Informa Healthcare; 2010.

20

Fungal and Algal Cutaneous Infections

J. Olufemi Ogunbiyi / Mark R. Wick

The cutaneous mycoses are fungal diseases of the hair, nails, and skin. They may be further separated into superficial dermatophytoses and deep mycoses.

SUPERFICIAL DERMATOPHYTOSES

Definition and Epidemiology

Superficial dermatophytoses are fungal infections of the skin, hair, and nails. They have a worldwide occurrence, but are more prevalent in tropical climates. The prevalence of the causative fungi differs in various geographical locations, but modern travel patterns have altered the distribution of these infections. People of virtually all ages and both sexes can be affected, but some clinical variants—such as tinea capitis—are more common in children.

Etiology

Dermatophytes belong to the genera *Microsporum, Trichophyton,* and *Epidermophyton.* These fungi can also be classified by the source of infection: *anthropophilic*—acquired from humans; *zoophilic*—acquired from animals; and *geophilic*—acquired from the soil. The organisms may be transmitted by direct contact or through a fomite intermediary. They invade the epidermis by adhering to surface keratinocytes and penetrating between the cells. A host response is variable and depends on several potential modifying factors. They include the presence of sebum, immunosuppression, and the specific source of the infection. As examples, nonanthrophilic organisms elicit a robust inflammatory reaction, and the prevalence of tinea capitis is lower in adolescents than in younger children because sebum—produced in greater quantity during puberty—has fungistatic properties. Particular clinical presentations of the dermatophytoses depend on the specific fungal organism, the immune status of the host, previous treatment, if any, and the site of skin involvement (Table 20-1) (Figure 20-1).

TABLE 20-1.	Diagnostic terms for forms of tinea
Scalp	Tinea capitis
Glabrous skin	Tinea corporis
Feet	Tinea pedis
Hands	Tinea manum
Groin	Tinea cruris
Face	Tinea barbae
Nails	Tinea unguium

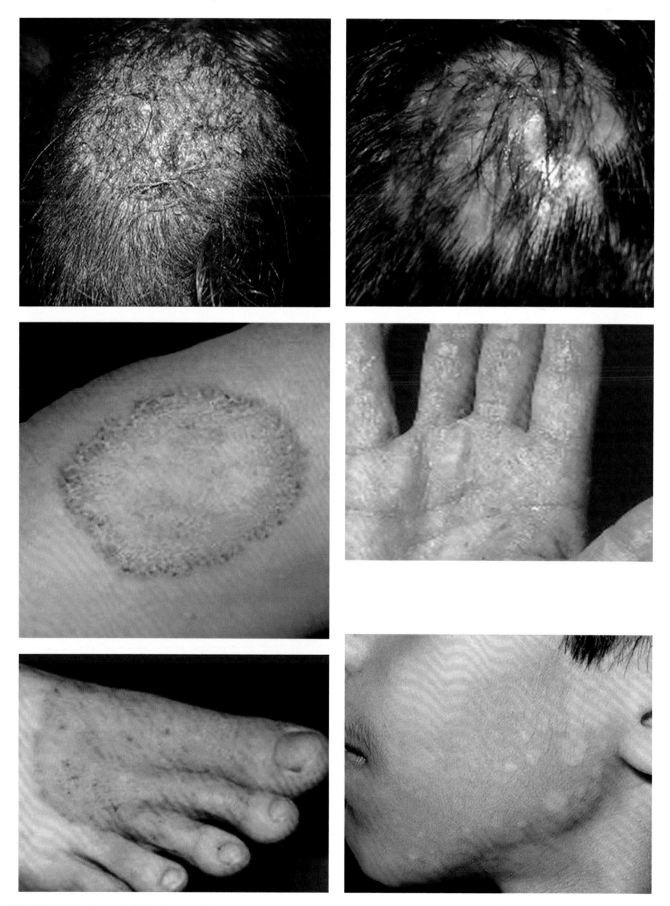

FIGURE 20-1. Several clinical forms of tinea are shown here. Beginning at the top left and moving clockwise, they are represented by tinea capitis, inflammatory tinea capitis (kerion), tinea corporis, tinea versicolor, tinea pedis, and tinea manum.

Tinea Infections

TINEA CAPITIS

Clinical Presentation

Tinea capitis is seen predominantly in the first decade of life. Responsible organisms include *Microsporum audouinii*, *Trichophyton schoenleinii*, and *Tricholosporum violaceum*. Involvement of the hair shafts may include the cortex, ecto-thrix, or endothrix. Clinical features include widespread scaling on the scalp with a seborrheic dermatitis–like pattern, as well as patchy alopecia. An inflammatory form of the disease, known as kerion, results from infection by zoophillic organisms such as *Trichophyton verrucosum* or *Trichophyton mentagrophytes*. Favus is a particularly severe form of kerion, usually caused by *T. schoenleinii*. Dermoscopic findings in tinea capitis include comma-shaped hairs with black dots.

Histologic Findings

The causative organisms invade the stratum corneum and then involve hair follicles, extending into the shafts to the level of the mid-follicle. Endothrix infections are defined as those showing intrapiliary hyphae or arthrospores. Endo-ectothrix infections are those that exhibit fungal elements within and around altered hair shafts. In the superficial dermis, the inflammatory response varies from scant perivascular lymphocytic infiltration to dense and diffuse effacement of the corium by acute and chronic inflammatory cells in kerion (Figure 20-2). Neutrophils are commonly seen in the stratum corneum. Rupture of hair follicles may provoke a granulomatous response.

TINEA CORPORIS

Clinical Presentation

Tinea corporis presents as a pruritic annular rash with an active border that is studded with papules and vesicles. The lesional center shows postinflammatory dyspigmentation, scaling, and scarring. In children with fair skin, the lesions may be erythematous.

Histologic Findings

The histopathologic images that are seen most commonly in tinea corporis are those of subacute or chronic spongiotic dermatitis or erythema perstans. The expanding edges of the lesions show acanthosis and parakeratosis, with inflammatory cell exocytosis, including neutrophils, in the parakeratotic crust. Fungal hyphae are demonstrable in the stratum corneum with periodic acid–Schiff (PAS) stains. Occasionally, idiosyncratic inflammatory reactions can resemble those of erythema multiforme, granuloma faciale, and nodular granulomatous parafolliculitis, and subepidermal bullae may also be seen (Figure 20-3).

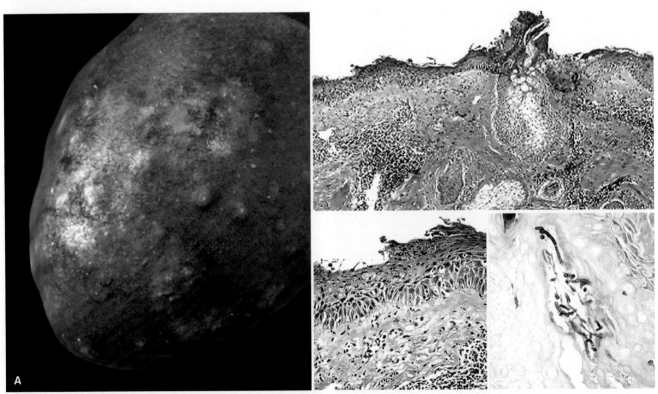

FIGURE 20-2. A, This adolescent patient has tinea capitis (left panel). Microscopically, the lesions show parakeratosis with intracorneal neutrophilia (top right panel and first bottom right panel). A Gomori methenamine-silver (GMS) stain demonstrates the dermatophytes.

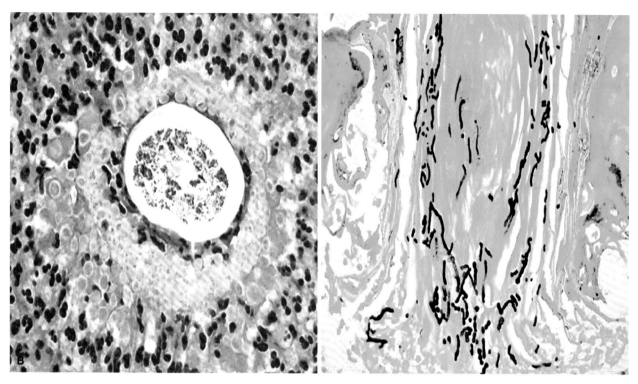

FIGURE 20-2. (*continued*) B, Acute and chronic inflammation surrounds infected hair follicles in kerion (left panel). A GMS stain demonstrates intrafollicular fungal organisms.

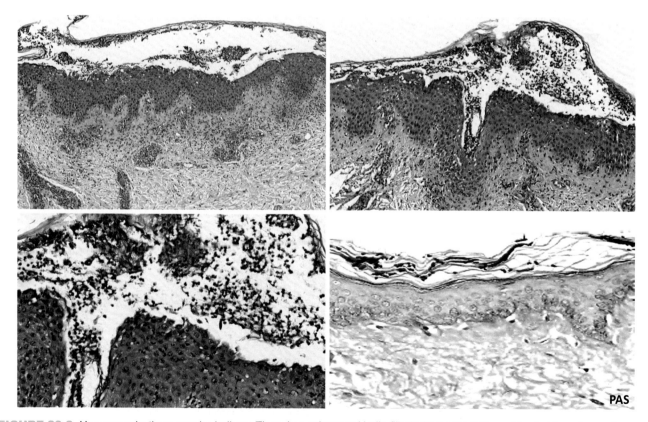

FIGURE 20-3. Uncommonly, tinea may be bullous. There is a subcorneal bulla filled with neutrophils, and hyphal fungal organisms are seen in the right lower panel with a digested Periodic acid–Schiff stain.

TINEA PEDIS

Clinical Presentation

Tinea pedis, or "athlete's foot," is usually caused by anthropophilic fungi such as *Trichophyton rubrum*, *Trichophyton mentagrophytes*, and *Epidermophyton floccosum*. The most common form of this condition features interdigital lesions that are characterized by peeling, maceration, and fissuring. The fourth interdigital cleft is often affected, and lesions may also involve the plantar surfaces of the toes. Chronic hyperkeratotic tinea pedis is typified by diffuse scaling or hyperkeratosis of both feet. Typically, the dorsal surfaces are unaffected, but, in severe cases, lesions may involve the entire foot. Inflammatory and vesicular tinea pedis produces painful, pruritic vesicles or bullae, most often on the instep or the sole. Complications of tinea pedis include cellulitis, lymphangitis, and lymphadenopathy. A hypersensitivity reaction to the dermatophytosis (dermatophytids) may subsequently develop on the palms of one or both hands and the sides of the fingers. Papules, vesicles, bullae, or pustules may develop, often symmetrically. The resulting eruption may mimic dyshidrotic eczema (pompholyx).

Histologic Findings

Tinea pedis is commonly complicated by a secondary bacterial infection, with neutrophilic infiltrates and intracorneal pustules. In ordinary cases, the histopathologic images are those of acute vesicular dermatitis or chronic psoriasiform dermatitis. PAS stains will show the causative organisms in the stratum corneum.

TINEA NIGRA

This is a form of superficial dermatophyte infection caused by *Hortaea werneckii*.

Clinical Presentation

Patients present with asymptomatic brown macules or patches on the palms, soles, neck, and trunk. The lesions have a darker pigment at the advancing borders, unlike acral nevi.

Histologic Findings

This form of infection has minimal to no inflammation. The epidermis and dermis of the acral skin infected with tinea nigra are largely unremarkable at low-power magnification. In the superficial aspects of the stratum corneum, numerous short, segmented hyphae and spores are seen. These organisms have a characteristic brown-yellow color on routine hematoxylin and eosin sections (Figure 20-4).

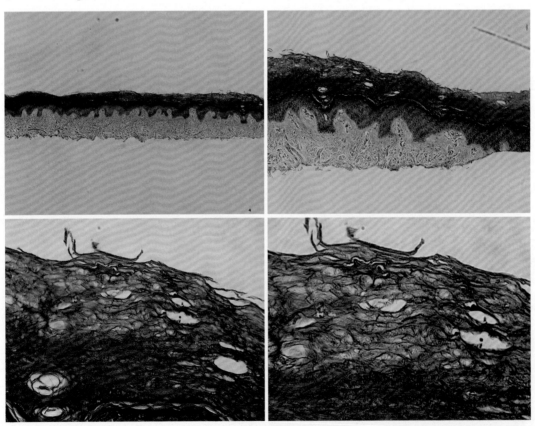

FIGURE 20-4. A case of tine nigra. The epidermis and dermis of the acral skin infected with tinea nigra are largely unremarkable at low-power magnification. In the superficial aspects of the stratum corneum, numerous short, segmented hyphae and spores are seen. These organisms have a characteristic brown-yellow color on routine hematoxylin and eosin sections.

The hyphae can be proven with the use of special stains (Gomori methenamine-silver [GMS] and PAS). Melanin pigment is confined to the stratum corneum and can be demonstrated with the use of Fontana-Masson stain.

TINEA (PITYRIASIS) VERSICOLOR

Definition and Epidemiology

Pityriasis versicolor (PV) is a superficial fungal infection of the skin caused by *Malassezia* organisms. It is characterized by hypo- or hyperpigmented scaly macules. PV is seen internationally, but usually in tropical climates. It occurs most often in adolescents, but also has been seen in a few preteen children. Some reports have suggested an increased prevalence in females.

Etiology

Malassezia is a part of the normal skin flora. It is a dimorphic lipophilic fungus that can exist as both yeasts and mycelia. The latter is the pathogenic form. Environmental factors and host susceptibility have been implicated in the development of skin lesions. The genus *Malassezia* has been subdivided into seven species—*Malassezia globosa, M. sympodialis, M. furfur, M. slooffiae, M. pachydermatis, M. restricta,* and *M. obtusa.* It would appear that the predominant species for PV is geographically determined.

Clinical Presentation

Characteristic lesions of PV are hypopigmented or hyperpigmented scaly macules that are initially perifollicular but then coalesce to form larger macules. Most lesions are asymptomatic, but they may be pruritic. Stretching the lesions on examination makes scaling obvious. Pigmentary changes are most apparent in dark-skinned persons. The Woods lamp examination is useful in delineating the borders of the lesions. Seborrheic areas of the face, chest, and upper back are commonly affected, although lesions may also extend to the extremities or be mainly located on them ("inverse" distribution). Extensive skin involvement may suggest an underlying immunosuppressive state. Mild erythema or inflammation may be seen around a few hypopigmented lesions.

Residual hypopigmentation persists after treatment, especially in covered areas; those in sun-exposed skin fields recolor faster. Diagnosis is usually based on clinical findings, together with the results of potassium hydroxide (KOH)-digested microscopic studies of skin scrapings.

Histologic Findings

In hematoxylin and eosin (H&E) sections, the causative organisms are usually seen as short wavy hyphae in the stratum corneum, associated with clusters of spores. The hyphae can be entrapped within the cornified layer (the "sandwich sign"). They are best seen with PAS or GMS stains, with associated parakeratosis and intracorneal neutrophilia (Figure 20-5). Epidermal spongiosis is variably present, but is often seen in lesions of the feet. In chronic lesions, one may see psoriasiform epidermal hyperplasia with papillary dermal chronic inflammatory cell infiltrates that are predominantly perivascular.

CAPSULE SUMMARY

TINEAS

The forms of tinea are caused by Microsporum, Trichophyton, Epidermophyton, and Malassezia, which are acquired from the soil or animal intermediaries. The specific names of the Tineas depend on the skin regions that they affect or their clinical appearances. The histopathologic image in all of the Tineas is identical, featuring epidermal parakeratosis, intracorneal neutrophilia, and the presence of fungal organisms in the stratum corneum. Chronic lesions may have a psoriasiform appearance.

CANDIDIASIS

Definition and Epidemiology

A spectrum of skin disorders is caused by yeasts in the genus *Candida.* They represent the commonest mucocutaneous fungal infections in children. Cutaneous candidiasis occurs worldwide, but the organisms especially thrive in a warm, humid environment. Neonates and immunocompromised children are preferentially affected.

Etiology

The most frequently seen *Candida* species in mucocutaneous disease is *Candida albicans,* which is dimorphic. Its yeast phase predominates, but the mycelial form is the invasive one. The other species of *Candida* include *C. tropicalis, C. dubliniensis, C. parapsilosis, C. guilliermondii, C. krusei, C. pseudotropicalis, C. lusitaniae, C. zeylanoides,* and *C. glabrata* (formerly *Torulopsis glabrata*). The dominant species varies with the geographical location. Colonization with *C. albicans* may occur during birth or infancy. Its mechanism of tissue invasion is unclear, but it is believed that the organism produces enzymes that encourage adhesion to epithelium. The pertinent defect in host defense mechanisms appears to be a loss of integrity in the stratum corneum via maceration or frictional damage. Malnutrition, endocrine dysfunction, and prolonged use of antibiotics are other predisposing factors.

Clinical Presentation

Clinical features of cutaneous candidiasis are variable; they are dependent on patient age, anatomic site, and immune status. Pruritus is common in all forms of cutaneous

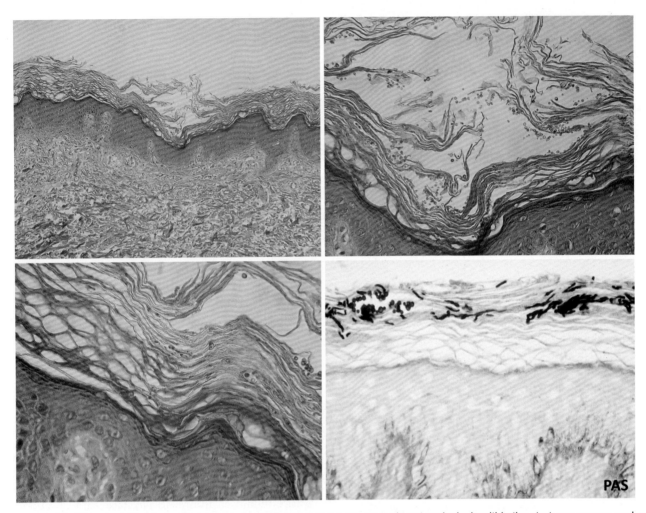

FIGURE 20-5. Tinea versicolor. In pityriasis versicolor, the organisms are seen almost exclusively within the stratum corneum and are readily seen on hematoxylin and eosin sections. The characteristic spores and short "cigar-butt" hyphae of Malassezia furfur are likened to spaghetti and meatballs. A mild superficial perivascular lymphocytic infiltrate, rarely with plasma cells is seen.

candidiasis, and it commonly assumes an "angry" erythematous appearance. In *congenital candidiasis*, an extensive eruption of pink-red macules and papules is present at birth or within a few hours thereafter. The rash is generalized, and palmoplantar surfaces may be involved. *Diaper dermatitis* is seen in the genitoperineal skin. Pruritus is common, subcorneal pustules are seen, and irregularly shaped lesions are encountered with satellitosis.

Vulvovaginitis presents in adolescents who complain of pruritus, vaginal soreness, and a whitish discharge. Vesicles and pustules may extend to the surrounding skin and perineum as well. It is common in girls who have taken antibiotics long term.

Candida balanitis is seen most often in uncircumcised boys, manifesting as transient tiny papules or pustules on the glans penis. They may rupture and leave a peeling edge. The lesions are associated with soreness and burning. In some individuals this condition is self-limiting, but it may also become chronic.

Intertriginous candidiasis is encountered in skin areas that are subject to friction, especially in obese children. Those include the groin, inframammary skin, and the intergluteal cleft. Lesional vesicles and pustules rupture and are associated with maceration and fissuring. The affected skin areas have a white rim that surrounds an erythematous and macerated base. Satellite lesions are commonly seen, and they may coalesce.

Candida paronychia is not common in children. It produces inflammatory, painful lesions of the nail bed that are usually painful. Persons who repeatedly dip their hands in water are preferentially affected. The nail beds are usually swollen and the nail cuticles are absent; a whitish discharge may be expressed from the nail bed. Several fingers may be involved.

Histologic Findings

Candida dermatitis may have an acute vesicular or subacute spongiotic appearance, or it may become psoriasiform if chronic. In acute infections the tissue reaction is purulent, with possible folliculitis. The fungi may be missed in H&E-stained sections, but they are readily identified in PAS or silver impregnation stains (Figure 20-6).

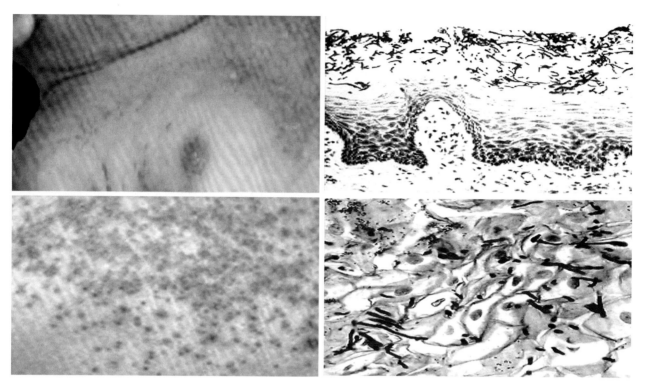

FIGURE 20-6. Moist, erythematous papules and pustules are present on the trunk of this infant with candidiasis (left panels). Numerous fungal organisms are seen in the epidermis with the Periodic acid–Schiff stain (right panels).

Candida are identified histologically by observing blastospores (yeast forms) in association with pseudohyphae. The blastospores are sharply defined, round, or oval structures, 3 to 4 microns in diameter; they may contain one or more vacuoles. Rarely, candidiasis may produce a granulomatous response, with pseudoepitheliomatous epidermal hyperplasia.

Differential Diagnosis

Contact dermatitis may be readily confused with *C. dermatitis*. Those conditions are easily separated by demonstrating the causative organisms histochemically.

CAPSULE SUMMARY

CANDIDIASIS

Candidiasis is a spectrum of superficial fungal infections caused by several Candida species. It is the most common mucocutaneous fungal disorder in children and presents with a rash that varies in appearance with patient age and anatomic site; it is almost always pruritic. Causative organisms can be labeled with the PAS method, and their presence separates candidiasis from its differential diagnostic alternatives histologically.

PITYROSPORUM FOLLICULITIS

Definition and Epidemiology

Pityrosporum folliculitis (PF) is inflammatory folliculitis of the chest and upper back of young adults due to infection with *Malassezia* organisms. PF has a worldwide occurrence, with the highest prevalence being in countries with a warm humid climate. It is seen commonly in adolescents and young adults.

Etiology

PF is caused by *Malassezia furfur*, a lipophilic yeast that was previously known as *Pityrosporum ovale* or *P. orbiculare*. *Malassezia* organisms are normal commensals in healthy people, but sebaceous gland activity during puberty may cause plugging of follicular ostia and facilitate colonization by the fungi. *Malassezia* can hydrolyze triglycerides into free fatty acids; this results in a cell-mediated response and activation of the alternate complement pathway with consequent inflammation.

Clinical Presentation

Multiple discrete 2 to 4 mm papules and pustules are seen, which are pruritic, erythematous, and monomorphic. Some may be hyperpigmented. PF favors the chest, upper back, and upper arms; facial involvement is uncommon. The lesions have a definite follicular pattern, which is best appreciated with the aid of a dermoscope. An absence of comedones helps rule out acne. Many patients have coexisting seborrheic dermatitis.

Histologic Findings

The histopathologic features are those of acute folliculitis and perifolliculitis with dilatation of the hair follicles and formation of keratin plugs. Rupture of the follicles may produce dermal abscesses. The fungi form colonies of yeasts within the follicles and dermal abscesses, surrounded by basophilic debris and neutrophils. The spores often have single buds and measure between 2 and 4 microns; they may be seen in H&E-stained sections, but are best demonstrated with the tissue Gram, PAS, and GMS methods (Figure 20-7).

Differential Diagnosis

The histologic differential diagnosis principally centers on bacterial folliculitis. Tissue Gram, PAS, and GMS stains will allow for a definite diagnosis of PF.

CAPSULE SUMMARY

PITYROSPORUM FOLLICULITIS

PF is folliculitis on the upper torso of children and young adults that is caused by infection with Malassezia species. Skin lesions are papulopustules that are pruritic and erythematous. Histopathologically, acute folliculitis and parafolliculitis are seen with dilation of hair follicles and follicular keratin plugs. Causative organisms can be labeled with tissue Gram, PAS, and GMS methods.

PIEDRA (TINEA NODOSA, TRICHOMYCOSIS NODULARIS, BEIGEL DISEASE, BLACK AND PIEDRA)

Definition and Epidemiology

Piedra is a fungal infection of the hair shafts, characterized by a hardening of the shafts and the development of nodules. There are two types—black piedra and white piedra. White piedra is more common in temperate and semitropical climates, such as Asia, Europe, Japan, and parts of the southern United States, whereas black piedra predominates in South America, East Asia, the Pacific islands, and sub-Saharan Africa. Both forms of piedra could conceivably exist in the same individual. Some reports have suggested a higher prevalence in females. Piedra can occur at any age; the incidence is greatest in young adults, but several reports have also been made of the disease in both preschool and school-age children.

Etiology

Black piedra is caused by infection with *Piedraia hortae* which is found in soil, stagnant water, and some vegetables. On the other hand, white piedra is caused by *Trichosporon asahii*, which is present in soil, water, sputum, and vegetables. Although the mode of infection in humans is not clear, the fungi invade hair shafts after colonization of the skin.

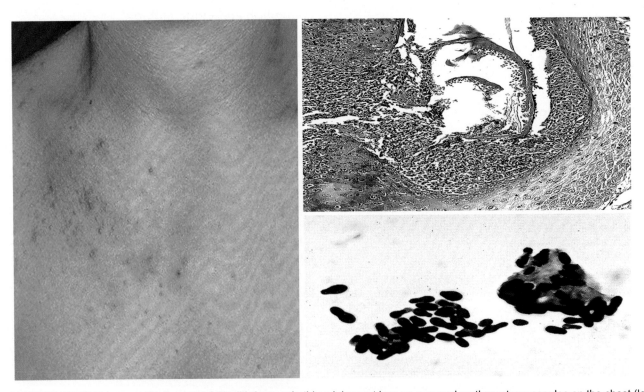

FIGURE 20-7. *Pityrosporum* (*Malassezia*) *folliculitis* is seen in this adolescent boy, as grouped erythematous papules on the chest (left panel). Histologically, acute folliculitis is present with follicular rupture (top right panel). The organisms can be labeled with the tissue Gram method (bottom right panel); Gomori methenamine-silver and Periodic acid–Schiff stains will also be positive.

Clinical Presentation

Black piedra is typified by firm, darkly pigmented nodules of variable sizes, especially on scalp hairs. The facial and pubic hair may also be affected. White piedra is characterized by lightly pigmented nodules that are soft in consistency, on hair shafts. It affects facial, axillary, and pubic hair, as well as the eyelashes and eyebrows. When white piedra is seen on the scalp, the disease may be extensive. Hair breakage occurs in both forms of piedra, but the surrounding skin is healthy.

Histologic Findings

There are large nodules along the hair shafts in both forms of piedra (Figure 20-8). Microscopic examination shows that they comprise masses of mycelia (loosely aggregated hyphae) as well as numerous ascospores. The latter forms are dematiaceous and can be labeled with the Fontana-Masson method. Transverse sections of the hair shafts show that they are surrounded by multiple arthrospores with a tendency for linear arrangement.

Differential Diagnosis

There is essentially no differential diagnosis, providing that direct microscopic examination of hairs is performed.

CAPSULE SUMMARY

PIEDRA

Piedra is a fungal infection of the hair shafts, caused by Piedraia hortae and Trichosporon asahii causing *black piedra* and *white piedra*, respectively, referring to the formation of dark or lightly pigmented nodules on the hair shafts as seen microscopically. Arthrospores surrounding the hair shafts can be labeled with the PAS or GMS methods, and those in black piedra are also Fontana-Masson-positive.

RHINOSPORIDIOSIS

Definition and Epidemiology

Rhinosporidiosis is (RS) a chronic granulomatous infection of the mucous membranes caused by the fungus *Rhinosporidium seeberi*. It is characterized by the growth of friable polyps on affected mucosal surfaces. RS is endemic in parts of India, Sri Lanka, South America, and Africa. However, it has also been reported in parts of North America. Males are most often affected, and the disease can be seen in either children or adults.

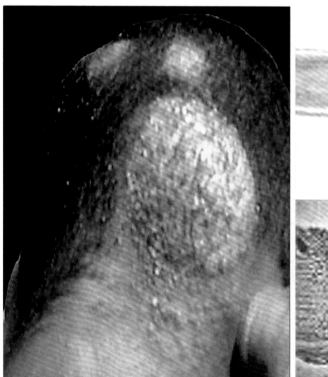
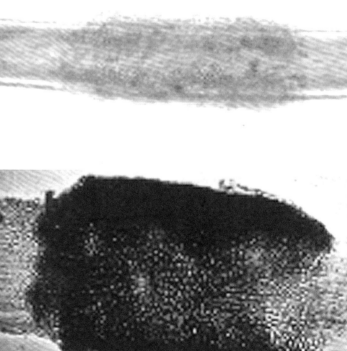

FIGURE 20-8. White Piedra is seen in an adolescent boy (left panel). Two forms of this disorder exist, depending on whether the causative fungi on hair shafts are pigmented or not (white and black Piedra) (right panels).

Etiology

Inoculation of *R. seeberi* occurs with trauma to mucosal surfaces. Local replication of the organism leads to hyperplasia of host tissue and a localized cell-mediated immune response. The commonest sites for RS are the nose, nasopharynx, and palpebral conjunctiva. Other mucosal areas are affected much more uncommonly, and dissemination to other organs is very rare.

RS is sporadic; although some authors have related the infection to contact with infected water, others have suggested a causal exposure to dust. Males are predominantly affected, and most patients are 13 to 40 years old.

Clinical Presentation

Symptoms of upper respiratory tract infection predate the development of soft polyps with a strawberry-like appearance, typically on the mucosal surfaces of the nose or eyes. The polyps are usually vascular and friable, and they bleed easily.

Histologic Findings

The skin lesions begin as papillomas that become more verrucoid with time and are associated with mucoid surface material. The surface epithelium and submucosa contain numerous globoid cysts that range from 10 to 200 microns in diameter (Figure 20-9). Some may be partially collapsed, assuming a semilunar shape. Spores are released from mature sporangia by rupture of their walls. They develop into small trophic cysts that contain a basophilic karyosome and distinct chitinous walls. H&E-stained sections clearly demonstrate the organisms, and they are stained by the PAS and GMS methods. The inner portion of the walls of larger sporangia may be birefringent.

Differential Diagnosis

The outer walls of the spores and the inner walls of the sporangia are well stained by Mayer's mucicarmine technique, but *R. seeberi* shows no morphologic resemblance to *Cryptococcus neoformans*. Occasionally, small collapsed cysts may contain degenerating small trophic forms that resemble empty spheroids of *Coccidioides immitis*. Finally, *R. seeberi* somewhat resembles *Emmonsia crescens* in size and appearance, but only the former of those organisms is labeled by mucicarmine.

CAPSULE SUMMARY

RHINOSPORIDIOSIS

RS is caused by infection of the mucous membranes of the eyes, nose, and oropharynx by *R. seeberi* and predominantly seen in India, Sri Lanka, South America, and Africa. Multiple soft polyps appear on the affected mucous membranes that are friable and bleed easily. Verrucoid papillomas are seen histologically, containing globoid cysts that represent sporangia with internal spores. These can be labeled with the PAS and GMS methods but are also easily seen in H&E stains.

Deep Mycoses

The "deep" mycoses are secondary cutaneous manifestations of fungal infections of the viscera. Many but not all use the lungs as the portal of entry.

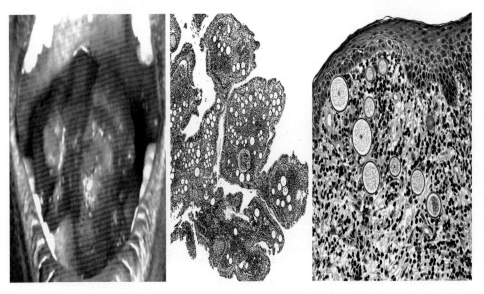

FIGURE 20-9. Rhinosporidiosis produces friable polypoid lesions in the mouth (left panel); other mucosal surfaces of the head and neck can be similarly affected. Microscopically, polypoid and inflammatory excrescences are present on the mucosa (middle panel), in which fungal sporangia are easily identified (right panel).

CRYPTOCOCCOSIS

Definition and Epidemiology

Cryptococcosis of the skin is caused by a dimorphous encapsulated yeast, *Cryptococcus neoformans*. It also has a predilection for growth in the lungs, brain, and meninges. Cutaneous involvement is seen in 10% to 15% of cases. *C. neoformans* has an international distribution. Spores of that fungal organism have been recovered from avian excreta, soil, and dust.

Etiology

C. neoformans has two variants—var. neoformans (serotypes A, D, and AD) and var. gattii (serotypes B and C). Neoformans is found most often in Europe and North America, particularly in HIV-infected patients. The gattii form is more prevalent in Africa. Both of the organismal variants are carried by airborne particulates that are inhaled. Localized lung disease is the most common, although systemic manifestations are possible depending on the host response, the size of the inoculum, and the virulence of the organism. Disseminated disease is usually seen in immunocompromised individuals. It occurs via hematogenous spread, leading to multiple organ involvement that can include the skin. Much less commonly, direct inoculation of *C. neoformans* into the skin may result in primary cutaneous disease.

Clinical Presentation

The rare primary lesions of cryptococcosis in the skin are usually single, predominantly situated on the extremities, and are accompanied by regional lymphadenopathy. They may manifest as ulcers, cellulitis, abscesses, or a sporotrichoid pattern of dermal involvement. Secondary skin involvement is the norm; it is associated with systemic (particularly pulmonary) symptoms and may affect any skin area. The lesions are initially papular, but then become pustular or ulcerated. Acneiform papules or pustules, warty or vegetating plaques and ulcers, hard infiltrated plaques or nodules, subcutaneous masses, abscesses, blisters, eczematous plaques, and vasculitis-like lesions are also possible.

Histologic Findings

In H&E-stained sections, *Cryptococcus* is usually relatively easy to identify. The organisms measure 4 to 7 microns in diameter, and they stain light blue. Their mucinous capsules appear as clear halos. Mucicarmine and colloidal-iron staining labels the capsular material (Figure 20-10), and the organisms may also be positive with the Masson-Fontana technique because they contain melanin precursors (Figure 20-11). The latter feature distinguishes *C. neoformans* from other yeasts. The surrounding tissue contains a mixture of acute and chronic inflammation, with variable formation of true granulomas. In overtly granulomatous

lesions, it may be more difficult to identify the organisms, and histochemical methods will figure more prominently into diagnosis.

Differential Diagnosis

Small forms of *C. neoformans* may resemble *Histoplasma*, and, on the other hand, large forms without capsules can mimic *Blastomyces*. The thick cell walls and multiple nuclei of *Blastomyces dermatitidis* distinguish it from *C. neoformans*. *Rhinosporidium* is regularly carminophilic, but its morphologic appearance is unlike that of *Cryptococcus*.

CAPSULE SUMMARY

CRYPTOCOCCOSIS

Cryptococcosis is caused by infection with Cryptococcus neoformans presenting with skin lesions that are typically secondary manifestations of distant spread from a primary pulmonary infection, usually in immunocompromised host. Lesions are popular, pustular, or ulcerated with possible progression to plaques, nodules, and vasculitis-like lesions. Yeast forms in the dermis are surrounded by clear halos with a neutrophilic and granulomatous inflammatory response. The organisms can be labeled with the PAS, colloidal iron, and Fontana-Masson technique.

BLASTOMYCOSIS

Definition and Epidemiology

Blastomycosis is a chronic granulomatous and suppurative deep mycosis, caused by infection with *B. dermatitidis*. This disease is seen globally, but it is commonest in northern parts of the United States and in sub-Saharan Africa. Blastomycosis is most prevalent in adult men, but it can be seen in children as well.

Etiology

B. dermatitidis is found in wood and soil, and some animal reservoirs (eg, dogs). Infection occurs is through inhalation of fungal spores, causing pulmonary disease with secondary involvement of the skin. Primary cutaneous infections are rare, and typically follow trauma with contamination of a wound by soil or wood. They have been documented in the Middle East, India, and Poland.

Clinical Presentation

Three forms of blastomycosis have been described—primary cutaneous, pulmonary, and disseminated. Primary cutaneous disease is rare, seen after an inoculation via skin puncture. A chancre develops at the wound site within 2 weeks and is often associated with lymphangitis and

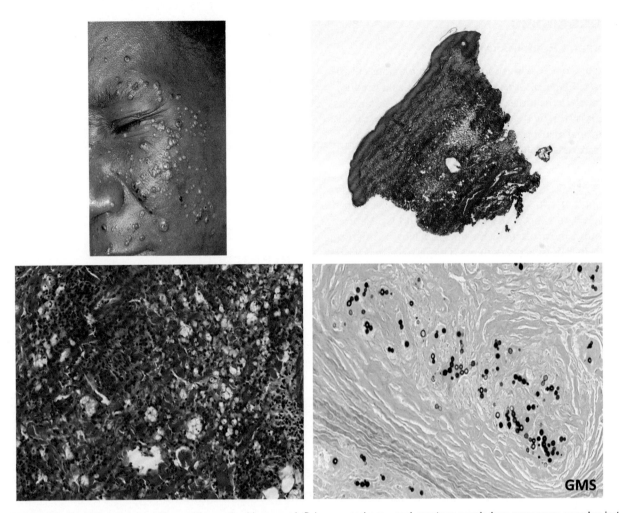

FIGURE 20-10. This adolescent boy with acquired immunodeficiency syndrome and cryptococcosis has numerous papules in the skin of the face (left panel). Histologically, they contain yeast-like fungi with mucoid capsules (middle panel), which can be labeled with the mucicarmine method (right panels).

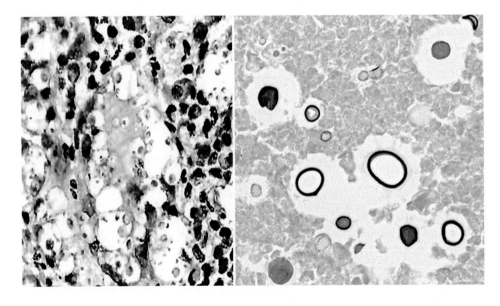

FIGURE 20-11. The capsules of *Cryptococcus* are well seen in the left panel. This organism can also be labeled with the Fontana-Masson method (right panel).

lymphadenopathy. Spontaneous recovery may occur without treatment. Pulmonary blastomycosis may be asymptomatic or produce symptoms like those of pulmonary tuberculosis. They include a persistent low-grade fever, chest pain, cough, and hemoptysis. Cavitary lesions and abscesses may develop in the lungs. Disseminated blastomycosis eventuates through the spread of a pulmonary infection via the bloodstream, to organs such as the skin, bones, and central nervous system. The pulmonary disease may be inapparent when the skin lesions appear.

Cutaneous involvement manifests with papules and nodules, which may ulcerate or become verrucoid. The lesions enlarge peripherally and show central clearing. A serpiginous appearance with a violaceous margin may be seen. The diagnosis can be confirmed with KOH preparations, formal culture, and biopsy.

Histologic Findings

Skin lesions of blastomycosis are characterized by pseudoepitheliomatous hyperplasia, intraepidermal microabscesses, and a mixture of acute and granulomatous inflammation in the corium, with the formation of giant cells (Figure 20-12). The epidermal hyperplasia may be so marked that it simulates the appearance of squamous cell carcinoma. The intraepidermal abscesses contain abundant neutrophils and the fungal organisms, which are best seen with the PAS stain. The yeasts in the dermis are extracellular for the most part, but also may be seen in the cytoplasm of giant cells, where they appear as "punched-out" holes. The organisms have the appearance of a thick-walled round structure, with broad-based budding.

Differential Diagnosis

The microscopic differential diagnosis of blastomycotic skin lesions can include squamous carcinoma, mycobacterioses, sarcoidosis, actinomycosis, and other fungal infections. It is obvious that several histochemical studies are necessary to address these possibilities, including tissue Gram, PAS, Ziehl-Neelsen, Fite-Faraco, and GMS methods.

The multiple nuclei seen in *B. dermatitidis* distinguish it from *Histoplasma capsulatum, Cryptococcus neoformans, and Paracoccidioides brasiliensis.* Even though a few blastomycotic cells may stain faintly with mucicarmine, separating them from *C. neoformans* is usually not difficult on morphologic grounds.

CAPSULE SUMMARY

BLASTOMYCOSIS

This cutaneous disease is usually caused by systemic spread from a primary pulmonary infection by *B. dermatitidis.* Skin lesions are papulonodular initially and may become verrucoid or ulcerated. Some have a serpiginous appearance with violaceous borders. Histologically, prominent epidermal hyperplasia is present with intraepidermal and dermal neutrophilic and granulomatous inflammation. Intralesional yeast forms are extracellular for the most part but may be seen within giant cells. They are best labeled with the PAS technique.

COCCIDIOIDOMYCOSIS

Definition and Epidemiology

Coccidioidomycosis (CM) comprises a spectrum of diseases that are caused by soil-dwelling fungi in the genus *Coccidioides* (*C. immitis* and *C. posadasii*). CM is endemic in the southwestern states of the United States and in some areas of South and Central America. Different serotypes of *Coccidioides* have dissimilar geographical distributions, with *C. posadasii* being found predominantly in North America. CM is

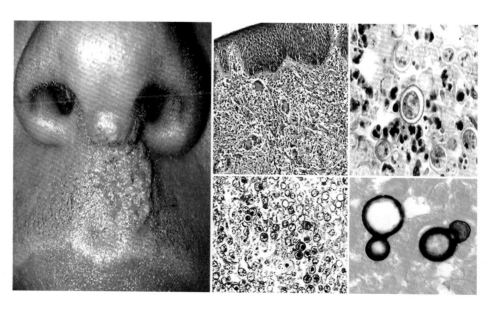

FIGURE 20-12. A teenage boy with cutaneous blastomycosis has an irregular, verrucoid plaque in the skin of the upper lip (left panel). Microscopically, granulomatous inflammation is seen in the dermis, with the formation of multinucleated giant cells (top middle panel). The fungi are large, broad-based budding yeast forms (top right panel) that are labeled with the Periodic acid–Schiff stain (bottom middle panel) and the Gomori methenamine-silver technique (bottom right panel).

most common in individuals who are repeatedly exposed to aerosolized arthroconidia. They include agricultural workers, hunters, and soil-diggers. Epidemics of CM have been associated with earthquakes and windstorms. The disease may affect children, but it is much more common in adults.

Etiology

CM is caused by inhalation of dust that contains *Coccidioides* arthroconidia. Direct infection of the skin has been reported, but only very rarely. Most persons do not develop any disease after exposure to the fungal spores. Risk factors for doing so include Asian or African ancestry, and immunosuppression. CM usually takes the form of mild-to-severe symptomatic pulmonary infection, and only occasionally becomes disseminated.

Clinical Presentation

The spectrum of diseases caused by coccidioidomycosis ranges from mild upper respiratory tract infections to disseminated and potentially fatal involvement of several organ sites. The primary pulmonary form of CM may be asymptomatic, in which case it can be mistaken for a neoplastic process on chest radiographs, or it can simulate tuberculosis. Erythema multiforme and erythema nodosum have been reported in some female patients as unusual secondary cutaneous reactions to CM.

Primary fungus-containing skin lesions in CM are rare. They are painless, firm, indurated nodules that usually follow cutaneous injury with contamination by soil. Spontaneous healing often follows after a few weeks.

The disseminated form of CM is also uncommon and may affect the skin, subcutaneous tissue, bones, joints, and visceral organs. Secondary cutaneous lesions may take the form of abscesses, granulomas, ulcers, or draining sinuses. Serologic testing, biopsy, and formal cultures can establish the diagnosis.

Histologic Findings

In tissue samples, pus from skin lesions, and sputum, *C. immitis* can be identified microscopically quite readily. It is represented by large globular sporangia that contain many endospores. The sporangia are easily demonstrated by H&E staining (Figure 20-13), but endospores may require labeling with PAS or GMS methods to be visible. The intact sporangia usually elicit a granulomatous reaction comprising histiocytes, lymphocytes, neutrophils, and giant cells of the foreign body or Langhans types.

CAPSULE SUMMARY

COCCIDIOIDOMYCOSIS

These cutaneous lesions are usually the result of secondary skin involvement from a primary pulmonary infection with *Coccidioides immitis*. Skin lesions may be represented by abscesses, ulcers, nodules, or draining sinuses. Histologic examination shows large intradermal globular sporangia with thick walls surrounded by neutrophilic and granulomatous inflammation. The organisms are easily seen in H&E stains, but can also be labeled with the PAS and GMS methods.

HISTOPLASMOSIS

Definition and Epidemiology

Histoplasmosis (HP) is a highly infectious disease caused by infection with the dimorphic fungus *Histoplasma capsulatum*.

Two varieties of Histoplasma have been described, both of which are seen internationally. Recent studies suggest that a separation between them may not be phylogenetically important, but there are morphologic and epidemiologic differences between them. *H. capsulatum* is widely

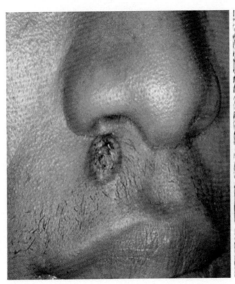
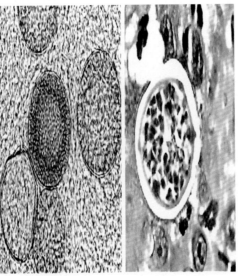

FIGURE 20-13. This adolescent boy with coccidioidomycosis has a nodular lesion in the skin of the upper lip (left panel). The causative fungi are seen as large sporangia that contain endospores (middle and right panels).

distributed, but it predominates in North America. *H. duboisii*, which causes "African HP" or "large-form HP," has been reported only in Africa. Patients of all ages may be infected, and, in adults, African HP is best represented in male agricultural workers. There is no gender difference in children.

Histoplasma duboisii is particularly common in Central and West Africa and on the island of Madagascar. African-type HP is rarely seen in the United States, except in persons who have previously lived in, or traveled to, Africa.

H. capsulatum inhabits soil that is contaminated with chicken or bat droppings, and usually causes human disease when the soil is aerosolized and inhaled. As true of other deep mycoses, primary cutaneous HP may follow trauma to the skin after contamination with soil.

Clinical Presentation

HP may be acute or chronic and localized to the lungs or disseminated. Patients usually present with lymphadenopathy, and mucocutaneous lesions may be ulcerated. Disseminated disease can involve the bones, liver, spleen, intestine, and lymphoreticular system, and is especially prevalent in immunocompromised patients. Mucocutaneous lesions are seen in the context of systemic infection. They may take the form of papulonodules, ulcers, or abscesses. In chronic disseminated HP, oral ulcers may be seen.

Primary cutaneous HP is very rare. The skin lesion in that condition is a nodule or an ulcer, often associated with regional lymphadenopathy. Erythema nodosum may complicate the clinical picture as a secondary phenomenon.

Histologic Findings

Histoplasma incites a histiocytic reaction, which may or may not be organized into granulomas. If the latter are seen, they can be either necrotizing or nonnecrotizing. Dystrophic calcification is a characteristic feature of long-standing lesions. Dermal granulomas contain macrophages that are laden with dot-like intracellular organisms that have a pseudocapsule. They are relatively evenly distributed within the macrophage cytoplasm. *Histoplasma* are often visible with H&E stains, but PAS and GMS stains are particularly helpful in their delineation (Figure 20-14). The lesions caused by *H. duboisii* contain large foreign body-type giant cells in which numerous large, round, thick-walled yeast forms can be seen. *H. duboisii* is also distinguished from *H. capsulatum* by its much larger size, averaging 2 to 4 μm in diameter. Both of them can be highlighted with the calcofluor white stain (Figure 20-15). In African HP, the organisms have thick walls and bud with a relatively narrow base. "Hourglass" and "double-cell" forms may evolve as budding takes place.

Differential Diagnosis

Toxoplasma may resemble *Histoplasma* superficially, but it is smaller and usually not seen in macrophages. Any of the special stains for fungi will distinguish the two organisms from one another. The size and thick walls of *H. duboisii* are somewhat similar to those of *B. dermatitidis*, but nuclei are typically single in *Histoplasma*. Moreover, budding cells of *H. duboisii* characteristically have an hourglass shape, as opposed to the broad-based budding of *Blastomyces*.

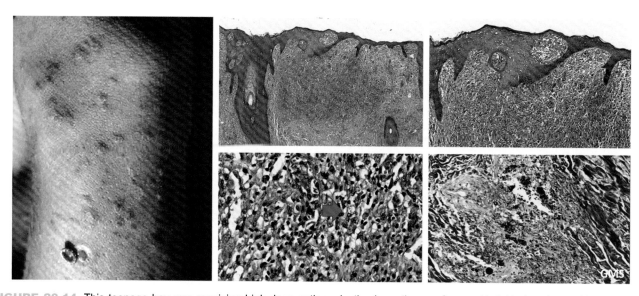

FIGURE 20-14. This teenage boy was receiving high-dose antineoplastic chemotherapy for non-Hodgkin lymphoma. He developed papulonodules in the arm (left panel), representing cutaneous involvement by histoplasmosis. Microscopically, the lesions comprise dermal collections of lymphocytes and histiocytes. The histiocytes are "parasitized" by many fungal yeast forms in the cytoplasm (arrow head), which can be labeled with the Gomori methenamine-silver method (bottom right panel).

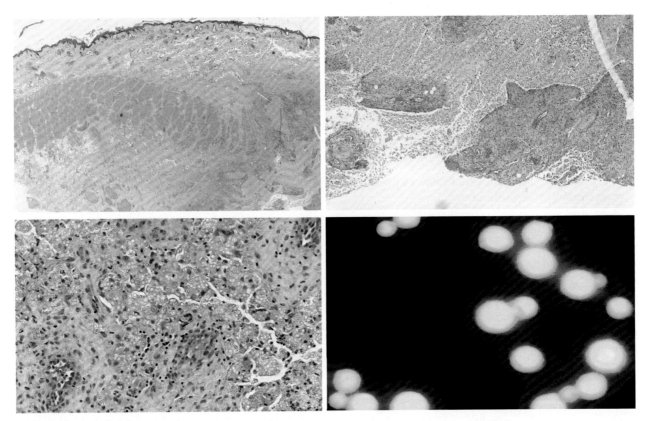

FIGURE 20-15. African histoplasmosis is caused by *Histoplasma duboisii*. The spherical to oval fungal cells are uninucleate and 8 to 15 μm in diameter, have thick walls, and bud by a relatively narrow base. Classical "hourglass" and "double-cell" forms are created when budding daughter cells enlarge until they equal the size of the parent cells, to which they remain connected by a narrow base. The yeasts can also be labeled histochemically with the calcofluor white method, as shown here (bottom right panel).

CAPSULE SUMMARY

HISTOPLASMOSIS

As is true of other deep mycoses, cutaneous histoplasmosis (CHP) is usually a secondary infection that follows primary pulmonary disease. A primary form is caused by injuring the skin with an object that is contaminated with soil. Many patients with secondary CHP are immunocompromised. Cutaneous lesions can be papulonodules, ulcers, or abscesses.

Histologically, CHP produces a histiocytic response to the fungal organisms that may or may not be overtly granulomatous, and a neutrophilic infiltrate is sometimes present as well. The organisms are seen in the cytoplasm of histiocytes as *dot-like* inclusions that can be highlighted with the PAS or GMS stains. Attention to the size of the organisms in CHP, which measure between 2 and 4 μm, allows for a distinction from Toxoplasma and Blastomyces.

PARACOCCIDIOIDOMYCOSIS

Definition and Epidemiology

Paracoccidioidomycosis (PCM) has also been called "Brazilian blastomycosis." It is caused by the fungus *Paracoccidioides brasiliensis*, an organism that is very different from *B. dermatitidis*.

PCM is an autochthonous disease that is seen in a broad region, from southern Mexico to northern Argentina, being particularly present in Brazil, Colombia, Venezuela, and Argentina. Rare if any cases have been reported outside of that geographic area. The disease can affect patients of any age, and it is especially associated with individuals who live in rural settings.

Etiology

P. brasiliensis is a dimorphic organism. Its habitats are still not clearly defined, but this fungus appears to be principally aquatic. It is a polygemulating yeast, and it infects hosts by inhalation into the respiratory tract. Pathologic lesions involve the mucous membranes, skin, lymph nodes, bones, and lungs. PCM is unlike many other mycoses in that it rather commonly occurs in immunocompetent hosts. However, immunosuppression does increase the severity of the disease. PCM is rarely seen in females once they reach reproductive age, probably because of a protective effect by estradiol.

Clinical Presentation

Pulmonary PCM is associated with shortness of breath, cough, and hemoptysis, as well as involuntary weight loss, fever, and fatigue. Chest films show the presence of pneumonia or pleural effusions. Secondary mucocutaneous lesions are often situated on the face, lips, and oral mucosa, as painful and potentially ulcerating papulonodules of various sizes with a violaceous hue. Primary infection is exceptionally rare. In children, a progressive form of PCM produces high fevers, generalized lymphadenopathy, miliary pulmonary lesions, and multifocal mucocutaneous involvement. It has an adverse prognosis, even with treatment.

Histologic Findings

Diagnosis is made by conventional cultures of the lesions or by visualization of the yeast cells in tissue. Seen in the context of a mixed granulomatous and neutrophilic inflammatory dermal infiltrate, they have an appearance like that of a "mariner's wheel," as seen with GMS stains (Figure 20-16).

Differential Diagnosis

Some forms of *P. brasiliensis* may resemble *B. dermatitidis* in tissue sections, but they vary more in size and shape, have thinner walls, and are not multinucleated.

Small variant forms of this organism may be mistaken for *Histoplasma*, and a large variant can simulate *Coccidioides* to some degree. However, attention to morphologic detail is effective in avoiding those misinterpretations.

CAPSULE SUMMARY

PARACOCCIDIOIDOMYCOSIS OF THE SKIN

This is predominantly seen in South America, especially Brazil, and cutaneous lesions usually follow primary pulmonary infection. Histologically, mixed granulomatous and neutrophilic dermal infiltrates are seen in which the organisms are dispersed. They have the appearance of a *mariner's wheel* on PAS and GMS stains.

SPOROTRICHOSIS

Definition and Epidemiology

Sporotrichosis (ST) is a chronic mycosis of the skin, subcutaneous tissues, regional lymph nodes, and, in some instances, the visceral organs. It is caused by the fungus *Sporothrix schenckii (Sporotrichum schenckii)*.

ST is seen worldwide, but its greatest prevalence is in tropical and subtropical locales. Epidemics have been reported in Peru, Brazil, Northeast China, Malaysia, and the mining areas of South Africa. Males are more affected, especially those with outdoor occupations. Cutaneous infections have been seen in children as well.

Etiology

The fungus grows on decaying matter and is found in the soil, plants, and hay. It can also be carried by animals (eg cats, armadillos). Cutaneous infection is acquired through puncture by thorns, splinters, and wounds contaminated with soil. The initial lesion is a pustule that ulcerates. Subsequently, nodules develop centrifugally along the lymphatics draining the primary pustule. Involvement of the viscera from a skin source of infection is rare except in individuals

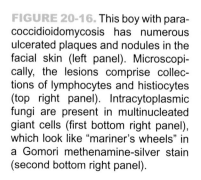
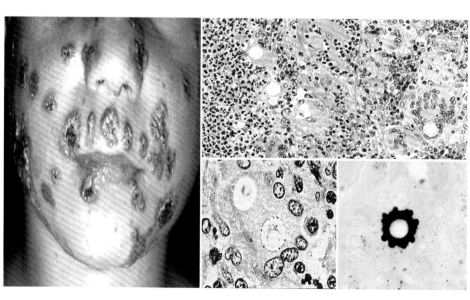

FIGURE 20-16. This boy with paracoccidioidomycosis has numerous ulcerated plaques and nodules in the facial skin (left panel). Microscopically, the lesions comprise collections of lymphocytes and histiocytes (top right panel). Intracytoplasmic fungi are present in multinucleated giant cells (first bottom right panel), which look like "mariner's wheels" in a Gomori methenamine-silver stain (second bottom right panel).

who are immunosuppressed. Primary inhalation of *Sporothrix* in aerosolized form may produce pulmonary disease as the initial manifestation.

Clinical Presentation

Cutaneous ST has two varieties: a localized, fixed form and a chronic lymphatic variant. The second is the more common. The initial inoculation site is usually on the exposed areas of the arms and hands. After implantation of the fungal spores, an ulcerated pustule forms, followed by satellitotic, nodular, and lymphangitic skin lesions with regional lymphadenopathy. The secondary nodules may ulcerate as well. Primary lesions may also develop in the mucous membranes of the nose, mouth, and pharynx.

The localized fixed variety of ST is uncommon, being represented by plaques, nodules, ulcers, or acneiform or verrucous lesions, with no lymphatic spread. Why the latter phenomenon does not occur in such cases is unknown.

Histologic Findings

Skin biopsies in ST show pseudoepitheliomatous epidermal hyperplasia and possible ulceration. Superficial and deep dermal stellate microabscesses are also present, surrounded by epithelioid granulomas that may contain giant cells. In fortuitous H&E preparations or PAS stains, one may see asteroid bodies that contain a central yeast-like cell (Figure 20-17). Macrophages may also contain small, round fungal forms that passingly resemble *Histoplasma*. It should be noted that PAS stains are much more likely to demonstrate the microbes than GMS preparations do.

Additional histochemical stains for fungi may reveal many extracellular forms that are characteristic of *S. schenckii*, with "cigar-shaped" forms, round yeasts, or variously shaped budding forms. The search for fungi should be concentrated in the microabscesses of the lesions rather than granulomas. A large variant of *S. Schenckii* differs from the conventional form in that it replicates by hyphal septation.

Differential Diagnosis

The organisms in some examples of blastomycosis, HP, leishmaniasis, nocardiosis, and PCM may resemble those of ST. Careful attention to the morphologic aspects of the fungi is sufficient to make a distinction between them.

CAPSULE SUMMARY

CUTANEOUS SPOROTRICHOSIS

These skin lesions are caused by puncture wounds with objects that are contaminated with soil.

Localized *fixed* and chronic lymphangitic patterns may be seen. Histologically, pseudoepitheliomatous epidermal hyperplasia is common with dermal stellate microabscesses. They may contain budding yeast forms or asteroid bodies, seen best with the PAS method.

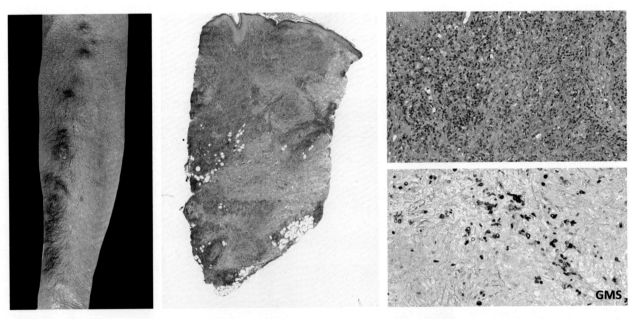

FIGURE 20-17. This adolescent boy was working as a gardener. He developed roughly linear aggregates of erythematous papulonodules in the skin of the forearm (left panel), representing sporotrichosis. Histologically, the lesions show epidermal acanthosis (top and central panel), with underlying lymphohistiocytic inflammation. A Gomori methenamine-silver stain shows the presence of intralesional fungal organisms (second bottom right panel).

CHROMO(BLASTO)MYCOSIS

Definition and Epidemiology

Chromomycosis (CM), also known as chromoblastomycosis, phaeohyphomycosis, cladosporiosis, and verrucous dermatitis, is a chronic fungal infection of the skin and subcutaneous tissues. It is characterized by verrucoid, crusted, or ulcerated lesions.

CM is international in its distribution and is especially seen in rural areas of subtropical and tropical locales. The prevalence of the disease is highest in adult males who are agricultural workers or farmers. The disease has also been reported in children.

Etiology

CM is potentially caused by several dematiaceous fungi, the most common of which are *Phialophora verrucosa, Fonsecaea pedrosoi, F. compacta,* and *Cladophialophora carrionii* (a.k.a. *Cladosporium carrionii*). Those agents are found on wood and in the soil. Infection follows their inoculation into the skin, usually by puncture wounds with wood splinters and thorns.

Clinical Presentation

The lesions of CM are usually found on exposed skin sites, particularly the feet, legs, arms, face, and neck (Figures 20-18 and 20-19). They may be ulcerated or papulonodular. Five clinical types have been described, including nodular, tumoral, plaque-like, warty, and cicatricial. Early lesions are skin-colored, pale pink, or purple. Their surfaces may be smooth or warty. Tumoral lesions have a tumefactive,

verrucoid, cauliflower-like appearance, and may resemble those of verruca vulgaris. Plaque-type lesions usually have scaly surfaces. Cicatricial forms of CM are often annular with heaped-up borders and central clearing. Lesions of CM are painful only if they become secondarily infected. Scratching produces satellite lesions through the Koebner phenomenon, and lymphatic spread is also possible. Untreated disease may eventuate in lymphatic stasis after the passage of time, with possible elephantiasis. Hematogenous spread to other organs is also possible, especially in immunocompromised patients.

Histologic Findings

The lesions of CM are hyperkeratotic with pseudoepitheliomatous epidermal hyperplasia. A diffuse dermal infiltrate is also present, comprising lymphocytes, plasma cells, neutrophils, histiocytes, and multinucleated giant cells. The causative fungal organisms are round, thick-walled, and brown (dematiaceous). They are known as sclerotic bodies, muriform cells, or medlar bodies, measuring 5 to 12 μm in diameter and predominantly situated in giant cells or in the centers of suppurative granulomas (Figure 20-20). Intraepidermal abscesses may be present in some cases, and transepithelial elimination of the organisms may occur as well.

Differential Diagnosis

Infection with any of the other fungi that can cause deep mycoses represents the differential diagnosis of CM. However, recognition of the characteristic pigmented organisms, and their affinity for the Fontana-Masson stain, is sufficient to establish a confident interpretation.

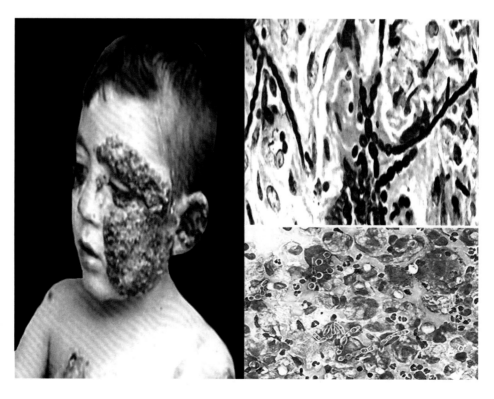

FIGURE 20-18. This boy with Wiskott-Aldrich syndrome has large verrucoid plaques in the facial skin, representing chromomycosis. The causative organism in this case was *Phialophora verrucosum*, seen in the lesions as Fontana-Masson-positive hyphal forms (top right panel). A Tzanck preparation of the lesions stained with the Giemsa method also demonstrates the fungi (bottom right panel).

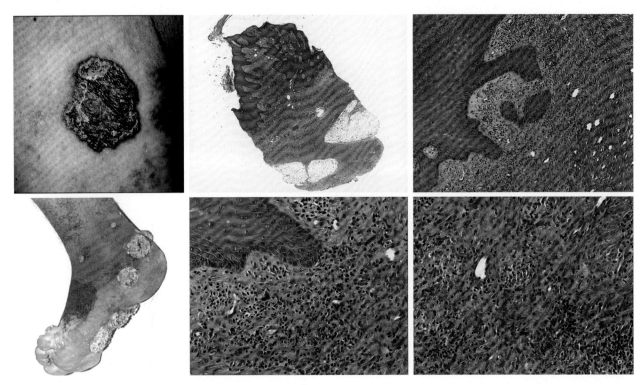

FIGURE 20-19. Another adolescent patient with chromomycosis has fungating, verruciform lesions on the leg and foot (bottom left panel) and thigh (top left panel). Pseudoepitheliomatous changes are present. Microscopically, they comprise dermal collections of lymphocytes and histiocytes, in which rounded fungal "medlar bodies" are present.

CAPSULE SUMMARY

CHROMOMYCOSIS

The highest incidence is in farmers and other agricultural workers, predominantly in subtropical or tropical locales. Skin lesions are seen in exposed skin sites and may be ulcerated, papulonodular, plaque-like, warty, or cicatricial, with variable coloration. Histologically, the image of chromomycosis is similar to that of sporotrichosis, except that the causative fungi are easily visible in H&E sections as round, brown structures that resemble *copper pennies*. They can be labeled with the Fontana-Masson method.

MYCETOMA (MADURA FOOT)

Definition and Epidemiology

Madura foot (MF) may be caused by fungi (the eumycotic form) or bacteria (the actinomycotic form), principally involving soil-dwelling organisms. Eumycetoma is a chronic subcutaneous infection caused by various genera of fungi, constituting about 40% of cases of MF.

Mycetoma is common among people who are usually barefoot, living in rural areas around the world. It is felt to be caused by puncture wounds to the foot and inoculation of the causative fungi. Children may be affected.

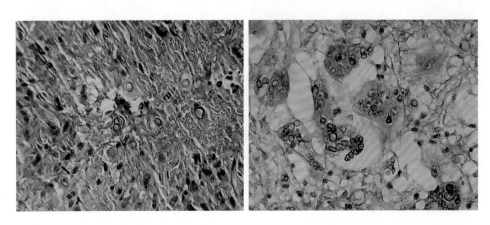

FIGURE 20-20. Closer magnification of the distinctive "Medlar" bodies of chromoblastomycosis.

Etiology

Possible causative fungal organisms for MF include *Acremonium strictum, Aspergillus nidulans, Noetestudina rosatii, Phaeoacremonium krajdenii, Pseudallescheria boydii, Aspergillus terreus, Curvularia lunata, Cladophialophora bantiana, Exophiala jeanselmei, Leptosphaeria senegalensis, Leptosphaeria tompkinsii, Madurella grisea, Madurella mycetomatis,* and *Pyrenochaeta romeroi.*

Clinical Presentation

The classic clinical constellation seen with MF is painless soft tissue swelling with a formation of sinus tracts and a discharge of macroscopic *grains,* which represent aggregates of the lesional organisms. If the condition is untreated, substantial swelling of the infected area occurs, with induration and sinus tract formation. Old sinuses may close, to be replaced by new ones. Regional lymphadenopathy is unusual. Secondary distant (usually pulmonary) mycetomas are principally seen in immunosuppressed persons.

Histologic Findings

Histopathologic evaluation allows for a distinction between actinomycotic and eumycotic MF. In H&E sections, mycetomas manifest the formation of dermal and subcutaneous microabscesses that contain large, dense masses of microorganisms, surrounded by an infiltrate of polymorphonuclear leukocytes. Actinomycotic lesions show amorphous eosinophilic material around clumps of filamentous bacteria (the Splendore-Hoeppli phenomenon) (Figure 20-21). Surrounding the microabscess, one sees a poorly defined zone of chronic inflammation containing epithelioid and giant cells, as well as granulation tissue. In long-standing lesions, fibrosis may be marked. Tissue Gram-staining labels only the actinomycotic form of MF, whereas fungal elements in eumycetomas are demonstrable with the PAS and GMS methods (Figure 20-22).

Differential Diagnosis

The most commonly implicated fungus in mycetomas is *Nocardia brasiliensis.*

Other organisms responsible for MF can include *Aspergillus, Botryomyces,* fungi that cause chromoblastomycosis, and *Sporothrix.*

CAPSULE SUMMARY

MYCETOMA (MADURA FOOT)

This is common in areas of the world where people are barefoot much of the time. It is caused by various fungi or filamentous bacteria that enter the skin through puncture wounds and contamination by soil. Clinical swelling and induration of the foot is present with the formation of draining sinus tracts that elaborate macroscopic *grains.* The microscopic image again resembles that of sporotrichosis, except that numerous microorganisms are present in the lesions. These can be visualized with the tissue Gram stain (in bacterial infections) or the PAS and GMS stains (in fungal lesions)

CUTANEOUS ASPERGILLOSIS

Definition and Epidemiology

Cutaneous aspergillosis (CA) is an opportunistic fungal infection caused by *Aspergillus* species. It is principally seen in immunocompromised patients. CA has a worldwide distribution and may affect patients of any age.

Etiology

Aspergillosis of the skin is a secondary complication of pulmonary infection, resulting from inhalation of fungal spores of the organism. The latter typically takes the form

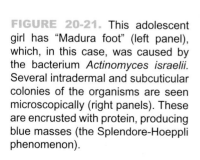

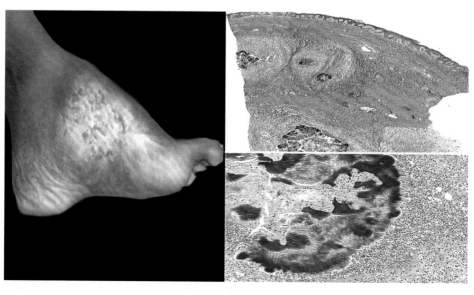

FIGURE 20-21. This adolescent girl has "Madura foot" (left panel), which, in this case, was caused by the bacterium *Actinomyces israelii.* Several intradermal and subcuticular colonies of the organisms are seen microscopically (right panels). These are encrusted with protein, producing blue masses (the Splendore-Hoeppli phenomenon).

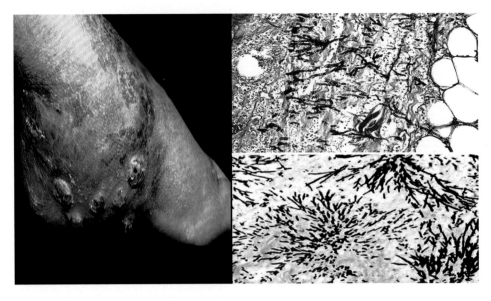

FIGURE 20-22. Another teenage girl has fungal "Madura foot" (left panel), caused by *Madurella grisea*. Hyphal organisms are present in the dermis and subcutis (top right panel), and they are labeled with the Gomori methenamine-silver stain method (bottom right panel).

of invasive aspergillosis of the lungs. Hematogenous dissemination results in colonization of other organ systems. Primary cutaneous disease is very rare and is most commonly caused by *Aspergillus fumigatus* and *Aspergillus flavus*. They are soil-dwelling organisms and are introduced into the skin at sites of trauma that are contaminated with dirt. Colonization of burn eschars by *Aspergillus* has also been reported.

Clinical Presentation

Cutaneous lesions of secondary aspergillosis begin as erythematous or violaceous, indurated, tender papules, or plaques. Subsequently, these develop central pustules, hemorrhagic vesicles, and, black eschars. Primary cutaneous infections originate as foci of localized cellulitis that later develops into necrotic ulcers and eschars.

Histologic Findings

Characteristic septated hyphae are identifiable in necrotic tissue (Figure 20-23). They show uniform, dichotomous, acute-angle branching, admixed with an inflammatory infiltrate comprising neutrophilic microabscesses and granulomas. Angioinvasion in aspergillosis is common, with potential vascular thrombosis and necrosis. Polarizable calcium oxalate deposits may be seen in the lesions as well (Figure 20-24).

Differential Diagnosis

In tissue sections, it is necessary to distinguish *Aspergillus* from organisms in the phylum *Zygomycetes* and the genus *Fusarium*. Zygomycetes generally have broader hyphae with no septation and more irregular branching patterns. However, *Fusarium* is morphologically indistinguishable from *Aspergillus* species.

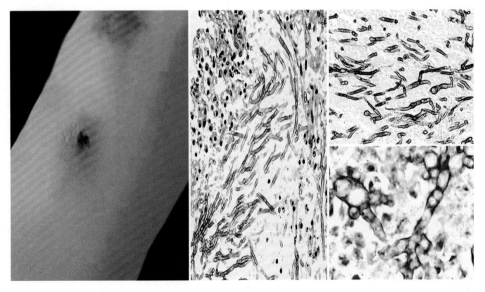

FIGURE 20-23. This adolescent girl was receiving chemotherapy for acute leukemia, when she developed erythematous and ulcerating lesions in the skin of the arms, some of which were covered with eschars (left panel). These represent cutaneous aspergillosis. Numerous septated hyphal organisms are present histologically in the lesions (middle panel). They are labeled with the Gomori methenamine-silver (top right panel) and Periodic acid–Schiff (bottom right panel) stains.

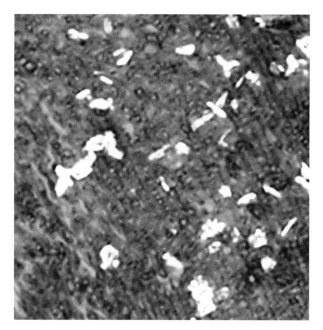

FIGURE 20-24. Crystals of calcium oxalate are also deposited in the lesions of cutaneous aspergillosis, as shown here by polarization microscopy.

CAPSULE SUMMARY

CUTANEOUS ASPERGILLOSIS

CA is typically seen in immunosuppressed individuals who have primary pulmonary infections with Aspergillus species. Skin lesions may be erythematous or violaceous papules or plaques that develop secondary ulceration or vesiculation and progress to eschar formation. Characteristic branching, septated hyphal fungal forms are seen in H&E stains in the dermis and subcutis microscopically, often with vascular invasion and secondary thrombosis. These can be accentuated with the GMS method.

ZYGOMYCOSIS (MUCORMYCOSIS)

Definition and Epidemiology

Zygomycosis, also known as mucormycosis, refers to several different angioinvasive diseases caused by infection with fungi in the order *Mucorales*, a subset of *Zygomycetes*.

Mucormycosis is rare but is seen internationally. Affected patients are either poorly controlled diabetics or others with immune compromise.

Etiology

Rhizopus species are the most common causative organisms in this group of infections. Other potentially responsible genera include *Mucor, Cunninghamella, Apophysomyces, Lichtheimia* (formerly *Absidia), Saksenaea,* and *Rhizomucor.* These fungi are found in soil and decaying organic matter,

such as moldy bread. The major route of cutaneous infection is secondary hematogenous spread to the skin after inhalation of conidia and subsequent primary pulmonary zygomycosis. Primary cutaneous disease is exceptionally rare, but it has been reported after the use of nonsterile tape in treating wounds, or injuries with contaminated wooden splinters.

Clinical Presentation

Cutaneous zygomycosis usually begins with the appearance of cellulitis, which progresses to ulceration and eschar formation. Affected patients with skin disease usually have obvious pulmonary infection, or they have had previous trauma to the skin with soil contamination. Rarely, primary skin lesions have occurred at catheter sites or illicit drug injection sites.

Histologic Findings

Rhizopus, Mucor, and *Lichtheimia* cannot be readily distinguished from one another morphologically in H&E sections (Figure 20-25). They cause histologic lesions that are essentially identical to those described previously for aspergillosis.

Differential Diagnosis

Folds in the hyphae of the zygomycetes are sometimes mistaken for septa microscopically. Thus, ultimately, formal cultures are necessary to distinguish such organisms from *Aspergillus* species, or *Fusarium.* Immunostains are available commercially for the recognition of *Aspergillus,* but they have not been tested rigorously for specificity.

CAPSULE SUMMARY

ZYGOMYCOSIS OF THE SKIN

Zygomycosis is seen in poorly controlled diabetes mellitus or other forms of immunocompromise. Skin involvement is typically secondary following primary pulmonary infection. Cutaneous lesions resemble those of aspergillosis grossly and microscopically, except that fungal hyphae in zygomycosis are nonseptated.

ALGAL INFECTION OF THE SKIN—PROTOTHECOSIS

Definition and Epidemiology

Protothecosis (PT) is rare human infection with an achlorophyllic algae of the genus *Prototheca.* It may present with localized infections of the skin, olecranon bursitis, or disseminated multiorgan disease. PT has been reported globally with no age or gender predilection.

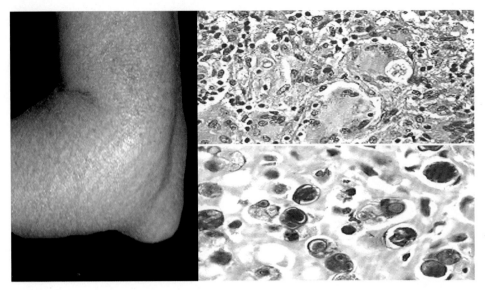

FIGURE 20-25. This adolescent boy has subacute combined immunodeficiency syndrome. He developed ulcerating plaques and nodules in the skin of the extremities, representing zygomycosis (mucormycosis) (left panel). A mixed inflammatory infiltrate in the dermis contains numerous broad, ribbon-like, nonseptated hyphal organisms (top right panel), representing *Rhizopus*. They are labeled with the Gomori methenamine-silver stain (bottom right panel).

Etiology

Infection of the skin is felt to occur through direct inoculation of the dermis or subcutaneous tissue by a puncture wound that is contaminated with brackish water. Although person-to-person transmission has not been reported, *Prototheca* has also been cultured from beneath the fingernails in healthy individuals. Infections in immunocompetent people may be self-limiting, but the majority of reported cases are seen in immunocompromised patients.

Clinical Presentation

Skin manifestations are common in PT, and the extremities are most commonly affected. The lesions are variable in appearance, including eczematous plaques and nodules. Other lesions may be atrophic, herpetiform, bullous, verrucous, or hypopigmented, and some having the appearance of apple jelly have been reported. Erythema and pain may be present. In immunocompetent patients, the lesions may be subtle, with mildly erythematous papulonodules that are stable for long periods of time.

Histologic Findings

Cutaneous lesions typically have a necrotic center surrounded by granulation tissue, histiocytes, and multinucleated giant cells. The causative organisms are seen intracellularly, or they can be extracellular in foci of necrosis. The algae are represented by thick-walled spherical sporangia (Figure 20-26). Morulating forms have a soccer ball–like appearance, and nonmorulating forms resemble eyeballs. These can be labeled with PAS and GMS stains. The inflammatory infiltrate may demonstrate angiocentricity and adnexocentricity, and the overlying epidermis is acanthotic and parakeratotic.

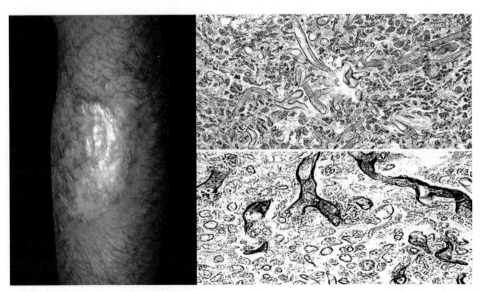

FIGURE 20-26. An adolescent girl developed olecranon bursitis (left panel). The lesion contained algal sporangia with refractile walls, representing *Prototheca* (right panels).

CAPSULE SUMMARY

PROTOTHECOSIS OF THE SKIN

PT is an algal infection, rather than a bacterial or fungal disease. It is usually caused by traumatic injury and contamination with brackish water; most patients are immunocompromised. Clinical lesions in the skin may be eczematous plaques, nodules, vesicobullous, verrucous, hypopigmented, or *apple jelly–like*. Histologically, the lesions of cutaneous protothecosis again resemble those of sporotrichosis, except featuring more necrosis. Spherical sporangia or morular algal forms may be seen in histiocytes or in areas of necrosis. Associated dermal inflammation is angiocentric or adnexocentric, and the epidermis is acanthotic. The organisms can be labeled with the PAS method.

REFERENCES

The Tineas

Admani S, Jinna S, Friedlander SF, Sloan B. Cutaneous infectious diseases: kids are not just little people. *Clin Dermatol.* 2015;33:657-671.

Alves R, Grimalt R. Hair loss in children. *Curr Probl Dermatol.* 2015;47:55-66.

Asz-Sigall D, Tosti A, Arenas R. Tinea unguium: diagnosis and treatment in practice. *Mycopathologia.* 2017;182:95-100.

Brito-Santos F, Figueiredo-Carvalho MHG, Coelho RA, Sales A, Almeida-Paes R. Tinea capitis by Microsporum audouinii: case reports and review of published global literature 2000-2016. *Mycopathologia.* 2017;182:1053-1060.

Canavan TN, Elewski BE. Identifying signs of tinea pedis: a key to understanding clinical variables. *J Drugs Dermatol.* 2015;14 (10 Suppl):S42-S47.

Coulibaly O, L'Ollivier C, Piarroux R, Ranque S. Epidemiology of human dermatophytoses in Africa. *Med Mycol.* 2018;56:145-161.

Eichenfield LF, Friedlander SF. Pediatric onychomycosis: the emerging role of topical therapy. *J Drugs Dermatol.* 2017;16:105-109.

Ferguson L, Fuller LC. Spectrum and burden of dermatophytes in children. *J Infect.* 2017;74(suppl 1):S54-S60.

Galadari I, El Komy M, Mousa A, Hashimoto K, Mehregan AH. Tinea versicolor: histologic and ultrastructural investigation of pigmentary changes. *Int J Dermatol.* 1992;31:253-256.

Hay RJ. Tinea capitis: current status. *Mycopathologia.* 2017;182:87-93.

Hube B, Hay R, Brasch J, Veraldi S, Schaller M. Dermatomycoses and inflammation: the adaptive balance between growth, damage, and survival. *J Mycol Med.* 2015;25:e44-e58.

John AM, Schwartz RA, Janniger CK. The kerion: an angry tinea capitis. *Int J Dermatol.* 2018;37:3-9.

Kaushik N, Pujalte GG, Reese ST. Superficial fungal infections. *Prim Care.* 2015;42:501-516.

Kutlubay Z, Yardımcı G, Kantarcıoğlu AS, Serdaroğlu S. Acral manifestations of fungal infections. *Clin Dermatol.* 2017;35:28-39.

LaSenna C, Miteva M. Special stains and immunohistochemical stains in hair pathology. *Am J Dermatopathol.* 2016;38:327-337.

Panthagani AP, Tidman MJ. Diagnosis directs treatment in fungal infections of the skin. *Practitioner.* 2015;259:25-29.

Rayala BZ, Morrell DS. Common skin conditions in children: skin Infections. *FP Essent.* 2017;453:26-32.

Rosen T. Assessment of dermatophytosis treatment studies: interpreting the data. *J Drugs Dermatol.* 2015;14(10 suppl):S48-S54.

Sahoo AK, Mahajan R. Management of tinea corporis, tinea cruris, and tinea pedis: a comprehensive review. *Indian Dermatol Online J.* 2016;7:77-86.

Solís-Arias MP, García-Romero MT. Onychomycosis in children. A review. *Int J Dermatol.* 2017;56:123-130.

Souza BD, Sartori DS, Andrade C, Weisheimer E, Kiszewski AE. Dermatophytosis caused by Microsporum gypseum in infants: report of four cases and review of the literature. *An Bras Dermatol.* 2016;91:823-825.

Tamburro J. Dermatology for the pediatrician: advances in diagnosis and treatment of common and not-so-common skin conditions. *Cleve Clin J Med.* 2015;82(11 suppl 1):S19-S23.

Verrier J, Monod M. Diagnosis of dermatophytosis using molecular biology. *Mycopathologia.* 2017;182:193-202.

Xu L, Liu KX, Senna MM. A practical approach to the diagnosis and management of hair loss in children and adolescents. *Front Med* (Lausanne). 2017;4:112. doi:10.3389/fmed.2017.00112. PMID: 28791288

Zampella JG, Kwatra SG, Blanck J, Cohen B. Tinea in tots: cases and literature review of oral antifungal treatment of tinea capitis in children under 2 years of age. *J Pediatr.* 2017;183:12-18.

Zhan P, Liu W. The changing face of dermatophytic infections worldwide. *Mycopathologia.* 2017;182:77-86.

Candidiasis

Agarwal S, Sharma M, Mehndirata V. Solitary ecthyma gangrenosum (EG)-like lesion consequent to Candida albicans in a neonate. *Indian J Pediatr.* 2007;74:582-584.

Aly R, Berger T. Common superficial fungal infections in patients with AIDS. *Clin Infect Dis.* 1996;22 (Suppl 2):S128-S132.

Bonifaz A, Rojas R, Tirado-Sanchez A, et al. Superficial mycoses associated with diaper dermatitis. *Mycopathologia.* 2016;181:671-679.

Campois TG, Zucoloto AZ, de Almeida Araujo EJ, et al. Immunological and histopathological characterization of cutaneous candidiasis. *J Med Microbiol.* 2015;64:810-817.

Chirac A, Brzezinski P, Chiriac AE, Foia L, Pinteala T. Autosensitisation (autoeczematisation) reactions in a case of diaper dermatitis candidasis. *Niger Med J.* 2014;55:274-275.

Diana A, Epiney M, Ecoffey M, Pfister RE. White dots on the placenta and red dots on the baby: congenital cutaneous candidiasis: a rare disease of the neonate. *Acta Paediatr.* 2004;93:996-999.

Gibney MD, Siegfried EC. Cutaneous congenital candidiasis: a case report. *Pediatr Dermatol.* 1995;12:359-363.

Hoppe JE. Treatment of oropharyngeal candidiasis and candidal diaper dermatitis in neonates and infants: review and reappraisal. *Pediatr Infect Dis J.* 1997;16:885-894.

Kränke B, Trummer M, Brabek E, Komericki P, Turek TD, Aberer W. Etiologic and causative factors in perianal dermatitis: results of a prospective study in 126 patients. *Wien Klin Wochenschr.* 2006;118:90-94.

Lim CS, Lim SL. New contrast stain for the rapid diagnosis of dermatophytic and candidal dermatomycoses. *Arch Dermatol.* 2008;144:1228-1229.

Mayer FL, Wilson D, Hube B. Candida albicans: pathogenicity mechanisms. *Virulence.* 2013;4:2.

Pappas PG, Kauffman CA, Andes DR, et al. Executive summary: clinical practice guideline for the management of candidiasis: 2016 update by the Infectious Diseases Society of America. *Clin Infect Dis.* 2016;62:409-417. [Medline]

Ramos-E-Silva M, Lima CM, Schechtman RC, Trope BM, Carneiro S. Superficial mycoses in immunodepressed patients. *Clin Dermatol.* 2010;28:217-225.

Raval DS, Barton LL, Hansen RC, Kling PJ. Congenital cutaneous candidiasis: case report and review. *Pediatr Dermatol.* 1995;12:355-358.

Shiraki Y, Ishibashi Y, Hiruma M, Nishikawa A, Ikeda S. *Candida albicans* abrogates the expression of interferon-gamma-inducible protein-10 in human keratinocytes. *FEMS Immunol Med Microbiol.* 2008;54:122-128.

Wang SM, Yang YJ, Chen JS, Lin HC, Chi CY, Liu CC. Invasive fungal infections in pediatric patients with leukemia: emphasis on pulmonary and dermatological manifestations. *Acta Paediatr Taiwan.* 2005;46:149-155.

Pityrosporum Folliculitis

Crespo Erchiga V, Delgado Florencio V. Malassezia species in skin diseases. *Curr Opin Infect Dis.* 2002;2:133-142.

Difonzo EM, Faggi E. Skin diseases associated with Malassezia species in humans: clinical features and diagnostic criteria. *Parassitologia.* 2008;50:69-71.

Difonzo EM, Faggi E, Bassi A, et al. Malassezia skin diseases in humans. *G Ital Dermatol Venereol.* 2013;148:609-619.

Gaitanis G, Magiatis P, Hantschke M, Bassukas ID, Velegraki A. The Malassezia genus in skin and systemic diseases. *Clin Microbiol Rev.* 2012;25:106-141.

Harada K, Saito M, Sugita T, Tsuboi R. Malassezia species and their associated skin diseases. *J Dermatol.* 2015;42:250-257.

Nenoff P, Krüger C, Mayser P. Cutaneous Malassezia infections and Malassezia associated dermatoses: an update. *Hautarzt.* 2015;66:465-484.

Prindaville B, Belazarian L, Levin NA, Wiss K. Pityrosporum folliculitis: a retrospective review of 110 cases. *J Am Acad Dermatol.* 2018;78:511-514.

Prohic A, Jovovic Sadikovic T, Krupalija-Fazlic M, Kuskunovic-Vlahovljak S. Malassezia species in healthy skin and in dermatological conditions. *Int J Dermatol.* 2016;55:494-504.

Rubenstein RM, Malerich SA. Malassezia (pityrosporum) folliculitis. *J Clin Aesthet Dermatol.* 2014;7:37-41.

Tragiannidis A, Bisping G, Koehler G, Groll AH. Minireview. Malassezia infections in immunocompromised patients. *Mycoses.* 2010;53:187-195.

Piedra

Gupta AK, Chaudhry M, Elewski B. Tinea corporis, tinea cruris, tinea nigra, and piedra. *Dermatol Clin.* 2003;21:395-400.

Kiken DA, Sekaran A, Antaya RJ, Davis A, Imaeda S, Silverberg NB. White Piedra in children. *J Am Acad Dermatol.* 2006;55:956-961.

Steinman HK, Pappenfort RB. White piedra: a case report and review of the literature. *Clin Exp Dermatol* 1984;9:591-598.

Rhinosporidiosis

Moréira Díaz EE, Milán Batista B, Eduardo Mayor González C, Yokoyama H. Rhinosporidiosis: a study of 33 cases diagnosed using biopsies at the Central Hospital of Maputo, since 1944 through 1986. *Rev Cubana Med Trop.* 1989;41:461-472.

Owor R, Wamukota WM. Rhinosporidiosis in Uganda: a review of 51 cases. *East Afr Med J.* 1978;55:582-586.

Pal DK, Mallick AA, Majhi TK, Biswas BK, Chowdhury MK. Rhinosporidiosis in southwest Bengal. *Trop Doct.* 2012;42:150-153.

Prabha N, Arora R, Chhabra N, Joseph W, Singh VY, Satpute SS, Nagarkar NM. Disseminated cutaneous Rhinosporidiosis. *Skinmed.* 2018;16(1):63-65.

Vallarelli AF, Rosa SP, Souza EM. Rhinosporidiosis: cutaneous manifestations. *An Bras Dermatol.* 2011;86:795-796.

Watve JK, Mane RS, Mohite AA, Patil BC. Lacrimal sac rhinosporidiosis. *Indian J Otolaryngol Head Neck Surg.* 2006;58:399-400.

Cryptococcosis

Chayakulkeeree M, Perfect JR. Cryptococcosis. *Infect Dis Clin North Am.* 2006;20:507-544.

Husain S, Wagener MM, Singh N. Cryptococcus neoformans infection in organ transplant recipients: variables influencing clinical characteristics and outcome. *Emerg Infect Dis.* 2001;7:375-381.

Maxson S, Jacobs RF. Community-acquired fungal pneumonia in children. *Semin Respir Infect.* 1996;11:196-203.

Negroni R: Cryptococcosis. *Clin Dermatol.* 2012;30:599-609.

Sarosi GA, Silberfarb PM, Tosh FE. Cutaneous cryptococcosis. *Arch Dermatol.* 1971;104:1-3.

Schupbach CW, Wheeler CE, Briggaman RA, Warner NA, Kanof EP. Cutaneous manifestations of disseminated cryptococcosis. *Arch Dermatol.* 1976;112:1734-1740.

Shah PM, Sharma KD: Cryptococcosis: report of a case with review of the literature. *Indian Pediatr.* 1964;1:181-189.

Blastomycosis

Bradsher RW, Chapman SW, Pappas PG. Blastomycosis. *Infect Dis Clin North Am.* 2003;17:21-40.

Carrasco-Zuber JE, Navarrete-Dechent C, Bonifaz A, Fich F, Vial-Letelier V, Berroeta-Mauriziano D. Cutaneous involvement in the deep mycoses: a review. Part II. Systemic mycoses. *Actas Dermosifiliogr.* 2016;107:816-822.

Elgart GW: Subcutaneous (deep) fungal infections. *Semin Cutan Med Surg.* 2014;33:146-150.

Emerson PA, Higgins E, Branfoot A. North American blastomycosis in Africans. *Br J Dis Chest.* 1984;78:286-291.

Gonzalez-Santiago TM, Pritt B, Gibson LE, Comfere NI. Diagnosis of deep cutaneous fungal infections: correlation between skin tissue culture and histopathology. *J Am Acad Dermatol.* 2014;71:293-301.

Guegan S, Lanternier F, Rouzaud C, Dupin N, Lortholary O. Fungal skin and soft tissue infections. *Curr Open Infect Dis.* 2016;29:124-130.

Larsh HW, Schwartz J. Accidental inoculation blastomycosis. *Cutis.* 1977;19:334-335.

Lopez-Martinez R, Mendez-Tovar LJ: Blastomycosis. *Clin Dermatol.* 2012;30:565-572.

McBride JA, Gauthier GM, Klein BS: Clinical manifestations and treatment of blastomycosis. *Clin Chest Med.* 2017;38:435-449.

Coccidioidomycosis

Barker BM, Jewell KA, Kroken S, Orbach MJ. The population biology of Coccidioides: epidemiologic implications for disease outbreaks. *Ann N Y Acad Sci.* 2007;1111:147-163.

DiCaudo DJ. Coccidioidomycosis. *Semin Cutan Med Surg.* 2014;33:140-145.

Galgiani JN, Ampel NM, Blair JE, et al. Coccidioidomycosis. *Clin Infect Dis.* 2005;41:1217-1223.

Garcia-Garcia SC, Salas-Alanis JC, Flores MG, Gonzalez-Gonzalez SE, Vera-Cabrera L, Ocampo-Candiani J. Coccidioidomycosis: a comprehensive review. *An Bras Dermatol.* 2015;90:610-619.

Werner SB, Pappagianis D, Heindl I, Mickel A. An epidemic of coccidioidomycosis among archeology students in northern California. *N Engl J Med.* 1972;286:507-512.

Histoplasmosis

Dijkstra JW. Histoplasmosis. *Dermatol Clin.* 1989;7:251-258.

Fischer GB, Mocelin H, Severo CB, Oliveira Fde M, Xavier MO, Severo LC. Histoplasmosis in children. *Paediatr Respir Rev.* 2009;10:172-177.

Jain A, Jain S, Rawat S. Emerging fungal infections among children: a review of clinical manifestations, diagnosis, and prevention. *J Pharm Bioallied Sci.* 2010;2:314-320.

Kurowski R, Ostapchuk M. Overview of histoplasmosis. *Am Fam Physician.* 2002;66:2247-2252.

McKinsey DS, McKinsey JP. Pulmonary histoplasmosis. *Semin Respir Crit Care Med.* 2011;32:735-744.

Wheat LJ, Kauffman CA. Histoplasmosis. *Infect Dis Clin North Am.* 2003;17:1-19.

Paracoccidioidomycosis

Bocca AL, Amaral AC, Teixeira MM, Sato PK, Shikanai-Yasuda MA, Soares-Felipe MS. Paracoccidioidomycosis: eco-epidemiology, taxonomy, and clinical & therapeutic issues. *Future Microbiol.* 2013;8:1177-1191.

Franco M, Del Negro G, Lacaz CDS, Restrepo-Moreno A. *Paracoccidioidomycosis.* Boca Raton, FL: CRC Press; 1994.

Marques SA. Paracoccidioidomycosis. *Clin Dermatol.* 2012;30:610-615.

Pereira RM, Tresoldi AT, da Silva MTN, Bucaretchi F. Fatal disseminated paracoccidioidomycosis in a two-year-old child. *Rev Do Instituto De Medicina Tropical De Sao Paulo.* 2004;46:37-39.

Sporotrichosis

Belknap BS. Sporotrichosis. *Dermatol Clin.* 1989;7:193-202.

Bullpitt P, Weedon D. Sporotrichosis: a review of 39 cases. *Pathology.* 1978;10:249-256.

da Rosa AC, Scroferneker ML, Vettorato R, Gervini RL, Vettorato G, Weber A. Epidemiology of sporotrichosis: a study of 304 cases in Brazil. *J Am Acad Dermatol.* 2005;52:451-459.

Ramos-e-Silva M, Vasconcelos C, Carneiro S, Cestari T. Sporotrichosis. *Clin Dermatol.* 2007;25:181-186.

Vieira-Dias D, Sena CM, Oréfice F, Tanure MA, Hamdan JS. Ocular and concomitant cutaneous sporotrichosis. *Mycoses.* 1997;40:197-201.

Chromomycosis

Caputo RV. Fungal infections in children. *Dermatol Clin.* 1986;4:137-149.

Carrion AL. Chromoblastomycosis and related infections. *Int J Dermatol.* 1975;14:27-32.

Currie BJ, Carapetis JR. Skin infections and infestations in Aboriginal communities in northern Australia. *Australas J Dermatol.* 2000;41:139-143.

Li R, Wang D, Dai W. Dematiaceous fungal infections in China. *Curr Top Med Mycol.* 1995;6:283-305.

López Martínez R, Méndez Tovar LJ. Chromoblastomycosis. *Clin Dermatol.* 2007;25:188-194.

Lu S, Lu C, Zhang J, Hu Y, Li X, Xi L: Chromoblastomycosis in Mainland China: a systematic review of clinical characteristics. *Mycopathologia.* 2013;175:489-495.

Mycetoma (Madura foot)

Al-Hatmi AM, Bonifaz A, Tirado-Sanchez A, Meis JF, de Hoog GS, Ahmed SA. Fusarium species causing eumycetoma: report of two cases and comprehensive review of the literature. *Mycoses.* 2017;60:204-212.

Arenas R, Fernandez-Martinez RF, Torres-Guerrero E, Garcia C. Actinomycetoma: an update on diagnosis and treatment. *Cutis.* 2017;99:e11-e15.

Mencarini J, Antonelli A, Scoccianti G, et al. Madura foot in Europe: diagnosis of an autochthonous case by molecular approach and review of the literature. *New Microbiol.* 2016;39:156-159.

Aspergillosis

Bernardeschi C, Foulet F, Ingen-Housz-Oro S, et al. Cutaneous invasive aspergillosis:retrospective multicenter study of the French Invasive-Aspergillosis Registry and literature review. *Medicine.* 2015;94:e1018.

Hasan RA, Abuhammour W. Invasive aspergillosis in children with hematologic malignancies. *Paediatr Drugs.* 2006;8:15-24.

Tatara AM, Mikos AG, Kontoyiannis DP. Factors affecting patient outcome in primary cutaneous aspergillosis. *Medicine.* 2016;95:e3747.

Zygomycosis

Gamaletsou MN, Sipsas NV, Roilides E, Walsh TJ. Rhino-orbital-cerebral mucormycosis. *Curr Infect Dis Rep.* 2012;14:423-434.

Kontoyiannis DP, Lewis RE. Agents of mucormycosis and entomophthoramycosis. In: Mandell GL, Bennett GE, Dolin R, eds. *Mandell, Douglas and Bennett's Principles and Practice of Infectious Diseases.* 7th ed. Philadelphia, PA: Churchill-Livingstone; 2010: 3257-3269.

Li H, Hwang SK, Zhou C, Du J, Zhang J. Gangrenous cutaneous mucormycosis caused by Rhizopus oryzae: a case report and review of primary cutaneous mucormycosis in China over the past 20 years. *Mycopathologia.* 2013:176:123-128.

Lowe CD, Sainato RJ, Stagliano DR, Morgan MM, Green BP. Primary cutaneous mucomycosis in an extremely preterm infant, successfully treated with liposomal amphotericin-B. *Pediatr Dermatol.* 2017;34:e116-e119.

Petrikkos G, Skiada A, Lortholary O, Roilides E, Walsh TJ, Kontoyiannis DP. Epidemiology and clinical manifestations of mucormycosis. *Clin Infect Dis.* 2012;(54 suppl 1):S23-S34.

Protothecosis

Hightower KD, Messina JL. Cutaneous prototothecosis: a case report and review of the literature. *Cutis.* 2007;80:129-131.

Hillesheim PB, Bahrami S. Cutaneous prototothecosis. *Arch Pathol Lab Med.* 2011;135:941-944.

Kantrow SM, Boyd AS. Prototothecosis. *Dermatol Clin.* 2003;21:249-255.

Lass-Flori C, Mayr A. Human prototothecosis. *Clin Microbiol Rev.* 2007;20:230-242.

Lee JS, Moon GH, Lee NY, Peck KR. Case report: protothecal tenosynovitis. *Clin Orthop Relat Res.* 2008;466:3143-3146.

Leimann BC, Monteiro PC, Lazéra M, Candanoza ER, Wanke B. Prototothecosis. *Med Mycol.* 2004;42:95-106.

Lu S, Xi L, Qin W, Luo Y, Lu C, Li X. Cutaneous prototothecosis: two new cases in China and literature review. *Int J Dermatol.* 2012;51:328-331.

Todd JR, King JW, Oberle A, et al. Prototothecosis: report of a case with 20-year follow-up, and review of previously published cases. *Med Mycol.* 2012;50:673-689.

Walsh SV, Johnson RA, Tahan SR. Prototothecosis: an unusual cause of chronic subcutaneous and soft tissue infection. *Am J Dermatopathol.* 1998;20:379-382.

Wirth FA, Passalacqua JA, Kao G. Disseminated cutaneous prototothecosis in an immunocompromised host: a case report and literature review. *Cutis.* 1999;63:185-188.

21

Parasite Infestations in Cutaneous Infections

J. Olufemi Ogunbiyi / Alejandro A. Gru

SCHISTOSOMIASIS

Definition and Epidemiology

Schistosomiasis is the most important trematode as a cause of dermatologic manifestations. It is also known as bilharzia or "snail fever," as the parasite is carried by freshwater snails.[1-5] It is caused by the human flukes *Schistosoma haematobium* (urogenital diseases), *Schistosoma mansoni,* and *Schistosoma japonicum* (gastrointestinal (GI) and liver disease), which are released by their snail intermediate hosts into freshwater. Humans get infected after recreational or occupational contact with freshwater that has free-swimming cercariae. The main types of exposure to infected water are connected to agricultural, fishing, domestic, and recreational activities.[6]

Etiology

S. haematobium and *S. mansoni* are endemic in Africa, Middle East, and Latin America, whereas *S. japonicum* is endemic in East Asia. *S. intercalatum* is found in parts of west and central Africa. In endemic areas, about 60% to 80% of cases are seen in children. It affects more than 200 million people worldwide.[2,3,5] All species are acquired by swimming and bathing in waters inhabited by schistosomes. The larvae emerge from the snails and swim in the water until they come in contact with an individual and penetrate the skin. Once inside the body, the larvae develop into adult male and female worms, which pair up and live together in the blood vessels from years, particularly in the venous system of the rectum and bladder. Female worms release thousands of eggs, which travel to the bladder and intestines, and are subsequently passed in the feces and urine. The eggs hatch and release the miracidia that swims in search of a member of the snail species that is specific for each schistosome species. The snail is an intermediary host, and within it, the cercariae develop into its infective form. The definitive hosts that are responsible for the disease are mammals or birds, where the cercariae complete their life cycle.

Clinical Presentation

Schistosomes produce cutaneous lesions at the site of skin penetration of the schistosomule (cercariae).[4,6-11] The typical lesion is referred to as the "swimmer's itch" (cercarial dermatitis)[4] and results from a cutaneous deposition of ova or hypersensitivity to the cercaria or ova of the parasite, leading to an urticarial reaction. Cercarial dermatitis is an acute itchy erythematous popular or urticarial rash that occurs within hours of cercarial penetration into the skin and it is usually followed by fever, headache, diarrhea, etc (also known as "*Katayama fever*").

Clinically, the most commonly affected areas include the genital and perineal sites forming multiple papular and nodular lesions (infrequently extragenital cutaneous depositions may be seen in children).[10-12] Widespread dissemination of the cercariae and/or ova could lead to an urticarial reaction to the parasite.

Histologic Findings

The histologic findings of cercarial dermatitis include the presence of a dermal suppurative acute inflammatory process with infiltration by neutrophils and a large proportion of eosinophils.[5,6,13] The ova of Schistosoma are usually seen in the dermis stimulating a granulomatous inflammation with variable eosinophilic infiltrates. In some occasions, eosinophilic flame figures can be present. Foreign body–type giant cells are seen attempting to ingest the ova. In older lesions, there is calcification of the ova. Species identification can be determined by the location of a spine or knob (terminal/apical spine for *S. haematobium*, a lateral spine for *S. mansoni* and a knob for *S. japonicum*)[6] (Figure 21-1).

The basic lesions of Schistosomiasis include (1) a circumscribed granuloma around eggs or (2) a diffuse cellular infiltrate around eggs. Eosinophils and neutrophils usually predominate in the diffuse dermal infiltrate, but plasma cells, lymphocytes, macrophages, and giant cells can also be present.[6] The circumoval granulomas, also called pseudotubercles, are primarily reactions of delayed hypersensitivity, but the immunologic mechanisms of the diffuse reactions are not known. The only pathognomonic finding is the presence of schistosomal eggs. Sometimes, the eggs can be surrounded by a layer of eosinophilic material, the so-called Splendore–Hoeppli phenomenon. Pseudoepitheliomatous changes can also be present (Figure 21-2).

CAPSULE SUMMARY

SCHISTOSOMIASIS

Schistosomiasis is the most important trematode that causes dermatological manifestations and is caused by the human flukes *S. haematobium* (urogenital diseases), *S. mansoni*, and *S. japonicum* (GI and liver disease). Schistosomes produce cutaneous lesions at the site of skin penetration of the schistosomule (cercariae) which is referred to as *swimmer's itch*, cutaneous deposition of ova or hypersensitivity to the schistosomule or ova of the parasite. Histopathologically, in cercarial dermatitis there is area of suppuration with collection of eosinophils and features of acute inflammation. The ova of Schistosoma are usually seen in the dermis with stimulation of granulomatous inflammation with variable eosinophilic infiltrates. Foreign body type giant cells are seen attempting to ingest the ova.

CYSTICERCOSIS

Definition and Epidemiology

Cysticercosis is the result of the infection with the larval stage (*cysticercosis cellulosae*) of the human pork tapeworm, *Tinea solium*, which results in the infection of multiple organ sites, but particularly the central nervous system (CNS) (neurocysticercosis).[14-16] The latter continues to be one of

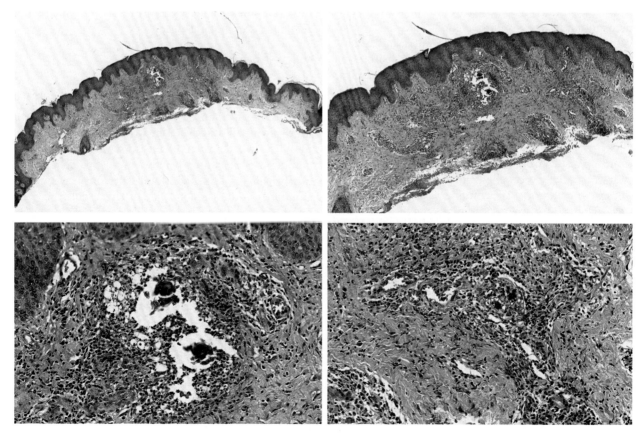

FIGURE 21-1. **Histology of schistosomiasis.** Digital slides courtesy of Path Presenter.com.

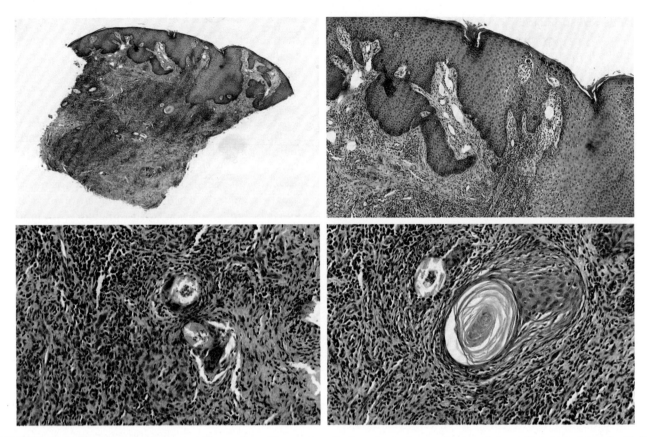

FIGURE 21-2. Chronic granulomatous inflammation with pseudoepitheliomatous changes in association with schistosomiasis. Digital slides courtesy of Path Presenter.com.

the most important causes of seizures in the world.[16] The disease is found in Eastern Europe, India, Pakistan, China, sub-Saharan Africa, South and Central America. It is usually more prevalent in low socioeconomic areas with poor hygiene and in areas where people live in proximity to pigs. It is not common in the United States, although it has been reported in immigrants.

Etiology

Cysticercosis results from a contamination of infected food and water, especially vegetables, with feces containing the eggs of the human pork tapeworm.[15-21] The parasite has a life cycle that includes two hosts: humans and pigs. Humans are the only host of the adult tapeworm, whereas humans and pigs can be intermediate hosts for the larval form, the cysticercus. Autoinoculation also occurs from dirty contaminated hands. The coat of the eggs is digested in the stomach and oncospheres are liberated. The oncospheres invade the intestinal wall and enter the blood stream after which they migrate and get lodged in various organs, particularly the eyes, skeletal muscle, subcutaneous tissue, and CNS where they mature to become a cysticercus. Eating food contaminated by human feces then infects pigs. In the pig, the embryo penetrates the intestinal wall, and via the bloodstream, reaches the skeletal muscle to become a cysticercus. When humans ingest undercooked pork meat, the cycle is completed. If human ingests organisms (not eggs),

the adult tapeworm develops into *T. solium*, which can measure up to 2 to 4 m in length.

Clinical Presentation

Cysticercosis has a peak incidence between the ages of 20 and 50. The cutaneous manifestations are characterized by the presence of subcutaneous nodules (*cysticercosis cellulosae cutis*), which are usually less than 2 cm in diameter (Figures 21-3 and 21-4).[18,22-24] Cystic lesions of most tapeworms do not evoke an immunologic response when the cyst is alive. The nodules are usually painless, firm, and round. There may be few or up to a hundred in the same individual. The nodules may remain unchanged for years. The skin nodules should prompt for the evaluation of involvement of other organ sites. Cutaneous cysticercosis is more common in Asia than in the Americas or Africa. In approximately 50% of patients the lesions have been present for a month. The remaining 50% can have lesions for several years. The lesions can also affect mucosal areas, such as the tongue. Approximately 20% of patients have an isolated skin lesion, and 70% have less than 10 lesions. The typically affected cutaneous sites include the trunk, scalp, eyelids, face, tongue, neck, breasts, upper limbs, and thighs. In some occasions, the patients might experience a "popping" sensation in the lesion than can correlate with a rupture of the cyst. Muscle pain is also frequent and 10% can show calcifications by x-ray. A diagnosis can be established by the biopsy of one of the nodules.

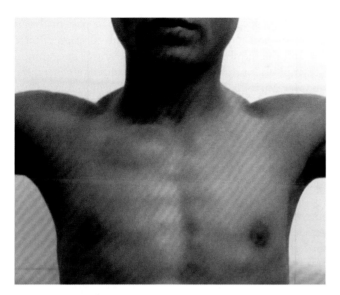

FIGURE 21-3. Photograph showing well-defined swelling in the right infraclavicular region. Obtained with permission from Chauhan S, Singh G, Khan I. Cysticercosis of the pectoralis major: a case report and review of literature. *Am J Dermatopathol.* 2017;39(3):e34-e37.

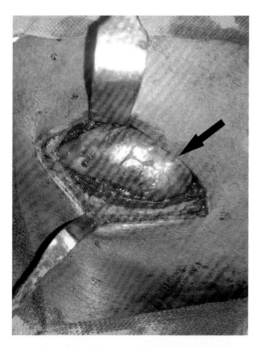

FIGURE 21-4. Intraoperative photograph showing a smooth-walled cyst within the muscle belly. Obtained with permission from Chauhan S, Singh G, Khan I. Cysticercosis of the pectoralis major: a case report and review of literature. *Am J Dermatopathol.* 2017;39(3):e34-e37.

Histologic Findings

Viable cysticerci may be seen in tissue, compressing adjacent structures, but causing virtually no inflammatory response. When the whole larva is present, it is seen as a cystic structure surrounded by a vesicular wall. The lumen

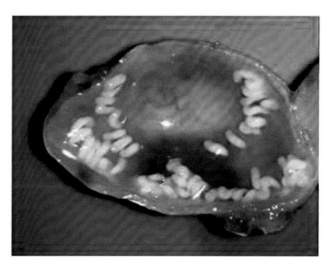

FIGURE 21-5. **Cysticercal larva.**

is folded and ribbon-like and contains the invaginated scolex. Occasionally, sucking discs and hooklets can be seen. Hooklets have a distinctive histologic appearance, as they appear as brown, refractile, sickle-shaped structures. However, when cysticerci degenerate, they elicit an inflammatory reaction with infiltration by neutrophils, histiocytes, and eosinophils. (Figures 21-5 and 21-6) A granulomatous reaction eventually develops, characterized by the presence of histiocytes, epithelioid cells, and foreign body giant cells. Ultimately, this leads to fibrosis and calcification.[17,23,25,26]

CAPSULE SUMMARY

CYSTICERCOSIS

Infection with the larval stage (*cystercicosis cellulosae*) of the human pork tapeworm, *T. solium*, results in the infection of multiple organ sites, but particularly the central nervous system. Cystercicosis results from contamination of infected food and water, especially vegetables, with feces containing the eggs of the human pork tapeworm. Autoinoculation also occurs from dirty contaminated hands. The oncospheres invade the intestinal wall and enter the blood stream after which they migrate and get lodged in various organs, particularly the eyes, skeletal muscle, subcutaneous tissue, and central nervous system.

ONCHOCERCIASIS

Definition and Epidemiology

Onchocerciasis is a filarial infection caused by the worm *Onchocerca volvulus*, leading to a variety of skin manifestation and blindness. It is endemic in some parts of sub-Saharan Africa especially West Africa, Yemen, Central, and South

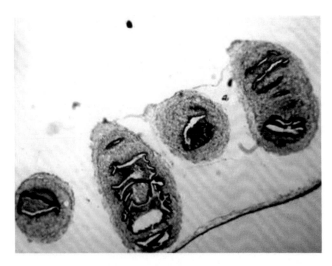

FIGURE 21-6. **Histology of cysticercosis.**

America. It is estimated that 18 million people are living with onchocerciasis and 99% of these reside in Africa.[27-31]

Onchocerciasis does not have any racial predilection, but it has been observed that the cutaneous findings are more common in the forested areas, whereas blindness is more common in the Savannah areas, possibly resulting from some type of genetic predisposition.[32]

Etiology

The vector of the disease is the *Simulium* (black fly), which is found around flowing water; hence Onchocerciasis is also known as "river blindness." *Simulium damnosum* is a species complex of 55 named cytoforms (cytospecies and cytotypes) and constitute the largest known species complex of any vector. It is distributed throughout sub-Saharan Africa and the Arabian Peninsula but is limited to being an onchocerciasis vector distributed in Uganda, Benin, Burkina Faso, Cameroon, Central African Republic, Ghana, Guinea, Guinea-Bissau, Ivory Coast, Liberia, Mali, Niger, Nigeria, Senegal, Sierra Leone, Sudan, and Togo.[30,31]

The *Simulium* fly takes a blood meal from an infected individual containing the microfilaria of *Onchocerca volvulus*. The microfilaria matures in the mouthparts of the fly to produce the larval stage. The larvae are introduced back into the humans by the bite of the *Simulium* fly. The larvae migrate to different parts of the body, but especially to the dermis, where adult *Onchocerca volvulus* worms develop (male and female). The worms reside in nodules known as *Onchocercomata*. The female and male worms mate and the fertilized female then produces microfilariae which move to different parts of the body, especially to the eyes and skin. They can also be eaten by the *Simulium* fly again.

Clinical Presentation

The cutaneous findings of onchocerciasis are variable.[33,34] Factors that affect the clinical features include the age,

geographical location, and immunity of the patient toward the microfilaria. Other factors include the duration of infection and the number of infecting organisms. The commonest symptom is pruritus that may be localized or generalized. However, microfilaria in the skin may be asymptomatic. Cutaneous findings of onchocerciasis include onchocercal dermatitis and skin nodules. Infected individuals may also become blind, especially when cutaneous findings occur on the head.

The clinical features can be different in accordance with the duration of the infection.[28,29,34,35] The acute findings include pruritus and inflammation of skin with edema, causing obliteration of the skin creases (the creases become less obvious). This presentation is more frequent in children. Vesicles and papules may be present. Nodules termed onchocercoma may be present at any stage especially on bony prominences. Patients with chronic disease have more papules, excoriation, lichenification, and postinflammatory hyperpigmentation. These are common on the covered areas, especially the trunk and buttocks. A distinct chronic form of the disease (with similar lichenification and postinflammatory dyspigmentation) with no skip areas affects the limb or contiguous sites and is also known as *Swoda* in Arabic-speaking countries. Enlarged regional lymphadenopathy may also be present, giving the hanging groin sign when the inguinal region is affected. Atrophy of the skin and hypopigmentation are also seen in long-standing cases, especially on the shins, even in the absence of microfilaria (Figure 21-7).

Diagnosis can be made clinically and confirmed by examination of skin snips or biopsy of nodules, which may reveal active microfilaria. ELISA can also be performed as an ancillary technique when it is difficult to demonstrate the organisms.

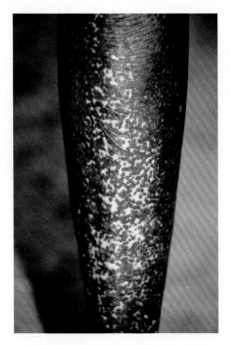

FIGURE 21-7. **Skin in onchocerciasis (clinical).**

Histologic Findings

Onchocercal nodules usually contain several adult worms in the dermis surrounded by an inflammatory reaction that varies from suppurative to granulomatous, with fibrosis[36] (Figures 21-8 and 21-9). The organizing inflammatory process can also be associated with calcification and ossification. A layer of fibrinoid material may be seen covering the worms. The overlying epidermis shows hyperpigmentation with acanthosis and melanin pigment incontinence.

Dermal changes are minimal in the early stage and are characterized by edema and the presence of a chronic inflammatory infiltrate with scattered lymphocytes, histiocytes, plasma cells, and eosinophils around vessels and skin appendages.

It is the degenerating microfilaria that tends to provoke a granulomatous reaction and a rich infiltrate of eosinophils. Proliferating fibroblasts and mast cells may be seen, but neutrophils are typically absent. Microfilariae are most numerous in the upper dermis; they may be scant or abundant and are sometimes present within dermal lymphatics. In more advanced lesions, acanthosis, hyperkeratosis, focal parakeratosis, and melanophages are noted in the upper dermis, with dilated lymphatics, tortuous dermal vessels, and interstitial dermal mucin seen between dermal collagen fibers (which can be proven by a colloidal iron and alcian blue stains). The advanced fibrosis leads to a concentric layering of collagen around dermal vessels.

In onchocerciasis, fibrosis begins early in the disease, is persistent and, ultimately, fibrous tissue replaces the specialized structures of the skin. The papules of *gale filarienne* are intraepidermal abscesses, which contain microfilariae. These are also called *craw craw*. There are, sometimes, subcutaneous fibrous nodules containing microfilaria or adult worms in a background of a mixed population of inflammatory cells that include eosinophils, lymphocytes, and giant cells. The microfilaria may be gravid.

CAPSULE SUMMARY

ONCHOCERCIASIS

Onchocerciasis is a filarial infection caused by the worm *Onchocerca volvulus*, leading to a variety of skin manifestation and blindness. It is endemic in some parts of sub-Saharan Africa especially West Africa, Yemen, Central and South America. It is estimated that 18 million people are living with onchocerciasis and 99% of these reside in Africa. Cutaneous findings of onchocerciasis include onchocercal dermatitis and skin nodules. Onchocercal nodules usually contain several adult worms in the dermis surrounded by an inflammatory reaction that varies from suppurative to granulomatous, with fibrosis.

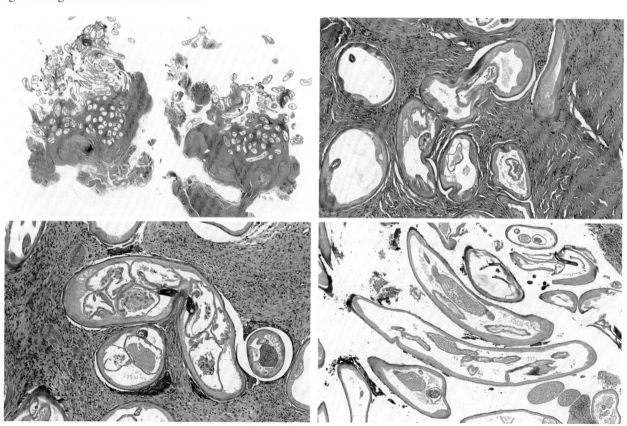

FIGURE 21-8. **Histology of the skin in onchocerciasis.** The transverse sections of the onchocerca demonstrate a prominent cuticle. Digital slides courtesy of Path Presenter.com.

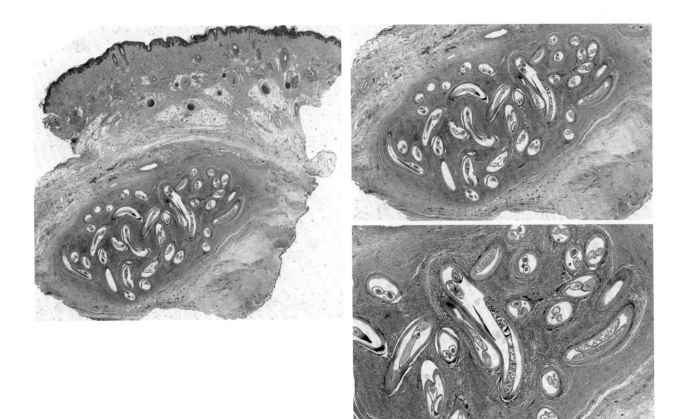

FIGURE 21-9. **Histology of the skin in onchocercoma.** Digital slides courtesy of Path Presenter.com.

CUTANEOUS LARVA MIGRANS

Definition and Epidemiology

This is a cutaneous parasitic infestation, resulting from the migration of parasites through the skin. This disease occurs worldwide.[37,38] However, it is seen more frequently in tropical climates where it affects children who play with soil contaminated with feces, especially on the beach, and in adults with soil-related occupations. In some areas of the world, the problem has led to the banning of pets from beaches. Cases of cutaneous larva migrans (CLM) have been reported at any age or sex.[39-41] The prevalence and infection can be as high as 4% of adults and 15% of children. One-third of those children can develop superimposed bacterial infections. The disease is also known as "creeping eruption," "creeping verminous dermatitis," "sandworm eruption," and "plumber's itch."

Etiology

The causative agents are larvae of nematodes, especially those of dog hookworms *Ancylostoma braziliense*, *Ancylostoma Caninum*, *Uncinaria stenocephala*, *Bunostomum phlebotomum*, and *Necator americanus*.[36] However, the term also encompasses infections produced by other helminths, including trematodes (*Fasciola*) and cestodes (*Spirometra*). Humans are accidental hosts, so the life cycle of the worms cannot be completed in them. The eggs in the feces-contaminated soil hatch when the environment is conducive and the larvae penetrate the skin

through fissures, follicles, or intact skin upon direct contact. The presence of the larvae and their products produce an immunologic response manifested by itching. In the appropriate host (animals), enzymes released by the worms enable them to penetrate into the dermis, blood vessels, and lungs, following a retrograde pathway through the trachea, larynx, and down the intestines to complete the cycle. In humans, the larvae are unable to pass through the basement membrane, and remain in the epidermis until they finally die over a period of weeks to months.

Clinical Presentation

The commonly affected sites include the hands, feet, buttocks, and trunk.[38,42,43] The disease is more commonly associated with walking on a sandy beach either barefoot or in sandals. The initial penetration of the larvae may produce itching and an eczematous rash in the affected areas. The first clinical lesion is a papule, whereas the creeping aspect develops later. The larvae subsequently move in the skin, usually for short distances, producing significant itching, a serpiginous tract or tracts accompanied by erythema and vesicular eruptions, depending on the number of larvae involved.[39,44] The larvae movement ranges across the different species, but it has an average of 2.7 mm/d (Figures 21-10 to 21-14). Secondary lesions and bacterial overinfection (impetiginization) may occur. The lesions are usually self-limiting. The diagnosis is usually clinical and can be facilitated with the use of a dermoscope.

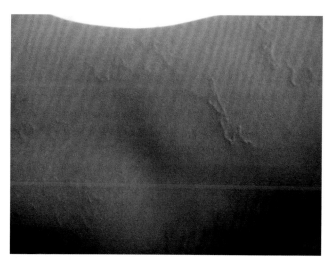

FIGURE 21-10. Clinical picture of cutaneous larva migrans.

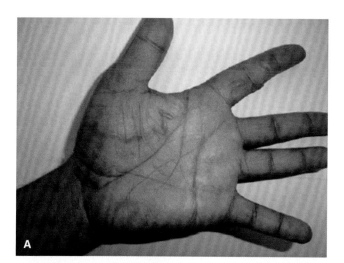

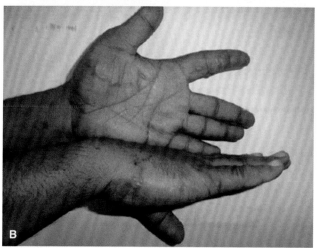

FIGURE 21-11. Multiple serpiginous tracks with a vesicle at the advancing end, one hand (A), both hands (B) in cutaneous larva migrans. Reprinted with permission from Podder I et al. Loeffler's Syndrome Following Cutaneous Larva Migrans: An Uncommon Sequel. *Indian J Dermatol.* 2016;61(2):190-192.

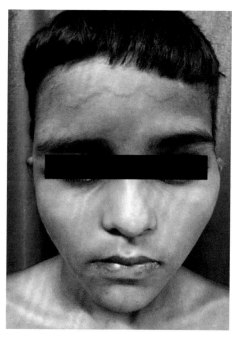

FIGURE 21-12. Single erythematous, curvilinear, track over the forehead. Obtained with permission from Kaur S, Jindal N, Sahu P, Jairath V, Jain VK. Creeping eruption on the move: a case series from Northern India. *Indian J Dermatol.* 2015;60(4):422.

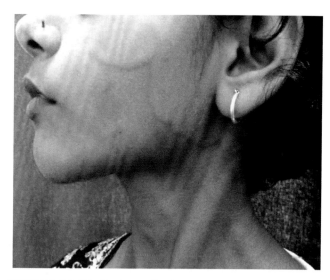

FIGURE 21-13. Single curvilinear track encircling the neck and sides of bilateral cheeks. Obtained with permission from Kaur S, Jindal N, Sahu P, Jairath V, Jain VK. Creeping eruption on the move: a case series from Northern India. *Indian J Dermatol.* 2015;60(4):422.

Histologic findings

The diagnosis is usually based on the clinical appearance of the lesions (the presence of parasitic galleries and identification of parasites within the skin tunnels) and, therefore, biopsies are not usually taken.[45] However, biopsies

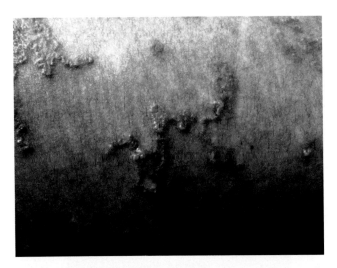

FIGURE 21-14. Multiple disseminated serpiginous tracks on the abdomen. Obtained with permission From Kaur S, Jindal N, Sahu P, Jairath V, Jain VK. Creeping eruption on the move: a case series from Northern India. *Indian J Dermatol.* 2015;60(4):422.

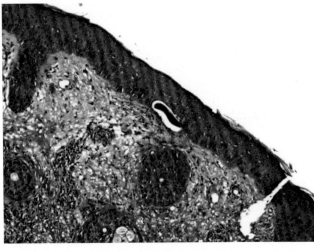

FIGURE 21-16. Cutaneous larva migrans. There is a nematode larva in the lower part of the epidermis. Obtained with permission from Mercado R, González-Chávez J, Sánchez JL, Figueroa LD. Erythematous plaque in the cheek of an HIV patient. *Am J Dermatopathol.* 2016;38(7):531-532.

may allow for differentiation from other creeping eruptions such as gnathostomiasis. Most biopsy specimens show only a sparse infiltrate of lymphocytes and eosinophils in the upper dermis and do not contain larvae. The larvae are usually present in burrows in the deeper layers of the epidermis. Biopsies taken from just beyond the leading edge of the track are the ones that most likely will reveal the larvae (Figures 21-15 and 21-16). The tracks of the larva form small epidermal cavitations and show a mixed population of inflammatory cell infiltrates

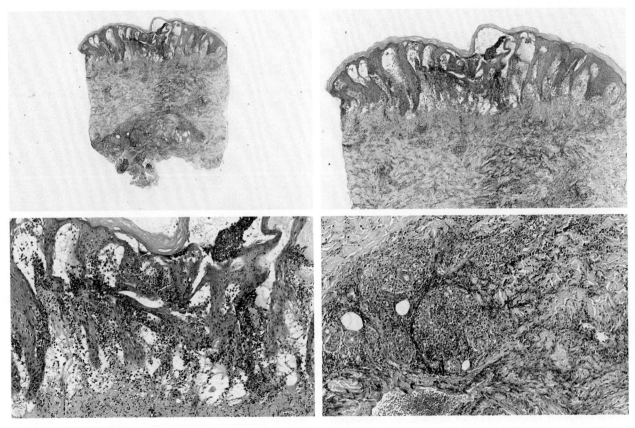

FIGURE 21-15. Cutaneous larva migrans. Marker intra- and subepidermal vesiculation is noted. A very intense eosinophilic inflammatory infiltrate is present. No larvae are seen. Digital slides courtesy of Path Presenter.com.

comprising eosinophils, neutrophils, lymphocytes, and plasma cells. There are intraepidermal vesicular lesions with associated eosinophilic spongiosis.

Identification of the species of the parasite is not readily done in tissue sections. Further penetration and invasion of the human dermis is not usually seen. The adult parasite is not seen in standard sections. The larva from hookworm-related CLM is small when compared with the larvae of *Gnathostoma*: the diameter of the formers is not wider than three keratinocytes, whereas *Gnathostoma* larvae are 0.3 mm in diameter and can be present in the dermis or subcutis. The former can be similar in size to the larvae of *Strongyloides*, but the latter usually presents in the dermis. Follicular localization has also been reported, and postulated as the point of entrance to the skin.

CAPSULE SUMMARY

CUTANEOUS LARVA MIGRANS

CLM is a cutaneous parasitic infestation, resulting from the migration of parasites through the skin. The disease is seen more frequently in tropical climates where is affects children who play with soil contaminated with feces, especially on the beach, and in adults with soil-related occupations. The commonly affected sites include the hands, feet, buttocks and trunk. The larvae moves within the skin, usually for short distances, producing significant itching, a serpiginous tract or tracts accompanied by erythema and vesicular eruptions, depending on the number of larvae involved. Biopsies are only rarely done.

GNATHOSTOMIASIS

Definition and Epidemiology

Gnathostomiasis is the infection produced by a larval stage of Gnanthostoma, a nematode that affects cats and dogs. It is associated with a migratory form of cellulitis or panniculitis. Several species have been identified in association with human disease. Most cases in Asia are associated with *Gnathostoma spinigerum*; other species include *G. doloresi*, *G. nipponicum*, and *G. binucleatum* (the latter responsible for the cases seen in Mexico and Ecuador).[46-49]

Etiology

The infection is commonly acquired after the ingestion of raw fish contaminated with the larva. All the countries with a diet rich in raw fish have a higher prevalence of this disease (Japan, Thailand, Cambodia, Laos, Myanmar, Indonesia, Philippines, Malaysia, China, Mexico, Ecuador, and Peru). In Asia, the infection is associated with the ingestion of sushi, sashimi, and eel dishes; in South America, it is associated with ceviche.[47,50,51] The life cycle begins in the adult nest, located in the stomach of cats and dogs. Eggs produced by the female in the nest are expelled into the animal feces. When the feces reach the water of nearby rivers or flowing water, the eggs evolve into the first larvarial stage. The worm is ingested by a copepod, a water flea of the genus Cyclops. The evolution into the second larvarial state occurs in the second host. Large predators (fish, eels, birds, frogs, or reptiles) ingest the copepod, and it is in the second host that the larva migrates to internal organs, such as the liver or muscle, evolving into the third stage. Any mammal feeding on the contaminated second host may become infected. In the definitive host, the larva reaches the GI tract to evolve into the adult worms, completing the cycle. Humans are accidental hosts, where the larva begins by adhering into the intestinal mucosa, peritoneal cavity, and potentially the skin. In some cases, CNS involvement occurs.

Clinical Presentation

The cutaneous manifestations usually appear 3 to 4 weeks after the ingestion of the larva. There are four different forms of skin disease: migratory panniculitis (Figure 21-17), creeping eruption, foruncular, and mixed forms.[48,49] Migratory panniculitis is the most common and more classic presentation of gnathostomiasis. This presentation shows red, indurated nodules, with or without itching or pain, on the trunk and extremities. The lesions can resolve upon treatment with antibiotics for a suspected abscess to reappear back, days to weeks later, either a few centimeters beyond the original location, or more distantly. This migratory pattern is classic for the disease; the speed of migration has been established in the range of 1 cm/h. The nodules can have an erythematous appearance and simulate the so-called peau d'orange. The creeping eruption is indistinguishable from the eruption caused by CLM. The mixed patterns result from a combination of the migratory

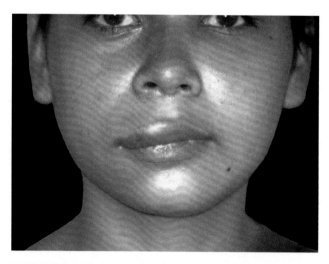

FIGURE 21-17. Gnathostomiasis. Nodular migratory panniculitis on the face. From Magana M, Messina M, Bustamante F, Cazarín J. Gnathostomiasis: clinicopathologic study. *Am J Dermatopathol.* 2004;26(2):91-95.

panniculitis and creeping eruption forms; sometimes they occur in continuity. The foruncular type presents typically after treatment, and is characterized by the presence of a papule or pustule, a consequence of the movement of the larva into the superficial dermis, and can sometimes be associated with the expulsion of the larva through the epidermis. Visceral forms of gnathostomiasis can occur with involvement of the lungs, genitourinary system, eyes, and CNS. The mortality associated with the CNS involvement can be as high as 8% to 25%, leaving frequent sequelae. Gnathostomiasis has been reported in children, with a prevalence of 15% among all cases of the disease.[48,49,52,53]

Histologic findings

Some histopathologic features present can suggest this disease, and these include variable amounts of eosinophilic inflammation in the adipose tissue or reticular dermis. Other inflammatory cells that can be present include lymphocytes, neutrophils, histiocytes, and plasma cells. Associated granulomatous inflammation can also be present. When a panniculitis is present, it is typically lobular. Because of the massive number of eosinophils present in some cases, eosinophilic flame figures, vasculitis, eosinophilic spongiosis, intraepidermal vesicles, and marked dermal edema can be encountered. The presence of the larva is considered diagnostic, but this is more of an exception than the rule.[48,49] The worm is typically found in the deep dermis or adipose tissue (Figure 21-18). The foruncular forms are the ones with a higher likelihood of identifying the worm. The tubular structure of the larvae is seen on tangential sections, with a diameter ranging from 200 to 300 μm. In addition to the hooks of the head bulb, tegumental structures (cuticle, cuticular spines, hypodermis, muscles, ventral and lateral cords) can be seen.

Differential diagnosis

Gnathostoma larvae should be distinguished from those of *Ancylostoma, Uncinaria,* and *Strongyloides.* The latter three worms mentioned are smaller in size and only *Strongyloides* can reach the dermis. *Ancylostoma* and *Uncinaria* are located at the level of the epidermis. Sparganosis can also have a similar size to that of Gnathostoma, but lacks a celomic cavity and tubular intestine.

CAPSULE SUMMARY

GNATHOSTOMIASIS

Gnathostomiasis is the infection produced by a larval stage of Gnathostoma, a nematode that affects cats and dogs. It's associated with a migratory form of cellulitis or panniculitis. The infection is commonly acquired after the ingestion of raw fish contaminated with the larva. There are four different forms of skin disease: migratory panniculitis, creeping eruption, foruncular, and mixed forms. Migratory panniculitis is the most common and more classic presentation of gnathostomiasis. Some histopathologic features present can suggest this disease, and those include variable amounts of eosinophilic inflammation in the adipose tissue or reticular dermis. The presence of the larva is considered diagnostic, but this is more of an exception than the rule.

STRONGYLOIDIASIS

Definition and Epidemiology

This is a parasitic disease that primarily affects the GI tract, but in some occasions, it can also involve the skin. The etiologic agent is the nematode *Strongyloides stercoralis.* It is believed that approximately 30 million people are infected worldwide, most of whom are living in developing countries. The disease can also affect migrants, refugees, and travelers from endemic regions. The infection is particularly important in individuals with an impaired immunologic response: elderly, institutionalized psychiatric patients, alcoholics, immunosuppressed, HIV/AIDS, and people with malignant hematologic disorders.[54-57]

Etiology

The adult form of *S. stercoralis* colonizes the GI tract, where the female worm has the capability to produce eggs (even without the need for a male partner). As a result, the worm in its first larvarial state (rhabditiform larva) is eliminated in the feces. The larva then can have two pathways: it evolves either into the second and third larvarial stages (filariform larva) with the potential to cause infection or into the adult

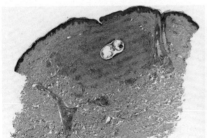
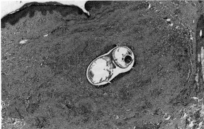
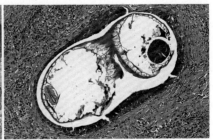

FIGURE 21-18. Gnathostomiasis. Histopathologic findings. Digital slides courtesy of Path Presenter.com.

form, either male or female. The adult forms reproduce in the soil, giving rise to organisms in the three larvarial stages. The filariform larva has the capability to infect humans by penetrating the skin. Once in the skin, they enter the circulation, reach the lung, and in a retrograde fashion, the trachea and larynx. They can be ingested from there and reach the duodenum. Another possible pathway of maturation occurs when the L1 form matures in the intestinal lumen into the L2 and L3 larvae, then penetrates the intestinal wall, and reaches the perineal skin. The latter pathway allows the organism to complete the cycle without leaving the human body.[54,58-60]

Clinical Presentation

The most common symptoms are related to the GI tract infection (diarrhea, abdominal pain, nausea, loss of appetite). Pulmonary symptoms include cough and shortness of breath. The cutaneous manifestations include itching and a popular eruption at the site of the larva entering the skin (feet or perianal region). In chronic infections, there is a nonspecific papular rash, and more frequently, the changes of larva currens form. The latter is a severely pruritic creeping eruption that moves faster than any other parasite at a rate of 5 to 15 cm/h. The lesions can be single or multiple, last from hours to days, and can have an urticarial appearance. The affected sites include the perianal area, buttocks, groin, and trunk. In some severe cases, the lesions can have a purpuric appearance with hemorrhagic area. The purpuric lesions can coalesce to form larger lesions, the "thumbprint purpura" (Figure 21-19). The lesions can spread in a centrifugal fashion across the abdomen and thighs. The purpuric presentations are associated with very high mortality, particularly in cancer patients.[58,59,61-63]

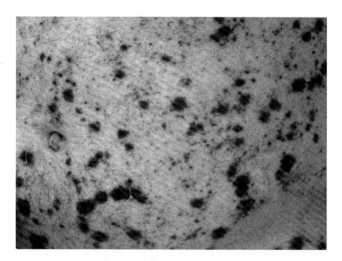

FIGURE 21-19. Strongyloidiasis. Periumbilical purpura resembling multiple thumbprints. Obtained with permission from Osio A, Demongeot C, Battistella M, Lhuillier E, Zafrani L, Vignon-Pennamen MD. Periumbilical purpura: challenge and answer. Diagnosis: strongyloides stercoralis hyperinfection. *Am J Dermatopathol.* 2014;36(11):899-900.

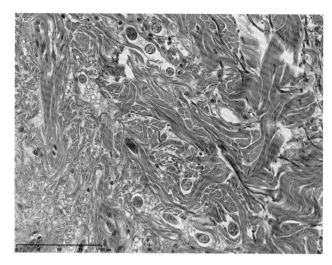

FIGURE 21-20. Strongyloidiasis. A sparse perivascular infiltrate is seen with numerous larvae in the dermis. From Osio A, Demongeot C, Battistella M, Lhuillier E, Zafrani L, Vignon-Pennamen MD. Periumbilical purpura: challenge and answer. Diagnosis: strongyloides stercoralis hyperinfection. *Am J Dermatopathol.* 2014;36(11):899-900.

Histologic findings

The larva of *S. stercoralis* can be detected in the reticular dermis among the collagen fibers or inside the capillaries, particularly in those individuals who are immunosuppressed. It is associated with some degree of vascular damage. Granulomatous inflammation can also be present.[59,60,62] The size of the larva is similar to that of the larva migrans–associated nematodes, but the latter are located in the epidermis and not in the dermis. In those suffering from severe immunosuppression, an immune reaction to the organism might be completely absent, and the organisms are more numerous in number (Figures 21-20 and 21-21).

CAPSULE SUMMARY

STRONGYLOIDIASIS

Strongyloidiasis is a parasitic disease that primarily affects the GI tract, but in some occasions it can also involve the skin. The etiologic agent is the nematode *Strongyloides stercoralis*. It's believed that approximately 30 million people are infected worldwide, most of which are living in developing countries. The cutaneous manifestations include itching and a popular eruption at the site of the larva entering the skin (feet or perianal region). In chronic infections, there is a nonspecific papula rash, and more frequently, the larva currens form. The latter is a severely pruritic creeping eruption, that moves faster than any other parasite, at a rate of 5 to 15 cm/h.

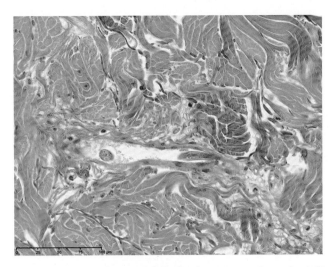

FIGURE 21-21. Strongyloidiasis. A sparse perivascular infiltrate is seen with numerous larvae in the dermis. From Osio A, Demongeot C, Battistella M, Lhuillier E, Zafrani L, Vignon-Pennamen MD. Periumbilical purpura: challenge and answer. Diagnosis: strongyloides stercoralis hyperinfection. *Am J Dermatopathol.* 2014;36(11):899-900.

ARTHROPOD BITES

Definition and Epidemiology

Arthropod bites from hematophagic organisms serve as vectors for diseases including (but not limited to) lyme disease and relapsing fever. Inoculation of toxins during feeding is usually the reason for the pathologic manifestations. The tick bites occur worldwide, although the tick species vary according to different geographical locations. Ticks could be found in woods, grass, farms, and cattle ranches.[64-67]

Etiology

Members of the venomous arthropods include the classes Insecta, Diplopoda, Chilopoda, and Arachnida. The classes Insecta and Arachnida are the two most important ones. The class Insecta is responsible for 60% of the arthropod species. These venomous insects belong to the orders of Lepidoptera (moths and caterpillars), Hymenoptera (ants and bees), Coleoptera (beetles), Diptera (true flies), Hemiptera (true bugs), and Siphonaptera (fleas). Spiders and scorpions belong to the class Arachnida. Arthropod bites and stings are very common, affect individuals across all ages, and have an increased susceptibility for toxic and systemic events in the very young and very old. Infestations by true bugs (order Hemiptera) are very common. Giant water bugs are usually found in freshwater habitats. Their saliva contains a mixture of enzymes that cause liquefaction of tissues, increased clotting, hemolysis, and paralysis of muscles of their prey. In humans, they cause painful lesions and infections. Bedbugs act more like parasites. True flies (Diptera) have the ability to bite and act as vectors of onchocerciasis and

trypanosomiasis. Some of the fly larvae (maggots) have the ability to feed on necrotic or live tissue (myasis).[68-72]

Spider bites (arachnida) can produce death. Although most are harmful, those belonging to the genus *Atrax* (funnel web spider of Australia), *Phoneutria* (armadeira), *Latrodectus* (black widow spider), and *Loxosceles* (brown recluse spider) can produce major tissue damage and sometimes be fatal.[65,68,73-77]

There are two main types of ticks: the hard ticks (*Ixodidae*) and the soft ticks (*Argasidase*). They have mouthparts that are able to puncture the skin and attach to it. The ticks tend to feed over several days and inoculation of the toxins causing systemic illness occur toward the end of the feed.[67,78]

Clinical Presentation

Cutaneous reactions to caterpillars and moths include limited papular eruptions, urticarial lesions, and scaly erythematous lesions in the affected areas (Figure 21-22).[66,69] The severity of the cutaneous reaction depends mainly on the extent of the contact. In some cases, necrosis of the skin can occur, and regional lymphadenopathy can also be present. Ant and bee stings typically produce a burning and painful sensation at the site of the injury. This is followed by a wheal that can be large and last for approximately 1 week. Generalized systemic reactions can occur in <5% of the patients and can potentially include anaphylactic shock. The manifestations of ant stings are similar to the ones from the bees, but differ on the formation of a sterile pustule that goes away between 48 and 72 hours. Giant water bugs and bed bugs cause burning and pruritic erythematous urticarial papules that can potentially become infected. The clinical manifestations of true fly bites include urticarial, vesicular, eczematous, or granulomatous lesions.[65-68,70,72,79,80]

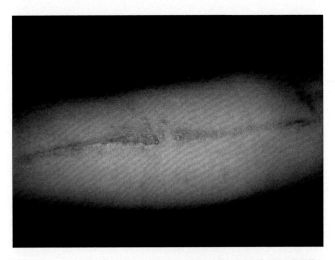

FIGURE 21-22. Forearm of the patient showing linear distribution of paederus dermatitis caused by blister beetle. Obtained with permission from Kar S, Dongre A, Krishnan A, Godse S, Singh N. Epidemiological study of insect bite reactions from central India. *Indian J Dermatol.* 2013;58(5):337-341.

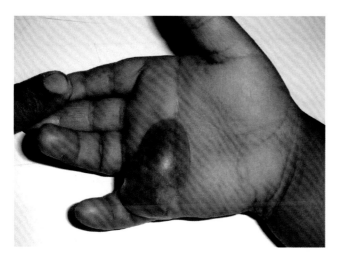

FIGURE 21-23. Hemorrhagic bulla following insect bite in a child. Obtained with permission from Kar S, Dongre A, Krishnan A, Godse S, Singh N. Epidemiological study of insect bite reactions from central India. *Indian J Dermatol.* 2013;58(5):337-341.

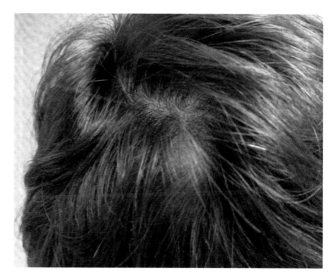

FIGURE 21-24. Tick bite alopecia. Obtained with permission from Lynch MC, Milchak MA, Parnes H, Ioffreda MD. Tick bite alopecia: a report and review. *Am J Dermatopathol.* 2016;38(11):e150-e153.

Venomous spider bites can lead to serious injuries primarily because of the neurotoxic events. Brown recluse bites can lead to death if not treated with the specific antiserum. After the initial injury and following the pain and burning at the site, a severe painful ischemic area develops. The area shows pallor, cyanosis, and erythema. Within 7 days, a full area of necrosis develops, which leads to the formation of a black scar. In approximately 5% of patients, there is hemolysis and acute renal failure. The venom of the black widow spider can also cause myalgias, muscle spasms, drooling, nausea, vomiting, hypotension, and potentially death.[73-77]

Adult or younger ticks can be seen attached to the skin. Pruritic papules and papular urticarial-like reactions have been reported. Other documented features include eczematous eruptions, nodules, bullae (Figure 21-23), and temporary alopecia (Figure 21-24). The African tick bite fever has been associated with multiple inoculation eschars on the legs. Other features will differ on the basis of the offending tick. Tick paralysis and Lyme disease are not uncommon.

Histologic findings and Differential Diagnosis

The histopathologic findings present in association with arthropod bites are variable[65,66,71,78,81-84]: those depend on the arthropod subtype, the duration, of the clinical lesion, the immunologic response, the presence or absence of arthropod parts, and the discharge of toxins. Changes due to tick bites involve both the epidermis and the dermis. In the epidermis, there is variable acanthosis, which in some cases, can be exuberant and have a pseudoepitheliomatous appearance. Epidermal spongiosis can also be seen, particularly in the acute phases. The spongiotic reaction can be localized to the site of the bite, or more extensive, with multiple intraepidermal vesicles and sometimes frank necrosis. Eosinophilic spongiosis can be a particular feature seen in arthropod bites. The dermal reaction is characterized by wedge-shaped dense foci of inflammatory cells consisting of lymphocytes,

histiocytes, plasma cells, and eosinophils, especially in the periappendageal region. Secondary lymphoid follicles with germinal centers are formed in some lesions. Mouth parts of the tick can be sometimes present, typically in the mid dermis and covered by a down-growth of the epidermis (Figures 21-25 and 21-26). The arthropod parts can be polarizable. Reactions to fleas, fire ants, mosquitoes, and spider envenomation show a predominance of neutrophils with vasculitic foci. Hemorrhage and edema can also be prominent.

Pseudolymphomatous changes can also be seen[85-89]: the pleomorphism of the mononuclear infiltrate may simulate mycosis fungoides or other lymphomas of the skin including Hodgkin disease, especially when accompanied by eosinophils. Cells resembling the Sternberg–Reed cells may sometimes be present. Usually, the clinical history and the presence of a single lesion help exclude lymphoma, but, when lesions are numerous, differentiation may be difficult. The abundance of plasma cells in the insect bite may aid in the differentiation.

CAPSULE SUMMARY

ARTHROPOD BITES

Histopathological changes due to tick bites include variable acanthosis, which may be so marked as to represent pseudoepitheliomatous hyperplasia, a dermal reaction characterized by dense foci of inflammatory cells consisting of lymphocytes, histiocytes, plasma cells and eosinophils, especially in the periappendageal region, as well as secondary lymphoid follicles with germinal centers in some lesions. The pleomorphism of the mononuclear infiltrate in association with eosinophils may simulate mycosis fungoides or other lymphomas of the skin including Hodgkin's disease, but the abundance of plasma cells in the insect bite may aid in the differentiation.

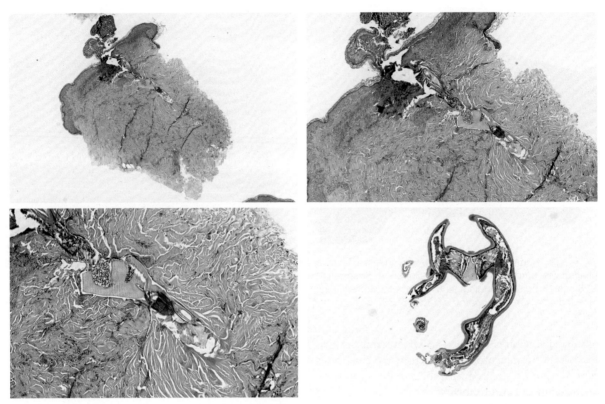

FIGURE 21-25. Tick bite. An arthropod is seen in the epidermis and dermis. The parts of an arthropod are seen on histologic examination (bottom right figure). Digital slides courtesy of Path Presenter.com.

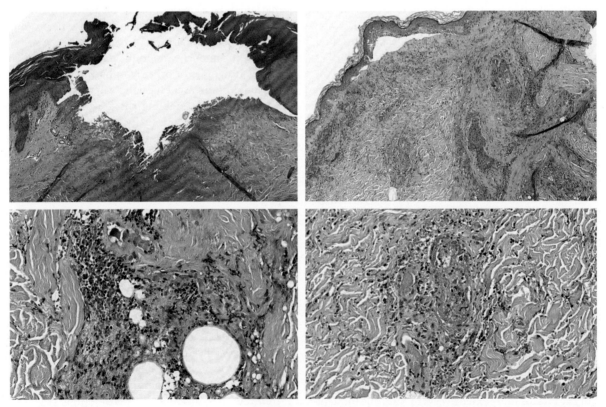

FIGURE 21-26. In the absence of the arthropod, a surface and wedge-shaped ulcer is seen ("punctum"). Within the dermis, a rich eosinophilic infiltrate (superficial and deep) is present. Vasculitic changes are seen with fibrin thrombi in some of the vessels. Digital slides courtesy of Path Presenter.com.

SCABIES

Definition and Epidemiology

Scabies is due to infestation of the human skin by the mite *Sarcoptes scabiei*. This infestation occurs worldwide, but is more common in the underdeveloped countries where there is overcrowding. It is seen in all age groups but is more frequent in children and in elderly people.[1] Some reports have suggested increased prevalence in females. Over 300 million cases are reported annually worldwide.[90-92]

Etiology

The infecting organism, Sarcoptes scabiei, is a mite that is transferred by close contact, that is, holding hands or sexual intercourse with an infected person. Upon contact with the skin, the mite burrows down into the epidermis, leaving a track ("burrow"), typically avoiding pilosebaceous structures. The female mite lays eggs in the burrows, which subsequently hatch over a few weeks. Thereafter, young mites are born. The organism is transferred by contact and hardly survives outside the body for more than 36 hours.[90,92-95] The transmission of the organism via infested objects is still a matter of controversy.

Clinical Presentation

Pruritus is the more frequent clinical manifestation that is particularly worse during the night.[14,91,93-98] This is particularly common in children and may be the only presenting symptom. It is believed to be secondary to a hypersensitivity reaction to the presence of the mites, which are usually between 12 and 20 in number. However, pruritus may be absent in those who are immunosuppressed (Norwegian scabies) despite the very large number of mites.[99-101] The typical lesion of scabies is the burrow that is linear and may have scaling. However, secondary lesions are more common on presentation due to the scratching (lichenification), and these include excoriation, pustules, papules, and sometimes nodules. Vesicles and bullae may be seen.

The sites of predilection for scabies include the wrists, hand borders, finger sides, web spaces between the fingers, the feet, buttocks, and genitalia. In children, the palms, soles, nails, and rarely the scalp may also be involved[102,103] (Figures 21-27 and 21-28).

Histologic findings

Biopsies from children with scabies demonstrate the changes of a dermal hypersensitivity reaction. Within the stratum corneum, small foci of parakeratosis and serum may be the first clue to the diagnosis. A "spiky" appearance of the epidermis has also been reported as a diagnostic clue.[14,95] The mites and ova could be difficult to find in ordinary scabies, hence the need to perform several levels on biopsies when there is a clinical suspicion for scabies. In Norwegian scabies, in counterpart, the stratum corneum may be virtually filled with mites and ova (Figure 21-29). Some authors have

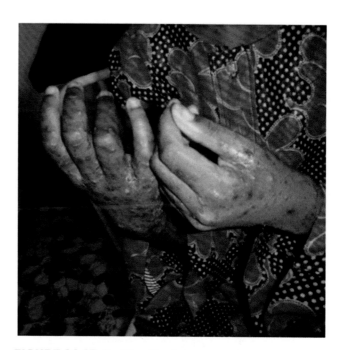

FIGURE 21-27. **Scabies.** Hand changes.

advocated that a shave biopsy is the most sensitive method to detect mites or their eggs. It is extraordinarily unusual to find organisms beneath the stratum corneum. Foo et al. described the use of polarizable light (from the detached spines and scybala—fecal material) in the diagnosis of scabies.[104] Persistent or nodular scabetic reactions that remain after the organisms are treated can show a superficial and sometimes deep inflammatory infiltrate of lymphocytes, histiocytes, and eosinophils. Such inflammation can extend into the adipose tissue (Figure 21-30). In some cases, the infiltrate can take a pseudolymphomatous appearance, including exuberant reactions with abundant CD30+ cells.[105] Marked Langerhans cell hyperplasia, mimicking Langerhans cell histiocytosis, can also be seen.[106-108] Persistent itching produces a chronic inflammatory response with eosinophils. This response is most prominent around cutaneous vessels and sweat glands.

Differential Diagnosis

A differential diagnosis can sometimes include Langerhans cell histiocytosis, particularly given the marked proliferation of Langerhans cells in reactive dermatoses in children. The presence of scabies mites can easily allow in establishing the

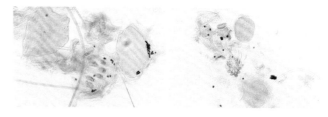

FIGURE 21-28. **Scabies, scraping.** Digital slides courtesy of Path Presenter.com.

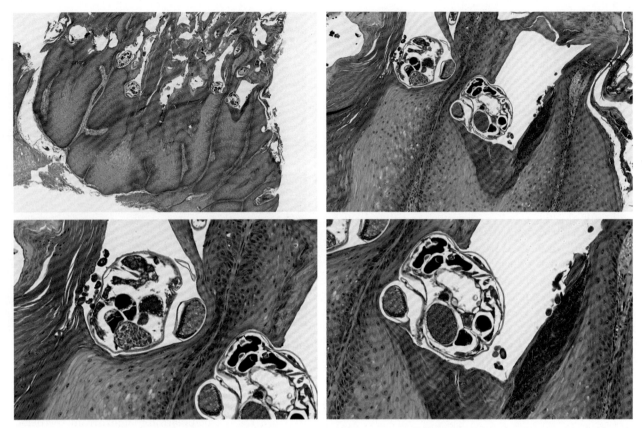

FIGURE 21-29. Norwegian scabies, histopathologic findings. Numerous scabies mites are seen in the stratum corneum in association with marked hyperkeratosis. The feces from the organisms can also be identified (scibala). Digital slides courtesy of Path Presenter.com.

correct diagnosis. Acropustulosis of infancy can also mimic scabies, but the latter is predominantly neutrophilic in nature.

CAPSULE SUMMARY

SCABIES

Mites and ova are difficult to find in ordinary scabies; more commonly seen are burrows, primarily in the stratum corneum, below which, there is often a mild predominantly lymphocytic response with edema in the Malpighian layer (spongiosis). Tissue eosinophilia is most prominent around cutaneous vessels and sweat glands.

PEDICULOSIS

Definition and Epidemiology

Pediculosis results from the infestation by *Pediculus humanus capitis,* also referred to as "sucking body louse." The infestation occurs worldwide, especially in areas of overcrowding and poor hygiene. It is more frequently encountered in children 3 to 11 years of age, and it is reported to have a female preponderance. Approximately 6 to 12 million children in the United States are estimated to have head lice infestation.[109-113] Another kind of body lice that are commonly found worldwide is crab lice or pubic lice. These produce infestation in the hair-bearing genital or pubic area.[114]

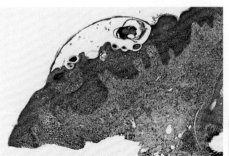
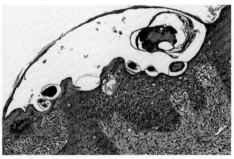

FIGURE 21-30. Bullous scabies. Digital slides courtesy of Path Presenter.com.

Etiology

After finding its way to the scalp, the female mite lays eggs ("nits") that are cemented to the hair shaft. The eggs hatch after 7 to 10 days and more mites are available for transmission. The empty egg cases remain attached to the hair shafts.

Clinical Presentation

Head lice may be asymptomatic, but pruritus of the scalp is the most common feature. This usually leads to excoriation and secondary bacterial infection with localized lymphadenopathy especially in the occipital region. Pruritic papular eruptions may be seen on the base of the neck. The eggs appear as grains on the hair, although frequently they may be empty, especially around the occipital and parietal areas. Dermoscopy may reveal adult mites. Combing through the hair may also dislodge mites. After treatment, the empty eggs may remain for a while.[113,115-117]

Histologic findings

It is rare that the lesions of pediculosis are biopsied. Diagnosis is primarily made by identification of the lice and their eggs. On the rare occasion of biopsy, the chitinous arthropod may be seen in the stratum corneum and epidermis. Erythrocytes can be present in the insect gut, and insect-striated muscle can be apparent. A pseudolymphomatous reaction with an abundance of CD30+ cells has been reported. Chronic itching will likely produce the same general features in the skin as with mite infestations except that the burrows are not expected to be seen.

MYIASIS

Definition and Epidemiology

Cutaneous myiasis results from an ectoparasitic infestation of the skin by the fly larvae of arthropods of the order Diptera. Myiasis occurs worldwide, but it is more frequent in the tropical and subtropical underdeveloped countries. It is also associated with traveling to endemic areas. Myiasis occurs more frequently in children in sub-Saharan Africa.[66,118-122]

Etiology

Cutaneous Myiasis is due to the infestation of flies especially from the human botfly (*Dermatobia hominis*) and the Tumbu fly (*Cordylobia anthropophaga*). The etiologic agents differ in different geographical locations; although the *D. hominis* is more frequent in South America, *C. anthropophaga* is more common in sub-Saharan Africa. The eggs of *d. hominis* are attached to other vectors such as mosquitoes and hatch when the eggs come in contact of human skin while the mosquito is sucking blood. The Tumbu fly is usually found in shady areas where babies are kept while their mothers are farming in several parts of Africa.[4,5] The fly also lays its eggs on clothes hung outside to dry. The eggs or larvae can remain viable for a few days on soil or on drying clothes, especially when not ironed. When activated by the warmth of human contact, the larvae burrow into the skin. The larvae grow to 13 to 15 mm and eventually fall out or are evacuated.[119,123-130]

The anatomic system classifies the infestation in relation to the location on the host and is the most useful clinically: bloodsucking, cutaneous myasis (foruncular and migratory), wound myasis, and cavitary myiasis (depends on the location of the larvae: cerebral, aural, nasal, ocular).

Clinical Presentation

This varies with the causative agents and characteristics of the larvae.[123,124,127,129-132] Cutaneous and wound infestations are the most frequent forms of myiasis. More frequently, the infestation is subcutaneous (Figures 21-31 and 21-32). Risk factors for the disease are poor hygiene, low socioeconomic status, and exposed preexistent suppurative lesions that attract the female insect allowing to deposit the eggs. Although more than a hundred species of Diptera are reported to cause human disease, essentially there are two main types of cutaneous myiasis: follicular and wound myiasis.[3] *D. hominis* (human botfly) and *C. anthropophaga* (Tumbu fly) cause follicular myiasis, whereas *Cochliomyia hominivorax* (America) and *Chrysomyia bezziana* (Africa, Australia, Asia) can produce wound myiasis. *Hypoderma bovis* (infested cattle) and *Gasterophilus intestinalis* (infested horses) may sometimes be important as they both cause creeping (migratory) myiasis.

The follicular (also called furuncular or "warble") form is the more frequent type. The lesions appear as painful furuncles, sometimes with a central punctum through which there is a serious discharge. The posterior end of the larvae may be seen clinically (Figure 21-33). The furuncle may be associated by lymphangitis and regional lymphadenopathy. The lesions are usually seen on the face, scalp, and extremities. In babies, the buttocks may be involved. Patients typically complain of pruritus, pain, and movement sensation, usually during the night. The lesions tend to heal without significant complications. However, scarring and bacterial infection can occur. Migratory myiasis occurs when the larvae migrate through the skin.

The wound form is as a result of eggs of the flies deposited on wounds/ulcers. The presence of necrosis is a main factor that predisposes to the infestation. Wound myiasis can be caused by facultative or obligatory parasites. Obligatory myiasis is usually secondary to infestation from *Muscidae, Sarcophagidae,* and *Calliphoridae* (the latter being the most frequent in the United States). Facultative myiasis is caused by *Cochliomyia hominivorax, Chrysomya bezziana,* and *Wohlfahrtia magnifica.*

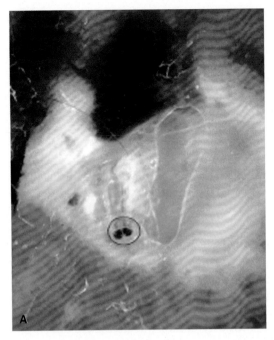

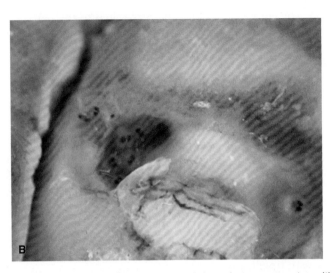

FIGURE 21-31. Myiasis. A, Dermatoscopic examination of the larvae of *Phormia regina* showing caudal respiratory apparatus with two oval openings representing dorsal tracheal trunks in the posterior segment (red circle). Incomplete peritreme and prominent slit in each of the three spiracles can be appreciated (×10), B, Multiple larvae in the nail fold (×10). Obtained with permission from Vinay K, Handa S, Khurana S, Agrawal S, De D. Dermatoscopy in diagnosis of cutaneous myiasis arising in pemphigus vulgaris lesions. *Indian J Dermatol.* 2017;62(4):440.

Cavitary myiasis occurs with infestation affecting body cavities, and it is given the name of the affected anatomic region (oculomyiasis, oral myiasis, otomyiasis—ear infestation which is particularly common in children, nasal myiasis, and urogenital form).

Histologic findings

Generally, pathologic changes of myiasis depend on the feeding habits of the larvae.[124] The species affecting wounds tend to be particularly troublesome by depositing their eggs in around the head region, with the feeding larvae causing

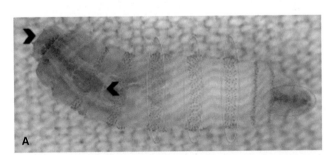

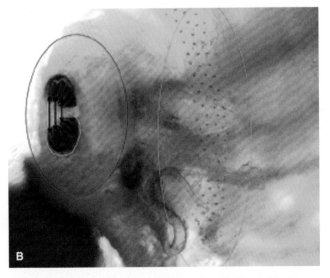

FIGURE 21-32. Myiasis. A, Dermatoscopic image of the third instar larva of *Phormia regina* showing dorsal tracheal trunk in the posterior segment (between solid arrowheads), multiple tiny spines on the body surface (green circles), and mouth parts (orange circle), (×10). B, Light microscopy of the third instar larva of *P. regina* showing caudal respiratory apparatus and posterior spiracle (red circle) and multiple tiny spines on the body surface (green circles). Incomplete peritreme (blue arc) and prominent slit in each of the three spiracles (black arrows) can be appreciated (×40). Obtained with permission from Vinay K, Handa S, Khurana S, Agrawal S, De D. Dermatoscopy in diagnosis of cutaneous myiasis arising in pemphigus vulgaris lesions. *Indian J Dermatol.* 2017;62(4):440.

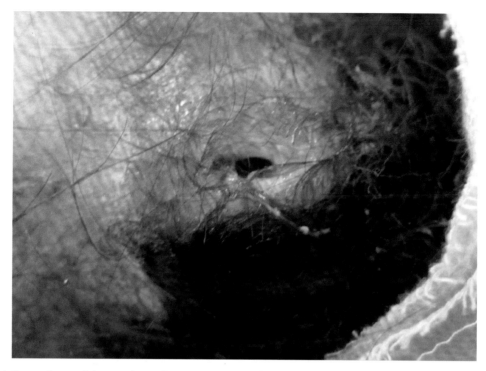

FIGURE 21-33. Inflammatory nodule over the scalp with a central discharging pore. Obtained with permission from Verma P. Cutaneous myiasis in an infant with cerebral palsy. *Indian J Dermatol.* 2014;59(3):310-311.

destruction of the nose, ears, and eyes with consequent secondary infection. The pharynx and palate are commonly involved, and fistulous tracts often develop in the process.

Nodules containing larval cysts may be seen with tracts lined by squamous epithelium. Regardless of specie, the histologic changes are similar and consist of the larva surrounded by

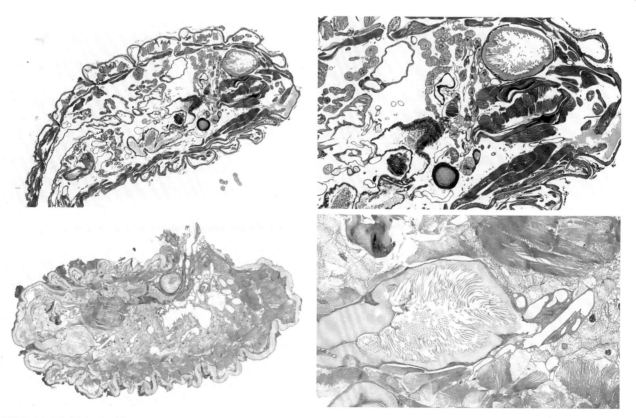

FIGURE 21-34. Myiasis. Histologic examination of the larvae. Digital slides courtesy of Path Presenter.com.

an intense inflammatory infiltrate composed of neutrophils, eosinophils, plasma cells, and lymphocytes. A dermal sinus tract can be present. The larva is more likely to be seen if the biopsy is taken from skin ahead of the advancing burrow (Figure 21-34), the burrow itself being either intraepidermal or immediately subepidermal and containing debris and desquamated cells. Bot fly larvae are characterized by the presence of an external cuticle covered with spines, with striated muscle underneath. In some cases, when the parasite is preserved, anatomic structures can be easily identified. The respiratory tract is identified by the presence of small tubular structures, as well as pigmented posterior respiratory spiracle.

Differential diagnosis

In the absence of the larva, burrows and subepidermal infiltrate will suggest any of the other creeping infestations such as Scabies and Larva migrans. Foruncular myiasis may mimic a wide spectrum of cutaneous entities, including arthropod bites, epidermal inclusion cysts, cellulitis, MRSA infection, impetigo, herpes zoster infection, and other parasitic infestations. In the case of migratory myiasis, CLM should be considered in the differential diagnosis. Migratory myiasis moves more slowly, and the cutaneous extension is more localized when compared with CLM.

CAPSULE SUMMARY

CUTANEOUS MYIASIS

Nodules containing larval cysts may be seen with tracts lined by squamous epithelium. The burrow is either intraepidermal or immediately subepidermal and containing debris and desquamated cells. The larva surrounded by an intense inflammatory infiltrate composed of neutrophils, eosinophils, plasma cells and lymphocytes. In the absence of the larva, burrows and subepidermal infiltrate will suggest any of the other creeping infestations such as Scabies and Larva migrans.

REFERENCES

1. Abdel-Aziz AH. Cutaneous bilharzial granulomas: a histopathologic study. *Cutis.* 1976;18(4):516-519.
2. Bergquist NR. Schistosomiasis vaccine development: progress and prospects. *Mem Inst Oswaldo Cruz.* 1998;93(suppl 1):95-101.
3. Bergquist NR, Colley DG. Schistosomiasis vaccine: research to development. *Parasitol Today.* 1998;14(3):99-104.
4. González E. Schistosomiasis, cercarial dermatitis, and marine dermatitis. *Dermatol Clin.* 1989;7(2):291-300.
5. Lucey DR, Maguire JH. Schistosomiasis. *Infect Dis Clin North Am.* 1993;7(3):635-653.
6. Amer M. Cutaneous schistosomiasis. *Dermatol Clin.* 1994;12(4):713-717.
7. Davis-Reed L, Theis JH. Cutaneous schistosomiasis: report of a case and review of the literature. *J Am Acad Dermatol.* 2000;42(4):678-680.
8. Diallo M, Niang SO, Faye PM, et al. [Schistosoma-induced granulomatous panniculitis. An unusual presentation of cutaneous schistosomiasis]. *Ann Dermatol Venereol.* 2012;139(2):132-136.
9. Farrell AM, Woodrow D, Bryceson AD, Bunker CB, Cream JJ. Ectopic cutaneous schistosomiasis: extragenital involvement with progressive upward spread. *Br J Dermatol.* 1996;135(1):110-112.
10. Poderoso WL, Santana WB, Costa EF, Cipolotti R, Fakhouri R. Ectopic schistosomiasis: description of five cases involving skin, one ovarian case and one adrenal case. *Rev Soc Bras Med Trop.* 2008;41(6):668-671.
11. Traore A, Barro-Traore F, Goumbri-Lompo O, et al. [Cutaneous schistosomiasis: six cases]. *Ann Dermatol Venereol.* 2008;135(1):71-72.
12. Adeyemi-Doro FA, Osoba AO, Junaid TA. Perigenital cutaneous schistosomiasis. *Br J Vener Dis.* 1979;55(6):446-449.
13. Perez E, Gazin P, Furtado A, et al. [Intestinal parasite infections and schistosomiasis in a poor urban area, in townships of the sugar cane belt and in villages of the semi-arid area of North-East Brazil]. *Sante.* 2000;10(2):127-129.
14. Eichenlaub D, Eichenlaub S. [Detection of parasites and symptoms of parasitic diseases. 2: Parasites of the gastrointestinal tract, tissue and organ parasites, ecto-and skin parasites]. *Internist (Berl).* 2003;44(4):449-456, 58-69;quiz 71-2.
15. Ekong PS, Juryit R, Dika NM, Nguku P, Musenero M. Prevalence and risk factors for zoonotic helminth infection among humans and animals-Jos, Nigeria, 2005-2009. *Pan Afr Med J.* 2012;12:6.
16. Garcia HH, Nash TE, Del Brutto OH. Clinical symptoms, diagnosis, and treatment of neurocysticercosis. *Lancet Neurol.* 2014;13(12):1202-1215.
17. Amatya BM, Kimula Y. Cysticercosis in Nepal: a histopathologic study of sixty-two cases. *Am J Surg Pathol.* 1999;23(10):1276-1279.
18. Khandpur S, Kothiwala SK, Basnet B, Nangia R, Venkatesh HA, Sharma R. Extensive disseminated cysticercosis. *Indian J Dermatol Venereol Leprol.* 2014;80(2):137-140.
19. Kraft R. Cysticercosis: an emerging parasitic disease. *Am Fam Physician.* 2007;76(1):91-96.
20. Rastogi S, Arora P, Devi P, Wazir SS, Kapoor S. Importance of ultrasonography and magnetic resonance imaging in diagnosis of cysticercosis of temporalis muscle mimicking temporal space infection. *Contemp Clin Dent.* 2013;4(4):504-508.
21. Trung DD, Praet N, Cam TD, et al. Assessing the burden of human cysticercosis in Vietnam. *Trop Med Int Health.* 2013;18(3):352-356.
22. Balaji BS, Kalpana S. Isolated cutaneous cysticercosis mimicking tubercular lymphadenitis. *Indian Pediatr.* 2015;52(8):715.
23. Lakhey M, Hirachand S, Akhter J, Thapa B. Cysticerci in palpable nodules diagnosed on fine needle aspiration cytology. *JNMA J Nepal Med Assoc.* 2009;48(176):314-317.
24. Uthida-Tanaka AM, Sampaio MC, Velho PE, et al. Subcutaneous and cerebral cysticercosis. *J Am Acad Dermatol.* 2004;50(2 suppl):S14-S17.
25. Handa U, Garg S, Mohan H. Fine needle aspiration in the diagnosis of subcutaneous cysticercosis. *Diagn Cytopathol.* 2008;36(3):183-187.
26. Kamal MM, Grover SV. Cytomorphology of subcutaneous cysticercosis. A report of 10 cases. *Acta Cytol.* 1995;39(4):809-812.
27. Boatin BA, Richards FO, Jr. Control of onchocerciasis. *Adv Parasitol.* 2006;61:349-394.
28. Richards F, Jr., Rizzo N, Diaz Espinoza CE, et al. One hundred years after its discovery in guatemala by rodolfo robles, onchocerca volvulus transmission has been eliminated from the central endemic zone. *Am J Trop Med Hyg.* 2015;93(6):1295-1304.
29. Vlaminck J, Fischer PU, Weil GJ. Diagnostic tools for onchocerciasis elimination programs. *Trends Parasitol.* 2015;31(11):571-582.
30. Coffeng LE, Pion SD, O'Hanlon S, et al. Onchocerciasis: the pre-control association between prevalence of palpable nodules and skin microfilariae. *PLoS Negl Trop Dis.* 2013;7(4):e2168.
31. Coffeng LE, Stolk WA, Zoure HG, et al. African Programme for Onchocerciasis Control 1995-2015: model-estimated health impact and cost. *PLoS Negl Trop Dis.* 2013;7(1):e2032.
32. Timmann C, van der Kamp E, Kleensang A, et al. Human genetic resistance to Onchocerca volvulus: evidence for linkage to chromosome 2p from an autosome-wide scan. *J Infect Dis.* 2008;198(3):427-433.
33. Ezzedine K, Malvy D, Dhaussy I, et al. Onchocerciasis-associated limb swelling in a traveler returning from Cameroon. *J Travel Med.* 2006;13(1):50-53.

34. Murdoch ME, Hay RJ, Mackenzie CD, et al. A clinical classification and grading system of the cutaneous changes in onchocerciasis. *Br J Dermatol.* 1993;129(3):260-269.

35. Thiele EA, Cama VA, Lakwo T, et al. Detection of onchocerca volvulus in skin snips by microscopy and real-time polymerase chain reaction: implications for monitoring and evaluation activities. *Am J Trop Med Hyg.* 2016;94(4):906-911.

36. Beaver PC, Jung RC, Craig CF, Cupp EW. *Clinical Parasitology.* 9th ed. Philadelphia, PA: Lea & Febiger; 1984.

37. Loukas A, Hotez PJ, Diemert D, et al. Hookworm infection. *Nat Rev Dis Primers.* 2016;2:16088.

38. Veraldi S, Persico MC, Francia C, Schianchi R. Chronic hookworm-related cutaneous larva migrans. *Int J Infect Dis.* 2013;17(4):e277-e279.

39. Blackwell V, Vega-Lopez F. Cutaneous larva migrans: clinical features and management of 44 cases presenting in the returning traveller. *Br J Dermatol.* 2001;145(3):434-437.

40. Caumes E, Danis M. From creeping eruption to hookworm-related cutaneous larva migrans. *Lancet Infect Dis.* 2004;4(11):659-660.

41. Chiriac A, Chiriac AE, Pinteala T, et al. Cutaneous larva migrans in a temperate area. *Arch Dis Child.* 2016;101(9):813.

42. Purdy KS, Langley RG, Webb AN, Walsh N, Haldane D. Cutaneous larva migrans. *Lancet.* 2011;377(9781):1948.

43. Siddalingappa K, Murthy SC, Herakal K, Kusuma MR. Cutaneous larva migrans in early infancy. *Indian J Dermatol.* 2015;60(5):522.

44. Hosseini-Safa A, Mousavi SM, Bahadoran Bagh Badorani M, Ghatreh Samani M, Mostafaei S, Yousofi Darani H. Seroepidemiology of toxocariasis in children (5-15 yr Old) referred to the Pediatric Clinic of Imam Hossein Hospital, Isfahan, Iran. *Iran J Parasitol* 2015;10(4):632-637.

45. Balfour E, Zalka A, Lazova R. Cutaneous larva migrans with parts of the larva in the epidermis. *Cutis.* 2002;69(5):368-370.

46. Bussaratid V, Dekumyoy P, Desakorn V, et al. Predictive factors for Gnathostoma seropositivity in patients visiting the Gnathostomiasis Clinic at the Hospital for Tropical Diseases, Thailand during 2000-2005. *Southeast Asian J Trop Med Public Health.* 2010;41(6):1316-1321.

47. Herman JS, Chiodini PL. Gnathostomiasis, another emerging imported disease. *Clin Microbiol Rev.* 2009;22(3):484-492.

48. Laga AC, Lezcano C, Ramos C, et al. Cutaneous gnathostomiasis: report of 6 cases with emphasis on histopathological demonstration of the larva. *J Am Acad Dermatol.* 2013;68(2):301-305.

49. Magana M, Messina M, Bustamante F, Cazarin J. Gnathostomiasis: clinicopathologic study. *Am J Dermatopathol.* 2004;26(2):91-95.

50. Chai JY, Han ET, Shin EH, et al. An outbreak of gnathostomiasis among Korean emigrants in Myanmar. *Am J Trop Med Hyg.* 2003;69(1):67-73.

51. Maek ANW, Bussaratid V, Phonrat B, Pakdee W, Nuamtanong S, Dekumyoy P. Diagnosis of gnathostomiasis by skin testing using partially purified specific antigen and total IgE levels. *Trans R Soc Trop Med Hyg.* 2014;108(2):71-76.

52. Bunyaratavej K, Pongpunlert W, Jongwutiwes S, Likitnukul S. Spinal gnathostomiasis resembling an intrinsic cord tumor/myelitis in a 4-year-old boy. *Southeast Asian J Trop Med Public Health.* 2008;39(5):800-803.

53. Kulkarni S, Sayed R, Garg M, Patil V. Neurognathostomiasis in a young child in India: A case report. *Parasitol Int.* 2015;64(5):342-344.

54. Marcos LA, Terashima A, Canales M, Gotuzzo E. Update on strongyloidiasis in the immunocompromised host. *Curr Infect Dis Rep.* 2011;13(1):35-46.

55. Basile A, Simzar S, Bentow J, et al. Disseminated Strongyloides stercoralis: hyperinfection during medical immunosuppression. *J Am Acad Dermatol.* 2010;63(5):896-902.

56. Clyti E, Reynier C, Couppie P, et al. [Infective dermatitis and recurrent strongyloidiasis in a child]. *Ann Dermatol Venereol.* 2004;131(2):191-193.

57. Kaminsky RL, Reyes-Garcia SZ, Zambrano LI. Unsuspected Strongyloides stercoralis infection in hospital patients with comorbidity in need of proper management. *BMC Infect Dis.* 2016;16:98.

58. Luna OB, Grasselli R, Ananias M, et al. [Disseminated strongyloidiasis: diagnosis and treatment]. *Rev Bras Ter Intensiva.* 2007;19(4):463-468.

59. Ly MN, Bethel SL, Usmani AS, Lambert DR. Cutaneous Strongyloides stercoralis infection: an unusual presentation. *J Am Acad Dermatol.* 2003;49(2 suppl Case Reports):S157-S160.

60. Montes M, Sawhney C, Barros N. Strongyloides stercoralis: there but not seen. *Curr Opin Infect Dis.* 2010;23(5):500-504.

61. Nozais JP, Thellier M, Datry A, Danis M. [Disseminated strongyloidiasis]. *Presse Med.* 2001;30(16):813-818.

62. Ronan SG, Reddy RL, Manaligod JR, Alexander J, Fu T. Disseminated strongyloidiasis presenting as purpura. *J Am Acad Dermatol.* 1989;21(5 Pt 2):1123-1125.

63. Salluh JI, Bozza FA, Pinto TS, Toscano L, Weller PF, Soares M. Cutaneous periumbilical purpura in disseminated strongyloidiasis in cancer patients: a pathognomonic feature of potentially lethal disease? *Braz J Infect Dis.* 2005;9(5):419-424.

64. Goddard J. *Physician's Guide to Arthropods of Medical Importance.* 5th ed. Boca Raton, FL: CRC Press/Taylor & Francis; 2007.

65. Haddad V, Jr., Cardoso JL, Lupi O, Tyring SK. Tropical dermatology: Venomous arthropods and human skin: Part II. Diplopoda, Chilopoda, and Arachnida. *J Am Acad Dermatol.* 2012;67(3):347 e1-e9;quiz 55.

66. Haddad V, Jr., Cardoso JL, Lupi O, Tyring SK. Tropical dermatology: Venomous arthropods and human skin: Part I. Insecta. *J Am Acad Dermatol.* 2012;67(3):331e1-14;quiz 45.

67. Steen CJ, Carbonaro PA, Schwartz RA. Arthropods in dermatology. *J Am Acad Dermatol.* 2004;50(6):819-842, quiz 42-4.

68. Hunt GR. Bites and stings of uncommon arthropods. 1. Spiders. *Postgrad Med.* 1981;70(2):91-102.

69. Hunt GR. Bites and stings of uncommon arthropods. 2. Reduviids, fire ants, puss caterpillars, and scorpions. *Postgrad Med.* 1981;70(2):107-114.

70. Vetter RS, Swanson DL. Arthropods in dermatology: errors in arachnology. *J Am Acad Dermatol.* 2005;52(5):923.

71. Villada G, Hafeez F, Ollague J, Nousari CH, Elgart GW. Imported fire ant envenomation: a clinicopathologic study of a recognizable form of arthropod assault reaction. *J Cutan Pathol.* 2017;44(12):1012-1017.

72. Wirtz RA. Allergic and toxic reactions to non-stinging arthropods. *Annu Rev Entomol.* 1984;29:47-69.

73. Camp NE. Black widow spider envenomation. *J Emerg Nurs.* 2014;40(2):193-194.

74. Diaz JH, Leblanc KE. Common spider bites. *Am Fam Physician.* 2007;75(6):869-873.

75. Isbister GK, Fan HW. Spider bite. *Lancet.* 2011;378(9808):2039-2047.

76. Kang JK, Bhate C, Schwartz RA. Spiders in dermatology. *Semin Cutan Med Surg.* 2014;33(3):123-127.

77. Siemens J, Zhou S, Piskorowski R, et al. Spider toxins activate the capsaicin receptor to produce inflammatory pain. *Nature.* 2006;444(7116):208-212.

78. McArdle DJ, McArdle JP. Tick bite reaction: caught in the act. *Int J Surg Pathol.* 2016;24(4):334-335.

79. Radmanesh M. Cutaneous manifestations of the Hemiscorpius lepturus sting: a clinical study *Int J Dermatol.* 1998;37(7):500-507.

80. Daly JS, Scharf MJ. *Bites and Stings of Terrestrial and Aquatic Life.* 6th ed. New York, NY: McGraw-Hill, Medical Pub. Division; 2003.

81. Elston DM, Eggers JS, Schmidt WE, et al. Histological findings after brown recluse spider envenomation. *Am J Dermatopathol.* 2000;22(3):242-246.

82. Lynch MC, Milchak MA, Parnes H, Ioffreda MD. Tick bite alopecia: a report and review. *Am J Dermatopathol.* 2016;38(11):e150-e153.

83. Miteva M, Elsner P, Ziemer M. A histopathologic study of arthropod bite reactions in 20 patients highlights relevant adnexal involvement. *J Cutan Pathol.* 2009;36(1):26-33.

84. Tatsuno K, Fujiyama T, Matsuoka H, Shimauchi T, Ito T, Tokura Y. Clinical categories of exaggerated skin reactions to mosquito bites and their pathophysiology. *J Dermatol Sci.* 2016;82(3):145-152.

85. Mitteldorf C, Kempf W. Cutaneous pseudolymphoma. *Surg Pathol Clin.* 2017;10(2):455-476.

86. Hussein MR. Cutaneous pseudolymphomas: inflammatory reactive proliferations. *Expert Rev Hematol.* 2013;6(6):713-733.

87. Reisman RE. Unusual reactions to insect stings. *Curr Opin Allergy Clin Immunol.* 2005;5(4):355-358.

88. Yalcin AD, Bisgin A, Akman A, Erdogan G, Ciftcioglu MA, Yegin O. Jessner lymphocytic infiltrate as a side effect of bee venom immunotherapy. *J Investig Allergol Clin Immunol.* 2012;22(4):308-309.

89. Castelli E, Caputo V, Morello V, Tomasino RM. Local reactions to tick bites. *Am J Dermatopathol.* 2008;30(3):241-248.

90. Arlian LG, Runyan RA, Achar S, Estes SA. Survival and infectivity of Sarcoptes scabiei var. canis and var. hominis. *J Am Acad Dermatol.* 1984;11(2 Pt 1):210-215.

91. Friedman R. *Scabies—Civil and Military; Its Prevalence, Prevention and Treatment.* New York, NY: Froben Press; 1941.

92. Mellanby K. Transmission of scabies. *Br Med J.* 1941;2(4211):405-406.

93. Dupuy A, Dehen L, Bourrat E, et al. Accuracy of standard dermoscopy for diagnosing scabies. *J Am Acad Dermatol.* 2007;56(1):53-62.

94. Heukelbach J, Wilcke T, Winter B, Feldmeier H. Epidemiology and morbidity of scabies and pediculosis capitis in resource-poor communities in Brazil. *Br J Dermatol.* 2005;153(1):150-156.

95. Sardana K, Mahajan S, Sarkar R, et al. The spectrum of skin disease among Indian children. *Pediatr Dermatol.* 2009;26(1):6-13.

96. Hossain D. Atypical scabies presenting as annular patches. *Pediatr Dermatol.* 2014;31(3):408-409.

97. Royer M, Latre CM, Paul C, Mazereeuw-Hautier J, Societe Francaise de Dermatologie P. [Infantile scabies]. *Ann Dermatol Venereol.* 2008;135(12):876-881;quiz 5.

98. Worth C, Heukelbach J, Fengler G, Walter B, Liesenfeld O, Feldmeier H. Impaired quality of life in adults and children with scabies from an impoverished community in Brazil. *Int J Dermatol.* 2012;51(3):275-282.

99. Barnes L, McCallister RE, Lucky AW. Crusted (Norwegian) scabies. Occurrence in a child undergoing a bone marrow transplant. *Arch Dermatol.* 1987;123(1):95-97.

100. Mantero NM, Jaime LJ, Nijamin TR, Laffargue JA, De Lillo L, Grees SA. [Norwegian scabies in a pediatric patient with Down syndrome, a case report]. *Arch Argent Pediatr.* 2013;111(6):e141-e143.

101. McLucas P, Fulchiero GJ, Jr., Fernandez E, Miller JJ, Zaenglein AL. Norwegian scabies mimicking onychomycosis and scalp dermatitis in a child with IPEX syndrome. *J Am Acad Dermatol.* 2007;56(2 suppl):S48-S49.

102. Finon A, Desoubeaux G, Nadal M, Georgescou G, Baran R, Maruani A. [Scabies of the nail unit in an infant]. *Ann Dermatol Venereol.* 2017;144(5):356-361.

103. Luo ZY, Zeng M, Gao Q, et al. Case Report: bullous scabies in two children below 10 years. *Am J Trop Med Hyg.* 2017;97(6):1746-1748.

104. Foo CW, Florell SR, Bowen AR. Polarizable elements in scabies infestation: a clue to diagnosis. *J Cutan Pathol.* 2013;40(1):6-10.

105. Werner B, Massone C, Kerl H, Cerroni L. Large CD30-positive cells in benign, atypical lymphoid infiltrates of the skin. *J Cutan Pathol.* 2008;35(12):1100-1117.

106. Drut R, Peral CG, Garone A, Rositto A. Langerhans cell hyperplasia of the skin mimicking Langerhans cell histiocytosis: a report of two cases in children not associated with scabies. *Fetal Pediatr Pathol.* 2010;29(4):231-238.

107. Thappa DM, Karthikeyan K. Exaggerated scabies: a marker of HIV infection. *Indian Pediatr.* 2002;39(9):875-876.

108. Tidman MJ, Adamson B, Allan S, Wallace WH. Childhood scabies mistaken for Langerhans cell histiocytosis. *Clin Exp Dermatol.* 2003;28(1):111-112.

109. Do-Pham G, Monsel G, Chosidow O. Lice. *Semin Cutan Med Surg.* 2014;33(3):116-118.

110. Faber WR, Hay RJ, Naafs B. *Imported Skin Diseases.* 2nd ed. Chichester, West Sussex, UK: Wiley-Blackwell; 2013:1 online resource.

111. Feldmeier H. Pediculosis capitis: new insights into epidemiology, diagnosis and treatment. *Eur J Clin Microbiol Infect Dis.* 2012;31(9):2105-2110.

112. Feldmeier H. [Pediculosis capitis-an update]. *MMW Fortschr Med.* 2017;159(7):39-42.

113. Hansen RC. Overview: the state of head lice management and control. *Am J Manag Care.* 2004;10(9 suppl):S260-S263.

114. Puri PK, House NS, Williams L, Elston D. The histopathology of Phthirus pubis. *J Cutan Pathol.* 2009;36(1):80-81.

115. Leung AK, Fong JH, Pinto-Rojas A. Pediculosis capitis. *J Pediatr Health Care.* 2005;19(6):369-373.

116. Veracx A, Raoult D. Biology and genetics of human head and body lice. *Trends Parasitol.* 2012;28(12):563-571.

117. Wadowski L, Balasuriya L, Price HN, O'Haver J. Lice update: new solutions to an old problem. *Clin Dermatol.* 2015;33(3):347-354.

118. Gunther S. Clinical and epidemiological aspects of the dermal Tumbu-fly-myiasis in Equatorial-Africa. *Br J Dermatol.* 1971;85(3):226-231.

119. Hall M, Wall R. Myiasis of humans and domestic animals. *Adv Parasitol.* 1995;35:257-334.

120. Hall MJ. Trapping the flies that cause myiasis: their responses to host-stimuli. *Ann Trop Med Parasitol.* 1995;89(4):333-357.

121. Hall MJ, Farkas R, Kelemen F, Hosier MJ, el-Khoga JM. Orientation of agents of wound myiasis to hosts and artificial stimuli in Hungary. *Med Vet Entomol.* 1995;9(1):77-84.

122. Lodi A, Bruscagin C, Gianni C, Mancini LL, Crosti C. Myiasis due to Cordylobia anthropophaga (Tumbu-fly). *Int J Dermatol.* 1994;33(2):127-128.

123. Caissie R, Beaulieu F, Giroux M, Berthod F, Landry PE. Cutaneous myiasis: diagnosis, treatment, and prevention. *J Oral Maxillofac Surg.* 2008;66(3):560-568.

124. Francesconi F, Lupi O. Myiasis. *Clin Microbiol Rev.* 2012;25(1):79-105.

125. Hakeem MJ, Bhattacharyya DN. Exotic human myiasis. *Travel Med Infect Dis.* 2009;7(4):198-202.

126. Lachish T, Marhoom E, Mumcuoglu KY, Tandlich M, Schwartz E. Myiasis in travelers. *J Travel Med.* 2015;22(4):232-236.

127. McGraw TA, Turiansky GW. Cutaneous myiasis. *J Am Acad Dermatol.* 2008;58(6):907-926;quiz 27-29.

128. Mohrenschlager M, Mempel M, Weichenmeier I, Engst R, Ring J, Behrendt H. Scanning electron microscopy of Dermatobia hominis reveals cutaneous anchoring features. *J Am Acad Dermatol.* 2007;57(4):716-718.

129. Robbins K, Khachemoune A. Cutaneous myiasis: a review of the common types of myiasis. *Int J Dermatol.* 2010;49(10):1092-1098.

130. Solomon M, Lachish T, Schwartz E. Cutaneous myiasis. *Curr Infect Dis Rep.* 2016;18(9):28.

131. Fydryszewski NA. Myiasis: diagnosis, treatment and medical use of maggots. *Clin Lab Sci.* 2013;26(2):76-81.

132. Hohenstein EJ, Buechner SA. Cutaneous myiasis due to Dermatobia hominis. *Dermatology.* 2004;208(3):268-270.

22

Melanocytic-Nevocellular Lesions

Louis P. Dehner / Esteban Fernandez Faith

Melanocytic neoplasms of one type or another are common in the pediatric population presenting as a birthmark or as a later acquired lesion(s). One-third or more of skin biopsies or excisions seen in dermatopathology laboratories from children are melanocytic lesions. Many of these lesions follow a stable course, whereas others are more dynamic in behavior with growth, changes in the clinical appearance, and, in some cases, spontaneous regression, on the basis of a suspected immunologic reaction.

As some measure of the frequency of cutaneous melanocytic lesions in children, we reviewed our experience over a recent 2-year period and found that one-third of all skin biopsies and excisions obtained during the first two decades of life were melanocytic proliferations.[1] Verruca vulgaris and squamous-lined cysts together comprised almost 20% of cases in the same age group and time period so that pediatric and dermatopathologists alike are more than familiar with these lesions in their practice.

Melanocytic nevus is a generic designation for a broad category of lesions that can be characterized clinically and pathologically into a number of subtypes in both children and adults, and several of these are seen predominantly in children and adolescents and are clustered in children 10 years old or less.

It is accepted today, though not consistently in the past, that the melanocyte is one of many derivatives of the neural crest (NC).[2] Progenitor melanocytes are one of the few NC-derived cells that arise from the four major axial designated sites: cranial, vagal, truncal, and lumbosacral; NC cells behave in many respects like stem cells. As NC cells initiate the process of migration, they undergo an epithelial to mesenchymal transition with the development of various differentiated tissue types.[3] Through a study of human embryos, Holbrook and associates determined that proto-melanocytes begin their migration to the epidermis at estimated gestational age of 40 to 50 days.[4] Melanocytes are also present in the mucosal basal layer in sites from the oral cavity, nasal mucosa, and genitourinary tract. It is thought that some melanoblasts fail to arrive at their epithelial destination as a defect in migration to explain some of the uncommon and unusual sites for melanocytic nevi and melanomas.

Given the commonality of the melanocytic nevus, there remain many unanswered questions despite the rather thorough evaluation of these lesions from the molecular genetic perspective.[5] Three competing hypotheses on the histogenesis of melanocytic or nevocellular nevus have been proposed over the last 100 years and still maintain an element of currency in the literature.[6] The oldest of these is the so-called "trickling down" hypothesis of Unna, which postulated that nevi arise from melanocytes in the dermoepidermal junction from a junctional nevus that migrates vertically into the dermis as the intermediate compound nevus and finally as a dermal nevus (DN) with the arrest of junctional proliferation, but Unna thought that the melanocyte arose in the epidermis.[6] It was well into the mid-twentieth century that the origin of the melanocyte remained a puzzle as articulated by Masson[7]: "Whatever their origin, schwannian or melanoblasts, all nevus cells share the properties, which are seen only as characteristics of the schwannian syncytium." It is as though Masson was anticipating the histogenetic relationship of these two cell types as derivatives of the

NC. Later Cramer,[8] acknowledging the NC origin of the melanocyte, also invoked peripheral nerve elements, especially the perineurial cell in an analogous fashion to Masson's hypothesis, in reference to the histogenesis of the congenital melanocytic nevus (CMN). The plasticity of melanocytes and Schwann cells has been discussed by others.[9] Migration of melanocytes arrested in the dermis explains the family of blue nevi (BN) and dermal melanocytosis (DM). Possibly the pure dermal melanoma is another clinical expression of arrested migration of progenitor preneoplastic cells.[10]

ACQUIRED MELANOCYTIC NEVUS

Epidemiology and Etiology

The several determinants in the development of acquired melanocytic nevus (AMN) are lifelong factors that include hereditary, skin type, and sun exposure in the form of ultraviolet light radiation (UVR). The latter is clearly the main environmental factor in the pathogenesis of most AMNs and melanomas. The interplay among these several factors in the development of AMNs is appreciated in the geographic and ethnic variation of these lesions.[11-13] The initial appearance of AMNs occurs in early childhood and then increases in number into the third decade of life. Among fair-skinned children, the mean nevus count is 15 to 30, whereas in children with skin of color, the total count is often less than 15. It is during the first decade of life when the greatest accumulation of AMNs is seen and the need for UVR prevention is maximum.[14-18] Yet another variable in UVR exposure is related to the latitude at which a sunburn occurs at seaside or an on-land site.[19] The numerical density of AMNs is greatest on the trunk compared to other body sites.[20] Those individuals with Fitzpatrick skin type 2 and dark hair have the highest nevus count, except in those with the "red hair phenotype" who appear to have a lower density of nevi. The greater the number of AMNs in childhood and a positive family history for cutaneous melanoma maximize the risk for the melanoma.[21]

Specific genetic mutations have been associated with the development of AMNs.[22] *BRAF* and much less frequently *NRAS* mutations are detected in these lesions; *BRAF* mutations are present in 60% to 90% of AMNs.[23,24] The same mutations are found in melanomas to serve as a pathogenetic linkage with AMNs.

Clinical and Pathologic Features

The designation of AMN includes the common melanocytic nevus whose three clinicopathologic types are the junctional, compound, and DN, but within this simplified scheme, there are a number of subtypes based upon clinical and morphologic features such as the so-called halo nevus with its intense lymphocytic infiltration; Spitz nevus (SN) with its spindle, epithelioid, and atypical features; spindle cell nevus of Reed; and deep penetrating nevus (DPN). Each of these latter entities is discussed subsequently, but the point is that there is a broad and overlapping clinicopathologic spectrum of AMNs. This is also appreciated in the different dermoscopic patterns including reticular, globular, and homogeneous patterns in children; the globular pattern is the most commonly detected one in childhood.[25]

Those with a higher density of nevi often develop them with a similar clinical pattern, which is referred to as a "signature nevus."[26] The patterns include solid pink, solid brown, "fried egg," "eclipse," pink eclipse, cockade (target) nevus, nevus with perifollicular hypopigmentation, multiple halo nevi, and lentiginous nevus (Figure 22-1A-C).

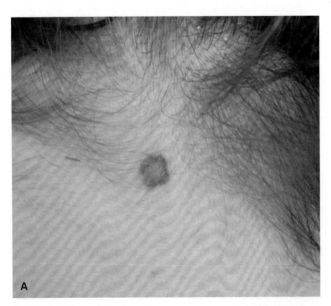
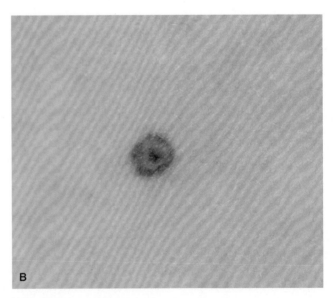

FIGURE 22-1. Various patterns of acquired melanocytic nevi. A, Eclipse nevus with central light tan color with brown rim. B, Cockade or target nevus with central brown papule followed by light tan area and outermost brown rim.

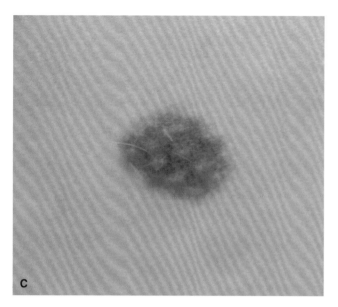

FIGURE 22-1. (*continued*) C, Perifollicular hypopigmentation in this nevus.

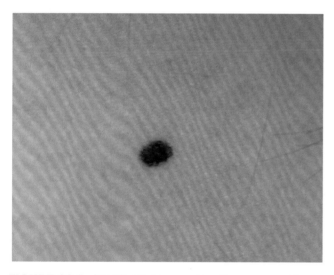

FIGURE 22-2. **Junctional nevus presenting as an oval macule with homogeneous dark brown pigmentation.**

Junctional Nevus

Junctional nevus initially appears as a hyperpigmented macule with rounded to oval contours; the coloration ranges from pink to brown to black (Figure 22-2). Microscopically, the nests of nevus cells are located along the dermoepidermal junctions with a more or less regular pattern of periodicity and usually a rather abrupt transition to uninvolved skin with sharply demarcated lateral borders without a trailing edge or border (Figure 22-3). The latter features differentiate the common junctional nevus from the architecturally disorder or dysplastic nevus.

Compound Nevus

Compound nevus has a papulonodular appearance and may be flesh colored or pigmented depending in part upon the degree of pigmentation of the junctional

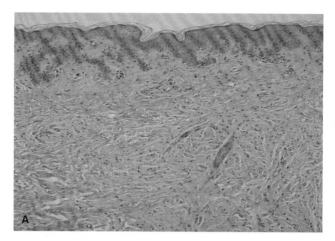

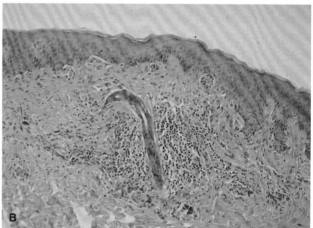

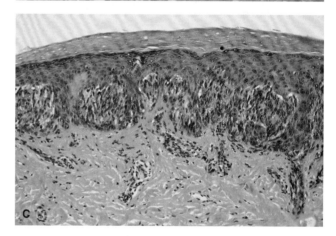

FIGURE 22-3. **Junctional melanocytic nevus.** A, A lesion from the back of a 7-year-old male with small, regularly distributed junctional nests. Note the diffuse neurofibroma in the dermis. B, Junctional nests with an irregular pattern and an accompanying lymphocytic reaction from the scalp of a 5-year-old female. This lesion may have some special site features. C, Nests of spindle cells at the junction from the dorsal hand of a 1-year-old female. This lesion was not appreciably pigmented, but the question is a junctional Spitz versus Reed nevus.

component and/or pigmentary incontinence (Figure 22-4). A dense lymphocytic infiltrate may obscure the nevus cells throughout and may be accompanied by a clinical halo (Figure 22-5). Multiple halo nevi can be seen in association

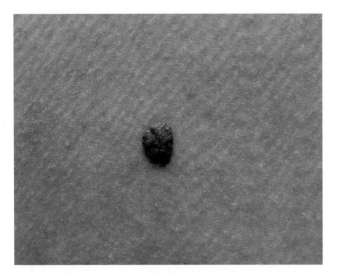

FIGURE 22-4. Compound melanocytic nevus as a light brown fleshy papule.

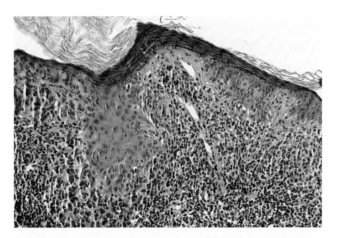

FIGURE 22-5. Compound melanocytic nevus from the posterior shoulder of a 14-year-old male showing a dense lymphocytic infiltrate obscuring in part the junctional and dermal nevus cells. This "halo" phenomenon is not always accompanied by a clinical halo.

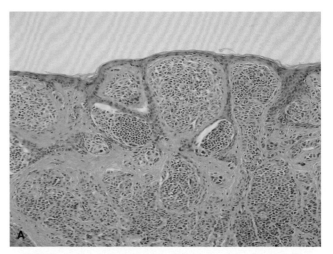

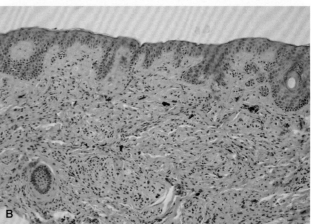

FIGURE 22-6. **Compound melanocytic nevus.** A, Compactly arranged nevus cells at the junction and in the dermis maintain a nested pattern. Note that the nevus cells are rounded and angulated with some spitzoid features. B, This lesion from the brow of a 9-year-old female shows small junctional nests and variably sized dermal nests with a plexiform-like pattern and scattered pigmented cells. The abundant eosinophilic background suggested neurotization or a combined nevus.

with Turner syndrome. The number of junctional nests can be quite variable from case to case but seem to diminish with the age of the child at the time of biopsy/excision (Figure 22-6A & B). The dermal component may retain its nested pattern or acquires a more diffuse pattern as individual nevus cells, which trickle through the dermis and convey the impression that the cells are smaller with depth in the dermis compared to those nevus cells at or beneath the dermoepidermal junction; this phenomenon is referred to correctly or incorrectly as so-called maturation or senescence with depth (Figure 22-7). Among the junctional and superficial DN cells, the nuclei are larger with an open chromatin pattern and a micronucleolus and with depth into the dermis, the nevus cells are smaller including the nucleus with its more dense chromatin. Those nevi whose nuclei do not undergo this transition and whose nucleoli persist within the depths should be evaluated carefully and if need be shared with colleagues.

Any mitotic activity in a compound nevus should be noted with the acknowledgment that 1 to 2 mitotic figures are found in a range of otherwise benign melanocytic lesions. Mitotic figures, when present, are generally confined to the nevus cells at the junction and/or papillary dermis.[27] Deep mitotic figures should be viewed with greater concern than the more superficial ones except if those mitotic figures are atypical. It appears that mitotic figures are found more commonly in those nevi from children and from special anatomic sites.[28,29] Of course, other features are incorporated into any pathologic assessment of an atypical melanocytic lesion.

Scattered enlarged individual nevus cells with densely aggregated nuclei in a background of multinucleated nevus cell can convey concern, but in most cases represent so-called senescent changes; multinucleated nevus cells are more commonly seen in benign lesions and can serve to ameliorate concern about the particular lesion (Figure 22-6B).

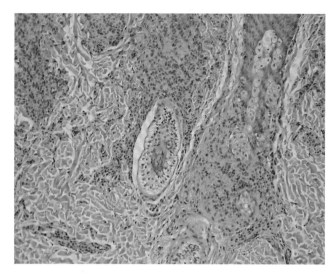

FIGURE 22-7. **Compound melanocytic nevus.** This lesion from the postauricular region of a 9-year-old female shows the small individual nevus cells compared to the larger more superficial nevus cells. Also note the loss of the nesting pattern around the hair follicle with congenital-like features.

TABLE 22-1.	Types of melanocytic lesions in the first two decades of life (2012–2016)	
Type	**Number**	**%**
Compound nevus	719	62
Dermal nevus	229	20
Spitz nevus	103	9
Junctional nevus	47	4
Blue nevus	22	2
Spindle cell nevus of Reed	15	1
Halo nevus	12	1
Atypical spitzoid tumor	7	1
Deep penetrating nevus	5	<1
Malignant melanoma	5	<1
Total	1164	~100

Compiled from the files of the Lauren V. Ackerman Laboratory of Surgical Pathology, Washington University Medical Center, St. Louis, Missouri.

From Yang C, Gru A, Dehner LP. Common and not so common melanocytic lesions in children and adolescents. *Pediatr Dev Pathol.* 2018;21(2):252-270.

Dermal Nevus

DN is defined as a melanocytic lesion without a junctional component. It is often characterized as a soft dome-shaped lesion whose differential diagnosis may include neurofibroma. Both the compound nevus and DN may be associated with alterations in the overlying epidermis including marked acanthosis or seborrheic keratosis–like architecture. With the loss of the junctional component, DN often appears lighter in color. Although we generally do not divide DN into the so-called Unna and Miescher patterns, the former is recognized by a widened papillary dermis, whereas the latter has a more diffuse infiltrative growth into the reticular dermis (Figure 22-8A-C).[30] Those DNs with the diffuse pattern can have a prominent fibrillary matrix or stroma and tactile body–like formations that have been referred to as neurotization with a resemblance to a neurofibroma. Adipose tissue and heterotopic bone (osteonevus of nanta) are other less common findings whose presence reflects the range of mesenchymal differentiation in NC-derived proliferations. Though uncommon in DNs from children, so called ancient changes can be mistaken for melanoma.[31] Exclusively dermal-based melanocytic nevi are seen in several other specific contexts including the SN, DPN, BN, and CMN.

Most AMNs are straightforward lesions in terms of the histologic features, which generally do not require any special or specific qualifications in the pathologic diagnosis whether in a child or adult. In the practice of one of us (LPD), 90% of AMNs were in descending order of frequency: compound (62%), dermal (20%), and junctional nevi (4%) (Table 22-1). The remaining nevocellular lesions (14%) represented specific pathologic types such as the SN. Most compound nevus and DN were seen in biopsies or excisions from children 8 years of age or older.

CAPSULE SUMMARY

ACQUIRED MELANOCYTIC NEVI

AMN initially appear in early childhood and etiologic factors include heredity (possible mutations in *BRAF* or *NRAS* genes), skin type, and sun exposure in the form of UVR. There are three forms: junctional, intradermal, and compound. Mitotic activity may be seen in AMN in young children. "Ancient" nuclear atypia should not be misconstrued as melanoma.

ATYPICAL MELANOCYTIC NEVUS

Atypical melanocytic nevus is a generic category based in part upon the clinical appearance and the pathologic features of the nevocellular proliferation. An irregular distribution of junctional nests, lentiginous (single-cell) junctional pattern, and nuclear alterations such as enlargement, density and coarseness of the chromatin, prominence of the nucleoli and mitotic figures, and their location are some of the qualifying histologic features of an "atypical nevus." In a sense, it does not imply a specific subtype of nevus because these findings occur across the broad spectrum of lesions. Less than 10% of atypical nevi are diagnosed in the first two decades of life in one epidemiologic study.[32] The most common context of an atypical melanocytic nevus in our experience is the so-called dysplastic or architecturally disordered nevus whose basic morphologic features include the following: (1) architecture with bridging of rete ridges; (2) nested nevus cells at the tips of the rete and single or lentiginous cells along the rete ridges; (3) continuous lamellar pattern of fibroplasia outlining the superficial papillary dermis; and (4) a shoulder of junctional nevus cells without an underlying

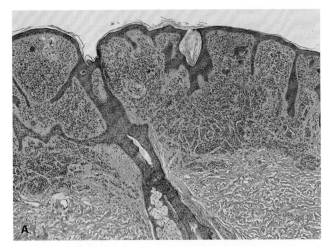

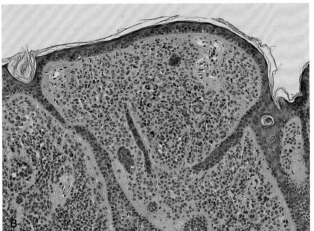

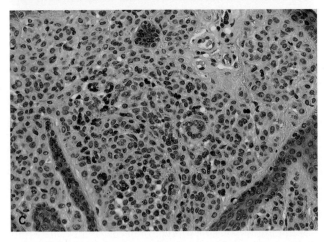

FIGURE 22-8. A, Dermal melanocytic nevus from the trunk of a 17-year-old female. Note the alterations of the overlying epidermis and the expansion of the papillary dermis. B, The nevus cells even in this obviously benign lesion show variations of cell size and scattered dense nuclei that may represent pyknosis rather than atypia. C, Nuclear pseudoinclusions and multinucleated nevus cells are present in this field.

dermal component (Figure 22-9).[33] The preference of one of us (LPD) is "melanocytic nevus with architectural disorder," rather than dysplastic or Clark's nevus. Despite the efforts of several convened consensus conferences, there is still a lack

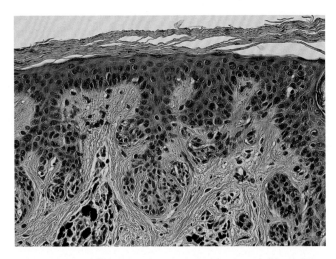

FIGURE 22-9. **Compound melanocytic nevus with architectural disorder (dysplastic nevus) in a 14-year-old male.** Note the irregular junctional nests and bridging of rete ridges focally. Nuclear atypia is evident in the junctional melanocytes, with maturation in the dermal nests with smaller nevus cells.

of consensus on many aspects of these lesions including the grading of atypia, its significance, and management.[34-38] So-called dysplastic features are not confined to the common AMN, but are seen in other nevocellular lesions such as the SN and combined nevus.[39-41]

Another category of AMNs with atypical features includes those from the so-called anatomic special sites such as the scalp, genital area, hand/foot, flexural sites, ear, breast, and lower extremity.[42-44] There is overlap in the histopathologic features of the special site AMN and the architecturally disordered or dysplastic nevus. AMNs can also be seen in association with pregnancy which particularly have a higher number of mitotic figures and in association with lichen sclerosus.

Scalp Nevus

Scalp nevus presenting in children and adolescents may herald the development of additional AMNs on the vertex and parietal scalp and elsewhere.[45-47] It has been noted that scalp nevi in children are accompanied by an increased number of nevi elsewhere than in children without scalp lesions.[48] The scalp nevus is often elliptical, is variably pigmented, and may have irregular borders. The presence of large, atypical nevus cells, dusty cytoplasmic melanin, and large, irregular nests, and lentiginous proliferation along and between rete ridges are some of the atypical features.[49] Pagetoid spread of nevus cells and dyscohesion of individual nevus cells within the nests are additional features.[50]

Genital AMN

Genital AMNs were detected in 35% of children in the experience of one pediatric dermatology practice.[51] These lesions are generally recognized at or before 5 years of age and even at or shortly after birth. A medium to dark brown symmetrical nevus(s) on the labia majora and minora or penile shaft or scrotum is the clinical appearance. Like the scalp nevus, the genital nevus has a compound pattern with architecturally disordered or dysplastic features.[52,53]

Acral Nevocellular Lesions

Acral nevocellular lesions include the acral nevus of acquired or congenital types and longitudinal melanonychia. One cohort study of individuals 18 years of age and older noted acral pigmentary lesions in 30% of cases.[54] Skin-of-color individuals are more likely to have acral melanocytic lesions, but when seen in non-Hispanic fair-skinned children, there is also an increased overall count of melanocytic nevi. A study of school-aged children in Colombia revealed 42% had at least one acral melanocytic lesion.[55] Kim et al[56] reported that the most common site of an acral lesion in children was the forefoot of the sole followed by the volar toe, together accounting for almost 85% of cases, whereas approximately 15% of pigmented lesions were found on the volar palm and finger.

Histopathologically, virtually all cutaneous acral lesions have architecturally disordered features and 60% to 65% are junctional proliferations and 25% to 30% are compound nevi with mixed lentiginous and nested patterns (Figure 22-10).[57] Cytologic atypia is generally mild in most cases. Pagetoid spread through the epidermis and transepidermal elimination of nevus nests are other findings. SN and BN are also present in acral sites.[58] Eruptive nevi are reported on the sole and/or palm in children after chemotherapy, but their histopathologic features are not unique from other acral nevi in children. In some cases, the pagetoid spreading can be very prominent, particularly in young patients. The term *MANIAC* nevus (melanocytic acral nevus with intraepidermal ascent of cells) has been used to described such findings.

Longitudinal Melanonychia (Melanonychia Striata)

Longitudinal melanonychia, like the cutaneous acral nevus, occurs more commonly in skin-of-color than fair-skinned children. The finger(s), especially the thumb, is the most common site of the longitudinal pigmented band in children and rarely in neonates.[59,60] Melanocytic activation with increased pigmentation in the basal–parabasal layer without an increased number of melanocytes, melanocytic hyperplasia with an increase in the number of melanocytes, and a disordered junctional melanocytic nevus are the range of histologic findings.[39,61] Subungual melanoma is rarely reported in children, but apparent progression of longitudinal melanonychia discovered in childhood to a melanoma in adults has been reported.[62,63]

CAPSULE SUMMARY

ATYPICAL MELANOCYTIC NEVI

Architecturally disordered (formerly "dysplastic") nevus is the most common form.

Atypical melanocytic nevi are defined histologically and typified by irregular distribution of junctional nests, prominent lentiginous proliferation, nuclear atypia, and mitotic activity. Architectural disorder can also be observed in some SNs and "special site" nevi of scalp, genital skin, and acral skin.

OTHER AMN

Several of the other AMNs are accompanied by a variety of eponyms, which is not altogether surprising because clinical dermatology is replete with these.[64] For those interested in the topic of melanocytic nevus–associated eponyms, the latter is an informative resource.

Meyerson Nevus (Phenomenon)

Meyerson nevus is an AMN that is accompanied by a spongiotic dermatitis, which is rich in CD4+ T-lymphocytes and histiocytes with accompanying clinical erythema and a centrally positioned nevus of either the congenital or acquired type in a child[65] (Figure 22-11A & B). The trunk or proximal extremities is the favored site.

Nevus Spilus (Speckled Lentiginous Nevus)

Speckled lentiginous nevus (SLN) is a clinical designation for a brownish macule or patch that is studded with hyperpigmented speckles[66] (Figure 22-12). A similar lesion with a papular appearance may present in association with the epidermal nevus or nevus sebaceous syndromes (phacomatosis pigmentokeratotica).[67] The syndromic SLN is a manifestation of HRAS mosaicism and is considered one of RASopathies.[68,69] The brownish macule is composed of an increased number of pigmented melanocytes with the so-called lentigo simplex pattern or with various nevocellular patterns in hyperpigmented foci whose histologic features are those of a disordered (dysplastic) junctional, compound nevus or SN.

Spitz Nevus Spectrum

SN spectrum represents a category of nevocellular proliferations that share similar clinicopathologic features. The characteristic presentation of a SN is solitary, often amelanotic, flesh-colored or erythematous, smooth dome-shaped papule measuring less than 10 mm in diameter in most cases; the head and neck region and lower extremities are the sites of predilection (Table 22-2; Figure 22-13).[70] The paradox of the "melanoma of childhood" as Spitz referred to the lesion known today as the SN was apparent to her in the initial study of 13 children with lesions in which she observed that "malignant melanoma . . . in children has clinical behavior rarely . . . that of a malignant tumor."[71] One of the original 13 cases in a 12-year-old behaved as a malignancy with metastases and death. Other than the presence of multinucleated nevus cells according to Spitz, the "histologic appearance (9 of 13 cases) . . . in most respects was indistinguishable from adult type of malignant melanomas."[71] It is now 70 years later, and we are arguably little better in some respects than over three generations ago in the reliable

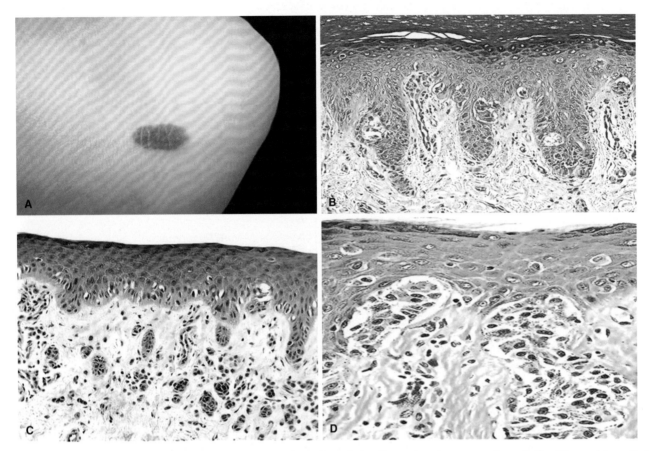

FIGURE 22-10. **Compound melanocytic nevus, acral type.** A, This clinical illustration shows some irregularity at the periphery. B, An alternating junctional lentiginous and nested melanocytic proliferation. C, This focus demonstrates the acrolentiginous pattern. D, This focus shows the atypical junctional nests composed of nevus cells with prominent nucleoli.

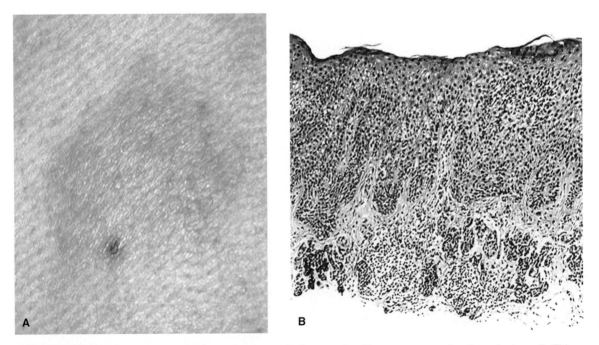

FIGURE 22-11. **Meyerson (spongiotic) melanocytic nevus.** A, A zone of erythema accompanies these lesions. B, This compound melanocytic nevus has a spongiotic and acanthotic epidermis.

TABLE 22-2.	Anatomic distribution of Spitz, atypical spitzoid tumor, and spitzoid melanoma		
Type	Spitz Nevus Number (%)	Atypical Spitzoid Tumor Number (%)	Spitzoid Melanoma Number (%)
Head and neck	264 (35)	13 (35)	12 (48)
Upper extremity	193 (26)	11 (30)	8 (32)
Lower extremity	186 (25)	9 (24)	5 (20)
Trunk	102 (13)	4 (11)	–
Perineum (penis 2, scrotum 1, vulva 1)	5 (<1)	–	–
Not stated	6 (<1)	–	–
Total	756 (~100)	37 (100)	25 (100)

Compiled from the files of the Lauren V. Ackerman Laboratory of Surgical Pathology, Washington University Medical Center, St. Louis, Missouri, 1990 to 2017.

From Yang C, Gru A, Dehner LP. Common and not so common melanocytic lesions in children and adolescents. *Pediatr Dev Pathol.* 2018;21(2):252-270.

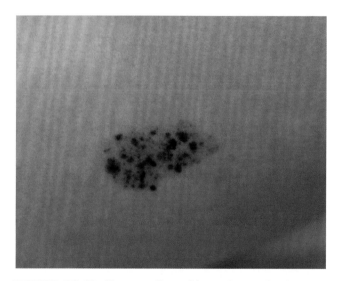

FIGURE 22-12. **Nevus spilus with tan-brown background speckled with dark brown macules.**

separation of one worrisome Spitz lesion from another.[72-74] Despite the seemingly endless discussions and controversies that are recounted in some of the latter cited references, we are still challenged by some but certainly not all SNs.

Spitz Nevus

SN in most cases and with experience can be recognized and diagnosed histopathologically as a benign lesion. Among cutaneous nevocellular lesions in individuals 20 years of age or less, SN represented almost 10% of nevocellular lesions in our experience (Table 22-1). Slightly over 80% of cases were examples of the compound SN (Table 22-2). Over 65% of SN are diagnosed in children 10 years old or less, with a near equal number of males and females. The head and neck and upper extremities were the sites of predilection, followed by the trunk (Table 22-2). With the infrequent exception, virtually all SNs were solitary lesions, with the exception of one case of agminated SN in our review.

Multifocal lesions are variably known as grouped (agminated) and eruptive disseminated SN whose estimated frequency is 0.3% of all SN.[75] Clustered or agminated SN are seen on the face, back, and extremities.[76] Eruptive disseminated SN have occurred in association with nevus spilus or as nodules in a large CMN.[77-79] Multiple epithelioid SN are the hallmark of the BAP1 syndrome with loss of germline *BAP1*.[80]

Pathologically, the SN is most often a nonpigmented nodule measuring 1 cm or less. The surface is smooth, but in some cases has a more irregular, verrucous appearance. An erythematous nodule may convey the clinical appearance of a pyogenic granuloma. There are several basic histologic features that characterize the SN, but these are not necessarily coincident in any one case. Most lesions are compound nevi with a junctional and dermal component in addition to the less common junctional and dermal SN (Figure 22-14A & B; Table 22-3). One series of SN, including both children and adults, reported the following distribution of lesions: compound 46%, junctional 33%, and dermal 21%.[81]

The histopathologic features of the SN include the following: (1) spindle and/or epithelioid melanocytes with prominent nucleoli more commonly seen in cells with an epithelioid morphology; (2) symmetric growth; (3) epidermal hyperplasia with verruciform features in some cases; (4) vascular ectasias prominent in the suprapapillary dermis to account for the clinical resemblance to a pyogenic granuloma; (5) junctional proliferation of epithelioid and/or spindle nevus cells with intercellular clefting and vertically oriented nests; (6) Kamino bodies (Periodic acid–Schiff–positive diastase-resistant eosinophilic globules above the tips of the papillae); (7) nested and/or confluent patterns in dermis with reduction of cell size including nuclei and nucleoli with dermal depth; (8) enlarged nuclei without appreciable pleomorphism; (9) mitotic figures, if present, mainly confined to the junctional and superficial dermal population, but exceptions exist of the isolated deep dermal mitosis (not to exceed 1 mitosis); and (10) multinucleated nevus cells usually with epithelioid features. Any atypical mitotic

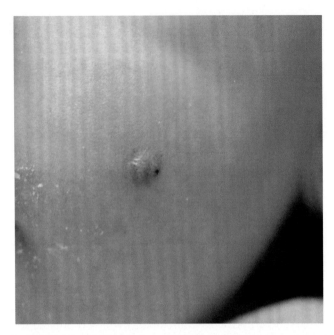

FIGURE 22-13. Spitz nevus presenting as a dome-shaped pink papule on the cheek of this child.

TABLE 22-3.	Spitz, spitzoid, and other spindle cell melanocytic lesions in first two decades	
Type	**Number (%)**	
Typical Spitz nevus (compound)	620 (82)	
Atypical Spitz nevus tumor	37 (5)	
Combined nevus with Spitz features	35 (5)	
Spitzoid melanoma	25 (3)	
Dermal Spitz nevus	14 (2)	
Pigmented spindle cell nevus (Reed)	12 (2)	
Junctional Spitz nevus	7 (<1)	
Cellular blue nevus	6 (<1)	
Total	756 (100)	

Compiled from the files of the Lauren V. Ackerman Laboratory of Surgical Pathology, Washington University Medical Center, St. Louis, Missouri, 1990 to 2017.

From Yang C, Gru A, Dehner LP. Common and not so common melanocytic lesions in children and adolescents. *Pediatr Dev Pathol.* 2018;21(2):252-270.

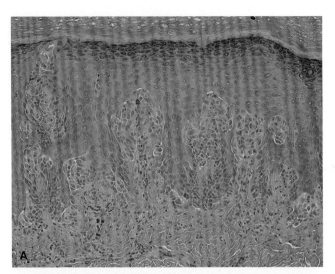

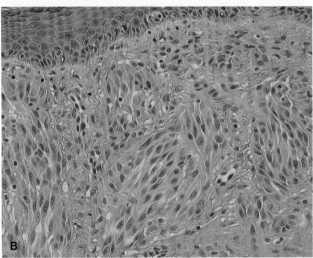

FIGURE 22-14. A, Spitz nevus from the finger of an 8-year-old female shows the mixture of spindle and epithelioid nevus cells. Note the mitotic figure that can be seen in the junctional and papillary dermal nevus cells. B, This field from a Spitz nevus of the cheek in a 5-year-old male shows the spindle and epithelioid nevus cells, intercellular clefts, and vertically oriented nests. The presence of a fascicular growth and spindle cell morphology should raise the possibility of an ALK translocation.

figures should be viewed with caution about a potentially aggressive lesion. Among these various microscopic features, the only uniform finding is the presence of spindle/epithelioid morphology, with the spindled nevus cell as the predominant feature in almost 50% of cases.[81]

In addition to the basic microscopic findings, a mucinous or myxoid stroma is presented as an uncommon feature, as well as a desmoplastic stroma, lymphocytic reaction as in a halo nevus, or a polypoid growth rather than a dome-shaped nodule.[82] A pagetoid pattern of individual nevus cells is uncommon in our experience, but is well-documented in SN and is seen more often in the junctional SN in our experience (Figure 22-15).[83,84] Rosette-like profiles and an intense inflammatory response with granulomatous-like features are other infrequent findings.[85,86] An angiomatoid variant of SN has also been described.[87] Just as the recurrent common melanocytic nevus may present with melanoma-like features with an altered pattern of junctional proliferation and an asymmetrical dermal pattern due in part to the scar, similar findings may be seen in the recurrent or persistent SN.[88] Combined nevus often includes SN and another nevocellular pattern, usually a common compound nevus with or without architecture disorder (Figure 22-16A-C).[40,89] Other combinations of SN in children include those accompanied by a hemangioma, leiomyoma, and epidermal nevus syndrome.[90-92]

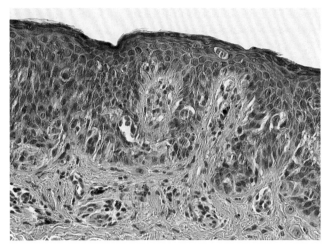

FIGURE 22-15. **Spitz nevus presenting on the arm of a 1-year-old male.** The epithelioid nevus cells are largely confined to the epidermis as junctional nests and as individual cells with a pagetoid pattern.

Intradermal SN

Intradermal SN is less common than the compound pattern SN, accounting for 15% to 20% of cases in our experience (Table 22-3).[81] The histologic pattern is that of individual spindled and/or epithelioid nevus cells in a hyalinized or sclerotic stroma or a stroma with a cellular, scar-like appearance with its designation of desmoplastic SN (Figure 22-17A and B).[93-95] Those lesions with a desmoplastic stroma may be mistaken for a dermatofibroma or desmoplastic melanoma; the latter is virtually unknown in children. Some are of the opinion that the desmoplastic nevus is a distinct lesion from both the SN and the BN.[96]

CAPSULE SUMMARY

SPITZ NEVI

SNs are most common in children and adolescents, as solitary, flesh-colored or reddish, dome-shaped papules, usually <1 cm in diameter, on the head and neck, trunk, or legs. The prototypical histologic profile includes a mixture of epithelioid and fusiform melanocytes, compound growth, sharp peripheral borders, associated epidermal hyperplasia, cleft-like spaces around nevus nests at the epidermal base, permeative involvement of the dermis, possible multinucleation, and the possible presence of "Kamino" bodies (eosinophilic inclusions) at or above the dermoepidermal junction. Mitotic figures can be seen in prepubertal children, and multiple SN with a purely epithelioid cell constituency are a hallmark of the constitutional *BAP1* mutation syndrome. SN may be one component of a combined nevus.

Atypical SN (Tumor)

Atypical Spitz nevus (tumor) (ASNT) in its simplest terms is a nevocellular lesion with the basic histopathologic features

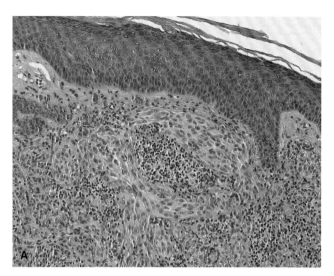

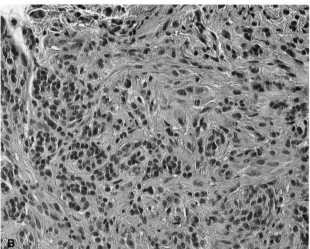

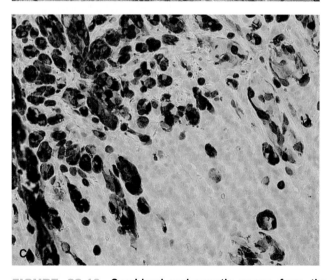

FIGURE 22-16. **Combined melanocytic nevus from the shoulder of a 4-year-old male.** A, This focus shows the spindle and epithelioid nevus cells. B, An adjacent field is composed of distinct dermal nests of nevus cell (common dermal nevus) with the intermixture of the larger epithelioid nevus cells. C, p16 immunostain shows strong nuclear reactivity of the epithelioid nevus cells, whereas the smaller nevus cells are nonreactive in the background.

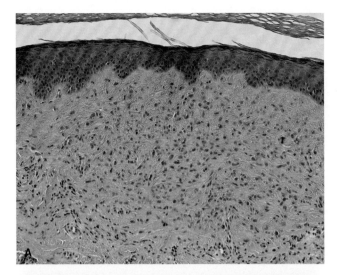

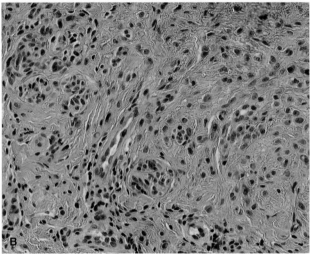

FIGURE 22-17. **Spitz nevus of the dermis presented as a firm nodule on the arm of a 4-year-old female.** A, Individual epithelioid nevus cells are embedded in a fibrous stroma. B, Elsewhere in the same lesion, distinct nests of a common nevus are present. The differential diagnosis is a desmoplastic or combined nevus.

of a SN, but with sufficient histopathologic variance to cause concern about the possibility of a melanoma with spitzoid features.[97] It should be recalled that Spitz regarded all the lesions in her series as atypical to the degree that she considered them all "melanomas of childhood."[71] Another expression of the challenge of the SN is the reference to them as the "everlasting diagnostic challenge."[98] Mones and Ackerman[99] considered ASNT as nothing more than an evasion from a straightforward diagnosis.

Approximately 5% of all Spitz lesions in children that were basically defined by the presence of spindle and/or epithelioid nevus cells were examples of so-called ASNTs in our series (Table 22-3). The age at diagnosis and the male-to-female ratio were the same as the typical SN. Others have reported a male predilection in the case of ASNTs,

fewer ASNTs presenting in the head and neck compared to the typical SN, and more frequent on the extremities.[100]

Pathologic criteria for the diagnosis of an ASNT have been proposed, but their application remains problematic in terms of reproducibility even for the "experts," which is not all that surprising in the case of any borderline melanocytic lesions regardless of type.[73,101] Even the appropriate nomenclature for these spitzoid lesions has not been standardized.[99,102]

The following are some of the applied morphologic features of a ASNT: (1) lesions greater than 1 cm; (2) solid rather than nested growth pattern extending to the deep reticular dermis and into the subcutis with exceptions; (3) asymmetrical growth into dermis; and (4) cytologic atypia in the form of enlarged nuclei with pleomorphism and dense irregular chromatin.[72,100] Nuclear atypia and its degree are subjective from one observer to another to account in part for the inter- and intraobserver variability. We have found it helpful to review the last "typical" SN and compare it to the current case where there is concern about an ASNT. Marked atypia is usually present throughout all levels of an ASNT, and mitotic figures, if present, should be counted with a threshold of greater or less than 6 mitoses per mm (Figure 22-18A and B).[2] The emphasis on mitotic figures in the evaluation of any melanocytic lesion is usually focused upon those mitoses in the mid-to-deep reticular dermis. However, numerous mitotic figures wherever they are identified should be integrated into the overall assessment with the other histopathologic findings, which is the case in any nevocellular proliferation.

Spitzoid Melanoma

Spitzoid melanoma (SM) represented 3% of all Spitz lesions in our review (Table 22-3). In simple terms, the SM is "worse" looking than the ASNT. Barnhill[72] made the point that the diagnosis of SM should only be made in retrospect in a young individual when a metastasis or other aggressive clinical behavior ensues; he discouraged "the use of the term spitzoid melanoma." Despite the latter recommendation, it has not in any way altered the fact that the diagnosis of SM is made in children and is included in any number of studies on melanoma in children where they account from 10% to 40% of all melanomas in this age group.[103-106]

Clinically, the SM has many overlapping features with the SN and ASNT except for size (generally greater than 1 cm), some irregularity in the shape and borders (both asymmetrical) and coloration (more often pigmentary variation), than the amelanotic and/or erythematous appearance of the SN.[107]

Though there is no standardization of the histopathologic criteria for the diagnosis of SM, nonetheless, some basic features of a non-SM are applicable such as deep, often clustered mitotic figures or dispersed, atypical mitotic figures asymmetrical, infiltrative growth, nuclear pleomorphism at all levels in the dermis, and failure of maturation

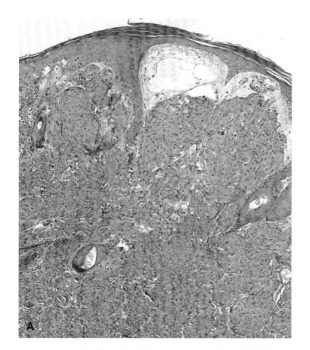

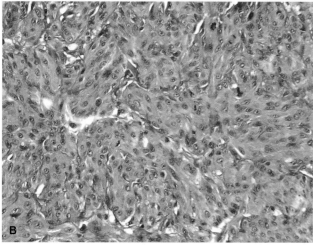

FIGURE 22-18. Atypical Spitz tumor presented on the cheek of a 3-year-old male. A, A nested pattern is present superficially but is less apparent with depth. B, There is no convincing maturation with depth and this microscopic field contains five mitotic figures, but none are overtly atypical. Following a reexcision, the patient has done well almost 3 years postexcision.

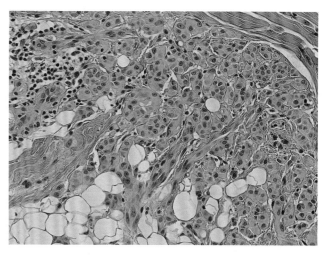

FIGURE 22-19. Atypical Spitz tumor. Nests of epithelioid nevus cells extending into superficial subcutis. Note that these cells retain their nucleoli without features of maturation with depth, but neither pleomorphism nor mitotic figures were apparent at this level.

Considerable attention has been directed to the genomic aberrations within the morphologic spectrum of Spitz lesions; these melanocytic lesions are in many respects unique when compared to the common AMN, CMN, and nonspitzoid cutaneous melanomas (Table 22-4).[108-110] Most AMNs have a *BRAF* mutation (80%), whereas 50% to 60% of cutaneous, non-SMs have a *BRAF* mutation. *HRAS* mutations are present in 6% to 20% of SN and ASNT. Translocation and kinase fusions are detected in *ROS1, ALK, NTRK1, RET,* and *MET* in approximately 50% of all Spitz lesions, whereas they are not found in the common AMN (Figure 22-21A-C; Table 22-4). Deficiency in BAP-1 characterizes a subset of epithelioid SNs that occur as sporadic solitary lesions or multiple nodules in the BAP-1 deficiency syndrome.[108,111]

Copy number aberrations by comparative genomic hybridization are more limited among the Spitz lesions than in non-Spitz melanomas.[112] In the SN, gain in 11p (+11p) is present in 20% of cases and less frequently in 2q (+2q). Gains in 6p (+6p) and 11q (+11q) and losses in 9p (−9p) and 6q (−6q) are detected in ASNT and a similar profile is identified in SM.[22,110,112]

Immunohistochemistry can be helpful in the differential diagnosis with the three stain panel of p16, Ki-67, and HMB-45; loss of p16 (cell cycle regulating protein as a product of CDKN2A loss in melanoma), Ki-67 nuclear expression in deep nevus cells, and loss of HMB-45 gradient are the findings in the ASNT and SM.[109,113,114]

Management and follow-up recommendations of Spitz lesions in children have been discussed from various perspectives.[115,116] If a Spitz lesion is suspected, an excisional biopsy is generally recommended, and though the SN is regarded as a benign lesion, complete excision is widely practiced.[115] Wide local excision with careful examination of the margins is the recommendation for the ASNT and

or zonation as a corollary to the diffuse, nuclear pleomorphism. Infiltration into the subcutis is a more frequent feature of SM in contrast to its less frequent presence in the classic SN and to a more limited degree in the ASNT (Figure 22-19). At the level of the epidermodermal interface, Barnhill[72] has enumerated some features present more often in SM than SN: (1) disordered junctional nesting pattern; (2) absence of intercellular clefting; (3) more frequent pagetoid pattern; (4) less prominent or absent epidermal hyperplasia; and (5) absence of defined symmetry (Figure 22-20A-C).

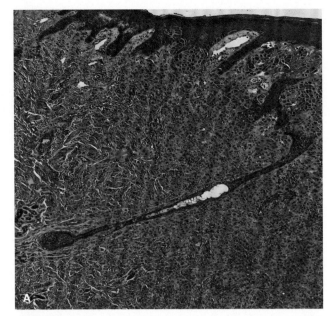
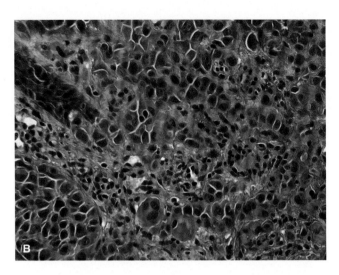
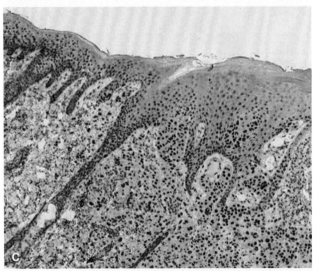

FIGURE 22-20. A, Spitzoid melanoma presented on the cheek of a 1-year-old male. This low-magnification field shows diffuse asymmetrical infiltration of the dermis. B, Highly pleomorphic epithelioid cells show the clefting intercellular spaces of a Spitz nevus, but atypical mitotic figures were present throughout all dermal levels. C, Ki-67 immunostain demonstrates diffuse nuclear reactivity throughout all levels of the dermis.

TABLE 22-4.	Genetic landscape of melanocytic lesions in children				
Gene	Congenital Melanocytic Nevus (%)	Common Acquired Nevus (%)	Spitz Nevus (%)	Atypical Spitz Tumor (%)	Spitz-Like (Spitzoid) Melanoma (%)
BRAF	5-15	~80	5-6	5-6	10 (50-60)[a]
NRAS	70-90	2-3	2-3	2-3	Rare
HRAS	N/A	N/A	10-20	15-16	Rare
ROS, ALK, NTRK1, RET, ROS1, MET	N/A	N/A	50-55	55-60	35-40

[a]Compiled from the following references: Roh MR, Eliades P, Gupta S, Tsao H. Genetics of melanocytic nevi. *Pigment Cell Melanoma Res.* 2015;28(6):661-672; Tschandl P, Berghoff AS, Preusser M, et al. NRAS and BRAF mutations in melanoma-associated nevi and uninvolved nevi. *PLoS One.* 2013;8:e369639; Wiesner T, Kutzner H, Cerroni L, Mihm MC Jr, Busam KJ, Murali R. Genomic aberrations in spitzoid melanocytic tumours and their implications for diagnosis, prognosis and therapy. *Pathology.* 2016;48(2):113-131; van Engen-van Grunsven AC, Kusters-Vandevelde H, Groenen PJ, Blokx WA. Update on molecular pathology of cutaneous melanocytic lesions: what is new in diagnosis and molecular testing for treatment? *Front Med (Lausanne).* 2014;1:39; Blokx WA, van Dijk MC, Ruiter DJ. Molecular cytogenetics of cutaneous melanocytic lesions: diagnostic, prognostic and therapeutic aspects. *Histopathology.* 2010;56(1):121-132; Ross AL, Sanchez MI, Grichnik JM. Molecular nevogenesis. *Dermatol Res Pract.* 2011;2011:463184; Yang C, Gru A, Dehner LP. Common and not so common melanocytic lesions in children and adolescents. *Pediatr Dev Pathol.* 2018;21(2):252-270.

SM.[116] The role of sentinel lymph node biopsy (SLNB) and its application have been thoroughly reviewed elsewhere.[117] A positive SLNB does not necessarily correlate with an unfavorable outcome in the case of ASNTs or SMs.

CAPSULE SUMMARY

ATYPICAL SPITZ TUMORS AND SPITZOID MELANOMAS

These lesions have the general clinicopathologic image of SNs, but with the following differentiating features: size greater than 1 cm, solid rather than nested cellular growth extending to the deep reticular dermis and even the subcutis, asymmetrical growth in the dermis, and cytologic atypia in the form of enlarged nuclei, nuclear pleomorphism, and dense irregular chromatin throughout all levels. When present, mitotic figures should be counted. Definitive histologic criteria for separation of atypical Spitz tumor and SM are still unsettled, but deep mitotic activity with >6 per mm² favors melanoma, as does loss of immunohistochemical labeling for p16.

Pigmented Spindle Cell Nevus of Reed

Pigmented spindle cell nevus of Reed (PSCNR) accounted for 2% of Spitz and other spindle cell melanocytic lesions in our survey of cases that were diagnosed in individuals less than 20 years old (Table 22-3). There is general agreement that PSCNR is a distinctive lesion, but is still considered in the "large spectrum of spindle-epithelioid nevi."[118,119] Some regard PSCNR as an unequivocal variant of the SN.[120] Approximately 30% of cases present in the first two decades of life as an intensely dark brown to black dome-shaped lesion with a predilection for the lower extremity and trunk (Figure 22-22). The deeply pigmented uniform spindle nevus cells have either a parallel or perpendicular orientation to the epidermis with a variable degree of epidermal hyperplasia. The proliferation is either confined to the epidermis or extends as a front of spindle cells into the papillary dermis; it is difficult in some cases to determine whether the lesion has a pure junctional or compound pattern without immunohistochemical staining (Figure 22-23A and B). Epithelioid nevus cells are usually not seen in the typical PSCNR.[119] Symmetrical growth and uniformity of nests are features that differentiate the PSCNR from a spindle cell melanoma, which is rarely encountered in children.[121] It has been observed that S100A6 protein is underexpressed in PSCNR in contrast to the SN.[122]

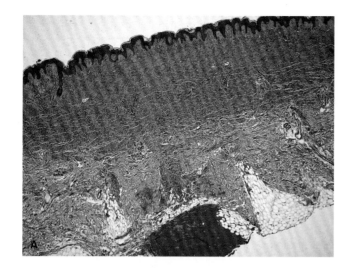
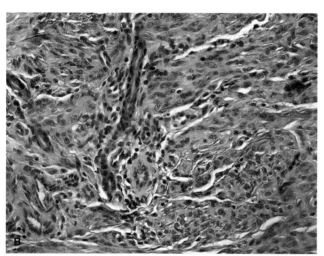
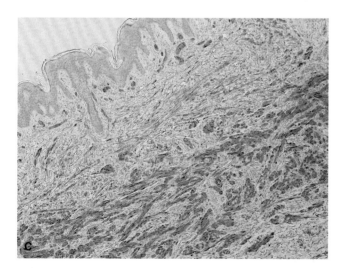

FIGURE 22-21. A, Spitz nevus from the neck of a 7-year-old female, with a spindle, fusiform pattern. B, The spindle nevus cells form into vaguely arranged fascicles. C, ALK membranocytoplasmic immunostaining of this lesion.

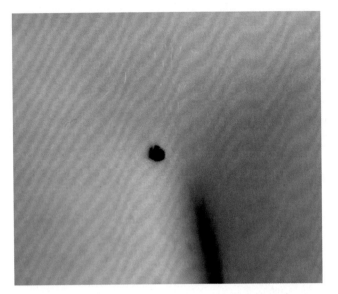

FIGURE 22-22. **Pigmented spindle cell nevus of Reed presenting as a dark brown-black papule on buttocks.**

CAPSULE SUMMARY

PIGMENTED SPINDLE CELL NEVUS OF REED

Generally this is considered to be a special variant of SN with marked cellular pigmentation. These lesions are confined to the epidermis or the papillary dermis. Constituent spindle cells may be aligned in parallel with or vertical to the epidermal surface. Lesions are histologically symmetric and cytologically uniform.

Deep Penetrating Nevus

DPN, like the PSCNR, is typically a heavily pigmented papule or nodule that is centered in the dermis and is a wedge-shaped, well-circumscribed focus of spindle and epithelioid nevus cells (Figure 22-24A-D).[123] Approximately 40% of cases are diagnosed in the first two decades of life, with a slight female predilection and a preference for the head and neck and trunk (60% of cases).[124] A junctional and papillary-upper dermal nevoid component has been noted in 50% or more of cases with the qualifying features of a combined nevus.[125] Extension of the DPN along neurovascular bundles and adnexal structures may result in the presence of nodules of pigmented nevus cells with or without epithelioid features in the subcutis. The latter pattern may convey the impression of a plexiform growth pattern, and a distinction from plexiform spindle cell nevus (PXSCN) and cellular epithelioid BN (EBN) is somewhat arbitrary.[125,126] However, the PXSCN has a more diffuse or dispersed pattern of dermal involvement consisting of small nodules and bundles of spindle cells radiating through the dermis in

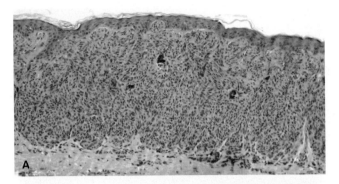

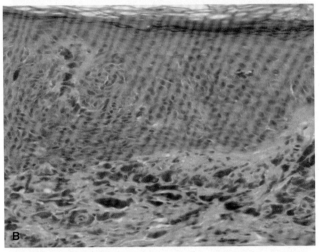

FIGURE 22-23. **Pigmented spindle cell nevus of Reed.** A, A lesion from the chest of a 9-year-old male shows a compound melanocytic pattern of compact, uniform spindle cells with scattered deeply pigmented melanocytes. B, A deeply pigmented lesion from the flank of a 10-year-old male demonstrates a predominantly junctional spindle cell proliferation with densely pigmented cells concentrated beneath the spindle nevus cells.

contrast to the wedge-shaped growth of the DPN. Mitotic activity and nuclear pleomorphism are atypical features of PXSCN.[126] Together with the atypical DPN, the latter lesion and ASNT are examples of dermal-based borderline melanocytic tumors.[127]

CAPSULE SUMMARY

DEEP PENETRATING NEVUS

This lesion is a deeply pigmented nodule, often on the head and neck or the trunk. Subcutaneous extension may be present in some cases. Histologic features include epithelioid and fusiform cells with obvious cytoplasmic pigmentation that are wedge-shaped, with the superficial aspect of the lesion being broadest. Microscopic similarity to plexiform nevus and cellular EBN may be evident. Mitotic activity and nuclear pleomorphism are typically absent.

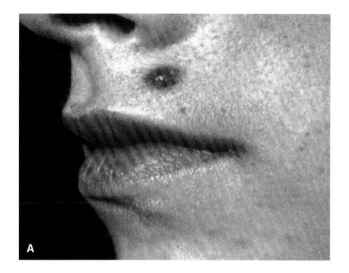

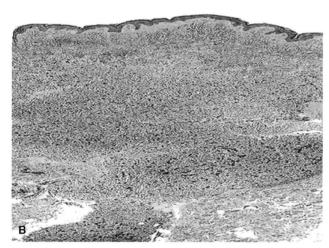

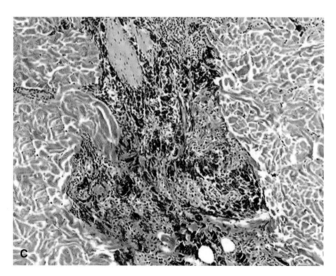

FIGURE 22-24. **Deep penetrating nevus.** A, A firm, deeply pigmented papule shows some variation in the shades of coloration. B, A broad base of nevus cells abuts the epidermis and becomes more restricted toward the deep apex. C, Pigmentation intensifies toward the apex as the overall cellularity diminishes.

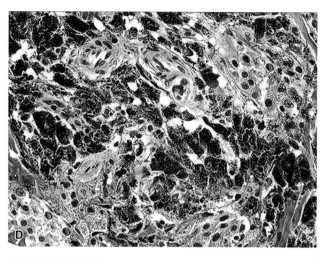

FIGURE 22-24. (*continued*) D, Nevus cells at the apex may appear larger than the more superficial nevus cells. Nodules may protrude into the subcutis as in the case of the cellular blue nevus.

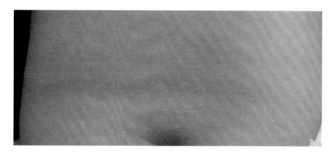

FIGURE 22-25. **Mongolian spots as a faint blue-gray ill-defined patches on the buttocks and lower back.**

DERMAL-BASED MELANOCYTIC LESIONS

Dermal Melanocytosis

DM in children is represented by three congenital pigmentary disorders: the so-called Mongolian spot(s), nevus of Ota, and nevus of Ito.[128] A prospective study of skin findings or birthmarks in neonates in one community in southern California revealed DM on average in 20% of infants with ethnic variations.[129] By contrast, only 2.4% of infants in the same study had CMNs. The buttock and sacrum (Mongolian spot) were the most common sites of congenital Mongolian spots that during later childhood gradually disappear in terms of clinical pigmentation, but remain microscopically as dermal, nonpigmented dendritic melanocytes (Figure 22-25). Mongolian spots may be encountered in the presence of a vascular anomaly (phacomatosis pigmentovascularis) as well as in several heritable metabolic disorders including gangliosidosis 1 and Hurler disease, which are just two examples.[130,131] Mongolian spots are found on other body surfaces. Nevus of Ota has a unilateral distribution along the first and second branches of the trigeminal nerve, whereas the nevus of Ito presents as a unilateral pigmentation in the distribution of the posterior supraclavicular and lateral brachial nerves[128,132] (Figure 22-26A and B). Both of the latter nevi are present at birth in 60% of cases and tend to persist clinically unlike most Mongolian spots.

It is generally uncommon in our experience to encounter DM in a biopsy, but the histologic features are those of dendritic melanocytes at various levels of the reticular dermis.[133] Dendritic melanocytes as individual spindle cells are present within the lower reticular dermis and without the sclerotic reaction of the Mongolian spots. The upper and lower reticular dermis and upper reticular dermis are the preferred locations for dendritic melanocytes in nevus of Ota and Ito, respectively. Sclerosis may accompany the dendritic melanocytes in the latter two nevi. Unlike the BN, DM does not form a localized, sclerotic aggregate of dendritic melanocytes.

CAPSULE SUMMARY

DERMAL MELANOCYTOSIS

These are macular lesions that are represented by so-called Mongolian spot, nevus of Ota, and nevus of Ito. They appear in variable anatomic locations and are potentially associated with vascular anomalies and metabolic storage disorders. Uncommonly biopsied, they demonstrate cytologically bland and pigmented dendritic melanocytes throughout the reticular dermis with variable associated sclerosis.

Blue Nevus

BN represented 2% of all cutaneous melanocytic lesions in our review of cases from our files (Table 22-1). The common BN may be recognized at or soon after birth with a predilection for acral sites, lower extremity, and scalp.[134,135] An intensely pigmented macule or papule measuring 5 mm or less is the typical clinical appearance (Figure 22-27). Multiple lesions may be a sign of Carney complex (CNC).

Histologically, a symmetrical focus of pigmented fusiform nevus cells with a variably prominent sclerotic stroma is usually found in the mid-to-deep reticular dermis or even the subcutis. However, the BN is found as well in the superficial dermis (Figure 22-28A-C).

The challenge in the diagnosis of the BN category of lesions occurs in those cellular lesions composed of spindled or epithelioid cells whose differential diagnoses include cellular BN, DPN, EBN–melanocytoma, and combined nevus with common acquired or Spitz-like features.[136] Some have included the DPN as a type of BN, but DPN does not have mutations in either *GNAQ* or *GNAII* as in the case of the BN.[137] Cellular BN (CBN) is more consistently a nodular lesion than is the BN (Figure 22-29A-D). The initial clinical presentation may be as early as in the neonatal period,

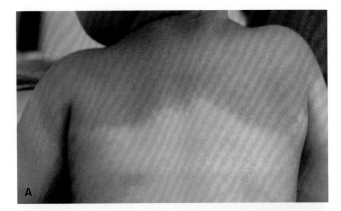

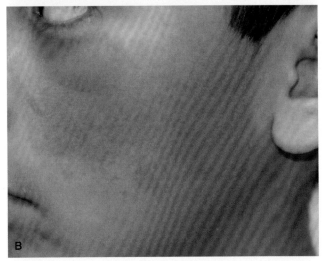

FIGURE 22-26. A, Nevus of Ito showing blue-gray pigmentation on scapular area and shoulder. B, Nevus of Ota presenting as a brown patch with irregular borders on maxillary area.

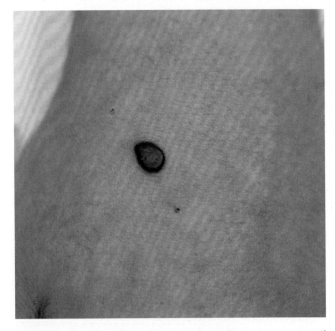

FIGURE 22-27. Blue nevus presenting as a smooth blue-black papule on the dorsum of the hand.

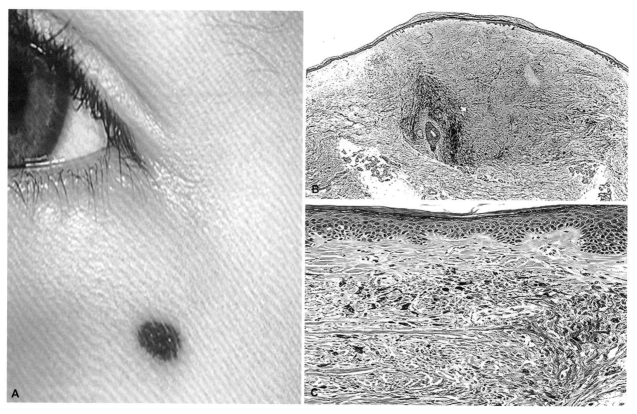

FIGURE 22-28. A, Blue nevus on the face of this young patient shows the dark bluish coloration with a slight erythematous halo. B, Low magnification demonstrates the dense sclerosis. C, Dendritic melanocytes as scattered heavily pigmented cells in the background. Note the sclerosis that is not seen in dermal melanocytosis.

but most lesions are encountered in older children and adolescents. The gluteal-sacral region and the scalp are the favored sites for a bluish-black nodule generally measuring 2 cm or less in diameter, but the cellular BN has the potential for larger growth and is seen in a wide range of sites.[134] At low magnification the lesion is well-circumscribed with smooth peripheral contours (Figure 22-29B). The degree of cellularity of the spindled to more epithelioid cells is generally more apparent in the deep reticular dermis and subcutis in a bulging nodule. The cellular foci are finely pigmented or have clear cytoplasm (Figure 22-29C and D). More superficially, delicate dendritic melanocytes and a sclerotic stroma often dominate where the lesion is considerably less cellular and has a BN-like appearance (Figure 22-30A and B). Any degree of nuclear enlargement, pleomorphism, and mitotic activity should alert to the possibility of a so-called atypical or malignant cellular BN or cellular BN-like melanoma.[138] Amelanotic cellular BN may display nuclear atypia as well as the challenge to arrive at the appropriate interpretation.[139]

Epithelioid Blue Nevus and Pigmented Epithelioid Melanocytoma

EBN and *pigmented epithelioid melanocytoma* (PEM) are seemingly related melanocytic lesions, both of which are manifestations of the CNC or present as a nonsyndromic sporadic lesion. Multifocal BN and/or EBN is seen in approximately 40% of cases of CNC, an autosomal dominant disorder with inactivating mutations or deletion in *PRKAR1A* gene (17q 22-24).[140] Large epithelioid nevus cells characterize the EBN and PEM, but dense coarse pigmentation of the polygonal nevus cells to the point of obscuring cellular detail is typical of PEM (Figure 22-31A-D). EBN lacks the intense pigmentation of PEM, but otherwise shares many features with the latter as well as the DPN and SN.[141] The presence of a BN pattern is found in some EBNs, which facilitates the proper interpretation. Both EBN and PEM tend to have a more diffuse growth pattern than the circumscribed CBN. The EBN and PEM are low-grade nevocellular tumors with a favorable prognosis in most cases even in the presence of a positive sentinel lymph node.[142,143]

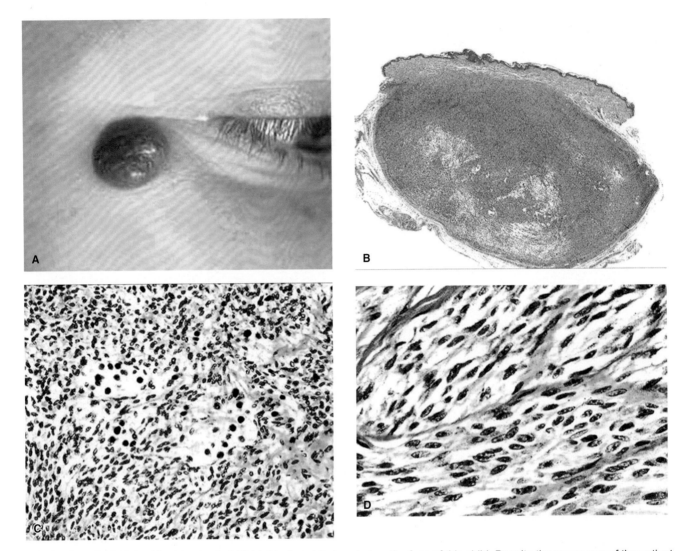

FIGURE 22-29. Cellular blue nevus. A, A bluish-black nodule is noted on the face of this child. Despite the young age of the patient, this pigmented lesion has a resemblance to a nodular melanoma. B, The characteristic, well-circumscribed nodule fills the dermis and bulges into the subcutis. C, A uniform spindle cell proliferation and interspersed more epithelioid cells are noted. D, Note the nested and fasciculated pattern that has a resemblance to cellular neurothekeoma and clear cell sarcoma of tendon sheath. There is minimal pigmentation of these cells.

CAPSULE SUMMARY

BLUE NEVI AND PIGMENTED EPITHELIOID MELANOCYTOMA

Ordinary BNs have a predilection for acral sites and the scalp, represented by darkly pigmented macules or papules that are usually <5 mm in size. Multiple BN may be seen in the CNC. Histologically, BN are symmetrical aggregates of pigmented spindle cells in the dermis. Cellular BN are histologic special variants, showing much greater cell density, a "dumbbell"-shaped configuration, and common growth into the subcutis. Central myxoid degenerative change is common. Uncommonly, obvious melanoma may emerge from cellular BN by clonal evolution. EBN are likely related to PEM and have a good prognosis even when regional lymph nodes contain tumor.

Neurocristic Hamartoma

Neurocristic hamartoma (NCH) is a rare, somewhat perplexing neuroectodermal tumor centered in the dermis, which is reported in children and adults alike with a predilection for the head and neck region.[144,145] These tumors may be locally aggressive with bone invasion and distant metastasis in rare cases.[146,147] Pigmented dendritic melanocytes like the BN or CBN, Schwann cells, and neuroid and plexiform bundles are the composite histologic features (Figure 22-32A-D). There is infiltration around adnexal structures, small nerves, and blood vessels like the CMN.[147] It is not surprising that the NCH may give rise to ambiguous, often descriptive interpretations.[148] These tumors are seemingly unique in that they do not have some of the more common mutations associated with the other nevocellular lesions.[147] In addition to being diffusely positive for S100, SOX-10 and HMB-45, they are also positive for CD34.

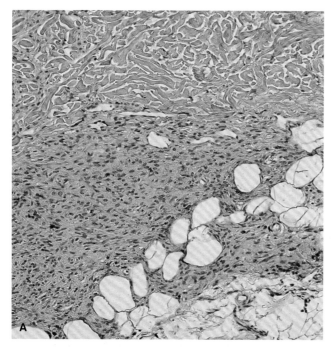

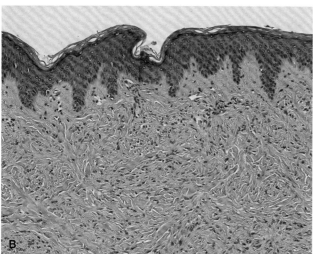

FIGURE 22-30. **Cellular blue nevus from the gluteal region of a 17-year-old female showing two additional features.** A, A spindle cell focus is pushing from the reticular dermis into the subcutis. When heavily pigmented, a wedge-shaped focus resembles the deep penetrating nevus. B, Some cellular blue nevi have dense sclerosis, either superficially with a resemblance to a desmoplastic blue nevus or a sclerotic dermatofibroma.

CONGENITAL MELANOCYTIC NEVUS

Epidemiology and Etiology

Incidence studies on cutaneous lesions in neonates have been conducted in countries across the globe with some ethnocultural variations especially in the prevalence of DM (Mongolian spot).[129,149-152] In terms of the CMN, 1% to 3% of neonates in all ethnic groups have a solitary lesion measuring 7 mm or less in most cases.[129] It has been

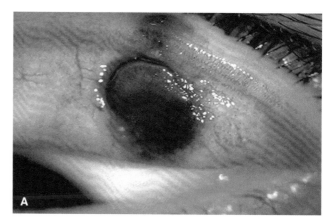

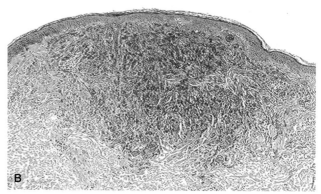

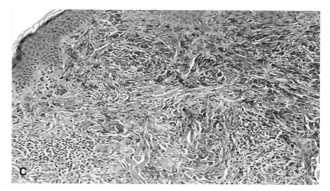

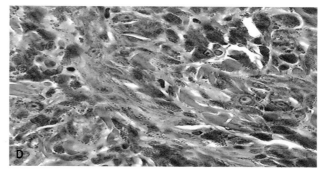

FIGURE 22-31. **Pigmented epithelioid melanocytoma.** A, A well-circumscribed, intensely pigmented nodule arising from the conjunctival mucous membrane. Note the pigmentation in the immediately surrounding mucosa, mainly on the basis of pigmentary incontinence. B, At low magnification, the circumscription is less apparent than in the cellular blue nevus. C, The densely pigmented epithelioid nevus cells are accompanied by spindle cells. D, Both epithelioid and spindle nevus cells are heavily pigmented.

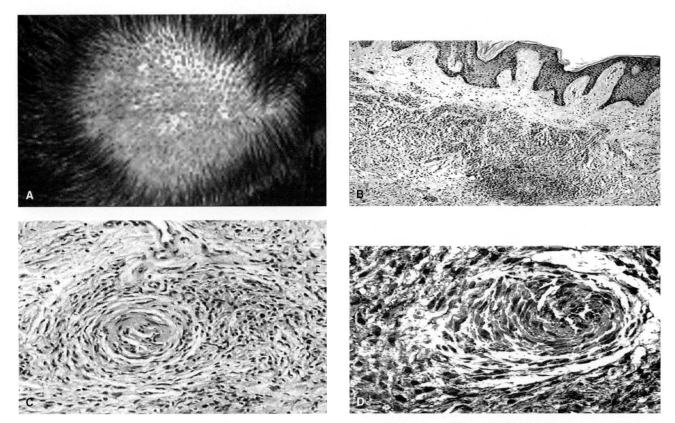

FIGURE 22-32. **Neurocristic hamartoma in an adolescent patient.** A, A faintly pigmented, indurated plaque is noted on the shaved scalp. B, The dermis contains a variable dense population of dendritic nevus cells. C, Concentric arrayed spindle cells surround a small cutaneous peripheral nerve. D, S-100 protein shows strong positivity as the peripheral spindle cells blend into a small nerve.

suggested that the incidence may be higher because some small CMNs may not come to clinical attention until later in childhood.[153] Those CMNs identified later in childhood have been termed "tardive" CMNs.[48]

Just as DM is regarded as a migratory defect of NC-derived melanocytes, so likewise is the pathogenesis of the CMN with specific mutations, which correlate with size classification. For instance, the small CMNs (<1.5 cm) have *BRAF* and *NRAS* mutations, whereas the medium (1.5–19.9 cm), large (>20 cm), and giant (>40 cm) nevi have an increased prevalence of *NRAS* mutations.[154-158] The size of a CMN is projected on the anticipated ultimate dimensions in an adult. Large and giant CMNs are seen far less commonly than smaller lesions, with a frequency variably reported as 1:20 000 to 50 000 newborns.[159,160]

Clinical and Pathologic Features

At birth, CMNs typically present as sharply demarcated macules or patches of different shapes ranging from round and oval to geographic with irregular borders. The color also varies from light tan-brown resembling a café au lait

spot to brown or black. When present on the scalp, CMNs may already have dark terminal hair with increased density and length.

Alterations occur in CMNs with age, including an increase in size relative to the patient's growth, color variegation from darkening or lightening, surface texture changes, and increased terminal hair growth (Figure 22-33). A globular pattern on dermoscopy is common in CMNs located on the head, neck, and trunk, whereas a reticular pattern predominates in those on the lower extremities. Other common dermoscopic findings in CMNs include milia-like cysts, perifollicular pigmentary changes, hypertrichosis, and vascular structures.[25]

Larger CMNs may develop nodularity, eczematous changes, and erosions or ulcerations; these findings may be evident early and eventually resolve spontaneously (Figure 22-34). Persistence of these findings should raise concern about an underlying malignant transformation.

Satellite nevi refer to the presence of multiple, smaller melanocytic nevi, typically in association with a large or giant CMN (Figure 22-34). The number of satellite nevi is variable, and these may be distributed in close proximity or distant from the larger CMN. Multiple small- and

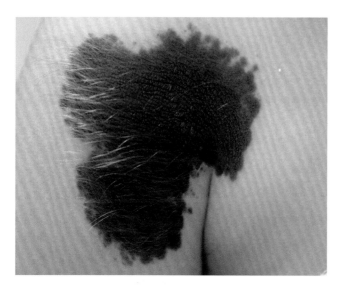

FIGURE 22-33. Congenital melanocytic nevus with hypertrichosis and increased rugosity.

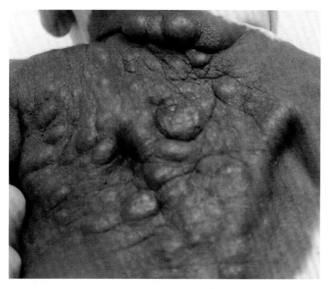

FIGURE 22-34. Congenital melanocytic nevus with multiple proliferative nodules.

medium-sized CMNs in the absence of a large or giant lesion are seen less commonly.

As with other melanocytic lesions, melanoma may develop in association with a CMN whose risk is directly associated with the size of the nevus. Small and medium CMN have an estimated incidence of melanoma of <1%.[160] On the other hand, the approximate lifetime risk of melanoma is 2% to 5% in larger CMNs, with other estimates indicating a risk of 10% to 15% in those CMNs greater than 40 cm (projected adult size).[161-163] Truncal lesions may be at a higher risk for melanomas.[164] Melanoma in CMN commonly presents as a new nodule or lump, typically arising in the dermis or subcutaneous tissues.[163] The deep origin of

some melanomas makes dermoscopy less useful in this setting. It is important for the clinician and pathologist to be aware of the proliferative nodule(s) that are entirely benign despite the worrisome clinical appearance of one or more nodules arising in any sized CMN.[165,166]

Neurocutaneous melanosis (NCM) occurs in the setting of a large or giant CMN in approximately 10% or more of cases; NCM is characterized by the presence of melanocytic lesions in the leptomeninges and brain parenchyma.[167-169] Satellite nevi and a giant CMN with a posterior axial distribution are one of the 6B patterns in association with NCM.[164,168,170] These children in general have a poor outcome with the development of melanoma of the central nervous system.

Histologic Findings and Differential Diagnosis

The specific histopathologic features to differentiate a CMN from an AMN would appear to be straightforward but some have argued that point.[171] In general, a skin biopsy that only includes papillary and the upper reticular dermis may provide few clues to the specific diagnosis of a CMN; one possible clue is the dispersion of a nested dermal pattern of nevus cells into a single pattern of nevus cells around the hair follicle(s), but this pattern is seen in the so-called CMN-like nevus, which is probably an AMN.[172] It is below the level of the hair follicles that a particular nevus demonstrates the generally acknowledged congenital features, with infiltration of the deep reticular dermis by small, individual nevus cells that can be difficult to differentiate at times from small lymphocytes without some accompanying small nests of nevus cells. Lymphovascular and perineural spaces, eccrine sweat glands, and arrector pili muscle may be involved in addition to the adipose tissue and septa of the subcutis (Figure 22-35A-C). Migration through the lymphovascular spaces accounts for the presence of nevus cells with a metastatic pattern in regional lymph nodes.

The junctional pattern of a CMN may display architecturally disordered or dysplastic features with or without substantial cytologic atypia. Pagetoid spread through the epidermis may be seen. In one series, 40% of CMNs were combined nevi with patterns of BN, SN, and DPNs.[173]

Proliferating nodule(s) (PN) is present in a variable proportion of CMNs, but more commonly in large or giant CMNs in 3% to 20% of cases.[174] This highly cellular nodule(s) is notably distinct from the surrounding CMN as an expansile focus (Figure 22-36A-C). The population of monotonous cells may be nevoid as small cells, spindled or epithelioid in appearance (Figure 22-37). Mitotic activity is inapparent in most, but not all cases, in which the distinction from a dermal melanoma can be challenging; the melanoma has a more infiltrative, overgrowth pattern than the PN.[166,175] Both immunohistochemistry (three stain panel—HMB-45, p16, and Ki-67) and genomic studies may be required in the problematic case in addition to consultation.[166,176,177]

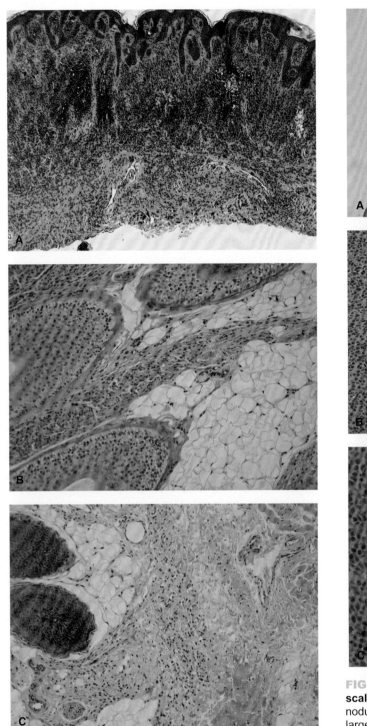

FIGURE 22-35. Congenital melanocytic nevus. A, Large congenital lesion from the trunk of this child showing the full thickness, dense pattern of nevus cells without apparent nest formation. B, Extension of individual nevus cells into connective tissue septum as individual lymphocytic-like nevus cells. C, Nevus cells infiltrating into connective tissues in this congenital nevus in the scalp.

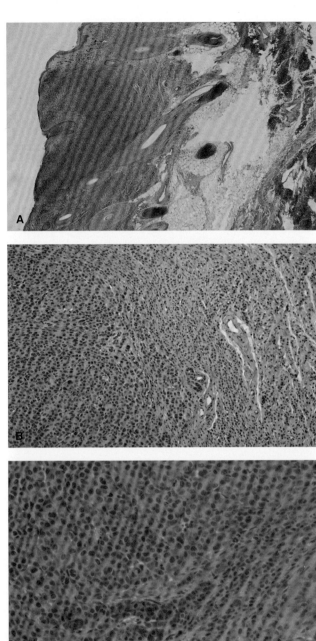

FIGURE 22-36. Congenital melanocytic nevus from the scalp of a 3-month-old female. A, A circumscribed proliferative nodule is distinct in the background of small nevus cells. B, The large atypical nevus cells of this proliferative nodule demonstrate an abrupt interface from the small nevus cells. C, Larger atypical polygonal cells and the surrounding large cells are not accompanied by mitotic figures.

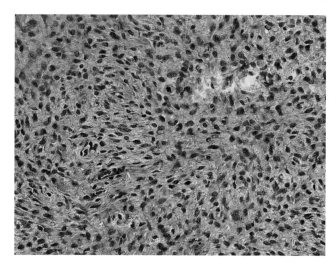

FIGURE 22-37. **Congenital melanocytic nevus with prolifer-ating nodule.** This nodule is composed of ovoid to spindle-shaped cells. An isolated mitotic figure is present.

CAPSULE SUMMARY

CONGENITAL MELANOCYTIC NEVI

These lesions are seen in 1% to 3% of all newborn children as solitary lesions that are usually 7 mm or less in diameter. However, occasional examples are several cm in greatest dimension and may be associated with localized hypertrichosis. Benign proliferative nodules may be seen clinically and histologically in large CMN. The risk for development of secondary melanoma is related to their sizes; surgical resection is usually attempted only for "giant" lesions that occupy greater than 2% of the overall body surface area. Approximately 10% of large CMN are associated with leptomeningeal or cerebral melanosis. Microscopic features include large melanocytic nests at the dermoepidermal junction; growth of nevus cells within dermal appendages and the perineurium; and "tracking" of nevus cells along neurovascular plexuses or along adnexal structures.

MALIGNANT MELANOMA

Epidemiology and Etiology

The topic of malignant melanoma (MM) in children has been discussed previously in the context of the SN spectrum. Though MM is a rare malignancy in the first two decades of life, it is the most common primary cutaneous malignancy of childhood and adolescence.[178] Various epidemiologic studies of MM in the pediatric population have reported some discordant results of rising, stable, or decreasing trends in incidence in the United States.[179-181]

Where efforts have been made to discourage UVR exposure in young individuals as in Australia, the incidence of MM has been on the decline.[182] The lowest incidence of MM is in the first 4 years of life and the highest between the ages of 15 and 19 years.[183,184]

Superficial spreading MM represents the largest category of all melanomas in the first two decades of life where they are diagnosed in older children and adolescents in contrast to those cases occurring in the previously discussed special clinical categories. Beyond the age of 15 years, there is a particularly steep rise in the incidence among females.[179,180,183] With increasing age from 15 years into the fourth decade of life, the incidence of MM increases by a factor of 9 to 10.[185] Truncal superficial spreading MM is the most common anatomic site and pathologic subtype in those tumors occurring in the second decade of life.[183] Almost 60% of MMs are less than 1 mm in thickness in older children and adolescents, whereas children less than 10 years have more advanced local disease in nontruncal sites.[183]

Risk factors in the occurrence of melanomas are similar to those in adults including family history of melanoma, number of melanocytic nevi, and history of intermittent and intense UVR exposure. There is a select group of conditions in the pediatric population that predispose this age group to melanoma; these conditions include: (1) large or giant CMNs, (2) genetic photosensitivity disorders (eg, xeroderma pigmentosum), and (3) immunosuppression (genetic and acquired).

Clinical Presentation and Pathogenesis

Melanomas in pediatric patients have distinct characteristics, particularly in the preadolescent population. In contrast, melanomas in adolescents tend to share the clinical characteristics of those melanomas in adults. Preadolescent melanomas are more likely to be amelanotic, have uniform color, regular borders, a size of 6 mm or less, and present as a papule or nodule (Figure 22-38).[186,187] This is in direct contrast to melanomas in adolescents and adult patients, which are more likely to present as a pigmented lesion with color variegation, irregular borders, and a diameter of 6 mm or larger.

As noted, MM has several unique clinical and pathologic settings in children in addition to MM arising in a giant CMN with or without NCM. Congenital/neonatal MM is defined as the vertical, transplacental spread to an infant from maternal MM or the equally rare "de novo" congenital melanoma. In fact, MM is the most common maternal malignancy to metastasize to the placenta (Figure 22-39) and infant where the infant skin is the common site of involvement.[188-190] De novo congenital melanoma is far less common than the maternal to fetal metastatic melanoma.[191-193] There is a seeming predilection for the head and neck and in particular the scalp in the case of de novo

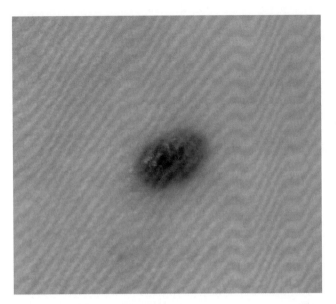

FIGURE 22-38. Amelanotic melanoma as a symmetric, smooth pink papule with regular borders.

MM. Most of these tumors have a nodular pattern with its anticipated poor prognosis.[194]

CMNs giving rise to MM are large or giant lesions in most cases on the trunk, especially posterior, and are accompanied by satellite melanocytic nevi.[195] With the recognition of the nonmalignant PN(s), the risk of MM has fallen to 5% or less at 2% to 3% compared to the pre-PN estimates of 20% to 40%.[196,197] The age at diagnosis of a MM in a CMN is reportedly later in childhood, 10 to 12 years, and from a truncal lesion.[195] In another study, the greatest period of incidence for MM was the first 3 years of life and 70% of tumors were diagnosed by puberty.[196] In addition to skin (60%–70%), MM also arise in visceral sites including the brain in NCM, deep soft tissues, or unknown primary site in approximately 10% of cases.[162] Unlike the conventional cutaneous MM, melanomas in CMN arise within the depths of the nevus and are "thick" (Figures 22-40 to 22-42); the prognosis is invariably poor in these children. Applying standard Breslow thickness is difficult in some cases, but generally the depth of the tumor can be determined. In one study in adults with MM arising in a giant CMN, the tumors were thicker when compared with superficial spreading MM and had comparable survivals.[198] SLNBs contain nodal nevi more often in those with CMNs.[199,200]

Familial melanoma predisposition is found in 5% to 10% of MM cases within all age groups.[201,202] The first melanoma susceptibility gene to be identified was *CDKN2A* in 20% to 40% of familial melanomas.[203] In addition to *CDKN2A*, other high-penetrance melanoma predisposition genes include *CDK4, BAP1, POT1, ACD, TERF21P,* and *TERT*; these genes in aggregate account for 50% of all familial melanomas.[202]

CAPSULE SUMMARY

MALIGNANT MELANOMAS IN CHILDREN AND ADOLESCENTS

Although rare lesions overall, they are the most common primary malignant skin tumors in the pediatric population. Predisposing conditions include giant CMNs, xeroderma pigmentosum, and immunodeficiency syndromes. Congenital MM may represent transplacental metastasis from the mother. MM arising in CMN typically develops in the dermis, rather than at the dermoepidermal junction, but other MMs in children are comparable in every histologic respect to those seen in adults. Childhood melanoma may be part of familial melanoma predisposition syndromes, involving hereditary abnormalities of the *CDKN2A, CDK4, BAP1, POT1, ACD, TERF21P,* and *TERT* genes.

PIGMENTARY DISORDERS

There are a number of disorders whose clinical manifestations are cutaneous hyper- or hypopigmentation or a mixed pattern. In adults more often than children, these non-nevoid lesions include seborrheic keratosis, basal cell carcinoma, and solar lentigo, to note some of the more common examples. Many of the hyperpigmentary and hypopigmentary disorders in children have an underlying gene mutation as in the case of multiple café au lait spots in neurofibromatosis type 1 (NF1) or multiple pigmentary spots in CNC as two examples. Attention is directed to the comprehensive review by Yamaguchi and Hearing of hereditary pigmentary disorders.[204] For the purpose of this discussion, café au lait macule (CALM) or spot, acanthosis nigricans (AN), Becker nevus (BEN), and postinflammatory hyperpigmentation (PIH) are considered.

Café Au Lait Macule or Spot

CALM is a uniformly pigmented, well-circumscribed macule or patch that can range in size from 1 to 2 mm to more than 20 cm.[205] It is estimated that 2% to 2.5% neonates and up to 25% of older children have at least one CALM.[206] Six or more CALMs in a child has an 80% probability for NF1.[207,208] Several other disorders are also accompanied by CALMs including NF2, Noonan syndrome, McCune-Albright syndrome, Jaffe-Campanacci syndrome (possibly a variant of NF1), and cardiofaciocutaneous syndrome.[206,209,210] Considerable interest at one time existed in the specificity of giant melanosomes in CALMs in NF1, but several studies have shown that giant melanosomes are not consistently present in NF1 as well as their presence in other melanocytic lesions.[211-215]

Basal hyperpigmentation with or without an increase in melanocytes or giant melanosomes is the rather modest histologic finding. Multiple agminated SNs have been reported in a CALM in a 16-year-old female.[216]

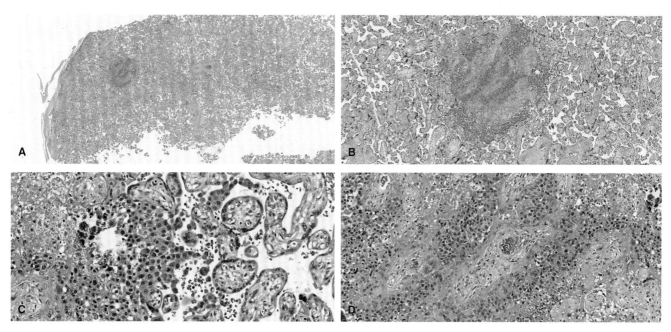

FIGURE 22-39. A small nodule in the placenta is present (A and B). The nodule contains malignant epithelioid cells with vesicular nuclei and prominent nucleoli. Melanin pigment is present (C and D). Digital slide courtesy of Path Presenter.

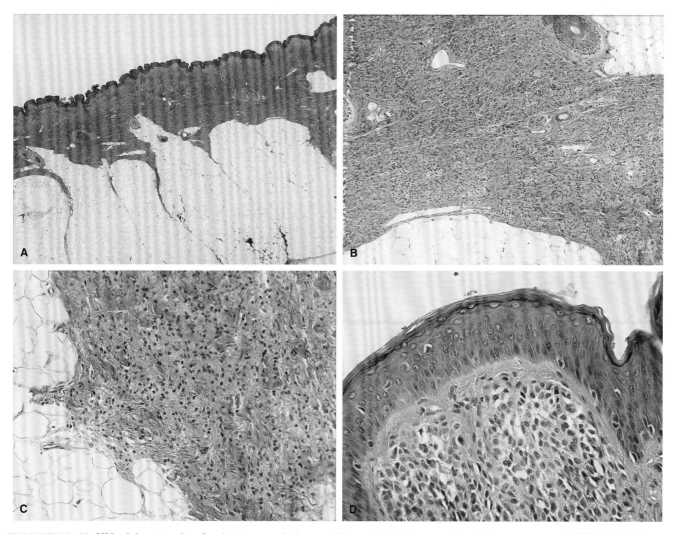

FIGURE 22-40. MM arising at a site of a giant congenital nevus. The patient is 18 years old and the nevus covered 90% of the body surface. The nevus is mostly centered in the dermis (A and B) and has diffuse extension along adnexae and into the adipose tissue (C and D).

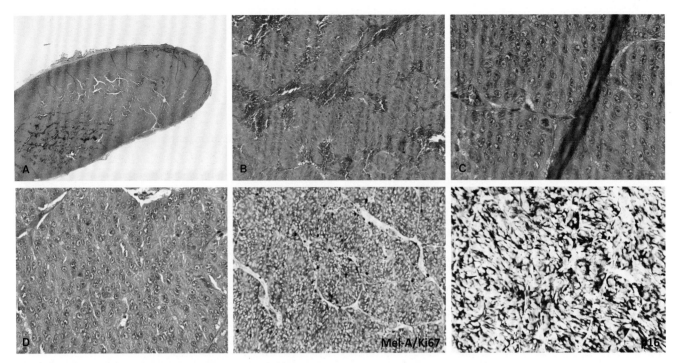

FIGURE 22-41. **The patient developed a nodular lesion in the back that was suspected to be a cyst.** An encapsulated tumor was seen histologically (A). The tumor was composed of highly pleomorphic cells (B). The neoplastic cells show frequent mitotic figures (C and D). A dual Melan-A and Ki67 shows prominent increased proliferation, p16 was mostly retained within the tumor.

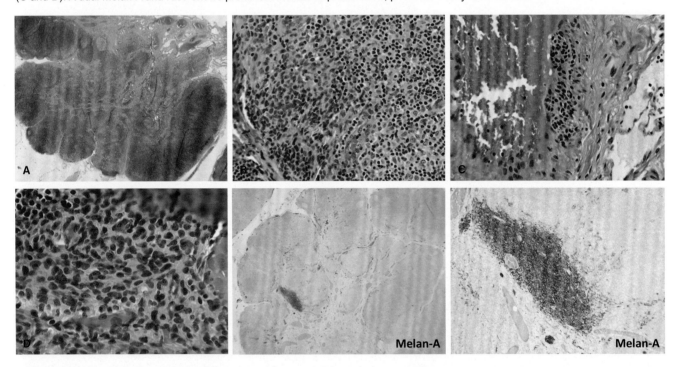

FIGURE 22-42. A sentinel lymph node biopsy was done. The architecture of the lymph node was retained (A). Several small aggregates of melanocytes were present, some with an intraparenchymal distribution (B and D) and some with features of nevus rests around vessels (C). The aggregates are highlighted by a Melan-A immunostain.

Acanthosis Nigricans

AN presents as hyperpigmented, symmetrical, "velvety" brownish lesions in intertriginous sites but not to the exclusion of other locations.[217] The incidence is increased in skin of color individuals including children and adolescents. Older children (10–14 years) with AN are more often obese and have an increased risk for insulin-resistant type 2 diabetes.[218,219]

The rarely performed biopsy shows the presence of epidermal papillomatosis with basal hyperpigmentation on the basis of an increased number of melanocytes. Pseudohorn cysts in AN can convey an impression of a pigmented seborrheic keratosis (uncommon in a child) or epidermal nevus in the absence of clinical correlation.[220,221] Pigmented hyperkeratosis is also seen.

Becker Nevus (Melanosis)

BEN is a pigmented epidermal nevus that may occur sporadically as a solitary lesion or less commonly in a syndromic setting with ipsilateral hypoplasia of the breast and skeletal muscle, lipoatrophy, and various skeletal anomalies.[222-224] It has been variably reported that 5% to 25% of BEN are recognized at birth.[224] There is a male predilection in some, but not all studies.[225]

A large hyperpigmented patch with irregular or geographic borders characterizes BEN. This is typically unilateral, located on the upper trunk (chest, shoulder, upper back) or proximal upper extremity.

A biopsy shows some acanthosis with elongation of rete ridges and hyperpigmentation of the basal layer without an increase in melanocytes. Pigment incontinence may be seen in the papillary dermis. An increase in arrector pili smooth muscle is not present in every case, but in some cases, the smooth muscle is increased to the point of a resemblance to a smooth muscle hamartoma.[225-227]

Postinflammatory Hyperpigmentation

PIH is one category of acquired hyperpigmentation.[228] Pigmentation occurs at the site of an inflammatory process and in children. Atopic dermatitis, acne, impetigo, lichen simplex chronicus, transient neonatal pustulosis, and insect bites are among the more common initiating disorders.[229] The latter group of conditions does not exhaust other causes of PIH.[230] The face and trunk are the sites of predilection. Skin of color children is more likely to develop PIH.[229]

The histopathologic findings include basal cell hyper- or hypopigmentation and melanophages in the superficial papillary dermis, with a variably prominent accompanying lymphocytic infiltrate and, in some cases, a perivascular collection of lymphocytes.[231]

CAPSULE SUMMARY

OTHER PIGMENTARY CUTANEOUS DISORDERS IN CHILDREN

This category of lesions is represented by CALM, AN, BEN, and PIH. CALM are potential markers of neurofibromatosis, Noonan syndrome, McCune-Albright syndrome, Jaffe-Campanacci syndrome, and cardiofaciocutaneous syndrome. They typically show basal epidermal hyperpigmentation with no melanocytic hyperplasia histologically.

AN appears as hyperpigmented, symmetric, velvety brown patches, usually in intertriginous skin areas. Many children with this condition are obese with

diabetes mellitus. Microscopically, AN shows epidermal papillomatosis and basal epidermal hyperpigmentation, with slight melanocytic hyperplasia. Pseudohorn cysts may be present.

BEN are pigmented epidermal nevi that may be sporadic or part of congenital syndromes that also involve malformations of the breasts, skeletal muscle, and bones. They are usually unilateral and located on the trunk or shoulders. Histologically, BEN shows epidermal acanthosis and basal hyperpigmentation. Hyperplasia of underlying arrector pili muscle bundles is often seen as well. PIH is caused by spillage of epidermal melanin into the dermis, with melanophagocytosis. It is principally seen on the face and trunk, as a consequence of previous atopic dermatitis, acne, impetigo, lichen simplex chronicus, transient neonatal pustulosis, or insect bites.

REFERENCES

1. Dehner LP, Gru AA. Nonepithelial tumors and tumor-like lesions of the skin and subcutis in children. *Pediatr Dev Pathol.* 2018;21:1-56.
2. Bronner ME, LeDouarin NM. Development and evolution of the neural crest: an overview. *Dev Biol.* 2012;366(1):2-9.
3. Noisa P, Raivio T. Neural crest cells: from developmental biology to clinical interventions. *Birth Defects Res C Embryo Today.* 2014;102(3):263-274.
4. Holbrook KA, Underwood RA, Vogel AM, Gown AM, Kimball H. The appearance, density and distribution of melanocytes in human embryonic and fetal skin revealed by the anti-melanoma monoclonal antibody, HMB-45. *Anat Embryol (Berl).* 1989;180(5):443-455.
5. Rogers T, Marino ML, Raciti P, et al. Biologically distinct subsets of nevi. *G Ital Dermatol Venereol.* 2016;151(4):365-384.
6. Tokuda Y, Saida T, Murata H, Murase S, Oohara K. Histogenesis of congenital and acquired melanocytic nevi based on histological study of lesion size and thickness. *J Dermatol.* 2010;37(12):1011-1018.
7. Masson P. My conception of cellular nevi. *Cancer.* 1951;4(1):9-38.
8. Cramer SF. The histogenesis of acquired melanocytic nevi. Based on a new concept of melanocytic differentiation. *Am J Dermatopathol.* 1984;6 suppl:289-298.
9. Dupin E. Phenotypic plasticity of neural crest-derived melanocytes and Schwann cells [in French]. *Biol Aujourdhui.* 2011;205(1):53-61.
10. Sidiropoulos M, Obregon R, Cooper C, Sholl LM, Guitart J, Gerami P. Primary dermal melanoma: a unique subtype of melanoma to be distinguished from cutaneous metastatic melanoma: a clinical, histologic, and gene expression-profiling study. *J Am Acad Dermatol.* 2014;71(6):1083-1092.
11. Harrison SL, MacLennan R, Buettner PG. Sun exposure and the incidence of melanocytic nevi in young Australian children. *Cancer Epidemiol Biomarkers Prev.* 2008;17(9):2318-2324.
12. Gallagher RP, McLean DI. The epidemiology of acquired melanocytic nevi. A brief review. *Dermatol Clin.* 1995;13(3):595-603.
13. Levy R, Lara-Corrales I. Melanocytic nevi in children: a review. *Pediatr Ann.* 2016;45(8):e293-e298.
14. Oliveria SA, Saraiya M, Geller AC, Heneghan MK, Jorgensen C. Sun exposure and risk of melanoma. *Arch Dis Child.* 2006;91(2):131-138.
15. Mahe E, Beauchet A, de Paula Correa M, et al. Outdoor sports and risk of ultraviolet radiation-related skin lesions in children: evaluation of risks and prevention. *Br J Dermatol.* 2011;165(2):360-367.
16. Moreno S, Soria X, Martinez M, Marti RM, Casanova JM. Epidemiology of melanocytic naevi in children from Lleida, Catalonia, Spain:

protective role of sunscreen in the development of acquired moles. *Acta Derm Venereol*. 2016;96(4):479-484.

17. Aalborg J, Morelli JG, Byers TE, Mokrohisky ST, Crane LA. Effect of hair color and sun sensitivity on nevus counts in white children in Colorado. *J Am Acad Dermatol*. 2010;63(3):430-439.

18. de Maleissye MF, Beauchet A, Saiag P, et al. Sunscreen use and melanocytic nevi in children: a systematic review. *Pediatr Dermatol*. 2013;30(1):51-59.

19. Rodvall Y, Wahlgren CF, Ullen H, Wiklund K. Common melanocytic nevi in 7-year-old schoolchildren residing at different latitudes in Sweden. *Cancer Epidemiol Biomarkers Prev*. 2007;16(1):122-127.

20. Autier P, Boniol M, Severi G, et al. The body site distribution of melanocytic naevi in 6-7 year old European children. *Melanoma Res*. 2001;11(2):123-131.

21. Gallus S, Naldi L, Oncology Study Group of the Italian Group for Epidemiologic Research in Dermatology. Distribution of congenital melanocytic naevi and congenital naevus-like naevi in a survey of 3406 Italian schoolchildren. *Br J Dermatol*. 2008;159(2):433-438.

22. Roh MR, Eliades P, Gupta S, Tsao H. Genetics of melanocytic nevi. *Pigment Cell Melanoma Res*. 2015;28(6):661-672.

23. Takata M, Saida T. Genetic alterations in melanocytic tumors. *J Dermatol Sci*. 2006;43(1):1-10.

24. Bastian BC. The molecular pathology of melanoma: an integrated taxonomy of melanocytic neoplasia. *Annu Rev Pathol*. 2014;9:239-271.

25. Haliasos EC, Kerner M, Jaimes N, et al. Dermoscopy for the pediatric dermatologist part III: dermoscopy of melanocytic lesions. *Pediatr Dermatol*. 2013;30(3):281-293.

26. Suh KY, Bolognia JL. Signature nevi. *J Am Acad Dermatol*. 2009;60(3):508-514.

27. O'Rourke EA, Balzer B, Barry CI, Frishberg DP. Nevic mitoses: a review of 1041 cases. *Am J Dermatopathol*. 2013;35(1):30-33.

28. Glatz K, Hartmann C, Antic M, Kutzner H. Frequent mitotic activity in banal melanocytic nevi uncovered by immunohistochemical analysis. *Am J Dermatopathol*. 2010;32(7):643-649.

29. Lu D, Levin EC, Dehner LP, Lind AC. Proliferative activity in melanocytic nevi from patients grouped by age with clinical follow-up. *J Cutan Pathol*. 2015;42(12):959-964.

30. Yus ES, del Cerro M, Simon RS, Herrera M, Rueda M. Unna's and Miescher's nevi: two different types of intradermal nevus: hypothesis concerning their histogenesis. *Am J Dermatopathol*. 2007;29(2):141-151.

31. Kerl H, Soyer HP, Cerroni L, Wolf IH, Ackerman AB. Ancient melanocytic nevus. *Semin Diagn Pathol*. 1998;15(3):210-215.

32. Adaji A, Gaba P, Lohse CM, Brewer JD. Incidence of atypical nevi in Olmsted County: an epidemiological study. *J Cutan Pathol*. 2016;43(7):557-563.

33. Rosendahl CO, Grant-Kels JM, Que SK. Dysplastic nevus: fact and fiction. *J Am Acad Dermatol*. 2015;73(3):507-512.

34. Shapiro M, Chren MM, Levy RM, et al. Variability in nomenclature used for nevi with architectural disorder and cytologic atypia (microscopically dysplastic nevi) by dermatologists and dermatopathologists. *J Cutan Pathol*. 2004;31(8):523-530.

35. Barnhill RL, Cerroni L, Cook M, et al. State of the art, nomenclature, and points of consensus and controversy concerning benign melanocytic lesions: outcome of an international workshop. *Adv Anat Pathol*. 2010;17(2):73-90.

36. Duncan LM, Berwick M, Bruijn JA, Byers HR, Mihm MC, Barnhill RL. Histopathologic recognition and grading of dysplastic melanocytic nevi: an interobserver agreement study. *J Invest Dermatol*. 1993;100(3):318S-321S.

37. Pozo L, Naase M, Cerio R, Blanes A, Diaz-Cano SJ. Critical analysis of histologic criteria for grading atypical (dysplastic) melanocytic nevi. *Am J Clin Pathol*. 2001;115(2):194-204.

38. Arumi-Uria M, McNutt NS, Finnerty B. Grading of atypia in nevi: correlation with melanoma risk. *Mod Pathol*. 2003;16(8):764-771.

39. Toussaint S, Kamino H. Dysplastic changes in different types of melanocytic nevi. A unifying concept. *J Cutan Pathol*. 1999;26(2):84-90.

40. Ko CJ, McNiff JM, Glusac EJ. Melanocytic nevi with features of Spitz nevi and Clark's/dysplastic nevi ("Spark's" nevi). *J Cutan Pathol*. 2009;36(10):1063-1068.

41. Buonaccorsi JN, Lynott J, Plaza JA. Atypical melanocytic lesions of the thigh with spitzoid and dysplastic features: a clinicopathologic study of 29 cases. *Ann Diagn Pathol*. 2013;17(3):265-269.

42. Wick MR. Selected benign cutaneous lesions that may simulate melanoma histologically. *Semin Diagn Pathol*. 2016;33(4):174-190.

43. Ahn CS, Guerra A, Sangueza OP. Melanocytic nevi of special sites. *Am J Dermatopathol*. 2016;38(12):867-881.

44. Hosler GA, Moresi JM, Barrett TL. Nevi with site-related atypia: a review of melanocytic nevi with atypical histologic features based on anatomic site. *J Cutan Pathol*. 2008;35(10):889-898.

45. De Giorgi V, Sestini S, Grazzini M, Janowska A, Boddi V, Lotti T. Prevalence and distribution of melanocytic naevi on the scalp: a prospective study. *Br J Dermatol*. 2010;162(2):345-349.

46. Tcheung WJ, Bellet JS, Prose NS, Cyr DD, Nelson KC. Clinical and dermoscopic features of 88 scalp naevi in 39 children. *Br J Dermatol*. 2011;165(1):137-143.

47. Hofmann-Wellenhof R. Special criteria for special locations 2: scalp, mucosal, and milk line. *Dermatol Clin*. 2013;31(4):625-636, ix.

48. Schaffer JV. Update on melanocytic nevi in children. *Clin Dermatol*. 2015;33(3):368-386.

49. Fisher KR, Maize JC Jr, Maize JC Sr. Histologic features of scalp melanocytic nevi. *J Am Acad Dermatol*. 2013;68(3):466-472.

50. Fabrizi G, Pagliarello C, Parente P, Massi G. Atypical nevi of the scalp in adolescents. *J Cutan Pathol*. 2007;34(5):365-369.

51. Hunt RD, Orlow SJ, Schaffer JV. Genital melanocytic nevi in children: experience in a pediatric dermatology practice. *J Am Acad Dermatol*. 2014;70(3):429-434.

52. Ribe A. Melanocytic lesions of the genital area with attention given to atypical genital nevi. *J Cutan Pathol*. 2008;35(suppl 2):24-27.

53. Gleason BC, Hirsch MS, Nucci MR, et al. Atypical genital nevi. A clinicopathologic analysis of 56 cases. *Am J Surg Pathol*. 2008;32(1):51-57.

54. Madankumar R, Gumaste PV, Martires K, et al. Acral melanocytic lesions in the United States: Prevalence, awareness, and dermoscopic patterns in skin-of-color and non-Hispanic white patients. *J Am Acad Dermatol*. 2016;74(4):724-730.

55. Jaramillo-Ayerbe F, Vallejo-Contreras J. Frequency and clinical and dermatoscopic features of volar and ungual pigmented melanocytic lesions: a study in schoolchildren of Manizales, Colombia. *Pediatr Dermatol*. 2004;21(3):218-222.

56. Kim NH, Choi YD, Seon HJ, Lee JB, Yun SJ. Anatomic mapping and clinicopathologic analysis of benign acral melanocytic neoplasms: a comparison between adults and children. *J Am Acad Dermatol*. 2017;77(4):735-745.

57. Evans MJ, Gray ES, Blessing K. Histopathological features of acral melanocytic nevi in children: study of 21 cases. *Pediatr Dev Pathol*. 1998;1(5):388-392.

58. Iriarte C, Rao B, Haroon A, Kirkorian AY. Acral pigmented Spitz nevus in a child with transepidermal migration of melanocytes: dermoscopic and reflectance confocal microscopic features. *Pediatr Dermatol*. 2018;35:e99-e102.

59. Goettmann-Bonvallot S, Andre J, Belaich S. Longitudinal melanonychia in children: a clinical and histopathologic study of 40 cases. *J Am Acad Dermatol*. 1999;41(1):17-22.

60. Skornsek N, Oresic Barac T, Marko PB. Congenital longitudinal melanonychia: a case report. *Acta Dermatovenerol Alp Pannonica Adriat*. 2017;26(4):119-120.

61. Cooper C, Arva NC, Lee C, et al. A clinical, histopathologic, and outcome study of melanonychia striata in childhood. *J Am Acad Dermatol*. 2015;72(5):773-779.

62. Antonovich DD, Grin C, Grant-Kels JM. Childhood subungual melanoma in situ in diffuse nail melanosis beginning as expanding longitudinal melanonychia. *Pediatr Dermatol*. 2005;22(3):210-212.

63. Nguyen JT, Bakri K, Nguyen EC, Johnson CH, Moran SL. Surgical management of subungual melanoma: mayo clinic experience of 124 cases. *Ann Plast Surg*. 2013;71(4):346-354.

64. Fernandez-Flores A. Eponyms, morphology, and pathogenesis of some less mentioned types of melanocytic nevi. *Am J Dermatopathol.* 2012;34(6):607-618.

65. Rolland S, Kokta V, Marcoux D. Meyerson phenomenon in children: observation in five cases of congenital melanocytic nevi. *Pediatr Dermatol.* 2009;26(3):292-297.

66. Happle R. Speckled lentiginous naevus: which of the two disorders do you mean? *Clin Exp Dermatol.* 2009;34(2):133-135.

67. Mendes M, Costa I. Speckled lentiginous nevus syndrome. *Int J Dermatol.* 2016;55(11):e602-e604.

68. Li JY, Berger MF, Marghoob A, Bhanot UK, Toyohara JP, Pulitzer MP. Combined melanocytic and sweat gland neoplasm: cell subsets harbor an identical HRAS mutation in phacomatosis pigmentokeratotica. *J Cutan Pathol.* 2014;41(8):663-671.

69. Om A, Cathey SS, Gathings RM, et al. Phacomatosis pigmentokeratotica: a mosaic rasopathy with malignant potential. *Pediatr Dermatol.* 2017;34(3):352-355.

70. Luo S, Sepehr A, Tsao H. Spitz nevi and other Spitzoid lesions part I. Background and diagnoses. *J Am Acad Dermatol.* 2011;65(6):1073-1084, 1087-1092.

71. Spitz S. Melanomas of childhood. *Am J Pathol.* 1948;24(3):591-609.

72. Barnhill RL. The Spitzoid lesion: rethinking Spitz tumors, atypical variants, "Spitzoid melanoma" and risk assessment. *Mod Pathol.* 2006;19(suppl 2):S21-S33.

73. Barnhill RL, Argenyi ZB, From L, et al. Atypical Spitz nevi/tumors: lack of consensus for diagnosis, discrimination from melanoma, and prediction of outcome. *Hum Pathol.* 1999;30(5):513-520.

74. Dika E, Ravaioli GM, Fanti PA, Neri I, Patrizi A. Spitz nevi and other spitzoid neoplasms in children: overview of incidence data and diagnostic criteria. *Pediatr Dermatol.* 2017;34(1):25-32.

75. Zayour M, Bolognia JL, Lazova R. Multiple Spitz nevi: a clinicopathologic study of 9 patients. *J Am Acad Dermatol.* 2012;67(3):451-458, 458.e1-2.

76. Ricci F, Paradisi A, Annessi G, Paradisi M, Abeni D. Eruptive disseminated Spitz nevi. *Eur J Dermatol.* 2017;27(1):59-62.

77. Feito-Rodriguez M, de Lucas-Laguna R, Bastian BC, et al. Nodular lesions arising in a large congenital melanocytic naevus in a newborn with eruptive disseminated Spitz naevi. *Br J Dermatol.* 2011;165(5):1138-1142.

78. Torti DC, Brennick JB, Storm CA, Dinulos JG. Spitz nevi arising in speckled lentiginous nevus: clinical, histologic, and molecular evaluation of two cases. *Pediatr Dermatol.* 2011;28(5):561-567.

79. Porubsky C, Teer JK, Zhang Y, Deschaine M, Sondak VK, Messina JL. Genomic analysis of a case of agminated Spitz nevi and congenital-pattern nevi arising in extensive nevus spilus. *J Cutan Pathol.* 2018;45(2):180-183.

80. Busam KJ, Wanna M, Wiesner T. Multiple epithelioid Spitz nevi or tumors with loss of BAP1 expression: a clue to a hereditary tumor syndrome. *JAMA Dermatol.* 2013;149(3):335-339.

81. Requena C, Requena L, Kutzner H, Sanchez Yus E. Spitz nevus: a clinicopathological study of 349 cases. *Am J Dermatopathol.* 2009;31(2):107-116.

82. Fernandez-Flores A, Riveiro-Falkenbach E, Cassarino DS. Myxoid Spitz nevi: report of 6 cases. *Am J Dermatopathol.* 2018;40(1):30-35.

83. Haupt HM, Stern JB. Pagetoid melanocytosis. Histologic features in benign and malignant lesions. *Am J Surg Pathol.* 1995;19(7):792-797.

84. Fernandez AP, Billings SD, Bergfeld WF, Ko JS, Piliang MP. Pagetoid Spitz nevi: clinicopathologic characterization of a series of 12 cases. *J Cutan Pathol.* 2016;43(11):932-939.

85. Arps DP, Harms PW, Chan MP, Fullen DR. Rosette-like structures in the spectrum of spitzoid tumors. *J Cutan Pathol.* 2013;40(9):788-795.

86. Sabater Marco V, Escutia Munoz B, Morera Faet A, Mata Roig M, Botella Estrada R. Pseudogranulomatous Spitz nevus: a variant of Spitz nevus with heavy inflammatory infiltrate mimicking a granulomatous dermatitis. *J Cutan Pathol.* 2013;40(3):330-335.

87. Tetzlaff MT, Xu X, Elder DE, Elenitsas R. Angiomatoid Spitz nevus: a clinicopathological study of six cases and a review of the literature. *J Cutan Pathol.* 2009;36(4):471-6.

88. Harvell JD, Bastian BC, LeBoit PE. Persistent (recurrent) Spitz nevi: a histopathologic, immunohistochemical, and molecular pathologic study of 22 cases. *Am J Surg Pathol.* 2002;26(5):654-661.

89. Baran JL, Duncan LM. Combined melanocytic nevi: histologic variants and melanoma mimics. *Am J Surg Pathol.* 2011;35(10):1540-1548.

90. Fernandez-Flores A, Saeb-Lima M. Spitz nevus intermingling with a hemangioma. *Am J Dermatopathol.* 2016;38(10):780-783.

91. Ieremia E, Taylor M, Calonje E. Desmoplastic Spitz nevus combined with cutaneous leiomyoma: a rare collision tumor. *Am J Dermatopathol.* 2015;37(9):732-733.

92. Kishida ES, Muniz Silva MA, da Costa Pereira F, Sanches JA Jr, Sotto MN. Epidermal nevus syndrome associated with adnexal tumors, Spitz nevus, and hypophosphatemic vitamin D-resistant rickets. *Pediatr Dermatol.* 2005;22(1):48-54.

93. Barr RJ, Morales RV, Graham JH. Desmoplastic nevus: a distinct histologic variant of mixed spindle cell and epithelioid cell nevus. *Cancer.* 1980;46(3):557-564.

94. Harris GR, Shea CR, Horenstein MG, Reed JA, Burchette JL Jr, Prieto VG. Desmoplastic (sclerotic) nevus: an underrecognized entity that resembles dermatofibroma and desmoplastic melanoma. *Am J Surg Pathol.* 1999;23(7):786-794.

95. Plaza JA, De Stefano D, Suster S, et al. Intradermal Spitz nevi: a rare subtype of Spitz nevi analyzed in a clinicopathologic study of 74 cases. *Am J Dermatopathol.* 2014;36(4):283-294;quiz 95-97.

96. Sherrill AM, Crespo G, Prakash AV, Messina JL. Desmoplastic nevus: an entity distinct from spitz nevus and blue nevus. *Am J Dermatopathol.* 2011;33(1):35-39.

97. Harms KL, Lowe L, Fullen DR, Harms PW. Atypical Spitz tumors: a diagnostic challenge. *Arch Pathol Lab Med.* 2015;139(10):1263-1270.

98. Situm M, Bolanca Z, Buljan M, Tomas D, Ivancic M. Nevus Spitz—everlasting diagnostic difficulties—the review. *Coll Antropol.* 2008;32(suppl 2):171-176.

99. Mones JM, Ackerman AB. "Atypical" Spitz's nevus, "malignant" Spitz's nevus, and "metastasizing" Spitz's nevus: a critique in historical perspective of three concepts flawed fatally. *Am J Dermatopathol.* 2004;26(4):310-333.

100. Massi D, Tomasini C, Senetta R, et al. Atypical Spitz tumors in patients younger than 18 years. *J Am Acad Dermatol.* 2015;72(1):37-46.

101. Gerami P, Busam K, Cochran A, et al. Histomorphologic assessment and interobserver diagnostic reproducibility of atypical spitzoid melanocytic neoplasms with long-term follow-up. *Am J Surg Pathol.* 2014;38(7):934-940.

102. Zhao G, Lee KC, Peacock S, et al. The utilization of Spitz-related nomenclature in the histological interpretation of cutaneous melanocytic lesions by practicing pathologists: results from the M-Path study. *J Cutan Pathol.* 2017;44(1):5-14.

103. Paradela S, Fonseca E, Pita-Fernandez S, et al. Prognostic factors for melanoma in children and adolescents: a clinicopathologic, single-center study of 137 Patients. *Cancer.* 2010;116(18):4334-4344.

104. Ferrari A, Bisogno G, Cecchetto G, et al. Cutaneous melanoma in children and adolescents: the Italian rare tumors in pediatric age project experience. *J Pediatr.* 2014;164(2):376-82.e1-2.

105. Reguerre Y, Vittaz M, Orbach D, et al. Cutaneous malignant melanoma in children and adolescents treated in pediatric oncology units. *Pediatr Blood Cancer.* 2016;63(11):1922-1927.

106. Offenmueller S, Leiter U, Bernbeck B, et al. Clinical characteristics and outcome of 60 pediatric patients with malignant melanoma registered with the German Pediatric Rare Tumor Registry (STEP). *Klin Padiatr.* 2017;229(6):322-328.

107. Massi D, De Giorgi V, Mandala M. The complex management of atypical Spitz tumours. *Pathology.* 2016;48(2):132-141.

108. Wiesner T, Kutzner H, Cerroni L, Mihm MC Jr, Busam KJ, Murali R. Genomic aberrations in spitzoid melanocytic tumours and their implications for diagnosis, prognosis and therapy. *Pathology.* 2016;48(2):113-131.

109. Cho-Vega JH. A diagnostic algorithm for atypical spitzoid tumors: guidelines for immunohistochemical and molecular assessment. *Mod Pathol.* 2016;29(7):656-670.

110. Gerami P, Busam KJ. Cytogenetic and mutational analyses of melanocytic tumors. *Dermatol Clin.* 2012;30(4):555-566, v.

111. Murali R, Wiesner T, Scolyer RA. Tumours associated with BAP1 mutations. *Pathology.* 2013;45(2):116-126.

112. Yang C, Gru AA, Dehner LP. Common and not so common melanocytic lesions in children and adolescents. *Pediatr Dev Pathol.* 2018;21(2):252-270.

113. Al Dhaybi R, Agoumi M, Gagne I, McCuaig C, Powell J, Kokta V. p16 expression: a marker of differentiation between childhood malignant melanomas and Spitz nevi. *J Am Acad Dermatol.* 2011;65(2):357-363.

114. Harms PW, Hocker TL, Zhao L, et al. Loss of p16 expression and copy number changes of CDKN2A in a spectrum of spitzoid melanocytic lesions. *Hum Pathol.* 2016;58:152-160.

115. Tlougan BE, Orlow SJ, Schaffer JV. Spitz nevi: beliefs, behaviors, and experiences of pediatric dermatologists. *JAMA Dermatol.* 2013;149(3):283-291.

116. Sreeraman Kumar R, Messina JL, Reed D, Navid F, Sondak VK. Pediatric melanoma and atypical melanocytic neoplasms. *Cancer Treat Res.* 2016;167:331-369.

117. Lallas A, Kyrgidis A, Ferrara G, et al. Atypical Spitz tumours and sentinel lymph node biopsy: a systematic review. *Lancet Oncol.* 2014;15(4):e178-e183.

118. Sau P, Graham JH, Helwig EB. Pigmented spindle cell nevus: a clinicopathologic analysis of ninety-five cases. *J Am Acad Dermatol.* 1993;28(4):565-571.

119. Barnhill RL, Barnhill MA, Berwick M, Mihm MC Jr. The histologic spectrum of pigmented spindle cell nevus: a review of 120 cases with emphasis on atypical variants. *Hum Pathol.* 1991;22(1):52-58.

120. Aung PP, Mutyambizi KK, Danialan R, Ivan D, Prieto VG. Differential diagnosis of heavily pigmented melanocytic lesions: challenges and diagnostic approach. *J Clin Pathol.* 2015;68(12):963-970.

121. Diaz A, Valera A, Carrera C, et al. Pigmented spindle cell nevus: clues for differentiating it from spindle cell malignant melanoma. A comprehensive survey including clinicopathologic, immunohistochemical, and FISH studies. *Am J Surg Pathol.* 2011;35(11):1733-1742.

122. Puri PK, Elston CA, Tyler WB, Ferringer TC, Elston DM. The staining pattern of pigmented spindle cell nevi with S100A6 protein. *J Cutan Pathol.* 2011;38(1):14-17.

123. Sade S, Al Habeeb A, Ghazarian D. Spindle cell melanocytic lesions: part II—an approach to intradermal proliferations and horizontally oriented lesions. *J Clin Pathol.* 2010;63(5):391-409.

124. Strazzula L, Senna MM, Yasuda M, Belazarian L. The deep penetrating nevus. *J Am Acad Dermatol.* 2014;71(6):1234-1240.

125. Luzar B, Calonje E. Deep penetrating nevus: a review. *Arch Pathol Lab Med.* 2011;135(3):321-326.

126. Hung T, Yang A, Mihm MC, Barnhill RL. The plexiform spindle cell nevus nevi and atypical variants: report of 128 cases. *Hum Pathol.* 2014;45(12):2369-2378.

127. Magro CM, Crowson AN, Mihm MC Jr, Gupta K, Walker MJ, Solomon G. The dermal-based borderline melanocytic tumor: a categorical approach. *J Am Acad Dermatol.* 2010;62(3):469-479.

128. Stanford DG, Georgouras KE. Dermal melanocytosis: a clinical spectrum. *Australas J Dermatol.* 1996;37(1):19-25.

129. Kanada KN, Merin MR, Munden A, Friedlander SF. A prospective study of cutaneous findings in newborns in the United States: correlation with race, ethnicity, and gestational status using updated classification and nomenclature. *J Pediatr.* 2012;161(2):240-245.

130. Happle R. Phacomatosis pigmentovascularis revisited and reclassified. *Arch Dermatol.* 2005;141(3):385-388.

131. Gupta D, Thappa DM. Mongolian spots: how important are they? *World J Clin Cases.* 2013;1(8):230-232.

132. Alshami M, Bawazir MA, Atwan AA. Nevus of Ota: morphological patterns and distribution in 47 Yemeni cases. *J Eur Acad Dermatol Venereol.* 2012;26(11):1360-1363.

133. Zembowicz A, Mihm MC. Dermal dendritic melanocytic proliferations: an update. *Histopathology.* 2004;45(5):433-451.

134. Zembowicz A, Phadke PA. Blue nevi and variants: an update. *Arch Pathol Lab Med.* 2011;135(3):327-336.

135. Zembowicz A. Blue nevi and related tumors. *Clin Lab Med.* 2017;37(3):401-415.

136. Murali R, McCarthy SW, Scolyer RA. Blue nevi and related lesions: a review highlighting atypical and newly described variants, distinguishing features and diagnostic pitfalls. *Adv Anat Pathol.* 2009;16(6):365-382.

137. Bender RP, McGinniss MJ, Esmay P, Velazquez EF, Reimann JD. Identification of HRAS mutations and absence of GNAQ or GNA11 mutations in deep penetrating nevi. *Mod Pathol.* 2013;26(10):1320-1328.

138. Daltro LR, Yaegashi LB, Freitas RA, Fantini BC, Souza CD. Atypical cellular blue nevus or malignant blue nevus? *An Bras Dermatol.* 2017;92(1):110-112.

139. Zembowicz A, Granter SR, McKee PH, Mihm MC. Amelanotic cellular blue nevus: a hypopigmented variant of the cellular blue nevus: clinicopathologic analysis of 20 cases. *Am J Surg Pathol.* 2002;26(11):1493-1500.

140. Correa R, Salpea P, Stratakis CA. Carney complex: an update. *Eur J Endocrinol.* 2015;173(4):M85-M97.

141. Groben PA, Harvell JD, White WL. Epithelioid blue nevus: neoplasm Sui generis or variation on a theme? *Am J Dermatopathol.* 2000;22(6):473-488.

142. Zembowicz A, Carney JA, Mihm MC. Pigmented epithelioid melanocytoma: a low-grade melanocytic tumor with metastatic potential indistinguishable from animal-type melanoma and epithelioid blue nevus. *Am J Surg Pathol.* 2004;28(1):31-40.

143. Bax MJ, Brown MD, Rothberg PG, Laughlin TS, Scott GA. Pigmented epithelioid melanocytoma (animal type melanoma): an institutional experience. *J Am Acad Dermatol.* 2017;77(2):328-332.

144. Pearson JP, Weiss SW, Headington JT. Cutaneous malignant melanotic neurocristic tumors arising in neurocristic hamartomas. A melanocytic tumor morphologically and biologically distinct from common melanoma. *Am J Surg Pathol.* 1996;20(6):665-677.

145. Smith KJ, Mezebish D, Williams J, Elgart ML, Skelton HG. The spectrum of neurocristic cutaneous hamartoma: clinicopathologic and immunohistochemical study of three cases. *Ann Diagn Pathol.* 1998;2(4):213-223.

146. Goyal S, Arora VK, Gupta L, Singal A, Kaur N. Neurocristic hamartoma with lymph node involvement: a diagnostic dilemma. *Am J Dermatopathol.* 2015;37(7):e87-e92.

147. Linskey KR, Dias-Santagata D, Nazarian RM, et al. Malignant neurocristic hamartoma: a tumor distinct from conventional melanoma and malignant blue nevus. *Am J Surg Pathol.* 2011;35(10):1570-1577.

148. Garcia-Rabasco A, Marin-Bertolin S, Esteve-Martinez A, Alegre-de-Miquel V. Dermal melanocytosis of the scalp associated to intracranial melanoma: malignant blue nevus, neurocutaneous melanosis, or neurocristic cutaneous hamartoma? *Am J Dermatopathol.* 2012;34(2):177-181.

149. Rivers JK, Frederiksen PC, Dibdin C. A prevalence survey of dermatoses in the Australian neonate. *J Am Acad Dermatol.* 1990;23(1):77-81.

150. Moosavi Z, Hosseini T. One-year survey of cutaneous lesions in 1000 consecutive Iranian newborns. *Pediatr Dermatol.* 2006;23(1):61-63.

151. Ferahbas A, Utas S, Akcakus M, Gunes T, Mistik S. Prevalence of cutaneous findings in hospitalized neonates: a prospective observational study. *Pediatr Dermatol.* 2009;26(2):139-142.

152. Reginatto FP, DeVilla D, Muller FM, et al. Prevalence and characterization of neonatal skin disorders in the first 72h of life. *J Pediatr (Rio J).* 2017;93(3):238-245.

153. Cramer SF, Salgado CM, Reyes-Mugica M. The high multiplicity of prenatal (congenital type) nevi in adolescents and adults. *Pediatr Dev Pathol.* 2016;19(5):409-416.

154. Guegan S, Kadlub N, Picard A, et al. Varying proliferative and clonogenic potential in NRAS-mutated congenital melanocytic nevi according to size. *Exp Dermatol.* 2016;25(10):789-796.

155. Price HN. Congenital melanocytic nevi: update in genetics and management. *Curr Opin Pediatr.* 2016;28(4):476-482.

156. van Engen-van Grunsven AC, Kusters-Vandevelde H, Groenen PJ, Blokx WA. Update on molecular pathology of cutaneous melanocytic lesions: what is new in diagnosis and molecular testing for treatment? *Front Med (Lausanne)*. 2014;1:39.

157. Zhang D, Ighaniyan S, Stathopoulos L, et al. The neural crest: a versatile organ system. *Birth Defects Res C Embryo Today*. 2014;102(3):275-298.

158. Mort RL, Jackson IJ, Patton EE. The melanocyte lineage in development and disease. *Development*. 2015;142(4):620-632.

159. Kinsler VA, Birley J, Atherton DJ. Great Ormond Street Hospital for Children Registry for congenital melanocytic naevi: prospective study 1988-2007. Part 1-epidemiology, phenotype and outcomes. *Br J Dermatol*. 2009;160(1):143-150.

160. Alikhan A, Ibrahimi OA, Eisen DB. Congenital melanocytic nevi: where are we now? Part I. Clinical presentation, epidemiology, pathogenesis, histology, malignant transformation, and neurocutaneous melanosis. *J Am Acad Dermatol*. 2012;67(4):495 e1-17.

161. Bett BJ. Large or multiple congenital melanocytic nevi: occurrence of cutaneous melanoma in 1008 persons. *J Am Acad Dermatol*. 2005;52(5):793-797.

162. Krengel S, Hauschild A, Schafer T. Melanoma risk in congenital melanocytic naevi: a systematic review. *Br J Dermatol*. 2006;155(1):1-8.

163. Kinsler VA, O'Hare P, Bulstrode N, et al. Melanoma in congenital melanocytic naevi. *Br J Dermatol*. 2017;176(5):1131-1143.

164. Marghoob AA, Dusza S, Oliveria S, Halpern AC. Number of satellite nevi as a correlate for neurocutaneous melanocytosis in patients with large congenital melanocytic nevi. *Arch Dermatol*. 2004;140(2):171-175.

165. Herron MD, Vanderhooft SL, Smock K, Zhou H, Leachman SA, Coffin C. Proliferative nodules in congenital melanocytic nevi: a clinicopathologic and immunohistochemical analysis. *Am J Surg Pathol*. 2004;28(8):1017-1025.

166. Phadke PA, Rakheja D, Le LP, et al. Proliferative nodules arising within congenital melanocytic nevi: a histologic, immunohistochemical, and molecular analyses of 43 cases. *Am J Surg Pathol*. 2011;35(5):656-669.

167. Foster RD, Williams ML, Barkovich AJ, Hoffman WY, Mathes SJ, Frieden IJ. Giant congenital melanocytic nevi: the significance of neurocutaneous melanosis in neurologically asymptomatic children. *Plast Reconstr Surg*. 2001;107(4):933-941.

168. DeDavid M, Orlow SJ, Provost N, et al. Neurocutaneous melanosis: clinical features of large congenital melanocytic nevi in patients with manifest central nervous system melanosis. *J Am Acad Dermatol*. 1996;35(4):529-538.

169. Sibbald C, Randhawa H, Branson H, Pope E. Neurocutaneous melanosis and congenital melanocytic naevi: a retrospective review of clinical and radiological characteristics. *Br J Dermatol*. 2015;173(6):1522-1524.

170. Martins da Silva VP, Marghoob A, Pigem R, et al. Patterns of distribution of giant congenital melanocytic nevi (GCMN): The 6B rule. *J Am Acad Dermatol*. 2017;76(4):689-694.

171. Cribier BJ, Santinelli F, Grosshans E. Lack of clinical-pathological correlation in the diagnosis of congenital naevi. *Br J Dermatol*. 1999;141(6):1004-1009.

172. Rivers JK, MacLennan R, Kelly JW, et al. The eastern Australian childhood nevus study: prevalence of atypical nevi, congenital nevus-like nevi, and other pigmented lesions. *J Am Acad Dermatol*. 1995;32(6):957-963.

173. Simons EA, Huang JT, Schmidt B. Congenital melanocytic nevi in young children: Histopathologic features and clinical outcomes. *J Am Acad Dermatol*. 2017;76(5):941-947.

174. Wood BA. Paediatric melanoma. *Pathology*. 2016;48(2):155-165.

175. Nguyen TL, Theos A, Kelly DR, Busam K, Andea AA. Mitotically active proliferative nodule arising in a giant congenital melanocytic nevus: a diagnostic pitfall. *Am J Dermatopathol*. 2013;35(1):e16-e21.

176. Yelamos O, Arva NC, Obregon R, et al. A comparative study of proliferative nodules and lethal melanomas in congenital nevi from children. *Am J Surg Pathol*. 2015;39(3):405-415.

177. Vergier B, Laharanne E, Prochazkova-Carlotti M, et al. Proliferative nodules vs melanoma arising in giant congenital melanocytic nevi during childhood. *JAMA Dermatol*. 2016;152(10):1147-1151.

178. Senerchia AA, Ribeiro KB, Rodriguez-Galindo C. Trends in incidence of primary cutaneous malignancies in children, adolescents, and young adults: a population-based study. *Pediatr Blood Cancer*. 2014;61(2):211-216.

179. Wong JR, Harris JK, Rodriguez-Galindo C, Johnson KJ. Incidence of childhood and adolescent melanoma in the United States: 1973-2009. *Pediatrics*. 2013;131(5):846-854.

180. Lowe GC, Brewer JD, Peters MS, Davis DM. Incidence of melanoma in children: a population-based study in Olmsted County, Minnesota. *Pediatr Dermatol*. 2015;32(5):618-620.

181. Campbell LB, Kreicher KL, Gittleman HR, Strodtbeck K, Barnholtz-Sloan J, Bordeaux JS. Melanoma incidence in children and adolescents: decreasing trends in the United States. *J Pediatr*. 2015;166(6):1505-1513.

182. Wallingford SC, Iannacone MR, Youlden DR, et al. Comparison of melanoma incidence and trends among youth under 25 years in Australia and England, 1990-2010. *Int J Cancer*. 2015;137(9):2227-2233.

183. Austin MT, Xing Y, Hayes-Jordan AA, Lally KP, Cormier JN. Melanoma incidence rises for children and adolescents: an epidemiologic review of pediatric melanoma in the United States. *J Pediatr Surg*. 2013;48(11):2207-2213.

184. LaChance A, Shahriari M, Kerr PE, Grant-Kels JM. Melanoma: kids are not just little people. *Clin Dermatol*. 2016;34(6):742-748.

185. Weir HK, Marrett LD, Cokkinides V, et al. Melanoma in adolescents and young adults (ages 15-39 years): United States, 1999-2006. *J Am Acad Dermatol*. 2011;65(5 suppl 1):S38-S49.

186. Cordoro KM, Gupta D, Frieden IJ, McCalmont T, Kashani-Sabet M. Pediatric melanoma: results of a large cohort study and proposal for modified ABCD detection criteria for children. *J Am Acad Dermatol*. 2013;68(6):913-925.

187. Ferrari A, Bono A, Baldi M, et al. Does melanoma behave differently in younger children than in adults? A retrospective study of 33 cases of childhood melanoma from a single institution. *Pediatrics*. 2005;115(3):649-654.

188. Baergen RN, Johnson D, Moore T, Benirschke K. Maternal melanoma metastatic to the placenta: a case report and review of the literature. *Arch Pathol Lab Med*. 1997;121(5):508-511.

189. Valenzano Menada M, Moioli M, Garaventa A, et al. Spontaneous regression of transplacental metastases from maternal melanoma in a newborn: case report and review of the literature. *Melanoma Res*. 2010;20(6):443-449.

190. Alomari AK, Glusac EJ, Choi J, et al. Congenital nevi versus metastatic melanoma in a newborn to a mother with malignant melanoma—diagnosis supported by sex chromosome analysis and imaging mass spectrometry. *J Cutan Pathol*. 2015;42(10):757-764.

191. Singh K, Moore S, Sandoval M, et al. Congenital malignant melanoma: a case report with cytogenetic studies. *Am J Dermatopathol*. 2013;35(8):e135-e138.

192. Enam SF, Waqas M, Rauf MY, Bari ME. Congenital malignant melanoma of the scalp in a 25-day-old neonate. *BMJ Case Rep*. 2014;2014. doi:10.1136/bcr-2013-202588.

193. Su A, Low L, Li X, Zhou S, Mascarenhas L, Barnhill RL. De novo congenital melanoma: analysis of 2 cases with array comparative genomic hybridization. *Am J Dermatopathol*. 2014;36(11):915-919.

194. Richardson SK, Tannous ZS, Mihm MC Jr. Congenital and infantile melanoma: review of the literature and report of an uncommon variant, pigment-synthesizing melanoma. *J Am Acad Dermatol*. 2002;47(1):77-90.

195. Vourc'h-Jourdain M, Martin L, Barbarot S, aRED. Large congenital melanocytic nevi: therapeutic management and melanoma risk: a systematic review. *J Am Acad Dermatol*. 2013;68(3):493-8.e1-14.

196. Watt AJ, Kotsis SV, Chung KC. Risk of melanoma arising in large congenital melanocytic nevi: a systematic review. *Plast Reconstr Surg.* 2004;113(7):1968-1974.

197. Shah KN. The risk of melanoma and neurocutaneous melanosis associated with congenital melanocytic nevi. *Semin Cutan Med Surg.* 2010;29(3):159-164.

198. Turkeltaub AE, Pezzi TA, Pezzi CM, Dao H Jr. Characteristics, treatment, and survival of invasive malignant melanoma (MM) in giant pigmented nevi (GPN) in adults: 976 cases from the National Cancer Data Base (NCDB). *J Am Acad Dermatol.* 2016;74(6):1128-1134.

199. Fontaine D, Parkhill W, Greer W, Walsh N. Nevus cells in lymph nodes: an association with congenital cutaneous nevi. *Am J Dermatopathol.* 2002;24(1):1-5.

200. Holt JB, Sangueza OP, Levine EA, et al. Nodal melanocytic nevi in sentinel lymph nodes. Correlation with melanoma-associated cutaneous nevi. *Am J Clin Pathol.* 2004;121(1):58-63.

201. Nagore E, Botella-Estrada R, Garcia-Casado Z, et al. Comparison between familial and sporadic cutaneous melanoma in Valencia, Spain. *J Eur Acad Dermatol Venereol.* 2008;22(8):931-936.

202. Read J, Wadt KA, Hayward NK. Melanoma genetics. *J Med Genet.* 2016;53(1):1-14.

203. Aoude LG, Wadt KA, Pritchard AL, Hayward NK. Genetics of familial melanoma: 20 years after CDKN2A. *Pigment Cell Melanoma Res.* 2015;28(2):148-160.

204. Yamaguchi Y, Hearing VJ. Melanocytes and their diseases. *Cold Spring Harb Perspect Med.* 2014;4(5). doi:10.1101/cshperspect.a017046.

205. Shah KN. The diagnostic and clinical significance of cafe-au-lait macules. *Pediatr Clin North Am.* 2010;57(5):1131-1153.

206. Madson JG. Multiple or familial cafe-au-lait spots is neurofibromatosis type 1: clarification of a diagnosis. *Dermatol Online J.* 2012;18(5):4.

207. Ben-Shachar S, Dubov T, Toledano-Alhadef H, et al. Predicting neurofibromatosis type 1 risk among children with isolated cafe-au-lait macules. *J Am Acad Dermatol.* 2017;76(6):1077-1083.e3.

208. Bernier A, Larbrisseau A, Perreault S. Cafe-au-lait macules and neurofibromatosis type 1: a review of the literature. *Pediatr Neurol.* 2016;60:24-29.e1.

209. Takenouchi T, Shimizu A, Torii C, et al. Multiple cafe au lait spots in familial patients with MAP2K2 mutation. *Am J Med Genet A.* 2014;164A(2):392-396.

210. Stewart DR, Brems H, Gomes AG, et al. Jaffe-Campanacci syndrome, revisited: detailed clinical and molecular analyses determine whether patients have neurofibromatosis type 1, coincidental manifestations, or a distinct disorder. *Genet Med.* 2014;16(6):448-459.

211. Silvers DN, Greenwood RS, Helwig EB. Cafe au lait spots without giant pigment granules. Occurrence in suspected neurofibromatosis. *Arch Dermatol.* 1974;110(1):87-88.

212. Takahasi M. Studies on cafe au lait spots in neurofibromatosis and pigmented macules of nevus spilus. *Tohoku J Exp Med.* 1976;118(3):255-273.

213. Jimbow K, Horikoshi T. The nature and significance of macromelanosomes in pigmented skin lesions: their morphological characteristics, specificity for their occurrence, and possible mechanisms for their formation. *Am J Dermatopathol.* 1982;4(5):413-420.

214. Hull MT, Epinette WW. Giant melanosomes in the dysplastic nevus syndrome. Electron microscopic observations. *Dermatologica.* 1984;168(3):112-116.

215. Bhawan J, Purtilo DT, Riordan JA, Saxena VK, Edelstein L. Giant and "granular melanosomes" in Leopard syndrome: an ultrastructural study. *J Cutan Pathol.* 1976;3(5):207-216.

216. Boer A, Wolter M, Kneisel L, Kaufmann R. Multiple agminated Spitz nevi arising on a cafe au lait macule: review of the literature with contribution of another case. *Pediatr Dermatol.* 2001;18(6):494-497.

217. Kutlubay Z, Engin B, Bairamov O, Tuzun Y. Acanthosis nigricans: a fold (intertriginous) dermatosis. *Clin Dermatol.* 2015;33(4):466-470.

218. Sinha S, Schwartz RA. Juvenile acanthosis nigricans. *J Am Acad Dermatol.* 2007;57(3):502-508.

219. Brickman WJ, Huang J, Silverman BL, Metzger BE. Acanthosis nigricans identifies youth at high risk for metabolic abnormalities. *J Pediatr.* 2010;156(1):87-92.

220. Curth HO. Unilateral epidermal naevus resembling acanthosis nigricans. *Br J Dermatol.* 1976;95(4):433-436.

221. Ersoy-Evans S, Sahin S, Mancini AJ, Paller AS, Guitart J. The acanthosis nigricans form of epidermal nevus. *J Am Acad Dermatol.* 2006;55(4):696-698.

222. Happle R, Koopman RJ. Becker nevus syndrome. *Am J Med Genet.* 1997;68(3):357-361.

223. Patel P, Malik K, Khachemoune A. Sebaceus and Becker's nevus: overview of their presentation, pathogenesis, associations, and treatment. *Am J Clin Dermatol.* 2015;16(3):197-204.

224. Asch S, Sugarman JL. Epidermal nevus syndromes. *Handb Clin Neurol.* 2015;132:291-316.

225. Kim YJ, Roh MR, Lee JH, et al. Clinicopathologic characteristics of early-onset Becker's nevus in Korean children and adolescents. *Int J Dermatol.* 2018;57(1):55-61.

226. Panizzon R, Brungger H, Vogel A. Becker nevus. A clinico-histologic-electron microscopy study of 39 patients [in German]. *Hautarzt.* 1984;35(11):578-584.

227. Sheng P, Cheng YL, Cai CC, et al. Clinicopathological features and immunohistochemical alterations of keratinocyte proliferation, melanocyte density, smooth muscle hyperplasia and nerve fiber distribution in Becker's nevus. *Ann Dermatol.* 2016;28(6):697-703.

228. Cestari TF, Dantas LP, Boza JC. Acquired hyperpigmentations. *An Bras Dermatol.* 2014;89(1):11-25.

229. Hearns R. Disorders of pigmentation. In: Irvine AD, Yan AC, eds. *Harper's Textbook of Pediatric Dermatology.* 3rd ed. Chichester, England: Wiley-Blackwell; 2011:104-114.

230. Silpa-Archa N, Kohli I, Chaowattanapanit S, Lim HW, Hamzavi I. Postinflammatory hyperpigmentation: a comprehensive overview: epidemiology, pathogenesis, clinical presentation, and noninvasive assessment technique. *J Am Acad Dermatol.* 2017;77(4):591-605.

231. Park JY, Park JH, Kim SJ, et al. Two histopathological patterns of postinflammatory hyperpigmentation: epidermal and dermal. *J Cutan Pathol.* 2017;44(2):118-124.

23

Epidermal and Adnexal Proliferations and Tumors

Nima Mesbah Ardakani / Ellen Koch / Jonathan J. Lee / Alejandro A. Gru / Benjamin Wood

Epidermal Proliferations

EPIDERMAL NEVUS

Definition and Epidemiology

"Epidermal nevus" refers to a benign developmental malformation of the epidermis. These lesions may present in isolation or in association with other developmental anomalies, thereby constituting an "epidermal nevus syndrome." Six major clinically distinct syndromes, with systemic anomalies that most frequently affect the musculoskeletal and neurologic systems, are currently recognized (Table 23-1).

Epidermal nevus may be present at birth or become more noticeable during early childhood (80% within the first year of life) with an estimated incidence of 1 in 1000 infants.[1] Initial recognition in adulthood has been reported.[2] Males and females appear to be equally affected, and there is no racial predilection. Familial cases with autosomal dominant inheritance patterns have been reported.[3-5]

Etiology

Mosaicism at specific genetic loci may underlie particular clinicopathologic subtypes of epidermal nevi. Genetic mosaicism, with activating *FGFR3* mutations at codon 248 (R248C) in the epidermis, caused by postzygotic mutations early in embryonic development are thought to cause the "common," nonorganoid, nonepidermolytic epidermal nevi.[1] In contrast, mosaicism in the genes encoding suprabasilar keratins 1 and 10 (*KRT1, KRT10*) has been shown to underlie the epidermolytic, hyperkeratotic subtype of epidermal nevi.[6] Importantly, the offspring of affected individuals may develop generalized epidermolytic ichthyosis (bullous congenital ichthyosiform erythroderma). Additional genetic abnormalities associated with epidermal nevi include activating mutations in *PIK3CA* (phosphoinositide-3-kinase, which functions downstream of FGFR3), as well as mutations in *KRAS*.[7,8]

Clinical Presentation

Epidermal nevus presents as an asymptomatic, occasionally pigmented, well-circumscribed papillomatous linear plaque comprised of numerous densely grouped fleshy papules (Figure 23-1). There is a predilection for the trunk, extremities, and neck, but any cutaneous surface can be affected. They most commonly occur as an isolated lesion, but multiple unilateral or bilateral plaques may be seen. Not infrequently, the lesion follows Blaschko's lines, and there may be midline demarcation. Importantly, early epidermal nevi may present with macular morphology and can mimic linear and whorled nevoid hypermelanosis. Over time, they may thicken and develop a verrucous surface texture, particularly in intertriginous areas. The *nevus verrucosus* subtype refers to localized epidermal nevus (EN) with a wart-like appearance. *Nevus unius lateris* is typified by a large epidermal nevus with extensive unilateral involvement of the trunk. The *ichthyosis hystrix* subtype refers to the clinical subtype with extensive bilateral involvement, typically on the trunk.

TABLE 23-1. **Key Features of the Major Epidermal Nevus Syndromes**

EN-Associated Condition	Key Features
Schimmelpenning syndrome	• Unilateral nevus sebaceus of head and neck • Cerebral, ocular, cardiac, vascular, skeletal abnormalities • Coloboma and lipodermoid of conjunctiva • Vitamin D–resistance hypophosphatemic rickets
Nevus comedonicus syndrome	• Nevus comedonicus • Electroencephalogram abnormalities, cataracts and skeletal defects
Becker's nevus syndrome	• Becker's nevus • Ipsilateral hypoplasia of breast, skeletal anomalies
Proteus syndrome	• Nonepidermolytic keratinocytic epidermal nevi • Asymmetric overgrowth syndrome due to activating mutations in *AKT1* • Limb gigantism, asymmetric macrodactyly, scoliosis • Visceral overgrowth (spleen) • Vascular malformations, palmoplantar cerebriform hyperplasia • Lipomas, regional lipohypoplasia
CHILD syndrome	• X-linked dominant disorder due to inactivating mutations in *NSDHL* • Congenital or neonatal unilateral erythema with sharp midline demarcation and facial sparing, closely resembling ILVEN (see Section "Inflammatory Linear Verrucous Epidermal Nevus") • Linear alopecia, claw-like nail dystrophy
Phakomatosis pigmentokeratotica	• Nevus sebaceous (with relatively increased risk of basal cell carcinoma) • Papular nevus spilus • CNS anomalies, hyperhidrosis, weakness • Vitamin D–resistant, hypophosphatemic rickets

CHILD, congenital hemidysplasia with ichthyosiform nevus and limb defects; CNS, central nervous system.

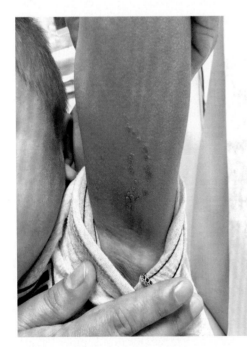

FIGURE 23-1. An epidermal nevus on the inner aspect of the arm presenting as a linear plaque formed by confluent fleshy papules.

Histologic Findings

Epidermal nevus typically demonstrates orthokeratosis, papillomatosis, acanthosis, and elongation of the epidermal rete (Figure 23-2). The histology is often subtle and not

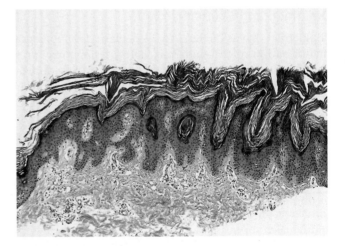

FIGURE 23-2. Epidermal nevus frequently resembles seborrheic keratosis histologically, with orthokeratotic hyperkeratosis, papillomatosis, and epidermal acanthosis.

infrequently mimics that of acanthosis nigricans or seborrheic keratosis.[9] Occasionally, epidermal nevus may show cornoid lamella formation. In addition, epidermal nevi may contain areas demonstrating features of epidermolytic hyperkeratosis. This finding should prompt the clinician to counsel the patient regarding the possibility of transmission of bullous congenital ichthyosiform erythroderma, as noted earlier.[10,11] Several reports have described focal acantholytic dyskeratosis within epidermal nevi, which some consider as a manifestation of segmental or zosteriform Darier disease.[12-14] Rare cases display a distinctive pattern of rectangular elongation of the rete ridges with palisading of basal keratinocytes and are referred to as papular epidermal nevus with skyline basal cell layer (PENS).[15] These are associated with extracutaneous findings (neurologic, in particular) in approximately 50% of cases.[16]

Basal cell carcinomas (BCCs), squamous cell carcinomas (SCCs), and keratoacanthomas are rarely reported in association with epidermal nevi, with a lower frequency than in the related nevus sebaceus.

Differential Diagnosis

The clinical differential diagnosis for nonorganoid, keratinocytic epidermal nevi includes nevus sebaceus, lichen striatus, porokeratotic eccrine ostial and dermal duct nevus, and other nevoid conditions distributed along Blaschko's lines. Linear lichen planus might also be considered. Histologically, seborrheic keratosis, acanthosis nigricans, verruca vulgaris, and other conditions characterized by hyperkeratosis and papillomatosis may enter the differential diagnosis. These latter conditions are usually clinically distinct.

CAPSULE SUMMARY

EPIDERMAL NEVUS

Epidermal nevus is a benign epidermal proliferation present at birth or becoming apparent in early childhood. The lesion typically presents as a linear papillomatous plaque and is characterized histologically by hyperkeratosis, papillomatosis, and a range of other epidermal alterations. It is important to consider the possibility of coexisting developmental abnormalities (epidermal nevus syndrome).

INFLAMMATORY LINEAR VERRUCOUS EPIDERMAL NEVUS

Definition and Epidemiology

Inflammatory linear verrucous epidermal nevus (ILVEN) was first described in 1971 by Altman and Mehregan and is thought to represent a distinct variant of epidermal nevus.[17]

ILVEN is uncommon, representing approximately 6% of epidermal nevi.[18] The majority arise in individuals before the age of 5 years and most commonly before the age of 6 months. There is a slight female predilection. Onset in adulthood has been reported, which may be associated with a familial predisposition.[5,19]

Etiology

The cause of ILVEN is not known. Some authors propose that this linear psoriasiform eruption may be due to clonal dysregulation of keratinocyte growth.[20] Distinction of ILVEN from linear psoriasis may be difficult. Proposed distinguishing biologic features include differential expression of involucrin, which is limited to the orthokeratotic stratum corneum in the former, whereas it is increased in all layers of the epidermis but the basal layer in the latter.[20] In addition, quantitative immunohistochemical studies indicate a significantly lower number of T-cell subpopulations relevant to the pathogenesis of psoriasis in ILVEN.[21]

Clinical Presentation

ILVEN presents as pruritic, erythematous, scaly, occasionally verrucous papules that often coalesce into a linear plaque, often following the lines of Blaschko (Figure 23-3).[22] It most frequently occurs on an extremity, with a propensity for the thigh and buttock. Given its pruritic nature, superimposed lichenification and excoriation are frequently present. On occasion, ILVEN coexists with psoriasis, may present as a part of an epidermal nevus syndrome, or may exceptionally be associated with underlying arthritis.[23-25]

Histologic Findings

ILVEN is characterized by psoriasiform acanthosis, with overlying alternating orthokeratotic and parakeratotic hyperkeratosis (Figure 23-4). Underneath the orthokeratosis, there is hypergranulosis, which alternates with hypogranulosis below the parakeratotic areas. There is typically mild spongiosis and a moderate superficial perivascular lymphocytic infiltrate.

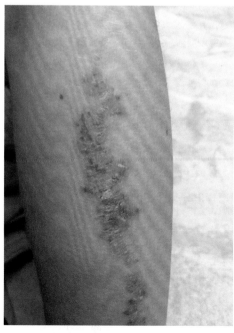

FIGURE 23-3. Inflammatory linear verrucous epidermal nevus (ILVEN) presents as an erythematous and scaly linear plaque, resembling linear psoriasis.

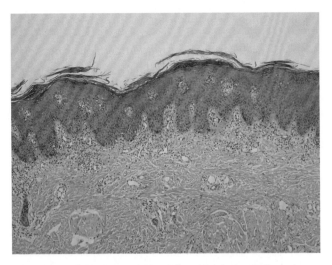

FIGURE 23-4. Horizontal alternation of orthokeratotic and parakeratotic hyperkeratosis is characteristic of inflammatory linear verrucous epidermal nevus (ILVEN), although the histologic features can be difficult to separate from psoriasis.

Differential Diagnosis

On routine dermatopathologic examination, ILVEN may be indistinguishable from psoriasis. Alternating orthokeratotic and parakeratotic areas may be a clue to the former diagnosis, but clinicopathologic integration is critical, because similar features may be seen in the eruption of pityriasis rubra pilaris. Dermatophyte infection and a wide range of spongiotic and psoriasiform dermatoses may also be considered on microscopic examination.

CAPSULE SUMMARY

INFLAMMATORY LINEAR VERRUCOUS EPIDERMAL NEVUS

ILVEN is an uncommon variant of epidermal nevus characterized by linear psoriasis-like clinical and histologic features.

ACANTHOSIS NIGRICANS

Definition and Epidemiology

Acanthosis nigricans presents as symmetric, hyperpigmented areas of velvety skin thickening that typically affects the dorsolateral neck and flexural areas and is commonly associated with an underlying metabolic disorder. Less common associations include an underlying malignancy, genetic predisposition, or association with medications.

The prevalence of acanthosis nigricans in children is not precisely known, but this condition is found in a significant fraction of those with obesity or insulin resistance. Acanthosis nigricans is more commonly seen among Native American, African American, and Hispanic individuals than

in those of Caucasian or Asian descent. A cross-sectional study of 1730 patients aged 7 to 65 years in the primary care setting across various sites in the United States found a 19% prevalence of acanthosis nigricans.[26] The incidence of acanthosis nigricans associated with other less common conditions, as discussed below, is not known.

Etiology

Acanthosis nigricans is most commonly associated with an underlying metabolic disease, inherited predisposition, or malignancy. However, other important associations must be recognized, including medications,[27] connective tissue disease,[28-30] and rare genetic syndromes.[31] Table 23-2 summarizes the underlying associated conditions.

The precise pathogenic pathways that lead to acanthosis nigricans are not well understood, but abnormalities related to tyrosine kinase receptors, including insulin-like growth factor receptor-1 (*IGFR1*), fibroblast growth factor receptors (*FGFR*), and epidermal growth factor receptor (*EGFR*), may be contributing factors. Of interest, activating mutations in *FGFR3* have been linked to several inherited syndromes that present with acanthosis nigricans, such as Crouzon syndrome, *s*evere *a*chondroplasia with *d*evelopmental *d*elay and *a*canthosis *n*igricans (SADDAN), and thanatophoric dysplasia *d*warfism.[32] In the setting of malignancy, elevated levels of transforming growth factor-α, which exerts proliferative effects on the epidermis via EGFR, may contribute to acanthosis nigricans.

Clinical Presentation

Acanthosis nigricans presents as a symmetric eruption, consisting of brown to gray, hyperpigmented, velvety

TABLE 23-2.	Conditions Associated With Acanthosis Nigricans
Hereditary benign	Epidermal nevus variant; may be inherited in autosomal dominant fashion
Metabolic or endocrinologic	Most common; insulin-resistant states, including metabolic syndrome and type II diabetes mellitus, polycystic ovarian syndrome
Malignancy	Underlying gastrointestinal adenocarcinoma, head and neck malignancy, carcinoma of the lung
Genetic syndromes	Bloom syndrome, Crouzon syndrome, Prader-Willi syndrome, Lawrence-Seip syndrome, Bear-Stevenson syndrome
Medications	Niacin, corticosteroids, oral contraceptives, others
Connective tissue (collagen vascular) disease	Systemic lupus erythematosus, dermatomyositis, scleroderma; note: may be medication related

plaques that primarily involves skin folds. The posterior and lateral folds of the neck are commonly affected. Early acanthosis nigricans may be heralded by slight hyperpigmentation that later eventuates into thickening of the skin. Other affected areas include the dorsal knuckles, genitalia, perineum, face, thighs, breast, and axillae. *Generalized acanthosis nigricans* may occur, which can present with involvement of the oral mucosa, lips, and eyelids and may herald an underlying malignancy.[33] Similarly, the finding of "tripe palms," or velvety thickening of the palms and dorsal hand, may also be paraneoplastic.[34] Rarely, acanthosis nigricans may present in the form of an epidermal nevus, which may be heritable in autosomal dominant fashion and can present at birth, childhood, or puberty.[35]

Histologic Findings

Despite the name, acanthosis nigricans is characterized by fine epidermal papillomatosis (rather than acanthosis), with overlying orthokeratotic hyperkeratosis (Figure 23-5). Basal keratinocyte pigmentation is typically readily identifiable, but there is no obvious increase in melanin pigmentation throughout the epidermis.

Differential Diagnosis

The histologic features of acanthosis nigricans show significant overlap with those of some epidermal nevi and confluent and reticulated papillomatosis (CARP). The prototypical clinical presentation of each of these conditions is distinct, but in some cases overlap may occur. Similar histologic features may be seen in conditions such as nevoid hyperkeratosis of the nipple and some examples of seborrheic keratosis.

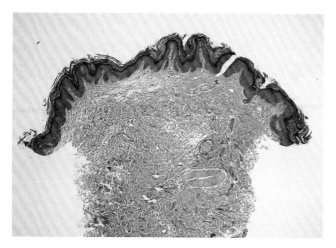

FIGURE 23-5. Acanthosis nigricans is characterized by hyperkeratosis and papillomatosis. The appearances are similar to those of confluent and reticulated papillomatosis (CARP) and some cases of epidermal nevus.

CAPSULE SUMMARY

ACANTHOSIS NIGRICANS

Acanthosis nigricans is a condition characterized by hyperpigmented velvety plaques in flexural areas, frequently associated with an underlying metabolic disorder. The histologic features are those of orthokeratotic hyperkeratosis and delicate papillomatosis.

CONFLUENT AND RETICULATED PAPILLOMATOSIS

Definition and Epidemiology

CARP of Gougerot and Carteaud was first described in 1927 and represents an idiopathic condition that clinicopathologically resembles acanthosis nigricans.

Although its precise incidence is unknown, CARP is a disorder seen primarily in adolescents and young adults, with females affected more than twice as often as males. It may be more common among African American as well as East and South Asian populations.[36] The vast majority of cases are sporadic, with familial occurrence limited to isolated case reports.[37,38]

Etiology

The etiopathogenesis of CARP is unknown, but several hypotheses have been proposed. Given its resemblance to acanthosis nigricans, an underlying endocrine imbalance has been postulated, which is supported by isolated case reports in patients having underlying obesity and insulin resistance.[39-42] Of interest, the majority of these cases occurred in individuals of East Asian descent. Historically, CARP was thought to be caused by an abnormal host response to *Malassezia furfur,* given its superficial clinical resemblance to tinea versicolor, reports of response to topical or oral antifungals, and the presence of yeast-like spores within the stratum corneum noted histologically.[43] However, recent reports have implicated a newly discovered and described Actinomycete species known as *Dietzia papillomatosis* in the pathogenesis of CARP.[44-46] This latter, novel hypothesis is consistent with clinical response to minocycline as well as other tetracyclines and macrolide antibiotics.[47]

Clinical Presentation

Early lesions of CARP consist of 1 to 2 mm hyperpigmented papules favoring the intermammary, interscapular, or epigastric skin that enlarge and coalesce into large brown, hyperkeratotic, reticulate patches or thin plaques (Figure 23-6). Other less common areas of involvement include the neck and shoulders. This benign dermatosis is usually asymptomatic, but can be associated with mild pruritus.

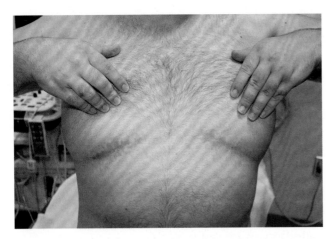

FIGURE 23-6. Confluent and reticulated papillomatosis (CARP) frequently presents in adolescent patients as hyperpigmented papules in the inframammary region, which coalesce to form thin reticulate plaques.

Histologic Findings

CARP shows orthokeratotic hyperkeratosis, slight papillomatosis, and delicate elongation of the rete ridges (Figure 23-7). Malassezia and gram positive bacteria are frequently identified on the surface.[48,49]

Differential Diagnosis

The histologic appearances of CARP can closely mimic epidermal nevus and acanthosis nigricans. Although acanthosis nigricans is described as showing more basal pigmentation, and more prominent epidermal acanthosis and papillomatosis, the discriminatory value in many cases is likely to be limited. Clinicopathologic correlation represents the mainstay of distinction.[49]

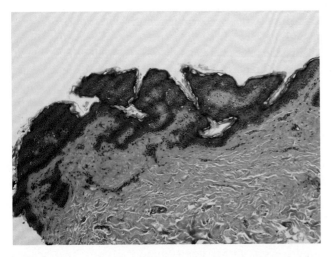

FIGURE 23-7. The histologic features of confluent and reticulated papillomatosis (CARP) include orthokeratotic hyperkeratosis and slight papillomatosis. Fungal yeast forms are often identifiable on the surface.

CAPSULE SUMMARY

CONFLUENT AND RETICULATED PAPILLOMATOSIS

CARP is a condition characterized by brown to gray papules that coalesce to form a reticulate eruption, usually involving the trunk. The condition frequently develops in adolescent patients. Although the typical distribution differs, and the association with metabolic abnormalities is less striking than for acanthosis nigricans, there are significant clinical and pathologic points of similarity.

PEDIATRIC BASAL CELL CARCINOMA AND HERITABLE BASAL CELL CARCINOMA SYNDROMES

Definition and Epidemiology

Basal cell carcinoma (BCC) is a typically nonmetastasizing, slowly growing, invasive, malignant neoplasm of the skin primarily caused by mutations acquired through exposure to ultraviolet radiation. Although the vast majority of cases are sporadic (nonsyndromic), a small subset arises in familial form (basal cell nevus syndrome, BCNS, or Gorlin syndrome).

BCC is the most frequent cancer diagnosed in the United States. Although older adults are typically afflicted, younger adults are increasingly being diagnosed with sporadic BCC.[50] Moreover, there are over 100 individual case reports of de novo BCC arising in children and adolescents, in whom there was no evidence of an underlying heritable, cancer predisposition syndrome or immunosuppressive disorder.[51] Age of onset of childhood BCC ranges from 2 to 18 years (median age of 12 years), with most cases occurring in fair-skinned patients, although occurrence in Hispanic and African-American patients, in whom pigmented variants are more common, is recognized.[51] Well-established risk factors for the development of sporadic, nonsyndromic BCC include extensive recreational and occupational exposure to ultraviolet radiation (UVR),[52] chemical exposures (ie, arsenic), immunosuppression with or without solid organ transplant, and smoking.[53] In addition to basal cell nevus syndrome (BCNS), or Gorlin syndrome, see Etiology), several heritable disorders also predispose to the development of BCC, including Bazex and Rombo syndrome, nevus sebaceus, xeroderma pigmentosum, and oculocutaneous albinism.[51]

Etiology

BCCs are thought to arise from the malignant transformation of basal keratinocytes. Several lines of evidence support the role of intermittent, recreational UVR exposure in pathogenesis.[54] In particular, activation of the sonic hedgehog (SHH)-Patched (*PTCH*) signaling pathway is thought to play a role, which may be achieved by homozygous inactivation of *PTCH* (9q22) or activating mutations of its target Smoothened (*SMO*, 7q32). Germline mutations in *PTCH1* are associated with autosomal dominantly inherited basal cell nevus syndrome (BCNS).[55,56] Mutations in the gene encoding tumor suppressor *p53* (17p13.1) as well as *CDKN2A* (9p21) may also play a role. Recent data suggest that a single-nucleotide polymorphism in mismatch repair genes *MSH2* (2p) and *MLH1* (Chr. 3) as well as variants in the melanocortin 1 receptor (*MC1R*, 16q) gene may predispose individuals to BCC.[57,58] A novel hereditary BCC syndrome, wherein patients develop multiple hereditary infundibulocystic variant BCCs, has recently been attributed to heterozygous splice site mutations in one copy of the tumor suppressor known as suppressor of fused gene (*SUFU*, 10q), a component of the sonic hedgehog pathway.[59,60]

Clinical Presentation

Sporadic pediatric BCC is rare.[51,61] Clinically, they present as a pink to flesh-colored, occasionally pigmented papule or nodule having a smooth surface with or without ulceration favoring the head (>90%), followed by the back, chest, and neck.[51] On the face, in order of decreasing frequency, childhood BCCs are more commonly identified on the cheek, nose, eyelid, scalp, chin, and lip.[51] Afflicted patients may note a recent increase in size, tenderness, bleeding, or change in color to the lesion.[51]

Individuals with the BCNS develop childhood onset of numerous BCCs, in addition to keratocystic odontogenic tumor of the jaw, bifid ribs, calcifications of the falx cerebri, and palmar or plantar pits.[62] Additional findings include childhood medulloblastoma, cardiac or ovarian fibromas, ocular abnormalities, macrocephaly, and polydactyly.[62] Afflicted individuals develop, on average, approximately 100 to 300 BCCs, although many more can occur, that tend to favor the face, neck, back, trunk, and upper extremities.[63] Over a 2-year period, these patients may develop from zero to 250 new BCCs (on average, approximately 10–25).[63] They present as variably sized flesh to pink dome–shaped papules, which less commonly demonstrate secondary features such as ulceration, crusting, or bleeding. Additional clues to diagnosis include coarse facies with broad nasal root, hypertelorism, milia, comedones, epidermal cysts, lipomas, fibromas, and café-au-lait macules.

Multiple hereditary infundibulocystic BCC syndrome (MHIBCC) has to date demonstrated a striking female predominance of middle age in whom multiple dome-shaped flesh-colored asymptomatic papules present on the face and vulva. Its predilection for the nasolabial folds may clinically mimic facial trichoepitheliomas, trichilemmomas, or adenoma sebaceum.[59,60]

Histologic Findings

The histologic appearances of BCC in children are similar to those in adults (Figure 23-8). Common patterns include superficial, nodular, and infiltrative growth of basaloid

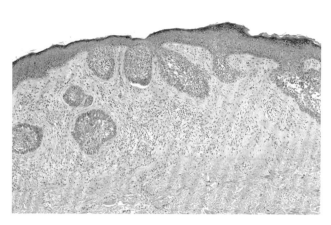

FIGURE 23-8. Basal cell carcinoma in children shows similar features to those seen in adults, although background solar elastosis is typically absent. This sporadic lesion arose on the shoulder of a 14-year-old patient.

epithelial cells. There is typically peripheral palisading, with clefting separation from the adjacent stroma and extracellular connective tissue mucin. Apoptosis, mitoses, and mucin deposition are also characteristic findings.

The palmar pits in the BCNS show hypokeratosis with crowding of the underlying basal cells, in some examples resembling superficial BCC, although the development of authentic BCC at this site is very uncommon.[64]

The infundibulocystic BCCs of MHIBCC syndrome often demonstrate hybrid morphology composed of conventional features of nodular BCC admixed with numerous, occasionally dilated infundibular cysts.[60]

Differential Diagnosis

In the pediatric setting, the principal differential diagnostic consideration is with trichoepithelioma/trichoblastoma. These lesions are discussed in greater detail below. Trichoepithelioma/trichoblastoma typically shows a symmetrical and noninfiltrative growth pattern, with a prominent stromal component and stromal-stromal clefting. The distinction of desmoplastic trichoepithelioma from infiltrating BCC can be problematic, particularly in small biopsy samples. Although the clinical presentation and relatively subtle morphologic features (eg, the characteristic "wrapping" of epithelial nests by thickened collagen; the presence of CK20-positive Merkel cells) may be helpful, in practice it is usually wise to ensure that lesions in which there is differential diagnostic difficulty are completely excised. Another problematic differential diagnosis with infiltrative BCCs is with microcystic adnexal carcinomas (MACs), also reported in the pediatric age group. As opposed to BCCs, MAC are negative for Ber-EP4 immunostain.

CAPSULE SUMMARY

BCC AND HERITABLE BCC SYNDROMES

Sporadic BCC is uncommon in children, with the majority of cases developing in later adolescence and showing features similar to those of adult BCC.

SQUAMOUS CELL CARCINOMA

Definition and Epidemiology

SCC is a malignant tumor of squamous keratinocytes that can arise on both cutaneous and mucosal surfaces.

Pediatric cutaneous or mucosal SCCs are exceedingly rare,[65] with most reported cases identified in children or adolescents with an underlying predisposition. Conditions with marked photosensitivity, such as xeroderma pigmentosum, oculocutaneous albinism,[66] PIBIDS (photosensitivity, ichthyosis, brittle hair, impaired physical and mental development, decreased fertility, and short stature) syndrome,[67] as well as medication-induced photosensitivity (particularly with voriconazole[68]) put the pediatric patient at the greatest risk for developing SCC. Those with a history of epidermolysis bullosa,[66] particularly dystrophic epidermolysis bullosa, and individuals with the related Kindler syndrome (*FERMT1*, 20p)[69] are also at increased risk. Pediatric SCCs may rarely arise from chronic wounds, including adjacent to gastrostomy tube sites,[70] in addition to scars, including within lesions of pansclerotic morphea.[71] Immunosuppression associated with organ transplantation,[72] chemotherapy treatment, or an underlying heritable immunodeficiency syndrome, such as the interferon-γ receptor-2 (*IFNGR2*, 21q) deficiency may also confer increased risk.[73] A higher incidence of pediatric SCC may also be seen in individuals predisposed to human papillomavirus (HPV) infection.[74]

Etiology

The precise etiology of SCC in the pediatric patient population is poorly understood. On the basis of studies of patients known to be at risk, such as those with photosensitivity conditions as well as epidemiologic and molecular studies of adult patients with SCCs, ultraviolet radiation exposure likely plays a key role in the pathogenesis of pediatric SCC.[75,76] The role of HPV has not been clearly delineated but is an active area of investigation. Although observed in the adult transplant patient population, diversity of β-HPV strains and greater β-HPV viral DNA load was found to predispose individuals to cutaneous SCCs.[77]

Clinical Presentation

Pediatric SCC most commonly arises on sun-exposed areas of the face, head, and neck region (particularly the lower lip and pinna of ear) as well as the hands and forearms. An indurated, scaly red papule or plaque may be observed, with or without associated telangiectasia, ulceration, and/or hemorrhagic crust. Lesions are usually solitary but rarely, particularly in the immunocompromised, may be multiple.[73]

Histologic Findings

The histologic appearances of SCC in children are similar to those seen in adults. Infiltrative growth of squamous keratinocytes displaying cytologic atypia is sine qua non for the diagnosis. Because of the extreme rarity of this neoplasm, careful consideration should be given to alternative diagnoses, as discussed later, particularly in the absence of a clear precipitating risk factor.

Differential Diagnosis

The differential diagnosis of SCC in the pediatric patient includes benign proliferations such as verruca vulgaris and adnexal tumors. In regard to the latter, lesions such as proliferating trichilemmal tumor and benign adnexal tumors with a "desmoplastic" pattern (eg, desmoplastic tricholemmoma, desmoplastic trichoepithelioma) or with squamous metaplasia and "pseudoinfiltrative" growth (eg, hidradenoma) should be considered. Extensive pseudoepitheliomatous (pseudocarcinomatous) epidermal hyperplasia can be seen secondary to infections, in the context of inflammatory conditions or associated with other neoplasms such as granular cell tumor and may closely mimic SCC. In general, the diagnosis of pediatric cutaneous SCC should be made with great caution, even more so in the absence of a predisposing risk factor.

CAPSULE SUMMARY

SQUAMOUS CELL CARCINOMA

SCC is extremely rare in children.[78] Many cases are associated with underlying conditions or exposures, including xeroderma pigmentosum, epidermolysis bullosa, and prior irradiation. The clinical and histologic features are otherwise similar to those seen in adults.

WHITE SPONGE NEVUS

Definition and Epidemiology

White sponge nevus, also known as *leukoedema exfoliativum mucosae oris* or *familial white folded dysplasia of mouth*, is a rare, heritable dermatologic condition that afflicts nonkeratinized stratified squamous epithelium and is clinically characterized by mucosal overgrowth.

This is a rare condition limited to individual case reports and pedigree series.[79-81] All ethnicities may be affected.

Etiology

White sponge nevus is autosomal dominantly inherited. The underlying genetic cause has been traced to mutations in the helical domain of mucosa-specific keratins K4 (12q) and K13 (17q).[82,83] Specifically, heterozygous deletions, missense mutations, and insertions involving these genes have been described.[84] Given the importance of keratins 4 and 13 to the epithelia of the oropharynx, anogenital, and esophageal mucosa, involvement of these sites is most commonly seen.

Clinical Presentation

White sponge nevus presents as an asymptomatic, exuberant diffuse, spongy, ragged-appearing white-to-gray folded plaque that affects the oral buccal mucosa but can also affect the tongue, gingiva, palate, floor of mouth, as well as the anogenital, nasal, esophageal, and conjunctival mucosa. The latter may be associated with coloboma.[75] Lesions may be noted at birth or develop anytime during childhood and adolescence.

Histologic Findings

White sponge nevus shows parakeratosis, acanthosis, and vacuolation of keratinocytes above the basal layer (Figure 23-9).[85] There are perinuclear accumulations of eosinophilic material, which correspond to tonofilament aggregation.[86]

Differential Diagnosis

The histologic features are quite striking, but other disorders with similar clinical appearances (eg, hereditary benign intraepithelial dyskeratosis) may enter the differential diagnosis. Much more common nonspecific reactive changes,

as seen in leukoedema and/or chronic bite injury, include prominent clear cell change. Infectious conditions such as oral hairy leukoplakia or Heck disease may enter the differential diagnosis. The combination of clinical presentation, vacuolization, and abnormal keratinization should allow separation.

CAPSULE SUMMARY

WHITE SPONGE NEVUS

White sponge nevus is a rare hereditary cause of oral leukoplakia associated with mutations in the keratin 4 and 13 genes.[82,83] The lesions clinically resemble oral candidiasis and are typically present from birth, although recognition may be delayed. Histologically, there is acanthosis with cytoplasmic clearing and perinuclear accumulation of eosinophilic material.

Adnexal Proliferations

NEVUS SEBACEUS

Definition and Epidemiology

Nevus sebaceus (of Jadassohn), also known as organoid nevus, is a common congenital hamartoma composed of epidermal, sebaceous, and apocrine elements that can, on occasion, give rise to secondary benign and malignant neoplasms. Nevus sebaceus has been described in up to 0.3% of neonates with an equal incidence in males and females.[87] Lesions are often noted at birth, but patients may not seek medical attention for decades.[88] Although most cases are sporadic, familial cases,[89] including with Schimmelpenning syndrome, have been reported.

Etiology

Recent molecular studies have identified postzygotic activating mutations, predominantly in *HRAS* as well as in *KRAS*, in lesional keratinocytes of nevus sebaceus.[90,91] These cause constitutive activation of the MAPK and PI3K-Akt signaling pathways, which lead to the clinical phenotype. Consistent with these findings, mosaicism in *HRAS* and *KRAS* was found in individuals with Schimmelpenning syndrome.[91]

Clinical Presentation

Nevus sebaceus most commonly presents on the head and neck region, favoring the scalp and, less commonly, involving the face (Figure 23-10). Lesions can also occur on the ears, trunk, extremities, oral, perianal, and genital (labial)

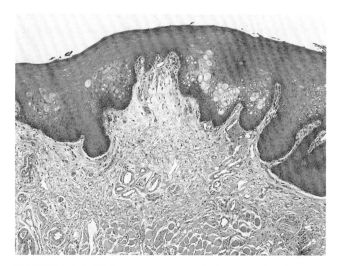

FIGURE 23-9. White sponge nevus displays parakeratosis, acanthosis, and prominent clearing of suprabasal keratinocytes.

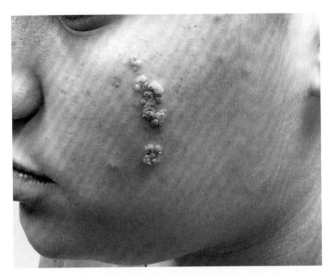

FIGURE 23-10. Nevus sebaceus presenting as a plaque with a pebbled appearance on the face of an adolescent patient.

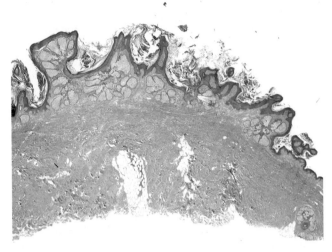

FIGURE 23-11. Nevus sebaceus displaying papillomatous epidermal hyperplasia and abnormal sebaceous glands. Note the absence of terminal hairs in this biopsy from the scalp, which can be a useful diagnostic clue.

mucosa.[92-96] A single, round to oval, sharply circumscribed, yellow to flesh-colored, pebbly thin plaque is often noted at birth and slowly thickens during childhood, while also assuming a more yellow-orange hue. Around adolescence, as a result of hormonal stimulation of lesional sebaceous glands, a more prominent thickening occurs, leaving a verrucous to cerebriform waxy smooth surface. Behind the ear, a linear configuration is often noted. Importantly, multiple lesions accompanied by seizures; intellectual impairment; and ocular, craniofacial, or skeletal abnormalities should raise suspicion for *Schimmelpenning syndrome*. The additional presence of a speckled lentiginous nevus along with skeletal and neurologic defects should raise concern for *phakomatosis pigmentokeratotica*.

Histologic Findings

Nevus sebaceus exhibits disorganized hamartomatous growth of both the epidermal and the adnexal structures (Figure 23-11). The epidermis is papillomatous and may contain distinctive areas of clear cell change. The sebaceous glands are usually hyperplastic, particularly in early infancy and puberty, but may be attenuated later in life. In addition, there is disorganization of sebaceous units, including superficial location of the glands, with incomplete lipidization and direct opening to the epidermal surface. The hair follicles are often decreased in number and miniaturized. An area of follicular absence in a scalp biopsy is an important low-power clue to the diagnosis. Abortive hair papillae are commonly present. Eccrine coils may be attenuated and occasionally cystically dilated. Ectopic apocrine glands may be seen in the deep dermis, particularly in adolescence and beyond. The dermis may be thickened and contains a mild lymphoplasmacytic inflammatory infiltrate. Benign proliferations

known as "basaloid follicular hamartoma" are frequently present, manifesting as strands and islands of basaloid cells with minimal cytologic atypia and low mitotic activity, associated with a loose follicular stroma with no retraction artifact.

Secondary benign or malignant neoplasms arise in approximately one fifth of cases of nevus sebaceus.[97-99] In decreasing order of frequency, trichoblastoma, syringocystadenoma papilliferum (SCP), and trichilemmoma are the most common benign secondary neoplasms. Others include poroma as well as both sebaceous and apocrine adenomas. Multiple neoplasms or overlapping lesions that are difficult to classify may be seen. Malignant neoplasms such as BCC, SCC, and sebaceous carcinoma are very rarely encountered in children.[99,100]

Differential Diagnosis

Epidermal nevus shows similar epidermal alterations; however, the abnormalities of pilosebaceous units are not present. Other than as a transient physiologic response to maternal hormones in the neonate, sebaceous proliferations are seldom seen in children. Sebaceous hyperplasia is characterized by lobular hyperplasia of normal-appearing sebaceous glands, without the other components of nevus sebaceus. Sebaceous adenoma is a lobular proliferation of abnormal sebaceous glands with expanded peripheral immature sebocytes with a basaloid appearance, and direct opening of the glands onto the epidermal surface. It also lacks the additional follicular and epidermal alterations seen in a nevus sebaceous. Rudimentary meningocele often occurs on the scalp. The morphologic features can show similarities to nevus sebaceous, with the additional feature of a proliferation of meningothelial cells.

CAPSULE SUMMARY

NEVUS SEBACEUS

CAPSULE SUMMARY

NEVUS SEBACEUS

Nevus sebaceus is a hamartoma, often present at birth, affecting mainly the head and neck area, particularly the scalp. It is histologically characterized by a complex disorganized proliferation of epidermal, folliculosebaceous, and sweat gland (eccrine and apocrine) elements. A variety of benign and malignant cutaneous neoplasms may arise from a nevus sebaceus, most commonly in adults.

NEVUS COMEDONICUS

Definition and Epidemiology

Also known as "comedo nevus," the nevus comedonicus is an uncommon, benign hamartoma of the folliculosebaceous unit, presenting as a plaque composed of numerous, dilated, keratin-filled comedones.

There does not appear to be any racial or sexual predilection. Approximately half of nevi comedonicus are present at birth, with the remaining cases noted during childhood before the age of 10. Adult onset is noted and, in such cases, may be related to cutaneous friction and/or trauma or, rarely, paraneoplastic.[101]

Etiology

Recent genomic analysis of nevus comedonicus demonstrated somatic mutations in the gene encoding the serine/threonine protein kinase Nek9 (*NEK9*), which may serve as an important regulator of follicular homeostasis and give rise to the clinical and histologic findings.[102] Somatic mutations in keratin 10 (*KRT10*) have been associated with epidermolytic nevus comedonicus associated with extensive lentigo simplex and linear epidermolytic nevus.[103] Mutations in *FGFR2* have also been described.[104]

Clinical Presentation

Nevus comedonicus presents as an asymptomatic, curvilinear plaque composed of hyperkeratotic papular comedones, some containing horny keratin plugs, with varying degrees of surrounding erythema (Figure 23-12). Lesions typically involve the face, neck, or upper trunk but can also extensively involve the hands bilaterally, with a predilection for the palms and wrists.[105-107] Occasionally, nevus comedonicus can assume a zosteriform configuration or present along the lines of Blaschko. Exceptional cases of secondary neoplasms, including SCC, keratoacanthoma, and BCC arising within nevus comedonicus have been described in adult patients.[108-110]

Most commonly, nevus comedonicus is an isolated anomaly, but it may be associated with syndromic features such as skeletal and dental defects (oligodontia)[111] or cerebral, skeletal defects and cataracts.[112] Rarely, nevus comedonicus may also occur in association with linear morphea and lichen striatus.[113]

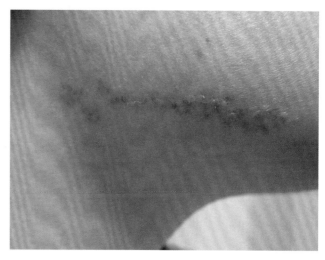

FIGURE 23-12. Nevus comedonicus presenting as a linear arrangement of papular comedones.

Histologic Findings

Nevus comedonicus is composed of multiple comedones, with cystically dilated follicular structures containing keratin debris with attached normal-appearing or attenuated sebaceous glands. The epidermis is usually acanthotic with surface hyperkeratosis. Additional findings include an adjacent fibro-inflammatory reaction with subsequent dermal scarring due to intermittent follicular rupture, areas of epidermolytic hyperkeratosis and, occasionally, formation of cornoid lamellae or epithelial proliferation similar to that seen in the dilated pore of Winer.[114]

Differential Diagnosis

Familial dyskeratotic comedones is a rare condition in which multiple comedones develop during childhood or adolescence, affecting mainly the trunk and limbs. Histologically, there are multiple follicle-like structures filled with keratin, showing scattered dyskeratotic cells in the lining of squamous epithelium often associated with subtle acantholysis.[115] Nodular solar elastosis with cysts and comedones (Favre-Racouchot syndrome) affects older patients and shows prominent solar elastosis histologically.

CAPSULE SUMMARY

NEVUS COMEDONICUS

Nevus comedonicus is a clinically distinct condition manifesting at birth or during the first two decades of life. It is characterized by a unilateral linear or grouped comedonal plaque composed of multiple cystically dilated hair follicles with attenuated epithelium and abundant keratin debris.

TRICHOEPITHELIOMA/TRICHOBLASTOMA

Definition and Epidemiology

Trichoepithelioma is a variant of trichoblastoma, representing a benign adnexal tumor with predominant differentiation toward the follicular bulb. Trichoepithelioma was historically used to refer to both the solitary lesion and familial multiple presentation (*epithelioma adenoides cysticum*) seen in the autosomal dominant Brooke-Spiegler syndrome.

These tumors are typically seen in early adult life but on occasion also during childhood. The incidence is unknown, but they are probably the second most common adnexal tumor in children after pilomatricoma.[100]

Etiology

Mutations in the gene encoding ubiquitin-specific protease *CYLD* (16q) are known to cause Brooke-Spiegler syndrome. Missense and nonsense mutations as well as deletions have been described.[116-119] Of interest, a mutational hotspot in *CYLD*, which is the specific *p.R758X* recurrent nonsense mutation, has been detected in patients with varying phenotypes, including multiple familial trichoepithelioma type 1 as well as familial cylindromatosis or Brooke-Spiegler syndrome.[117]

Clinical Presentation

Trichoepitheliomas are only rarely identified clinically as an isolated lesion, occurring primarily on the face. Multiple trichoepitheliomas present in early childhood as small, flesh-colored to translucent, firm papules and nodules favoring the central face, particularly involving the nasolabial folds, nose, forehead, upper lip, and eyelids. Rarely, the scalp, neck, trunk, scrotum, perianal area may be involved. Admixed telangiectasias are occasionally noted. Lesions may be numerous and coalesce into nodular aggregates on the face.[120] Linear and dermatomal variants have been described.[121] The presence of multiple lesions should raise suspicion of an inherited process.

Multiple familial trichoepithelioma type 1 is inherited in autosomal dominant fashion, with multiple lesions typically present by puberty.[122] Systemic associations are unusual, but renal and pulmonary cysts as well as parotid lesions have been described, as have adjacent BCCs, although the latter occurred in adult patients.[123-125] Brooke-Spiegler syndrome is characterized by multiple facial trichoepitheliomas in addition to numerous cylindromas (particularly of the scalp, so-called turban tumor syndrome), spiradenomas, and milia. Malignant transformation occurring within trichoepitheliomas has been described in adults.[126] Of clinical and pathologic importance, lesions with desmoplastic histologic features may induce epidermal surface changes that clinically and histologically mimic SCC.[127]

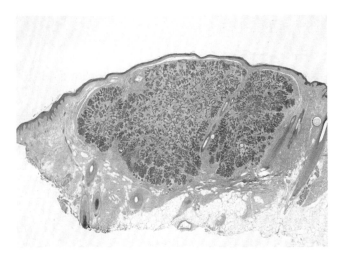

FIGURE 23-13. Trichoepithelioma/trichoblastoma appears as a circumscribed nodule of basaloid epithelial cells. Note the characteristic stromal component, with stromal-stromal clefting.

Histologic Findings

Trichoepithelioma is a dermal-based tumor composed of lobules and islands of basaloid epithelial cells forming thin radiating strands and cords within a distinctive stroma resembling normal follicular mesenchyme (Figure 23-13). The stroma often protrudes focally into the epithelial lobules, forming characteristic papillary mesenchymal bodies (Figure 23-14). Focal peripheral palisading may be seen, mimicking BCC; however, there is generally no tumor–stromal clefting or mucinous stromal alteration. Other typical findings include the presence of small keratin horn cysts, which may rupture and incite a local granulomatous reaction, abortive hair follicles, areas of calcifications, and,

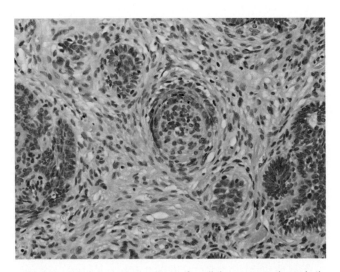

FIGURE 23-14. Invagination of cellular mesenchymal tissue into epithelial structures with a "ball-in-mitt" appearance, recapitulating the follicular bulb, is typical of trichoepithelioma/trichoblastoma.

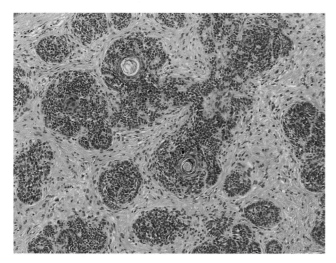

FIGURE 23-15. Melanin pigmentation can be seen in some examples of trichoepithelioma/trichoblastoma.

less commonly, amyloid deposition or melanin pigmentation (Figure 23-15). By immunohistochemistry, sparse CK20-positive Merkel cells can be detected among the basaloid cells and may help distinguish trichoepithelioma from BCC. The lesional cells are often positive for CK15 and PHLDA1.[128]

Histologic variants include "desmoplastic trichoepithelioma," "cutaneous lymphadenoma" (lymphotropic adamantinoid trichoblastoma) and "trichoadenoma (of Nikolowski)." Desmoplastic trichoepithelioma is a well-delineated dermal-based tumor, composed of thin strands and nests of basaloid cells in a desmoplastic stroma (Figure 23-16). Keratinous horn cysts and syringoma-like "tadpoles" are frequently seen. An admixed component of melanocytic nevus is not uncommon.[129] CK20-positive Merkel cells are often

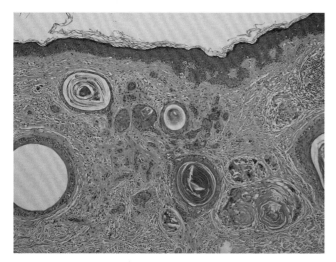

FIGURE 23-16. Desmoplastic trichoepithelioma is characterized by comma- and tadpole-shaped epithelial structures with keratocystic structures in a dense collagenous stroma. Granulomatous reaction to extruded keratin is frequently present.

present. Lesional cells are positive for PHLDA1, and stromal cells show focal strong positivity for CD34. These markers are useful in the separation of this lesion from its mimics. Deep, infiltrative growth is not seen in desmoplastic or conventional trichoepithelioma. Very focal invasion of small nerve twigs may be seen in desmoplastic trichoepithelioma, although a cautious approach to diagnosis of such cases is warranted.[130] Trichoadenoma (of Nikolowski) is composed mainly of dilated keratinous cysts with epidermoid keratinization and attenuated basaloid islands. Lymphotropic adamantinoid trichoblastoma shows a prominent component of admixed lymphocytes and a readily identifiable population of larger epithelioid cells.

Differential Diagnosis

BCC is a rare tumor in children, and when it does occur, the patient is typically in the later years of adolescence. BCC can closely mimic both conventional and desmoplastic trichoepithelioma. There is frequently significant cytologic atypia of basaloid cells, scattered mitoses, single cell apoptosis, as well as occasional necrosis. BCC has a mucinous stroma and exhibits characteristic tumor–stromal cleft formation. BCC lacks CK20-positive Merkel cells and is negative for PHLDA1; however, it is often positive for androgen receptor (AR). Syringoma can mimic desmoplastic trichoepithelioma; however, the lack of keratinous cysts, luminal secretory material, and the presence of ductal structures in syringoma (which can be highlighted by carcinoembryonic antigen, or CEA, immunohistochemistry) distinguish this entity from trichoepithelioma. MAC can show cytomorphologic features very similar to desmoplastic trichoepithelioma; however, the typical clinical presentation (a progressive infiltrative plaque on sun-damaged skin in an elderly patient) and the architecture on an adequate biopsy specimen are entirely different. MAC shows infiltrative growth, frequently with deep extension to the subcutaneous tissue and perineural invasion. In addition, MAC is often positive for CK19, whereas trichoepithelioma is largely negative.[128] MAC also lacks staining for Ber-EP4 as opposed to BCC and trichoepitheliomas.

CAPSULE SUMMARY

TRICHOEPITHELIOMA/TRICHOBLASTOMA

Trichoepithelioma is the second most common adnexal tumor in children, manifesting either as a sporadic and solitary lesion or as multiple lesions because of familial predisposition associated with *CYLD* gene mutations. Histologically, it is a dermal-based tumor, composed of lobules, islands, and strands of bland basaloid cells with follicular differentiation, manifesting as papillary mesenchymal bodies and abortive hair follicles, surrounded by a distinctive perifollicular stroma.

TRICHILEMMOMA

Definition and Epidemiology

Trichilemmoma is a benign follicular neoplasm with outer root sheath differentiation. These neoplasms are usually seen as an isolated lesion but, when numerous, may indicate Cowden syndrome (multiple hamartoma syndrome).

The incidence of trichilemmomas in the pediatric patient population is not known, but they are only rarely reported in children.[131] The incidence of Cowden syndrome is estimated at 1:200 000.[132] The syndrome is associated with an increased risk of malignancies, particularly of the breast, thyroid, and endometrium.[133]

Etiology

Cowden disease is caused by alterations in *PTEN* tumor suppressor gene (mapped to chromosome 10q22-23), which encodes phosphatase and tensin homolog (PTEN) protein and serves as a key regulator of the PI3K/AKT signaling.[134,135] The vast majority of Cowden disease patients harbor germline loss-of-function mutations in this key tumor suppressor. The condition is an autosomal dominantly inherited condition with nearly complete penetrance.

Although the precise etiopathogenesis of trichilemmoma is not understood, loss of PTEN is usually identified immunohistochemically in Cowden syndrome–associated trichilemmomas, but not in sporadic trichilemmomas.[136] The pathogenesis of sporadic and nevus sebaceous–associated trichilemmomas may be related to underlying mutations in *HRAS* (11p).[137]

Clinical Presentation

Trichilemmomas may present in solitary or multiple fashion as a small verrucous, hyperkeratotic, or smooth-surfaced, skin-colored papule with a predilection for the nose, mouth, ears, periorbital (eyelid, eyebrow), and genital skin.[138] Cowden syndrome is also associated with acral punctate keratoses; papillomatous papules; and oral mucosal papillomatosis of the tongue, cheek, or gingiva.[139] Vitiligo, hemangiomas, neurofibromas, schwannomas, xanthomas, and lipomas are additional cutaneous findings. More recently, multiple clear cell acanthomas were found arising in a patient with Cowden syndrome and may represent a *forme fruste*.[138] Additional major criteria for the diagnosis include macrocephaly (megalencephaly), breast carcinoma, thyroid carcinoma (follicular thyroid carcinoma, especially), Lhermitte-Duclos disease (dysplastic cerebellar gangliocytoma), endometrial carcinoma.[139] Cowden syndrome patients may also develop benign thyroid lesions (adenomas, multinodular goiter), mental retardation, gastrointestinal hamartomas, fibrocystic disease of the breast, fibromas, and genitourinary neoplasms.[139]

Histologic Findings

Trichilemmoma is characterized by one or multiple lobules of squamoid polygonal cells in the dermis, with attachment

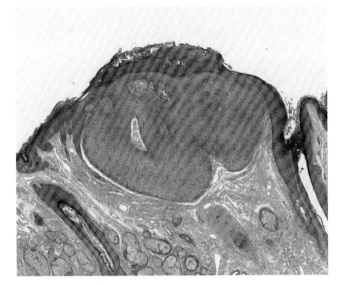

FIGURE 23-17. Trichilemmoma is an endophytic lobulated proliferation attached to the undersurface of the epidermis.

to the epidermis and sometimes to the follicular infundibulum (Figure 23-17). There is at least focal outer root sheath differentiation, visualized as clear cells containing abundant cytoplasmic glycogen and showing nuclear palisading at the periphery of the lobules (Figure 23-18). The lobules are partly surrounded by thick eosinophilic PAS-positive basement membrane–type material. Focal keratinization, squamous eddies, and keratinous cysts may be seen. The overlying epidermis is acanthotic and hyperkeratotic. The constituent clear cells show positive membranous staining with CD34.

Desmoplastic trichilemmoma is a histologic variant characterized by peripheral lobules of epithelial cells, similar to that seen in conventional trichilemmoma, and central sclerotic areas. Cords and strands of bland epithelial cells are present within the central desmoplastic and sometimes inflamed stroma.

Differential Diagnosis

Inverted follicular keratosis (IFK) is a hair follicle–based lesion, showing architectural similarity to trichilemmoma. IFK displays frequent squamous eddies without well-developed peripheral palisading or prominent basement membrane material. Clear cell change may occasionally develop in the IFK. There is probably significant diagnostic, and possibly biologic, overlap between IFK and trichilemmoma. The constituent epithelial cells in poroma are smaller and exhibit a monomorphous appearance, without peripheral palisading. In addition, eccrine duct structures are typically present in poroma, although they may be sparse. Focal trichilemmal differentiation is occasionally seen in other tumors such as squamous cell carcinoma or BCC; however, these epithelial tumors are extremely rare in children and often show more typical areas allowing for their distinction from trichilemmoma.

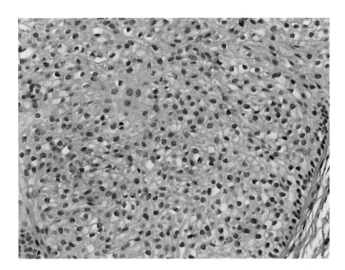

FIGURE 23-18. Cytoplasmic clearing and thick eosinophilic basement membrane are both characteristic of trichilemmoma, although often present only focally.

CAPSULE SUMMARY

TRICHILEMMOMA

Trichilemmoma is a rare follicular neoplasm in children with outer root sheath differentiation. It often presents as a sporadic single papular lesion on the face; however, multiple lesions may be encountered in patients with Cowden syndrome. Histologically, it is a lobulated dermal proliferation, which connects to the epidermis or follicular infundibulum. It is composed of squamoid to clear epithelial cells with peripheral palisading and is partially surrounded by thick eosinophilic basement membrane–type material.

TRICHOFOLLICULOMA

Definition and Epidemiology

Trichofolliculoma is an uncommon, benign follicular hamartoma characterized by the presence of radiating, small, but fully formed follicular structures surrounding a central follicular canal. There is morphologic and conceptual overlap between lesions described as hair follicle nevus, sebaceous trichofolliculoma, and folliculosebaceous cystic hamartoma.[140]

Trichofolliculomas are uncommon in the pediatric patient population. They may rarely present congenitally.[141]

Etiology

The underlying pathogenesis of the trichofolliculoma is not known. This hamartoma does not appear to be associated with any underlying systemic or other dermatologic diseases.[142]

Clinical Presentation

Trichofolliculoma typically presents as a dome-shaped, flesh-colored to reddish nodule containing a central pore from which numerous vellus hairs protrude. There is a

predilection for the head and neck regions, including the face, scalp, and neck. Trichofolliculoma may rarely involve the vulva and, in the adult patient, may be associated with vulvar intraepithelial neoplasia.[143]

Histologic Findings

On histologic examination, there is a cystically dilated follicle filled with keratin debris and hair shaft material, which may show attachment to the epidermal surface. There are numerous smaller hair follicles budding from the periphery of the lesion. The central canal may not be visualized in many planes of section. Attached sebaceous lobules may be present, and if prominent, the term "sebaceous trichofolliculoma" has been applied. Additional features that may be occasionally encountered include focal granulomatous reaction in the surrounding dermis as well as areas of acantholytic dyskeratosis.

Differential Diagnosis

Folliculosebaceous cystic hamartoma shows numerous small sebaceous lobules connecting to a central cystic cavity via sebaceous ducts and an intimate fibrovascular and fatty stroma showing cleft-like spaces between the stroma and the adjacent dermis. The lesion probably represents a form of trichofolliculoma. Dermoid cyst, often located on the face in children, is a dermal-based cystic lesion lined by a stratified squamous epithelium with a granular layer and attached folliculosebaceous units with or without eccrine and apocrine glands. Typically, there is no connection to the epidermis. Dilated pore of Winer lacks attached fully formed hair follicles.

CAPSULE SUMMARY

TRICHOFOLLICULOMA

Trichofolliculoma is a hamartomatous follicular lesion on the face with a central pore. It is histologically characterized by a central dilated hair follicle and numerous radiating small follicular structures with or without attached sebaceous lobules.

PILOMATRICOMA (PILOMATRIXOMA)

Definition and Epidemiology

Also known as the calcifying epithelioma of Malherbe, pilomatricoma is a benign tumor showing predominant follicular matrical differentiation.

Pilomatricoma is by far the most common cutaneous adnexal tumor in children, representing more than 90% of all adnexal tumors in patients younger than 18 years.[100] The lesion typically develops within the first two decades, with the median age at resection of 6 years.[144] There may be a slight female predilection.[144,145]

Etiology

Mutations in β-catenin (*CTNNB1*, 3p22) and trisomy 18 have been demonstrated in pilomatricomas and may play a role in its pathogenesis.[146,147]

Clinical Presentation

Pilomatricoma typically presents as a slowly growing, flesh-colored to pale, firm papulonodule with an overlying pink to blue hue ranging in size from 0.5 to greater than 5 cm (usually approximately 1.5 cm).[144] Lesions may be solitary or multiple. Particularly when multiple, they may be associated with an underlying disorder such as myotonic dystrophy, Rubinstein-Taybi syndrome, familial adenomatous polyposis (ie, Gardner syndrome), Lynch syndrome, Turner's syndrome, trisomy 9, Soto's syndrome, spina bifida, and Kabuki syndrome.[145,148-153]

The most commonly involved anatomic regions are the head and neck, especially the cheek, periorbital, and preauricular skin. Other less common locations include upper limbs, trunk, and lower limbs. Rarely, the paratesticular region may be involved. The "teeter-totter sign" may be elicited by using downward pressure at one end of the lesion to elicit an upward bulge on the opposing end. Pilomatricomas may also demonstrate the "tent sign," where multiple, subtle triangular bulges may be visualized on stretching the skin surface. These correspond to underlying chalky cystic debris enclosed within the tumor, which may be confirmed with radiologic or ultrasonic studies. Clinically, these lesions may mimic a parotid mass or masquerade as an infantile hemangioma.[154,155] Rapid growth due to hemorrhage or rupture may be encountered occasionally. Malignant transformation is exceedingly rare and usually limited to older adult patients.

Histologic Findings

Pilomatricoma is typically a dermally based tumor with a well-circumscribed nodular architecture, often located in the lower dermis, with or without extension to the subcutaneous tissue (Figure 23-19). It is composed of a variable volume of sheets and lobules of basaloid matrical and supramatrical cells. There is matrical keratinization, manifesting as eosinophilic shadow/ghost cells (Figure 23-20), with a heterogeneous connective tissue stroma. The latter includes varying proportions of vessels and inflammatory cells, including foreign body–type giant cells with areas of hyalinization, calcification, and bone formation in some cases. Melanin, hemosiderin, or amyloid deposition may be seen. Mitotic figures can be numerous (Figure 23-21). The shadow cells show a pink-orange polygonal appearance, with no nuclear staining, representing terminal differentiation of matrical cells. Cystic changes and calcification are common findings. Burned-out pilomatricoma with extensive calcification and/or ossification and little to no extant epithelial component

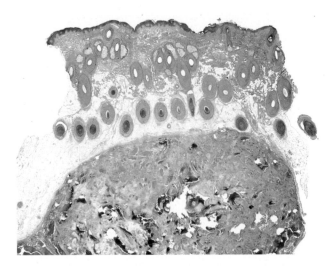

FIGURE 23-19. Pilomatricoma frequently presents as a circumscribed and partially calcified nodule in the deep dermis or superficial subcutis.

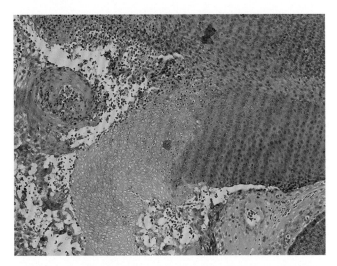

FIGURE 23-20. Matrical keratinization manifests as the formation of shadow/ghost cells.

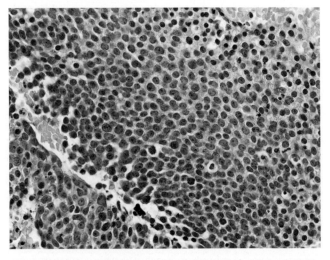

FIGURE 23-21. Mitotic figures are frequently abundant in the cellular portions of pilomatricoma.

may be encountered. By immunohistochemistry, the matrical cells show nuclear and cytoplasmic expression of β-catenin.

The terms "proliferating pilomatricoma" and "matricoma" have been used to describe dermal-based multilobular matrical tumors predominantly composed of solid nodules of basaloid matrical cells with focal aggregates of shadow cells and scant stroma. "Melanocytic matricoma" is histologically akin to matricoma with the addition of a prominent population of admixed bland, lightly pigmented dendritic melanocytes and heavy tumor melanization.[156] "Pigmented pilomatricoma" features abundant melanin pigmentation in the epithelial cells and stroma, with no significant melanocytic proliferation.[156]

Differential Diagnosis

Pilomatrix (matrical) carcinoma is exceedingly rare in children.[157,158] Pilomatrix carcinoma is often ulcerated, asymmetrical, and shows poor circumscription with infiltrative borders. The constituent basaloid matrical cells show nuclear pleomorphism, with prominent nucleoli, and frequent mitoses including atypical forms. Necrosis is also suggestive of malignancy. BCC with matrical differentiation may mimic pilomatricoma but is very uncommon in the pediatric age group; the typical features of BCC such as peripheral palisading of basaloid cells, tumor-stromal clefting, extracellular mucin, and immunostaining for BerEP4 should allow for recognition of this lesion. Proliferating trichilemmal tumor may be confused with pilomatricoma because of some architectural similarity and focal presence of matrical keratinization; however, the constituent cells in proliferating trichilemmal tumor show squamoid features with abundant eosinophilic cytoplasm. Matrical differentiation may be rarely seen in epidermoid cysts, a phenomenon that has been reported in patients with Gardner syndrome[159]; however, such hybrid cysts are predominantly lined by a stratified squamous epithelium with a granular layer, and matrical differentiation is only focal. Other follicular neoplasms such as trichoepithelioma and trichilemmoma may show focal matrical keratinization with formation of shadow cells; however, they lack sheets of basaloid matrical cells, which allows distinction from pilomatricoma.

CAPSULE SUMMARY

PILOMATRICOMA (PILOMATRIXOMA)

Pilomatricoma is the most common adnexal neoplasm in children, often presenting as a solitary soft or calcified nodule on the head and neck area and upper limbs. Histologically, the tumor has a well-circumscribed silhouette and is composed of varying proportions of basaloid matrical and supramatrical cells, shadow cells, multinucleated giant cells, and inflammatory cells within a hyalinized or calcified stroma.

SYRINGOCYSTADENOMA PAPILLIFERUM

Definition and Epidemiology

SCP is a hamartoma or benign neoplasm with a branching, glandular, and papillary architecture opening to the skin surface and a variable intradermal ductal component. The characteristic epithelial component includes a bilayer of cells, with luminal cuboidal cells showing features of apocrine differentiation.

The population incidence of SCP is unknown. The lesion typically occurs in children and adolescents, with occasional congenital examples reported.[160,161] Around one-third of cases are associated with nevus sebaceus.

Etiology

BRAF V600E mutation has been reported in some cases of SCP.[162] Rare loss of heterozygosity (LOH) of CDKN2A and/or PTCH1 genes has been reported in a subset of cases.[163]

Clinical Presentation

SCP occurs as raised, red to gray, linear papules or papillomatous plaque, often on the forehead and scalp. When occurring on the scalp, it is commonly associated with or arising within a nevus sebaceus. It is occasionally seen on other anatomic sites such as the proximal extremities, neck, trunk, breast, and scrotum. It can reach a size of 3 cm. Linear and segmental variants, occasionally following Blaschko's line may be seen.

Histologic Findings

The tumor typically exhibits an exophytic and endophytic growth pattern with a solid to cystic appearance. It is composed of duct-like invaginations from the epidermis as well as papillary structures lined by a dual layer of luminal columnar apocrine cells and basal cuboidal myoepithelial cells. Focal squamous lining is often observed. The papillary cores show a densely packed lymphoplasmacytic infiltrate, which is a characteristic finding. The lesion commonly merges with the overlying epidermis. Underlying cystically dilated eccrine and apocrine glands may be seen in the dermis. By immunohistochemistry, the luminal cells show variable positivity for GCDFP-15 as well as CK7 and CK19. The myoepithelial cells are positive for myoepithelial markers such as Calponin and SMA.

An unusual keratotic lesion termed "apocrine acrosyringeal keratosis" has been reported in association with SCP.[164] This lesion is characterized by tiers of hyperkeratosis encompassed by a hyperplastic epidermis showing trichilemmal keratinization.

Differential Diagnosis

Hidradenoma papilliferum shows some similarities to SCP; however, hidradenoma papilliferum typically occurs in the anogenital region, usually lacks epidermal connection, and exhibits solid-cystic growth with delicate papillary structures lacking a plasma cell–rich stroma. Apocrine tubular adenoma is a closely related entity, showing a tubular, cribriform, and solid architecture, lacking epidermal connection and a plasma cells–rich stroma. Areas with this appearance are frequently seen at the base of conventional SCP. Syringocystadenocarcinoma papilliferum is not usually seen in children. It shows an infiltrative solid to cystic growth with multilayering of the glandular epithelium showing significant cytologic atypia, frequent mitoses, and focal necrosis.

CAPSULE SUMMARY

SYRINGOCYSTADENOMA PAPILLIFERUM

SCP is a relatively common apocrine tumor in children,[100] which can be present at birth or can develop during childhood. SCP is common in nevus sebaceus. Histologically, it has an exophytic and endophytic solid to cystic architecture that opens to the epidermal surface and typically exhibits papillary structures lined by a dual layer of apocrine epithelial and myoepithelial cells with a plasma cell–rich stromal core.

SYRINGOMA

Definition and Epidemiology

Syringoma is a benign adnexal neoplasm showing differentiation toward the acrosyringium.

Syringomas are uncommon benign adnexal neoplasms, seen mostly in adolescent to middle-aged adult females and more commonly those of Asian descent. Some previous studies have identified an earlier childhood onset between the ages of 4 and 10 years.[165] There is an association with Down syndrome. The clear cell syringoma variant may be associated with underlying diabetes mellitus.[166]

Etiology

Although the underlying etiopathogenesis of syringoma is poorly understood, the syndrome of autosomal dominant multiple syringomas was found to be linked to chromosome 16q22, which encodes the zinc finger homeobox 3 (*ZFHX3*) gene.[167] Syringomas may develop as a reactive proliferative phenomenon, such as after pubic waxing.[168]

Clinical Presentation

Syringomas present most commonly as multiple, 1 to 3 mm pink, flesh-colored, yellow to brown papules that are usually symmetric in distribution and characteristically favor the periorbital (lower eyelid) skin as well as the upper cheeks (Figure 23-22).[169] This presentation is often seen

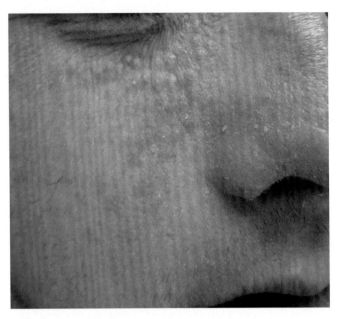

FIGURE 23-22. Multiple syringomas beneath the eye in a patient with Down syndrome.

among Japanese women. Of importance, involvement of the eyelid may be a clue to an underlying familial syringomatosis.[169] The second most common location in a recent literature review was the vulva,[169] where so-called giant syringomas, measuring anywhere from 1 to 3 cm in solitary or multiple fashion have also been described.[170,171] Syringomas may also present as plaques that can clinically and histologically mimic MAC.[172,173] In addition, eruptive[174] and segmental[175] presentations have been described, as has familial inheritance of eruptive and multiple syringomas. Familial syringomas may also be associated with steatocystoma multiplex.[176] Rarely, subclinical, incidental syringomas of the scalp, noted during the histologic evaluation of scalp biopsies for alopecia, have been described, although it is not clear whether it represents a causal or reactive phenomenon (such as in the setting of lichen planopilaris).[177] A congenital linear variant has also been described.[178]

Syringomas are uncommonly associated with underlying conditions. The most commonly associated include Down syndrome[179] and diabetes mellitus, the latter of which may be associated with the clear cell histologic subtype. Isolated reports of syringomas have also been observed in association with Brooke-Spiegler syndrome,[180] Nicolau-Balus syndrome,[181] and Costello syndrome.[182]

Histologic Findings

On microscopic examination, syringomas are dermal-based tumors with a relatively well-defined architecture and lacking extension to the subcutaneous tissue. They are composed of multiple, small tubular duct-like structures, often with comma-shaped tails, apparently streaming within a collagenous stroma (Figure 23-23). The tubules are lined by

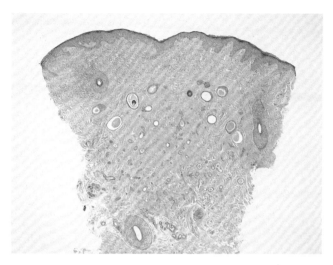

FIGURE 23-23. Syringomas show some architectural similarities to desmoplastic trichoepithelioma, with comma- and tadpole-shaped epithelial formations, generally confined to the upper- and middermis.

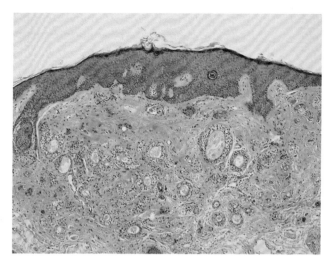

FIGURE 24-25. Clear cell syringoma shows ductal structures lined by epithelial cells with glycogenated cytoplasm.

a layer of cuboidal to columnar epithelial cells surrounded by sparse and often barely discernible myoepithelial cells (Figure 23-24). Solid nests and strands of basaloid cells may also be identifiable. Importantly, perineural invasion does not occur and, if identified, should raise suspicion for MAC. The clear cell variant of syringoma is characterized by ductal structures lined by more voluminous, epithelial cells containing abundant, clear, glycogen-rich cytoplasm (Figure 23-25).

Differential Diagnosis

Reactive syringomatous, eccrine ductal proliferations are characterized by reactive haphazard proliferation of normal-appearing eccrine ducts secondary to an inflammatory or neoplastic process, particularly on the scalp. In contrast,

true syringomas are well circumscribed, and there is generally no associated neoplastic or inflammatory process in the vicinity of the tumor. MAC can closely mimic syringoma, particularly on small and/or superficial biopsy samples, but the former tends to show more infiltrative growth, extending deeply into the subcutaneous fat and is frequently associated with perineural invasion. Importantly, occasional cases of syringoma of the vulvar region may exhibit deeper growth.[183] Morpheaform BCC, unlike syringoma, also shows an infiltrative deep dermal and sometimes subcutaneous growth. The tumor cords and islands exhibit mild to moderate cytologic atypia, frequent mitoses and apoptosis. Perineural invasion can be seen in this variant of BCC. Desmoplastic trichoepitheliomas can also enter into the differential diagnosis. As opposed to syringomas, desmoplastic trichoepitheliomas are positive for Ber-EP4 and lack expression of CEA.

CAPSULE SUMMARY

SYRINGOMA

Syringomas often occur as multiple skin-colored papules on the periorbital skin of an Asian female. They are rare in children, although a congenital linear variant has been described. An association with Down syndrome and diabetes mellitus (with the clear cell variant) has been described. Histologically, syringoma is characterized by a well-defined superficial dermal proliferation of small comma-shaped tubular and ductal structures lacking deep infiltration.

CYLINDROMA

Definition and Epidemiology

Cylindroma is a benign neoplasm of likely eccrine or apocrine derivation that can arise in solitary or multiple fashion. The latter is suggestive of the autosomal

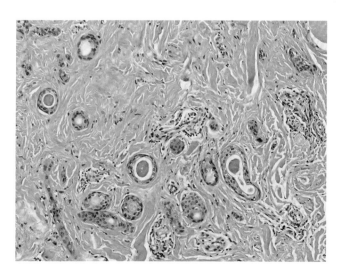

FIGURE 23-24. The luminal spaces in syringoma are lined by a bilayer of cells and frequently contain eosinophilic secretory material.

dominant Brooke-Spiegler syndrome (familial cylindro-matosis), which is also characterized by multiple spirad-enomas, trichoepitheliomas, follicular cysts, and milia. Affected individuals also develop hybrid tumors that show features of both cylindroma and spiradenoma. Multiple familial trichoepithelioma syndrome shows clinicopathologic and molecular overlap with Brooke-Spiegler syndrome.[184]

Cylindromas are an uncommon benign adnexal neo-plasm whose incidence is not known. Sporadic cylindromas typically arise in middle-aged or elderly individuals, with a predilection for women, while multiple, inherited cylindro-mas typically arise in adolescence or young adulthood.

Etiology

Brooke-Spiegler syndrome is caused by germline muta-tions in the gene encoding tumor suppressor ubiquitin carboxyl-terminal hydrolase CYLD (*CYLD*, 16q12-q13).[185] Loss-of-function mutations are observed in syndromic and solitary (sporadic) tumors. CYLD functions as a deubiqui-tinating protein that plays a predominant role in the regu-lation of NF-κB, a transcription factor that promotes cell survival and oncogenesis.[186-188]

Clinical Presentation

Cylindromas occur predominantly on the scalp and face as a solitary, pink to blue, firm to rubbery papulonodule that ranges in size from millimeters to several centimeters. In the autosomal dominant Brooke-Spiegler syndrome, mul-tiple cylindromas, clinically likened to bunches of grapes or small tomatoes, arise soon after puberty as numerous round masses on the scalp, and less commonly on the trunk or extremities. Malignant variants of adnexal tumors can arise in Brooke-Spiegler syndrome.[189,190]

Histologic Findings

Cylindromas are often present in the dermis and may extend to the subcutaneous tissue. They are composed of multiple irregular basaloid nodules and islands sur-rounded by densely eosinophilic basement membrane material, imparting a jigsaw puzzle or giraffe skin–like ap-pearance (Figure 23-26). Droplets of similar hyaline mate-rial can be seen within the nodules. The nodules contain two populations of basaloid cells. The peripheral cells ex-hibit small dark nuclei with a tendency to palisade. The central cells show larger pale nuclei. The surrounding stroma has a cellular collagenous appearance. Occasional duct-like structures are seen. Cylindromas with focal apocrine differentiation can be seen (Figure 23-27). Cyl-indroma with hybrid features of spiradenoma or tricho-epithelioma may be seen, particularly in patients with Brooke-Spiegler syndrome.

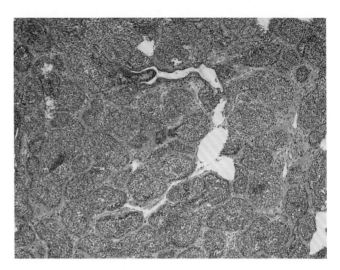

FIGURE 23-26. The cellular nodules of cylindroma are arranged in a pattern likened to a jigsaw or giraffe skin and rimmed by eo-sinophilic basement membrane.

Differential Diagnosis

Spiradenoma shows significant histologic overlap with cylindroma, and admixed components are common. The former is typically composed of a single large nodule with occasional smaller satellite nodules, rather than the typical jigsaw appearance seen in cylindroma. A lymphocytic infil-trate is commonly seen. Trichoblastoma lacks the basement membrane material seen in cylindroma and includes a char-acteristic stromal component, as well as showing features of follicular differentiation such as papillary mesenchymal bodies and abortive hair follicles.

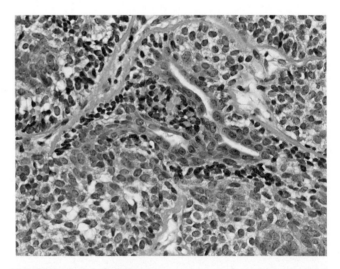

FIGURE 23-27. Cylindroma is composed of small basaloid cells periphery of the lobules and larger pale central cells. There are frequently areas of ductal differentiation.

CAPSULE SUMMARY

CYLINDROMA

Cylindroma is a benign adnexal neoplasm, often present as a solitary lesion on the head and neck area; however, multiple lesions are seen in association with autosomal dominant familial syndromes such as Brooke-Spiegler syndrome and familial cylindromatosis. Histologically, it has a multinodular jigsaw puzzle–like appearance and is composed of two types of basaloid cells surrounded by dense basement membrane–type material.

SPIRADENOMA

Definition and Epidemiology

Spiradenoma is a benign adnexal tumor related to cylindroma, which presents as dermal or subcutaneous nodules composed of small darker cuboidal cells, larger pale epithelial cells, and lymphocytes. Tubular structures are, on close inspection, apparent within the cellular nodules.

Spiradenoma usually occurs in adults; however, it can occasionally occur at birth or early childhood, particularly in association with a nevus sebaceus.

Etiology

The etiology is likely to be similar to that of cylindroma (see Capsule Summary—Cylindroma).

Clinical Presentation

Spiradenoma usually presents as a tender solitary gray, pink to bluish nodule on the head and neck, trunk, and limbs, ranging from 0.3 to 5 cm in size. Giant spiradenomas with a clinical size greater than 5 cm have been reported.[191] Whereas spiradenoma tends to be single, multiple lesions or lesions with linear arrangement have been reported sporadically or in familial syndromes such as Brooke-Spiegler syndrome.[192-194]

Histologic Findings

The constituent cells in spiradenoma are similar to cylindroma; however, the architecture is different. Spiradenoma is usually composed of a large dermal-based nodule or nodules, with no attachment to the epidermis (Figure 23-28). Smaller satellite nodules may be present and can extend into the subcutis. Droplets of eosinophilic basement membrane–type material may be seen throughout the lesion; however, the presence of this material at the periphery of the nodules is uncommon. Often, there are numerous small

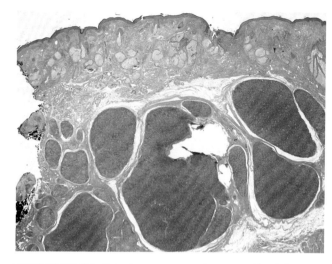

FIGURE 23-28. Spiradenoma presents as a multinodular tumor within the deep dermis, frequently extending into the subcutis.

lymphocytes, admixed or "peppered" between peripherally located small basaloid cells and central larger cells with pale nuclei (Figure 23-29). Frequent ductal structures are seen. Areas of stromal vascularization, lymphedema, hemorrhage, and cystic degeneration with or without infarction are sometimes present.

Differential Diagnosis

There is histologic overlap between spiradenoma and cylindroma, with architectural differences, which have been discussed earlier. Hybrid features of both entities are encountered in patients with familial syndromes. Such hybrid tumors are often referred to as spiradenocylindroma.

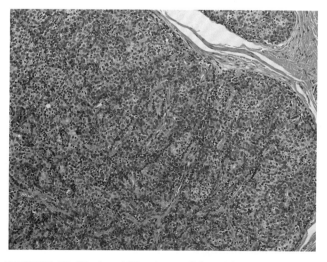

FIGURE 23-29. In addition to small basaloid and larger epithelial cells, an admixed population of lymphocytes is typical of spiradenoma.

CAPSULE SUMMARY

SPIRADENOMA

Spiradenoma usually presents as a tender solitary gray, pink to bluish nodule on the head and neck, trunk, and limbs, ranging from 0.3 to 5 cm in size. Histologically, spiradenoma is usually composed of a large dermal-based nodule or nodules, with no attachment to the epidermis. Droplets of eosinophilic basement membrane-type material may be seen throughout the lesion. Often, there are numerous small lymphocytes, admixed or "peppered" between peripherally located small basaloid cells and central larger cells with pale nuclei.

POROMA

Definition and Epidemiology

The group of poroid tumors encompasses an architecturally diverse spectrum of benign adnexal neoplasms arising from the sweat duct ridge and lower acrosyringium.[195] The lesions within this group are composed primarily of small uniform cuboidal cells (poroid cells), with smaller numbers of larger eosinophilic cells (cuticular cells). Formation of tubular structures lined by a cuticle and early ductal differentiation in the form of vacuolization of the cuticular cells is seen on close inspection.

The incidence of poroma is unknown, although they are rare in the pediatric population.[196,197] A recent review identified only nine reported cases in children.[198]

Etiology

The etiology of poroma is unknown. LOH of the *APC* gene was reported in three of seven cases of poroma in one study and may play a role in tumorigenesis.[199]

Clinical Presentation

Poromas commonly occur on the distal lower extremities as a red to pink to skin-colored raised wet-appearing papule or nodule, sometimes resembling pyogenic granuloma. Although the plantar or lateral aspects of the foot are the most common anatomic location, involvement of the head and neck, scalp, and trunk can occur. Lesions are often slow growing and solitary. However, multiple lesions do occur and have been described in adults following chemo- or radiotherapy.[200] There is no known familial predisposition or syndromic association.

Histologic Findings

Poroma is a well-circumscribed tumor composed of multiple acanthotic attachments to the epidermis, showing a sharp demarcation from adjacent keratinocytes (Figure 23-30). Descending into the dermis are broad columns and

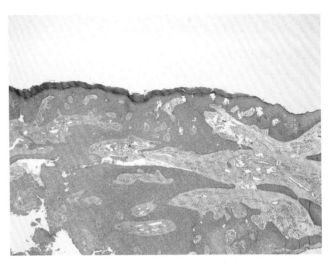

FIGURE 23-30. Poroma displays broad columns of small epithelial cells descending from the epidermis.

well-delineated lobules of small basaloid cells, with regular, round nuclei and moderately abundant cytoplasm, often with a pale, pink to clear appearance (Figure 23-31). Peripheral palisading of basaloid cells is not a feature. Mitoses are infrequent. Scattered ductal structures or cysts are often seen within the acanthotic lobules. Necrosis en masse is frequently seen in this lesion, being a useful diagnostic clue, and in this context does not imply malignancy. The surrounding stroma is vascular. Melanin pigmentation and colonization with dendritic melanocytes may be seen. Differentiation toward folliculosebaceous–apocrine unit, with the presence of sebaceous cells or sebaceous duct-like structures may be encountered, and such lesions can be referred to as apocrine poroma.

Dermal duct tumor is a dermal-based poroma with no connection to the epidermis at first glance; however, evaluation of multiple levels may reveal focal epidermal connections. Clear cell dermal duct tumor is a similar tumor with diffuse cytoplasmic clearing of the constituent poroid cells.

Hidroacanthoma simplex, on the other hand, is a poroma that is entirely confined within the epidermis. The adjacent nonlesional epidermis is often acanthotic with surface keratosis. Syringoacanthoma (of Rahbari) is an acrosyringeal tumor similar to hidroacanthoma simplex but with a papillomatous architecture and irregular intraepidermal nests of poroid cells.[201] Syringofibroadenoma (of Mascaro) is a variant that may rarely occur as multiple lesions (syringofibroadenomatosis) in conditions such as hidrotic ectodermal dysplasia (Clouston's syndrome and Schöpf syndrome) or familial syndromes with ophthalmologic abnormalities.[202,203] It has also been reported as a reactive phenomenon adjacent to an inflammatory or neoplastic process.[114] Histologically, it is characterized by elongated and anastomosing thin bands and cords of basaloid poroid cells radiating down from the epidermis and encompassed by a rich fibrovascular stroma. Occasional ductal structures and clear cell change may be evident.

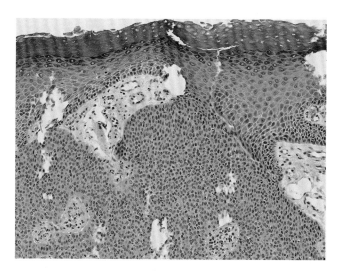

FIGURE 23-31. The population of small cuboidal poroid cells in poroma frequently shows sharp demarcation from larger adjacent epidermal keratinocytes.

Differential Diagnosis

Hidradenoma is a somewhat related tumor that may mimic poroma. Hidradenoma often exhibits a heterogeneous appearance with variable cell types, including squamoid cells, poroid cells, as well as clear cells, and often shows a deep dermal/subcutaneous location, with no attachment to the epidermis. Some variants of seborrheic keratosis (clonal seborrheic keratosis) may mimic poroma but lack ductal differentiation and typically show pseudohorn cysts.

CAPSULE SUMMARY

POROMA

Poromas commonly occur on the distal lower extremities as a red to pink to skin-colored raised wet-appearing papule or nodule, sometimes resembling pyogenic granuloma. Poroma is a well-circumscribed tumor, composed of multiple acanthotic attachments to the epidermis, showing a sharp demarcation from adjacent keratinocytes. Descending into the dermis are broad columns and well-delineated lobules of small basaloid cells, with regular, round nuclei and moderately abundant cytoplasm, often with a pale, pink to clear appearance. Ductular structures lined by "poroid" cells are seen at the periphery of the lesion.

HIDRADENOMA

Definition and Epidemiology

Hidradenoma is a benign sweat gland neoplasm characterized by a variably solid and cystic nodular growth within the dermis. Differing combinations of the various histologic features have led to a plethora of names, including nodular hidradenoma, acrospiroma, clear cell hidradenoma, solid-cystic hidradenoma, and apocrine hidradenoma.

The population incidence of hidradenoma is unknown, but they are generally rare in the pediatric age group.[100] A recent review identified 14 case reports of hidradenoma in children.[204]

Etiology

A t(11;19) chromosomal translocation resulting in a fusion of the *CRTC1* and *MAML2* genes has been recently identified in up to 50% of hidradenomas.[205] In addition, another translocation, t(6;22), involving the *EWS* and *POU5F1* genes has been reported in a subset of cases.[206] No familial predisposition has been reported.

Clinical Presentation

Hidradenoma typically presents as a solitary reddish-blue nodule with no particular anatomic site predilection at an average size of 2 cm with a slight female predominance. The tumors may be occasionally symptomatic with associated burning, tenderness, oozing, and/or hemorrhage.

Histologic Findings

Hidradenoma is a well-circumscribed dermal-based tumor with a solid, solid and cystic, or largely cystic appearance and diverse cellular composition (Figure 23-32). It is composed of variable proportions of squamoid epithelial cells with abundant eosinophilic cytoplasm, basaloid cells, poroid cells, and clear cells, often merging indistinctly in between each phenotypic zone (Figure 23-33). Apocrine-type cells with decapitation secretion, sebaceous cells and mucin-containing goblet cells may be seen occasionally. The constituent cells show an overall bland appearance. Occasional mitoses may be present, but mitotic activity is generally low. Duct-like structures are frequently present. Large cystic cavities lined by flattened cells may exist, and on occasion

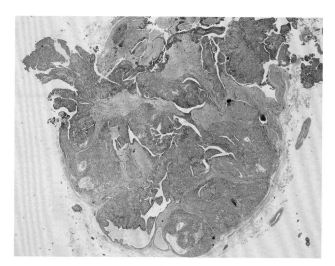

FIGURE 23-32. Hidradenoma is a variably solid and cystic dermal tumor with variable cellular composition.

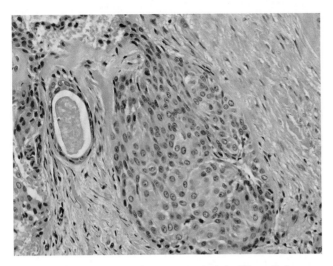

FIGURE 23-33. Squamoid and ductal differentiation are among the multiple cytologic components that may be seen in hidradenoma.

a tumor is largely or entirely cystic (Figure 23-34). Focal attachment to the epidermis or extension to the subcutaneous tissue may be encountered. The surrounding stroma ranges from loose and fibrovascular to a more collagenous and densely hyalinized. Tumor cells variably express different types of cytokeratins as well as EMA and CEA by immunohistochemistry. "Clear cell hidradenoma" is a variant that is predominantly composed of clear cells with small dark nuclei. The term "poroid hidradenoma" has been applied to tumors with a predominant poroid cell population and architectural features of hidradenoma with solid and cystic areas without epidermal attachment.

Differential Diagnosis

Cutaneous mixed tumor may show similar cytologic and architectural features; however, the stroma in mixed tumor is typically chondromyxoid, and there are clusters and islands

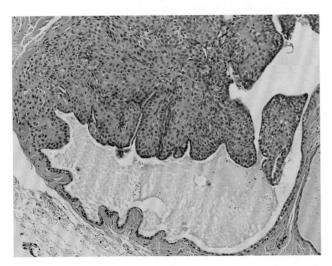

FIGURE 23-34. Cystic spaces in hidradenoma may be lined by a flattened layer of epithelial cells.

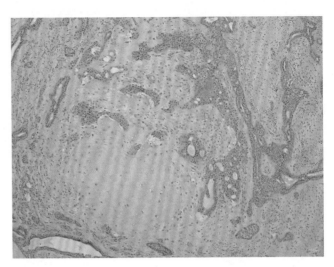

FIGURE 23-35. Apocrine mixed tumor shows chondroid or chondromyxoid stroma, in contrast to hidradenoma.

of myoepithelial cells with variable morphology, including plasmacytoid, spindle and clear cell appearance, indistinctly merging into the stroma (Figure 23-35). On cursory examination, glomus tumor may mimic hidradenoma. However, the former shows arrangement of cuboidal cells around vascular spaces, a component of cells with a myoid appearance, and frequently admixed nerve fibers. Immunohistochemistry for smooth muscle actin and cytokeratins will easily resolve this differential diagnosis.

CAPSULE SUMMARY

HIDRADENOMA

Hidradenoma is a benign adnexal tumor that usually presents as a solitary red to blue nodule, with no site predilection. It is a dermal-based tumor, with a solid to cystic appearance and a heterogeneous cellular composition including squamoid cells, basaloid cells, poroid cells, clear cells, apocrine cells, and, less commonly, sebaceous and mucin-containing epithelial cells.

MICROCYSTIC ADNEXAL CARCINOMA

Definition and Epidemiology

MAC, also known as sclerosing sweat duct (syringomatous) carcinoma, or malignant syringoma, is a locally aggressive combined adnexal carcinoma displaying ductal, glandular, and follicular differentiation. If incompletely excised, the recurrence rate is high. Lymph node metastasis is uncommon, and systemic spread or mortality is exceptionally rare.

This uncommon malignant tumor typically afflicts individuals in their 50s to 60s.[207-210] It may affect children very rarely. [208,209] An isolated example of congenital MAC has been described.[211]

Etiology

The etiopathogenesis of MAC is poorly understood. Several reports describe antecedent therapeutic radiation years before the onset of MAC.[210,212] A rare familial incidence of MAC involving two sisters has been described.[213] Immunodeficiency may also play a role.[214,215] Deletions of the long arm of 6q, reminiscent of malignant salivary gland tumors, have been reported in MAC.[216] An uncommon case of metastatic MAC was shown to harbor loss-of-function mutations in *TP53* and *CDKN2A*.[217]

Clinical Presentation

MAC typically presents as a slowly growing, flesh-colored to yellow, erythematous firm plaque or nodule on the face, scalp, and/or head and neck region, with a predilection for the central face, periorbital area, and upper lip (which is involved significantly more often than the lower lip). Tumors range in size from 0.5 to greater than 10 cm. A central dell or overlying hyperkeratosis may be noted. Although mostly asymptomatic, some may cause pain, burning, or paresthesia, which may be a harbinger of perineural infiltration.[218] This locally aggressive tumor can invade through subcutaneous fat and into bone.[219] Locoregional and distant metastases are exceptional.[220] Periorbital involvement with perineural invasion has been associated with cavernous sinus and brainstem metastases.[221]

Histologic Findings

The histologic diagnosis can be challenging on superficial biopsies. MAC originates from the dermis, and often involves the subcutis, skeletal muscle, and fascia. Superficially, the tumor is composed of multiple keratinous cysts, small tubular structures, as well as narrow cords and strands of epithelial cells with a basaloid to squamoid appearance. The constituent epithelial cells are deceptively bland to mildly atypical in appearance; however, a high-grade variant with marked cytologic atypia and squamous pearl formation has been reported.[222] Mitotic figures are infrequent. Intracytoplasmic lumina are sometimes present. An attenuated external layer of myoepithelial cells is frequently identifiable. The deep aspect of the tumor often exhibits an infiltrative growth pattern and a desmoplastic stroma. Areas of perineural invasion are commonly encountered. Focal folliculosebaceous differentiation, apocrine differentiation, or clear cell change may be seen.

By immunohistochemistry, the tumor cells are often positive for cytokeratins such as AE1/3, CK19, CK7, as well as EMA. CEA highlights ductal structures and intracytoplasmic lumina. BerEP4 shows variable staining, with both positive and negative results having been described in the literature.[128,223,224]

Entities such as "syringoid eccrine carcinoma" and "solid carcinoma" show marked histologic similarities and are probably best regarded as histologic variants of MAC. Syringoid eccrine carcinoma is composed of cytologically bland-appearing basaloid to squamoid cells forming cords, strands, and comma-shaped tubular structures within a dense hyalinized stroma with focal ductal differentiation. Keratinous cysts or follicular differentiation are not a prominent feature. The tumor often extends to the subcutis as well as underlying skeletal muscle and fascia. Solid carcinoma is characterized by numerous cords and nests of basaloid cells, showing a solid sheet-like growth with focal ductal differentiation and associated desmoplastic stroma and perineural invasion.[114]

Differential Diagnosis

Syringoma differs from MAC by being confined to the upper dermis and the absence of cytologic atypia, keratinous cysts, and perineural invasion. This distinction, however, can be very challenging or impossible in superficial or partial biopsies, and, thus, a deep punch or incisional biopsy when MAC is in the differential diagnosis is mandatory. Desmoplastic trichoepithelioma can mimic MAC. The former distinctly lacks ductal differentiation and does not demonstrate deep subcutaneous or perineural invasion. By immunohistochemistry, trichoepithelioma is positive for CK15 and PHLDA1, whereas they are often negative in MAC. Morpheaform BCC can be distinguished from MAC by the presence of focal extracellular mucin and tumor–stroma clefting. The presence of the occasional, admixed prototypical islands of nodular or superficial BCC (if present) also helps in this distinction. Ductal differentiation can occasionally be seen in BCC. Squamoid eccrine duct carcinoma is a rare malignant adnexal neoplasm that can be distinguished from MAC by its focal attachment to the epidermis or hair follicle, cytologic atypia, and prominent superficial squamous differentiation resembling SCC. However, the deep aspect of the tumor may be identical to MAC.

CAPSULE SUMMARY

MICROCYSTIC ADNEXAL CARCINOMA

MAC is a locally aggressive malignant tumor that is extremely rare in children and demonstrates a predilection for the face and lip with high recurrence rates following incomplete excision. Histologically, it is characterized by multiple keratinous cysts, cords, strands, and tubular structures with focal ductal differentiation, deep dermal, and subcutaneous extension, and frequent perineural invasion.

ANGIOFIBROMA (FIBROUS PAPULE OF THE FACE)

Definition and Epidemiology

Angiofibroma is a benign fibrovascular proliferation within the upper dermis, often showing a concentric perivascular and perifollicular growth pattern, which may be derived from perifollicular mesenchyme[225] or may represent a reactive proliferation of dermal dendrocytes. A variety of histologic variants are recognized.[226] Lesions occurring on the face (particularly when solitary) are described as *fibrous papule* of the face or nose, whereas multiple lesions in the setting of tuberous sclerosis are described (incorrectly) as *adenoma sebaceum*. Analogous lesions occur on acral sites (referred to as *Koenen's tumor* in the setting of tuberous sclerosis) and on genital skin (*pearly penile papules*).

The incidence of facial angiofibroma is unknown. Multiple facial angiofibromas develop in most patients with tuberous sclerosis, frequently in childhood.[227] They can also develop in Birt-Hogg-Dube syndrome [228] (with concurrent trichofolliculomas and trichodiscomas).

Etiology

Tuberous sclerosis is an autosomal dominant disorder characterized by hamartomas in multiple organ systems. Tuberous sclerosis 1 (OMIM 191100) is caused by mutations in the *TSC1* gene on chromosome 9q34, whereas tuberous sclerosis 2 (OMIM 613254) is caused by mutations in the *TSC2* gene on chromosome 16p13.[229]

Clinical Presentation

Angiofibroma usually presents as a solitary dome-shaped skin-colored papule on the nose or face of adults. In children, angiofibromas often occur as multiple lesions in association with familial syndromes such as tuberous sclerosis. [230,231]

Histologic Findings

Angiofibroma is characterized by superficial dermal proliferation of mononuclear or multinuclear spindle to stellate fibrohistiocytic cells often associated with dilated dermal vessels and a collagenous stroma. Concentric perivascular or periadnexal fibrosis is typically observed. Epidermal changes such as obliteration of rete ridges and junctional melanocytic hyperplasia may be seen. Several histologic variants have been described that can occasionally cause diagnostic confusion. These variants include cellular, clear cell, granular cell, inflammatory, pleomorphic, and epithelioid fibrous papule.[226]

Differential Diagnosis

The frequent presence of a subtle increase in plump single melanocytes over angiofibroma was formerly used to infer that the lesion represented a sclerosed melanocytic process, and this remains an occasional differential diagnosis, particularly for epithelioid fibrous papule. It is easily resolved with immunohistochemistry. Parenthetically, MITF usually stains the cells of fibrous papule (unpublished observation). Dermatofibroma is rare on the face. It is often more cellular and associated with thickened collagen fibers.

The constituent cells show a storiform rather than perivascular or perifollicular arrangement. The mesenchymal portion of fibrofolliculoma/trichodiscoma shows a significant overlap with fibrous papule, although the former entities include a malformed pilosebaceous component.

CAPSULE SUMMARY

ANGIOFIBROMA (FIBROUS PAPULE OF THE FACE)

Angiofibroma (*fibrous papule* of the nose or face, *adenoma sebaceum*) is a well-defined proliferation of spindle to epithelioid cells cuffing vascular and follicular structures in the superficial dermis. It can present as multiple facial lesions in children in association with familial syndromes such as tuberous sclerosis and Birt-Hogg-Dube syndrome. There are several histologic variants such as cellular, epithelioid, and granular cell angiofibroma, which may mimic other fibrohistiocytic or melanocytic neoplasms.

REFERENCES

1. Hafner C, van Oers JM, Vogt T, et al. Mosaicism of activating FGFR3 mutations in human skin causes epidermal nevi. *J Clin Invest.* 2006;116:2201-2207.
2. Adams BB, Mutasim DF. Adult onset verrucous epidermal nevus. *J Am Acad Dermatol.* 1999;41:824-826.
3. Meschia JF, Junkins E, Hofman KJ. Familial systematized epidermal nevus syndrome. *Am J Med Genet.* 1992;44:664-667.
4. Alsaleh QA, Nanda A, Hassab-el-Naby HM, Sakr MF. Familial inflammatory linear verrucous epidermal nevus (ILVEN). *Int J Dermatol.* 1994;33:52-54.
5. Goldman K, Don PC. Adult onset of inflammatory linear verrucous epidermal nevus in a mother and her daughter. *Dermatology.* 1994;189:170-172.
6. Paller AS, Syder AJ, Chan YM, et al. Genetic and clinical mosaicism in a type of epidermal nevus. *N Engl J Med.* 1994;331:1408-1415.
7. Bourdeaut F, Herault A, Gentien D, et al. Mosaicism for oncogenic G12D KRAS mutation associated with epidermal nevus, polycystic kidneys and rhabdomyosarcoma. *J Med Genet.* 2010;47:859-862.
8. Hafner C, Lopez-Knowles E, Luis NM, et al. Oncogenic PIK3CA mutations occur in epidermal nevi and seborrheic keratoses with a characteristic mutation pattern. *Proc Natl Acad Sci U S A.* 2007;104:13450-13454.
9. Su WP. Histopathologic varieties of epidermal nevus. A study of 160 cases. *Am J Dermatopathol.* 1982;4:161-170.
10. Reddy BS, Thadeus J, Kumar SK, Jaishanker T, Garg BR. Generalized epidermolytic hyperkeratosis in a child born to a parent with systematized epidermolytic linear epidermal nevus. *Int J Dermatol.* 1997;36:198-200.
11. Tsubota A, Akiyama M, Sakai K, et al. Keratin 1 gene mutation detected in epidermal nevus with epidermolytic hyperkeratosis. *J Invest Dermatol.* 2007;127:1371-1374.
12. Goldberg EI, Lefkovits AM, Sapadin AN. Zosteriform Darier's disease versus acantholytic dyskeratotic epidermal nevus. *Mt Sinai J Med.* 2001;68:339-341.
13. Munro CS, Cox NH. An acantholytic dyskeratotic epidermal naevus with other features of Darier's disease on the same side of the body. *Br J Dermatol.* 1992;127:168-171.

14. Cambiaghi S, Brusasco A, Grimalt R, Caputo R. Acantholytic dyskeratotic epidermal nevus as a mosaic form of Darier's disease. *J Am Acad Dermatol*. 1995;32:284-286.

15. Torrelo A, Colmenero I, Kristal L, et al. Papular epidermal nevus with "skyline" basal cell layer (PENS). *J Am Acad Dermatol*. 2011;64:888-892.

16. Zahn CA, Itin P. Papular epidermal nevus with "Skyline" basal cell layer syndrome—natural course: case report and literature review. *Case Rep Dermatol*. 2017;9:1-5.

17. Altman J, Mehregan AH. Inflammatory linear verrucose epidermal nevus. *Arch Dermatol*. 1971;104:385-389.

18. Rogers M, McCrossin I, Commens C. Epidermal nevi and the epidermal nevus syndrome. A review of 131 cases. *J Am Acad Dermatol*. 1989;20: 476-488.

19. Kawaguchi H, Takeuchi M, Ono H, Nakajima H. Adult onset of inflammatory linear verrucous epidermal nevus. *J Dermatol*. 1999;26:599-602.

20. Welch ML, Smith KJ, Skelton HG, et al. Immunohistochemical features in inflammatory linear verrucous epidermal nevi suggest a distinctive pattern of clonal dysregulation of growth. Military Medical Consortium for the Advancement of Retroviral Research. *J Am Acad Dermatol*. 1993;29:242-248.

21. Vissers WH, Muys L, Erp PE, de Jong EM, van de Kerkhof PC. Immunohistochemical differentiation between inflammatory linear verrucous epidermal nevus (ILVEN) and psoriasis. *Eur J Dermatol*. 2004;14:216-220.

22. Lee SH, Rogers M. Inflammatory linear verrucous epidermal naevi: a review of 23 cases. *Australas J Dermatol*. 2001;42:252-256.

23. Oram Y, Arisoy AE, Hazneci E, Gurer I, Muezzinoglu B, Arisoy ES. Bilateral inflammatory linear verrucous epidermal nevus associated with psoriasis. *Cutis*. 1996;57:275-278.

24. Golitz LE, Weston WL. Inflammatory linear verrucous epidermal nevus. Association with epidermal nevus syndrome. *Arch Dermatol*. 1979;115:1208-1209.

25. Al-Enezi S, Huber AM, Krafchik BR, Laxer RM. Inflammatory linear verrucous epidermal nevus and arthritis: a new association. *J Pediatr*. 2001;138:602-604.

26. Kong AS, Williams RL, Rhyne R, et al. Acanthosis nigricans: high prevalence and association with diabetes in a practice-based research network consortium: a PRImary care Multi-Ethnic network (PRIME Net) study. *J Am Board Fam Med*. 2010;23:476-485.

27. Stals H, Vercammen C, Peeters C, Morren MA. Acanthosis nigricans caused by nicotinic acid: case report and review of the literature. *Dermatology*. 1994;189:203-206.

28. Baird JS, Johnson JL, Elliott-Mills D, Opas LM. Systemic lupus erythematosus with acanthosis nigricans, hyperpigmentation, and insulin receptor antibody. *Lupus*. 1997;6:275-278.

29. Tuna Castro MA, Garcia Kutzbach A. Acanthosis nigricans associated with longstanding dermatomyositis. *J Rheumatol*. 1996;23:1487-1488.

30. Kura MM, Sanghavi SA. Acral Acanthosis nigricans in a case of scleroderma. *Indian J Dermatol*. 2015;60:423.

31. Schwartz RA. Acanthosis nigricans. *J Am Acad Dermatol*. 1994;31:1-19; quiz 20-22.

32. Berk DR, Spector EB, Bayliss SJ. Familial acanthosis nigricans due to K650T FGFR3 mutation. *Arch Dermatol*. 2007;143:1153-1156.

33. Wang L, Long H, Wen H, Liu Z, Ling T. Image gallery: generalized mucosal and cutaneous papillomatosis, a unique sign of malignant acanthosis nigricans. *Br J Dermatol*. 2017;176:e99.

34. Gungor S, Topal I. Images in clinical medicine. Tripe palms. *N Engl J Med*. 2014;370:558.

35. Ersoy-Evans S, Sahin S, Mancini AJ, Paller AS, Guitart J. The acanthosis nigricans form of epidermal nevus. *J Am Acad Dermatol*. 2006;55: 696-698.

36. Huang W, Ong G, Chong WS. Clinicopathological and diagnostic characterization of confluent and reticulate papillomatosis of Gougerot and Carteaud: a retrospective study in a South-East Asian population. *Am J Clin Dermatol*. 2015;16:131-136.

37. Henning JP, de Wit RF. Familial occurrence of confluent and reticulated papillomatosis. *Arch Dermatol*. 1981;117:809-810.

38. Inaloz HS, Patel GK, Knight AG. Familial confluent and reticulated papillomatosis. *Arch Dermatol*. 2002;138:276-277.

39. Fukumoto T, Kozaru T, Sakaguchi M, Oka M. Concomitant confluent and reticulated papillomatosis and acanthosis nigricans in an obese girl with insulin resistance successfully treated with oral minocycline: case report and published work review. *J Dermatol*. 2017;44:954-958.

40. Lim JH, Tey HL, Chong WS. Confluent and reticulated papillomatosis: diagnostic and treatment challenges. *Clin Cosmet Investig Dermatol*. 2016;9:217-223.

41. Lee E, Kang BS, Cho SH, Lee JD. Three cases of concomitant acanthosis nigricans with confluent and reticulated papillomatosis in obese patients. *Ann Dermatol*. 2008;20:94-97.

42. Hirokawa M, Matsumoto M, Iizuka H. Confluent and reticulated papillomatosis: a case with concurrent acanthosis nigricans associated with obesity and insulin resistance. *Dermatology*. 1994;188:148-151.

43. Tamraz H, Raffoul M, Kurban M, Kibbi AG, Abbas O. Confluent and reticulated papillomatosis: clinical and histopathological study of 10 cases from Lebanon. *J Eur Acad Dermatol Venereol*. 2013;27:e119-e123.

44. Scheinfeld N. Confluent and reticulated papillomatosis: a review of the literature. *Am J Clin Dermatol*. 2006;7:305-313.

45. Jones AL, Koerner RJ, Natarajan S, Perry JD, Goodfellow M. Dietzia papillomatosis sp. nov., a novel actinomycete isolated from the skin of an immunocompetent patient with confluent and reticulated papillomatosis. *Int J Syst Evol Microbiol*. 2008;58:68-72.

46. Natarajan S, Milne D, Jones AL, Goodfellow M, Perry J, Koerner RJ. Dietzia strain X: a newly described Actinomycete isolated from confluent and reticulated papillomatosis. *Br J Dermatol*. 2005;153:825-827.

47. Davis MD, Weenig RH, Camilleri MJ. Confluent and reticulate papillomatosis (Gougerot-Carteaud syndrome): a minocycline-responsive dermatosis without evidence for yeast in pathogenesis. A study of 39 patients and a proposal of diagnostic criteria. *Br J Dermatol*. 2006;154: 287-293.

48. Yesudian P, Kamalam S, Razack A. Confluent and reticulated papillomatosis (Gougerot-Carteaud). An abnormal host reaction to Malassezia furfur. *Acta Derm Venereol*. 1973;53:381-384.

49. Park YJ, Kang HY, Lee ES, Kim YC. Differentiating confluent and reticulated papillomatosis from acanthosis nigricans. *J Cutan Pathol*. 2015;42(12):944-952.

50. Barton DT, Zens MS, Nelson HH, et al. Distinct histologic subtypes and risk factors for early onset basal cell carcinoma: a population-based case control study from New Hampshire. *J Invest Dermatol*. 2016;136: 533-535.

51. Griffin JR, Cohen PR, Tschen JA, et al. Basal cell carcinoma in childhood: case report and literature review. *J Am Acad Dermatol*. 2007;57: S97-S102.

52. Corona R, Dogliotti E, D'Errico M, et al. Risk factors for basal cell carcinoma in a Mediterranean population: role of recreational sun exposure early in life. *Arch Dermatol*. 2001;137:1162-1168.

53. Bakos RM, Kriz M, Muhlstadt M, Kunte C, Ruzicka T, Berking C. Risk factors for early-onset basal cell carcinoma in a German institution. *Eur J Dermatol*. 2011;21:705-709.

54. Armstrong BK, Kricker A. The epidemiology of UV induced skin cancer. *J Photochem Photobiol B*. 2001;63:8-18.

55. Binkley GW, Johnson HH Jr. Epithelioma adenoides cysticum; basal cell nevi, agenesis of the corpus callosum and dental cysts; a clinical and autopsy study. *AMA Arch Derm Syphilol*. 1951;63:73-84.

56. Johnson RL, Rothman AL, Xie J, et al. Human homolog of patched, a candidate gene for the basal cell nevus syndrome. *Science*. 1996;272: 1668-1671.

57. da Silva Calixto P, Lopes OS, Dos Santos Maia M, et al. Single-nucleotide polymorphisms of the MSH2 and MLH1 genes, potential molecular markers for susceptibility to the development of basal cell carcinoma in the Brazilian population. *Pathol Oncol Res*. 2018;24(3):489-496.

58. Ferrucci LM, Cartmel B, Molinaro AM, et al. Host phenotype characteristics and MC1R in relation to early-onset basal cell carcinoma. *J Invest Dermatol*. 2012;132:1272-1279.

59. Schulman JM, Oh DH, Sanborn JZ, Pincus L, McCalmont TH, Cho RJ. Multiple hereditary infundibulocystic basal cell carcinoma syndrome associated with a germline SUFU mutation. *JAMA Dermatol.* 2016;152:323-327.

60. Requena L, Farina MC, Robledo M, et al. Multiple hereditary infundibulocystic basal cell carcinomas: a genodermatosis different from nevoid basal cell carcinoma syndrome. *Arch Dermatol.* 1999;135:1227-1235.

61. Zoccali G, Pajand R, Giuliani M. Basal cell carcinoma in childhood: a case report. *Pediatr Dermatol.* 2013;30:144-145.

62. Gorlin RJ. Nevoid basal cell carcinoma syndrome. *Dermatol Clin.* 1995;13:113-125.

63. Solis DC, Kwon GP, Ransohoff KJ, et al. Risk factors for basal cell carcinoma among patients with basal cell nevus syndrome: development of a basal cell nevus syndrome patient registry. *JAMA Dermatol.* 2017;153(2):189-192.

64. North JP, McCalmont TH, LeBoit P. Palmar pits associated with the nevoid basal cell carcinoma syndrome. *J Cutan Pathol.* 2012;39:735-738.

65. de la Luz Orozco-Covarrubias M, Tamayo-Sanchez L, Duran-McKinster C, Ridaura C, Ruiz-Maldonado R. Malignant cutaneous tumors in children. Twenty years of experience at a large pediatric hospital. *J Am Acad Dermatol.* 1994;30:243-249.

66. Fogel AL, Sarin KY, Teng JMC. Genetic diseases associated with an increased risk of skin cancer development in childhood. *Curr Opin Pediatr.* 2017;29:426-433.

67. Charles CA, Connelly EA, Aber CG, Herman AR, Schachner LA. A rare presentation of squamous cell carcinoma in a patient with PIBIDS-type trichothiodystrophy. *Pediatr Dermatol.* 2008;25:264-267.

68. Wong JY, Kuzel P, Mullen J, et al. Cutaneous squamous cell carcinoma in two pediatric lung transplant patients on prolonged voriconazole treatment. *Pediatr Transplant.* 2014;18:E200-E207.

69. Mizutani H, Masuda K, Nakamura N, Takenaka H, Tsuruta D, Katoh N. Cutaneous and laryngeal squamous cell carcinoma in mixed epidermolysis bullosa, kindler syndrome. *Case Rep Dermatol.* 2012;4:133-138.

70. Oh PS, Gill KZ, Lynch LJ, Cowles RA. Primary squamous cell carcinoma arising at a gastrostomy tube site. *J Pediatr Surg.* 2011;46:756-758.

71. Petrov I, Gantcheva M, Miteva L, Vassileva S, Pramatarov K. Lower lip squamous cell carcinoma in disabling pansclerotic morphea of childhood. *Pediatr Dermatol.* 2009;26:59-61.

72. Euvrard S, Kanitakis J, Cochat P, Claudy A. Skin cancers following pediatric organ transplantation. *Dermatol Surg.* 2004;30:616-621.

73. Toyoda H, Ido M, Nakanishi K, et al. Multiple cutaneous squamous cell carcinomas in a patient with interferon gamma receptor 2 (IFN gamma R2) deficiency. *J Med Genet.* 2010;47:631-634.

74. Weitzner JM, Fields KW, Robinson MJ. Pediatric bowenoid papulosis: risks and management. *Pediatr Dermatol.* 1989;6:303-305.

75. Wright S, Levy IS. White sponge naevus and ocular coloboma. *Arch Dis Child.* 1991;66:514-516.

76. Schmitt J, Seidler A, Diepgen TL, Bauer A. Occupational ultraviolet light exposure increases the risk for the development of cutaneous squamous cell carcinoma: a systematic review and meta-analysis. *Br J Dermatol.* 2011;164:291-307.

77. Bouwes Bavinck JN, Feltkamp MCW, Green AC, et al. Human papillomavirus and post-transplant cutaneous squamous-cell carcinoma: a multicenter, prospective cohort study. *Am J Transplant.* 2018;18(5):1220-1230.

78. Pearce MS, Parker L, Cotterill SJ, Gordon PM, Craft AW. Skin cancer in children and young adults: 28 years' experience from the Northern Region Young Person's Malignant Disease Registry, UK. *Melanoma Res.* 2003;13:421-426.

79. Sanjeeta N, Nandini DB, Premlata T, Banerjee S. White sponge nevus: report of three cases in a single family. *J Oral Maxillofac Pathol.* 2016;20:300-303.

80. Liu X, Li Q, Gao Y, Song S, Hua H. Mutational analysis in familial and sporadic patients with white sponge naevus. *Br J Dermatol.* 2011;165:448-451.

81. Lopez Jornet P. White sponge nevus: presentation of a new family. *Pediatr Dermatol.* 2008;25:116-117.

82. Richard G, De Laurenzi V, Didona B, Bale SJ, Compton JG. Keratin 13 point mutation underlies the hereditary mucosal epithelial disorder white sponge nevus. *Nat Genet.* 1995;11:453-455.

83. Rugg EL, McLean WH, Allison WE, et al. A mutation in the mucosal keratin K4 is associated with oral white sponge nevus. *Nat Genet.* 1995;11:450-452.

84. de Haseth SB, Bakker E, Vermeer MH, et al. A novel keratin 13 variant in a four-generation family with white sponge nevus. *Clin Case Rep.* 2017;5:1503-1509.

85. Songu M, Adibelli H, Diniz G. White sponge nevus: clinical suspicion and diagnosis. *Pediatr Dermatol.* 2012;29:495-497.

86. Frithiof L, Banoczy J. White sponge nevus (leukoedema exfoliativum mucosae oris): ultrastructural observations. *Oral Surg Oral Med Oral Pathol.* 1976;41:607-622.

87. Alper J, Holmes LB, Mihm MC Jr. Birthmarks with serious medical significance: nevocullular nevi, sebaceous nevi, and multiple cafe au lait spots. *J Pediatr.* 1979;95:696-700.

88. Morioka S. The natural history of nevus sebaceus. *J Cutan Pathol.* 1985;12:200-213.

89. Sahl WJ Jr. Familial nevus sebaceus of Jadassohn: occurrence in three generations. *J Am Acad Dermatol.* 1990;22:853-854.

90. Aslam A, Salam A, Griffiths CE, McGrath JA. Naevus sebaceus: a mosaic RASopathy. *Clin Exp Dermatol.* 2014;39:1-6.

91. Groesser L, Herschberger E, Ruetten A, et al. Postzygotic HRAS and KRAS mutations cause nevus sebaceous and Schimmelpenning syndrome. *Nat Genet.* 2012;44:783-787.

92. Kavak A, Ozcelik D, Belenli O, Buyukbabani N, Saglam I, Lazova R. A unique location of naevus sebaceus: labia minora. *J Eur Acad Dermatol Venereol.* 2008;22:1136-1138.

93. Yamane N, Kato N, Yanagi T, Osawa R. Naevus sebaceus on the female breast accompanied with a tubular apocrine adenoma and a syringocystadenoma papilliferum. *Br J Dermatol.* 2007;156:1397-1399.

94. Bothwell NE, Willard CC, Sorensen DM, Downey TJ. A rare case of a sebaceous nevus in the external auditory canal. *Ear Nose Throat J.* 2003;82:38-41.

95. Kanekura T, Kawahira M, Kanzaki T. Three cases of organoid nevus on the trunk and extremity. *J Dermatol.* 1994;21:771-775.

96. Morency R, Labelle H. Nevus sebaceus of Jadassohn: a rare oral presentation. *Oral Surg Oral Med Oral Pathol.* 1987;64:460-462.

97. Hsu MC, Liau JY, Hong JL, et al. Secondary neoplasms arising from nevus sebaceus: a retrospective study of 450 cases in Taiwan. *J Dermatol.* 2016;43:175-180.

98. Idriss MH, Elston DM. Secondary neoplasms associated with nevus sebaceus of Jadassohn: a study of 707 cases. *J Am Acad Dermatol.* 2014;70:332-337.

99. Cribier B, Scrivener Y, Grosshans E. Tumors arising in nevus sebaceus: a study of 596 cases. *J Am Acad Dermatol.* 2000;42:263-268.

100. Ireland AM, Harvey NT, Berry BD, Wood BA. Paediatric cutaneous adnexal tumours: a study of 559 cases. *Pathology.* 2017;49:50-54.

101. Polat M, Altunay Tuman B, Sahin A, Dogan U, Boran C. Bilateral nevus comedonicus of the eyelids associated with bladder cancer and successful treatment with topical tretinoin. *Dermatol Ther.* 2016;29:479-481.

102. Levinsohn JL, Sugarman JL, McNiff JM, Antaya RJ, Choate KA; Yale Center for Mendelian Genomics. Somatic mutations in NEK9 cause nevus comedonicus. *Am J Hum Genet.* 2016;98:1030-1037.

103. Samuelov L, Sarig O, Gat A, Halachmi S, Shalev S, Sprecher E. Extensive lentigo simplex, linear epidermolytic naevus and epidermolytic naevus comedonicus caused by a somatic mutation in KRT10. *Br J Dermatol.* 2015;173:293-296.

104. Munro CS, Wilkie AO. Epidermal mosaicism producing localised acne: somatic mutation in FGFR2. *Lancet.* 1998;352:704-705.

105. Ganjoo S, Mohanan S, Kumari R, Thappa DM, Rajesh NG. Extensive nevus comedonicus involving the palm: questionable role of the pilosebaceous unit in pathogenesis. *Pediatr Dermatol.* 2014;31:e96-e99.

106. Harper KE, Spielvogel RL. Nevus comedonicus of the palm and wrist. Case report with review of five previously reported cases. *J Am Acad Dermatol*. 1985;12:185-188.

107. Wood MG, Thew MA. Nevus comedonicus. A case with palmar involvement and review of the literature. *Arch Dermatol*. 1968;98:111-116.

108. Zarkik S, Bouhllab J, Methqal A, Afifi Y, Senouci K, Hassam B. Keratoacanthoma arising in nevus comedonicus. *Dermatol Online J*. 2012;18:4.

109. Alpsoy E, Durusoy C, Ozbilim G, Karpuzoglu G, Yilmaz E. Nevus comedonicus syndrome: a case associated with multiple basal cell carcinomas and a rudimentary toe. *Int J Dermatol*. 2005;44:499-501.

110. Walling HW, Swick BL. Squamous cell carcinoma arising in nevus comedonicus. *Dermatol Surg*. 2009;35:144-146.

111. Kaliyadan F, Nampoothiri S, Sunitha V, Kuruvilla VE. Nevus comedonicus syndrome: nevus comedonicus associated with ipsilateral polysyndactyly and bilateral oligodontia. *Pediatr Dermatol*. 2010;27:377-379.

112. Patrizi A, Neri I, Fiorentini C, Marzaduri S. Nevus comedonicus syndrome: a new pediatric case. *Pediatr Dermatol*. 1998;15:304-306.

113. Sinha A, Natarajan S. Linear morphea, nevus comedonicus, and lichen striatus in a 5-year-old girl. *Pediatr Dermatol*. 2011;28:72-74.

114. Weedon D, Strutton G, Rubin A. *Weedon's skin pathology*. Edinburgh, Scotland: Churchill Livingstone/Elsevier; 2010.

115. Hall JR, Holder W, Knox JM, Knox JM, Verani R. Familial dyskeratotic comedones: a report of three cases and review of the literature. *J Am Acad Dermatol*. 1987;17:808-814.

116. Aguilera CA, De la Varga Martinez R, Garcia LO, Jimenez-Gallo D, Planelles CA, Barrios ML. Heterozygous cylindromatosis gene mutation c.1628_1629delCT in a Family with Brook-Spiegler syndrome. *Indian J Dermatol*. 2016;61:580.

117. Farkas K, Deak BK, Sanchez LC, et al. The CYLD p.R758X worldwide recurrent nonsense mutation detected in patients with multiple familial trichoepithelioma type 1, Brooke-Spiegler syndrome and familial cylindromatosis represents a mutational hotspot in the gene. *BMC Genet*. 2016;17:36.

118. Almeida S, Maillard C, Itin P, Hohl D, Huber M. Five new CYLD mutations in skin appendage tumors and evidence that aspartic acid 681 in CYLD is essential for deubiquitinase activity. *J Invest Dermatol*. 2008;128:587-593.

119. Liang YH, Gao M, Sun LD, et al. Two novel CYLD gene mutations in Chinese families with trichoepithelioma and a literature review of 16 families with trichoepithelioma reported in China. *Br J Dermatol*. 2005;153:1213-1215.

120. Oh DH, Lane AT, Turk AE, Kohler S. A young boy with a large hemifacial plaque with histopathologic features of trichoepithelioma. *J Am Acad Dermatol*. 1997;37:881-883.

121. Geffner RE, Goslen JB, Santa Cruz DJ. Linear and dermatomal trichoepitheliomas. *J Am Acad Dermatol*. 1986;14:927-930.

122. Anderson DE, Howell JB. Epithelioma adenoides cysticum: genetic update. *Br J Dermatol*. 1976;95:225-232.

123. Inatomi Y, Yonehara T, Fujioka S, Urata J, Ohyama K, Uchino M. Familial multiple trichoepithelioma associated with subclavian-pulmonary collateral vessels and cerebral aneurysm: case report. *Neurol Med Chir (Tokyo)*. 2001;41:556-560.

124. Wallace ML, Smoller BR. Trichoepithelioma with an adjacent basal cell carcinoma, transformation or collision? *J Am Acad Dermatol*. 1997;37:343-345.

125. Autio-Harmainen H, Paakko P, Alavaikko M, Karvonen J, Leisti J. Familial occurrence of malignant lymphoepithelial lesion of the parotid gland in a Finnish family with dominantly inherited trichoepithelioma. *Cancer*. 1988;61:161-166.

126. Schulz T, Proske S, Hartschuh W, Kurzen H, Paul E, Wunsch PH. High-grade trichoblastic carcinoma arising in trichoblastoma: a rare adnexal neoplasm often showing metastatic spread. *Am J Dermatopathol*. 2005;27:9-16.

127. Rossi AM, Busam KJ, Mehrara B, Nehal KS. Desmoplastic trichoepithelioma with overlying pseudoepitheliomatous hyperplasia mimicking squamous cell carcinoma in a pediatric patient. *Dermatol Surg*. 2014;40:477-479.

128. Sellheyer K, Nelson P, Kutzner H, Patel RM. The immunohistochemical differential diagnosis of microcystic adnexal carcinoma, desmoplastic trichoepithelioma and morpheaform basal cell carcinoma using BerEP4 and stem cell markers. *J Cutan Pathol*. 2013;40:363-370.

129. Brownstein MH, Starink TM. Desmoplastic trichoepithelioma and intradermal nevus: a combined malformation. *J Am Acad Dermatol*. 1987;17:489-492.

130. Harvey NT, Leecy T, Beer TW, Wood BA. Desmoplastic trichoepitheliomas with perineural involvement. *Pathology*. 2013;45:196-198.

131. Ng DW. Trichilemmoma in childhood. *J Pediatr Health Care*. 2016;30:491-494.

132. Salem OS, Steck WD. Cowden's disease (multiple hamartoma and neoplasia syndrome). A case report and review of the English literature. *J Am Acad Dermatol*. 1983;8:686-696.

133. Ngeow J, Stanuch K, Mester JL, Barnholtz-Sloan JS, Eng C. Second malignant neoplasms in patients with Cowden syndrome with underlying germline PTEN mutations. *J Clin Oncol*. 2014;32:1818-1824.

134. Nelen MR, Padberg GW, Peeters EA, et al. Localization of the gene for Cowden disease to chromosome 10q22-23. *Nat Genet*. 1996;13:114-116.

135. Liaw D, Marsh DJ, Li J, et al. Germline mutations of the PTEN gene in Cowden disease, an inherited breast and thyroid cancer syndrome. *Nat Genet*. 1997;16:64-67.

136. Al-Zaid T, Ditelberg JS, Prieto VG, et al. Trichilemmomas show loss of PTEN in Cowden syndrome but only rarely in sporadic tumors. *J Cutan Pathol*. 2012;39:493-499.

137. Tsai JH, Huang WC, Jhuang JY, et al. Frequent activating HRAS mutations in trichilemmoma. *Br J Dermatol*. 2014;171:1073-1077.

138. Potenziani S, Applebaum D, Krishnan B, Gutierrez C, Diwan AH. Multiple clear cell acanthomas and a sebaceous lymphadenoma presenting in a patient with Cowden syndrome: a case report. *J Cutan Pathol*. 2017;44:79-82.

139. Eng C. Will the real Cowden syndrome please stand up: revised diagnostic criteria. *J Med Genet*. 2000;37:828-830.

140. Karabulut YY, Senel E, Karabulut HH, Dolek Y. Three different clinical faces of the same histopathological entity: hair follicle nevus, trichofolliculoma and accessory tragus. *An Bras Dermatol*. 2015;90:519-522.

141. Ishii N, Kawaguchi H, Takahashi K, Nakajima H. A case of congenital trichofolliculoma. *J Dermatol*. 1992;19:195-196.

142. Wu YH. Follicolusebaceous cystic hamartoma or trichofolliculoma? A spectrum of hamartomatous changes inducted by perifollicular stroma in the follicular epithelium. *J Cutan Pathol*. 2008;35:843-848.

143. Peterdy GA, Huettner PC, Rajaram V, Lind AC. Trichofolliculoma of the vulva associated with vulvar intraepithelial neoplasia: report of three cases and review of the literature. *Int J Gynecol Pathol*. 2002;21:224-230.

144. Hassan SF, Stephens E, Fallon SC, et al. Characterizing pilomatricomas in children: a single institution experience. *J Pediatr Surg*. 2013;48:1551-1556.

145. Cigliano B, Baltogiannis N, De Marco M, et al. Pilomatricoma in childhood: a retrospective study from three European paediatric centres. *Eur J Pediatr*. 2005;164:673-677.

146. Lazar AJ, Calonje E, Grayson W, et al. Pilomatrix carcinomas contain mutations in CTNNB1, the gene encoding beta-catenin. *J Cutan Pathol*. 2005;32:148-157.

147. Agoston AT, Liang CW, Richkind KE, Fletcher JA, Vargas SO. Trisomy 18 is a consistent cytogenetic feature in pilomatricoma. *Mod Pathol*. 2010;23:1147-1150.

148. Bendelsmith CR, Skrypek MM, Patel SR, Pond DA, Linabery AM, Bendel AE. Multiple pilomatrixomas in a survivor of WNT-activated medulloblastoma leading to the discovery of a germline APC mutation and the diagnosis of familial adenomatous polyposis. *Pediatr Blood Cancer*. 2018; 65(1):e26756.

149. Chmara M, Wernstedt A, Wasag B, et al. Multiple pilomatricomas with somatic CTNNB1 mutations in children with constitutive mismatch repair deficiency. *Genes Chromosomes Cancer*. 2013;52:656-664.

150. Hamahata A, Kamei W, Ishikawa M, Konoeda H, Yamaki T, Sakurai H. Multiple pilomatricomas in Kabuki syndrome. *Pediatr Dermatol.* 2013;30:253-255.

151. Chan JJ, Tey HL. Multiple pilomatricomas: case presentation and review of the literature. *Dermatol Online J.* 2010;16:2.

152. Wood S, Nguyen D, Hutton K, Dickson W. Pilomatricomas in Turner syndrome. *Pediatr Dermatol.* 2008;25:449-451.

153. Cambiaghi S, Ermacora E, Brusasco A, Canzi L, Caputo R. Multiple pilomatricomas in Rubinstein-Taybi syndrome: a case report. *Pediatr Dermatol.* 1994;11:21-25.

154. Cozzi DA, d'Ambrosio G, Cirigliano E, et al. Giant pilomatricoma mimicking a malignant parotid mass. *J Pediatr Surg.* 2011;46:1855-1858.

155. Hassanein AH, Alomari AI, Schmidt BA, Greene AK. Pilomatrixoma imitating infantile hemangioma. *J Craniofac Surg.* 2011;22:734-736.

156. Ardakani NM, Palmer DL, Wood BA. Malignant melanocytic matricoma: a report of 2 cases and review of the literature. *Am J Dermatopathol.* 2016;38:33-38.

157. Otero MN, Trujillo CP, Parra-Medina R, Morales SD. Metastatic malignant pilomatrixoma in an 8-year-old girl misdiagnosed as a recurrent pilomatrixoma. *Am J Dermatopathol.* 2017;39:e41-e43.

158. Joshi A, Sah SP, Agrawal CS, Jacob M, Agarwalla A. Pilomatrix carcinoma in a child. *Acta Derm-Venereol.* 1999;79:476-477.

159. Cooper PH, Fechner RE. Pilomatricoma-like changes in the epidermal cysts of Gardner's syndrome. *J Am Acad Dermatol.* 1983;8:639-644.

160. Karg E, Korom I, Varga E, Ban G, Turi S. Congenital syringocystadenoma papilliferum. *Pediatr Dermatol.* 2008;25:132-133.

161. Jordan JA, Brown OE, Biavati MJ, Manning SC. Congenital syringocystadenoma papilliferum of the ear and neck treated with the CO_2 laser. *Int J Pediatr Otorhinolaryngol.* 1996;38:81-87.

162. Levinsohn JL, Sugarman JL, Bilguvar K, McNiff JM, Choate KA, The Yale Center For Mendelian G. Somatic V600E BRAF mutation in linear and sporadic syringocystadenoma papilliferum. *J Invest Dermatol.* 2015;135:2536-2538.

163. Böni R, Xin H, Hohl D, Panizzon R, Burg G. Syringocystadenoma papilliferum: a study of potential tumor suppressor genes. *Am J Dermatopathol.* 2001;23:87-89.

164. Kishimoto S, Wakabayashi S, Yamamoto M, Noda Y, Takenaka H, Yasuno H. Apocrine acrosyringeal keratosis in association with syringocystoadenoma papilliferum. *Br J Dermatol.* 2000;142:543-547.

165. Pruzan DL, Esterly NB, Prose NS. Eruptive syringoma. *Arch Dermatol.* 1989;125:1119-1120.

166. Furue M, Hori Y, Nakabayashi Y. Clear-cell syringoma. Association with diabetes mellitus. *Am J Dermatopathol.* 1984;6:131-138.

167. Wu WM, Lee YS. Autosomal dominant multiple syringomas linked to chromosome 16q22. *Br J Dermatol.* 2010;162:1083-1087.

168. Garrido-Ruiz MC, Enguita AB, Navas R, Polo I, Rodriguez Peralto JL. Eruptive syringoma developed over a waxing skin area. *Am J Dermatopathol.* 2008;30:377-380.

169. Williams K, Shinkai K. Evaluation and management of the patient with multiple syringomas: a systematic review of the literature. *J Am Acad Dermatol.* 2016;74:1234.e9-1240.e9.

170. Sadeghian G, Ziaei H. Multiple giant vulvar syringoma: an extraordinary report. *Skinmed.* 2013;11:305-306.

171. Blasdale C, McLelland J. Solitary giant vulval syringoma. *Br J Dermatol.* 1999;141:374-375.

172. Wallace JS, Bond JS, Seidel GD, Samie FH. An important mimicker: plaque-type syringoma mistakenly diagnosed as microcystic adnexal carcinoma. *Dermatol Surg.* 2014;40:810-812.

173. Suwattee P, McClelland MC, Huiras EE, et al. Plaque-type syringoma: two cases misdiagnosed as microcystic adnexal carcinoma. *J Cutan Pathol.* 2008;35:570-574.

174. Soler-Carrillo J, Estrach T, Mascaro JM. Eruptive syringoma: 27 new cases and review of the literature. *J Eur Acad Dermatol Venereol.* 2001;15:242-246.

175. Ceulen RP, Van Marion AM, Steijlen PM, Frank J, Poblete-Gutierrez P. Multiple unilateral skin tumors suggest type 1 segmental manifestation of familial syringoma. *Eur J Dermatol.* 2008;18:285-288.

176. Marzano AV, Fiorani R, Girgenti V, Crosti C, Alessi E. Familial syringoma: report of two cases with a published work review and the unique association with steatocystoma multiplex. *J Dermatol.* 2009;36:154-158.

177. Deen K, Curchin C, Wu J. Incidental syringomas of the scalp in a patient with scarring alopecia. *Case Rep Dermatol.* 2015;7:171-177.

178. White J, Short K, Salisbury J, Fuller L. A novel case of linear syringomatous hamartoma. *Clin Exp Dermatol.* 2006;31:222-224.

179. Urban CD, Cannon JR, Cole RD. Eruptive syringomas in Down's syndrome. *Arch Dermatol.* 1981;117:374-375.

180. Uede K, Yamamoto Y, Furukawa F. Brooke-Spiegler syndrome associated with cylindroma, trichoepithelioma, spiradenoma, and syringoma. *J Dermatol.* 2004;31:32-38.

181. Dupre A, Carrere S, Bonafe JL, Christol B, Lassere J, Touron P. Eruptive generalized syringomas, milium and atrophoderma vermiculata. Nicolau and Balus' syndrome (author's transl) [in French]. *Dermatologica.* 1981;162:281-286.

182. Nguyen V, Buka RL, Roberts BJ, Eichenfield LF. Cutaneous manifestations of Costello syndrome. *Int J Dermatol.* 2007;46:72-76.

183. Kazakov DV, Bouda J Jr, Kacerovska D, Michal M. Vulvar syringomas with deep extension: a potential histopathologic mimic of microcystic adnexal carcinoma. *Int J Gynecol Pathol.* 2011;30:92-94.

184. Kazakov DV, Vanecek T, Zelger B, et al. Multiple (familial) trichoepitheliomas: a clinicopathological and molecular biological study, including CYLD and PTCH gene analysis, of a series of 16 patients. *Am J Dermatopathol.* 2011;33:251-265.

185. Bignell GR, Warren W, Seal S, et al. Identification of the familial cylindromatosis tumour-suppressor gene. *Nat Genet.* 2000;25:160-165.

186. Sun SC. CYLD: a tumor suppressor deubiquitinase regulating NF-kappaB activation and diverse biological processes. *Cell Death Differ.* 2010;17:25-34.

187. Leonard N, Chaggar R, Jones C, Takahashi M, Nikitopoulou A, Lakhani SR. Loss of heterozygosity at cylindromatosis gene locus, CYLD, in sporadic skin adnexal tumours. *J Clin Pathol.* 2001;54:689-692.

188. Trompouki E, Hatzivassiliou E, Tsichritzis T, Farmer H, Ashworth A, Mosialos G. CYLD is a deubiquitinating enzyme that negatively regulates NF-kappaB activation by TNFR family members. *Nature.* 2003;424:793-796.

189. Durani BK, Kurzen H, Jaeckel A, Kuner N, Naeher H, Hartschuh W. Malignant transformation of multiple dermal cylindromas. *Br J Dermatol.* 2001;145:653-656.

190. Pizinger K, Michal M. Malignant cylindroma in Brooke-Spiegler syndrome. *Dermatology.* 2000;201:255-257.

191. Cotton D, Slater D, Rooney N, Goepel J, Mills P. Giant vascular eccrine spiradenomas: a report of two cases with histology, immunohistology and electron microscopy. *Histopathology.* 1986;10:1093-1099.

192. Gupta S, Radotra B, Kaur I, Handa S, Kumar B. Multiple linear eccrine spiradenomas with eyelid involvement. *J Eur Acad Dermatol Venereol.* 2001;15:163-166.

193. Ikeya T. Multiple linear eccrine spiradenoma associated with multiple trichoepithelioma. *J Dermatol.* 1987;14:48-53.

194. Gordon S, Styron BT, Haggstrom A. Pediatric segmental eccrine spiradenomas: a case report and review of the literature. *Pediatr Dermatol.* 2013;30:e285-286.

195. Battistella M, Langbein L, Peltre B, Cribier B. From hidroacanthoma simplex to poroid hidradenoma: clinicopathologic and immunohistochemic study of poroid neoplasms and reappraisal of their histogenesis. *Am J Dermatopathol.* 2010;32:459-468.

196. Orlandi C, Arcangeli F, Patrizi A, Neri I. Eccrine poroma in a child. *Pediatr Dermatol.* 2005;22:279-280.

197. Valverde K, Senger C, Ngan BY, Chan HS. Eccrine porocarcinoma in a child that evolved rapidly from an eccrine poroma. *Med Pediatr Oncol.* 2001;37:412-414.

198. Majmudar V, Schollenberg E, Fish J, Lara-Corrales I. Pediatric dermatology photoquiz: an ulcerated nodule on the abdomen of a child. Eccrine poroma. *Pediatr Dermatol.* 2016;33:87-88.

199. Ichihashi N, Kitajima Y. Loss of heterozygosity of adenomatous polyposis coli gene in cutaneous tumors as determined by using polymerase chain reaction and paraffin section preparations. *J Dermatol Sci.* 2000;22:102-106.

200. Mayo TT, Kole L, Elewski B. Eccrine poromatosis: case report, review of the literature, and treatment. *Skin Appendage Disord.* 2015;1:95-98.

201. Rahbari H. Syringoacanthoma: acanthotic lesion of the acrosyringium. *Arch Dermatol.* 1984;120:751-756.

202. Starink TM. Eccrine syringofibroadenoma: multiple lesions representing a new cutaneous marker of the Schöpf syndrome, and solitary nonhereditary tumors. *J Am Acad Dermatol.* 1997;36:569-576.

203. Carlson JA, Rohwedder A, Daulat S, Schwartz J, Schaller J. Detection of human papillomavirus type 10 DNA in eccrine syringofibroadenomatosis occurring in Clouston's syndrome. *J Am Acad Dermatol.* 1999;40:259-262.

204. Ahmed A, Kim W, Speiser J. Mucinous hidradenoma in a child: a case report and review of the literature. *J Cutan Pathol.* 2017;44(7):643-646.

205. Winnes M, Mölne L, Suurküla M, et al. Frequent fusion of the CRTC1 and MAML2 genes in clear cell variants of cutaneous hidradenomas. *Genes Chromosomes Cancer.* 2007;46:559-563.

206. Möller E, Stenman G, Mandahl N, et al. POU5F1, encoding a key regulator of stem cell pluripotency, is fused to EWSR1 in hidradenoma of the skin and mucoepidermoid carcinoma of the salivary glands. *J Pathol.* 2008;215:78-86.

207. Green M, Mitchum M, Marquart J, Bowden LP III, Bingham J. Microcystic adnexal carcinoma in the axilla of an 18-year-old woman. *Pediatr Dermatol.* 2014;31:e145-e148.

208. Friedman PM, Friedman RH, Jiang SB, Nouri K, Amonette R, Robins P. Microcystic adnexal carcinoma: collaborative series review and update. *J Am Acad Dermatol.* 1999;41:225-231.

209. McAlvany JP, Stonecipher MR, Leshin B, Prichard E, White W. Sclerosing sweat duct carcinoma in an 11-year-old boy. *J Dermatol Surg Oncol.* 1994;20:767-768.

210. Borenstein A, Seidman DS, Trau H, Tsur H. Microcystic adnexal carcinoma following radiotherapy in childhood. *Am J Med Sci.* 1991;301:259-261.

211. Smart DR, Taintor AR, Kelly ME, et al. Microcystic adnexal carcinoma: the first reported congenital case. *Pediatr Dermatol.* 2011;28:35-38.

212. Antley CA, Carney M, Smoller BR. Microcystic adnexal carcinoma arising in the setting of previous radiation therapy. *J Cutan Pathol.* 1999;26:48-50.

213. Abbate M, Zeitouni NC, Seyler M, Hicks W, Loree T, Cheney RT. Clinical course, risk factors, and treatment of microcystic adnexal carcinoma: a short series report. *Dermatol Surg.* 2003;29:1035-1038.

214. Lei JY, Wang Y, Jaffe ES, et al. Microcystic adnexal carcinoma associated with primary immunodeficiency, recurrent diffuse herpes simplex virus infection, and cutaneous T-cell lymphoma. *Am J Dermatopathol.* 2000;22:524-529.

215. Carroll P, Goldstein GD, Brown CW Jr. Metastatic microcystic adnexal carcinoma in an immunocompromised patient. *Dermatol Surg.* 2000;26:531-534.

216. Wohlfahrt C, Ternesten A, Sahlin P, Islam Q, Stenman G. Cytogenetic and fluorescence in situ hybridization analyses of a microcystic adnexal carcinoma with del(6)(q23q25). *Cancer Genet Cytogenet.* 1997;98:106-110.

217. Chen MB, Laber DA. Metastatic microcystic adnexal carcinoma with DNA sequencing results and response to systemic antineoplastic chemotherapy. *Anticancer Res.* 2017;37:5109-5111.

218. Hodgson TA, Haricharan AK, Barrett AW, Porter SR. Microcystic adnexal carcinoma: an unusual cause of swelling and paraesthesia of the lower lip. *Oral Oncol.* 2003;39:195-198.

219. Nagatsuka H, Rivera RS, Gunduz M, et al. Microcystic adnexal carcinoma with mandibular bone marrow involvement: a case report with immunohistochemistry. *Am J Dermatopathol.* 2006;28:518-522.

220. Rotter N, Wagner H, Fuchshuber S, Issing WJ. Cervical metastases of microcystic adnexal carcinoma in an otherwise healthy woman. *Eur Arch Otorhinolaryngol.* 2003;260:254-257.

221. Gomez-Maestra MJ, Espana-Gregori E, Avino-Martinez JA, Mancheno-Franch N, Pena S. Brainstem and cavernous sinus metastases arising from a microcystic adnexal carcinoma of the eyebrow by perineural spreading. *Can J Ophthalmol.* 2009;44:e17-e18.

222. Fernández-Figueras M-T, Montero M-A, Admella J, de la Torre N, Quer A, Ariza A. High (nuclear) grade adnexal carcinoma with microcystic adnexal carcinoma-like structural features. *Am J Dermatopathol.* 2006;28:346-351.

223. Hoang MP, Dresser KA, Kapur P, High WA, Mahalingam M. Microcystic adnexal carcinoma: an immunohistochemical reappraisal. *Mod Pathol.* 2008;21:178.

224. Krahl D, Sellheyer K. Monoclonal antibody Ber-EP4 reliably discriminates between microcystic adnexal carcinoma and basal cell carcinoma. *J Cutan Pathol.* 2007;34:782-787.

225. Misago N, Kimura T, Narisawa Y. Fibrofolliculoma/trichodiscoma and fibrous papule (perifollicular fibroma/angiofibroma): a revaluation of the histopathological and immunohistochemical features. *J Cutan Pathol.* 2009;36:943-951.

226. Bansal C, Stewart D, Li A, Cockerell CJ. Histologic variants of fibrous papule. *J Cutan Pathol.* 2005;32:424-428.

227. Webb DW, Clarke A, Fryer A, Osborne JP. The cutaneous features of tuberous sclerosis: a population study. *Br J Dermatol.* 1996;135:1-5.

228. Dutta A, Ghosh SK, Mandal RK. Facial angiofibromas. *Indian Pediatr.* 2015;52(7):634.

229. Schwartz RA, Fernandez G, Kotulska K, Jozwiak S. Tuberous sclerosis complex: advances in diagnosis, genetics, and management. *J Am Acad Dermatol.* 2007;57:189-202.

230. Choudhuri S, Mishra J, Singh GP, Hota D. Tuberous sclerosis with bilateral renal cell carcinoma in a child: a case report. *Pediatr Urology Case Rep.* 2014;2:1-6.

231. Kukreja R, Mital M, Gupta P, Rathee N. A case series of tuberous sclerosis complex: clinico-radiological study and review of the literature. *West African J Radiol.* 2017;24:109.CAPSULE SUMMARY

24

Soft Tissue Tumors of Skin and Subcutis

Louis P. Dehner / Alejandro A. Gru / Aimee C. Smidt / Emma F. Johnson

The designation of soft tissue tumors as applied to the skin and subcutis of children and adults alike include a broad range of neoplasms and malformations that are composed of a single or multiple mesenchymal tissues. In a review of skin biopsies and excision from the institution of one of us during a 1-year period, approximately 15% of all cases were soft tissue tumors in a time interval when one-third of all lesions were melanocytic proliferations.[1] The most common category of the mesenchymal lesions was vascular anomalies, both neoplastic and malformational types (see Chapter 25).

Many of the soft tissue tumors of the skin and/or subcutis are a challenge to pathologists and dermatopathologists often as a spindle cell, fibrous-appearing tumor, which is centered in the dermis or involves both the dermis and subcutis as a contiguous mass.

Peripheral Nerve Sheath and Other Neurogenic Tumors

A review of our experience with soft tissue tumors of the skin in children during a recent 2-year period revealed slightly less than 50% of lesions were vascular anomalies, but the next most common category was neurogenic tumors of various types comprising approximately 20% of cases (Table 24-1).

Peripheral nerve sheath tumors (PNSTs) are represented by a group of soft tissue tumors that are composed of one or more cell types such as Schwann cells in the case of schwannoma, perineurial cells in the perineurioma, or a mixture of neural elements including neurites, Schwann cells, and perineurial cells in the neurofibroma (NF) or hybrid PNSTs.[2] Granular cell tumor (GCT) is considered a Schwannian neoplasm in almost all cases except for the congenital epulis arising from the gingival soft tissues of an infant. Other neural lesions presenting in the skin and underlying soft tissues in children include the neural lipofibromatous hamartoma (NFH), ectopic meningothelial hamartoma, and neuromas of various types that are either developmental anomalies or a disordered reactive-regenerative process.

NEUROFIBROMA

NF was the most common of the PNSTs presenting in the skin and subcutis of children and represented 75% of cases (Table 24-1). Unlike most cutaneous NFs in adults that are typically sporadic and solitary, the clinical context in children is quite the contrary, with multiple tumors in superficial and deep soft tissue sites; these patients all have NF type 1 (NF1).[3] In general, the cutaneous NFs in NF1 are just one feature in which café au lait spots and axillary freckles are also seen.[4,5] Less frequently, NFs are seen in NF type 2 (NF2), but with many fewer lesions, and are often more subtle in their clinical presentation.[6-8] Schwannomas arising in the skin and soft tissues are seen in the setting of NF2 or schwannomatosis.[9,10] The salient features of NF1,

TABLE 24-1.	Mesenchymal tumor and tumor-like lesions of the dermis and subcutis

Vascular	Number
Lobular capillary hemangioma (PG)	77
Malformation	48
Infantile hemangioma	24
Others	37
Total	**186 (49%)**
Nerve/Nerve Sheath	
Neurofibroma	61
Schwannoma	6
Ependymal rests	5
Ganglioneuroma	3
Granular cell tumor	2
Plexiform palisaded neuroma	1
Soft tissue glioma	1
Meningothelial hamartoma	1
Total	**80 (21%)**
Others	
Dermatofibroma (cutaneous fibrous histiocytoma)	13
Sarcoma[a]	9
Angiofibroma	8
Plexiform fibrohistiocytic tumor	5
Dermatofibrosarcoma protuberans-giant cell fibroblastoma	2
Cellular neurothekeoma	2
Leiomyosarcoma	1
Myxoinflammatory fibroblastic sarcoma	1
Myxoma (multiple)	1
Total	**42 (11%)**
Fibrous/Myofibrous	
Fibromatosis including desmoid tumor	13
Myofibroma	8
Infantile subcutaneous fibromatosis	6
Fibrous hamartoma of infancy	5
Nodular fasciitis	5
Digital fibroma	3
Myopericytoma	1
Total	**41 (11%)**
Lipomatous	
Lipoma	19
Lipoblastoma	5
Myxoid liposarcoma	1
Nevus lipomatosis	1
Angiolipoma	1
Total	**27 (7%)**
Grand total	**376**

From the files of the Lauren V. Ackerman Laboratory of Surgical Pathology and Dermatopathology, Washington University Medical Center, St. Louis, MO, for the years of 2015 and 2016.

[a]Ewing sarcoma (3), clear cell sarcoma (1), rhabdomyosarcoma (3), histiocytic sarcoma (1), extraskeletal myxoid chondrosarcoma (1).

Abbreviation: PG, pyogenic granuloma.
From Dehner LP, Gru AA. Non-epithelial tumor and tumor-like lesions of the skin and subcutis in children. *Pediatr Dev Pathol.* 2018;21(2):150-207.

NF2, and schwannomatosis are summarized in Table 24-2. Virtually all of those with NF1 develop NFs, and 50% of children with NF1 have at least one, if not more, NF by the age of 10 years. In children under 10 years of age, NFs often have exclusive plexiform features.

NF1 is caused by mutation in the *NF1* gene that encodes the tumor suppressor protein neurofibromin.[11] Specifically, NFs are characterized by biallelic inactivation of the *NF1* gene in a subpopulation of Schwann cells within the lesion.[11] NF2 is caused by a loss of function of the *NF2* gene that encodes the cell membrane protein and tumor suppressor protein merlin.[12] Schwannomatosis is caused by a mutation in the *SMARCB1* gene.[13]

NFs present as protuberant to pedunculated, flesh-colored to pinkish papules or nodules (Figure 24-1). They are soft on palpation and can demonstrate the "buttonhole sign" in which the lesion can be invaginated into the subcutis with pressure and reappear after release of pressure.[14]

In the setting of NF1, NFs occur in young adults and continue to develop over time.[4] Patients can have tens, hundreds, or even thousands of cutaneous NFs.[4] Cutaneous NFs occur in 99% of patients with NF1. Two or more NFs or one plexiform NF (Figure 24-2) is included in the diagnostic criteria for NF1. Other diagnostic criteria, of which the patient needs two to confirm the diagnosis, are six café au lait spots greater than 5 mm in diameter in prepubertal children and greater than 15 mm in postpubertal children (Figure 24-3); freckling in the axillary or inguinal region; optic glioma; two or more iris hamartomas (Lisch nodules); a distinctive osseous lesion (sphenoid dysplasia or thinning of long bones); and a first-degree relative with NF1.[15] Approximately one-third of NF1 patients develop plexiform NFs.[11,16]

Plexiform NFs are clinically distinct from cutaneous NFs as they are generally present at birth (congenital). They are associated with overlying hyperpigmentation and/or hypertrichosis and are often described as "bag of worms" on palpation.[16] Lesions are diffuse and can grow into large, disfiguring masses.[17]

TABLE 24-2	Clinical and pathologic features of neurofibromatoses		
	Neurofibromatosis Type 1	**Neurofibromatosis Type 2**	**Schwannomatosis**
Incidence, inheritance, and mutation	1:2500-3500, AD, neurofibromin 1 (17q11.2, RAS-GTPase)	1:25 000-60 000 AD (*de novo* mutation 50%), neurofibromin 2 (22q12.2, ERM cell membrane protein, merlin)	Incidence unknown, AD, INI1/ SMARCB1 (22q11.23, chromatin remodeling protein)
Cutaneous findings	Six or more CAL before puberty, skin-folding freckles, two or more NFs, 1 plexiform NF	One or more dermal plaque-like or subcutaneous schwannomas, 10 or more and less common NF	Two or more nondermal schwannomas
Other neoplasms	Embryonal rhabdomyosarcoma, 3 y or less; optic nerve glioma, MPNST (rare before adolescence)	Bilateral VIIIn schwannomas, one or more meningiomas, ependymomas	No evidence of VIIIn schwannomas

Abbreviations: AD, autosomal dominant; CAL, café au lait; ERM, ezrin, radixin, and moesin; MPNST, malignant peripheral nerve sheath tumor; NF, neurofibroma.

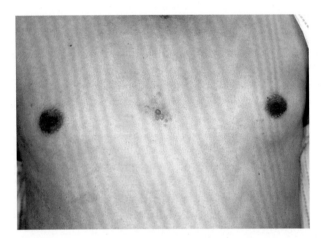

FIGURE 24-1. **Neurofibroma.** Small pedunculated papules on the trunk.

In the setting of NF2, NFs are significantly less common. NF2 is characterized by the development of acoustic nerve schwannomas, meningiomas, ependymomas, and ocular abnormalities. Studies have reported 70% of patients with NF2 have skin tumors, although only 10% have greater than 10 cutaneous lesions.[8] Cutaneous tumors in NF2 are most commonly schwannomas, although NFs do occur. Schwannomatosis has significant clinical overlap with NF2.[13]

Pathologically, the sporadic, solitary NF is characterized by a circumscribed dermal nodule, typically measuring 1 cm or less and with a differential diagnosis that includes a dermal melanocytic nevus. A pale-staining, uniform spindle cell proliferation has an eosinophilic background, with only a hint of stromal mucin. Scattered mast cells are present

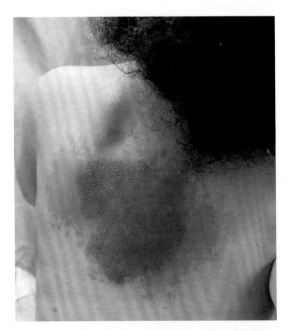

FIGURE 24-2. Plexiform neurofibroma in a patient with neurofibromatosis type 1.

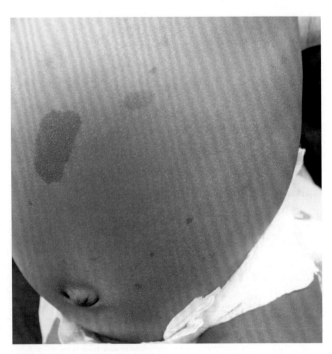

FIGURE 24-3. Large café au lait spots in a patient with neurofibromatosis type 1.

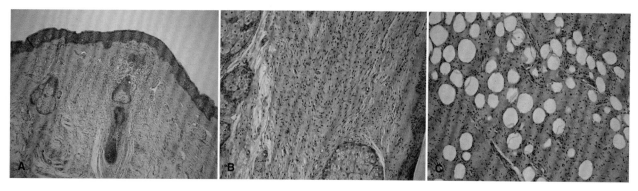

FIGURE 24-4. A-C, **Neurofibroma (NF) from the chin of a 12-year-old male with NF1.** A, The diffuse NF shows the growth between pilosebaceous units. B, The degree of cellularity can be quite variable from one focus of the same tumor to another. C, Extension into the subcutis demonstrates the so-called honeycomb pattern that is usually made in reference to dermatofibrosarcoma protuberans.

within the stroma. Nuclear pleomorphism and sclerosis are two uncommon features.[18,19] It is uncommon to encounter a solitary NF in an individual less than 20 years of age.

A contrasting histologic pattern of dermal and subcutaneous involvement is present in the NF1-associated NF where the tumor has a diffuse and/or plexiform appearance with growth through the dermis and replacement by bland spindle cells in a pale-staining eosinophilic stroma (Figure 24-4A-C). Adnexal structures in the dermis are surrounded, but not displaced, by the proliferation. The plexiform profiles may be present as one or more bundles of spindle cells within the background of diffuse NF or as separate distinct profiles in the dermis and/or subcutis (Figure 24-4A-C). Within the dermis, the short to fusiform spindle cells have elongated, bland nuclei; nuclear enlargement with hyperchromatism is uncommon in the dermal-based NFs, but may be seen in the deep soft tissue NFs in older children and young adults.[20] When the subcutis is involved as it often is, the growth is usually contiguous with a dermal component and the fat is overgrown in a manner similar to dermatofibrosarcoma protuberans (DFSP) and some of the fibrous tumors of childhood (Figure 24-4A-C).

The plexiform pattern of NF is characterized by multiple circumscribed bundles of pale-staining spindle cells in a myxoid background (Figure 24-5A-C). The contours of the plexiform bundles are sharply demarcated as distinct profiles in the deep dermis and subcutis. Nuclear enlargement and atypia are uncommon in the more superficial plexiform NFs but, if present, should not be viewed as indicative of sarcomatous transformation (Figures 24-5C and 24-6).

Other features found in NFs in the setting of NF1 include floret-type giant cells with similarities to those seen in the pleomorphic lipoma (rare in children) and giant cell fibroblastoma (GCF; typically presenting in children).[21] Melanin pigmentation is yet another uncommon histologic finding.[22]

The differential diagnosis of NF in the skin or subcutis includes the following in the presence of the diffuse, infiltrating pattern: infantile subcutaneous fibromatosis (ISF; lipofibromatosis), fibrous hamartoma of infancy (FHI), DFSP (including the pigmented Bednar tumor), cellular neurothekeoma (CNTK), and congenital melanocytic nevus with neurotization. Various immunohistochemical approaches can be applied with a combination of smooth muscle actin (mature fibrous areas of ISF and FHI), S-100 protein (NF and neurotized nevus), and CD34 (DFSP and NF, diffuse staining and immature nodules in FHI), collagen type IV (NF), and Melan-A (neurotized nevus and melanocytes in NF).[23] An additional challenge in the diagnosis

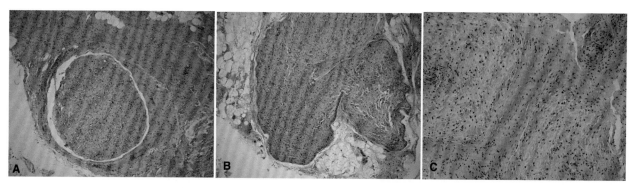

FIGURE 24-5. A-C, **Neurofibroma from the scalp of an 11-year-old female with NF1.** A, Plexiform profile is surrounded in part by diffuse neurofibroma. B, Serpentine architecture is displayed in these foci with a pure plexiform pattern. C, Mild degree of scattered nuclear enlargement and hyperchromatism without apparent sarcomatous overgrowth should not be a source of concern in most cases.

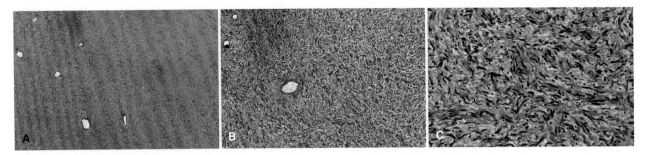

FIGURE 24-6. A-C, **Neurofibroma, degenerative atypia.** Such changes should not be viewed as an indication of malignancy.

of diffuse NF is the recently reported neural ISF-like tumor because it expresses CD34 and S-100 protein and has a recurrent *NTRK1* fusion.[24]

CAPSULE SUMMARY

NEUROFIBROMA

NFs are common, benign PNSTs that often occur as solitary lesions. Neurofibromatosis is the presence of multiple lesions in a segmental or widespread distribution. Most of these tumors are seen in adolescents or adults as a solitary nodule in the skin, which is well circumscribed, has a uniform population of small spindle cells in a pale myxoid background, and contains scattered mast cells.

SCHWANNOMA

Schwannoma is a purely Schwann cell neoplasm that occurs sporadically as a solitary mass in any number of anatomic sites or as multiple tumors in NF2, schwannomatosis, and Carney complex.[25] A review of the files of one of us (LPD) revealed that only 10% of schwannomas presented in the first two decades of life[1]; a schwannoma in an individual less than 20 years old is likely to have NF2 or schwannomatosis.[9,26] Cutaneous manifestations in NF2 occur less commonly in children with NF2 than with NF1.[27] Cutaneous schwannomas or cortical and posterior subcapsular or capsular cataracts are more common as initial presentations in prepubertal children with NF2 in contrast to adolescents and adults whose clinical presentation is more often related to the bilateral VIII nerve schwannomas.[28,29] However, congenital-infantile NF2 may present with bilateral acoustic neuromas or schwannomas with or without cutaneous schwannomas.[30] It is estimated that 70% of those with NF2 develop one or more skin tumors, generally less than 10.[8]

Schwannoma presents as one or more (uncommon) soft to firm nodular mass(es) measuring 1 to 2 cm in the dermis or subcutis. Approximately one-third of tumors are accompanied by pain and tenderness, unlike most NFs, and there is a predilection for the extremities where the tumor can measure in excess of 5 cm.[16]

Pathologically, the schwannoma is a well-circumscribed, encapsulated spindle cell neoplasm to be differentiated from the myriad of other similarly appearing related and unrelated tumors (Figure 24-7). In those schwannomas whose capsule is not apparent, the cellular variant with or without mitotic activity, nuclear enlargement, and hyperchromatism or one of the several less common variants including the plexiform (Figure 24-8), myxoid-reticular (Figure 24-9), and glandular subtypes can be a histopathologic challenge.

When a schwannoma presents in a child, it is often in the setting of NF2 and may present in the subcutis and less often in the dermis alone, with the exception of the plexiform schwannoma (PS) with its predilection for the skin and underlying soft tissues.[31] This tumor is seen in children and is associated with NF2 and schwannomatosis.[32-34] PS is often cellular and displays some nuclear pleomorphism and mitotic activity (5 or less per high-power field [HPF]); these features in the context of PS are not indicative of malignancy because this tumor behaves in an entirely benign fashion (Figure 24-8). Unlike the conventional schwannoma, a capsule is not present in most PSs. The encapsulated nature of PS may be inapparent.

The small, superficial schwannoma in a young individual is often moderately cellular and is composed of uniform fusiform cells often, but not always, without Verocay bodies, hyalinized vessels, macrophages, and myxoid or Antoni type B stroma.

In addition to the cellularity of the PS, the cellular variant of schwannoma is a problematic tumor because it must be differentiated from the malignant PNST (MPNST), an extremely rare tumor in the skin or subcutis of a child even in the presence of NF1.[35] Retained nuclear expression for SOX-10 and H3K27me, and diffuse expression of S-100 protein, collagen type IV, and calretinin all favor a schwannoma including the PS rather than MPNST.[20,36-38]

Melanotic schwannoma (MS) is a rare variant that typically presents in the paraspinal location, but not to the exclusion of other sites including the skin.[39] An MS should strongly suggest the likelihood of Carney complex.[40,41] The cause of Carney complex in most patients is a mutation in the *PRKAR1A* gene, a tumor suppressor gene.[42,43] *PRKAR1A* expression is lost in 35% to 40% of sporadic and Carney complex–associated psammomatous MSs.[44]

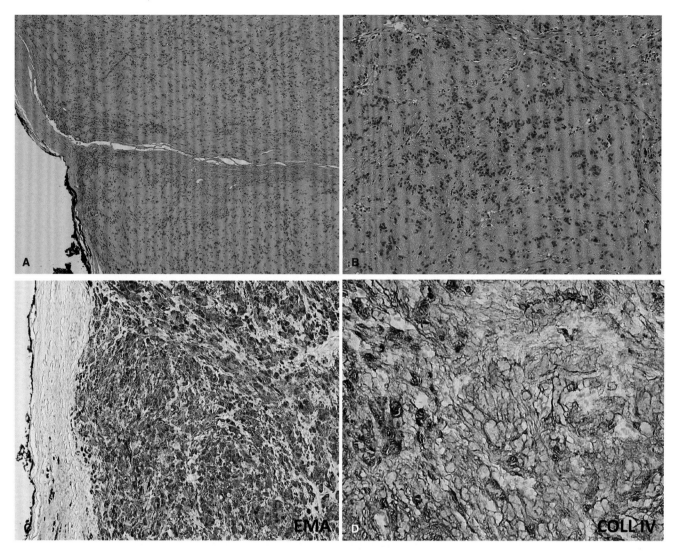

FIGURE 24-7. A-D, **Schwannoma presenting on the upper eyelid of an 11-year-old male with NF2.** A, The well-defined peripheral capsule is shown together with the inked margin. B, The fibrillary background is composed of cytoplasmic processes. The nuclei are arranged in small aggregates suggesting the formation of pseudorosettes. C, Unlike the neurofibroma, S100 protein is strongly and diffusely positive. D, Collagen type IV immunostain demonstrates the characteristic pattern of basement membrane positivity.

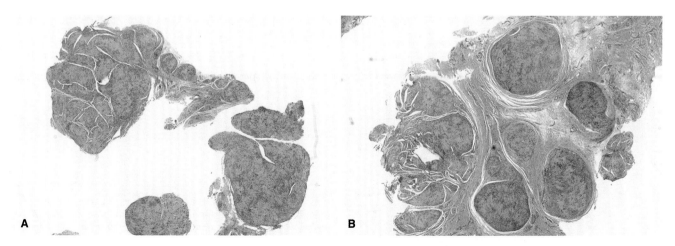

FIGURE 24-8. A-D, **Plexiform schwannoma.** Numerous plexiform profiles are composed of uniform spindle cells with focal Verocay body formation. Antoni A and Antoni B patterns are seen. Digital slides courtesy of Path Presenter.com.

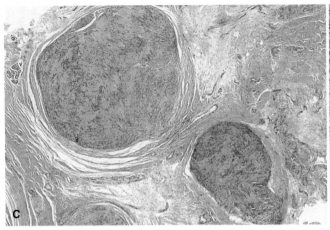

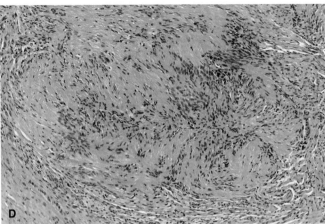

FIGURE 24-8. (*continued*)

Psammomatous MSs most commonly present on the posterior spinal nerve roots, alimentary tract, bone, and rarely skin.[40,45] Tumors can range between 1.4 and 7.0 cm, with an average of 3.2 cm. As lesions are most commonly deep, patients generally present with pain, muscle weakness, dysesthesias, and numbness.[44] The behavior of melanotic

psammomatous schwannomas is unpredictable, with metastases reported in 13% to 42% of patients (Figure 24-10).[44]

This heavily pigmented spindled to epithelioid neoplasm can have substantial nuclear atypia and may have psammomatous calcifications. In the absence of the latter findings, metastatic melanoma is an

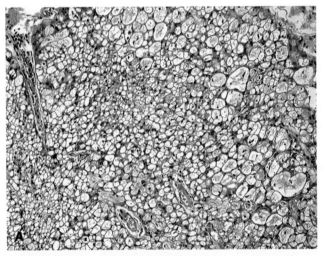

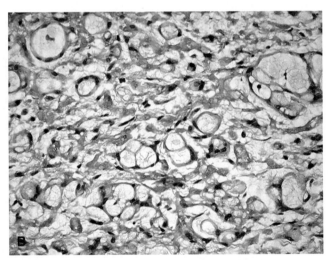

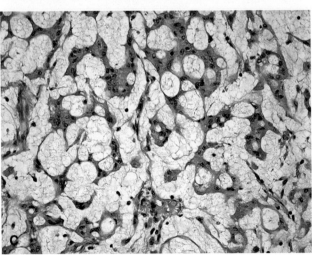

FIGURE 24-9. **Myxoid-reticular pattern in schwannoma.** Microcystic/reticular schwannoma. Views from three representative cases, highlighting the characteristically microcystic or reticular growth patterns. Obtained with permission Liegl B, Bennett MW, Fletcher CD. Microcystic/reticular schwannoma: a distinct variant with predilection for visceral locations. *Am J Surg Pathol.* 2008;32(7):1080-1087.

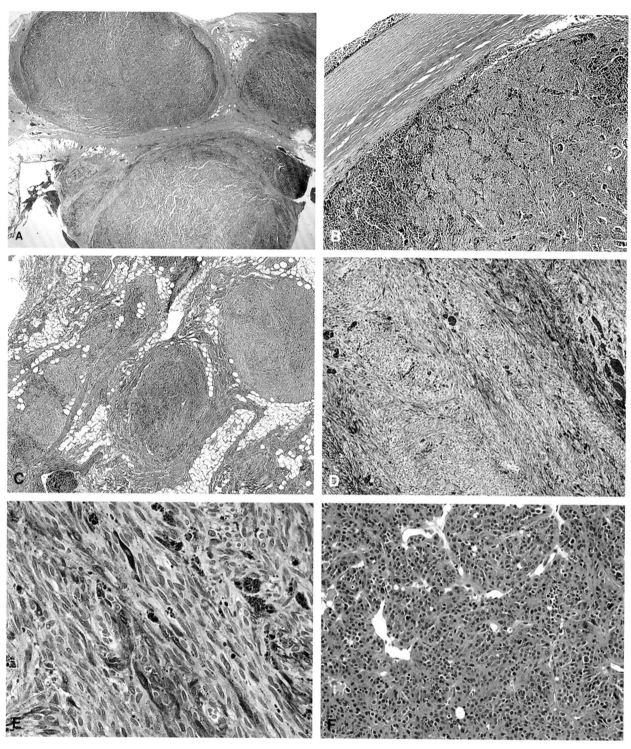

FIGURE 24-10. Psammomatous melanotic schwannoma. A, At low-power magnification, melanotic schwannoma typically grew as multinodular, generally circumscribed masses. A minority of cases showed at least partial encapsulation (B), but more often the tumors were unencapsulated and grew into surround fibroadipose tissue (C). D, At higher-power magnification, the tumors were most often composed of a fascicular proliferation of melanin-containing, moderately variable spindle cells, with an inconspicuous vasculature. E, Spindled melanotic schwannoma, showing elongated nuclei with small nucleoli. F, A minority of tumors were composed largely of epithelioid cells, resembling cutaneous melanoma. Obtained with permission Torres-Mora J, Dry S, Li X, Binder S, Amin M, Folpe AL. Malignant melanotic schwannian tumor: a clinicopathologic, immunohistochemical, and gene expression profiling study of 40 cases, with a proposal for the reclassification of "melanotic schwannoma". *Am J Surg Pathol.* 2014;38(1):94-105.

unavoidable consideration, but in the context of a child, it is very unlikely. Schwannoma may have a predominant epithelioid cellular composition or may resemble a neuroblastoma.[46,47]

Epithelioid schwannoma (Figure 24-11) presents in the skin and/or subcutis, and only a minority of cases occur in children, usually in older children and adolescents.[46,48] The challenge is differentiating the ES from the menu of other epithelioid neoplasms ranging from epithelioid sarcoma (ES) to hemangioendothelioma. A single cell pattern with the features of a classic schwannoma focally in those tumors with trabecular to nodular profiles of epithelioid cells in a myxohyaline, myxoid, or dense collagenous stroma is the spectrum of microscopic features.[46,48-54] In addition to the characteristic immunophenotype of the schwannoma, a CD34+ population of spindle cells may also be present.

Schwannomatosis is the "third" neurofibromatosis that is characterized by multiple, nonvestibular schwannomas in contrast to NF2.[1] Germline mutations in either *SMARCB1* or *LZTR1* tumor suppressor genes are found in almost 90% of familial cases (representing 15%-25% of all cases) and in 40% of sporadic cases (representing 75%-85% of all cases). Somatic mutations in both *NF2* alleles have been detected in the schwannomas.[55] In the presence of a germline mutation in *SMARCB1*, the risk of malignant rhabdoid tumor (MRT) may also exist.[56,57]

CAPSULE SUMMARY

SCHWANNOMA

Schwannoma is a purely Schwann cell neoplasm that occurs sporadically as a solitary mass in any number of anatomic sites or as multiple tumors in the NF2, schwannomatosis, and Carney complex. Schwannoma presents as one or more (uncommon) soft to firm nodular mass(es) measuring 1 to 2 cm in the dermis or subcutis. Pathologically, the schwannoma is a well-circumscribed, encapsulated spindle cell neoplasm to be differentiated from the myriad of other similarly appearing related and unrelated tumors. Variants of schwannoma include epithelioid, cellular, melanotic, plexiform, among others.

PERINEUROMA

Perineuroma (PN) is the third type of PNST that is composed of spindle cells with the immunophenotype of pia-arachnoid-meningeal cells with expression of vimentin and epithelial membrane antigen.[58] This tumor is well circumscribed, arises in the subcutis and dermis, has an intraneural localization in some cases, and has a predilection for the extremities. PN occurs more commonly in adults, but is seen in children, usually over 10 years of age.[59] Delicate fusiform cells resembling Schwann cells are arranged in fascicles and/or whorls of loosely arranged

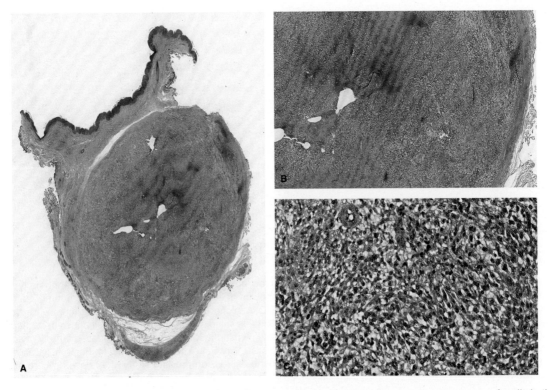

FIGURE 24-11. A-C, **Epithelioid schwannoma.** A single cell pattern with the features of a classic schwannoma focally in those tumors with trabecular to nodular profiles of epithelioid cells in a myxohyaline, myxoid, or dense collagenous stroma is the spectrum of microscopic features present in this tumor (A-C). Digital slides courtesy of Path Presenter.com.

spindle cells. A myxoid background or plexiform growth may be prominent in some cases (Figure 24-12).[2] Dense sclerosis is a feature in some cases. Epithelial membrane antigen reactivity is essential because the PN may also express CD34, smooth muscle actin, and S-100 protein (less than 10%).[58]

Hybrid PNST is a neoplasm that has challenged the concept of the single lineage nerve sheath tumor with the combination of patterns and the overlapping immunophenotype of the three major PNSTs.[60-62] These tumors have a preference for the subcutis and dermis of adults more commonly than older children. The PN and schwannoma hybrid is one of the more frequent combinations. Other neural tumors in the skin and superficial soft tissues include both neoplasms, reactive proliferations, and possibly a hamartoma or localized overgrowth process.

CAPSULE SUMMARY

PERINEUROMA

PN is the third type of PNST that is composed of spindle cells with the immunophenotype of pia-arachnoid-meningeal cells with expression of vimentin and epithelial membrane antigen. Hybrid PNST is a neoplasm that has challenged the concept of the single lineage nerve sheath tumor with the combination of patterns and the overlapping immunophenotype of the three major PNSTs.

GRANULAR CELL TUMOR

GCT is a neoplasm with a broad distribution of primary sites, with the skin as the most common location in children where 60% of lesions are found with a predilection for the head and neck region.[1] GCTs may be congenital, known by a variety of different names including congenital GCT, congenital epulis, congenital myoblastoma, or Neumann tumor.[63] Their incidence is suggested to be 6 per million children per year.[63] GCTs occur in adults between 20 and 60 years of age.[64] Females are affected more commonly than males in both congenital and adult lesions.[63,64]

GCTs arise most commonly as solitary asymptomatic, pale, or yellowish smooth nodules, rarely larger than 3 cm (Figure 24-13).[64,65] There is a predilection for the head and neck region. The congenital forms typically present on the gum pads.[63] In adults there is a predilection for the oral cavity, especially the tongue, and, when present in the skin, the upper extremities and upper torso.[64,66,67]

Because of almost universal S-100 protein immunopositivity, GCT is considered a Schwann cell–derived tumor except in the case of the congenital granular cell epulis arising in the oral-maxillofacial region.[68,69] Multifocal congenital GCTs and familial GCTs are other reported occurrences.[70,71] Both circumscribed and infiltrating growth patterns of granular cells with abundant eosinophilic granular cytoplasm with somewhat larger eosinophilic bodies are present in the biopsy or excision. In the GCT with infiltration of

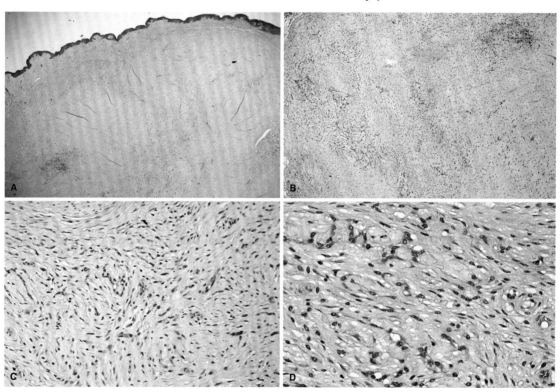

FIGURE 24-12. A-D, **Perineurioma.** Nodular and diffuse spindle cell tumor in the dermis that is well circumscribed on the edges (A and B). The lesion shows a storiform growth and myxoid background (C). Most of the cells show a cytoplasm with fibrillary features (D). Obtained with permission Dehner LP, Gru AA. Nonepithelial tumors and tumor-like lesions of the skin and subcutis in children. *Pediatr Dev Pathol.* 2018;21(2):150-207.

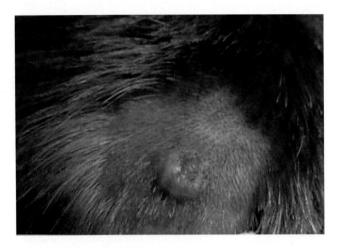

FIGURE 24-13. **Granular cell tumor.** Flesh-colored to slightly orange-hued soft nodule on the scalp of a young boy. Reprinted with permission from Olayiwola O, Hook K, Miller D, et al. Cutaneous granular cell tumors in children: case series and review of the literature. *Pediatr Dermatol.* 2017;34(4):e187-e190.

the dermis, the small groups of granular cells blend into the background of dermal collagen (Figure 24-14). The nuclei of the tumor cells are rounded to ovoid with fine to coarse chromatin, but infrequently the nuclei may appear larger

and hyperchromatic with an inconspicuous nucleolus. The granules are lysosomes that account for CD68 immunopositivity, in addition to characteristic S-100 protein reactivity (Figure 24-15). The congenital granular tumor or epulis has a densely cellular appearance as it forms a nodule or mass. With the rare exception, these tumors are nonreactive for S-100 protein.

CAPSULE SUMMARY

GRANULAR CELL TUMOR

GCT is a neoplasm with a broad distribution of primary sites, with the skin as the most common location in children where 60% of lesions are found with a predilection for the head and neck region. Both circumscribed and infiltrating growth patterns of granular cells with abundant eosinophilic granular cytoplasm with somewhat larger eosinophilic bodies are present in the biopsy or excision. Because of almost universal S-100 protein immunopositivity, GCT is considered a Schwann cell–derived tumor.

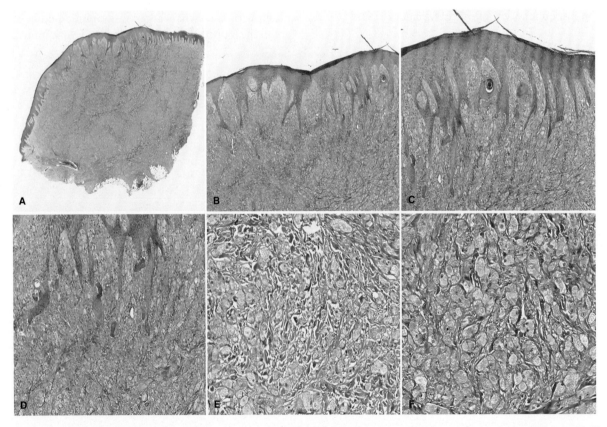

FIGURE 24-14. **Granular cell tumor.** Note the presence of pseudoepitheliomatous changes in the surface epidermis (A-C). Such changes can be confused with those of squamous cell carcinoma. Nested and diffuse sheets of uniform, pale rounded to ovoid to spindle shaped with abundant eosinophilic granular cytoplasm are the principal microscopic features of this tumor (D-F). Obtained with permission Dehner LP, Gru AA. Nonepithelial tumors and tumor-like lesions of the skin and subcutis in children. *Pediatr Dev Pathol.* 2018;21(2):150-207.

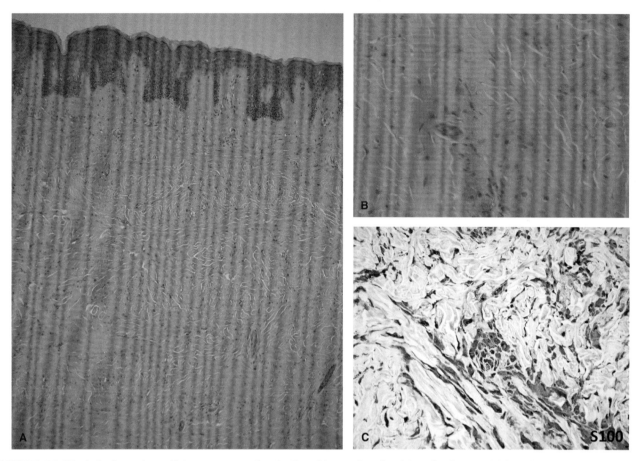

FIGURE 24-15. A-C, Granular cell tumor presenting in the skin on the shoulder of a 9-year-old female. A, The dermis at this magnification is seemingly unremarkable, which may be the initial impression in a granular cell tumor with a diffuse infiltrative pattern. B, Granular cells are infiltrating into superficial subcutaneous fat. C, S-100 protein immunostain demonstrates the striking number of granular cells in the dermis.

NERVE SHEATH MYXOMA

Nerve sheath myxoma (myxoid neurothekeoma) is a dermal and/or subcutaneous-based, circumscribed multinodular neoplasm typically presenting in the extremities or head and neck region of adolescents and young adults.[72] Septated lobules of spindle cells are suspended in a myxoid matrix (Figure 24-16); the spindle cells are S-100 protein immunopositive and presumably represent Schwann cells.[73,74] CD34 and epithelial membrane antigen are both nonreactive, but glial fibrillary acidic protein may be positive as in some schwannomas as well as NFs.[75] There is no apparent histogenetic relationship with the CNTK.[76]

NEUROMA

Neuroma is a generic designation for several lesions of neoplastic, hamartomatous, and traumatic nature.

Palisaded encapsulated neuroma (PEN) is a likely neoplasm presenting in the dermis or submucosa of the oral cavity, but it occurs in other sites such as the palms and soles in children.[77-79] Only 10% of cases occur in children. It has been suggested that a histogenetic relationship may exist between PEN and the mucocutaneous neuromas of multiple endocrine neoplasia 2B (MEN2B).[80] A solitary flesh-colored papule or nodules, generally measuring less than 2 cm, is the clinical presentation. A uniform, spindle cell population arranged in fascicles is surrounded by a delicate fibrous capsule (Figure 24-17). A contiguous peripheral nerve is present in some cases. As in the case of a schwannoma, the spindle cells are diffusely positive for S-100 protein, but unlike the latter tumor, neurofilament protein and epithelial membrane antigen are positive.[77,80]

Mucocutaneous neuroma of MEN2B is composed of smaller and less expansile circumscribed individual bundles of Schwann cells than the PEN. When these lesions initially develop in a young child on the tongue, palate, pharynx, and lip, they may be the first manifestation of MEN2B.[81-83] The multiple neural bundles are separated by a stromal background. The site of the neural bundles is somewhat circumscribed, but in the lip with progressive enlargement, the entire submucosa is occupied by these formations. Like the PEN and

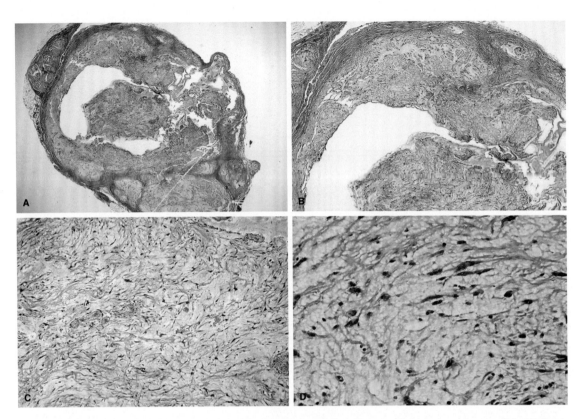

FIGURE 24-16. Dermal nerve sheath myxoma (myxoid neurothekeoma). A circumscribed, but nonencapsulated lesion is composed of multiple smaller nodules with a prominent myxoid or myomatous background containing dispersed spindle cells (A-D). Obtained with permission Dehner LP, Gru AA. Nonepithelial tumors and tumor-like lesions of the skin and subcutis in children. *Pediatr Dev Pathol.* 2018;21(2):150-207.

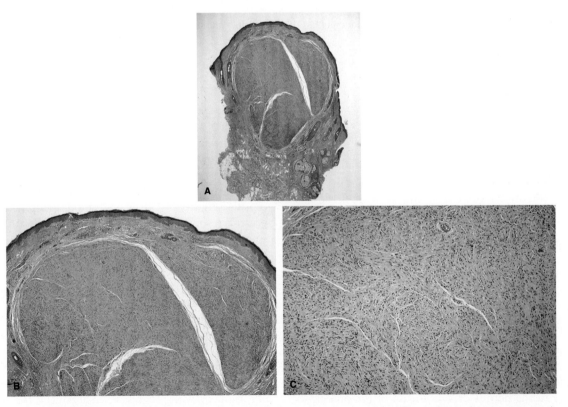

FIGURE 24-17. Palisaded encapsulated neuroma. Solitary well-circumscribed nodule with a schwannian appearance is present in the dermis (A-C). Obtained with permission Dehner LP, Gru AA. Nonepithelial tumors and tumor-like lesions of the skin and subcutis in children. *Pediatr Dev Pathol.* 2018;21(2):150-207.

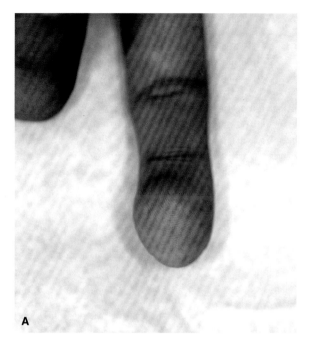

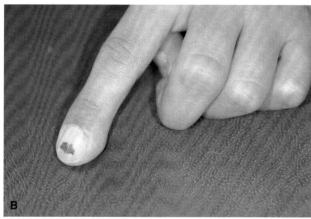

FIGURE 24-18. **Traumatic neuroma.** Nodule in the finger (A and B).

schwannoma, the spindle cells are uniformly S-100 protein positive and a peripheral capsule, if present, is at least focally positive for epithelial membrane antigen.

Traumatic neuroma occurs in the axilla of infants after neonatal brachial plexus palsy or the hand or foot in an older child after laceration of a digital nerve (Figure 24-18). A background of fibrosis (scar) contains numerous small peripheral nerve twigs in a more or less circumscribed focus. A mixture of axons, Schwann cells, and perineurial cells is the composition of the neuroma (Figure 24-19). A variation

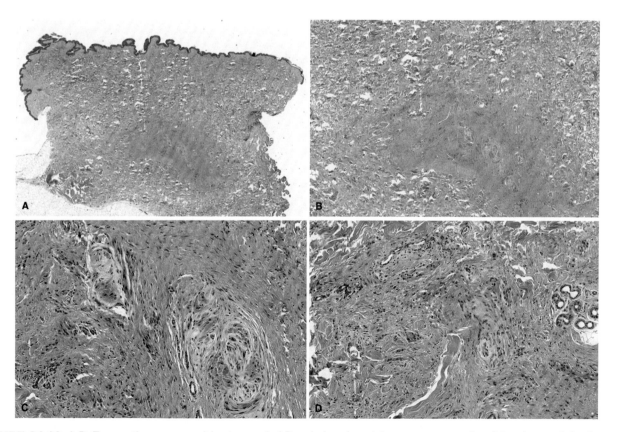

FIGURE 24-19. A-D, **Traumatic neuroma.** A background of fibrosis (scar) contains numerous small peripheral nerve twigs in a more or less circumscribed focus. A mixture of axons, Schwann cells, and perineurial cells is the composition of the neuroma. Digital slides courtesy of Path Presenter.com.

of the traumatic neuroma occurs after ligature amputation of a rudimentary digit in polydactyly, whereas this complication is avoided with surgical excision.[84,85]

CAPSULE SUMMARY

NEUROMA

Neuroma is a generic designation for several lesions of neoplastic, hamartomatous, and traumatic nature. PEN is a likely neoplasm presenting in the dermis or submucosa of the oral cavity, but it occurs in other sites such as the palms and soles in children. Mucocutaneous neuroma of MEN2B is composed of smaller and less expansile circumscribed individual bundles of Schwann cells than the PEN. Traumatic neuroma occurs in the axilla of infants after neonatal brachial plexus palsy or the hand or foot in an older child after laceration of a digital nerve.

NEURAL LIPOFIBROMATOUS HAMARTOMA

NFH (neural fibrolipoma), a nonneoplastic process, is likely a localized overgrowth of collagenous and adipocytic tissues around a major peripheral nerve in the upper or lower extremity. The median nerve is preferentially involved, with the formation of a mass on the volar aspect of the hand, wrist, and forearm often with accompanying macrodactyly.[86-88] Individual nerve bundles are infiltrated by mature adipocytes and are surrounded by dense fibrous connective tissue and embedded in a lipomatous mass. Bony overgrowth and osseous metaplasia are other findings. Somatic gain-of-function mutations in *PIK3CA* have been detected in the affected nerve, but not in the germline (Figure 24-20).[89]

NEUROGLIAL HETEROTOPIA

Neuroglial heterotopia constitutes a rare category of anomalies presenting as a mass, most commonly in children during the first decade of life. Not entirely surprising, these

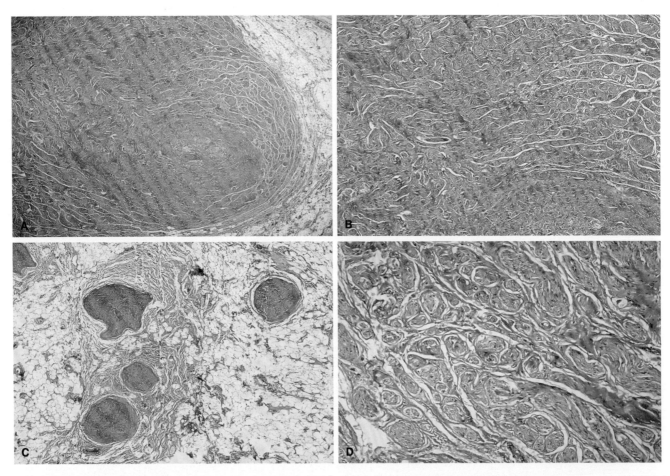

FIGURE 24-20. Neural fibrolipomatous hamartoma. Lobulated adipose tissue is evident and individual nerve bundles with perineural spindle cell proliferation composed of CD34 perineurial cells are encompassed by adipose tissue (A and B). Several contiguous nerve bundles may be surrounded by mature fat around the periphery of these nerves (C and D). Obtained with permission Dehner LP, Gru AA. Nonepithelial tumors and tumor-like lesions of the skin and subcutis in children. *Pediatr Dev Pathol.* 2018;21(2):150-207.

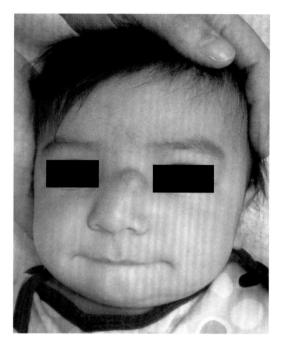

FIGURE 24-21. Nasal glioma.

masses have a predilection for the head and neck region, but not exclusively so.[90] Those lesions presenting in the skin and subcutis often come to the attention of the pediatrician and dermatologist, whereas a nasal or oronasopharyngeal lesion is more likely seen by the pediatrician. All of these lesions have a common histogenesis of a presumed extracranial sequestration of neuroectodermal tissue.

Nasal glioma (NG), a misnomer in terms of its "glioma" designation, is seen in 1:20 000 to 40 000 live births as an intranasal mass at or before 2 years of age (Figure 24-21).[91]

Unlike the encephalocele, NG lacks an intracranial component and is regarded as a so-called sequestered encephalocele. A firm mass is composed of dense fibrous stroma with embedded variably sized islands of more or less mature neuroglial tissue, which may contain an isolated neuron.

Other sites of heterotopic neuroglia are found in and around the oral cavity, oropharynx, and various other soft tissue sites in the head and neck region. Scalp lesions are potentially problematic when there is an underlying defect through the cranium.[92] An isolated nodule of neuroglial tissue with or without meningothelial elements or choroid plexus is the spectrum of microscopic findings.[93-98]

Myxopapillary ependymoma (MXPE) and rests are known to present as an extramedullary cutaneous and/or subcutaneous nodule or mass in the sacrococcygeal region of children.[99-101] This anatomic site is the embryonic consequential location of the primitive streak so that it is not entirely surprising that heterotopic nephrogenic rests, teratoma, and other anomalies present as a mass lesion, as an anal skin tag, or as an incidental microscopic finding (Figure 24-22).[102-106] These embryonic rests may be identified in a pilonidal sinus or skin tag.[107] The focus of the MXPE usually measures 1 cm or less, is well circumscribed, and is located in the dermis or more often in the subcutis. Papillary profiles with myxohyaline stroma supporting the papillae are the microscopic findings (Figure 24-23A-C).

Rudimentary meningocele (meningothelial hamartoma) is a lesion that may present with alopecia, tufted hairs, or soft mass of the scalp (20% or more of cases) in a young child.[108] Other sites include the spine and forehead. The age at clinical presentation ranges from the newborn period to later childhood.[109-111] The dermis and/

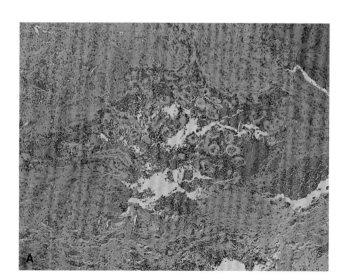

FIGURE 24-22. A, **Myxopapillary ependymal rest presenting as an anal skin tag in a 2-day-old female.** Note the myxohyaline vascular profiles surrounded in part by small primitive cells. A somewhat similar pseudovascular architecture is seen in the ectopic rudimentary meningocele. B, Another focus shows a circumscribed nodule of immature neuroglia.

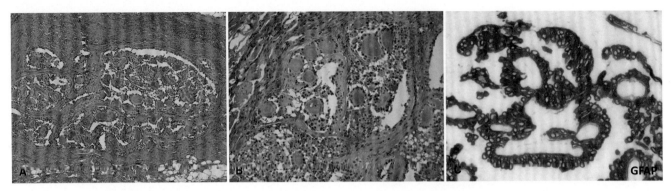

FIGURE 24-23. A-C, **Myxopapillary ependymoma presenting as a "gluteal cyst" in a 5-year-old female.** A, The tumor is composed of multiple circumscribed nodules of papillary profiles with central myxohyaline cores. B, The individual papillae are lined by low-grade cuboidal cells. C, Glial fibrillary acidic protein (GFAP) immunostaining shows strong diffuse positivity.

or subcutis is the location of a circumscribed focus of collapsed, irregular spaces with an inconspicuous lining and/or a small nest(s) of compact, bland-appearing round cells, calcifications (psammomatous in some cases), and giant cells. A solid glial nodule may be present in some cases to provide a clue to neurogenic process of some kind. The giant cells and a pseudoinfiltrative pattern may suggest GCF or a vascular anomaly.[112,113] The spaces are immunoreactive for vimentin and epithelial membrane antigen and nonreactive for CD31.

CAPSULE SUMMARY

NEUROGLIAL HETEROTOPIA

Neuroglial heterotopia constitutes a rare category of anomalies presenting as a mass, most commonly in children during the first decade of life. Not entirely surprising, these masses have a predilection for the head and neck region. All of these lesions have a common histogenesis of a presumed extracranial sequestration of neuroectodermal tissue.

Nonneurogenic Neoplasms

Like the previously discussed PNST and other neurogenic anomalies, this generic category of nonneurogenic tumors is a generally dominated lesion with a spindle cell morphology, which almost mandates the inclusion of these various other tumors in each other's differential diagnosis. Based upon a review of the files of one of us (LPD), a miscellaneous "other" category constituted 22% of the nonvascular mesenchymal neoplasms of which DFSP was the most common entity (Table 24-1).[1] There was an almost equal number of fibrous-myofibroblastic neoplasms.

Fibrohistiocytic and CD34⁺ Spindle Cell Tumors

DERMATOFIBROSARCOMA PROTUBERANS AND GIANT CELL FIBROBLASTOMA

DFSP and GCF are one in the same neoplasm with the identical recurrent translocation, t(17;22)(q22;q13).[114] This results in a specific cytogenetic reciprocal translocation of the collagen type-1 alpha 1 (COL1A1) gene at chromosome 17q21.3 with the second exon of the platelet-derived growth factor β (PDGFB) gene at chromosome 22q13.1, resulting in a COL1A1-PDGFB fusion gene.[115,116]

The exclusive GCF pattern is seen more commonly in children, but both patterns are seen in DFSPs or only the DFSP pattern in individuals less than 20 years old at diagnosis.[117] Only 2% to 5% of all DFSPs present in the first two decades of life, but it is the most common primary cutaneous sarcoma in children followed by Kaposi sarcoma.[118]

DFSP typically presents as an asymptomatic, indurated fibrous plaque or nodule that may be asymmetric in appearance.[119,120] DFSP is most commonly located on the trunk but can occur on the extremities, head and neck region, and acral sites (Figure 24-24).[120] Tumor size normally ranges from 1 to 5 cm, growing slowly over years and developing superimposed multiple nodules over time.[121] In the pediatric population there can be a variable morphology resembling vascular lesions, NFs, or atrophic plaques (Figure 24-25).[119] Children less than 5 years old are more likely to have a tumor with a predominant GCF or mixed pattern of GCF and DFSP.

Several challenges are offered in the pathologic diagnosis of DFSP in that this neoplasm is uncommon in children so that the diagnosis of DFSP may not arise initially and because the histopathologic pattern may suggest a fibrous, myxoid, neurogenic, or fibromyxoid neoplasm because all of these various patterns are encountered in a DFSP.

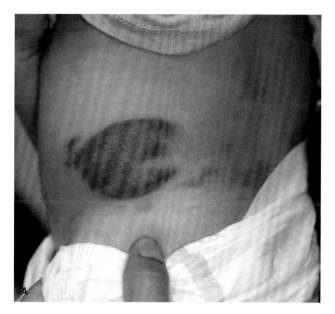
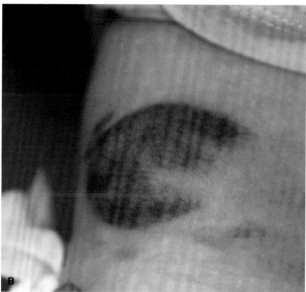

FIGURE 24-24. **Dermatofibrosarcoma protuberans.** Erythematous nodule on the trunk.

One of the consistent histologic features if the biopsy includes the subcutis is the near total replacement of the dermis and infiltration of the subcutaneous fat (Figure 24-26). The latter finding is not specific to DFSP because it is also present in diffuse NF and some of the fibrous tumors in an infant or young child. The classic pattern of DFSP consists of uniform, compactly arranged, spindle cells in fascicles and/or storiform profile, which replace the dermis and extend in a confluent fashion into the subcutis (Figure 24-27A-C). Fusiform cells have uniform nuclei with minimal pleomorphism and sparing mitotic activity. In addition to this basic pattern, myxoid and/or collagen-rich foci may be seen as adjoining foci with the classic pattern or as the exclusive pattern in some cases. The presence of scattered multinucleated

giant cells in clefted or pseudovascular spaces in a spindle cell background or loose fibrous stroma are the features of GCF (Figure 24-28A-C). The GCF pattern can be localized in a DFSP with classic or fibrous features, may represent the exclusive pattern, or is present as the initial histologic feature in a tumor that recurs with classic, myxoid, or fibrous features.[113] Pigmentation of tumor cells is uncommonly present in DFSP in the so-called Bednar tumor. Immunohistochemistry is a useful adjunct to the diagnosis of DFSP as long as it is understood that other dermal and subcutaneous spindle cell tumors are CD34+.[122] Typically, CD34 staining is uniformly and diffusely positive (Figures 24-29 and 24-30), but other markers have been reported to facilitate the diagnosis including CD99, D2-40, and apolipoprotein

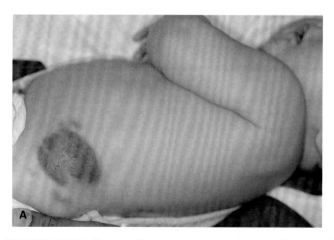
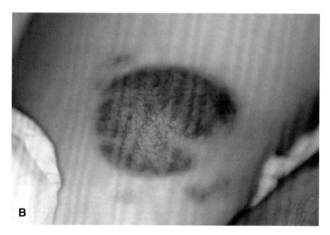

FIGURE 24-25. **Dermatofibrosarcoma protuberans.** Tumor on the flank.

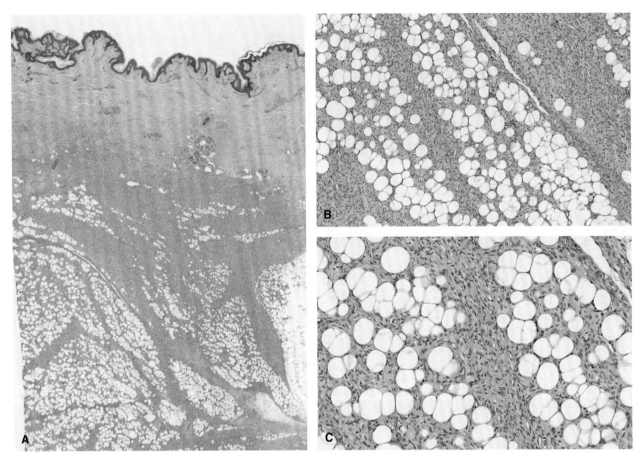

FIGURE 24-26. A-C, **Dermatofibrosarcoma protuberans.** Fibrohistiocytic proliferation with near total replacement of the dermis and infiltration of the subcutaneous fat (A). Uniform, compactly arranged, spindle cells in fascicles and/or storiform profiles that replace the dermis and extend in a confluent fashion into the subcutis (B and C). Digital slides courtesy of Path Presenter.com.

D.[121,123-126] Fluorescent in situ hybridization (FISH) is the most specific and sensitive method for the diagnosis.[115]

CD34 positivity does not distinguish DFSP from some of the other CD34+ spindle cell neoplasms; a similar pattern is present in the diffuse NFs in NF1, FHI, lipofibromatosis, and fibroblastic connective tissue nevus.

The prognosis of DFSP is essentially the same in children as in adults, with local recurrence as the principal unfavorable outcome.[127] Fibrosarcomatous (FS) or pleomorphic sarcomatous progression is seen in approximately 10% to 15% of cases and is seen in children but less often.[128,129] The overall favorable prognosis of DFSP is unfavorably altered by the presence of FS.[110] FS transformation is associated with higher grade cytology, numerous mitoses, necrosis, and particularly loss of CD34 staining. Cases of DFSP have been shown to occur more frequently in association with individuals diagnosed with adenosine deaminase–deficient severe combined immune deficiency. Such cases appear to be more frequently multifocal.[130]

CAPSULE SUMMARY

DERMATOFIBROSARCOMA PROTUBERANS AND GIANT CELL FIBROBLASTOMA

DFSP and GCF are one and the same neoplasm with the identical recurrent translocation, t(17;22)(q22;q13). The exclusive GCF pattern is seen more commonly in children, but both patterns are seen in DFSPs or only the DFSP pattern in individuals less than 20 years old at diagnosis. Only 2% to 5% of all DFSPs present in the first two decades of life, but it is the most common primary cutaneous sarcoma in children followed by Kaposi sarcoma. The classic pattern of DFSP consists of uniform, compactly arranged, spindle cells in fascicles and/or storiform profiles, which replace the dermis and extend in a confluent fashion into the subcutis. Diffuse CD34 immunoreactivity is characteristic of this tumor.

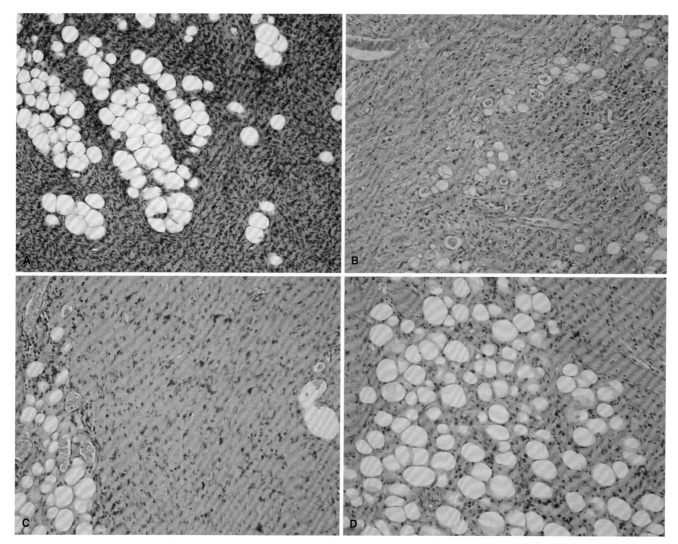

FIGURE 24-27. A-D, **Dermatofibrosarcoma protuberans on the trunk of a 4-year-old male.** A, Infiltration of tumor into the subcutis shows the overgrowth pattern. B, Another focus of this tumor shows a similar overgrown pattern, but note its more fibrous, hypocellular appearance. C, This focus shows scattered, enlarged tumor cells. D, The so-called honeycomb pattern of tumor growth is present in this focus.

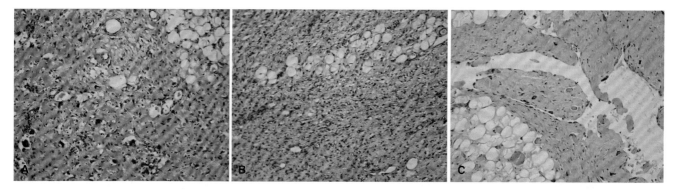

FIGURE 24-28. A-C, **Giant cell fibroblastoma (GCF) presenting in the breast of a 7-year-old female.** A, Numerous multinucleated giant cells with pericellular clear space are accompanied by a neoplastic fibrous stroma. B, Another area in the same neoplasm shows a diffuse fibrous pattern of this tumor. Most GCFs arise in a similar fibrous pattern. C, This GCF from the trunk of a 4-year-old male shows the exaggerated pseudoangiectoid pattern.

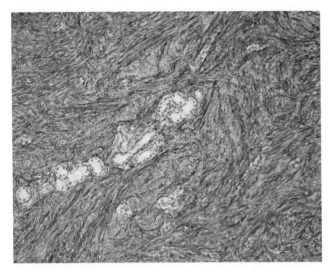

FIGURE 24-29. Dermatofibrosarcoma protuberans on the trunk of a 4-year-old male. Diffuse immunostaining for CD34 is characteristic of this neoplasm.

DERMATOFIBROMA AND FIBROUS HISTIOCYTOMAS

Dermatofibroma (DF) or fibrous histiocytoma of skin is one of the most common dermal-based mesenchymal tumors and is seen predominantly in adults between 20 and 40 years of age, with a predilection for the lower extremity (60%-70% of cases); it may present on any body surface and is infrequent in the head and neck region.[131,132] The origin of DF is unknown. There is debate if DFs represent a reactive or neoplastic process. Studies demonstrating clonal chromosomal abnormalities support the neoplastic nature of DFs.[133] Recently, recurrent gene fusion involving protein kinase C have been identified in a subset of fibrous histiocytomas.[134]

Among our cases of DF in children and adolescents between 5 and 19 years old at diagnosis, the trunk and lower extremities were the sites of presentation in over 60% of cases (Table 24-3). The mean and median age in our series (LPD)

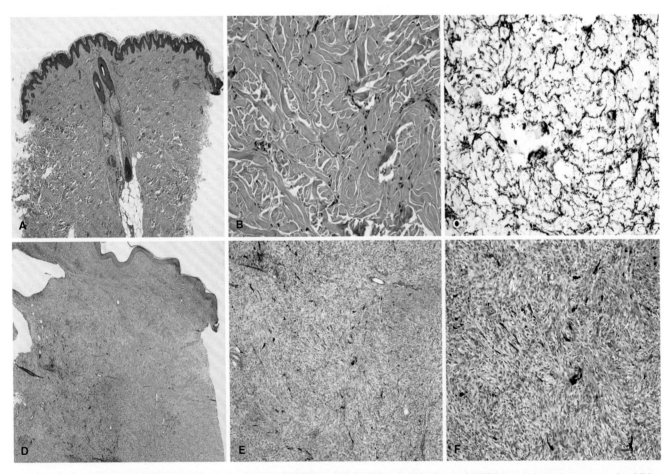

FIGURE 24-30. Dermatofibrosarcoma protuberans (DFSP) variants. The atrophic form of DFSP is particularly common in children and shows a very deceptive cytologic appearance (A and B). Diffuse CD34 staining (C) can be a clue to such diagnosis. The so-called medallion dermal dendrocyte hamartoma has identical histologic findings but lacks the *PDGFB* rearrangement seen in more than 90% of cases of DFSP. Pigmented DFSP (Bednar tumor) has the presence of deeply pigmented melanocytic cells admixed with the classic tumor cells of DFSP (D-F). Obtained with permission Dehner LP, Gru AA. Nonepithelial tumors and tumor-like lesions of the skin and subcutis in children. *Pediatr Dev Pathol.* 2018;21(2):150-207.

TABLE 24-3	Anatomic sites of dermatofibroma in 115 patients less than 20 years old
Site	Number (%)
Trunk (back and abdomen)	38 (32)
Lower extremity	37 (31)
Shoulder	20 (17)
Upper extremity	13 (11)
Head and neck	8 (7)
Breast	2 (2)
Total	118 (~100)[a]

From the files of Lauren V. Ackerman Laboratory of Surgical Pathology, St. Louis Children's Hospital, Washington University Medical Center, St. Louis, MO, 1998 to 2018; 62 females:53 males with mean and median ages: 13 years.

[a]Three patients had a second dermatofibroma.

was 13 years. Approximately 2% to 5% of DFs are diagnosed in the first two decades of life. A well-circumscribed, symmetric, round to ovoid, firm dermal nodule measures 2 cm or less in most cases.[135] On occasion, the nodule may be accompanied by tenderness or pain.[136] The overlying skin is often reddish-brown, shiny or scaly or darkly pigmented on the basis of so-called inductive changes in the epidermis.[137,138] A central dimple on lateral compression, the "button hole sign," is present in many cases. Multiple lesions are found in a small minority of cases where it was seen in 2% of children in our own series. Multiple DFs may present as congenital lesions, as eruptive nodules, or in children with trisomy 21.[139,140]

The histopathologic features of DF are relatively uniform in the majority of cases as a dermal-based spindle cell proliferation positioned in the mid-dermis, situated beneath the flattened epidermis or pushing into the underlying subcutis with absent or minimal infiltration into the subcutis, unlike the DFSP (Figure 24-31A-C). The lateral dermal borders typically demonstrate the spindle cells extending into the collagen with so-called collagen trapping. Within the body of the lesion, the spindle cells are arranged in short storiform or fascicular profiles. Some nuclear pleomorphism may be

present together with scattered mitotic figures. Lymphocytes and even eosinophils may be identified in the background. Variant patterns include those with blood-filled nonvascular spaces (aneurysmal DF), numerous macrophages with hemosiderin-laden cytoplasm, and xanthomatized macrophages. Touton giant cells in the latter setting presents the microscopic dilemma and distinction (if there is one) from the xanthogranuloma (Figure 24-32). More than one histologic pattern is present in a minority of DFs.[141]

Cellular variant of DF (cellular benign fibrous histiocytoma) is recognized by its relatively monotonous spindle cell composition and its fascicular architecture. These tumors are more mitotically active than the common DF, and focal necrosis may be present.[142] Extension into subcutis is a frequent finding and infrequently like the common DF may be centered in the subcutis.

It is unnecessary in most DFs to apply immunohistochemistry, but like the DFSP, these tumors are CD34[+]; the CD34 staining is usually localized to the periphery unlike the diffuse staining in DFSP (Figure 24-33). Unlike the DFSP, DF and its variants are diffusely reactive for CD163 in addition to factor XIIIa (Figure 24-33).[143] Cellular DF or cellular benign fibrous histiocytoma may be diffusely positive for CD34 in some cases, but desmin reactivity is present in the latter tumor in contrast to DFSP.[144]

The *atypical variants of DF* encompass a heterogeneous group of lesions that are characterized by a large size (>2 cm), more infiltrative borders, extension into the adipose tissue, frequent (>5 per 10 HPFs) or atypical mitoses, and extensive areas of necrosis.[145] Nonetheless, most of the lesions are characterized by areas of conventional DF. Within this group, the rate of local recurrence is higher (~15%) and on rare occasions metastases can be present. Horenstein et al also introduced the concept of "indeterminate fibrohistiocytic lesions" to highlight a group of neoplasms with a small size (<2.0 cm), low mitotic index (<4/10 HPF), a keloidal collagen pattern, a slight degree of pleomorphism, but honeycomb and deep infiltration into the adipose tissue. These lesions were partially immunoreactive for factor XIIIa and CD34.[145,146] This tumor type is seen in children.[147]

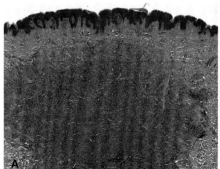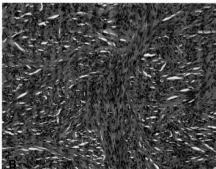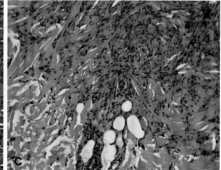

FIGURE 24-31. A-C, **Dermatofibroma presenting on the breast of a 17-year-old female.** A, The spindle cell tumor is centered in the dermis as a circumscribed nodule. Mild acanthosis noted in the overlying epidermis. B, This focus shows the uniform spindle cells arranged in a storiform profile. C, The periphery demonstrates the insinuation of spindle cells into adjacent dermis with collagen trapping. Note the limited extension.

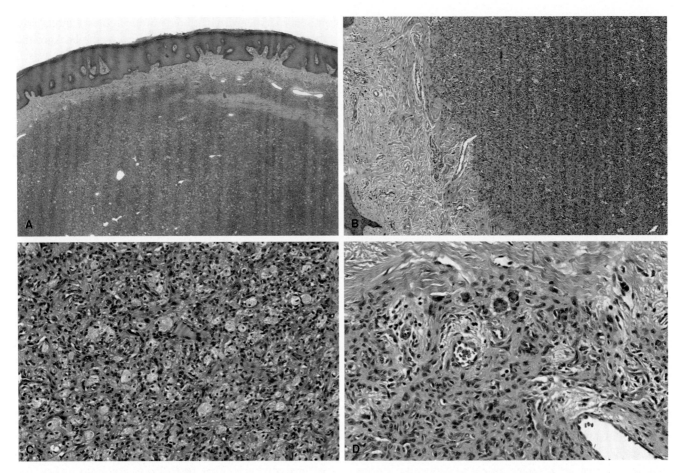

FIGURE 24-32. A-D, **Dermatofibroma versus juvenile xanthogranuloma.** Fibrohistiocytic lesion with epidermal induction changes (A). Collagen trapping at the periphery is seen (B). Xanthomatized cells (C) and Touton-type giant cells (D) are seen. Digital slides courtesy of Path Presenter.com.

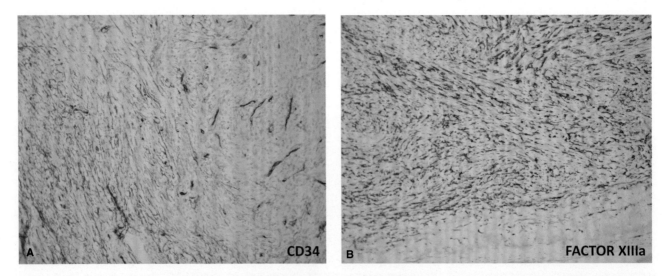

FIGURE 24-33. A and B, **Dermatofibroma presenting on the back of a 10-year-old male.** A, CD34 immunostaining demonstrates peripheral pattern of positivity, whereas only small blood vessels are highlighted in the body of the tumor. B, Factor XIIIa is diffusely positive within the tumor.

Epithelioid histiocytoma (EH, epithelioid fibrous histiocytoma) and reticulohistiocytoma are similar cutaneous neoplasms that may or may not be synonymous entities whose relationship to DF is in question because of the *ALK* rearrangement and expression, which distinguishes this tumor from DF and its variants.[148] This tumor presenting as a raised cutaneous nodule generally measures 2 cm or less.[149-151] Though mainly occurring in young to middle age adults, individual cases as young as 2 years old at presentation have been documented.[150] The predilection for the trunk and lower extremity is similar to the more common DF. A dense population of polygonal epithelioid cells with abundant pale to intensely eosinophilic cytoplasm form a nodule (Figure 24-34). Multinucleated cells vary from case to case as well as lymphocytes and plasma cells. The presence of emperipolesis and plasma cells is a feature in common with Rosai-Dorfman disease.[152] A spindle cell pattern may be seen in some cases. The differential diagnosis includes perivascular epithelioid cell tumor and BAP1-deficient epithelioid melanocytic nevus. In addition to ALK cytoplasmic positivity, EH is immunoreactive for CD163, TFE3, CD31, epithelial membrane antigen, and factor XIIIa.[149,150,153]

CAPSULE SUMMARY

DERMATOFIBROMA AND FIBROUS HISTIOCYTOMAS

DF or fibrous histiocytoma of skin is one of the most common dermal-based mesenchymal tumors. Approximately 2% to 5% of DFs are diagnosed in the first two decades of life. The histopathologic features of DF are relatively uniform in the majority of cases as a dermal-based spindle cell proliferation positioned in the mid-dermis, situated beneath the flattened epidermis or pushing into the underlying subcutis. The lateral dermal borders typically demonstrate the spindle cells extending into the collagen with so-called collagen trapping. Cellular and atypical variants have been recognized. The so-called EH might not be related to DF, as they harbor an ALK translocation.

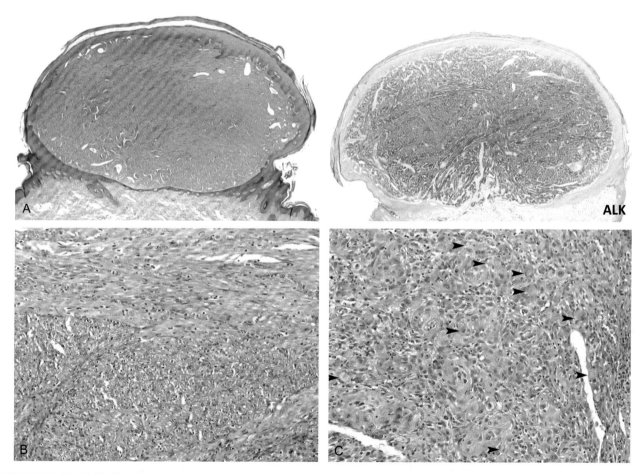

FIGURE 24-34. Epithelioid fibrous histiocytoma. Typical polypoid architecture (A) and composed of densely packed pale to clear spindle cells arranged in fascicles (B). Numerous mucinous cells are seen (C), arrow heads indicate the presence of mucinous cells. ALK is diffusely positive in the lesional cells. Adapted and obtained with permission from Kazakov DV, Kyrpychova L, Martinek P, et al. ALK Gene Fusions in Epithelioid Fibrous Histiocytoma: A Study of 14 Cases, With New Histopathological Findings. *Am J Dermatopathol.* 2018 Jan 11.

PLEXIFORM FIBROHISTIOCYTIC TUMOR

Plexiform fibrohistiocytic tumor (PFHT) is an uncommon neoplasm of the dermis and subcutis when compared to DF in individuals 20 years old or less at diagnosis. It represents a soft tissue tumor of intermediate malignancy.[154] Its etiology is unknown, but onset following local trauma has been reported.[155] Over 50% of cases present before 20 years of age with the rare congenital or early infancy occurrence, but the mean and median ages range from 14 to 20 years, respectively.[155-157] A slow-growing mass in the dermis-subcutis of the upper extremity (65%-70% of cases) or lower extremity (~15%-25%) measuring 1 to 3 cm is the clinical presentation.[155,158] The local recurrence rate is as high as 40% and metastasis to regional lymph nodes and/or lungs in 5% or less of cases, usually after one or more local recurrences.[157]

Wide local resection with tumor-free margins is generally acknowledged as the management of choice.

Because PFHT may present as a dermal-based spindle cell and/or fibrous proliferation (25%-30% of cases), as a deep dermal-subcutaneous lesion, or as a purely subcutaneous mass with a spindle cell-nodular pattern, the differential diagnosis in some cases may be a broad one.[159,160] Without the nodules of histiocytic mononuclear cells and multinucleated osteoclast-like giant cells, the lesion is another spindle cell tumor with a fibroblastic appearance (Figure 24-35A-D). It is the presence of the nodular formations with or without giant cells that is the critical clue to the diagnosis of PFHT rather than a fibrous tumor. The spindle cells are immunoreactive for smooth muscle actin, but the nodules are positive for CD68 and CD163 in PFHT (Figure 24-35D).

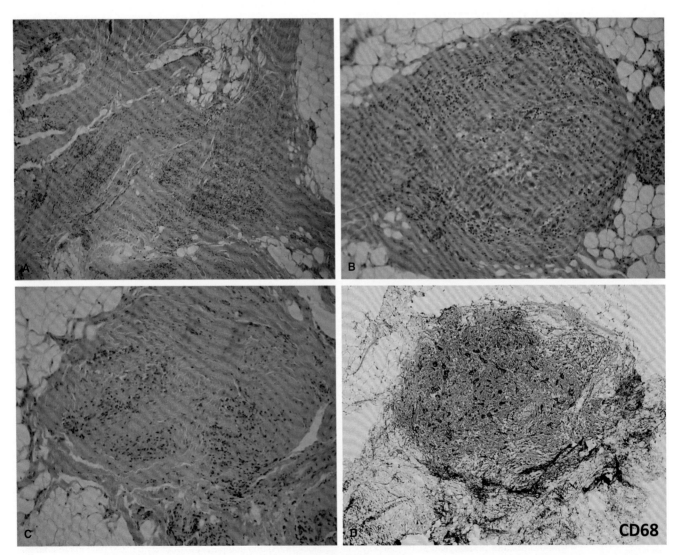

FIGURE 24-35. A-D, Plexiform fibrohistiocytic tumor presenting on the cheek of an 8-year-old male. A, Multiple nodules are present in a fibrous stromal background. B, The more cellular nodule has a granuloma-like appearance with a mixture of mononuclear and multinucleated cells. C, Here the nodules have a more fibrous appearance and may represent involution. D, CD68 immunostain shows intense positivity in the multinucleated cells.

The radiating pattern of spindle cells in the subcutis has a resemblance to FHI, lipofibromatosis, and diffuse NF. The immature mesenchymal nodules of FHI and the spindle cells of lipofibromatosis and NF are CD34⁺ in contrast to the spindle cells of PFHT.[22,23]

A problematic differential diagnosis is PFHT versus CNTK because of their overlapping histologic features and immunophenotype. These tumors are positive for CD68, NK1C3, CD10, and PAX2.[161] It has been suggested that MiTF, nonreactive in PFHT and reactive in CNTK, may be helpful in the separation of the lesions.[161] PGP9.5 is reportedly a more reliable marker of CNTK.[162] Possibly all this effort may support the hypothesis that PFHT and CNTK are related, if not the same entity.[158]

CAPSULE SUMMARY

PLEXIFORM FIBROHISTIOCYTIC TUMOR

PFHT is an uncommon neoplasm of the dermis and subcutis and represents a soft tissue tumor of intermediate malignancy (local recurrence of 40% and metastatic rate of 5%). It is the presence of the nodular formations with or without giant cells that is the critical clue to the diagnosis of PFHT rather than a fibrous tumor. Many authors consider CNTKs and PFHT histopathologic patterns that are common to a single neoplastic condition.

GIANT CELL ANGIOBLASTOMA

Giant cell angioblastoma (GCA) is an uncommon neoplasm of early infancy with rare exceptions whose nodular and spindle cell angiocentric formations, unlike PFHT, display an infiltrative pattern into the surrounding soft tissues and even bone where GCA has been reported as a primary osseous lesion.[163,164] The nodules are variably composed of mononuclear and multinucleated osteoclast-like giant cells.

CELLULAR NEUROTHEKEOMA

CNTK is an ambiguous tumor in terms of histogenesis, but is not related to the nerve sheath myxoma or myxoid neurothekeoma, which is S-100 protein and SOX-10 positive unlike the CNTK.[165] However, there is the question whether CNTK and PFHT are related histogenetic entities.[166] CNTK has the myogenic and histiocytic immunophenotype of DF and other cutaneous and soft tissue "histiocytic" tumors.[167,168] A cutaneous nodule measuring 2 cm or less arises in the arm including the shoulder or head and neck region in 60% to 70% of all cases.[169,170] Approximately 40% of patients are 20 years old or less at diagnosis including those as young as 4 to 5 years.

The range of features includes a solid, compact nodular or nested pattern or a combination of these (Figure 24-36A-D). The nests may have plexiform features composed of epithelioid and/or spindle cells and are separated by a myxohyaline or fibrous stroma. A predominant fasciculated spindle cell

pattern is yet another pattern. Within this range of patterns, the differential diagnosis includes a histiocytic or fibrohistiocytic or melanocytic neoplasm given the epithelioid and/or spindle cell morphology. Pleomorphism, mitotic activity, and infiltrative growth introduce the question of a malignancy. Like a fibrohistiocytic tumor, CNTK may be CD68 and smooth muscle actin immunopositive, but neuron-specific enolase and PGP9⁵ bring the discussion back to the neural histogenesis; these stains are generally regarded as more nonspecific than specific because S-100 protein is uniformly nonreactive, but CD10 and NK1-C3 are consistently immunopositive with focal or diffuse patterns.[170] A plausible argument can be made that CNTK, despite the misnomer, is more a fibrohistiocytic than neural immunophenotype.

ANGIOMATOID FIBROUS HISTIOCYTOMA

Angiomatoid fibrous histiocytoma (AFH) is a dermal and/or subcutaneous neoplasm with a number of less common variant sites including the lung, bone, and brain. AFH is a rare soft tissue neoplasm of intermediate biologic potential.[171] AFHs account for only 0.3% of all soft tissue tumors. Sexes are affected equally and tumors can occur in infants (including congenitally) and adults into the ninth decade of life. Most tumors present in the first three decades of life.[171]

The AFH together with several other tumors is characterized by an EWSR1 fusion transcript that includes EWSR1-ATF1 [t(12;22)(q13;q12)] as well as FUS-ATF1 [t(12;16)(q13;p11)] and EWSR1-CREB1 [t(2;22)(q33;q12)].[171-173] Most AFHs have the EWSR1 fusion.[174] A mass, generally measuring 4 cm or less, usually presents in the deep dermis and subcutis of the trunk, lower extremity, and head and neck region in patients during the first three decades of life, even in infants.[171]

A circumscribed, multinodular gray-tan to yellowish mass with or without multicystic hemorrhagic spaces is the gross appearance. A resemblance to a lymph node with hemorrhage is reflected in the microscopic features of lymphoid nodules distributed about a fibrous pseudocapsule (Figure 24-37A-D). The lymphoid nodules are an important prompt to the diagnosis of AFH, but are not present in all cases. Nodules of tumor are accompanied by dense bands of collagen. Uniform polygonal to ovoid cells with prominent pale cytoplasm and rounded to clefted or grooved nuclei comprise the nodules (Figure 24-37B). Mitotic figures are inconspicuous and nuclear pleomorphism is uncommon, but is seen in some cases without adverse prognostic implications. Osteoclast-like giant cells are far less common than in PFHT. However, these tumors may display a rather striking degree of nuclear atypia or have myxoid or spindle cell features, which may lead to other diagnostic considerations.[175-178] Among the various immunohistochemical markers, AFH is variably positive for desmin, epithelial membrane antigen, CD99, and CD68 (Figure 24-37D). Wide local excision is the recommended management with tumor-free margins because the local recurrence rate is 15% or so.[171] The metastatic potential is very low.

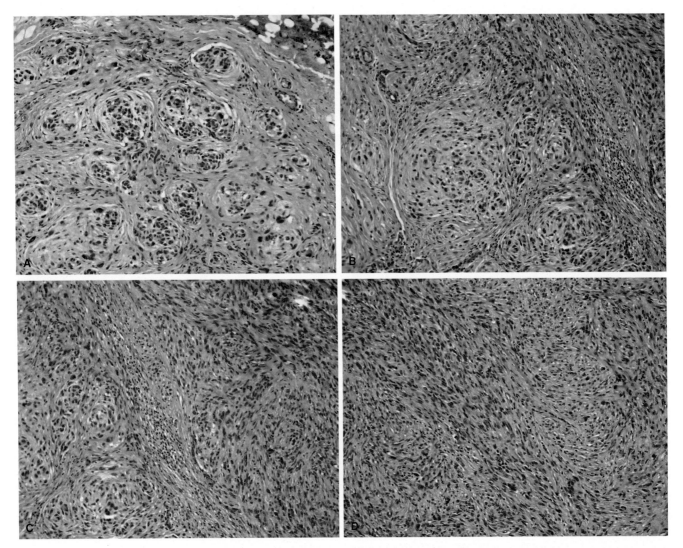

FIGURE 24-36. A-D, Cellular neurothekeoma presenting as a nodule on the face of a 16-year-old male. Several patterns of this one tumor are shown. A, A nodule is composed of multiple discrete nests with a resemblance to the nests of a plexiform fibrohistiocytic tumor. B, Several nests are shown and the larger one has a myxoid background. C, Contiguous foci show the nesting pattern and adjacent spindle cell focus. D, This focus of the same tumor has a predominant spindle cell pattern. The tumor was diffusely immunopositive for NK1-C3 (not shown).

CAPSULE SUMMARY

ANGIOMATOID FIBROUS HISTIOCYTOMA

AFH is a dermal and/or subcutaneous neoplasm of intermediate biologic potential. The AFH together with several other tumors is characterized by an *EWSR1* fusion transcript that includes *EWSR1-ATF1* [t(12;22)(q13;q12)] as well as *FUS-ATF1* [t(12;16)(q13;p11)] and *EWSR1-CREB1* [t(2;22)(q33;q12)]. A resemblance to a lymph node with hemorrhage is reflected in the microscopic features of lymphoid nodules distributed about a fibrous pseudocapsule. However, marked cellular pleomorphism is noted.

TENOSYNOVIAL GIANT CELL TUMOR

Tenosynovial giant cell tumor, although generally considered to be a "synovial"-derived neoplasm, is composed of mononuclear histiocyte-like cells with or without accompanying multinucleated osteoclast-like giant cells. The more common localized variant is the giant cell tumor of tendon sheath (GCT-TS, nodular tenosynovitis), which presents in older children and adolescents as a painless, but tender nodule in the digit, palm, or wrist as well as other sites.[179-183] The nodule, typically measuring less than 3 cm, is attached to the tendon or synovium. A multilobulated, gray to yellowish-orange mass is densely cellular and is composed of uniform mononuclear cells with or without accompanying xanthomatized cells resembling those of a xanthogranuloma and a more or less conspicuous population of multinucleated giant cells (Figure 24-38A-C).

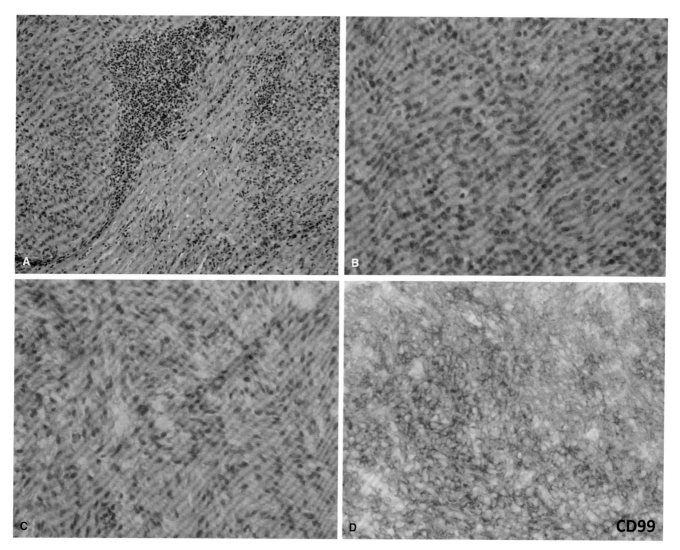

FIGURE 24-37. A-D, Angiomatoid fibrous histiocytoma presenting on the back of a 2-year-old female. A, The well-circumscribed nodule is surrounded in part by fibrous pseudocapsule with a prominent lymphocytic response. B, The tumor cells are rounded in this focus. C, Other foci of the same tumor have a more spindle cell appearance with an occasional enlarged, pleomorphic cell. D, The tumor cells are diffusely positive for CD99 as well as desmin and CD163 (not shown). EWSR1 break-apart was demonstrated by fluorescent in situ hybridization.

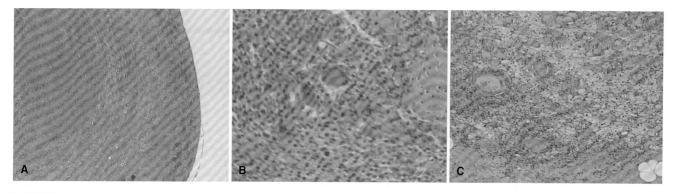

FIGURE 24-38. A-C, Giant cell tumor of tendon sheath (nodular tenosynovitis) around the knee of an 8-year-old female. A, The well-circumscribed uniformly cellular neoplasm is shown at low magnification. B, The predominant tumor cell is a mononuclear cell with scattered multinucleated giant cells. The number of giant cells within any one tumor is variable. Note the bland appearance of these cells. C, Xanthomatized mononuclear cells occupied portions of this tumor.

The tumor cells are immunoreactive for CD68 and CD163. Several molecular genetic abnormalities have been reported, in particular translocations involving 1p13, the location of macrophage colony-stimulating factor. In addition to GCT-TS, diffuse variants include pigmented villonodular synovitis and diffuse giant cell tumor arising as an intra-articular or deep soft tissue mass, respectively.

CD34⁺ DERMAL FIBROMA (MEDALLION-LIKE DERMAL DENDROCYTE HAMARTOMA)

CD34⁺ dermal fibroma (medallion-like dermal dendrocyte hamartoma) presents as an indurated plaque or nodule on the neck or upper trunk, which may be recognized soon after birth or early infancy (Figure 24-39).[184,185] Bland-appearing spindle cells replace the dermis and may extend into subcutis in a fashion resembling DFSP (Figure 24-40). Adnexal structures and blood vessels are surrounded by the bland-appearing spindle cells. In addition to CD34 immunopositivity, the spindle cells as dermal dendrocytes are reactive for factor XIIIa (Figure 24-41).

SOLITARY FIBROUS TUMOR

Solitary fibrous tumor (SFT) is a neoplasm with a number of primary sites beyond the pleura including the skin. One series of 10 cutaneous SFTs included a child, an 8-month-old male, with a forehead nodule.[186] These tumors are composed of uniform spindle cells forming into nodules or infiltrating into a fibrotic, hyalinized, or myxoid stroma (Figure 24-42). A prominent hemangioma-like or HPC-like vasculature is present in some, but not all cases. Because the SFT is immunopositive for CD34 like other similar-appearing spindle cell tumors with overlapping histologic features, nuclear expression of STAT6 is to date the only specific marker for these tumors as a manifestation of *NAB2-STAT6* gene fusion.[187-189]

FIBROUS AND MYOFIBROBLASTIC TUMORS

Fibrous and myofibroblastic tumors consist of several dermal and soft tissue neoplasms that are unique to children, with the occasional exception, especially in children less than 16 years old at diagnosis.[190] These neoplasms represented slightly more than 10% of all dermal and subcutaneous mesenchymal neoplasms among our cases (Table 24-2). However, over the two-year survey period of dermatopathologic specimens in children, only 2% of all cases were fibrous-myofibroblastic tumors (Table 24-1). In terms of morphology, most tumors are composed of spindle cells or those with a unique composition of spindle cells and adipocytes as in the case of FHI and ISF (lipofibromatosis). The differential diagnosis can be a challenging one at times with the need for immunohistochemistry and less often molecular genetics; one example is the distinction between a fibromatosis and a collagen-rich DFSP.

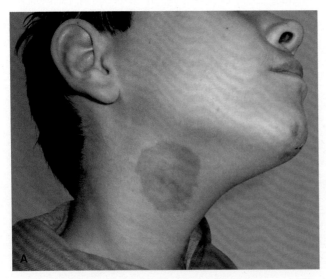
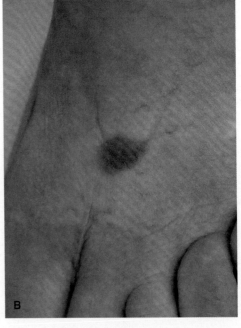

FIGURE 24-39. **Medallion-like dermal dendrocyte hamartoma.** Plaque-like dermal fibroma. Congenital lesion in a 9-year-old boy (A) and acquired lesion in an adult (B). Obtained with permission Kutzner H, Mentzel T, Palmedo G, et al. Plaque-like CD34⁺ dermal fibroma ("medallion-like dermal dendrocyte hamartoma"): clinicopathologic, immunohistochemical, and molecular analysis of 5 cases emphasizing its distinction from superficial, plaque-like dermatofibrosarcoma protuberans. *Am J Surg Pathol.* 2010;34(2):190-201.

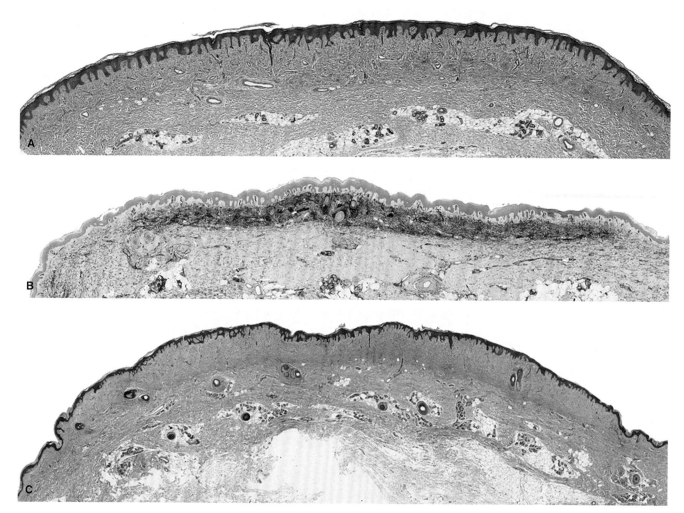

FIGURE 24-40. **Medallion-like dermal dendrocyte hamartoma.** Plaque-like dermal fibroma (scanning magnification). Richly vascularized tumor within the upper half of the dermis (A). The CD34$^+$ tumor characteristically spares the papillary body (B). The tumor always presents as a band-like fibroblastic proliferation, often covered by a hyperpigmented epidermis (C). Obtained with permission Kutzner H, Mentzel T, Palmedo G, et al. Plaque-like CD34$^+$ dermal fibroma ("medallion-like dermal dendrocyte hamartoma"): clinicopathologic, immunohistochemical, and molecular analysis of 5 cases emphasizing its distinction from superficial, plaque-like dermatofibrosarcoma protuberans. *Am J Surg Pathol.* 2010;34(2):190-201.

INCLUSION BODY FIBROMA (INFANTILE DIGITAL FIBROMA-FIBROMATOSIS) AND MYOFIBROMA/MYOFIBROMATOSIS

Inclusion body fibroma (IBF, infantile digital fibroma-fibromatosis) and *myofibroma* (MYF) are fibrous tumors of childhood that are centered in the dermis as a confluent diffuse growth into the subcutis in the case of IBF or a multinodular pattern in the MYF.[190,191] The fingers and toes are the near exclusive sites of IBF presenting as a firm nodule on the lateral and dorsal aspects of the digit(s) and measuring 2 cm or less in most cases (Figure 24-43). The extent of infiltration into the underlying tissues is difficult to appreciate from the clinical examination. Nodules on multiple fingers

and/or toes are present in 40% of cases in children less than 3 years of age and often discovered in the first year of life even in early infancy.[1] A dense collagenous and paucicellular fibrous proliferation fills the dermis with entrapment of sweat ducts and glands in the background (Figure 24-44A-C). A small paranuclear inclusion is found in all cases, but its presence in routine histologic sections may not be appreciated without a trichrome stain (Figure 24-44C). Smooth muscle actin, desmin, calponin, and CD99 are expressed in the absence of β-catenin (unlike desmoid fibromatosis). These lesions have a local recurrence rate of 40% to 70% whose growth can extend beyond the digit into the volar aspect of the hand and/or foot. Another somewhat similar-appearing acral tumor is digital fibromyxoma that

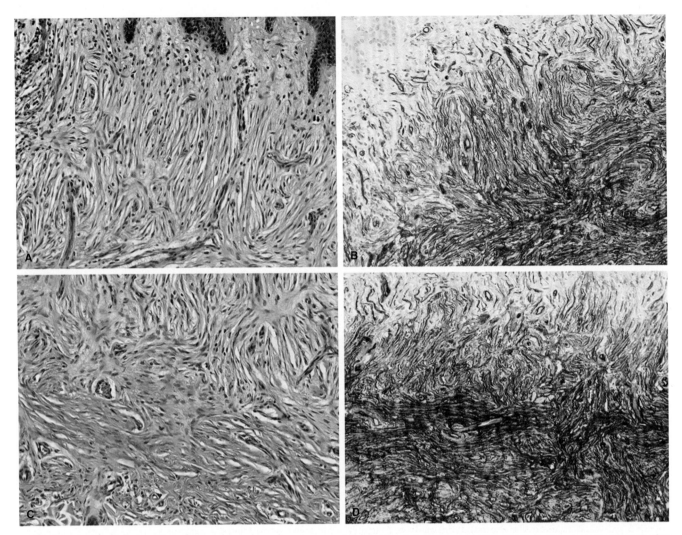

FIGURE 24-41. Medallion-like dermal dendrocyte hamartoma. Plaque-like dermal fibroma. Fibroblasts in the upper tumor part often are vertically oriented (A); vertical orientation is accentuated by the CD34 immunostain (B). Horizontally arranged fibroblasts in the lower tumor half, with steel-gray actinic elastotic material beneath (C); corresponding CD34 immunostain (D). Obtained with permission Kutzner H, Mentzel T, Palmedo G, et al. Plaque-like CD34+ dermal fibroma ("medallion-like dermal dendrocyte hamartoma"): clinicopathologic, immunohistochemical, and molecular analysis of 5 cases emphasizing its distinction from superficial, plaque-like dermatofibrosarcoma protuberans. *Am J Surg Pathol.* 2010;34(2):190-201.

occurs principally in adults, but is confined to the dermis and is CD34 immunopositive.[192] Unlike DF, fibrokeratoma, and angiofibroma with factor XIIIa positivity, the IDF is nonreactive for the latter marker. Surgical margins are not necessarily predictive of local recurrence. Paradoxically, IDF is also known to undergo spontaneous regression.[193]

The differential diagnosis of IDF is more challenging from the clinical perspective, but there are other histologically similar lesions presenting in the distal digits including the acquired digital fibrokeratoma, periungual fibroma of tuberous sclerosis, digital fibroma (noninclusion type), and digital fibromyxoma.[194-200]

Infantile MYF is one of the most common soft tissue tumors of childhood.[201] Because of the predilection of these tumors to present in young children, they are commonly referred to as infantile MYF, but the MYF is seen throughout childhood and adolescence, and even in adults.[202] Among our 175 cases in children, 92 (52%) were diagnosed at or before 1 year of age (Table 24-4). There was a male preference and almost 50% of cases presented in the head and neck region, especially the scalp with or without calvarial involvement as well as the lip and oral cavity, which is the experience of others.[202,203] Males are affected slightly more frequently than females.[204]

Infantile myofibromatosis can be sporadic or familial. Familial forms exhibit both autosomal dominant and autosomal recessive inheritance patterns.[205] Familial myofibromatosis is associated with mutations in *PDGFRB* and

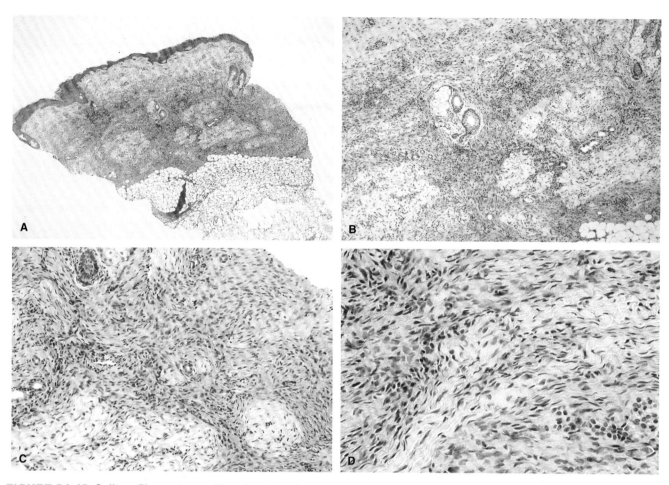

FIGURE 24-42. Solitary fibrous tumor. Short fascicles of delicate fusiform spindle cells separating bundles of dermal collagen are the histologic features present in this lesion (A-D). However, in other occasions, the tumors can have a more myxoid appearance. Obtained with permission Dehner LP, Gru AA. Nonepithelial tumors and tumor-like lesions of the skin and subcutis in children. *Pediatr Dev Pathol.* 2018;21(2):150-207.

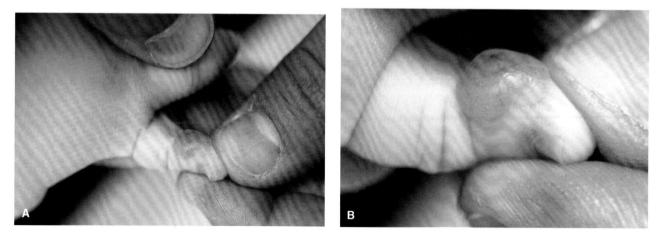

FIGURE 24-43. A and B, **Infantile digital fibroma (inclusion body fibroma [IBF]).** The fingers and toes are the near exclusive sites of IBF presenting as a firm nodule on the lateral and dorsal aspects of the digit(s) and measuring 2 cm or less in most cases.

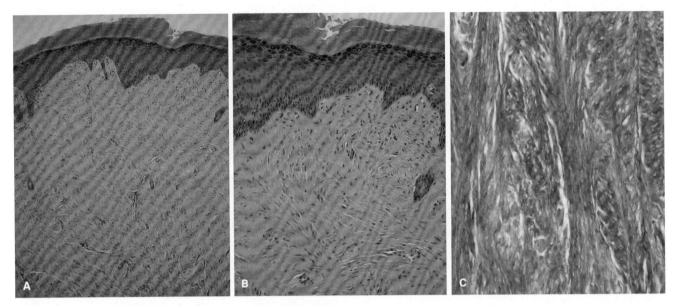

FIGURE 24-44. A-C, **Digital (inclusion) body fibromatosis presenting on the finger of a 2-year-old female.** A, The entire dermis is replaced by uniformly distributed spindle cells in a collagen-rich stroma. B, An isolated sweat duct has been enveloped by the fibrous proliferation. C, Paranuclear inclusions are optimally seen with the trichrome stain.

NOTCH3 genes.[205] Multicentric infantile myofibromatosis and some solitary lesions have also been found to have gain-of-function mutations in *PDGFRB* (a receptor tyrosine kinase).[201] MYFs are also reported in Kosaki overgrowth syndrome, also with PDGFRB germline mutations.[206] Recently, Antonescu et al identified the presence of *SRF-RELA* fusion transcripts in a subset of tumors with MYF/myopericytoma (MPC) morphology.[207]

Infantile MYF generally presents as painless, firm, flesh-colored, or purple nodules in the skin and subcutaneous tissue (Figure 24-45).[204] Tumors present in both solitary and multicentric forms (5%). The solitary form occurs in the head and neck region and upper extremity as a single cutaneous nodule. Multicentric infantile myofibromatosis involves the skin, subcutaneous tissue, muscles, and bones.[208] Multicentric and solitary forms both have a generally benign clinical course with spontaneous regression within 12 to 18 months. Generalized infantile myofibromatosis has visceral involvement and is associated with significant morbidity and mortality (Table 24-4).[1,204]

Multiple variably sized cellular to fibrohyaline nodules are present in the dermis with or without additional nodules in the subcutis. The smaller nodules may be contiguous to a small, compressed vascular space or the small vessels are accentuated by a concentric, spindle cell thickening (Figures 24-46 and 24-47). The degree of cellularity may resemble congenital-infantile fibrosarcoma, but the latter tumor has a uniformly spindle cell morphology unlike MYF. Clefted vascular spaces with a hemangiopericytoma (HPC)-like appearance is another feature that if present is usually noted in the larger, deeper nodules of tumor. Hemorrhage and necrosis may be accompanying features in the presence of the HPC-like focus. Smooth muscle actin is expressed in the myofibromatous and CD34 in the HPC-like foci. β-Catenin is not expressed by MYF, unlike desmoid fibromatosis including those presenting in infancy and Gardner-nuchal fibroma (GNF).

TABLE 24-4	Myofibroma in children and adolescents		
Anatomic Site	**Number (%)**	**M/F**	**Mean/ Median Age**
Head and neck (multifocal, 4)	76 (48)	46/30	3 y, 1 y
Trunk (multifocal, 5)	48 (27)	26/22	2.5 y, 1 y
Upper extremity	23 (13)	15/8	6 y, 1 y
Lower extremity (multifocal, 1)	21 (12)	12/9	2 y, 2 y
Other[a]	7 (4)	4/3	4 mo, 1 mo
Total	175 (100)	103/72	

Compiled from the files of the Lauren V. Ackerman Laboratory of Surgical Pathology, Washington University Medical Center, St. Louis, MO, 1989 to 2016.

[a]Small intestine (2), lung (2), kidney (1), retroperitoneum (1), posterior fossa (1).

From Dehner LP, Gru AA. Non-epithelial tumor and tumor-like lesions of the skin and subcutis in children. *Pediatr Dev Pathol.* 2018;21(2):150-207.

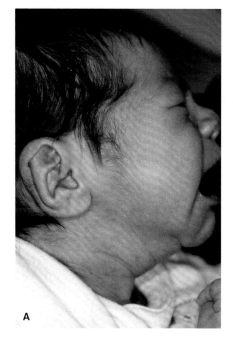
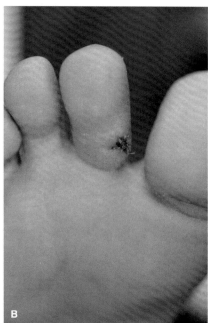

FIGURE 24-45. A and B, Infantile myofibroma generally presents as painless, firm, flesh-colored or purple nodules in the skin and subcutaneous tissue.

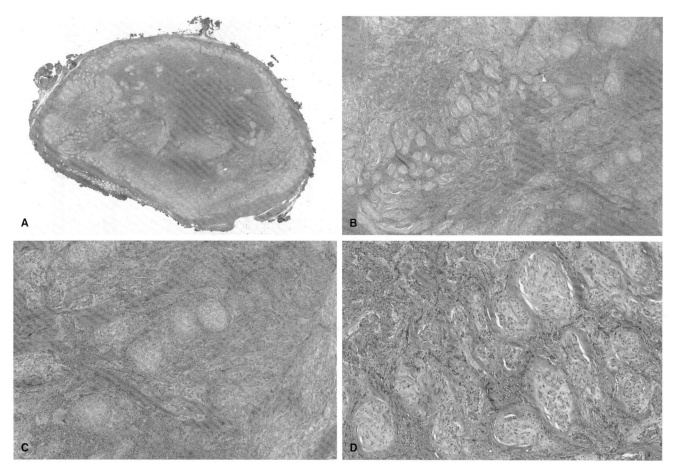

FIGURE 24-46. A-D, **Cutaneous myofibroma.** Multiple fibrohyaline nodules in the dermis are seen (A and B). Cellular areas with a sclerotic stroma are present (C). Some areas can have the appearance of hemangiopericytoma (D). Digital slides courtesy of Path Presenter.com.

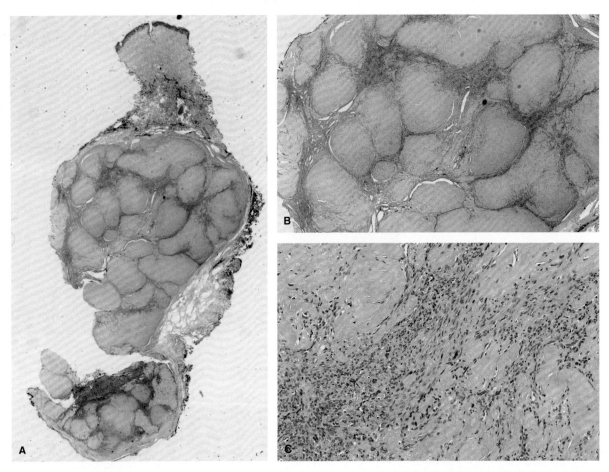

FIGURE 24-47. A-C, **Cutaneous myofibromatosis.** Well-defined nodules are noted (A and B). Bland spindle cell areas alternate with foci of dermal sclerosis (C). Digital slides courtesy of Path Presenter.com.

CAPSULE SUMMARY

INCLUSION BODY FIBROMA AND MYOFIBROMA

IBF, infantile digital fibroma-fibromatosis, and MYF are fibrous tumors of childhood that are centered in the dermis as a confluent diffuse growth into the subcutis in the case of IBF or a multinodular pattern in the MYF. The fingers and toes are the near exclusive sites of IBF presenting as a firm nodule on the lateral and dorsal aspects of the digit(s) and measuring 2 cm or less in most cases. A dense collagenous and paucicellular fibrous proliferation fills the dermis. The lesional cells show a small paranuclear trichrome-positive inclusion in all cases.

Infantile MYF is one of the most common soft tissue tumors of childhood. They have a male predominance, and almost 50% of cases present in the head and neck region, especially the scalp with or without calvarial involvement. Multiple variably sized cellular to fibrohyaline nodules are present in the dermis with or without additional nodules in the subcutis.

FIBROUS HAMARTOMA OF INFANCY

FHI and *ISF (lipofibromatosis)* are exclusively centered in the subcutis with only minimal involvement of the deep reticular dermis.[1,23,209,210] FHI affects mostly infants. Ninety percent of cases occur before the age of 2 years, 20% of cases are present at birth.[209] Boys are more commonly affected than girls. The cause of FHI is unknown. There is no established association with any familial or syndromic disorder. Recently, *EGFR* exon 20 insertion/duplication mutation has been reported, which may play a principal role in the pathogenesis.[211]

Fibrous hamartomas of infancy are characterized by solitary, enlarging tumors most commonly affecting the axilla, trunk, upper extremity, and groin area.[203] Neoplasms are generally painless and freely mobile.[212] Lesions are typically small, about 3 cm on average (Figure 24-48).[209] Rarely, overlying skin changes with discoloration, hypertrichosis, and skin tethering are reported. These tumors do not regress spontaneously, and surgical excision is generally the treatment of choice.[203]

Though FHI may appear well circumscribed by clinical evaluation, the resected specimen often fails to reflect the latter impression, but rather has a diffuse fatty and myxoid appearance. Microscopically, the subcutis is variably replaced

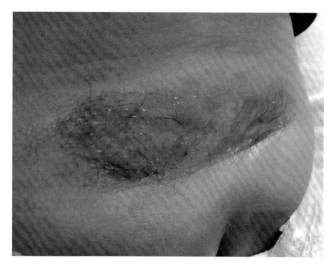

FIGURE 24-48. Fibrous hamartoma of infancy. Skin-colored plaque on the lumbar back with hypertrichosis and perspiration. Reprinted with permission from Melnick L, Berger EM, Elenitsas R, et al. Fibrous hamartoma of infancy: a firm plaque presenting with hypertrichosis and hyperhidrosis. *Pediatr Dermatol.* 2015;34(4):533-535.

by a fibrous spindle cell proliferation, myxoid foci of immature spindle to ovoid cells, and a background of adipose tissue; less the myxoid nodules, the pattern is very similar to ISF (lipofibromatosis) (Figure 24-49). The myxoid nodules of FHI may be identified as isolated small foci within the fat or at the periphery of the more fibrous fascicles where fibrous overgrowth and maturation convey the sense of a more fibromatosis-like appearance. Some cases have been found in association with a congenital nevus.[213] Foci of hypercellularity resembling congenital-infantile fibrosarcoma are found in a minority of cases similar to the same findings in the infantile MYF.[214] Pseudovascular and GCF-like areas may be encountered as well. If a skin ellipse accompanies the resected mass, extension of the fibrous spindle cells into the reticular dermis with compression of the eccrine sweat glands may be seen. Smooth muscle actin is expressed in the fibrous spindle cell component, and CD34 immunopositivity is detected in the immature myxoid nodules and GCF-like foci.[209]

Both tumor types have similar patterns of growth in the subcutis between lobules of fat, with expansive overgrowth of contiguous lobules rather than the so-called honeycomb

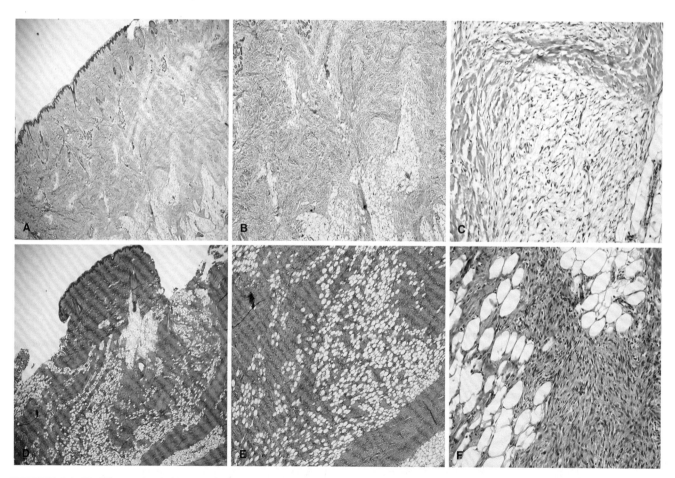

FIGURE 24-49. Fibrous hamartoma of infancy (FHI). In FHI, the subcutis is variably replaced by a fibrous spindle cell proliferation, myxoid foci of immature spindle to ovoid cells, and background of adipose tissue (A-C). The myxoid nodules of FHI may be identified as isolated foci within the fat or at the periphery of the more fibrous fascicles where fibrous overgrowth or maturation conveys the sense of incorporation into the more fibromatosis-like area (C). The example in the bottom images shows much resemblance to a dermatofibrosarcoma protuberans (D-F).

or infiltrative pattern of DFSP or diffuse NF (Figure 24-49). The differential diagnosis of ISF includes an aggressive tumor with similar histologic features, but is diffusely S-100 protein and CD34 immunopositive.

CAPSULE SUMMARY

FIBROUS HAMARTOMA OF INFANCY

FHI and ISF (lipofibromatosis) are exclusively centered in the subcutis with only minimal involvement of the deep reticular dermis. Fibrous hamartomas of infancy are characterized by solitary, enlarging tumors most commonly affecting the axilla, trunk, upper extremity, and groin area. Though FHI may appear well circumscribed by clinical evaluation, the resected specimen often fails to reflect the latter impression, but rather has a diffuse fatty and myxoid appearance. Microscopically, the subcutis is variably replaced by a fibrous spindle cell proliferation, myxoid foci of immature spindle to ovoid cells, and a background of adipose tissue.

NODULAR FASCIITIS

Nodular fasciitis (NoF) is regarded as a benign, self-limited neoplasm consisting of myofibroblasts and is one of several other lesions with a *MYH9-USP6* translocation, including aneurysmal bone cyst, myositis ossificans, and cellular tendon sheath fibroma.[215-217] A minority of NoFs present in the dermis, whereas most are found in the subcutis as a rubbery to cystic mass measuring 2 cm or less in most cases. NoF typically presents as an asymptomatic, solitary, firm, fast-growing nodule on the upper extremities, trunk, and head and neck region.[218-220] Tumors are generally 2 to 3 cm in size and are often described as fixed or immobile (Figure 24-50A and B).[221] Although surgical excision is often performed, lesions often regress spontaneously.[220]

Pathologically, NoF is composed of plump spindle cells in variable myxoid background with mucoid microcysts and patchy extravasation of erythrocytes (Figure 24-51A-D). Both the dermis and subcutis are occupied by circumscribed nodules in most cases with limited dermal involvement.[222-226] Cellular variant of tendon sheath fibroma has some overlapping histologic features to NoF, but is present in acral sites (Figure 24-51A and B). *Proliferative fasciitis*, far less common than NoF especially in younger individuals, arises in the subcutis and infrequently in the dermis (Figure 24-52).[223] Ganglion-like cells among spindle cells are characteristic of this lesion. Keratin AE1/AE3 is often expressed in the ganglion-like cells.[224]

CAPSULE SUMMARY

NODULAR FASCIITIS

NoF is regarded as a benign, self-limited neoplasm consisting of myofibroblasts and is one of several other lesions with a MYH9-USP6 translocation. NoF typically presents as an asymptomatic, solitary, firm, fast-growing nodule on the upper extremities, trunk, and head and neck region. Pathologically, NoF is composed of plump spindle cells in variable myxoid background with mucoid microcysts and patchy extravasation of erythrocytes.

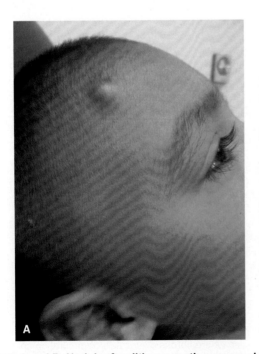
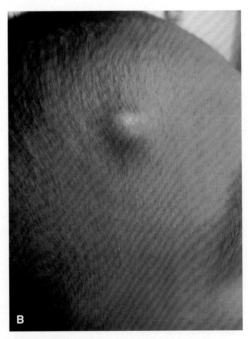

FIGURE 24-50. **A and B, Nodular fasciitis presenting as a nodule on the forehead.**

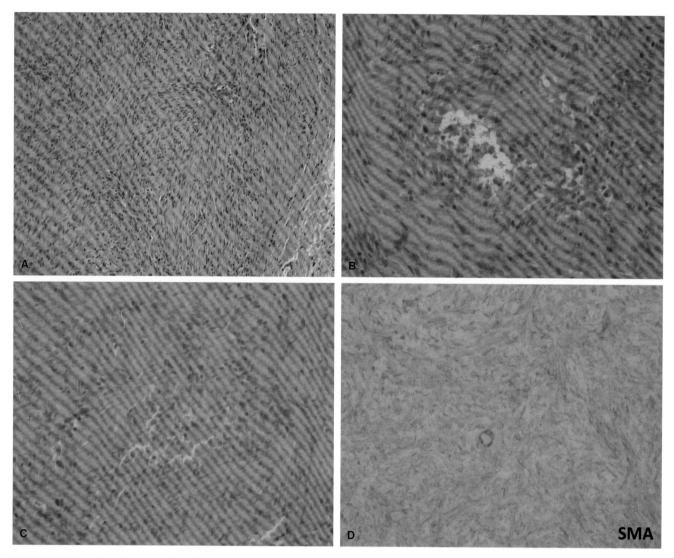

FIGURE 24-51. A-D, **Nodular fasciitis presenting on the forehead of a 1-year-old male.** A, The interface between the nodule and the adjacent subcutis is shown. This area is important in the differential diagnosis from myofibroma which often has small compressed vessels not seen in nodular fasciitis. B, Microcyst such as this one is important to the diagnosis. C, Interstitial hemorrhage is another characteristic feature. D, Smooth muscle actin (SMA) is diffusely positive.

DESMOPLASTIC FIBROBLASTOMA

Desmoplastic fibroblastoma (DFB, collagenous fibroma) is an uncommon fibrous neoplasm with some resemblance to the tendon sheath fibroma (Figure 24-53) with its nodular dense collagenous hypocellular appearance and its predilection for the hand and feet, but a wider distribution in nonacral sites as well.[227] Both superficial and deep soft tissues are sites of presentation for a firm mass that generally measures 2 cm or less in the subcutis. A few examples have been reported in children.[228,229] Circumscribed nodules without infiltrative borders are composed of dense, hypovascular collagen with an overall paucicellular appearance

(Figure 24-54A and B). Fusiform and stellate fibroblasts occupy the stroma without any particular architectural arrangement.[230] The fibroblasts may express smooth muscle actin, but are nonreactive for CD34. FOSL1 is overexpressed in the nuclei of DFB on the basis of the 11q12 rearrangement.[227] These tumors are known to locally recur.

The sclerotic nodular appearance of DFB has the differential diagnosis of sclerotic fibroma (SF), partially sclerotic dermatofibroma (SDF) and sclerotic SFT.[231-234] With the exception of the SFT, the SF and SDF are dermocentric tumors unlike DFB with its subcutaneous and deep soft tissue involvement.

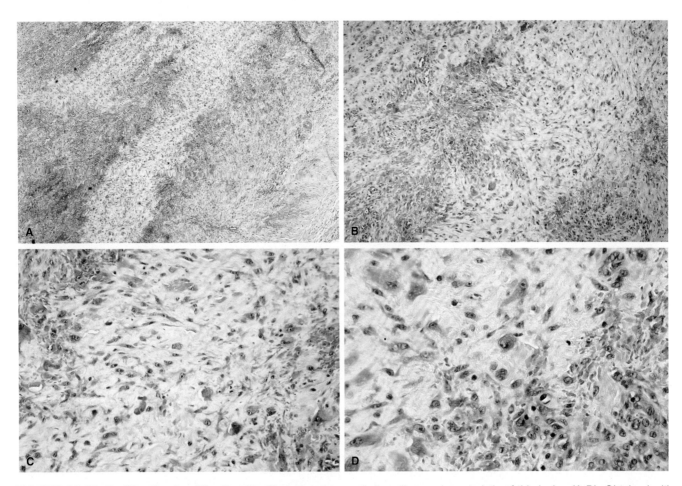

FIGURE 24-52. **Proliferative fasciitis.** Ganglion-like cells among spindle cells are characteristic of this lesion (A-D). Obtained with permission Dehner LP, Gru AA. Nonepithelial tumors and tumor-like lesions of the skin and subcutis in children. *Pediatr Dev Pathol.* 2018;21(2):150-207.

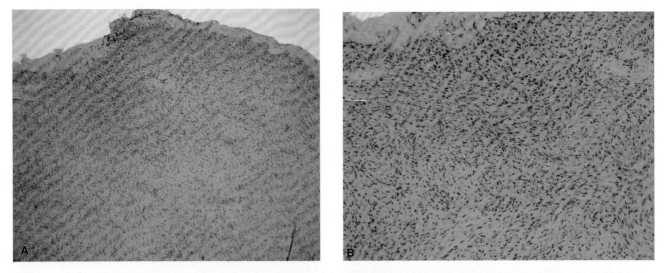

FIGURE 24-53. A and B, **Tendon sheath fibroma, cellular variant presenting on the finger of a 5-year-old female.** A, This encapsulated nodular lesion has a diffusely cellular appearance unlike the hypocellular collagenous appearance of the classic tendon sheath fibroma. B, The spindle cells have uniform benign features. This variant is reported to have a *USP6* gene rearrangement that is not found in the classic lesion.

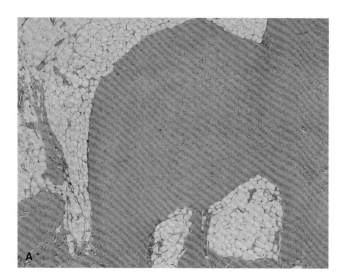 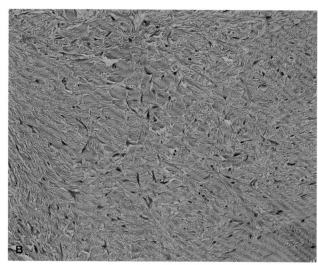

FIGURE 24-54. A and B, **Desmoplastic fibroblastoma presenting as a firm nodule on the back of an 18-year-old male.** A, Partial overgrowth of the subcutis by a collagen-rich, hypocellular fibrous proliferation is seen. B, Both spindle and stellate cells are separated by the dense collagen.

CAPSULE SUMMARY

DESMOPLASTIC FIBROBLASTOMA

DFB, collagenous fibroma, is an uncommon fibrous neoplasm with some resemblance to the tendon sheath fibroma with its nodular dense collagenous hypocellular appearance and its predilection for the hand and feet, but a wider distribution in nonacral sites as well.

GARDNER-NUCHAL FIBROMA

GNF is a fibrous neoplasm typically presenting in the posterior neck and/or trunk (paraspinal region) in 60% of cases, but not to the exclusion of other anatomic sites (Figures 24-55 and 24-56).[190,235] The GNF presents as a firm, plaque-like mass, and almost 80% of cases are recognized during the first decade of life and even before 1 year of age.[235] An association with familial adenomatous polyposis-Gardner syndrome (FAP-GS) is reported in 60% to 70% of cases. NGF in a child or young adult may be the first clinical manifestation

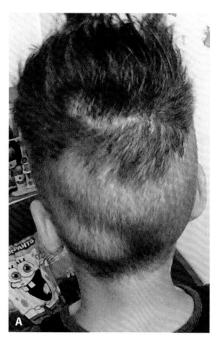 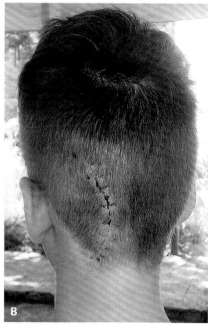

FIGURE 24-55. Gardner nuchal fibroma. Clinical presentation. A, Poorly circumscribed, firm, rubbery, plaque-like tumor formation, measuring approximately 4/5 cm, located on the left occipital region in an 8-year-old male patient. B, Postoperative findings. Wound is sutured after total surgical excision under general anesthesia. Obtained with permission Chokoeva AA, Patterson JW, Tchernev G, et al. Giant subcutaneous solitary Gardner fibroma of the head of a Bulgarian child. *Am J Dermatopathol.* 2017;39(12):950-952.

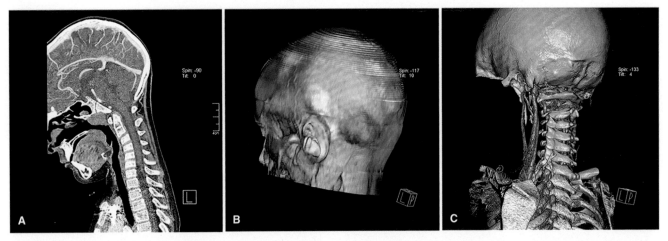

FIGURE 24-56. Gardner nuchal fibroma. A, A tumor formation measuring approximately 4 cm in thickness is observed through native scanning, located in the left occipital right area, with an inhomogeneous structure and sharp and smooth margins. Computerized tomography with contrast—the visible part of the aortic arch, extracranial vessels, and intracranial vessels are presented with preserved architecture. B, Extra- and intracranial venous vascular structures have preserved hemodynamics and architecture. A more extended arterial structure, representing a branch of occipitalis (A), is observed as a "feeder" vessel of the described tumor formation in the left occipital area. C, Small changes in progress, folded vessels, and early intravenous contrasting are observed with contrast saturation. In the venous phase, the described formation is highlighted more significantly. There are no visible changes in the underlying bone structure. Obtained with permission Chokoeva AA, Patterson JW, Tchernev G, et al. Giant subcutaneous solitary Gardner fibroma of the head of a Bulgarian child. *Am J Dermatopathol.* 2017;39(12):950-952.

of FAP-GS.[236] However, there are isolated examples of non–FAP-associated NGFs, but all children should be provided with the opportunity for genetic counseling.[237] Pathologically, the mass is poorly circumscribed, measures 2 to 10 cm, and has a dense, hypocellular, somewhat nodular-appearing collagen that occupies the subcutis with a fibrolipomatous or scar-like appearance (Figure 24-57A-C). It is estimated that approximately 25% of FAP-GS-associated desmoid-type fibromatosis has an accompanying GNF.[238] Recurrent GNF may have the histologic features of a desmoid-like fibromatosis. Like the latter tumor, there is diffuse nuclear expression of β-catenin in NGF.[235,239,240] There is also nuclear positivity for cyclin D1 and C-myc.[235] Immunostains are helpful in the problematic case of a scar-like mass in a child without a history of a previous procedure.

MYOPERICYTOMA

MPC is a spindle cell neoplasm with a predilection for the extremities and presents as a nodule in the dermis and/or subcutis. The age range is broader than infantile MYF, with cases reported in older children and adults.[241] One of the challenges is the differentiation of MPC from infantile MYF in a young child.[242] The presence of plump myoid or glomoid tumor cells around vascular spaces within the tumor is one of the distinctive features of the MPC, but otherwise there are many overlapping features with the infantile MYF (Figure 24-58).[243] Myxohyaline stroma, a characteristic of infantile MYF, is generally inconspicuous in the MPC, but we acknowledge that the distinction can be a subtle one. A malignant counterpart of MPC is recognized and has a

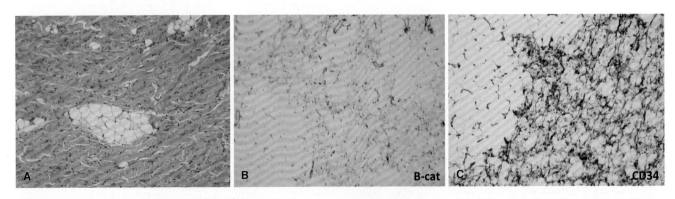

FIGURE 24-57. A-C, Gardner-nuchal fibroma presenting as a mass on the back of a 6-month-old male with no known history of Gardner syndrome. A, The subcutis is diffusely occupied by a fibrolipomatous lesion with uniformly dispersed cellularity. B, β-Catenin immunostains demonstrate nuclear positivity. C, The CD34 immunostain is also diffusely positive.

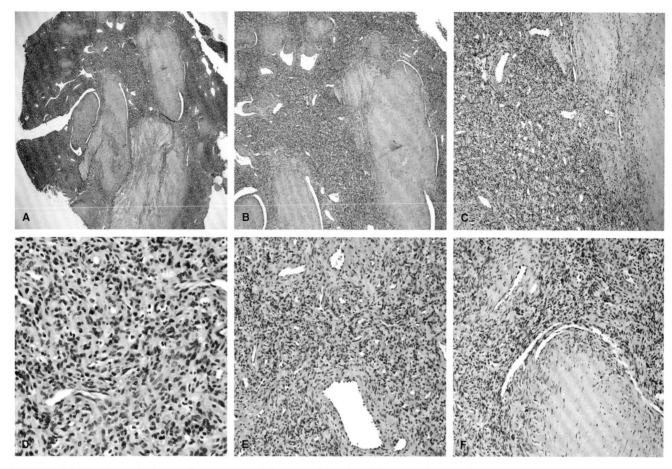

FIGURE 24-58. **Myopericytoma.** The presence of plump myoid or glomoid tumor cells around vascular spaces within the tumor mass is one of the distinctive features of the myopericytoma, but otherwise there are many overlapping features with the infantile myofibroma (A-F).

NTRK1 gene fusion.[244] The pediatric cases are more akin to infantile myofibromatosis/hemangiopericytoma.

Myogenic, Myxomatous, and Adipose Tumors

RHABDOMYOMATOUS MESENCHYMAL HAMARTOMA

Rhabdomyomatous mesenchymal hamartoma (RMH) is a well-documented, presumably anomalous lesion occurring in infants and young children as a nodule, plaque, or skin tag–like polypoid papule in the head and neck or sacral-perianal region.[245,246] Scattered individual fibrous or small clusters of mature and somewhat immature skeletal muscle are present in the dermis and/or superficial subcutis.[247-249] The degree of skeletal muscle differentiation in RMH is well beyond a cutaneous embryonal rhabdomyosarcoma (RMS) with its overtly malignant features (Figure 24-59).

SMOOTH MUSCLE HAMARTOMA

Smooth muscle hamartoma (SMH), usually discovered at or shortly after birth, is typically located in the lumbosacral region as a skin-colored plaque or, in association with hyperpigmentation, as in a Becker nevus, or capillary vascular anomaly, or hypertrichosis (Figure 24-60).[250-252] Vellus hairs are often an accompanying finding. Generalized SMHs have been reported to raise the question of an overgrowth syndrome.[253] Bundles of disorganized smooth muscle originating from the arrector pili muscle occupy the dermis with the formation of a dermal-occupying mass. The blue nevus and SMH are rarely seen together in the same lesion (Figure 24-61).

CUTANEOUS LEIOMYOMA

Leiomyoma (LM) of the skin is classified on the basis of the smooth muscle from which the tumor is derived, such as arrector pili (piloleiomyoma), anatomic site-specific smooth muscle (scrotum, vulva, nipple), or the media

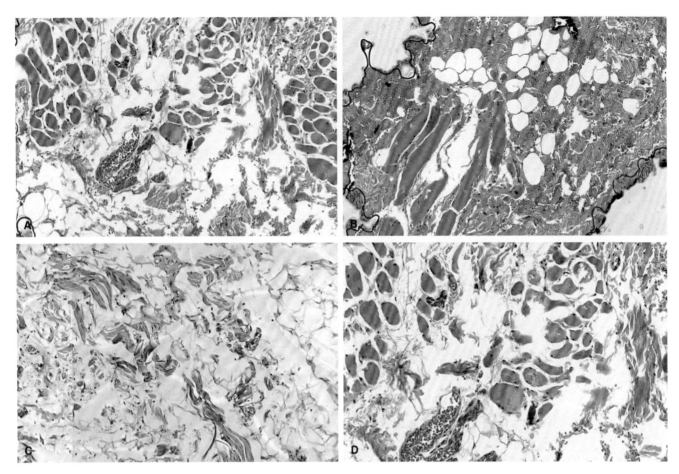

FIGURE 24-59. A-D, Rhabdomyomatous mesenchymal hamartoma. Scattered individual fibrous or small clusters of mature and somewhat immature skeletal muscle are present in the dermis and/or superficial subcutis. Digital slides courtesy of Path Presenter.com.

of blood vessels (angioleiomyoma).[254-256] Most LMs are solitary papulonodular tumors arising from arrector pili smooth muscle, but in the presence of multiple such lesions, the possibility of hereditary leiomyomatosis-renal cell carcinoma should be considered.[257-259]

LMs in the setting of hereditary leiomyomatosis and renal cell cancer occur most commonly in the second and third decade of life and affect approximately 75% of patients with this condition.[260] Hereditary leiomyomatosis and renal cell cancer, also known as Reed syndrome, is an

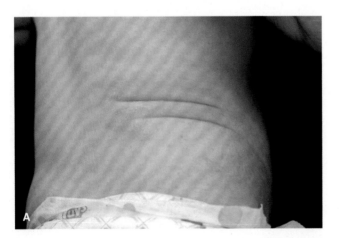
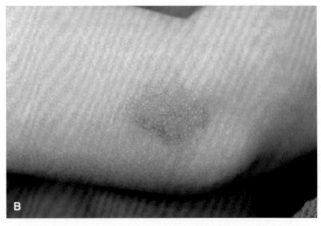

FIGURE 24-60. Smooth muscle hamartoma. Smooth muscle hamartoma. Yellow-to-light-brown hued, slightly verrucous plaques (A and B).

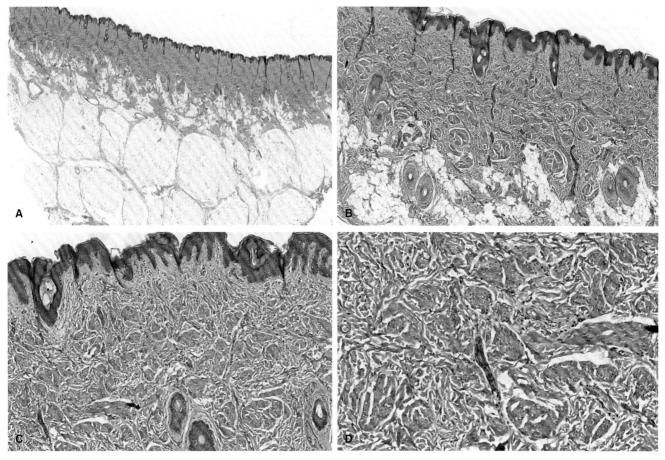

FIGURE 24-61. **Smooth muscle hamartoma.** Disorganized bands of mature smooth muscle fibers are noted in the dermis (A-D). Digital slides courtesy of Path Presenter.com.

autosomal dominant condition caused by mutation in the fumarate hydratase gene located on chromosome 1q.[260]

LMs present as grouped skin-colored to brownish-red, firm papules or nodules that slowly enlarge. The most common location is trunk and extremities. Lesions can be painful or hypersensitive.[260,261] In patients with multiple, progressive, and painful LMs, the diagnosis of hereditary leiomyomatosis and renal cell cancer should be considered.[262]

Piloleiomyoma is composed of multiple contiguous bundles of smooth muscle forming a mass. A distinctive feature is the presence of spindle cells with cigar-shaped nuclei and perinuclear halos. The cells are positive for smooth muscle actin, desmin, and h-caldesmon by immunohistochemistry (Figure 24-62).

Angioleiomyoma (vascular LM) is uncommon in children, but is seen in the third decade as a painful nodule, measuring 2 cm or less on the lower extremity (60%-80% of cases) and less commonly in other sites.[263-265] A circumscribed nodule with or without an attachment to the lower dermis is composed of spindle to epithelioid cells with conspicuous eosinophilic cytoplasm and slit-like vascular spaces (Figure 24-63A-C).[266]

CAPSULE SUMMARY

LEIOMYOMA

LM of the skin is classified on the basis of the smooth muscle from which the tumor is derived, such as arrector pili (piloleiomyoma), anatomic site-specific smooth muscle (scrotum, vulva, nipple), or the media of blood vessels (angioleiomyoma).[254-256] Most LMs are solitary papulonodular tumors arising from arrector pili smooth muscle, but in the presence of multiple such lesions, the possibility of hereditary leiomyomatosis-renal cell carcinoma should be considered.

Smooth Muscle Tumors of Indeterminant or Overtly Malignant Type (Leiomyosarcoma)

Another category of smooth muscle tumors are those that arise in a number of sites as a solitary or multiple lesions including the subcutis in immunocompromised individuals and

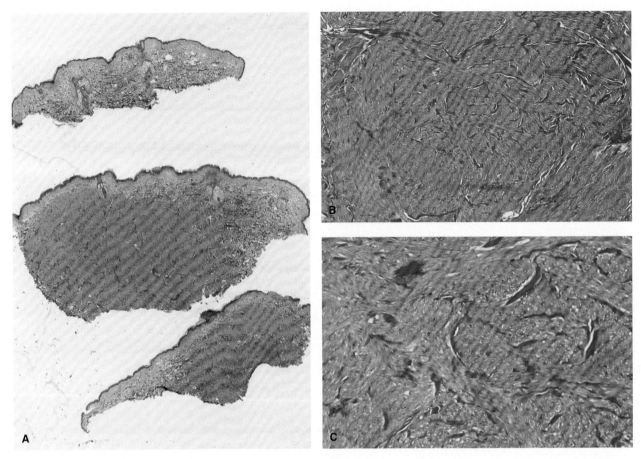

FIGURE 24-62. **Leiomyoma, pilar type.** Nodular spindle cell lesion in the dermis. The lesional cells have elongated, cigar-shaped nuclei, perinuclear vacuoles, and sclerotic bands of collagen in between (A-C). No mitotic figures are noted. Obtained with permission Dehner LP, Gru AA. Nonepithelial tumors and tumor-like lesions of the skin and subcutis in children. *Pediatr Dev Pathol.* 2018;21(2):150-207.

are associated with Epstein–Barr virus (EBV).[267,268] Initially, it was thought that these tumors were restricted to HIV-infected children because they are also seen in similarly infected adults. The skin and subcutis are just two sites among a number of other locations where these neoplasms may present, including the soft tissues and in various organs. Histopathologically, these tumors may have overtly malignant features with nuclear enlargement, pleomorphism, and mitotic activity to those with more benign features. The histologic features can vary from an immature mesenchymal neoplasm to a fasciculated spindle cell tumor with apparent smooth muscle differentiation as confirmed by immunohistochemistry (Figure 24-64).[269,270] One case has been reported in a young HIV-infected adult with the features of an angioleiomyoma.[202]

Myxomatous and lipomatous tumors together accounted for 10% or less of dermal and subcutaneous tumors in children.[1] Myxomatous or mucoid stroma is a feature in a number of tumors that have been discussed in prior sections. Neurogenic, fibrohistiocytic, and myofibroblastic neoplasms of various types can have a myxoid stroma as an accompanying or predominant feature as in the case of the myxoid neurothekeoma or nerve sheath myxoma with its lobulated myxoid nodules, myxomatous AFH, myxoid SFT, and NoF. The general topic of myxomatous and lipomatous tumors has been reviewed at length elsewhere.[1,271,272]

SUPERFICIAL ANGIOMYXOMA

Superficial angiomyxoma (SAM) may present throughout the life span, with some examples in children as young as 2 years old (5%-10% of SAM occur in children).[207,273] The trunk, head and neck, lower extremities, and perineum are the various sites of presentation.[274] The lesions have a very high rate of local recurrence, usually around 30% to 40% depending on the series. The recurrences are typically larger in size. However, such tumors do not show widespread metastasis. A papule, nodule, or polyp measuring less than 2 cm in most cases is represented by a poorly delineated myxoid nodule with small vascular structures and spindle cells in the background of this dermal-based lesion (Figure 24-65). The neutrophils are a very helpful clue to establish such diagnosis, as those cells are absent in other

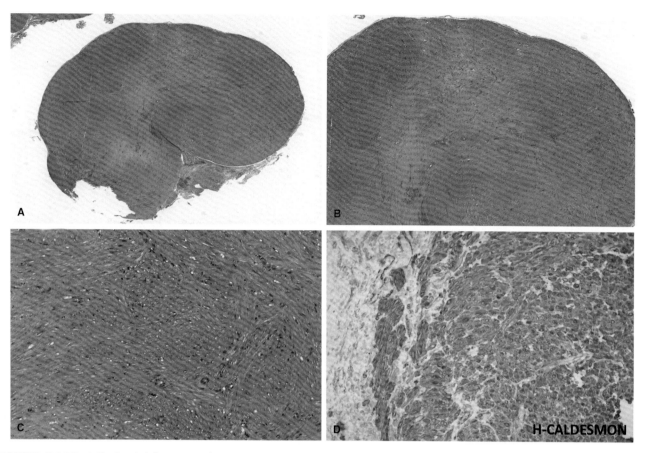

FIGURE 24-63. **A-D, Angioleiomyoma (vascular leiomyoma) presenting as a nodule on the scalp of a 4-month-old male.** A, The well-circumscribed nodule is composed of round and spindle cells. B and C, A suggested remnant of the vessel wall at the periphery blends into the cellular portion of the tumor with numerous small vascular spaces. D, The tumor cells are strongly and diffusely positive for Caldesmon (shown) and smooth muscle actin. A portion of the vessel wall is seen at the periphery.

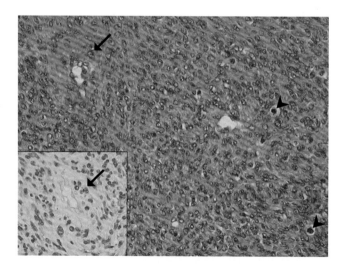

FIGURE 24-64. **Epstein–Barr virus+ leiomyosarcoma in an HIV+ child.** Diffuse round cell component with focal vascular mural cellular proliferation (arrow) and mitoses (arrowheads) (hematoxylin and eosin, 320×). Inset: diffuse nuclear EBER positivity of leiomyosarcoma and vascular mural cells (arrow) (480×). Obtained with permission Ramdial PK, Sing Y, Deonarain J, Hadley GP, Singh B. Dermal Epstein–Barr virus—associated leiomyosarcoma: tocsin of acquired immunodeficiency syndrome in two children. *Am J Dermatopathol.* 2011;33(4):392-396.

types of myxoid neoplasms. Entrapped adnexal structures are frequently seen.[274,275] The spindle cells and small vessels are immunopositive for CD34.[272] There is a variant of SAM that presents in the digits.[276] The presence of multiple SAMs is a manifestation of Carney complex or occurs sporadically.[277-279]

CUTANEOUS MYXOMAS

Myxoma of the skin, especially multiple myxomas, should initiate the inquiry about the possibility of Carney complex.[3] Mucocutaneous myxomas of Carney complex present as multiple sessile and pedunculated papules in the head and neck region, including the eyelids, earlobes, oral cavity, nipple, and perineum. These lesions are seen in the first two decades of life (Figure 24-66).[280] Cutaneous myxomas have been reported in more than 30% to 50% of patients with Carney complex.[42,281] Cutaneous myxomas are even more common in patients with Carney complex and cardiac myxomas (detected in 81% of patients with cardiac myxomas).[42] There are extraordinary examples of multiple cutaneous myxomas in children without apparent Carney complex. Within an individual myxomatous focus, the presence of

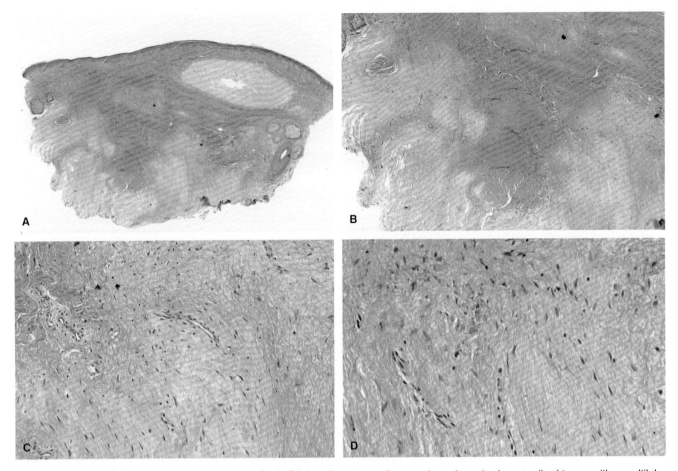

FIGURE 24-65. A-D, Superficial angiomyxoma. Superficial angiomyxoma shows a dermal poorly circumscribed tumor with a multilobular growth, composed of scattered bland, spindle-shaped to stellate cells in a copious amount of myxoid stroma (A and B). The cells lack significant cytologic atypia. Small, thin-walled vessels are prominent in the background (C and D). Digital slides courtesy of Path Presenter.com.

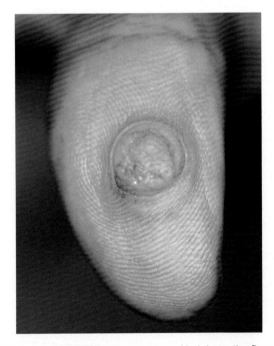

FIGURE 24-66. Cutaneous myxoma. Nodule on the finger.

fibroblast-like cells and small blood vessels may have some features of a SAM, but they are composed of multiple circumscribed myxoid nodules with minimal or modest cellularity in a fibrous background.[282]

A distinction should be made between a myxoma and focal dermal mucinosis. Sharply demarcated, hypocellular myxoid nodules are the composition of the myxoma with abundant pale staining to bluish mucoid matrix (Figure 24-67). The nodules occupy the dermis to a variable degree and extend into the subcutis. A fine network of reticulum fibers is present in the myxoma, whereas mucinosis forms a focus of mucin that separates but does not entirely displace the dermal collagen.

PRIMITIVE MYXOID MESENCHYMAL TUMOR OF INFANCY

Primitive myxoid mesenchymal tumor of infancy (PMMTI) is a neoplasm of early childhood from newborn to 3 years of age.[283] It can present as a superficial polyp or deep soft tissue mass measuring 1 cm or less to 15 cm.[284] A prominent, uniform myxoid background contains a population of

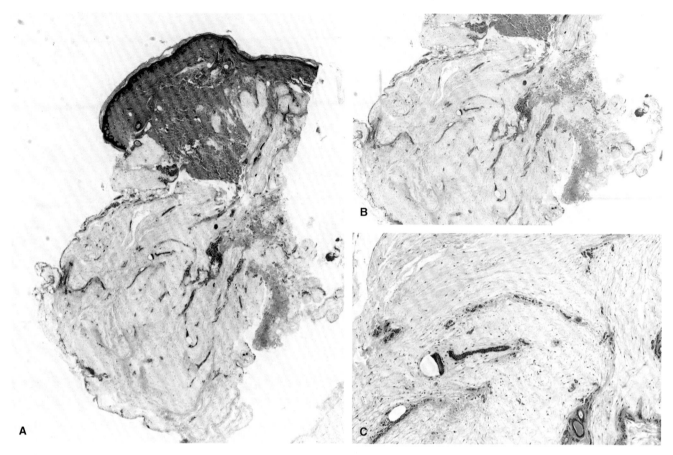

FIGURE 24-67. A-C, Cutaneous myxoma. Sharply demarcated, hypocellular myxoid nodules are the composition of the myxoma with abundant pale staining to bluish mucoid matrix. Digital slides courtesy of Path Presenter.com.

bland, small, rounded to ovoid to stellate-appearing cells with a more or less uniform distribution. A faintly nodular pattern and small mucoid cysts or pools have a resemblance to the lipoblastoma (LPB; Figure 24-68). Except for vimentin, the tumor cells are nonreactive for most other markers including desmin and myogenin. However, these tumors display nuclear BCL-6 immunostaining as a surrogate of BCOR internal tandem duplication.[285,286] Despite the rather innocuous appearance of PMMTI, this tumor is locally aggressive and has the potential to metastasize and undergo sarcomatous transformation.[287]

LIPOMAS AND VARIANTS

Lipomatous tumors are typically located in the subcutis or deeper soft tissues so that a punch biopsy is unlikely to sample only the superficial aspects of one of these tumors. A lipomatous tumor in a child may be nothing more than a solitary lipoma or it may be the entry lesion to one of many other manifestations of the PIK3CA/AKT-related overgrowth spectrum.[288] Several of these disorders are characterized by somatic activating mutations in the PIK3CA pathway, resulting in the development of lipomatous hyperplasia and multiple lipomas. In addition to the lipomas, vascular anomalies and connective tissue nevi are present in the various phenotype subtypes including the CLOVES and Proteus syndromes.[288-292] Facial infiltrating lipomatosis is another phenotypic expression of the PIK3CA spectrum.[293-295] Encephalocraniocutaneous lipomatosis not only has spinal and intracranial lipomas but also has aplasia cutis congenita with an associated localized lipoma.[296,297] Mosaic somatic mutations have been detected in KRAS and FGFR1.[298,299] PTEN hamartoma tumor syndrome is characterized by deep soft tissue masses, with a mixed mesenchymal pattern of mature adipose tissue, myxoid stroma, and abnormal appearing vessels.[300]

Angiolipoma frequently presents as one or more nodules, often on the forearm more so than other sites, in adolescents and young adults (Figure 24-69). Approximately 5% of cases are familial.[301] These tumors have been associated with capillary malformation.[302] A sharply demarcated nodule measuring 2 cm or less is composed of lobules of

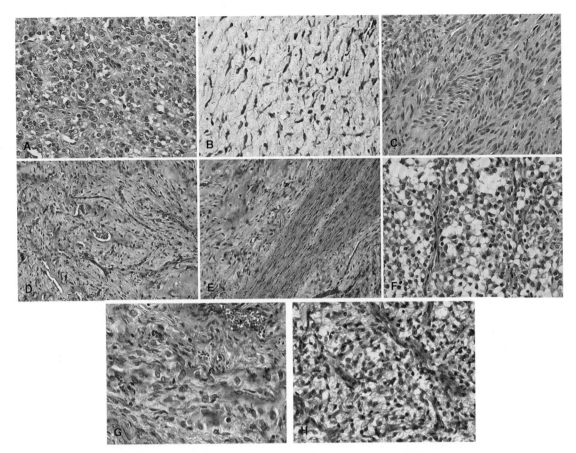

FIGURE 24-68. Morphologic spectrum of primitive myxoid mesenchymal tumor of infancy (PMMTI). The PMMTIs are associated with a monomorphic cytomorphology, ranging from round (A), stellate (B), to spindle (C). Overlapping histologic features with undifferentiated round cell sarcomas and clear cell sarcoma of the kidney were noted, including rich vascular network (D) and cellular fibrous septa (E). Other features included occasional cytoplasmic vacuoles (F) or rhabdoid cells (G). The only PMMTI lacking BCOR internal tandem duplication showed ovoid to stellate tumor cells, with slightly clumped chromatin and myxoid stroma (H). Obtained with permission Kao YC, Sung YS, Zhang L, et al. Recurrent BCOR internal tandem duplication and YWHAE-NUTM2B fusions in soft tissue undifferentiated round cell sarcoma of infancy: overlapping genetic features with clear cell sarcoma of kidney. *Am J Surg Pathol.* 2016;40(8):1009-1020.

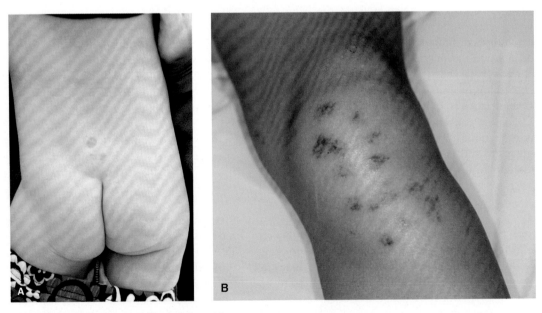

FIGURE 24-69. A and B, Angiolipomas on the trunk and knee.

mitotic fat and small vessels concentrated at the periphery of the lobules (Figure 24-70). The vessels may be so sparse as to be overlooked or cellular to the extreme that lobular fat is observed.[303] At either extreme, the diagnosis is facilitated by the presence of the fibrin thrombi (Figure 24-71).

Lipoma is the most common of all soft tissue tumors and is diagnosed in individuals between 30 and 60 years of age.[1] Most lipomas in children are sporadic and truncal in location (Figure 24-72). The histologic features are indistinguishable from their adult counterpart. In the presence of conspicuous lobulation and peripheral myxolipomatous features, the tumor may be a lipoma-like LPB with *PLAG* rearrangement rather than *HMGA2* and *HMGA1* rearrangements as found in lipomas in adults.[304]

Congenital lumbosacral lipomas are often linked to spinal dysraphism.[3] They are more common in girls and have a bimodal age distribution (peaks at 0-2 and 7-8 years).[305,306] Approximately 20% to 25% of patients with spinal dysraphism develop lipomas in the lumbosacral region, and intracanal extension is invariably present in all cases. The lumbosacral lipomas typically lack a capsule, have large amounts of fibrous tissue, and a variety of ectopic neuroectodermal and mesenchymal tissues including nephrogenic rests.

Angiomyxolipoma or vascular myxolipoma has a resemblance to the angiolipoma except for its myxoid stroma. This uncommon tumor has been reported in the subcutis or submucosa in children.[307-309] Multiple angiomyxomas have been reported in a child.[277]

CAPSULE SUMMARY

LIPOMAS AND VARIANTS

A lipomatous tumor in a child may be nothing more than a solitary lipoma or it may be the entry lesion to one of many other manifestations of the PIK3CA/AKT-related overgrowth spectrum. Most lipomas in children are sporadic and truncal in location. The histologic features are indistinguishable from their adult counterpart. Angiolipoma presents frequently as one or more nodules, often on the forearm more so than on other sites, in adolescents and young adults. Congenital lumbosacral lipomas are often linked to spinal dysraphism. Angiomyxolipoma or vascular myxolipoma has a resemblance to the angiolipoma except for its myxoid stroma.

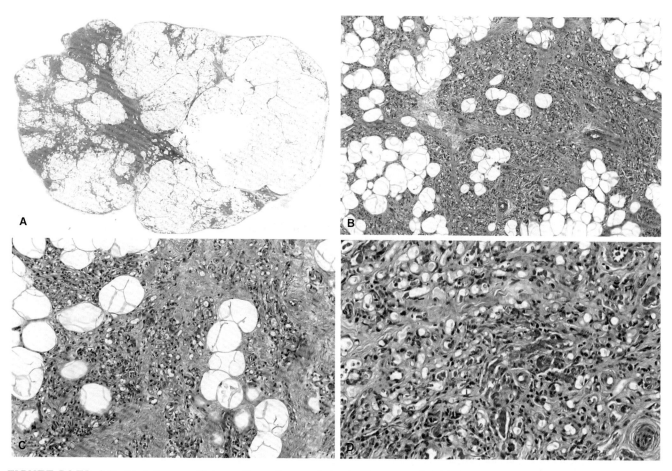

FIGURE 24-70. A-D, Angiolipoma. Mature adipose tissue admixed with a somewhat lobular vascular proliferation is present. Digital slides courtesy of Path Presenter.com.

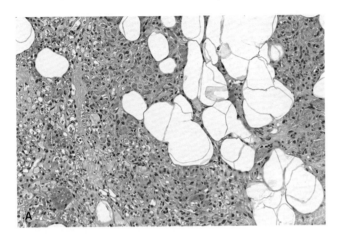
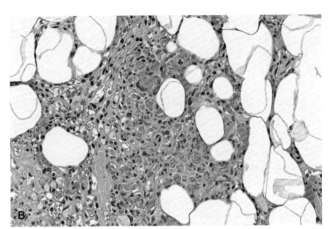

FIGURE 24-71. **A and B, Angiolipoma.** Multiple fibrin thrombi.

LIPOBLASTOMA

LPB is a benign tumor of the adipose tissue that differs from lipomas as they contain both mature and immature fat and are found exclusively in infancy and early childhood.[310] LPBs are the second most common adipose tumor after lipomas, accounting for 30% of adipose tumors in children. Typically children are affected within the first 3 years of life.[310] LPBs affect males more frequently than females.[304,311] The etiology of LPBs remains unknown. Recent cytogenetic studies have found rearrangement of the *PLAG1* gene as the most frequently encountered genetic alteration.[304]

They have a predilection for the superficial and deep soft tissues of the trunk (65%-70% of cases) and extremities (25%-30%) (Figures 24-73 and 24-74).[312,313] The smaller LPBs tend to occur in the superficial soft tissues and within reach of a deep punch biopsy or excision. In addition to the exquisite lobulation with prominent fibrous septa, the lobules may have a lipomatous, myxolipomatous, or a spindle cell

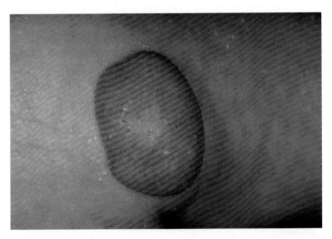

FIGURE 24-73. **Lipoblastoma.** Firm, pink tumor on the knee. Reprinted with permission from Shen LY, Amin SM, Chamlin SL, Mancini AJ. Varied presentation of pediatric lipoblastoma: case series and review of the literature. *Pediatr Dermatol.* 2017;34(2):180-186.

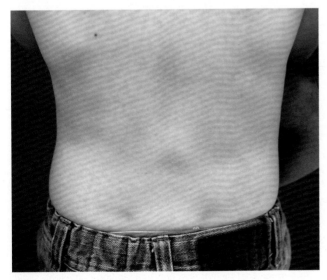

FIGURE 24-72. Lipoma on the trunk in an infant.

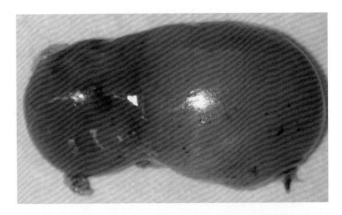

FIGURE 24-74. **This lipoblastoma is an encapsulated lobulated mass with a smooth external surface.** Obtained with permission Coffin CM, Lowichik A, Putnam A. Lipoblastoma (LPB): a clinicopathologic and immunohistochemical analysis of 59 cases. *Am J Surg Pathol.* 2009;33(11):1705-1712.

background within multiple myxoid or myxolipomatous foci. (Figure 24-75) Immature-appearing mesenchymal or spindle cells at the periphery of the lobules are commonly desmin-positive cells.[312,314] The tumor cells may be multivacuolated, signet ring like, multinucleated, or mature lipocyte like.[312] Mast cells are also common in these tumors. The vascular pattern may have a plexiform or branching configuration with a resemblance to myxoid liposarcoma. The immature adipocytes are positive for S-100 and CD34.[315] A primitive LPB is reported with features of PMMTI except with *PLAG1-HAS2* that is characteristic of LPB.[316] *PLAG1* rearrangement is a specific signature event in LPB except for an isolated case with HMGA1 rearrangement.[317]

CAPSULE SUMMARY

LIPOBLASTOMAS

LPBs are the second most common adipose tumor after lipomas, accounting for 30% of adipose tumors in children. Typically children are affected within the first 3 years of life. They have a predilection for the superficial and deep soft tissues of the trunk and extremities. In addition to the exquisite lobulation with prominent fibrous septa, the lobules may have a lipomatous, myxolipomatous, or spindle cell background within multiple myxoid or myxolipomatous foci. The tumor cells may be multivacuolated, signet ring like, multinucleated, or mature lipocyte like.

SARCOMAS

Sarcomas of the skin exclusive of DFSP and KS are very uncommon, and even the latter two neoplasms are rare in the age group between 0 and 20 years.[1] However, the skin is a known site of metastatic disease exclusive of hematolymphoid malignancies, with RMS as the most common sarcoma metastatic to the skin (40% of cases) in one pediatric series.[318] Other metastatic sarcomas to the skin in the latter series included osteosarcoma, MRT, and Ewing sarcoma.

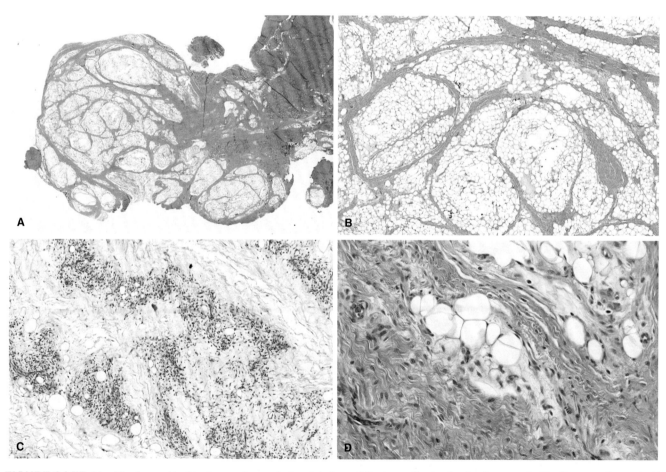

FIGURE 24-75. Lipoblastoma. Lipoblastomas demonstrate a lobular architecture with sheets of cells separated by fibrovascular septa (A and B). Myxoid areas with primitive mesenchymal cells are seen (C). The adipocytes have a spectrum of maturation, ranging from primitive stellate or spindle mesenchymal cells to multivacuolated or small signet ring cell–like lipoblasts (D). Digital slides courtesy of Path Presenter.com.

EWING SARCOMA-PRIMITIVE NEUROECTODERMAL TUMOR

Ewing sarcoma-primitive neuroectodermal tumor (EWS-PNET) is just one of the *EWSR1*-associated neoplasms presenting in the skin and/or subcutis as a primary neoplasm; the other EWSR1 tumors include not only the previously discussed AFH, but also clear cell sarcoma (CCS) and myoepithelial carcinoma (MC)/myoepithelioma.[172] Approximately 60% to 75% of all EWS-PNETs present in the bone, soft tissues (20%-25%), variety of organs, and skin and/or subcutis in a small minority of cases.[319,320] As an estimate, 1% to 3% of EWS-PNETs are primary cutaneous neoplasms, are seen in adolescents, and present on the extremity as a nodule measuring 3 to 4 cm.[321,322] The tumor is composed of uniform round cells forming a nodule(s) with or without an infiltrating pattern in the dermis and/or subcutis. A clear rim of cytoplasm is identified in well-prepared sections, reflecting the glycogen-rich cytoplasm. Nuclear pleomorphism and numerous mitotic figures are generally not apparent. Both vimentin and CD99 in a membrane-cytoplasmic pattern

are positive, and 90% or more of tumors have an *EWSR1* rearrangement by FISH using a break-apart probe. Cutaneous EWS-PNET has a generally more favorable outcome compared to the deep noncutaneous sites of this neoplasm (Figure 24-76).[319]

CLEAR CELL SARCOMA/MALIGNANT MELANOMA OF SOFT PARTS

CCS or melanoma of soft parts in the skin is seemingly less common than EWS-PNET in this location. The distal lower extremity is the site of predilection in adolescents or young adults who present with a faintly pigmented cutaneous nodule or more commonly with a deeper lesion.[323-325] Cutaneous CCS tends to be smaller (<3 cm) than those in the deeper soft tissue (~5-7 cm or larger), similar to the cutaneous EWS-PNET. The overlying epidermis is devoid of any junctional melanocytic proliferation. The nodule is composed of nested epithelioid cells with pale eosinophilic granular cytoplasm and identifiable fine melanin granules

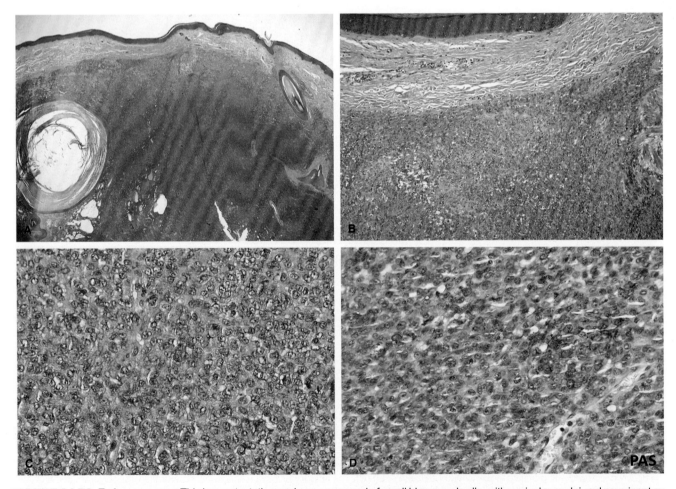

FIGURE 24-76. Ewing sarcoma. This is a metastatic neoplasm composed of small blue round cells, with vesicular nuclei and prominent nucleoli (A-C). A periodic acid–Schiff stain reveals positive cytoplasmic staining in a subset of the malignant cells (D). Obtained with permission. Dehner LP, Gru AA. Nonepithelial tumors and tumor-like lesions of the skin and subcutis in children. *Pediatr Dev Pathol.* 2018;21(2):150-207.

in some cases. The nests of tumor cells may be separated by a fibrous stroma. A more pleomorphic population of spindle cells with prominent nucleoli may dominate the histologic pattern. Multinucleated giant cells are infrequently noted. Malignant melanoma, poorly differentiated synovial sarcoma, and CNTK are some of the considerations in the differential diagnosis. Because CCS is immunoreactive for S-100 protein, HMB-45, and melanin-A, one can arrive at the diagnosis of melanoma without a second thought. CD99 and neuron-specific enolase are immunopositive in a minority of cases.[326] BRAF rearrangements have been reported in CCS.[327,328] The *EWSR1* break-apart is present in 70% to 90% of cases as a manifestation of the *EWSR1/AFT1* [t(12;22)(q13;q12)] fusion transcript.[323]

MYXOINFLAMMATORY FIBROBLASTIC SARCOMA

Myxoinflammatory fibroblastic sarcoma (MIFS) is a low-grade sarcoma with a predilection for the dorsal aspects of the extremities where it presents as a slow-growing superficial mass generally measuring less than 4 cm in children.[329,330] MIFS is recognized in other anatomic sites. Because the MIFS has a spectrum of microscopic features including neutrophils,

lymphocytes, fibromyxoid stroma, and vascular proliferation in the subcutis, a nonspecific inflammatory process may be the favored diagnosis. The pleomorphic spindle and epithelioid cells with nuclear pseudoinclusions and prominent nucleoli conveying a Reed-Sternberg cell–like experience may be obscured in the fibroinflammatory background (Figure 24-77).[331] Immunohistochemistry has limited utility. MIFS has a characteristic translocation, t(1;10)(p22;q24), whose fusion partners are *TGFBR3* and *MGEAS*.[332] *BRAF* rearrangements have been reported in MIFS.[333]

MYOEPITHELIOMA AND MYOEPITHELIAL CARCINOMA

MCs are extraordinarily rare. They are more frequent in individuals between the third and fifth decade of life. It has been described that 20% of myoepithelial neoplasms occur in children and, when they do, they are typically malignant. Myoepithelial tumor (myoepithelioma) and MC are a category of skin and soft tissue neoplasms that have in common, not necessarily morphologically, an immunophenotype associated with myoepithelial differentiation with cytokeratin (AE1/AE3, CAM 5.2), epithelial membrane antigen, S-100 protein, glial fibrillary acidic protein (27%-54%), calponin (86%), smooth

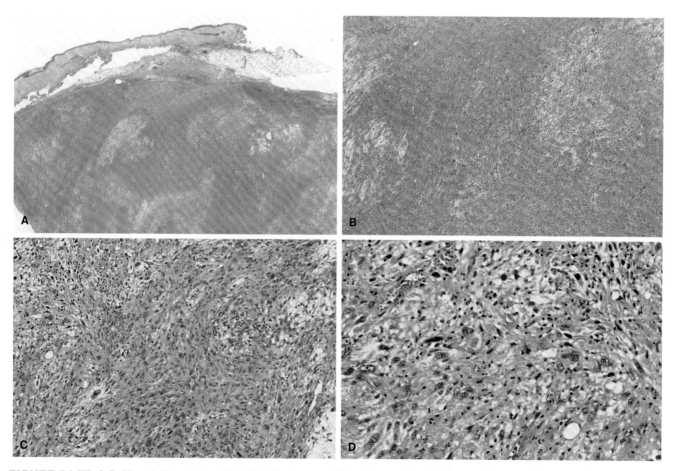

FIGURE 24-77. A-D, Myxoinflammatory fibroblastic sarcoma. The pleomorphic spindle and epithelioid cells with nuclear pseudoinclusions and prominent nucleoli conveying a Reed-Sternberg cell–like experience are contained within the fibroinflammatory background. Digital slides courtesy of Path Presenter.com.

muscle actin (36%-64%), p63 (7%-40%), and SOX-10 reactivity.[334] *EWSR1* is the fusion partner with *POUF1, PBX1, PBX3, ZN444,* and *AFT1* in 40% to 50% of cases, whereas *FUS* rearrangement and *SMARCB/IN1* deletion are found especially in undifferentiated MC with epithelioid/rhabdoid features especially in children (9%-22%).[334-336] Those superficial myoepithelial tumors with evidence of ductal differentiation have a *PLAG1* rearrangement like the pleomorphic adenoma of the salivary gland and LPB.[337] Myoepithelial tumors have a predilection for the dermis and/or subcutis of the extremities (60%-70% of cases), but no anatomic site or organ is seemingly spared. Older children and adolescents present with a dermal or subcutaneous nodule measuring 1 to 3 cm in greatest dimension. A circumscribed nodular or multinodular lesion occupies the dermis with some infiltration of the subcutis or is centered in the subcutis. Various patterns and tumor cell morphology exists from solid to nested to trabecular and strands; the tumor cells are epithelioid to plasmacytoid to spindled in the absence of a background stroma to those with a myxoid or dense hyaline stroma.[338-340] In approximately 15% of cases, foci of heterologous differentiation (chondro-osseous, adipocytic, squamous) are present (Figure 24-78). MCs are graded as low, intermediate, and high, based on the degree of nuclear atypia, mitoses, and necrosis. A sheet-like growth of round cells with scant cytoplasm is typical in the pediatric group. In other words, it is necessary to include a myoepithelial neoplasm in the differential diagnosis of a variety of neoplasms already and yet to be discussed.

CAPSULE SUMMARY

MYOEPITHELIOMA AND MYOEPITHELIAL CARCINOMA

These are extraordinarily rare and are more frequent in individuals between the third and fifth decade of life. It has been described that 20% of myoepithelial neoplasms occur in children and, when they do, they are typically malignant. Myoepithelial tumor (myoepithelioma) and MC are a category of skin and soft tissue neoplasms that have in common, not necessarily morphologically, an immunophenotype associated with myoepithelial differentiation. *EWSR1, FUS, and PLAG1* translocations are typical. Approximately 9% to 22% of cases are INI1 deficient.

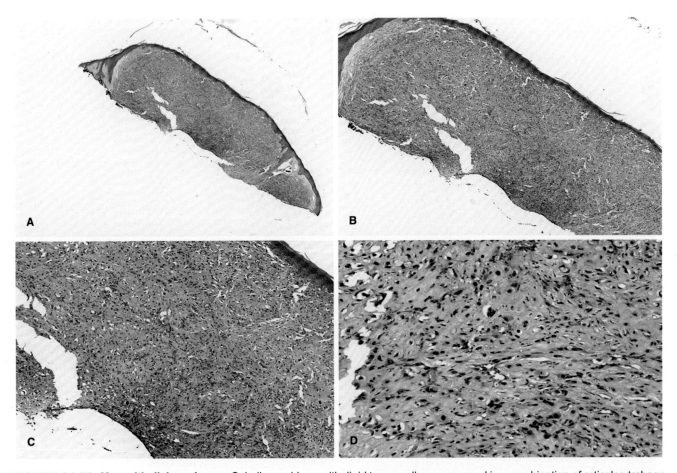

FIGURE 24-78. Myoepithelial carcinoma. Spindle, ovoid, or epithelioid tumor cells are arranged in a combination of reticular, trabecular, or nested growth, in a background of a chondromyxoid or hyalinized stroma (A-D). Such lesions frequently show a rearrangement of the *EWSR1* gene. Digital slides courtesy of Path Presenter.com.

EPITHELIOID SARCOMA

INI1-deficient neoplasms include *ES* and a subset of MCs.[341,342] ES represents 2% of soft tissue sarcomas in children and adolescents, which is a similar figure for liposarcoma and leiomyosarcoma (LMS) in the same age group.[343] Approximately 10% to 15% of ESs present at or before 20 years of age, mainly between the ages of 10 and 20 years.[344,345] This tumor presents in the dermis and/or subcutis (classic ES), but the proximal variant occurs in the deep soft tissues in and around the pelvis.[346] One or more slowly growing dermal nodules with or without epidermal ulceration in the distal extremities (upper > lower) is the most common clinical presentation. However, other peripheral sites in the axial soft tissues and even bone are documented as well.[345] The dermal-based ES is less than 5 cm in greatest dimension in contrast to the deep classic and proximal neoplasms. Nodules of large polygonal cells with abundant eosinophilic cytoplasm and a vesicular nucleus are the typical microscopic features. Dense filamentous cytoplasmic inclusions are variably prominent in individual tumors or within scattered microscopic fields within the

same tumor; these inclusions account for the designation of a cell having "rhabdoid" features. Rhabdoid inclusions, if inapparent by routine microscopy, are often demonstrable by vimentin and/or cytokeratin (CAM 5.2) immunostaining. One or more foci of necrosis and/or fibrosis is situated within or along the margins of the nodules.

Other histologic features of ES include spindle cell areas at the periphery of the epithelioid nodules.[346] In general, the tumor cells are relatively uniform, and mitotic activity is variable. Nuclear pleomorphism is generally not prominent in the newly diagnosed case, but may be striking in the recurrent or metastatic tumor. The differential diagnosis includes the other epithelioid/rhabdoid neoplasms.[347] The central necrosis in a dermal-based ES and the palisaded architecture may be mistaken for granuloma annulare (GA; Figure 24-79).[348]

In addition to coexpression of vimentin and one or more keratin, INI1 loss (absence of nuclear staining) is demonstrated in 70% to 90% of cases.[346] CD34 immunoreactivity is detected in 45% to 65% of cases. Because CD34, D2-40, ERG, and FLI1 are expressed in ES, there exists the possibility of a diagnosis of an epithelioid vascular tumor.[315,349]

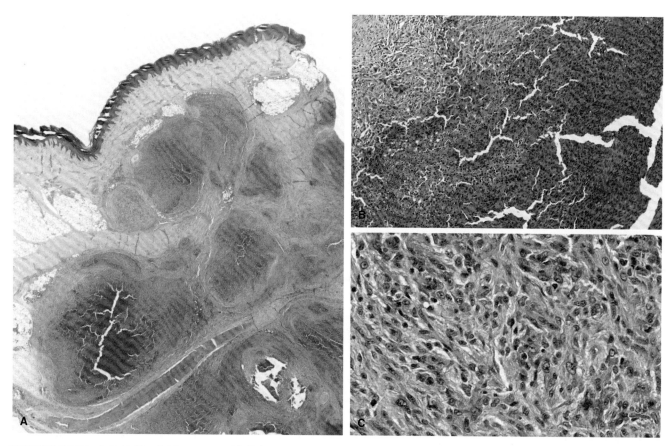

FIGURE 24-79. A-C, Epithelioid sarcoma. Multiple tumor nodules in the dermis and subcutis (A). In this case, the nodules show areas of central necrosis, a feature that can potentially mimic a granuloma annulare (B). The tumor cells are epithelioid, with versicular nuclei and prominent nucleoli (C). Digital slides courtesy of Path Presenter.com.

CAPSULE SUMMARY

EPITHELIOID SARCOMA

INI1-deficient neoplasms include ES and a subset of MCs. ES represents 2% of soft tissue sarcomas in children and adolescents. This tumor presents in the dermis and/or subcutis (classic ES), but the proximal variant occurs in the deep soft tissues in and around the pelvis. Nodules of large polygonal cells with abundant eosinophilic cytoplasm and a vesicular nucleus are the typical microscopic features. In addition to coexpression of vimentin and one or more keratin, INI1 loss (absence of nuclear staining) is demonstrated in 70% to 90% of cases.

MALIGNANT RHABDOID TUMOR

MRT, the other INI1-deficient neoplasm of childhood, may present primarily in the skin, as a metastasis from an as yet undetected tumor in the kidney or elsewhere, or as one of multiple tumors in congenital disseminated MRT.[350-353] A rapidly enlarging mass in the skin or one or more nodules in an infant 15 months or younger is the clinical presentation (Figure 24-80). An infiltrating round cell neoplasm in the dermis and subcutis may not have obvious rhabdoid features, but the nuclei are often the clue with enlarged vesicular nuclei and prominent nucleoli (Figure 24-81). A high-grade hematopoietic neoplasm, like a myeloid

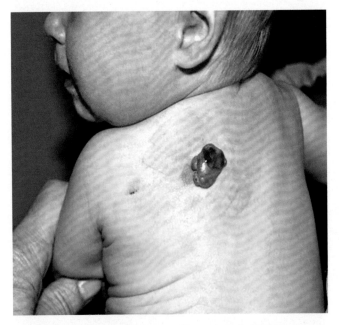

FIGURE 24-80. Cutaneous malignant rhabdoid tumor. Lesion on the back of a 6-month-old girl. Obtained with permission Chakrapani AL, White CR, Korcheva V, et al. Congenital extrarenal malignant rhabdoid tumor in an infant with distal 22q11.2 deletion syndrome: the importance of SMARCB1. *Am J Dermatopathol.* 2012;34(6):e77-e80.

sarcoma, in an infant, is one consideration in the differential diagnosis. Like ES, homozygous loss of function of INI1/SMARCB1/BAF47 or SMARCA4 (GBRG1) results in loss of nuclear immunoreactivity.[354] CD99 expression should not be confused with lymphoblastic leukemia/lymphoma and acute myeloid leukemia in which there is TdT nuclear staining.

MYOGENIC SARCOMAS

Myogenic sarcomas are represented by *LMS* and *RMS*, with the latter considerably more common than the former in children. RMS occurring in the skin of a child, as noted in the introduction to this section, is more likely a metastasis than a primary tumor. It has been estimated that less than 1% of all RMSs present as primary cutaneous neoplasm.[355] In infants, the so-called blueberry muffin syndrome with multiple violaceous lesions may be the clinical presentation of a disseminated alveolar RMS whose prognosis is poor.[356-361] A disproportionate number of these cases in infancy are alveolar RMS rather than embryonal RMS. The biopsy shows a high-grade malignant round cell infiltrate with overgrowth of the dermis and subcutis (Figure 24-82A-C). The desmin and myogenin immunostains are diffusely positive with cytoplasmic and nuclear staining, respectively (Figure 24-83). Embryonal RMS, in addition to skin metastasis, presents as a primary cutaneous neoplasm (Figure 24-84) in the setting of a large or giant congenital melanocytic nevus.[362,363]

LMSs of the dermis and subcutis are regarded as tumors arising from the arrector pilorum (dermis) or vascular smooth muscle (subcutis).[364,365] The former type of LMS has an indolent clinical course in contrast to the deeper LMS with its potential for metastatic behavior. When LMS presents in a child, it is usually in an older child or adolescent.[366] There are reports of dermal-based LMSs in HIV-infected children whose tumors are associated with EBV.[367,368] Given the benign behavior of dermal LMS, it has been suggested that this tumor should be designated as "an atypical intradermal smooth muscle tumor."[369]

CUTANEOUS EPITHELIOID MALIGNANT PERIPHERAL NERVE SHEATH TUMOR

Cutaneous epithelioid MPNST is a variant of MPNST occurring in the dermis and/or subcutis, composed predominantly (at least 50%) or exclusively of epithelioid tumor cells showing diffuse and at least a moderate degree of cytologic atypia. They represent approximately 5% of all cases of MPNST and have a much higher propensity to arise at superficial locations than in the deep soft tissues, as opposed to conventional MPNST. Its occurrence in children is very uncommon. The predilection sites include the lower extremities and trunk. As opposed to the conventional forms of MPNST, these tumors are not associated with neurofibromatosis. In approximately 14% of cases, the tumors arise in a preexistent

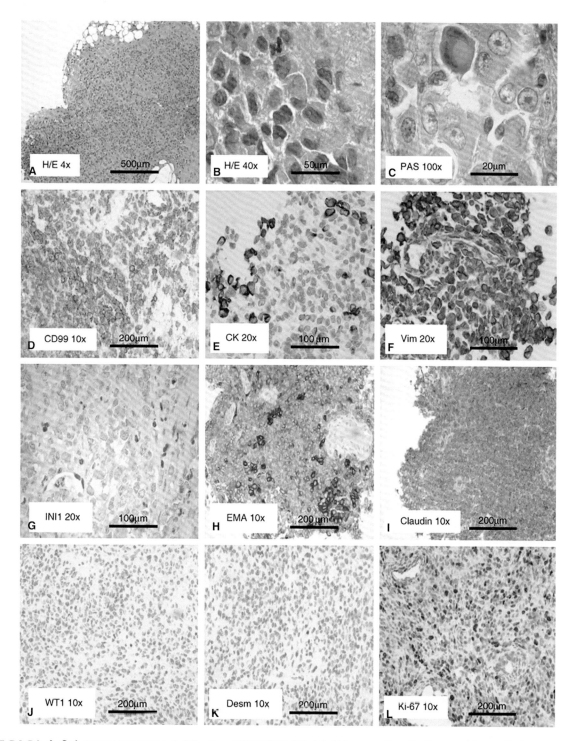

FIGURE 24-81. A, Subcutaneous tumor infiltration (H/E 4×). B, Rhabdoid tumor cells with pleomorphic morphology, mitotic figures, nuclear infolding, and prominent single nucleoli (H/E 40×). C, Rhabdoid tumor cells with eosinophilic cytoplasms and globular condensations (PAS 100×). D, CD99 cytoplasm and membrane staining (++) in tumor cells (10×). E, CK (AE1/AE3) cytoplasm staining (+++) in rhabdoid tumor cells (20×). F, Vimentin cytoplasm staining (+++) in rhabdoid tumor cells (20×). G, Absence of INI1 nuclear staining in tumor cells, positive nuclear INI1 staining in control cells (endothelial cells and fibroblastic nontumor cells) (20×). H, EMA membrane and cytoplasm staining (+++) in tumor cells (10×). I, Claudin cytoplasmic diffuse staining (+++) in tumor cells (10×). J, WT1 nuclear staining negative in tumor cells (10×). K, Absence of desmin cytoplasm staining in tumor cells (10×). L, High proliferation index +++, Ki-67 nuclear staining (10×). CK indicates cytokeratin; H/E, hematoxylin-eosin; PAS, periodic acid–Schiff. Obtained with permission Machado I, Noguera R, Santonja N, et al. Immunohistochemical study as a tool in differential diagnosis of pediatric malignant rhabdoid tumor. *Appl Immunohistochem Mol Morphol.* 2010;18(2):150-158.

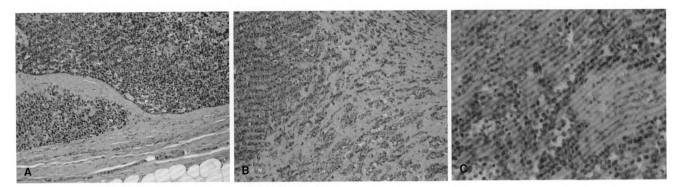

FIGURE 24-82. **A-C, Alveolar rhabdomyosarcoma presenting as a subcutaneous nodule on the hand of a 12-year-old female.** A, Broad nests of relatively uniform high-grade malignant cells are seen in the subcutis. B, Other foci are composed of discrete nests of tumor in pale myxoid background with the differential diagnosis of Ewing sarcoma and myoepithelial carcinoma. C, Other foci show the more typical alveolar pattern with tumor cells clinging to the stroma.

schwannoma. Approximately a third of patients develop disseminated disease. The lesions are smaller than conventional MPNST (1.6-5 cm) and are characterized by the presence of polygonal epithelioid cells, displaying a multinodular growth, and less often an infiltrative growth. The tumor cells tend to grow in cords, strands, nests, or sheets and are surrounded by hyalinized or myxoid stroma. Mitotic activity is very high, and heterologous elements can be present, but with a lower incidence than in conventional MPNST. As opposed to conventional MPNST, these tumors show strong and diffuse expression for S-100. EMA is expressed in 43% of cases and CK in 28.5% of cases. A single case has been shown to have the *BRAFV600E* mutation.[370,371]

ATYPICAL FIBROXANTHOMA AND PLEOMORPHIC DERMAL SARCOMA

Atypical fibroxanthoma (AFX) of skin and *pleomorphic dermal sarcoma* (PDS) are closely related neoplasms that typically arise in the head and neck in elderly individuals with chronic cutaneous ultraviolet injury.[372-375] These tumors have overlapping histologic and cytogenetic features, but PDS is the more aggressive tumor with deep invasion into

the subcutis, necrosis, and lymphovascular invasion.[375] Those few documented cases of AFX in children have been reported in those with xeroderma pigmentosum.[376,377]

Nonneoplastic Tumor-Like Lesions

Nonneoplastic tumefactive lesions in the skin and subcutis of children constitute a heterogeneous group of entities that are submitted as a neoplasm or "rule out" a neoplasm. Some of the more comprehensive reviews of these various lesions are found in the studies on the imaging features because these children are referred to the radiologist to further characterize the mass.[378,379] These lesions include one or another type of squamous-lined cyst, scar, or keloid. If a cyst has ruptured, a granulomatous and fibrous reaction contributes further to the mass effect. Another mass-producing, often necrotizing, granulomatous inflammatory process is atypical mycobacteriosis and Bartonella. These various cysts and granulomatous lesions have a predilection for the head and neck region of children, often less than 10 years of age.

Subcutaneous or deep GA (pseudorheumatoid nodule) often presents as a mass in the subcutis of children, often

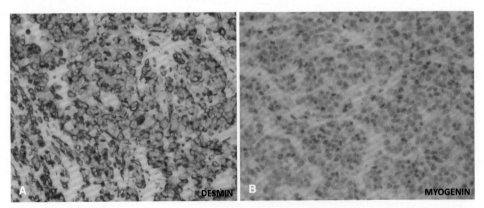

FIGURE 24-83. **Alveolar rhabdomyosarcoma.** The tumor cells are diffusely immunopositive for desmin (A). Diffuse nuclear positivity for myogenin (B) serves as a surrogate marker for FOX01 rearrangement which was identified by fluorescent in situ hybridization in this case.

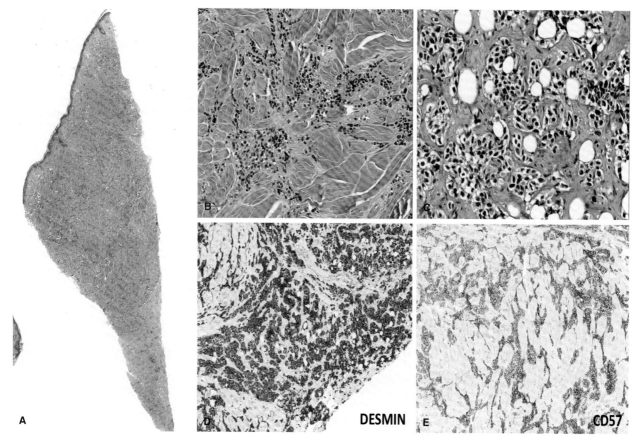

FIGURE 24-84. **Rhabdomyosarcoma, embryonal type.** A metastatic tumor is present in the dermis, composed of small, round, blue cells (A-C). The tumor shows nests of epithelioid cells in this example of embryonal rhabdomyosarcoma. The malignant cells are positive for desmin (D) and CD57 (E).

less than 10 years old, and adolescents on the distal lower extremity and head and neck region.[380] A rapidly enlarging, ill-defined mass without inflammatory signs, measuring from 1 to 6 cm, is the clinical presentation. Multiple lesions and local recurrences are known to occur as well as a more typical dermal GA.[381] A biopsy or more often in our experience a local resection is performed.

The subcutis has a more or less diffuse fibrous appearance with interspersed adipose tissue. Within the stroma, several circumscribed foci are characterized by central necrobiosis surrounded by a mantle of macrophages producing a necrobiotic granuloma (Figure 24-85A-C). The prominence of the macrophages can vary from one granuloma to the next. Apparent resolutions of the granuloma are recognized by central fibrosis with circumferential arcades of capillaries with a hemangioma-like appearance (Figure 24-85B).[380] CD68 and cytokeratin immunostaining are in order in those cases with the differential diagnosis of ES versus GA.[347,382-384]

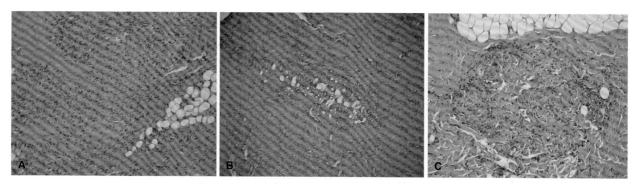

FIGURE 24-85. **A-C, Deep granuloma annulare often presents as a mass in the subcutis of the distal lower extremity or head and neck.** A, This pretibial lesion in a 4-year-old male shows the mantle of palisading macrophages with central necrobiosis. B, This lesion from the forearm of a 7-year-old female shows the clustering of small blood vessels adjacent to a central focus of fibrosis as features of an involuted focus of necrosis. C, Elsewhere in this forearm lesion, a small interstitial focus of granuloma annulare is present in lower reticular dermis.

REFERENCES

1. Dehner LP, Gru AA. Nonepithelial tumors and tumor-like lesions of the skin and subcutis in children. *Pediatr Dev Pathol.* 2018:1-56.
2. Rodriguez FJ, Stratakis CA, Evans DG. Genetic predisposition to peripheral nerve neoplasia: diagnostic criteria and pathogenesis of neurofibromatoses, Carney complex, and related syndromes. *Acta Neuropathol.* 2012;123(3):349-367.
3. Hirbe AC, Gutmann DH. Neurofibromatosis type 1: a multidisciplinary approach to care. *Lancet Neurol.* 2014;13(8):834-843.
4. Ehara Y, Yamamoto O, Kosaki K, Yoshida Y. Natural course and characteristics of cutaneous neurofibromas in neurofibromatosis 1. *J Dermatol.* 2018;45(1):53-57.
5. Cannon A, Chen MJ, Li P, et al. Cutaneous neurofibromas in Neurofibromatosis type I: a quantitative natural history study. *Orphanet J Rare Dis.* 2018;13(1):31.
6. Ruggieri M, Iannetti P, Polizzi A, et al. Earliest clinical manifestations and natural history of neurofibromatosis type 2 (NF2) in childhood: a study of 24 patients. *Neuropediatrics.* 2005;36(1):21-34.
7. Plana-Pla A, Bielsa-Marsol I, Carrato-Monino C, en representacion del grupo de Centros SyUdReF. Diagnostic and prognostic relevance of the cutaneous manifestations of neurofibromatosis type 2. *Actas Dermosifiliogr.* 2017;108(7):630-636.
8. Strowd RE, Strowd LC, Blakeley JO. Cutaneous manifestations in neuro-oncology: clinically relevant tumor and treatment associated dermatologic findings. *Semin Oncol.* 2016;43(3):401-407.
9. Mautner VF, Tatagiba M, Guthoff R, Samii M, Pulst SM. Neurofibromatosis 2 in the pediatric age group. *Neurosurgery.* 1993;33(1):92-96.
10. Dhamija R, Plotkin S, Asthagiri A, Messiaen L, Babovic-Vuksanovic D. Schwannomatosis. In: Adam MP, Ardinger HH, Pagon RA, et al, eds. *GeneReviews* [Internet]. Seattle, WA: University of Washington; 1993.
11. Jouhilahti EM, Peltonen S, Heape AM, Peltonen J. The pathoetiology of neurofibromatosis 1. *Am J Pathol.* 2011;178(5):1932-1939.
12. Le C, Bedocs PM. Neurofibromatosis. In: *StatPearls* [Internet]. Treasure Island, FL: StatPearls Publishing; 2017.
13. Kresak JL, Walsh M. Neurofibromatosis: a review of NF1, NF2, and Schwannomatosis. *J Pediatr Genet.* 2016;5(2):98-104.
14. Madke B, Nayak C. Eponymous signs in dermatology. *Indian Dermatol Online J.* 2012;3(3):159-165.
15. Little H, Kamat D, Sivaswamy L. Common neurocutaneous syndromes. *Pediatr Ann.* 2015;44(11):496-504.
16. Rodriguez-Peralto JL, Riveiro-Falkenbach E, Carrillo R. Benign cutaneous neural tumors. *Semin Diagn Pathol.* 2013;30(1):45-57.
17. Boyd KP, Korf BR, Theos A. Neurofibromatosis type 1. *J Am Acad Dermatol.* 2009;61(1):1-14; quiz 15-16.
18. Jokinen CH, Argenyi ZB. Atypical neurofibroma of the skin and subcutaneous tissue: clinicopathologic analysis of 11 cases. *J Cutan Pathol.* 2010;37(1):35-42.
19. Nakashima K, Yamada N, Yoshida Y, Yamamoto O. Solitary sclerotic neurofibroma of the skin. *Am J Dermatopathol.* 2008;30(3):278-280.
20. Miettinen MM, Antonescu CR, Fletcher CDM, et al. Histopathologic evaluation of atypical neurofibromatous tumors and their transformation into malignant peripheral nerve sheath tumor in patients with neurofibromatosis 1-a consensus overview. *Hum Pathol.* 2017;67:1-10.
21. Swick BL. Floret-like multinucleated giant cells in a neurofibromatosis type 1-associated neurofibroma. *Am J Dermatopathol.* 2008;30(6):632-634.
22. Fetsch JF, Michal M, Miettinen M. Pigmented (melanotic) neurofibroma: a clinicopathologic and immunohistochemical analysis of 19 lesions from 17 patients. *Am J Surg Pathol.* 2000;24(3):331-343.
23. Saab ST, McClain CM, Coffin CM. Fibrous hamartoma of infancy: a clinicopathologic analysis of 60 cases. *Am J Surg Pathol.* 2014;38:394-401.
24. Agaram NP, Zhang L, Sung YS, et al. Recurrent *NTRK1* gene fusions define a novel subset of locally aggressive lipofibromatosis-like neural tumors. *Am J Surg Pathol.* 2016;40:1407-1416.

25. Hilton DA, Hanemann CO. Schwannomas and their pathogenesis. *Brain Pathol.* 2014;24(3):205-220.
26. Mautner VF, Lindenau M, Baser ME, Kluwe L, Gottschalk J. Skin abnormalities in neurofibromatosis 2. *Arch Dermatol.* 1997;133(12):1539-1543.
27. Miyakawa T, Kamada N, Kobayashi T, et al. Neurofibromatosis type 2 in an infant with multiple plexiform schwannomas as first symptom. *J Dermatol.* 2007;34(1):60-64.
28. Ruggieri M, Pratico AD, Evans DG. Diagnosis, management, and new therapeutic options in childhood neurofibromatosis type 2 and related forms. *Semin Pediatr Neurol.* 2015;22(4):240-258.
29. Evans DG. Neurofibromatosis type 2. *Handb Clin Neurol.* 2015;132:87-96.
30. Ruggieri M, Gabriele AL, Polizzi A, et al. Natural history of neurofibromatosis type 2 with onset before the age of 1 year. *Neurogenetics.* 2013;14(2):89-98.
31. Woodruff JM, Scheithauer BW, Kurtkaya-Yapicier O, et al. Congenital and childhood plexiform (multinodular) cellular schwannoma: a troublesome mimic of malignant peripheral nerve sheath tumor. *Am J Surg Pathol.* 2003;27(10):1321-1329.
32. Ishida T, Kuroda M, Motoi T, Oka T, Imamura T, Machinami R. Phenotypic diversity of neurofibromatosis 2: association with plexiform schwannoma. *Histopathology.* 1998;32(3):264-270.
33. Reith JD, Goldblum JR. Multiple cutaneous plexiform schwannomas. Report of a case and review of the literature with particular reference to the association with types 1 and 2 neurofibromatosis and schwannomatosis. *Arch Pathol Lab Med.* 1996;120(4):399-401.
34. Val-Bernal JF, Figols J, Vazquez-Barquero A. Cutaneous plexiform schwannoma associated with neurofibromatosis type 2. *Cancer.* 1995;76(7):1181-1186.
35. Pekmezci M, Reuss DE, Hirbe AC, et al. Morphologic and immunohistochemical features of malignant peripheral nerve sheath tumors and cellular schwannomas. *Mod Pathol.* 2015;28(2):187-200.
36. Karamchandani JR, Nielsen TO, van de Rijn M, West RB. Sox10 and S100 in the diagnosis of soft-tissue neoplasms. *Appl Immunohistochem Mol Morphol.* 2012;20(5):445-450.
37. Miettinen M, McCue PA, Sarlomo-Rikala M, et al. Sox10—a marker for not only schwannian and melanocytic neoplasms but also myoepithelial cell tumors of soft tissue: a systematic analysis of 5134 tumors. *Am J Surg Pathol.* 2015;39(6):826-835.
38. Schaefer IM, Fletcher CD, Hornick JL. Loss of H3K27 trimethylation distinguishes malignant peripheral nerve sheath tumors from histologic mimics. *Mod Pathol.* 2016;29(1):4-13.
39. Kaehler KC, Russo PA, Katenkamp D, et al. Melanocytic schwannoma of the cutaneous and subcutaneous tissues: three cases and a review of the literature. *Melanoma Res.* 2008;18(6):438-442.
40. Carney JA, Stratakis CA. Epithelioid blue nevus and psammomatous melanotic schwannoma: the unusual pigmented skin tumors of the Carney complex. *Semin Diagn Pathol.* 1998;15(3):216-224.
41. Kaltsas G, Kanakis G, Chrousos G. Carney's complex. In: De Groot LJ, Chrousos G, Dungan K, et al, eds. *Endotext.* South Dartmouth, MA: MDText.com, Inc; 2000.
42. Carney JA, Headington JT, Su WP. Cutaneous myxomas. A major component of the complex of myxomas, spotty pigmentation, and endocrine overactivity. *Arch Dermatol.* 1986;122(7):790-798.
43. Wilkes D, McDermott DA, Basson CT. Clinical phenotypes and molecular genetic mechanisms of Carney complex. *Lancet Oncol.* 2005;6(7):501-508.
44. Torres-Mora J, Dry S, Li X, Binder S, Amin M, Folpe AL. Malignant melanotic schwannian tumor: a clinicopathologic, immunohistochemical, and gene expression profiling study of 40 cases, with a proposal for the reclassification of "melanotic schwannoma." *Am J Surg Pathol.* 2014;38(1):94-105.
45. Carney JA. Psammomatous melanotic schwannoma. A distinctive, heritable tumor with special associations, including cardiac myxoma and the Cushing syndrome. *Am J Surg Pathol.* 1990;14(3):206-222.

46. Laskin WB, Fetsch JF, Lasota J, Miettinen M. Benign epithelioid peripheral nerve sheath tumors of the soft tissues: clinicopathologic spectrum of 33 cases. *Am J Surg Pathol*. 2005;29(1):39-51.

47. Suchak R, Luzar B, Bacchi CE, Maguire B, Calonje E. Cutaneous neuroblastoma-like schwannoma: a report of two cases, one with a plexiform pattern, and a review of the literature. *J Cutan Pathol*. 2010;37(9):997-1001.

48. Hart J, Gardner JM, Edgar M, Weiss SW. Epithelioid schwannomas: an analysis of 58 cases including atypical variants. *Am J Surg Pathol*. 2016;40:704-713.

49. Rezanko T, Sari AA, Tunakan M, et al. Epithelioid schwannoma of soft tissue: unusual morphological variant causing a diagnostic dilemma. *Ann Diagn Pathol*. 2012;16:521-526.

50. Antonescu CR, Louis DN, Hunten S, et al, eds. *WHO Classification of Tumours of the Central Nervous System*. 4th ed. Lyon, France: IARC; 2016:214-218.

51. Yamada S, Kirshima M, Hiraki T, et al. Epithelioid schwannoma of the skin displaying unique histopathological features: a teaching case giving rise to diagnostic difficulties on a morphological examination of a resected specimen, with a brief literature review. *Diagn Pathol*. 2017;12:11.

52. Stratakis CA, Salpea P, Raygada M. Carney complex. In: Pagon RA, Adam MP, Ardinger HH, et al, eds. *GeneReview* [Internet]. Seattle, WA: University of Washington; 1993-2017.

53. Thomas AK, Egelhoff JC, Curran JG, Thomas B. Pediatric schwannomatosis, a rare but distinct form of neurofibromatosis. *Pediatr Radiol*. 2016;46:430-435.

54. Merker VL, Esparza S, Smith MJ, Stemmer-Rachamimov A, Plotkin SR. Clinical features of schwannomatosis: a retrospective analysis of 87 patients. *Oncologist*. 2012;17:1317-1322.

55. Kehrer-Sawatzki H, Farschtschi S, Mautner VF, Cooper DN. The molecular pathogenesis of schwannomatosis, a paradigm for the co-involvement of multiple tumor suppressor genes in tumorigenesis. *Hum Genet*. 2017;136:129-148.

56. Agaimy A. The expanding family of SMARCB1(INI1)-deficient neoplasia: implications of phenotypic, biological, and molecular heterogeneity. *Adv Anat Pathol*. 2014;21:394-410.

57. Kohashi K, Oda Y. Oncogenic roles of SMARCB1/INI1 and its deficient tumors. *Cancer Sci*. 2017;108(4):547-552.

58. Hornick JL, Fletcher CD. Soft tissue perineurioma: clinicopathologic analysis of 81 cases including those with atypical histologic features. *Am J Surg Pathol*. 2005;29(7):845-858.

59. Balarezo FS, Muller RC, Weiss RG, Brown T, Knibbs D, Joshi VV. Soft tissue perineuriomas in children: report of three cases and review of the literature [corrected]. *Pediatr Dev Pathol*. 2003;6(2):137-141.

60. Hornick JL, Bundock EA, Fletcher CD. Hybrid schwannoma/perineurioma: clinicopathologic analysis of 42 distinctive benign nerve sheath tumors. *Am J Surg Pathol*. 2009;33(10):1554-1561.

61. Montgomery BK, Alimchandani M, Mehta GU, et al. Tumors displaying hybrid schwannoma and neurofibroma features in patients with neurofibromatosis type 2. *Clin Neuropathol*. 2016;35(2):78-83.

62. Ud Din N, Ahmad Z, Abdul-Ghafar J, Ahmed R. Hybrid peripheral nerve sheath tumors: report of five cases and detailed review of literature. *BMC Cancer*. 2017;17(1):349.

63. Yuwanati M, Mhaske S, Mhaske A. Congenital granular cell tumor—a rare entity. *J Neonatal Surg*. 2015;4(2):17.

64. Carinci F, Piattelli A, Rubini C, et al. Genetic profiling of granular cell myoblastoma. *J Craniofacial Surg*. 2004;15(5):824-834.

65. Stemm M, Suster D, Wakely PE Jr, Suster S. Typical and atypical granular cell tumors of soft tissue: a clinicopathologic study of 50 patients. *Am J Clin Pathol*. 2017;148(2):161-166.

66. Richmond AM, La Rosa FG, Said S. Granular cell tumor presenting in the scrotum of a pediatric patient: a case report and review of the literature. *J Med Case Rep*. 2016;10(1):161.

67. Cardis MA, Ni J, Bhawan J. Granular cell differentiation: a review of the published work. *J Dermatol*. 2017;44(3):251-258.

68. Alemayehu H, Polites SF, Kats A, Ishitani MB, Moir CR, Iqbal CW. Granular cell tumors and congenital granular cell epulis in children: similar entities. *J Pediatr Surg*. 2015;50(5):775-778.

69. Childers EL, Fanburg-Smith JC. Congenital epulis of the newborn: 10 new cases of a rare oral tumor. *Ann Diagn Pathol*. 2011;15(3):157-161.

70. Park SH, Kim TJ, Chi JG. Congenital granular cell tumor with systemic involvement. Immunohistochemical and ultrastructural study. *Arch Pathol Lab Med*. 1991;115(9):934-938.

71. Sanford LJ, Gordon S, Travers JB. Familial granular cell tumors: a case report and review of the literature. *Pediatr Dermatol*. 2013;30(3):e8-e11.

72. Fetsch JF, Laskin WB, Miettinen M. Nerve sheath myxoma: a clinicopathologic and immunohistochemical analysis of 57 morphologically distinctive, S-100 protein-and GFAP-positive, myxoid peripheral nerve sheath tumors with a predilection for the extremities and a high local recurrence rate. *Am J Surg Pathol*. 2005;29(12):1615-1624.

73. Cribier B, Baran R, Varini JP. Nerve sheath myxoma of the hyponychium [in French]. *Ann Dermatol Venereol*. 2013;140(8-9):535-539.

74. Graadt van Roggen JF, Hogendoorn PC, Fletcher CD. Myxoid tumours of soft tissue. *Histopathology*. 1999;35(4):291-312.

75. Gray MH, Rosenberg AE, Dickersin GR, Bhan AK. Glial fibrillary acidic protein and keratin expression by benign and malignant nerve sheath tumors. *Hum Pathol*. 1989;20(11):1089-1096.

76. Sheth S, Li X, Binder S, Dry SM. Differential gene expression profiles of neurothekeomas and nerve sheath myxomas by microarray analysis. *Mod Pathol*. 2011;24(3):343-354.

77. Dakin MC, Leppard B, Theaker JM. The palisaded, encapsulated neuroma (solitary circumscribed neuroma). *Histopathology*. 1992;20(5):405-410.

78. Megahed M. Palisaded encapsulated neuroma (solitary circumscribed neuroma). A clinicopathologic and immunohistochemical study. *Am J Dermatopathol*. 1994;16(2):120-125.

79. Omori Y, Tanito K, Ito K, Itoh M, Saeki H, Nakagawa H. A pediatric case of multiple palisaded encapsulated neuromas of the palms and soles. *Pediatr Dermatol*. 2014;31(4):e107-e109.

80. Misago N, Toda S, Narisawa Y. The relationship between palisaded encapsulated neuroma and the mucocutaneous neuroma seen in multiple endocrine neoplasia 2b syndrome: a histopathologic and immunohistochemical study. *Am J Dermatopathol*. 2014;36(7):562-569.

81. Lee MJ, Chung KH, Park JS, Chung H, Jang HC, Kim JW. Multiple endocrine neoplasia type 2B: early diagnosis by multiple mucosal neuroma and its DNA analysis. *Ann Dermatol*. 2010;22(4):452-455.

82. Sallai A, Hosszu E, Gergics P, Racz K, Fekete G. Orolabial signs are important clues for diagnosis of the rare endocrine syndrome MEN 2B. Presentation of two unrelated cases. *Eur J Pediatr*. 2008;167(4):441-446.

83. Marquard J, Eng C. Multiple endocrine neoplasia type 2. In: Adam MP, Ardinger HH, Pagon RA, et al, eds. *GeneReviews* [Internet]. Seattle, WA: University of Washington; 1993.

84. Leber GE, Gosain AK. Surgical excision of pedunculated supernumerary digits prevents traumatic amputation neuromas. *Pediatr Dermatol*. 2003;20(2):108-112.

85. Mullick S, Borschel GH. A selective approach to treatment of ulnar polydactyly: preventing painful neuroma and incomplete excision. *Pediatr Dermatol*. 2010;27(1):39-42.

86. Bisceglia M, Vigilante E, Ben-Dor D. Neural lipofibromatous hamartoma: a report of two cases and review of the literature. *Adv Anat Pathol*. 2007;14(1):46-52.

87. Tahiri Y, Xu L, Kanevsky J, Luc M. Lipofibromatous hamartoma of the median nerve: a comprehensive review and systematic approach to evaluation, diagnosis, and treatment. *J Hand Surg Am*. 2013;38(10):2055-2067.

88. Venkatesh K, Saini ML, Rangaswamy R, Murthy S. Neural fibrolipoma without macrodactyly: a subcutaneous rare benign tumor. *J Cutan Pathol*. 2009;36(5):594-596.

89. Rios JJ, Paria N, Burns DK, et al. Somatic gain-of-function mutations in PIK3CA in patients with macrodactyly. *Hum Mol Genet*. 2013;22:444-451.

90. Bellet JS. Developmental anomalies of the skin. *Semin Perinatol.* 2013;37(1):20-25.

91. Adil E, Robson C, Perez-Atayde A, et al. Congenital nasal neuroglial heterotopia and encephaloceles: an update on current evaluation and management. *Laryngoscope.* 2016;126(9):2161-2167.

92. Rogers GF, Mulliken JB, Kozakewich HP. Heterotopic neural nodules of the scalp. *Plast Reconstr Surg.* 2005;115(2):376-382.

93. Aanaes K, Hasselby JP, Bilde A, Therkildsen MH, von Buchwald C. Heterotopic neuroglial tissue: two cases involving the tongue and the buccal region. *Oral Surg Oral Med Oral Pathol Oral Radiol Endod.* 2008;105(6):e22-e29.

94. Bass PS, Theaker JM, Griffiths DM, Fletcher CD. Subcutaneous, meningo-glial nodule—a novel lesion in the buttock of a neonate. *Histopathology.* 1993;22(2):182-184.

95. Chen D, Dedhia K, Ozolek J, Mehta D. Case series of congenital heterotopic neuroglial tissue in the parapharyngeal space. *Int J Pediatr Otorhinolaryngol.* 2016;86:77-81.

96. McDermott MB, Glasner SD, Nielsen PL, Dehner LP. Soft tissue gliomatosis. Morphologic unity and histogenetic diversity. *Am J Surg Pathol.* 1996;20(2):148-155.

97. Shepherd NA, Coates PJ, Brown AA. Soft tissue gliomatosis—heterotopic glial tissue in the subcutis: a case report. *Histopathology.* 1987;11(6):655-660.

98. Tambay MC, Rodriguez IZ, Gil YR, Garcia AR, Saez RS, Moreno JJ. Heterotopic neuroglial tissue as a congenital laterocervical mass: a case report. *Int J Oral Maxillofac Surg.* 2009;38(4):382-384.

99. Cimino PJ, Agarwal A, Dehner LP. Myxopapillary ependymoma in children: a study of 11 cases and a comparison with the adult experience. *Pediatr Blood Cancer.* 2014;61(11):1969-1971.

100. Helwig EB, Stern JB. Subcutaneous sacrococcygeal myxopapillary ependymoma. A clinicopathologic study of 32 cases. *Am J Clin Pathol.* 1984;81(2):156-161.

101. Pulitzer DR, Martin PC, Collins PC, Ralph DR. Subcutaneous sacrococcygeal ("myxopapillary") ependymal rests. *Am J Surg Pathol.* 1988;12(9):672-677.

102. Bale PM. Sacrococcygeal developmental abnormalities and tumors in children. *Perspect Pediatr Pathol.* 1984;8(1):9-56.

103. Cooke A, Deshpande AV, La Hei ER, Kellie S, Arbuckle S, Cummins G. Ectopic nephrogenic rests in children: the clinicosurgical implications. *J Pediatr Surg.* 2009;44(12):e13-e16.

104. Downs KM. The enigmatic primitive streak: prevailing notions and challenges concerning the body axis of mammals. *Bioessays.* 2009;31(8):892-902.

105. Herion NJ, Salbaum JM, Kappen C. Traffic jam in the primitive streak: the role of defective mesoderm migration in birth defects. *Birth Defects Res A Clin Mol Teratol.* 2014;100(8):608-622.

106. Ma Y, Zheng J, Feng J, Zhu H, Xiao X, Chen L. Ectopic nephrogenic rests in children: a series of 13 cases in a single institution. *Pediatr Blood Cancer.* 2018;65(6):e26985.

107. Patel RM, Embi CS, Bergfeld WF. 'Myxopapillary' ependymal rest presenting as a pre-sacral skin tag. *Pathology.* 2005;37(1):89-91.

108. Chan HH, Fung JW, Lam WM, Choi P. The clinical spectrum of rudimentary meningocele. *Pediatr Dermatol.* 1998;15(5):388-389.

109. El Shabrawi-Caelen L, White WL, Soyer HP, Kim BS, Frieden IJ, McCalmont TH. Rudimentary meningocele: remnant of a neural tube defect? *Arch Dermatol.* 2001;137(1):45-50.

110. Marrogi AJ, Swanson PE, Kyriakos M, Wick MR. Rudimentary meningocele of the skin. Clinicopathologic features and differential diagnosis. *J Cutan Pathol.* 1991;18(3):178-188.

111. Sibley DA, Cooper PH. Rudimentary meningocele: a variant of "primary cutaneous meningioma." *J Cutan Pathol.* 1989;16(2):72-80.

112. Suster S, Rosai J. Hamartoma of the scalp with ectopic meningothelial elements. A distinctive benign soft tissue lesion that may simulate angiosarcoma. *Am J Surg Pathol.* 1990;14(1):1-11.

113. Terrier-Lacombe MJ, Guillou L, Maire G, et al. Dermatofibrosarcoma protuberans, giant cell fibroblastoma, and hybrid lesions in children:

clinicopathologic comparative analysis of 28 cases with molecular data--a study from the French Federation of Cancer Centers Sarcoma Group. *Am J Surg Pathol.* 2003;27(1):27-39.

114. Kornik RI, Muchard LK, Teng JM. Dermatofibrosarcoma protuberans in children: an update on the diagnosis and treatment. *Pediatr Dermatol.* 2012;29(6):707-713.

115. Karanian M, Perot G, Coindre JM, Chibon F, Pedeutour F, Neuville A. Fluorescence in situ hybridization analysis is a helpful test for the diagnosis of dermatofibrosarcoma protuberans. *Mod Pathol.* 2015;28(2):230-237.

116. Llombart B, Monteagudo C, Sanmartin O, et al. Dermatofibrosarcoma protuberans: a clinicopathological, immunohistochemical, genetic (COL1A1-PDGFB), and therapeutic study of low-grade versus high-grade (fibrosarcomatous) tumors. *J Am Acad Dermatol.* 2011;65(3):564-575.

117. Jha P, Moosavi C, Fanburg-Smith JC. Giant cell fibroblastoma: an update and addition of 86 new cases from the Armed Forces Institute of Pathology, in honor of Dr. Franz M. Enzinger. *Ann Diagn Pathol.* 2007;11(2):81-88.

118. Senerchia AA, Ribeiro KB, Rodriguez-Galindo C. Trends in incidence of primary cutaneous malignancies in children, adolescents, and young adults: a population-based study. *Pediatr Blood Cancer.* 2014;61(2):211-216.

119. Tsai YJ, Lin PY, Chew KY, Chiang YC. Dermatofibrosarcoma protuberans in children and adolescents: clinical presentation, histology, treatment, and review of the literature. *J Plast Reconstr Aesthet Surg.* 2014;67(9):1222-1229.

120. Valdivielso-Ramos M, Torrelo A, Campos M, Feito M, Gamo R, Rodriguez-Peralto JL. Pediatric dermatofibrosarcoma protuberans in Madrid, Spain: multi-institutional outcomes. *Pediatr Dermatol.* 2014;31(6):676-682.

121. Llombart B, Serra-Guillen C, Monteagudo C, Lopez Guerrero JA, Sanmartin O. Dermatofibrosarcoma protuberans: a comprehensive review and update on diagnosis and management. *Semin Diagn Pathol.* 2013;30(1):13-28.

122. Tardio JC. CD34-reactive tumors of the skin. An updated review of an ever-growing list of lesions. *J Cutan Pathol.* 2009;36(1):89-102.

123. Bandarchi B, Ma L, Marginean C, Hafezi S, Zubovits J, Rasty G. D2-40, a novel immunohistochemical marker in differentiating dermatofibroma from dermatofibrosarcoma protuberans. *Mod Pathol.* 2010;23(3):434-438.

124. Kazlouskaya V, Malhotra S, Kabigting FD, Lal K, Elston DM. CD99 expression in dermatofibrosarcoma protuberans and dermatofibroma. *Am J Dermatopathol.* 2014;36(5):392-396.

125. Lisovsky M, Hoang MP, Dresser KA, Kapur P, Bhawan J, Mahalingam M. Apolipoprotein D in CD34-positive and CD34-negative cutaneous neoplasms: a useful marker in differentiating superficial acral fibromyxoma from dermatofibrosarcoma protuberans. *Mod Pathol.* 2008;21(1):31-38.

126. Thway K, Noujaim J, Jones RL, Fisher C. Dermatofibrosarcoma protuberans: pathology, genetics, and potential therapeutic strategies. *Ann Diagn Pathol.* 2016;25:64-71.

127. Rubio GA, Alvarado A, Gerth DJ, Tashiro J, Thaller SR. Incidence and outcomes of dermatofibrosarcoma protuberans in the US pediatric population. *J Craniofac Surg.* 2017;28(1):182-184.

128. Liang CA, Jambusaria-Pahlajani A, Karia PS, Elenitsas R, Zhang PD, Schmults CD. A systematic review of outcome data for dermatofibrosarcoma protuberans with and without fibrosarcomatous change. *J Am Acad Dermatol.* 2014;71(4):781-786.

129. Mentzel T, Beham A, Katenkamp D, Dei Tos AP, Fletcher CD. Fibrosarcomatous ("high-grade") dermatofibrosarcoma protuberans: clinicopathologic and immunohistochemical study of a series of 41 cases with emphasis on prognostic significance. *Am J Surg Pathol.* 1998;22(5):576-587.

130. Kesserwan C, Sokolic R, Cohen EW, et al. Multicentric dermatofibrosarcoma protuberans in patients with adenosine

deaminase-deficient severe combined immune deficiency. *J Allergy Clin Immunol.* 2012;129(3):762-769.

131. McCalmont TH. Everything you wanted to know about dermatofibroma but were afraid to ask. *J Cutan Pathol.* 2014;41(1):5-8.

132. Alves JV, Matos DM, Barreiros HF, Bartolo EA. Variants of dermatofibroma—a histopathological study. *An Bras Dermatol.* 2014;89(3):472-477.

133. Vanni R, Fletcher CD, Sciot R, et al. Cytogenetic evidence of clonality in cutaneous benign fibrous histiocytomas: a report of the CHAMP study group. *Histopathology.* 2000;37(3):212-217.

134. Plaszczyca A, Nilsson J, Magnusson L, et al. Fusions involving protein kinase C and membrane-associated proteins in benign fibrous histiocytoma. *Int J Biochem Cell Biol.* 2014;53:475-481.

135. Romano RC, Fritchie KJ. Fibrohistiocytic tumors. *Clin Lab Med.* 2017;37(3):603-631.

136. Han TY, Chang HS, Lee JH, Lee WM, Son SJ. A clinical and histopathological study of 122 cases of dermatofibroma (benign fibrous histiocytoma). *Ann Dermatol.* 2011;23(2):185-192.

137. Black J, Coffin CM, Dehner LP. Fibrohistiocytic tumors and related neoplasms in children and adolescents. *Pediatr Dev Pathol.* 2012;15(1 suppl):181-210.

138. Luzar B, Calonje E. Cutaneous fibrohistiocytic tumours-an update. *Histopathology.* 2010;56(1):148-165.

139. Honda M, Tomimura S, de Vega S, Utani A. Multiple dermatofibromas in a patient with Down syndrome. *J Dermatol.* 2016;43(3):346-348.

140. Pinto-Almeida T, Caetano M, Alves R, Selores M. Congenital multiple clustered dermatofibroma and multiple eruptive dermatofibromas—unusual presentations of a common entity. *An Bras Dermatol.* 2013;88(6 suppl 1):63-66.

141. Zelger BG, Sidoroff A, Zelger B. Combined dermatofibroma: co-existence of two or more variant patterns in a single lesion. *Histopathology.* 2000;36(6):529-539.

142. Mentzel T. Cutaneous mesenchymal tumours: an update. *Pathology.* 2014;46(2):149-159.

143. Sachdev R, Sundram U. Expression of CD163 in dermatofibroma, cellular fibrous histiocytoma, and dermatofibrosarcoma protuberans: comparison with CD68, CD34, and Factor XIIIa. *J Cutan Pathol.* 2006;33(5):353-360.

144. Volpicelli ER, Fletcher CD. Desmin and CD34 positivity in cellular fibrous histiocytoma: an immunohistochemical analysis of 100 cases. *J Cutan Pathol.* 2012;39(8):747-752.

145. Horenstein MG, Prieto VG, Nuckols JD, et al. Indeterminate fibrohistiocytic lesions of the skin: is there a spectrum between dermatofibroma and dermatofibrosarcoma protuberans? *Am J Surg Pathol.* 2000;24(7):996-1003.

146. Kaddu S, McMenamin ME, Fletcher CD. Atypical fibrous histiocytoma of the skin: clinicopathologic analysis of 59 cases with evidence of infrequent metastasis. *Am J Surg Pathol.* 2002;26(1):35-46.

147. Marrogi AJ, Dehner LP, Coffin CM, Wick MR. Atypical fibrous histiocytoma of the skin and subcutis in childhood and adolescence. *J Cutan Pathol.* 1992;19(4):268-277.

148. Doyle LA, Marino-Enriquez A, Fletcher CD, Hornick JL. ALK rearrangement and overexpression in epithelioid fibrous histiocytoma. *Mod Pathol.* 2015;28(7):904-912.

149. Kazakov DV, Kyrpychova L, Martinek P, et al. ALK gene fusions in epithelioid fibrous histiocytoma: a study of 14 cases, with new histopathological findings. *Am J Dermatopathol.* 2018. doi:10.1097/DAD.0000000000001085.

150. Miettinen M, Fetsch JF. Reticulohistiocytoma (solitary epithelioid histiocytoma): a clinicopathologic and immunohistochemical study of 44 cases. *Am J Surg Pathol.* 2006;30(4):521-528.

151. Singh Gomez C, Calonje E, Fletcher CD. Epithelioid benign fibrous histiocytoma of skin: clinico-pathological analysis of 20 cases of a poorly known variant. *Histopathology.* 1994;24(2):123-129.

152. Kutlubay Z, Bairamov O, Sevim A, Demirkesen C, Mat MC. Rosai-Dorfman disease: a case report with nodal and cutaneous

involvement and review of the literature. *Am J Dermatopathol.* 2014;36(4):353-357.

153. Doyle LA, Fletcher CD. EMA positivity in epithelioid fibrous histiocytoma: a potential diagnostic pitfall. *J Cutan Pathol.* 2011;38(9):697-703.

154. Leclerc-Mercier S, Pedeutour F, Fabas T, Glorion C, Brousse N, Fraitag S. Plexiform fibrohistiocytic tumor with molecular and cytogenetic analysis. *Pediatr Dermatol.* 2011;28(1):26-29.

155. Taher A, Pushpanathan C. Plexiform fibrohistiocytic tumor: a brief review. *Arch Pathol Lab Med.* 2007;131(7):1135-1138.

156. Leclerc S, Hamel-Teillac D, Oger P, Brousse N, Fraitag S. Plexiform fibrohistiocytic tumor: three unusual cases occurring in infancy. *J Cutan Pathol.* 2005;32(8):572-576.

157. Moosavi C, Jha P, Fanburg-Smith JC. An update on plexiform fibrohistiocytic tumor and addition of 66 new cases from the Armed Forces Institute of Pathology, in honor of Franz M. Enzinger, MD. *Ann Diagn Pathol.* 2007;11(5):313-319.

158. Elwood H, Taube J. Dermal and subcutaneous plexiform soft tissue neoplasms. *Surg Pathol Clin.* 2011;4(3):819-842.

159. Jacobson-Dunlop E, White CR Jr, Mansoor A. Features of plexiform fibrohistiocytic tumor in skin punch biopsies: a retrospective study of 6 cases. *Am J Dermatopathol.* 2011;33(6):551-556.

160. Zelger B, Weinlich G, Steiner H, Zelger BG, Egarter-Vigl E. Dermal and subcutaneous variants of plexiform fibrohistiocytic tumor. *Am J Surg Pathol.* 1997;21(2):235-241.

161. Fox MD, Billings SD, Gleason BC, et al. Expression of MiTF may be helpful in differentiating cellular neurothekeoma from plexiform fibrohistiocytic tumor (histiocytoid predominant) in a partial biopsy specimen. *Am J Dermatopathol.* 2012;34:157-160.

162. Wang GY, Nazarian RM, Zhao L, et al. Protein gene product 9.5 (PGP9.5) expression in benign cutaneous mesenchymal, histiocytic and melanocytic lesions: comparison with cellular neurothekeoma. *Pathology.* 2017;49:44-49.

163. Vargas SO, Perez-Atayde AR, Gonzalez-Crussi F, Kozakewich HP. Giant cell angioblastoma: three additional occurrences of a distinct pathologic entity. *Am J Surg Pathol.* 2001;25(2):185-196.

164. Yu L, Lao IW, Wang J. Giant cell angioblastoma of bone: four new cases provide further evidence of its distinct clinical and histopathological characteristics. *Virchows Arch.* 2015;467(1):95-103.

165. Fried I, Sitthinamsuwan P, Muangsomboon S, Kaddu S, Cerroni L, McCalmont TH. SOX-10 and MiTF expression in cellular and 'mixed' neurothekeoma. *J Cutan Pathol.* 2014;41(8):640-645.

166. Jaffer S, Ambrosini-Spaltro A, Mancini AM, Eusebi V, Rosai J. Neurothekeoma and plexiform fibrohistiocytic tumor: mere histologic resemblance or histogenetic relationship? *Am J Surg Pathol.* 2009;33(6):905-913.

167. Misago N, Satoh T, Narisawa Y. Cellular neurothekeoma with histiocytic differentiation. *J Cutan Pathol.* 2004;31(8):568-572.

168. Zelger BG, Steiner H, Kutzner H, Maier H, Zelger B. Cellular 'neurothekeoma': an epithelioid variant of dermatofibroma? *Histopathology.* 1998;32(5):414-422.

169. Hornick JL, Fletcher CD. Cellular neurothekeoma: detailed characterization in a series of 133 cases. *Am J Surg Pathol.* 2007;31(3):329-340.

170. Stratton J, Billings SD. Cellular neurothekeoma: analysis of 37 cases emphasizing atypical histologic features. *Mod Pathol.* 2014;27(5):701-710.

171. Thway K, Fisher C. Angiomatoid fibrous histiocytoma: the current status of pathology and genetics. *Arch Pathol Lab Med.* 2015;139(5):674-682.

172. Boland JM, Folpe AL. Cutaneous neoplasms showing EWSR1 rearrangement. *Adv Anat Pathol.* 2013;20(2):75-85.

173. Thway K, Fisher C. Tumors with EWSR1-CREB1 and EWSR1-ATF1 fusions: the current status. *Am J Surg Pathol.* 2012;36(7):e1-e11.

174. Tanas MR, Rubin BP, Montgomery EA, et al. Utility of FISH in the diagnosis of angiomatoid fibrous histiocytoma: a series of 18 cases. *Mod Pathol.* 2010;23(1):93-97.

175. Bohman SL, Goldblum JR, Rubin BP, Tanas MR, Billings SD. Angiomatoid fibrous histiocytoma: an expansion of the clinical and histological spectrum. *Pathology.* 2014;46(3):199-204.

176. Matsumura T, Yamaguchi T, Tochigi N, Wada T, Yamashita T, Hasegawa T. Angiomatoid fibrous histiocytoma including cases with pleomorphic features analysed by fluorescence in situ hybridisation. *J Clin Pathol*. 2010;63(2):124-128.

177. Schaefer IM, Fletcher CD. Myxoid variant of so-called angiomatoid "malignant fibrous histiocytoma": clinicopathologic characterization in a series of 21 cases. *Am J Surg Pathol*. 2014;38(6):816-823.

178. Thway K, Strauss DC, Wren D, Fisher C. 'Pure' spindle cell variant of angiomatoid fibrous histiocytoma, lacking classic histologic features. *Pathol Res Pract*. 2016;212(11):1081-1084.

179. Gholve PA, Hosalkar HS, Kreiger PA, Dormans JP. Giant cell tumor of tendon sheath: largest single series in children. *J Pediatr Orthop*. 2007;27(1):67-74.

180. Hwang JS, Fitzhugh VA, Gibson PD, Didesch J, Ahmed I. Multiple giant cell tumors of tendon sheath found within a single digit of a 9-year-old. *Case Rep Orthop*. 2016;2016:1834740.

181. Lucas DR. Tenosynovial giant cell tumor: case report and review. *Arch Pathol Lab Med*. 2012;136(8):901-906.

182. Tsujino S, Matsumoto S, Ae K. Tenosynovial giant cell tumour of the hand in children under 10 years of age. *J Hand Surg Eur Vol*. 2018;43(3):335-337.

183. Yun SJ, Hwang SY, Jin W, Lim SJ, Park SY. Intramuscular diffuse-type tenosynovial giant cell tumor of the deltoid muscle in a child. *Skeletal Radiol*. 2014;43(8):1179-1183.

184. Mutgi KA, Chitgopeker P, Ciliberto H, Stone MS. Hypocellular plaque-like CD34-positive dermal fibroma (medallion-like dermal dendrocyte hamartoma) presenting as a skin-colored dermal nodule. *Pediatr Dermatol*. 2016;33(1):e16-e19.

185. Stuart LN, Hiatt KM, Zaki Z, Gardner JM, Shalin SC. Plaque-like CD34-positive dermal fibroma/medallion-like dermal dendrocyte hamartoma: an unusual spindle cell neoplasm. *J Cutan Pathol*. 2014;41(8):625-629.

186. Erdag G, Qureshi HS, Patterson JW, Wick MR. Solitary fibrous tumors of the skin: a clinicopathologic study of 10 cases and review of the literature. *J Cutan Pathol*. 2007;34(11):844-850.

187. Doyle LA, Vivero M, Fletcher CD, Mertens F, Hornick JL. Nuclear expression of STAT6 distinguishes solitary fibrous tumor from histologic mimics. *Mod Pathol*. 2014;27(3):390-395.

188. Ouladan S, Trautmann M, Orouji E, et al. Differential diagnosis of solitary fibrous tumors: A study of 454 soft tissue tumors indicating the diagnostic value of nuclear STAT6 relocation and ALDH1 expression combined with in situ proximity ligation assay. *Int J Oncol*. 2015;46(6):2595-2605.

189. Tan SY, Szymanski LJ, Galliani C, Parham D, Zambrano E. Solitary fibrous tumors in pediatric patients: a rare and potentially overdiagnosed neoplasm, confirmed by STAT6 immunohistochemistry. *Pediatr Dev Pathol*. 2017; 21(4):389-400.

190. Coffin CM, Alaggio R. Fibroblastic and myofibroblastic tumors in children and adolescents. *Pediatr Dev Pathol*. 2012;15(1 suppl):127-180.

191. Laskin WB, Miettinen M, Fetsch JF. Infantile digital fibroma/fibromatosis: a clinicopathologic and immunohistochemical study of 69 tumors from 57 patients with long-term follow-up. *Am J Surg Pathol*. 2009;33(1):1-13.

192. McNiff JM, Subtil A, Cowper SE, Lazova R, Glusac EJ. Cellular digital fibromas: distinctive CD34-positive lesions that may mimic dermatofibrosarcoma protuberans. *J Cutan Pathol*. 2005;32(6):413-418.

193. Niamba P, Léauté-Labrèze C, Boralevi F, et al. Further documentation of spontaneous regression of infantile digital fibromatosis. *Pediatr Dermatol*. 2007;24:280-284.

194. Baykal C, Buyukbabani N, Yazganoglu KD, Saglik E. Acquired digital fibrokeratoma. *Cutis*. 2007;79:129-132.

195. Hwang S, Kim M, Cho BK, Park HJ. Clinical characteristics of acquired ungual fibrokeratoma. *Indian J Dermatol Venereol Leprol*. 2017;83(3):337-343.

196. Aldrich SL, Hong CH, Groves L, Olsen C, Moss J, Darling TN. Acral lesion in tuberous sclerosis complex: insights into pathogenesis. *J Am Acad Dermatol*. 2010;63:244-251.

197. Jóźwiak S, Schwartz RA, Janniger CK, Michalowicz R, Chmielik J. Skin lesions in children with tuberous sclerosis complex: their prevalence, natural course, and diagnostic significance. *Int J Dermatol*. 1998;37:911-917.

198. Drut R, Pedemonte L, Rositto A. Noninclusion-body infantile digital fibromatosis: a lesion heralding terminal osseous dysplasia and pigmentary defects syndrome. *Int J Surg Pathol*. 2005;13:181-184.

199. Izadpanah A, Hogeling M, Buka RL, Eichenfield LF, Bird LM. Digitocutaneous dysplasia. *J Am Acad Dermatol*. 2007;56:86-89.

200. Hollmann TJ, Bovée JV, Fletcher CD. Digital fibromyxoma (superficial acral fibromyxoma): a detailed characterization of 124 cases. *Am J Surg Pathol*. 2012;36:789-798.

201. Arts FA, Sciot R, Brichard B, et al. PDGFRB gain-of-function mutations in sporadic infantile myofibromatosis. *Hum Mol Genet*. 2017;26(10):1801-1810.

202. Chang JY, Wang CS, Hung CC, Tsai TF, Hsiao CH. Multiple Epstein-Barr virus-associated subcutaneous angioleiomyomas in a patient with acquired immunodeficiency syndrome. *Br J Dermatol*. 2002;147(3):563-567.

203. Netscher DT, Baumholtz MA, Popek E, Schneider AM. Non-malignant fibrosing tumors in the pediatric hand: a clinicopathologic case review. *Hand (N Y)*. 2009;4(1):2-11.

204. Mashiah J, Hadj-Rabia S, Dompmartin A, et al. Infantile myofibromatosis: a series of 28 cases. *J Am Acad Dermatol*. 2014;71(2):264-270.

205. Murray N, Hanna B, Graf N, et al. The spectrum of infantile myofibromatosis includes both non-penetrance and adult recurrence. *Eur J Med Genet*. 2017;60(7):353-358.

206. Gawlinski P, Pelc M, Ciara E, et al. Phenotype expansion and development in Kosaki overgrowth syndrome. *Clin Genet*. 2018;93(4):919-924.

207. Antonescu CR, Sung YS, Zhang L, Agaram NP, Fletcher CD. Recurrent SRF-RELA Fusions Define a Novel Subset of Cellular Myofibroma/Myopericytoma: A Potential Diagnostic Pitfall With Sarcomas With Myogenic Differentiation. *Am J Surg Pathol*. 2017;41(5):677-684.

208. Oudijk L, den Bakker MA, Hop WC, et al. Solitary, multifocal and generalized myofibromas: clinicopathological and immunohistochemical features of 114 cases. *Histopathology*. 2012;60(6B):E1-E11.

209. Al-Ibraheemi A, Martinez A, Weiss SW, et al. Fibrous hamartoma of infancy: a clinicopathologic study of 145 cases, including 2 with sarcomatous features. *Mod Pathol*. 2017;30(4):474-485.

210. Fetsch JF, Miettinen M, Laskin WB, Michal M, Enzinger FM. A clinicopathologic study of 45 pediatric soft tissue tumors with an admixture of adipose tissue and fibroblastic elements, and a proposal for classification as lipofibromatosis. *Am J Surg Pathol*. 2000;24(11):1491-1500.

211. Park JY, Cohen C, Lopez D, Ramos E, Wagenfuehr J, Rakheja D. EGFR exon 20 insertion/duplication mutations characterize fibrous hamartoma of infancy. *Am J Surg Pathol*. 2016;40(12):1713-1718.

212. Melnick L, Berger EM, Elenitsas R, Chachkin S, Treat JR. Fibrous hamartoma of infancy: a firm plaque presenting with hypertrichosis and hyperhidrosis. *Pediatr Dermatol*. 2015;32(4):533-535.

213. Müller CS, Pföhler C, Cerroni L, Meier CM, Vogt T. Fibrous hamartoma of infancy within a congenital nevus. *J Dtsch Dermatol Ges*. 2015;13:1282-1284.

214. Murphy CM, Grau-Massanes M, Sanchez RL. Multiple cutaneous myxomas. Report of a case without other elements of Carney's complex. *J Cutan Pathol*. 1995;22(6):556-562.

215. Bekers EM, Eijkelenboom A, Grunberg K, et al. Myositis ossificans-Another condition with USP6 rearrangement, providing evidence of a relationship with nodular fasciitis and aneurysmal bone cyst. *Ann Diagn Pathol*. 2018;34:56-59.

216. Carter JM, Wang X, Dong J, Westendorf J, Chou MM, Oliveira AM. USP6 genetic rearrangements in cellular fibroma of tendon sheath. *Mod Pathol*. 2016;29(8):865-869.

217. Oliveira AM, Chou MM. USP6-induced neoplasms: the biologic spectrum of aneurysmal bone cyst and nodular fasciitis. *Hum Pathol*. 2014;45(1):1-11.

218. Lu L, Lao IW, Liu X, Yu L, Wang J. Nodular fasciitis: a retrospective study of 272 cases from China with clinicopathologic and radiologic correlation. *Ann Diagn Pathol*. 2015;19(3):180-185.

219. Bemrich-Stolz CJ, Kelly DR, Muensterer OJ, Pressey JG. Single institution series of nodular fasciitis in children. *J Pediatr Hematol Oncol.* 2010;32(5):354-357.

220. Pandian TK, Zeidan MM, Ibrahim KA, Moir CR, Ishitani MB, Zarroug AE. Nodular fasciitis in the pediatric population: a single center experience. *J Pediatr Surg.* 2013;48(7):1486-1489.

221. Hseu A, Watters K, Perez-Atayde A, Silvera VM, Rahbar R. Pediatric nodular fasciitis in the head and neck: evaluation and management. *JAMA Otolaryngol Head Neck Surg.* 2015;141(1):54-59.

222. Erber R, Agaimy A. Misses and near misses in diagnosing nodular fasciitis and morphologically related reactive myofibroblastic proliferations: experience of a referral center with emphasis on frequency of *USP6* gene rearrangements. *Virchows Arch.* 2018. doi:10.1007/s00428-018-2350-0.

223. Magro G, Michal M, Alaggio R, D'Amore E. Intradermal proliferative fasciitis in childhood: a potential diagnostic pitfall. *J Cutan Pathol.* 2011;38:59-62.

224. Barak S, Wang Z, Miettinen M. Immunoreactivity for calretinin and keratins in desmoid fibromatosis and other myofibroblastic tumors: a diagnostic pitfall. *Am J Surg Pathol.* 2012;36:1404-1409.

225. Kumar E, Patel NR, Demicco EG, et al. Cutaneous nodular fasciitis with genetic analysis: a case series. *J Cutan Pathol.* 2016;43(12):1143-1149.

226. Magro G. Differential diagnosis of benign spindle cell lesions. *Surg Pathol Clin.* 2018;11(1):91-121.

227. Kato I, Yoshida A, Ikegami M, et al. FOSL1 immunohistochemistry clarifies the distinction between desmoplastic fibroblastoma and fibroma of tendon sheath. *Histopathology.* 2016;69(6):1012-1020.

228. Magro G, Venti C. Childhood desmoplastic fibroblastoma (collagenous fibroma) with a 12-year follow-up. *Pediatr Dev Pathol.* 1999;2(1):62-64.

229. Nishio J, Iwasaki H, Nishijima T, Kikuchi M. Collagenous fibroma (desmoplastic fibroblastoma) of the finger in a child. *Pathol Int.* 2002;52(4):322-325.

230. Hasegawa T, Shimoda T, Hirohashi S, Hizawa K, Sano T. Collagenous fibroma (desmoplastic fibroblastoma): report of four cases and review of the literature. *Arch Pathol Lab Med.* 1998;122(5):455-460.

231. Gonzalez-Vela MC, Val-Bernal JF, Martino M, Gonzalez-Lopez MA, Garcia-Alberdi E, Hermana S. Sclerotic fibroma-like dermatofibroma: an uncommon distinctive variant of dermatofibroma. *Histol Histopathol.* 2005;20(3):801-806.

232. High WA, Stewart D, Essary LR, Kageyama NP, Hoang MP, Cockerell CJ. Sclerotic fibroma-like change in various neoplastic and inflammatory skin lesions: is sclerotic fibroma a distinct entity? *J Cutan Pathol.* 2004;31(5):373-378.

233. Ramdial PK, Madaree A. Aggressive CD34-positive fibrous scalp lesion of childhood: extrapulmonary solitary fibrous tumor. *Pediatr Dev Pathol.* 2001;4(3):267-275.

234. Sohn IB, Hwang SM, Lee SH, Choi EH, Ahn SK. Dermatofibroma with sclerotic areas resembling a sclerotic fibroma of the skin. *J Cutan Pathol.* 2002;29(1):44-47.

235. Coffin CM, Hornick JL, Zhou H, Fletcher CD. Gardner fibroma: a clinicopathologic and immunohistochemical analysis of 45 patients with 57 fibromas. *Am J Surg Pathol.* 2007;31(3):410-416.

236. Vieira J, Pinto C, Afonso M, et al. Identification of previously unrecognized FAP in children with Gardner fibroma. *Eur J Hum Genet.* 2015;23(5):715-718.

237. LeBlanc KG Jr, Wenner M, Davis LS. Multiple nuchal fibromas in a 2-year-old without Gardner syndrome. *Pediatr Dermatol.* 2011;28(6):695-696.

238. Cates JM, Stricker TP, Sturgeon D, Coffin CM. Desmoid-type fibromatosis-associated Gardner fibromas: prevalence and impact on local recurrence. *Cancer Lett.* 2014;353(2):176-181.

239. Carlson JW, Fletcher CD. Immunohistochemistry for beta-catenin in the differential diagnosis of spindle cell lesions: analysis of a series and review of the literature. *Histopathology.* 2007;51(4):509-514.

240. Ferenc T, Wronski JW, Kopczynski J, et al. Analysis of APC, alpha-, beta-catenins, and N-cadherin protein expression in aggressive fibromatosis (desmoid tumor). *Pathol Res Pract.* 2009;205(5):311-324.

241. Mentzel T, Dei Tos AP, Sapi Z, Kutzner H. Myopericytoma of skin and soft tissues: clinicopathologic and immunohistochemical study of 54 cases. *Am J Surg Pathol.* 2006;30:104-113.

242. LeBlanc RE, Taube J. Myofibroma, myopericytoma, myoepithelioma and myofibroblastoma of skin and soft tissue. *Surg Pathol Clin.* 2011;4:745-759.

243. Dray MS, McCarthy SW, Palmer AA, et al. Myopericytoma: a unifying term for a spectrum of tumours that show overlapping features with myofibroma. A review of 14 cases. *J Clin Pathol.* 2006;59:67-73.

244. Haller F, Knopf J, Ackermann A, et al. Paediatric and adult soft tissue sarcomas with *NTRK1* gene fusions: a subset of spindle cell sarcomas unified by a prominent myopericytic/haemangiopericytic pattern. *J Pathol.* 2016;238:700-710.

245. Mazza JM, Linnell E, Votava HJ, Wisoff JH, Silverberg NB. Biopsy-proven spontaneous regression of a rhabdomyomatous mesenchymal hamartoma. *Pediatr Dermatol.* 2015;32(2):256-262.

246. Sampat K, Cheesman E, Siminas S. Perianal rhabdomyomatous mesenchymal hamartoma. *Ann R Coll Surg Engl.* 2017;99(6):e193-e195.

247. Fontecilla NM, Weitz NA, Day C, Golas AR, Grossman ME, Reiffel R. Rhabdomyomatous mesenchymal hamartoma presenting as a skin tag in a newborn. *JAAD Case Rep.* 2016;2(3):222-223.

248. McKinnon EL, Rand AJ, Selim MA, Fuchs HE, Buckley AF, Cummings TJ. Rhabdomyomatous mesenchymal hamartoma presenting as a sacral skin tag in two neonates with spinal dysraphism. *J Cutan Pathol.* 2015;42(10):774-778.

249. Solis-Coria A, Vargas-Gonzalez R, Sotelo-Avila C. Rhabdomyomatous mesenchymal hamartoma presenting as a skin tag in the sternoclavicular area. *Pathol Oncol Res.* 2007;13(4):375-378.

250. Johnson MD, Jacobs AH. Congenital smooth muscle hamartoma. A report of six cases and a review of the literature. *Arch Dermatol.* 1989;125(6):820-822.

251. Kim YJ, Roh MR, Lee JH, et al. Clinicopathologic characteristics of early-onset Becker's nevus in Korean children and adolescents. *Int J Dermatol.* 2018;57(1):55-61.

252. Schmidt CS, Bentz ML. Congenital smooth muscle hamartoma: the importance of differentiation from melanocytic nevi. *J Craniofac Surg.* 2005;16(5):926-929.

253. Janick EC, Nazareth MR, Rothman IL. Generalized smooth muscle hamartoma with multiple congenital anomalies without the "Michelin tire baby" phenotype. *Pediatr Dermatol.* 2014;31:731-733.

254. Bernett CN, Mammino JJ. Cutaneous leiomyomas. In: *StatPearls.* Treasure Island, FL: StatPearls Publishing; 2018.

255. Malik K, Patel P, Chen J, Khachemoune A. Leiomyoma cutis: a focused review on presentation, management, and association with malignancy. *Am J Clin Dermatol.* 2015;16(1):35-46.

256. Spencer JM, Amonette RA. Tumors with smooth muscle differentiation. *Dermatol Surg.* 1996;22(9):761-768.

257. Caliskan E, Bodur S, Ulubay M, et al. Hereditary leiomyomatosis and renal cell carcinoma syndrome: a case report and implications of early onset. *An Bras Dermatol.* 2017;92(5 suppl 1):88-91.

258. Costigan DC, Doyle LA. Advances in the clinicopathological and molecular classification of cutaneous mesenchymal neoplasms. *Histopathology.* 2016;68(6):776-795.

259. Lencastre A, Cabete J, Goncalves R, Joao A, Fidalgo A. Cutaneous leiomyomatosis in a mother and daughter. *An Bras Dermatol.* 2013;88(6 suppl 1):124-127.

260. Wofford J, Fenves AZ, Jackson JM, Kimball AB, Menter A. The spectrum of nephrocutaneous diseases and associations: Genetic causes of nephrocutaneous disease. *J Am Acad Dermatol.* 2016;74(2):231-244; quiz 245-236.

261. Holst VA, Junkins-Hopkins JM, Elenitsas R. Cutaneous smooth muscle neoplasms: clinical features, histologic findings, and treatment options. *J Am Acad Dermatol.* 2002;46(4):477-490; quiz, 491-474.

262. Patel VM, Handler MZ, Schwartz RA, Lambert WC. Hereditary leiomyomatosis and renal cell cancer syndrome: an update and review. *J Am Acad Dermatol.* 2017;77(1):149-158.

263. Arishima H, Takeuchi H, Kitai R, Yamauchi T, Kikuta K. Vascular leiomyoma of the scalp with a small deformity on the skull mimicking a dermoid cyst. *Pediatr Dermatol.* 2013;30(3):e27-e29.

264. Ramesh P, Annapureddy SR, Khan F, Sutaria PD. Angioleiomyoma: a clinical, pathological and radiological review. *Int J Clin Pract.* 2004;58(6):587-591.

265. Zhang JZ, Zhou J, Zhang ZC. Subcutaneous angioleiomyoma: clinical and sonographic features with histopathologic correlation. *J Ultrasound Med.* 2016;35(8):1669-1673.

266. Lau SK, Koh SS. Cutaneous smooth muscle tumors: a review. *Adv Anat Pathol.* 2018;25(4):282-290.

267. Deyrup AT, Lee VK, Hill CE, et al. Epstein-Barr virus-associated smooth muscle tumors are distinctive mesenchymal tumors reflecting multiple infection events: a clinicopathologic and molecular analysis of 29 tumors from 19 patients. *Am J Surg Pathol.* 2006;30(1):75-82.

268. Jossen J, Chu J, Hotchkiss H, et al. Epstein-Barr virus-associated smooth muscle tumors in children following solid organ transplantation: a review. *Pediatr Transplant.* 2015;19(2):235-243.

269. Hussein K, Rath B, Ludewig B, Kreipe H, Jonigk D. Clinico-pathological characteristics of different types of immunodeficiency-associated smooth muscle tumours. *Eur J Cancer.* 2014;50(14):2417-2424.

270. Petrilli G, Lorenzi L, Paracchini R, et al. Epstein-Barr virus-associated adrenal smooth muscle tumors and disseminated diffuse large B-cell lymphoma in a child with common variable immunodeficiency: a case report and review of the literature. *Int J Surg Pathol.* 2014;22(8):712-721.

271. Coffin CM, Alaggio R. Adipose and myxoid tumors of childhood and adolescence. *Pediatr Dev Pathol.* 2012;15(1 suppl):239-254.

272. Zou Y, Billings SD. Myxoid cutaneous tumors: a review. *J Cutan Pathol.* 2016;43(10):903-918.

273. Nakamura M, Tokura Y. Superficial angiomyxoma on the scrotum of a child. *Pediatr Dermatol.* 2011;28(2):200-201.

274. Calonje E, Guerin D, McCormick D, Fletcher CD. Superficial angiomyxoma: clinicopathologic analysis of a series of distinctive but poorly recognized cutaneous tumors with tendency for recurrence. *Am J Surg Pathol.* 1999;23(8):910-917.

275. Allen PW, Dymock RB, MacCormac LB. Superficial angiomyxomas with and without epithelial components. Report of 30 tumors in 28 patients. *Am J Surg Pathol.* 1988;12(7):519-530.

276. Prescott RJ, Husain EA, Abdellaoui A, et al. Superficial acral fibromyxoma: a clinicopathological study of new 41 cases from the U.K.: should myxoma (NOS) and fibroma (NOS) continue as part of 21st-century reporting? *Br J Dermatol.* 2008;159(6):1315-1321.

277. Marti N, Jorda E, Monteagudo C, Gamez L, Reig I, Calduch L. Multiple cutaneous angiomyxomas in a child. *Pediatr Dermatol.* 2011;28(4):462-464.

278. Takahashi H, Hida T. Carney complex: report of a Japanese case associated with cutaneous superficial angiomyxomas, labial lentigines, and a pituitary adenoma. *J Dermatol.* 2002;29(12):790-796.

279. Vandersteen A, Turnbull J, Jan W, et al. Cutaneous signs are important in the diagnosis of the rare neoplasia syndrome Carney complex. *Eur J Pediatr.* 2009;168(11):1401-1404.

280. Leventhal JS, Braverman IM. Skin manifestations of endocrine and neuroendocrine tumors. *Semin Oncol.* 2016;43(3):335-340.

281. Mateus C, Palangie A, Franck N, et al. Heterogeneity of skin manifestations in patients with Carney complex. *J Am Acad Dermatol.* 2008;59(5):801-810.

282. Briassoulis G, Quezado M, Lee CC, Xekouki P, Keil M, Stratakis CA. Myxoma of the ear lobe in a 23-month-old girl with Carney complex. *J Cutan Pathol.* 2012;39(1):68-71.

283. Foster JH, Vasudevan SA, John Hicks M, Schady D, Chintagumpala M. Primitive myxoid mesenchymal tumor of infancy involving chest wall in an infant: a case report and clinicopathologic correlation. *Pediatr Dev Pathol.* 2016;19(3):244-248.

284. Lam J, Lara-Corrales I, Cammisuli S, Somers GR, Pope E. Primitive myxoid mesenchymal tumor of infancy in a preterm infant. *Pediatr Dermatol.* 2010;27(6):635-637.

285. Kao YC, Sung YS, Zhang L, et al. Recurrent BCOR internal tandem duplication and YWHAE-NUTM2B fusions in soft tissue undifferentiated round cell sarcoma of infancy: overlapping genetic features with clear cell sarcoma of kidney. *Am J Surg Pathol.* 2016;40(8):1009-1020.

286. Santiago T, Clay MR, Allen SJ, Orr BA. Recurrent BCOR internal tandem duplication and BCOR or BCL6 expression distinguish primitive myxoid mesenchymal tumor of infancy from congenital infantile fibrosarcoma. *Mod Pathol.* 2017;30(6):884-891.

287. Guilbert MC, Rougemont AL, Samson Y, Mac-Thiong JM, Fournet JC, Soglio DB. Transformation of a primitive myxoid mesenchymal tumor of infancy to an undifferentiated sarcoma: a first reported case. *J Pediatr Hematol Oncol.* 2015;37(2):e118-e120.

288. Keppler-Noreuil KM, Rios JJ, Parker VER, et al. PIK3CA-related overgrowth spectrum (PROS): diagnostic and testing eligibility criteria, differential diagnosis and evaluation. *Am J Med Genet A.* 2015;167A:287-295.

289. Boybeyi O, Alanay Y, Kayikcioglu A, Karnak I. Hemihyperplasia-multiple lipomatosis syndrome: an underdiagnosed entity in children with asymmetric overgrowth. *J Pediatr Surg.* 2010;45:E19-E23.

290. Gucev ZS, Tasic V, Jancevska A, et al. Congenital lipomatous overgrowth, vascular malformations, and epidermal nevi (CLOVE) syndrome: CNS malformations and seizures may be a component of this disorder. *Am J Med Genet A.* 2008;146A:2688-2690.

291. Craiglow BG, Ko CJ, Antaya RJ. Two cases of hemihyperplasia-multiple lipomatosis syndrome and review of asymmetric hemihyperplasia syndromes. *Pediatr Dermatol.* 2014;31:507-510.

292. Beachkofsky TM, Sapp JC, Biesecker LG, Darling TN. Progressive overgrowth of the cerebriform connective tissue nevus in patients with Proteus syndrome. *J Am Acad Dermatol.* 2010;63:799-804.

293. Talamanca LF, Verdolotti T, Colafati GS, Bernadi B. Hemimegalencephaly associated with congenital infiltrating lipomatosis of the face: a case report. *Neuropediatrics.* 2012;43:349-352.

294. Couto JA, Vivero MP, Upton J, et al. Facial infiltrating lipomatosis contains somatic PIK3CA mutations in multiple tissues. *Plast Reconstr Surg.* 2015;136(4 suppl):72-73.

295. Serpa MS, Scully C, Molina Vivas AP, de Almeida OP, Costa FD, Alves FA. Infiltrating lipomatosis of the face: case series and literature review. *Oral Surg Oral Med Oral Pathol Oral Radiol.* 2017;123:e99-e105.

296. Bieser S, Reis M, Guzman M, et al. Grade II pilocytic astrocytoma in a 3-month-old patient with encephalocraniocutaneous lipomatosis [ECCL]: case report and literature review of low grade gliomas in ECCL. *Am J Med Genet Part A.* 2015;167A:878-881.

297. Ruggieri M, Pratico AD. Mosaic neurocutaneous disorders and their causes. *Semin Pediatr Neurol.* 2015;22:207-233.

298. Boppudi S, Bogershausen N, Hove HB, et al. Specific mosaic KRAS mutations affecting codon 146 cause oculoectodermal syndrome and encephalocraniocutaneous lipomatosis. *Clin Genet.* 2016;90:334-342.

299. Bennett JT, Tan TY, Alcantara D, et al. Mosaic activating mutations in FGFR1 cause encephalocraniocutaneous lipomatosis. *Am J Hum Genet.* 2016;98:579-587.

300. Kurek KC, Howard E, Tennant LB, et al. PTEN hamartoma of soft tissue: a distinctive lesion in PTEN syndromes. *Am J Surg Pathol.* 2012;36:671-687.

301. Garib G, Siegal GP, Andea AA. Autosomal-dominant familial angiolipomatosis. *Cutis.* 2015;95(1):E26-E29.

302. Lapidoth M, Ben Amitai D, Feinmesser M, Akerman L. Capillary malformation associated with angiolipoma: analysis of 127 consecutive clinic patients. *Am J Clin Dermatol.* 2008;9(6):389-392.

303. Sheng W, Lu L, Wang J. Cellular angiolipoma: a clinicopathological and immunohistochemical study of 12 cases. *Am J Dermatopathol.* 2013;35(2):220-225.

304. Dadone B, Refae S, Lemarie-Delaunay C, Bianchini L, Pedeutour F. Molecular cytogenetics of pediatric adipocytic tumors. *Cancer Genet.* 2015;208(10):469-481.

305. Pierre-Kahn A, Zerah M, Renier D, et al. Congenital lumbosacral lipomas. *Childs Nerv Syst.* 1997;13:298-334.

306. Morota N, Ihara S, Ogiwara H. New classification of spinal lipomas based on embryonic stage. *J Neurosurg Pediatr.* 2017;19:428-439.

307. Kim HJ, Yang I, Jung AY, Hwang JH, Shin MK. Angiomyxolipoma (vascular myxolipoma) of the knee in a 9-year-old boy. *Pediatr Radiol.* 2010;40(suppl 1):S30-S33.

308. Martinez-Mata G, Rocio MF, Juan LE, Paes AO, Adalberto MT. Angiomyxolipoma (vascular myxolipoma) of the oral cavity. Report of a case and review of the literature. *Head Neck Pathol.* 2011;5:184-187.

309. Pontes HA, Pontes FS, Cruz e Silva BT, et al. Angiomyolipomatous hamartoma of the upper lip: a rare case in an 8-month-old child and differential diagnosis. *J Craniomaxillofac Surg.* 2011;39:102-106.

310. Sheybani EF, Eutsler EP, Navarro OM. Fat-containing soft-tissue masses in children. *Pediatr Radiol.* 2016;46(13):1760-1773.

311. Shen LY, Amin SM, Chamlin SL, Mancini AJ. Varied presentations of pediatric lipoblastoma: case series and review of the literature. *Pediatr Dermatol.* 2017;34(2):180-186.

312. Coffin CM, Lowichik A, Putnam A. Lipoblastoma (LPB): a clinicopathologic and immunohistochemical analysis of 59 cases. *Am J Surg Pathol.* 2009;33(11):1705-1712.

313. Han JW, Kim H, Youn JK, et al. Analysis of clinical features of lipoblastoma in children. *Pediatr Hematol Oncol.* 2017;34(4):212-220.

314. Kubota F, Matsuyama A, Shibuya R, Nakamoto M, Hisaoka M. Desmin-positivity in spindle cells: under-recognized immunophenotype of lipoblastoma. *Pathol Int.* 2013;63(7):353-357.

315. Kohashi K, Yamada Y, Hotokebuchi Y, et al. ERG and SALL4 expressions in SMARCB1/INI1-deficient tumors: a useful tool for distinguishing epithelioid sarcoma from malignant rhabdoid tumor. *Hum Pathol.* 2015;46(2):225-230.

316. Warren M, Turpin BK, Mark M, Smolarek TA, Li X. Undifferentiated myxoid lipoblastoma with PLAG1-HAS2 fusion in an infant; morphologically mimicking primitive myxoid mesenchymal tumor of infancy (PMMTI)—diagnostic importance of cytogenetic and molecular testing and literature review. *Cancer Genet.* 2016;209(1-2):21-29.

317. Pedeutour F, Deville A, Steyaert H, Ranchere-Vince D, Ambrosetti D, Sirvent N. Rearrangement of HMGA2 in a case of infantile lipoblastoma without Plag1 alteration. *Pediatr Blood Cancer.* 2012;58(5):798-800.

318. Wesche WA, Khare VK, Chesney TM, Jenkins JJ. Non-hematopoietic cutaneous metastases in children and adolescents: thirty years' experience at St. Jude Children's Research Hospital. *J Cutan Pathol.* 2000;27(10):485-492.

319. Balamuth NJ, Womer RB. Ewing's sarcoma. *Lancet Oncol.* 2010;11(2):184-192.

320. Somers G. Ewing family tumours: a paediatric perspective. *Diagn Histopathol.* 2014;20(2):49-55.

321. Delaplace M, Lhommet C, de Pinieux G, Vergier B, de Muret A, Machet L. Primary cutaneous Ewing sarcoma: a systematic review focused on treatment and outcome. *Br J Dermatol.* 2012;166(4):721-726.

322. Di Giannatale A, Frezza AM, Le Deley MC, et al. Primary cutaneous and subcutaneous Ewing sarcoma. *Pediatr Blood Cancer.* 2015;62(9):1555-1561.

323. Dim DC, Cooley LD, Miranda RN. Clear cell sarcoma of tendons and aponeuroses: a review. *Arch Pathol Lab Med.* 2007;131(1):152-156.

324. Falconieri G, Bacchi CE, Luzar B. Cutaneous clear cell sarcoma: report of three cases of a potentially underestimated mimicker of spindle cell melanoma. *Am J Dermatopathol.* 2012;34(6):619-625.

325. Hantschke M, Mentzel T, Rutten A, et al. Cutaneous clear cell sarcoma: a clinicopathologic, immunohistochemical, and molecular analysis of 12 cases emphasizing its distinction from dermal melanoma. *Am J Surg Pathol.* 2010;34(2):216-222.

326. Hisaoka M, Ishida T, Kuo TT, et al. Clear cell sarcoma of soft tissue: a clinicopathologic, immunohistochemical, and molecular analysis of 33 cases. *Am J Surg Pathol.* 2008;32(3):452-460.

327. Park BM, Jin SA, Choi YD, et al. Two cases of clear cell sarcoma with different clinical and genetic features: cutaneous type with BRAF mutation and subcutaneous type with KIT mutation. *Br J Dermatol.* 2013;169(6):1346-1352.

328. Protsenko SA, Semionova AI, Komarov YI, et al. BRAF-mutated clear cell sarcoma is sensitive to vemurafenib treatment. *Invest New Drugs.* 2015;33(5):1136-1143.

329. Laskin WB, Fetsch JF, Miettinen M. Myxoinflammatory fibroblastic sarcoma: a clinicopathologic analysis of 104 cases, with emphasis on predictors of outcome. *Am J Surg Pathol.* 2014;38(1):1-12.

330. Weiss VL, Antonescu CR, Alaggio R, et al. Myxoinflammatory fibroblastic sarcoma in children and adolescents: clinicopathologic aspects of a rare neoplasm. *Pediatr Dev Pathol.* 2013;16(6):425-431.

331. Lucas DR. Myxoinflammatory fibroblastic sarcoma: review and update. *Arch Pathol Lab Med.* 2017;141(11):1503-1507.

332. Ieremia E, Thway K. Myxoinflammatory fibroblastic sarcoma: morphologic and genetic updates. *Arch Pathol Lab Med.* 2014;138(10):1406-1411.

333. Kao YC, Ranucci V, Zhang L, et al. Recurrent *BRAF* gene rearrangements in myxoinflammatory fibroblastic sarcomas, but not hemosiderotic fibrolipomatous tumors. *Am J Surg Pathol.* 2017;41(11):1456-1465.

334. Jo VY. Myoepithelial tumors: an update. *Surg Pathol Clin.* 2015;8(3):445-466.

335. Antonescu CR, Zhang L, Chang NE, et al. EWSR1-POU5F1 fusion in soft tissue myoepithelial tumors. A molecular analysis of sixty-six cases, including soft tissue, bone, and visceral lesions, showing common involvement of the *EWSR1* gene. *Genes Chromosomes Cancer.* 2010;49(12):1114-1124.

336. Flucke U, Palmedo G, Blankenhorn N, Slootweg PJ, Kutzner H, Mentzel T. *EWSR1* gene rearrangement occurs in a subset of cutaneous myoepithelial tumors: a study of 18 cases. *Mod Pathol.* 2011;24(11):1444-1450.

337. Antonescu CR, Zhang L, Shao SY, et al. Frequent *PLAG1* gene rearrangements in skin and soft tissue myoepithelioma with ductal differentiation. *Genes Chromosomes Cancer.* 2013;52(7):675-682.

338. Gleason BC, Fletcher CD. Myoepithelial carcinoma of soft tissue in children: an aggressive neoplasm analyzed in a series of 29 cases. *Am J Surg Pathol.* 2007;31(12):1813-1824.

339. Hornick JL, Fletcher CD. Cutaneous myoepithelioma: a clinicopathologic and immunohistochemical study of 14 cases. *Hum Pathol.* 2004;35(1):14-24.

340. Mentzel T, Requena L, Kaddu S, Soares de Aleida LM, Sangu0za OP, Kutzner H. Cutaneous myoepithelial neoplasms: clinicopathologic and immunohistochemical study of 20 cases suggesting a continuous spectrum ranging from benign mixed tumor of the skin to cutaneous myoepithelioma and myoepithelial carcinoma. *J Cutan Pathol.* 2003;30(5):294-302.

341. Le Loarer F, Zhang L, Fletcher CD, et al. Consistent SMARCB1 homozygous deletions in epithelioid sarcoma and in a subset of myoepithelial carcinomas can be reliably detected by FISH in archival material. *Genes Chromosomes Cancer.* 2014;53(6):475-486.

342. Pawel BR. SMARCB1-deficient tumors of childhood: a practical guide. *Pediatr Dev Pathol.* 2018;21(1):6-28.

343. Spunt S, million L, Coffin C. The non-rhabdomyosarcoma soft tissue sarcomas. In: Pizzo PA, ed. *Principles and Practice of Pediatric Oncology.* 7th ed. Philadelphia, PA: Wolters Kluwer; 2016:827-854.

344. Gasparini P, Facchinetti F, Boeri M, et al. Prognostic determinants in epithelioid sarcoma. *Eur J Cancer.* 2011;47(2):287-295.

345. Jawad MU, Extein J, Min ES, Scully SP. Prognostic factors for survival in patients with epithelioid sarcoma: 441 cases from the SEER database. *Clin Orthop Relat Res.* 2009;467(11):2939-2948.

346. Thway K, Jones RL, Noujaim J, Fisher C. Epithelioid sarcoma: diagnostic features and genetics. *Adv Anat Pathol.* 2016;23(1):41-49.

347. Cacciatore M, Dei Tos AP. Challenging epithelioid mesenchymal neoplasms: mimics and traps. *Pathology.* 2014;46(2):126-134.

348. Cancado CG, Vale FR, Bacchi CE. Subcutaneous (deep) granuloma annulare in children: a possible mimicker of epithelioid sarcoma. *Fetal Pediatr Pathol*. 2007;26(1):33-39.

349. Stockman DL, Hornick JL, Deavers MT, Lev DC, Lazar AJ, Wang WL. ERG and FLI1 protein expression in epithelioid sarcoma. *Mod Pathol*. 2014;27(4):496-501.

350. Assen YJ, Madern GC, de Laat PC, den Hollander JC, Oranje AP. Rhabdoid tumor mimicking hemangioma. *Pediatr Dermatol*. 2011;28(3):295-298.

351. Cobb AR, Sebire NJ, Anderson J, Dunaway D. Congenital malignant rhabdoid tumor of the scalp. *J Craniomaxillofac Surg*. 2012;40(8):e258-e260.

352. Hsueh C, Kuo TT. Congenital malignant rhabdoid tumor presenting as a cutaneous nodule: report of 2 cases with review of the literature. *Arch Pathol Lab Med*. 1998;122(12):1099-1102.

353. White FV, Dehner LP, Belchis DA, et al. Congenital disseminated malignant rhabdoid tumor: a distinct clinicopathologic entity demonstrating abnormalities of chromosome 22q11. *Am J Surg Pathol*. 1999;23(3):249-256.

354. Sredni ST, Tomita T. Rhabdoid tumor predisposition syndrome. *Pediatr Dev Pathol*. 2015;18(1):49-58.

355. Marburger TB, Gardner JM, Prieto VG, Billings SD. Primary cutaneous rhabdomyosarcoma: a clinicopathologic review of 11 cases. *J Cutan Pathol*. 2012;39(11):987-995.

356. Kitagawa N, Arata J, Ohtsuki Y, Hayashi K, Oomori Y, Tomoda T. Congenital alveolar rhabdomyosarcoma presenting as a blueberry muffin baby. *J Dermatol*. 1989;16(5):409-411.

357. Godambe SV, Rawal J. Blueberry muffin rash as a presentation of alveolar cell rhabdomyosarcoma in a neonate. *Acta Paediatr*. 2000;89(1):115-117.

358. Grundy R, Anderson J, Gaze M, et al. Congenital alveolar rhabdomyosarcoma: clinical and molecular distinction from alveolar rhabdomyosarcoma in older children. *Cancer*. 2001;91(3):606-612.

359. Holland KE, Galbraith SS, Drolet BA. Neonatal violaceous skin lesions: expanding the differential of the "blueberry muffin baby." *Adv Dermatol*. 2005;21:153-192.

360. Rodriguez-Galindo C, Hill DA, Onyekwere O, et al. Neonatal alveolar rhabdomyosarcoma with skin and brain metastases. *Cancer*. 2001;92(6):1613-1620.

361. Rekhi B, Qureshi SS, Narula G, Gujral S, Kurkure P. Rapidly progressive congenital rhabdomyosarcoma presenting with multiple cutaneous lesions: an uncommon diagnosis and a therapeutic challenge. *Pathol Res Pract*. 2014;210(5):328-333.

362. Christman MP, Kerner JK, Cheng C, et al. Rhabdomyosarcoma arising in a giant congenital melanocytic nevus. *Pediatr Dermatol*. 2014;31(5):584-587.

363. Hoang MP, Sinkre P, Albores-Saavedra J. Rhabdomyosarcoma arising in a congenital melanocytic nevus. *Am J Dermatopathol*. 2002; 24(1):26-29.

364. Fauth CT, Bruecks AK, Temple W, Arlette JP, DiFrancesco LM. Superficial leiomyosarcoma: a clinicopathologic review and update. *J Cutan Pathol*. 2010;37(2):269-276.

365. Winchester DS, Hocker TL, Brewer JD, et al. Leiomyosarcoma of the skin: clinical, histopathologic, and prognostic factors that influence outcomes. *J Am Acad Dermatol*. 2014;71(5):919-925.

366. Blaise G, Nikkels AF, Quatresooz P, Hermanns-Le T, Pierard GE. Childhood cutaneous leiomyosarcoma. *Pediatr Dermatol*. 2009;26(4): 477-479.

367. Ramdial PK, Sing Y, Deonarain J, Hadley GP, Singh B. Dermal Epstein–Barr virus—associated leiomyosarcoma: tocsin of acquired immunodeficiency syndrome in two children. *Am J Dermatopathol*. 2011;33(4):392-396.

368. Tetzlaff MT, Nosek C, Kovarik CL. Epstein–Barr virus-associated leiomyosarcoma with cutaneous involvement in an African child with human immunodeficiency virus: a case report and review of the literature. *J Cutan Pathol*. 2011;38(9):731-739.

369. Kraft S, Fletcher CD. Atypical intradermal smooth muscle neoplasms: clinicopathologic analysis of 84 cases and a reappraisal of cutaneous "leiomyosarcoma." *Am J Surg Pathol*. 2011;35(4):599-607.

370. Rekhi B, Kosemehmetoglu K, Tezel GG, Dervisoglu S. Clinicopathologic features and immunohistochemical spectrum of 11 cases of epithelioid malignant peripheral nerve sheath tumors, including INI1/SMARCB1 results and BRAF V600E analysis. *APMIS*. 2017;125(8):679-689.

371. Luzar B, Falconieri G. Cutaneous malignant peripheral nerve sheath tumor. *Surg Pathol Clin*. 2017;10(2):337-343.

372. Griewank KG, Schilling B, Murali R, et al. TERT promoter mutations are frequent in atypical fibroxanthomas and pleomorphic dermal sarcomas. *Mod Pathol*. 2014;27(4):502-508.

373. Hussein MR. Atypical fibroxanthoma: new insights. *Expert Rev Anticancer Ther*. 2014;14(9):1075-1088.

374. Lopez L, Velez R. Atypical fibroxanthoma. *Arch Pathol Lab Med*. 2016;140(4):376-379.

375. Miller K, Goodlad JR, Brenn T. Pleomorphic dermal sarcoma: adverse histologic features predict aggressive behavior and allow distinction from atypical fibroxanthoma. *Am J Surg Pathol*. 2012;36(9):1317-1326.

376. Dilek FH, Akpolat N, Metin A, Ugras S. Atypical fibroxanthoma of the skin and the lower lip in xeroderma pigmentosum. *Br J Dermatol*. 2000;143(3):618-620.

377. Shao L, Newell B, Quintanilla N. Atypical fibroxanthoma and squamous cell carcinoma of the conjunctiva in xeroderma pigmentosum. *Pediatr Dev Pathol*. 2007;10(2):149-152.

378. Navarro OM. Soft tissue masses in children. *Radiol Clin North Am*. 2011;49(6):1235-1259, vi-vii.

379. Navarro OM, Laffan EE, Ngan BY. Pediatric soft-tissue tumors and pseudo-tumors: MR imaging features with pathologic correlation: part 1. Imaging approach, pseudotumors, vascular lesions, and adipocytic tumors. *Radiographics*. 2009;29(3):887-906.

380. McDermott MB, Lind AC, Marley EF, Dehner LP. Deep granuloma annulare (pseudorheumatoid nodule) in children: clinicopathologic study of 35 cases. *Pediatr Dev Pathol*. 1998;1(4):300-308.

381. Requena L, Fernandez-Figueras MT. Subcutaneous granuloma annulare. *Semin Cutan Med Surg*. 2007;26(2):96-99.

382. Fisher C. Epithelioid sarcoma of Enzinger. *Adv Anat Pathol*. 2006; 13(3):114-121.

383. Stefanaki K, Tsivitanidou-Kakourou T, Stefanaki C, et al. Histological and immunohistochemical study of granuloma annulare and subcutaneous granuloma annulare in children. *J Cutan Pathol*. 2007;34(5):392-396.

384. Wick MR, Manivel JC. Epithelioid sarcoma and isolated necrobiotic granuloma: a comparative immunocytochemical study. *J Cutan Pathol*. 1986;13(4):253-260.

25

Vascular Lesions

Daniel D. Miller / Alejandro A. Gru / Sheilagh M. Maguiness

Introduction and Classification

The field of vascular anomalies has grown at a rapid pace over the past decade. The International Society for the Study of Vascular Anomalies (ISSVA) was first established in 1976 by Drs John Mulliken and Anthony Young. Since then, ISSVA has developed and updated the classification schema for vascular lesions, building from the initial biologic classification proposed by Mulliken and Glowacki in 1982.[1] The most recent classification for vascular anomalies was proposed in 2014[2] (Table 25-1). Genetic advances have led to an improved understanding of these conditions and paved the way for potential targeted therapies. Correct classification of vascular anomalies is of utmost importance, because although the lesions may clinically resemble one another, the prognosis and natural history of this heterogeneous group of conditions varies widely. Accurate and precise diagnosis is necessary and possible on the basis of the clinical appearance, natural history, imaging, and histopathologic features of the malformation or tumor. This chapter reviews the basic epidemiology, etiology, clinical manifestations, and histopathology for the most common pediatric vascular tumors and malformations.

Vascular tumors comprise a heterogeneous group of vascular lesions, many of which most commonly present during childhood. Table 25-2 lists the ISSVA basic classification of vascular tumors, of which infantile hemangioma is the most common, classic, pediatric vascular tumor.

INFANTILE HEMANGIOMA

Definition and Epidemiology

Infantile hemangiomas (IH) are present in about 4% of newborns.[3] They are an extremely common type of vascular tumor that have a distinctive natural history.

Etiology

Risk factors for the development of IH are well characterized and include female gender, low birth weight, and Caucasian skin type. The etiology of IH remains incompletely understood; however, experts believe that a somatic mutation may be responsible.

Clinical Presentation

IH are typically not present at birth. Rather, they may exist initially as a premonitory mark/precursor lesion, such as an

TABLE 25-1.	Classification of vascular anomalies: basic overview[2] (ISSVA, 2014)
Vascular Tumors	**Vascular Malformations**
Benign	Simple: CM, VM, LM, AVM, AVF (Table 25-3)
Locally aggressive/ Borderline	Combined: See Table 25-4
Malignant	Associated with other anomalies: See Table 25-5

Abbreviations: AVF, arteriovenous fistulae; AVM, arteriovenous malformations; CM, capillary malformations; ISSVA, International Society for the Study of Vascular Anomalies; LM, lymphatic malformations; VM, venous malformations.

TABLE 25-2.	Vascular tumors (ISSVA, 2014)
Category	**Specific Tumors**
Benign	• Infantile hemangioma • Congenital hemangiomas (RICH, NICH, PICH) • Tufted angioma • Spindle cell hemangioma • Epithelioid hemangioma • Pyogenic granuloma • Microvenular hemangioma
Locally Aggressive/ Borderline Tumors	• Kaposiform hemangioendothelioma • Retiform hemangioendothelioma • PILA, Dabska tumor • Composite hemangioendothelioma • Pseudomyogenic hemangioendothelioma • Kaposi sarcoma • Others
Malignant	• Angiosarcoma • Epithelioid hemangioendothelioma • Others

Abbreviations: NICH, noninvoluting congenital hemangioma; PICH, partially involuting congenital hemangioma; PILA, papillary intralymphatic angioendothelioma; RICH, rapidly involuting congenital hemangioma.

area of pallor or telangiectasia; initially, they may resemble a bruise. Hemangiomas may occur anywhere on the body but may have a predilection for the head and neck. Hemangiomas grow rapidly over the first 5 to 7 weeks of life, ultimately growth stabilizes, and IH involute or regress slowly over the course of years.[4] There are several clinical subtypes, including superficial, deep, mixed, and IH with minimal or arrested growth. All have a typical clinical appearance in the skin. Superficial IH are well-demarcated bright red vascular plaques. Deep IH are bluish-hued subcutaneous nodules. Mixed IH demonstrate both a red superficial component and a deeper underlying bluish tumor. IH with minimal or arrested growth tend to favor the lower body and are often flat or telangiectatic in their appearance, with proliferation occurring only in <20% of the lesion, most often at the periphery (Figure 25-1A-D clinical subtypes). IH may be solitary or multifocal in their presentation. When they appear to occupy a region or territory of the body, for example large facial hemangiomas on the frontotemporal area, they may be associated with underlying structural anomalies as seen in Posterior fossa anomalies, large facial Hemangioma, Arterial anomalies, Cardiac anomalies, Eye anomalies (PHACE).[5]

Histologic Findings

In its proliferative phase, IH exhibits lobules and sheets of capillaries lined by plump endothelial cells arranged in "back-to-back" fashion, with little intervening stroma (Figure 25-2A and B). IH may be centered superficially, deep or both. Occasional mitoses and scattered mast cells may be observed.[6,7] In the involutional phase, stromal fibrosis is increased between the vascular lobules. Endothelial cells are typically more flattened, basement membranes thicken, and mitotic activity is diminished. Biopsy of fully involuted IH demonstrates a "fibrofatty" residuum, with thinned epidermis, scar tissue (including loss of cutaneous appendages), and diminished dermal elastic fibers. The sparse remaining vessels appear small and "ghosted" with thickened basement membranes and often occluded lumens.[6]

The histopathologic differential diagnosis for IH includes congenital hemangiomas (see following paragraphs) and pyogenic granuloma; glucose transporter protein isoform 1 (GLUT1) immunostain readily distinguishes IH from other vascular anomalies, the majority of which exhibit negative staining. GLUT1 facilitates glucose transport across the cell membranes of erythrocytes and is widely expressed in fetal tissue.[8] GLUT1 immunostain labels IH endothelial cells in all phases of its evolution.

CAPSULE SUMMARY

INFANTILE HEMANGIOMA

IH is characterized microscopically by sheets of capillaries arranged in close proximity, with or without intervening fibrotic stroma, depending on the timing of biopsy in the life cycle of the lesion. GLUT1 immunostaining is sensitive and specific for IH, when the diagnosis is in question.

CONGENITAL HEMANGIOMAS

Definition and Epidemiology

Congenital hemangiomas (CH) are an uncommon but benign type of vascular tumor that present fully formed at birth. They are distinct from IH in many ways, including their natural history and histopathologic features. CH occur much less frequently than IH in only 0.3% of newborns, according to one prospective study.[3]

Etiology

CH may occur anywhere on the body and have no clear gender predilection. They are typically solitary, although multifocal variants have been reported. Clinical variants of CH include rapidly involuting congenital hemangioma (RICH), noninvoluting congenital hemangioma (NICH), and partially involuting congenital hemangioma (PICH).[9] These three subtypes share significant clinical and histopathologic overlap and also genetic etiology. Mutations in *GNAQ* and *GNA11* have been reported in both RICH and NICH.[10] Thus, many authors believe that these uncommon vascular tumors exist on a spectrum.

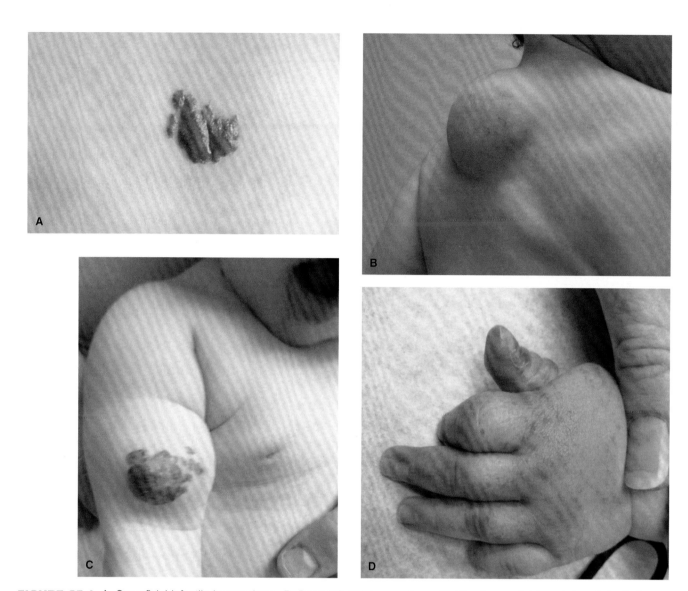

FIGURE 25-1. A, Superficial infantile hemangioma. B, Deep infantile hemangioma. C, Mixed, superficial, and deep infantile hemangioma. D, Infantile hemangioma with minimal or arrested growth.

Clinical Presentation

RICH is likely the most common variant. These tumors present right at birth as solitary, large, violaceous vascular tumors. They may be exophytic and often have a surrounding halo of vasoconstriction (Figure 25-3A). They are high-flow vascular tumors and demonstrate high flow on Doppler evaluation. Usually, they are asymptomatic, although rarely, ulceration, bleeding (much more high flow than an IH), or transient thrombocytopenia may occur. They involute rapidly over the first few months of life, leaving behind atrophic, anetoderma-like plaques with prominent veins (Figure 25-3B).

NICH are less common. They typically present as round or oval plaques or nodules with a bluish hue and overlying venules and telangiectasias (Figure 25-4). They also demonstrate a surrounding halo of pallor/vasoconstriction and high blood flow on Doppler evaluation. NICH are generally asymptomatic, although because they persist over time, they may become more symptomatic or bothersome. Pain is sometimes reported, and lesions may expand or worsen during times of hormonal excess such as puberty or pregnancy.[11]

Histologic Findings

RICH is comprised of small, mostly similar-sized dermal lobules of capillaries. Endothelial cells are plump and surrounded by layers of pericytes. Prominent fibrous tissue is typically present, surrounding individual capillary lobules. Centrally, RICH often has near-absence of these lobules but instead shows dense fibrosis and large, thickened draining veins with irregular muscular walls. Aneurysmally dilated vessels, interstitial hemosiderin, and calcification are also commonly present. Extramedullary hematopoiesis may also be seen[6,12] (Figure 25-5A and B).

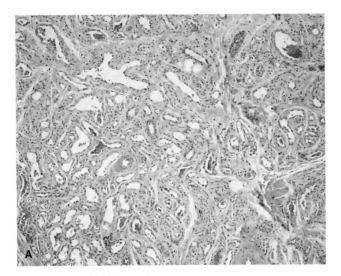
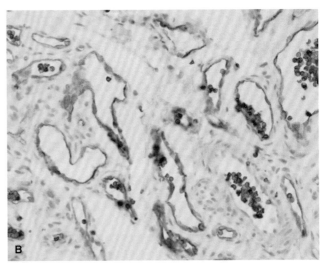

FIGURE 25-2. **Infantile hemangioma (IH).** A, Lobulated clusters of small, thin-walled vessels with minimal intervening stroma are present in the dermis (H&E-stained section, 100× magnification). B, Glucose transporter protein isoform 1 immunostain, with a positive labeling of the endothelium of lesional vessels in IH.

NICH exhibits larger, varying sized lobules of capillaries that may coalesce into larger masses (Figure 25-5C). These capillaries are lined by plump endothelial cells with little cytoplasm; some lobules may contain more dilated capillaries lined by hyperchromatic small nuclei that often hobnail into the vascular lumen. Cytoplasmic eosinophilic globules are occasionally present. The main differential diagnosis for RICH and NICH includes IH and pyogenic granuloma. GLUT1 immunostain is highly effective in distinguishing between IH and congenital hemangioma, because the latter is consistently negative.

CAPSULE SUMMARY

CONGENITAL HEMANGIOMAS

RICH and NICH are congenital vascular lesions characterized by lobular proliferations of small vessels seen prominently within the dermis. Although they may resemble IH, stromal features such as central fibrosis (indicative of involutional changes) and GLUT1 negativity on immunostaining typically permit differentiation.

4 weeks

11 weeks

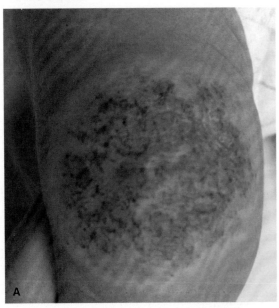
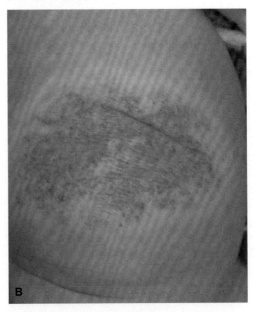

FIGURE 25-3. Rapidly involuting congenital hemangioma of the left leg (A) at 4 weeks (B) at 11 weeks.

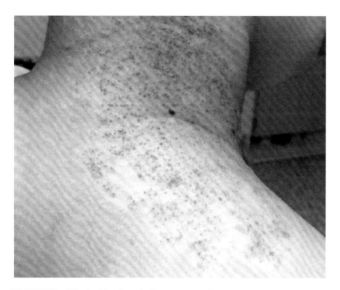

FIGURE 25-4. Noninvoluting congenital hemangioma of the neck.

PYOGENIC GRANULOMA ("LOBULAR CAPILLARY HEMANGIOMA")

Definition and Epidemiology

Pyogenic granuloma (PG) is one of the most commonly acquired vascular tumors in children. It is a benign tumor with a male predilection that can occur at any site on the body at any age, although the vast majority occur in children.

Etiology

Recently, the majority of PGs have been shown to arise secondary to mutations in *BRAF*, and in a smaller subset, to mutations in *RAS*.[13,14] In the case of the *BRAF* mutation, this is the same "hotspot" that is present in many human cancers, including melanoma, leading to a constitutive activation of RAS-MAPK signaling in mutated cells. Interestingly, PGs are also known to arise in the setting of treatment with BRAF inhibitors, which may represent a paradoxical activation of MAPK signaling in this setting.[15,16]

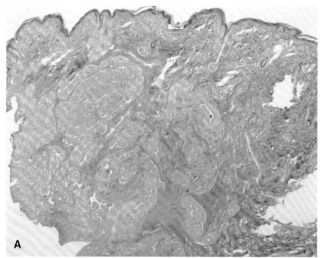

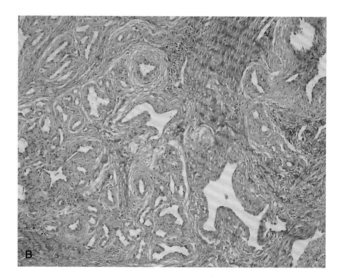

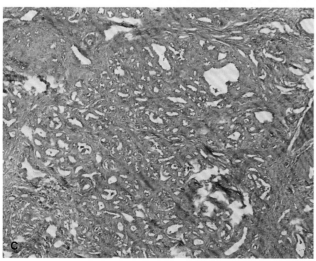

FIGURE 25-5. **Histopathology of congenital hemangiomas.** A, Rapidly involuting congenital hemangioma: Similar-sized lobules of capillaries fill and expand the dermis (H&E, 20× magnification). B, Partially involuting congenital hemangioma: Vascular lobules with intervening stromal fibrosis indicative of partial involution (100× magnification). C, Noninvoluting congenital hemangioma: Variably sized capillaries with hyperchromatic, occasionally hobnailing, endothelial cells (40× magnification).

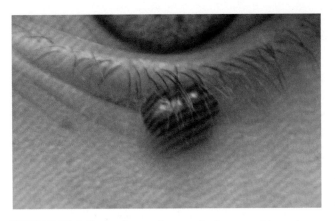

FIGURE 25-6. Pyogenic granuloma on the lower eyelid margin.

Clinical Presentation

Clinically, PG present as bright red, pedunculated papules varying in size from a few millimeters up to several centimeters, often with a surrounding collarette of scale (Figure 25-6). The overlying epidermis is often eroded or ulcerated. Thus, common complications include bleeding and infection. PGs may occur sporadically or arise secondarily. For example, there may be a history of antecedent trauma, such as an insect bite or scratch, hormonal or other factors involved. In addition, PGs are known to occur secondarily within several different types of vascular anomalies, including capillary malformations and arteriovenous malformations (AVMs), which may be directly related to their genetic etiology.[17]

Histologic Findings

PG exhibits an exophytic, polypoid tumor predominantly within the upper dermis, often with central shallow ulceration and an adjacent epidermal collarette (Figure 25-7A). Clusters of capillaries and venules are lined by plump endothelial cells and are typically organized into discrete lobules by interlacing strands of fibrotic stroma. Dermal edema and lymphocytes are commonly present, as are neutrophils in cases of ulceration. A larger feeding arterial vessel may be present at the base of the tumor. PG with partial regression

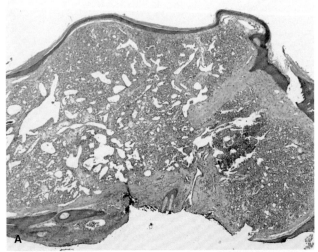

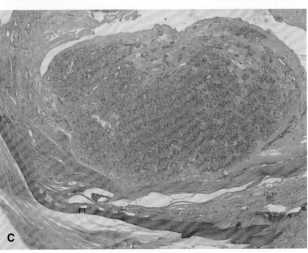

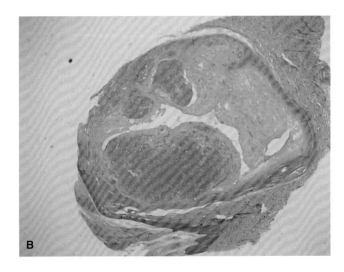

FIGURE 25-7. **Pyogenic granuloma (PG).** A, An epidermal collarette is seen surrounding an upper dermal proliferation of small, thin-walled vessels arranged in lobules and separated by thin fibrous septae (H&E-stained section, 40× magnification). B and C, Intravascular PG: clusters of small vessels with a lobulated architecture filling a dilated, thin-walled vessel (20× and 40× magnification, respectively).

demonstrates increased fibrosis and diminished vascular lobules. Deep dermal or subcutaneous presentations of PG are not uncommon and may be intravascular. Intravascular PG presents within the lumen of a vein or artery. Intravenous PG was originally described by Cooper et al. in 1979,[18] as an intraluminal polyp comprised by lobules of capillaries lined by flattened or rounded endothelial cells (Figure 25-7B). A surrounding fibrous stroma is also usually observed.[19,20]

The primary differential diagnosis for PG in a neonate or infant is a superficially sampled IH. Negative GLUT1 immunostaining will confirm the diagnosis in this situation. Deep PG may resemble other benign vascular tumors such as tufted angioma; the characteristic lymphatic structures in tufted angioma aid in differentiation.

CAPSULE SUMMARY

PYOGENIC GRANULOMA

PG is among the most common benign vascular proliferations in pediatric patients and demonstrates a characteristic lobulated pattern of small vessels. The common superficial variant is typically diagnosed easily, whereas deeper presentations may mimic other benign vascular anomalies. GLUT1 immunostain is helpful in excluding IH.

SPINDLE CELL HEMANGIOMA

Definition and Epidemiology

Spindle cell hemangioma (SCH) was originally described as a hemangioendothelioma, implying low-grade malignant potential.[21] As it is now understood to have benign biologic behavior, it is classified as a hemangioma.[22] SCH is one of the characteristic findings in Mafucci syndrome.

Etiology

The majority of SCH are known to arise because of mutations in *IDH1* or *IDH2*.[23] This mutation is common both to sporadic SCH and those found in Maffucci syndrome. *IDH* mutations appear to be specific to this vascular tumor and have not been observed in other vascular anomalies.[23]

Clinical Presentation

SCH presents as red-brown to blue nodules in the dermis or subcutaneous tissue. SCH is often multifocal and occurs most frequently on the distal extremities.[24] Lesions are often tender to palpation.

Histopathology

SCH is a tumor seen in both the dermis and the subcutis, which exhibits an admixture of thin-walled dilated venous channels, and nodules of spindled cells with extravasated erythrocytes, which resemble nodular Kaposi's sarcoma (KS)[21,22] (Figure 25-8). Microthrombi with organization may be seen within venous channels. A subpopulation of ovoid cells with readily visible cytoplasmic vacuoles may also be seen. This latter cell population and the presence of venous channels permit distinction from KS, as does negative HHV8 staining. Focal positivity with lymphatic immunostains including D2-40, Prox1, and Wilms tumor-1 (WT-1) in both the vascular structures and spindle cell population suggests a lymphatic origin.[25]

CAPSULE SUMMARY

SPINDLE CELL HEMANGIOMA

SCH may arise sporadically or in association with Mafucci syndrome, and microscopically exhibits thin-walled vascular channels with admixed spindle cell nodules, a pattern that may mimic nodular KS.

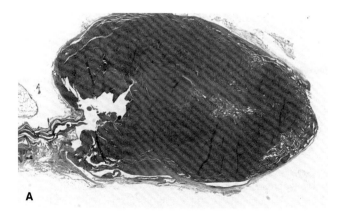
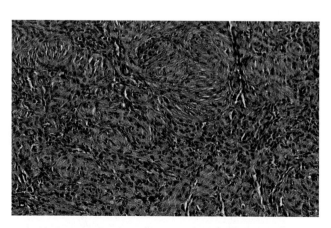

FIGURE 25-8. Spindle cell hemangioma. A, Well-circumscribed tumor with dense cellularity centrally and dilated thin-walled vessels peripherally (20× magnification). B, Sheets of spindled cells that may resemble nodular Kaposi's sarcoma (200× magnification). Digital slides courtesy of Path Presenter.com.

EPITHELIOID HEMANGIOMA

Definition and Epidemiology

Epithelioid hemangioma (EH) is a rare vascular tumor with highly variable histomorphology. Nonetheless, it is a distinctive vascular neoplasm displaying well-formed vascular channels lined by prominent epithelioid endothelial cells.[26]

EH has previously been described under numerous designations, including angiolymphoid hyperplasia with eosinophilia (ALHE), intravenous atypical vascular tumor, inflammatory angiomatous nodule, and histiocytoid hemangioma.[27] In the past, this tumor was believed to arise primarily in the skin of the head and neck. However, it is now recognized that EH may occur anywhere on the body in any tissue or organ, particularly in the bone.[28] Bony EH may lead to significant destruction, and thus, it is important to distinguish it from malignant vascular tumors or other neoplasms.

Etiology

Recently, *FOS* gene rearrangements have been observed in nearly one-third of EH in a variety of anatomic locations and histologic variants. Of note, bony EHs tended to harbor this rearrangement most frequently, whereas very few of the cutaneous ALHE-type EHs (ie, the head and neck-predominant variant) demonstrated this change.[27]

Clinical Presentation

Cutaneous variants of EH present as red-to-blue firm, round nodules or clustered papules that tend to itch; patients may also report a pulsatile sensation. As noted previously, the head and neck regions are the most common cutaneous locations, but EH may present at any anatomic site, including the penis.[27]

Histologic Findings

Cutaneous EH is typically centered within the dermis, with circumscribed borders and an often lobulated growth pattern. EH is composed of capillaries lined by epithelioid endothelial cells that are occasionally vacuolated (Figure 25-9A and B). These capillaries have patent lumens. The surrounding stroma contains a variably dense inflammatory infiltrate of eosinophils, lymphocytes, and occasionally plasma cells.

The differential diagnosis varies on the basis of EH presentation. ALHE-type lesions may be confused with Kimura disease; the latter tends to exhibit deeper tissue involvement and a predominantly inflammatory pattern (commonly with

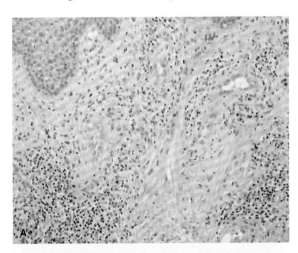

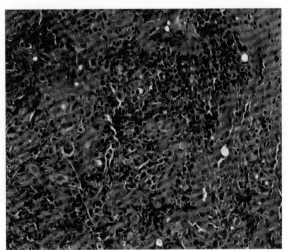

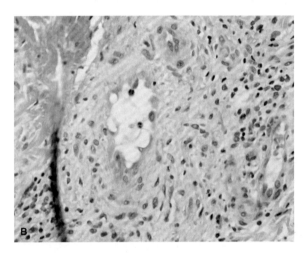

FIGURE 25-9. **Epithelioid hemangioma (EH).** A and B, Angiolymphoid hyperplasia with eosinophilia-type. Small vessels with epithelioid endothelial cells with vacuolated cytoplasm, and surrounding inflammation rich in eosinophils (100× and 200× magnification). C, Cellular EH variant that may mimic epithelioid hemangioendothelioma or angiosarcoma (200× magnification).

lymphoid follicles) and a lesser vascular element. More cellular EH types may mimic malignant tumors such as epithelioid hemangioendothelioma (EHE) or even epithelioid angiosarcoma (AS) (Figure 25-9C). Immunohistochemistry and molecular studies such as fluorescent in situ hybridization (FISH) can be helpful in ruling in these malignant tumors, because 90% of EHE demonstrate a characteristic *WWTR1-CAMTA1* fusion, which results from a t(1;3)(p36;q25) translocation,[29] and many ASs demonstrate *MYC* amplification on FISH and/or MYC-positivity on immunohistochemistry.[30]

CAPSULE SUMMARY

EPITHELIOID HEMANGIOMA

Cutaneous EH typically presents on the head and neck, but also on the extremities or penis, and exhibits epithelioid, often vacuolated endothelial cell morphology with a variable eosinophilic infiltrate. Distinction from malignant epithelioid vascular tumors is critical.

MICROVENULAR HEMANGIOMA

Definition and Epidemiology

Microvenular hemangioma is an uncommon, acquired benign vascular tumor; less than 100 cases have been reported in the medical literature. It typically presents as a solitary lesion in adulthood, with a slight female predominance and an average age of onset of 32, but occasionally may be seen in children.[31,32] A patient as young as 16 months of age has been reported.[31]

Etiology

As a sporadic, typically solitary tumor of adult onset, the pathogenesis of microvenular hemangioma is not well understood. A single patient with POEMS syndrome (*Poly*neuropathy, *O*rganomegaly, *E*ndocrinopathy, *M*onoclonal protein, *S*kin changes) presenting with multiple microvenular hemangiomas has been reported[33]; all other reported patients with multiple lesions have had no identifiable comorbidities.[34]

Clinical Presentation

Microvenular hemangioma presents in most cases as a solitary lesion, most commonly on the trunk or upper extremities, with a reddish brown papule or plaque less than 2 cm in diameter.[31] Most are asymptomatic.

Histologic Findings

The characteristic microscopic finding is of many small, thin-walled vessels interstitially arrayed, dissecting between collagen fibers in the mid-dermis (Figure 25-10A and B). Adnexocentricity may present. Endothelial cells are bland in appearance, with a visible surrounding pericyte layer. Surrounding stromal collagen may be mildly sclerotic, and mild lymphoplasmacytic inflammation is often present. Lesional cells uniformly stain with CD31, CD34, and ERG, and are negative on D2-40.[31] GLUT1 immunostaining is consistently negative.[35]

CAPSULE SUMMARY

MICROVENULAR HEMANGIOMA

Microvenular hemangioma is a benign, usually solitary tumor with occasional pediatric presentations. Microscopic findings of many slit-like vessels dissecting between dermal collagen fibers may mimic other vascular tumors such as patch-stage KS, or occasionally, a low-grade AS.

Tufted Angioma and Kaposiform Hemangioendothelioma

Definition and Epidemiology

Tufted angioma (TA) and kaposiform hemangioendothelioma (KHE) are classified according to ISSVA as vascular tumors with benign or aggressive characteristics, respectively. These lesions share many similar clinical and

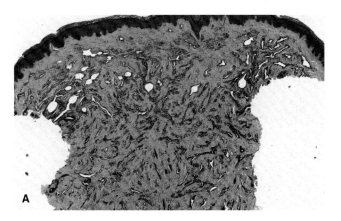
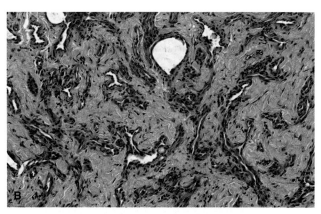

FIGURE 25-10. Microvenular hemangioma. A and B, Interstitially arrayed small, thin-walled vessels dissecting between dermal collagen fibers (40× and 100× magnification). Digital slides courtesy of Path Presenter.com.

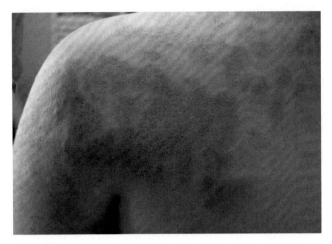

FIGURE 25-11. Tufted angioma on the left upper extremity in a 10–year-old female.

histopathologic features and thus it is felt that they may exist together on a spectrum. On one end, TAs are considered benign and tend to be smaller in size, whereas KHE is locally aggressive and potentially life threatening. Both may be associated with a consumptive coagulopathy known as Kasabach Merritt phenomenon (KMP), which is the main source of mortality in the setting of KHE. This phenomenon does not occur in the more common entity of IH. KMP occurs because of platelet trapping within the aberrant vessels of these two unique tumors. In extensive, infiltrative lesions, more commonly with KHE, this leads to profound thrombocytopenia, hypofibrinogenemia, elevated

D-dimer, and prolonged prothrombin time and activated partial thromboplastin time. Infants with KMP are at risk for life-threatening bleeding/hemorrhage.[36]

TUFTED ANGIOMA

Clinical Presentation

TAs are rare vascular tumors that are usually limited to the skin and subcutis and may occur anywhere on the body. TA tends to grow slowly and is unlikely to be infiltrative. It is usually solitary, and may appear clinically as an indurated, violaceous plaque with overlying hypertrichosis or hyperhidrosis (Figure 25-11). In the case of very extensive lesions, TA may also be associated with KMP; however, this is less common in the setting of TA than in that of KHE. The clinical course for TA is variable; some lesions may regress spontaneously, whereas others persist.

Histologic Findings

TA exhibits well-defined lobules of closely apposed capillaries within the dermis and upper subcutis. Given their notably round, blue appearance at scanning magnification, these lobules are colloquially referred to as "cannonballs" (Figure 25-12A and B). Endothelial cells are often subtly spindled.[37] Individual lobules exhibit a surrounding thin, crescentic lymphatic channel, which labels positively with lymphatic marker immunostains such as D2-40 and PROX-1. Spindled endothelial cells may demonstrate similar positivity, although most of the central portions of lobules are D2-40 negative.[38]

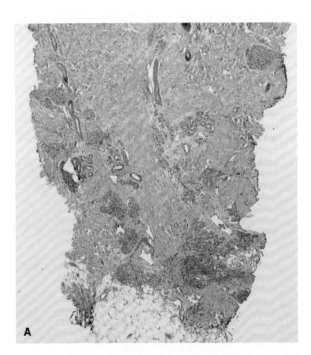

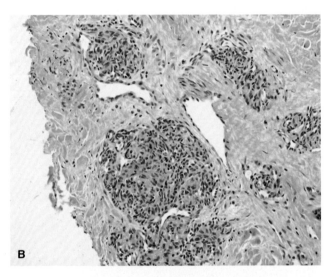

FIGURE 25-12. **Tufted angioma.** A, Rounded lobules of small, thin-walled vessels in the deep dermis, with minimal intervening stromal changes and absence of subcutaneous extension (H&E-stained section, 40× magnification). B, Crescentic lymphatic channels encircle individual lobules (H&E-stained section, 200× magnification).

The primary differential diagnosis is KHE. KHE and TA exhibit many overlapping features; in addition to the above-mentioned findings, both may also exhibit microthrombi, hemosiderin-laden endothelial cells, extravasated red blood cells, and a lymphatic immunoprofile. These overlapping features underscore the difficulty in conclusively differentiating TA and KHE on biopsy. Correlation with clinical and imaging features (deeper, multiplane involvement is more typical of KHE) is often required for definitive diagnosis between these two entities.

KAPOSIFORM HEMANGIOENDOTHELIOMA

Etiology

KHE is a rare, locally aggressive vascular tumor. In one study, the prevalence of KHE in New England was estimated at 0.91 cases per 100 000 children.[39] In the same study, authors estimated that KMP is present in up to 71% of children or infants presenting with KHE.

Clinical Presentation

KHE has a predilection for occurrence on the extremities, but may also occur in the retroperitoneum, head and neck, trunk or groin.[40] They present most commonly as a violaceous, indurated plaque or nodule in early infancy. Similar to TA, hypertrichosis or hyperhidrosis may be observed. As discussed earlier, KHE can develop into a KMP more commonly than in tufted hemangiomas. Rapid expansion, bruising, or purpura may be associated with lesions undergoing KMP (Figure 25-13). KHE are often deep and infiltrative; thus, if deep tissues such as muscle or fascia are involved, it may lead to fibrosis and chronic pain later in the course.

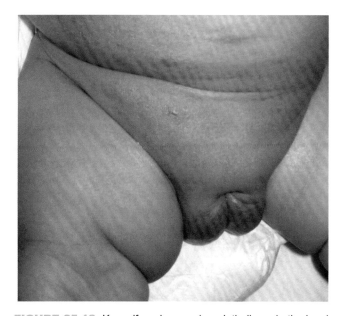

FIGURE 25-13. Kaposiform hemangioendothelioma in the inguinal region of an infant. Photo courtesy of Dr. Kristen Hook.

Histologic Findings

KHE demonstrates coalescent lobules of mostly poorly canalized vessels with rounded or spindled endothelial cells (Figure 25-14). Sheets and fascicles of spindled cells which form slit-like vessels resemble those seen in nodular KS. Clusters of cells with a glomeruloid appearance may be seen, similar to those in TA, although these tend to be larger and less circumscribed in KHE. Extension into the subcutis and deeper tissue planes is more common than in TA, and KHE tends to have a more infiltrating architectural pattern. Cytologic atypia is minimal, and mitotic figures are uncommon. Microthrombi are commonly present in capillaries, and hemosiderin may be seen within individual endothelial cells. The interlobular stroma of KHE commonly demonstrates fibrosis, edema, or mucin deposition.[41] Lesional cells stain positively for lymphatic markers including D2-40/podoplanin, PROX-1, and other vascular markers such as CD31.[41,42] As noted earlier, the differential diagnosis includes nodular KS, although HHV8 staining in KHE is consistently negative.[43]

CAPSULE SUMMARY

TUFTED ANGIOMA AND KAPOSIFORM HEMANGIOENDOTHELIOMA

TA and KHE may be closely related entities that exist on a histopathologic spectrum, and both can be involved in KMP. TA exhibits well-defined lobules of capillaries with surrounding lymphatic channels and typically little intervening stromal changes and tends to be centered in the dermis and superficial subcutis. KHE has similar vascular lobules, but also spindle cell–rich zones, more intervening stromal changes, and deeper extension. Caution should be observed, however, in distinguishing these two entities purely on histologic grounds.

PAPILLARY INTRALYMPHATIC ANGIOENDOTHELIOMA (FORMERLY DABSKA TUMOR)

Definition and Epidemiology

Papillary intralymphatic angioendothelioma (PILA or Dabska tumor) was first described in 1969 by Maria Dabska. This borderline malignant vascular tumor occurs almost exclusively in children and young adults.[44] PILA tumors are quite rare, and usually involve only the skin and subcutis, although deeper infiltrative PILA tumors have also been described.[44] Because of their rarity, their long-term behavior and overall prognoses are not understood. However, it should be noted that in some cases, regional lymph node involvement and at least one case of disseminated metastatic disease resulting in death have been reported.[45]

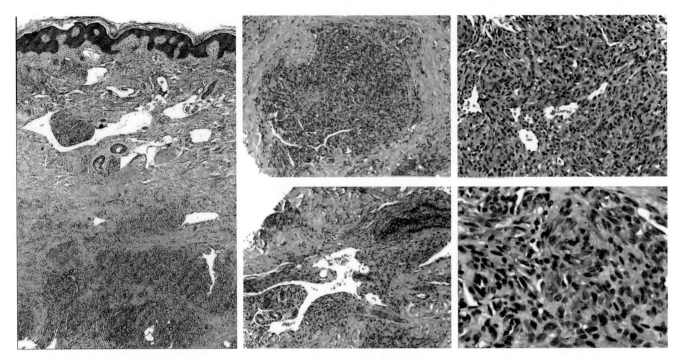

FIGURE 25-14. Kaposiform hemangioendothelioma. Tumor with lobulated zones that resemble those of tufted angioma, but also with increased interlobular vessels in a dissecting pattern similar to that of Kaposi's sarcoma.

Clinical Presentation

Lesions present as ill-defined, erythematous to violaceous vascular plaques or nodules. There are several reports of PILA/Dabska tumors arising in the setting of an underlying lymphatic malformation (LM) or other vascular anomalies.

Histologic Findings

PILA demonstrates both slit-like and widely dilated vascular channels lined by hyperchromatic endothelial cells with prominent hobnailing (Figure 25-15). The characteristic finding is of intravascular papillary clusters ("tufts") of endothelial cells surrounding a central hyaline core. These tufts may resemble glomeruli and can fill and occlude vascular channels. Dense lymphocytic inflammation may also be present adjacent to vascular structures.[22] The differential diagnosis includes papillary endothelial hyperplasia (Masson's phenomenon), retiform hemangioendothelioma, and the glomeruloid hemangioma associated with POEMS syndrome. The characteristic appearance of tufts in PILA, with eosinophilic cores and surrounding roundish endothelial cells, typically permits distinction.

CAPSULE SUMMARY

PAPILLARY INTRALYMPHATIC ANGIOENDOTHELIOMA

PILA is an intermediate-grade vascular neoplasm that can be locally destructive, and exhibits a distinctive histologic pattern of intravascular papillary projections of enlarged endothelial cells surrounding brightly eosinophilic cores.

COMPOSITE HEMANGIOENDOTHELIOMA

Definition and Epidemiology

Composite hemangioendothelioma, so named because it exhibits multiple histologically distinct components (originally described as demonstrating overlapping features of benign, low-grade, and malignant-appearing vascular tumors[46]), is considered to be a low-grade malignancy with frequent local recurrence and a low risk of lymph node or distant metastasis.[47] The majority of cases present in adulthood, although childhood (and rarely congenital[48]) presentations are described. The overall incidence is unknown, but it is believed to be quite rare; fewer than 40 cases have been reported.[49]

Etiology

A molecular basis for this rare tumor has not been established. Most are reported to arise sporadically, without underlying comorbidities, although rare associations with vascular malformations, Mafucci syndrome, lymphedema, or prior irradiation have been described. An aggressive variant of composite hemangioendothelioma that expresses neuroendocrine markers has recently been reported.[49]

Clinical Presentation

Tumors present as slow-growing, nodular masses or zones of ill-defined soft tissue swelling, most commonly on the lower extremities, up to 6 cm in diameter.[46] Patients may report pain. Surface skin changes may include purpura, a violaceous hue, or alopecia.[50]

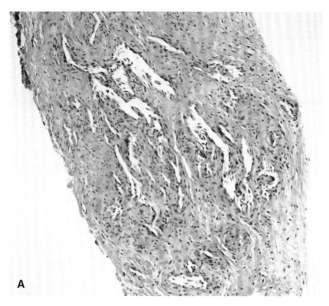
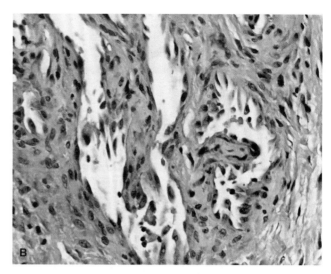

FIGURE 25-15. Papillary intralymphatic angioendothelioma. Tuft-like projections of endothelial cells surrounding a hyaline core into vascular lumens. This case exhibits overlapping features with retiform hemangioendothelioma (A and B) (H&E-stained section, 40× and 200× magnification).

Histologic Findings

Most tumors are centered within the deep dermis and subcutis, with infiltrative architecture and poor circumscription.[46] Overlying epidermal hyperplasia is common. Composite hemangioendothelioma, by definition, exhibits multiple distinct vascular tumor patterns, which may resemble benign angioma, PILA, retiform or EHE, or well-differentiated AS (Figure 25-16). Epithelioid and retiform are the most commonly reported hemangioendothelioma subtypes.[47] Tumor necrosis and low mitotic activity may be observed. Lesional cells stain positively with vascular endothelial markers such as CD31, von Willebrand factor, ERG, and FLI1.[46,49,50] Focal cytokeratin positivity may be observed.[47] As noted earlier, an aggressive subset of these tumors expresses neuroendocrine markers such as synaptophysin.[49]

CAPSULE SUMMARY

COMPOSITE HEMANGIOENDOTHELIOMA

Composite hemangioendothelioma is a rare low-grade malignant vascular tumor that may be difficult to differentiate from AS microscopically. It characteristically exhibits multiple morphologic patterns, including angiomatous zones, multiple different hemangioendothelioma subtypes, and areas resembling well-differentiated AS. Neuroendocrine marker expression portends a worse prognosis.

PSEUDOMYOGENIC HEMANGIOENDOTHELIOMA

Definition and Epidemiology

Pseudomyogenic hemangioendothelioma is an uncommon soft tissue tumor that was initially described as a suspected fibroma-like variant of epithelioid sarcoma (because it exhibits cytokeratin-positive spindled cells) in 1992,[51] but was recognized as endothelial cell-derived by Fletcher and colleagues in 2011.[52] Most tumors present in young adults (mean onset is at 31 years of age), occasionally in adolescents and teenagers,[53] with a notable male:female predominance of 4.5:1.[52] Currently, it is considered of indeterminate biologic potential.

Etiology

This tumor has a recently recognized consistent chromosomal translocation t(7;19)(q22;q13), with a SERPINE1-FOSB gene fusion product.[54,55] A similar FOSB gene fusion has also been reported in a subset of EHs with atypical clinical behavior.[56] FOSB is a transcription factor that, among other functions, regulates trophoblasts during placental growth, and is a recognized factor in ovarian and breast oncogenesis. SERPINE1 encodes the plasminogen activator inhibitor-1 protein product, which is expressed in endothelial cells.[57]

Clinical Presentation

Tumors commonly present within soft tissue on the extremities of young adults, typically with nodules that may

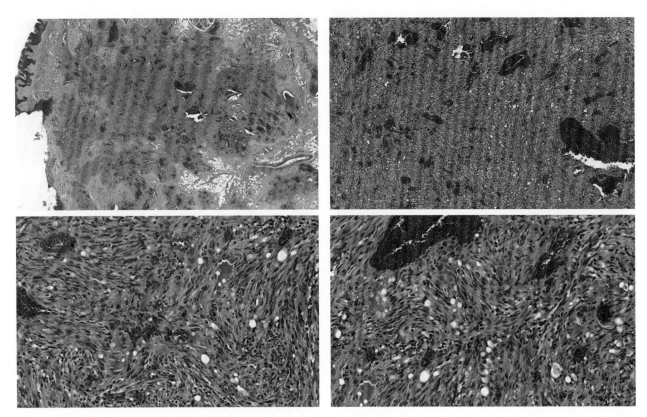

FIGURE 25-16. Composite hemangioendothelioma. Large tumor with deep extension into subcutaneous tissue, with both spindle cell and epithelioid zones. Areas resembling retiform and/or epithelioid hemangioendothelioma may be present, as may angiosarcoma-like zones. Digital slides courtesy of Path Presenter.com.

be painful. Multifocal lesions are present in two-thirds of patients; up to 15 discrete lesions have been reported.[52] Approximately half of all lesions involve the dermis and/or subcutis, and in those cases may demonstrate erythematous or purpuric skin surface changes.[58]

Histologic Findings

Histopathology demonstrates tumors of predominantly plump-appearing spindled cells with vesicular nuclei but minimal pleomorphism and low mitotic activity (with a mean of 2 mitoses per 10 high power fields) (Figure 25-17). Many cases exhibit a minor population of rhabdomyoblast-like cells.[58] Architectural features include infiltrative-appearing borders, fascicular and sheet-like growth with an often-plexiform low-power appearance, and a variable inflammatory infiltrate that may be rich in neutrophils. Tumors with dermal involvement commonly have overlying epidermal hyperplasia. On immunohistochemistry, tumors are consistently positive for cytokeratin AE1/AE3 and FLI1, and approximately half exhibit some CD31 positivity. Other cytokeratin stains are variably positive, and CD34 is negative. Unlike epithelioid sarcoma, INI1 expression is retained.[52] FOSB has recently been identified as a highly sensitive marker in the diagnosis of this tumor, although it is not entirely specific; diffuse nuclear positivity

was reported in 48 of 50 (96%) of pseudomyogenic hemangioendotheliomas, also with positivity in approximately half of tested EHs, and rarely in ASs and EHE.[57]

CAPSULE SUMMARY

PSEUDOMYOGENIC HEMANGIOENDOTHELIOMA

Pseudomyogenic hemangioendothelioma is a cutaneous and soft tissue tumor of young adults and may mimic epithelioid sarcoma in clinical presentation and histopathology; distinction between these two entities is critical, given their significant differences in malignant/metastatic potential. A *SERPINE1-FOSB* gene fusion is characteristic, and thus FOSB immunohistochemistry is a highly sensitive stain that can aid in confirming this diagnosis.

KAPOSI SARCOMA

Definition and Epidemiology

KS is a malignancy of endothelial cell origin occurring in the setting of immunosuppression. First described in elderly males of Eastern European and Mediterranean

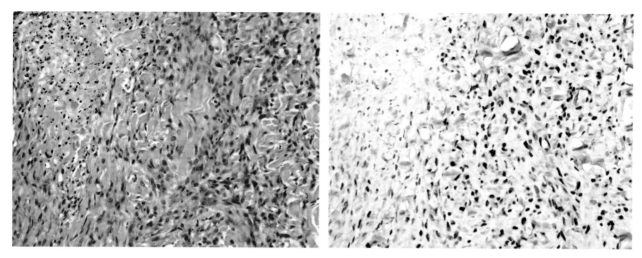

FIGURE 25-17. Pseudomyogenic hemangioendothelioma. A, Focal necrosis with neutrophilic infiltration and entrapment of collagen fibers, mimicking epithelioid sarcoma or cellular benign fibrous histiocytoma; B, Diffuse strong nuclear FOSB expression is present. Obtained with permission, Hung YP, Fletcher CD, Hornick JL. FOSB is a useful diagnostic marker for pseudomyogenic hemangioendothelioma. *Am J Surg Pathol.* 2017;41(5):596-606.

ancestry (classic KS), KS was later identified in an endemic form in portions of Africa, and in an epidemic form in patients infected with HIV/AIDS. All subtypes of KS have been reported in children. Prior to the late 1980s, endemic KS was the most common variant seen in children, but now HIV-associated (epidemic) KS predominates.[59] Pediatric KS has a predilection for males. The mean age of onset for either variant is 6 to 9 years of age.[60]

Etiology

Human herpesvirus 8 (HHV-8) is the defining pathogen in KS; HHV8 is identifiable in all HIV- and non-HIV-associated cases.[61,62] HHV8 infection alone is considered insufficient for tumor development, with a cofactor such as HIV or other immunosuppression typically required.

Clinical Presentation

The clinical presentation of pediatric KS varies by subtype. Skin and mucosal lesions, when present, begin as purple or brown-red patches that grow into plaques and nodules (Figure 25-18). Lesions are usually painless, but may koebnerize in areas of past trauma.[60] As in adults, classic KS in children has an acral predilection.

Histologic Findings

KS histopathology varies by stage, but is fundamentally characterized by aggregates of spindled cells and extravasated erythrocytes surrounding slit-like vascular spaces (Figure 25-19 histopathology of KS). In *patch-stage KS*, increased interstitial vasculature predominates, with only a minor (if any) spindle cell component. Irregularly sized and shaped thin-walled vessels are seen dissecting through dermal collagen and encircling background normal vessels and adnexal structures. Admixed lymphocytes, plasma

cells, and extravasated erythrocytes are commonly present. In *plaque-* and *nodular-stage KS*, fascicles of spindled cells are prominent and form large nodular aggregates within the dermis and subcutis. Abundant admixed erythrocytes form a "sieve-like" pattern. Slit-like vessels are present in these stages as well but are more evident at the periphery of solid nodules. Spindle cell nuclei may be pleomorphic, but generally do not exhibit high-grade atypia. Erythrophagocytosis is common, and results in intracytoplasmic hyaline globules in both spindle cells and histiocytes. Lymphocytes and plasma cells are also commonly seen.

The lesional cells of KS stain positively for the endothelial markers CD31, CD34, and factor VIII, as well as D2-40 and other lymphatic markers. The most definitive marker is HHV-8 latency–associated nuclear antigen, present in all KS clinical variants.[63] In patch KS, the differential diagnosis includes early low-grade AS, dermatofibroma, and other dermatoses with a so-called busy dermis, including interstitial granuloma annulare. Plaque and nodular tumors may resemble SCH, KHE, LMs, and PG (because both *lymphangioma-like* and *PG-like KS* have been described). HHV-8 immunostain is highly sensitive and specific to the diagnosis of KS and is indispensable in challenging cases.[64]

CAPSULE SUMMARY

KAPOSI SARCOMA

KS is a tumor of indeterminant malignant behavior that is closely associated with HHV8 infection and immunosuppression. Typical microscopic features include slit-like thin-walled vessels with a spindle cell component, extravasated erythrocytes, and lymphoplasmacytic inflammation. HHV-8 immunostain confirms the diagnosis in ambiguous cases.

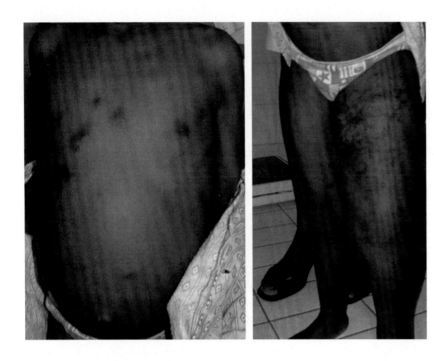

FIGURE 25-18. Child with Kaposi's sarcoma and associated lymphedema of the left lower extremity. Photo courtesy of Dr. Toby Maurer.

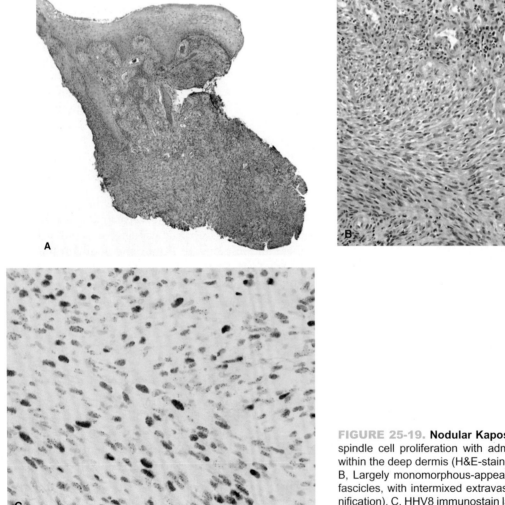

FIGURE 25-19. Nodular Kaposi's sarcoma (KS). A, A dense spindle cell proliferation with admixed small vessels is present within the deep dermis (H&E-stained section, 40× magnification). B, Largely monomorphous-appearing spindled cells arranged in fascicles, with intermixed extravasated erythrocytes (200× magnification). C, HHV8 immunostain labels nuclei of lesional spindled cells in KS, often in dot-like fashion.

EPITHELIOID HEMANGIOENDOTHELIOMA

Definition and Epidemiology

EHE is an uncommon, malignant vascular tumor derived from endothelial cells. Epithelioid hemangioendothelioma was first described in 1982 by Weiss and Enziger.[65] EHE are often multifocal and may involve internal organs such as lung, liver, and bone.

Etiology

Approximately 90% of EHE demonstrate a characteristic *WWTR1-CAMTA1* fusion, which results from a t(1;3)(p36;q25) translocation.[29] CAMTA1 is a transcription activator believed to be involved in the regulation of cell cycling, whereas WWTR1 is a downstream effector in the Hippo pathway that regulates cellular proliferation and programmed death. A small minority of EHE exhibit a *YAP1-TFE3* fusion gene.[66]

Clinical Presentation

Cutaneous involvement is rare but reported in children. Lesions appear as solitary or multiple, erythematous to violaceous plaques or nodules, some with ulceration.[67] They are more common in adults but can rarely present in the pediatric population. Metastases are reported in up to 25% of cases.[68]

Histologic Findings

Primary cutaneous tumors demonstrate dermal fibromyxoid nodules with solid and cord-like aggregates of ovoid and polygonal cells with abundant pale cytoplasm and frequently, intracytoplasmic vacuoles ("blister" cells) or primitive lumen-like structures[22] (Figure 25-20). Tumor stroma

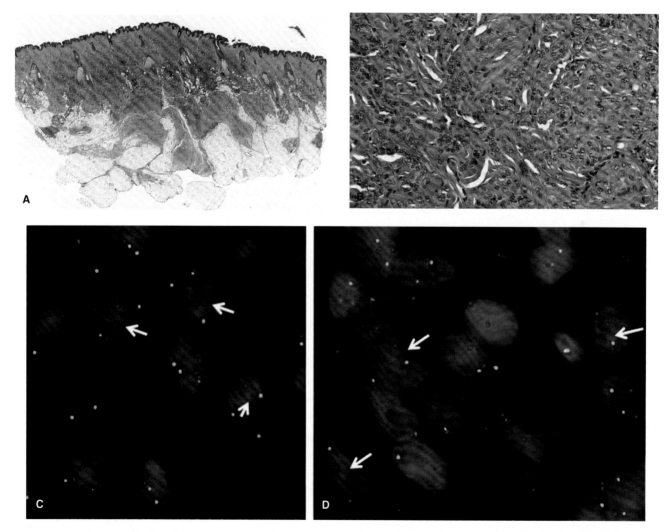

FIGURE 25-20. **Epithelioid endothelioma.** A and B, Dermally based tumor with sheets and cords of epithelioid endothelial cells with intracytoplasmic lumen-like structures but only minimal formation of vascular channels. C and D, Fluorescent in situ hybridization showing break-apart signals (white arrows) for CAMTA1 and *WWTR1* genes (red, centromeric; green, telomeric). A and B, Digital slides courtesy of Path Presenter.com. C and D, Obtained with permission, Anderson T, Zhang L, Hameed M, Rusch V, Travis WD, Antonescu CR. Thoracic epithelioid malignant vascular tumors: a clinicopathologic study of 52 cases with emphasis on pathologic grading and molecular studies of WWTR1-CAMTA1 fusions. *Am J Surg Pathol.* 2015;39(1):132-139.

is commonly characterized as "myxohyaline." Occasional mitoses may be seen. The differential diagnosis includes EH and epithelioid AS. In notable contrast to these, EHE tends to lack well-formed vascular channels. EHE exhibits well-circumscribed, nodular architecture at scanning magnification, whereas epithelioid AS exhibits a more infiltrative, destructive architectural pattern, as well as high-grade atypia, nuclear pleomorphism, atypical mitoses and necrosis. Cytokeratin expression patterns vary between EHE and epithelioid AS; CK7 expression is present in 50% of EHE and less frequently in AS, whereas 50% of epithelioid AS are positive for CK8, as against 10% of EHE.[69] CK18 expression is more common in EHE, because reported positivity approaches 100%. Recently, a CAMTA1 immunostain has been validated as highly sensitive and specific for EHE diagnosis; this stain may become an important tool in diagnosis as it becomes more widely available.[70] The vacuolated cells of EHE may also mimic a metastatic adenocarcinoma. Immunoreactivity for vascular- and lymphatic-specific markers (eg, CD31, podoplanin, LYVE-1) is helpful in such ambiguous cases.

CAPSULE SUMMARY

EPITHELIOID HEMANGIOENDOTHELIOMA

Epithelioid hemangioendothelioma is classified within the malignant spectrum of vascular tumors and is considered by many authors equivalent to a low-grade AS. Microscopically, it is characterized by strands of epithelioid cells with abundant eosinophilic cytoplasm that exhibit characteristic cytoplasmic vacuoles and primitive lumen-like structures that may contain red blood cells.

ANGIOSARCOMA

Definition and Epidemiology

AS is an uncommon, aggressive malignant vascular tumor with high morbidity and mortality. AS presents in the skin in one of three usual clinical scenarios: "idiopathic" (primary cutaneous) tumors of the head and neck in elderly patients (most commonly on sun-exposed sites), chronic lymphedema-associated AS, and postirradiation AS.[71] Presentation in childhood is rare, although reported, including a case of AS arising within an IH.[72]

Etiology

AS may arise primarily, or secondary to irradiation or chronic lymphedema. Amplification of the proto-oncogene *MYC* has recently been consistently identified in secondary AS,[73,74] and also to a lesser degree in primary cutaneous tumors.[75] MYC is a transcription factor with important regulatory roles in cell cycling and proliferation. Recently,

whole-genome and exome-sequencing studies have identified *PTPRB* and *PLCG1* as important driver mutations, primarily in secondary AS. Both genes are important players in angiogenesis; *PTPRB* is expressed in vascular endothelium and regulates vascular growth factors. *PLCG1* is involved in the vascular endothelial growth factor (VEGF) signaling pathway, and *PLCG*-deficient mice exhibit reduced angiogenesis.[76]

Clinical Presentation

AS presents as purpuric patches, plaques, nodules, or tumors, most commonly within zones of chronic lymphedema, prior ionizing radiation, or chronically sun-damaged skin. Ulceration and bleeding is common.

Histologic Findings

The various clinical subtypes of AS do not differ significantly microscopically. Tumors demonstrate infiltrative architecture and deep extension, often into the subcutis, with both interstitial anastomosing vessels and solid angiomatous areas. Vascular channels commonly dissect between collagen bundles and around hair follicles and sweat duct epithelium. Endothelial cells demonstrate variable cytologic atypia, crowding, and multilayering patterns. Individual cells may be ovoid to epithelioid, hyperchromatic, and highly pleomorphic. CD31 is considered to be the most helpful immunostain in diagnosing poorly differentiated tumors, although many tumors also stain with CD34 and Factor VIII-related antigen. Epithelioid AS is often positive for cytokeratin markers, including CK8 and 18. MYC immunostaining is an important tool in differentiating postirradiation AS from histologic mimics such as atypical vascular lesion of the breast, because this stain exhibits high sensitivity and specificity for AS diagnosis.[30]

CAPSULE SUMMARY

ANGIOSARCOMA

AS is an aggressive malignancy that is rare in children but may arise secondarily within other vascular anomalies. Architectural features including dissecting, anastomosing, and endothelial cell multilayering patterns are important findings for diagnosis.

Vascular Malformations

Vascular malformations represent a varied group of benign birthmarks and are divided into four main groups. In the updated ISSVA classification, these include simple, combined, or major named vessels and those associated with other anomalies. Vascular malformations are present at birth, persist throughout life, and may enlarge or worsen over time, secondary to trauma or because of the influence of hormonal changes. Simple malformations (Table 25-3) are comprised of predominantly one vessel type, for example, capillary malformations are made up almost entirely of capillaries in the mid and superficial dermis. However,

TABLE 25-3. Simple vascular malformations (adapted from ISSVA.org)

CMs
 CM cutaneous and/or mucosal CM
  CM with bone and/or soft tissue overgrowth
  CM with CNS and/or ocular anomalies (Sturge-Weber syndrome)
  CM of CM–AVM
  CM of MICCAP
  CM of MCAP
  Telangiectasia
  Cutis marmorata telangiectatica congenita
  Nevus simplex (also known as salmon patch/stork bite/angel's kiss, etc.)
  Others

LMs
 Common (cystic) LMs
  Macrocystic LM
  Microcystic LM
  Mixed cystic LM
 GLA
 LM in Gorham-Stout disease
 Channel-type LM
 Primary lymphedema
 Others

VMs
 Common VMs
 Familial VMCM
 Blue rubber bleb nevus (Bean) syndrome
 GVM
 CCM
 Others

AVMs
 Sporadic
 In HHT
 In CM–AVM

AVF
 Sporadic
 In HHT
 In CM–AVM
 Others

Abbreviations: AVF, arteriovenous fistulae; AVMs, arteriovenous malformations; CCM, cerebral cavernous malformation; CM, capillary malformations; CNS, central nervous system; GLA, generalized lymphatic anomaly; GVM, glomuvenous malformation; HHT, hereditary hemorrhagic telangiectasia; LM, lymphatic malformations; MCAP, megalencephaly-CM-polymicrogyria syndrome; MICCAP, microcephaly-capillary malformation syndrome; VM, venous malformations; VMCM, VM cutaneo-mucosal.

malformations can also arise because of multiple vessel types, and thus combined malformations are also fairly common (Table 25-4). Recent genetic advances have aided our understanding of the genetic basis and biology for vascular malformations, many of which arise because of postzygotic, somatic mutations in different genes within the Ras/MAP kinase pathway.

Vascular malformations may be sporadic, or they may exist in an individual as part of a clinical syndrome. For example, specific vascular malformations manifest as part of several overgrowth or neurocutaneous syndromes. Vascular malformations associated with other abnormalities are listed in Table 25-5. All tables are adapted from ISSVA Classification, 2014.

CAPILLARY MALFORMATIONS

Definition and Epidemiology

Capillary malformations (CMs) are the most common simple vascular malformations and sometimes referred to as "port-wine stains" because of their color. They are present in 0.3% of the population occurring on either the skin or mucosa.[77] CMs are slow-flow and present as erythematous, telangiectatic patches, most of which are confluent in color and of homogeneous thickness (Figure 25-21A).

Etiology

The etiology for CM has recently been elucidated. CMs arise because of somatic mutations in *GNAQ*, in both sporadic cases and those associated with Sturge-Weber syndrome (SWS).[78]

TABLE 25-4. Combined malformations (ISSVA, 2014)

CM + VM	Capillary-venous malformation	CVM
CM + LM	Capillary-lymphatic malformation	CLM
CM + AVM	Capillary-arteriovenous malformation	CAVM
LM + VM	Lymphatic-venous malformation	LVM
CM + LM + VM	Capillary-lymphatic-venous malformation	CLVM
CM + LM + AVM	Capillary-lymphatic-arteriovenous malformation	CLAVM
CM + VM + AVM	Capillary-venous-arteriovenous malformation	CVAVM
CM + LM + VM + AVM	Capillary-lymphatic-venous-arteriovenous malformation	CLVAVM

TABLE 25-5.	Vascular anomalies associated with other abnormalities (ISSVA, 2014)
Klippel-Trenaunay syndrome	CM + VM ± LM + limb overgrowth
Parkes Weber syndrome	CM + AVF + limb overgrowth
Servelle-Martorell syndrome	Limb VM + bone undergrowth
Sturge-Weber syndrome	Facial + leptomeningeal CM + eye anomalies ± bone and/or soft tissue overgrowth
Limb CM	+ Congenital nonprogressive limb hypertrophy
Mafucci syndrome	VM ± spindle cell hemangioma + enchondroma
M-CM/MCAP	Reticulated CM + pronounced nevus simplex + macrocephaly
MICAP	Reticulated CM with macrocephaly
CLOVES syndrome	LM + VM + CM ± AVM + lipomatous overgrowth
Proteus syndrome	CM, VM, and/or LM + asymmetrical somatic overgrowth
Bannayan-Riley-Ruvalcaba syndrome	AVM + VM + macrocephaly, lipomatous overgrowth

Abbreviations: AVF, arteriovenous fistulae; AVM, arteriovenous malformations; CLOVES, congenital lipomatous overgrowth, vascular anomalies, epidermal nevi, scoliosis; CM, capillary malformation; LM, lymphatic malformations; M-CM/MCAP, macrocephaly CM syndrome; MICAP, microcephaly CM syndrome; VM, venous malformations.

Clinical Presentation

Presenting as pink to erythematous to purple patches, CMs may darken or become thicker/nodular over time and may be associated with underlying soft tissue or bony overgrowth. CMs are most often unilateral, but may also be multifocal. Multifocal CMs with a rim of pallor and background of hyperpigmentation that are of thumbprint size should make one consider CM–AVM syndrome (CM–AVM) (Figure 25-21B). CMs may be associated with several different genetic syndromes, such as SWS, MCAP, and CM–AVM, or with asymmetric overgrowth of the extremities.[79]

Histologic Findings

Early in course, classic CM (including salmon patches and port-wine stains) demonstrates thin-walled, dilated vessels within the upper dermis (Figure 25-22). These structures resemble capillaries, but many may appear malformed.[80] In later lesions, increasing vessels are apparent in both the papillary and reticular dermis; these vessels tend to be arranged haphazardly, and more resemble dilated venules.[6] Endothelial cells appear flattened and are surrounded by an identifiable pericyte layer. Secondary changes may develop later in life. Pronounced skin thickening may occur on overlying facial port-wine stains in adults, and intralesional PGs may appear.[81,82] In these later phases, microscopic changes include epidermal hyperplasia, progressively dilated vessels, venule-type channels with thickened walls, and deep dermal, subcutaneous, and skeletal muscle involvement.[83] Fibrotic stromal changes may be present within the subcutaneous and fascial planes.

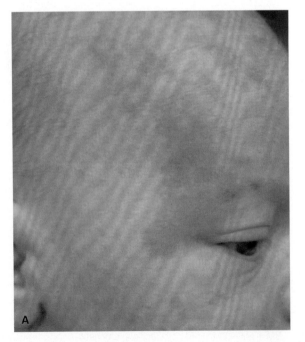
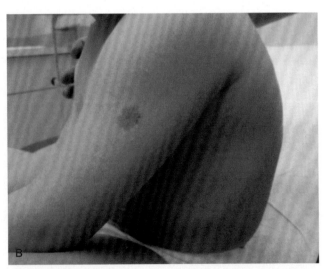

FIGURE 25-21. A, Capillary malformation of the right eyelid and forehead. Workup for the underlying Sturge-Weber syndrome was negative. B, Capillary malformation with rim of pallor and underlying hyperpigmentation classic for capillary malformation–arteriovenous malformation syndrome.

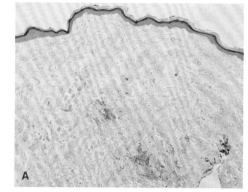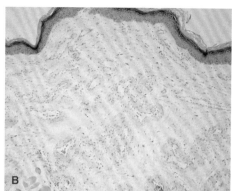

FIGURE 25-22. **Capillary malformation.** A and B, Many ectatic, somewhat malformed, capillaries with modestly thickened walls that fill the upper dermis (40× and 100× magnification).

CAPSULE SUMMARY

CAPILLARY MALFORMATIONS

CM involves malformed, dilated, thin-walled vessels mainly within the upper dermis. Various reactive stromal changes as well as secondary vascular proliferations such as PG may appear within CM later in life.

VENOUS MALFORMATIONS

Definition and Epidemiology

Venous malformations (VMs) are also slow-flow vascular malformations with an estimated incidence of 1 to 2 individuals per 10 000; thus, they are the second most common malformation following CM.

Etiology

VMs arise because of mutations in *TIE-2/TEK* gene and in some cases the *PIK3CA* gene.[84] Glomuvenous malformations arise because of mutations in *glomulin*. In familial cases, there is an autosomal dominant germline *glomulin* mutation that leads to multifocal involvement. Affected individuals may develop more glomuvenous malformations with time.

Clinical Presentation

Clinically, VMs appear as soft, compressible blue-hued nodules that swell with dependency (Figure 25-23). VMs can occur anywhere on the body, including the skin, mucous membrane, intramuscularly, or rarely, within the bone. VMs can be painful and enlarge over time. In the case of large, deep, and/or intramuscular VMs, an associated coagulopathy may be present (localized intravascular coagulopathy, LIC). In LIC, there is a tendency for clot formation and activated coagulation within the aberrant vessels which results in painful phlebolith formation and clotting diathesis. Elevated D-dimer levels are a sensitive indicator of LIC in the setting of a VM.[85]

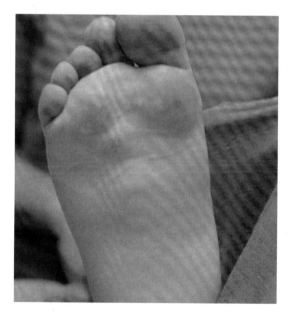

FIGURE 25-23. Venous malformation of the foot.

Glomuvenous malformations (GVMs) are a subtype of VM. Like classic VMs, they are blue to purple in color but are not compressible by palpation (Figure 25-24). GVMs are typically limited to the skin and subcutis and may have a cobblestoned appearance when the lesions aggregate. They are made up of glomus bodies and are more cellular than VMs, which accounts for their lack of compressability.[86]

Histologic Findings

VM exhibits widely dilated venous channels with irregular sizes and shapes that are haphazardly arranged in the dermis and subcutis (Figure 25-25A and B). These malformed veins are usually concentrically muscularized, with exceptions being VMs occurring in specific sites including periarticular locations, head and neck, and genitourinary regions. Irregular, malformed vessels may surround other normal vessels and nerve bundles and also dissect through muscular tissue planes. Endothelial cells

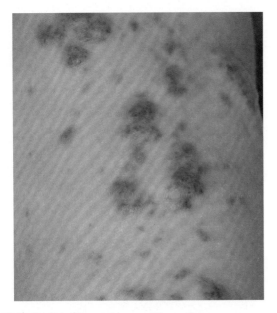

FIGURE 25-24. Glomuvenous malformation.

are small and flat, without notable cytologic atypia. Masson's phenomenon, with luminal thrombi with organization and papillary endothelial hyperplasia, is common. Thrombi may result in calcifications (ie, phleboliths) or as fibromyxoid nodules seen within vessel walls. Vascular markers such as CD31 highlight the lesional cells of VM, whereas D2-40/podoplanin and GLUT1 are negative. Ki-67 labeling rate is low.[6] The primary differential diagnosis is with other malformations of medium-sized vessels, including AVM, LM, and combined malformations. Lymphatic immunomarkers are helpful in excluding LM or a combined venous-LM.

GVM (synonymous with *glomangioma* for histopathologic purposes) demonstrates multiple layers of round, monomorphous glomus cells lining malformed veins[87] (Figure 25-25C and D). Glomus cells stain positively with smooth muscle actin and commonly with vimentin and desmin.

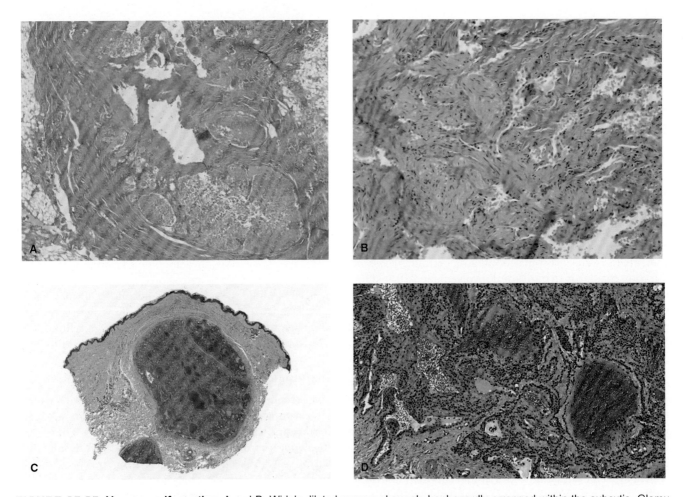

FIGURE 25-25. **Venous malformation.** A and B, Widely dilated venous channels haphazardly arranged within the subcutis. Glomuvenous malformation. C and D, Multilayered, monomorphous-appearing glomus cells surrounding malformed veins in the dermis. Digital slides courtesy of Path Presenter.com (C and D only).

CAPSULE SUMMARY

VENOUS MALFORMATIONS

VM is a common malformation that may present in the skin or the soft tissue. Microscopic features include malformed venous channels, often with many secondary changes, including thrombi, calcifications, and Masson's phenomenon. GVM exhibits characteristic multilayering of glomus cells surrounding similar malformed vessels.

ARTERIOVENOUS MALFORMATIONS

Definition and Epidemiology

Arteriovenous malformations are high-flow vascular anomalies that arise because of direct connections between arteries and veins without an intermediary capillary bed.

Etiology

AVMs are uncommon, and recently their genetic etiology has been attributed to mutations in *RASA1* in many cases.[88]

Clinical Presentation

AVMs may first be observed on the skin similar in appearance to a CM, a pink to red telangiectatic patch of variable size. If the AVM is deep or extensive, overgrowth of the affected area is common (Figure 25-26). For example, AVMs of the extremities are associated with hypertrophy of the affected limb. AVMs may be warm on palpation, pulsatile, and may be associated with an audible bruit on auscultation.

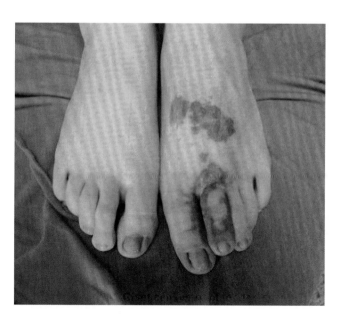

FIGURE 25-26. Arteriovenous malformation with associated overgrowth of the left foot.

Over time, AVMs may expand or worsen in the setting of hormonal changes and trauma or simply because of natural progression. As they worsen, they may cause serious complications including skin breakdown, ulceration and bleeding, bony erosion, and/or high-output cardiac failure.

Histologic Findings

AVMs are comprised of malformed veins and arteries with disrupted elastic laminae (Figure 25-27). Complete destruction of the arterial internal elastic lamina may occur, making the evaluation of the subtype of vessel involved difficult. Irregular myxoid degeneration is commonly present within vascular walls. AVMs often exhibit a reactive proliferative component in one of four patterns: scattered proliferating capillaries; PG-like proliferation, IH-like proliferation (GLUT1 negative), and pseudokaposiform proliferation.[87] The later type of proliferation has been associated with ulcerated nodular skin lesions and is also known as Stewart-Bluefarb syndrome. Abnormalities in elastic laminae can be highlighted by Verhoff Von Gieson stain.

CAPSULE SUMMARY

ARTERIOVENOUS MALFORMATIONS

AVM is a high-flow vascular anomaly with a high potential for morbidity, including overgrowth and/or eventual destruction of the surrounding tissue. Microscopic features include direct shunts between malformed arteries and veins, with significant elastic tissue alterations of these abnormal vessels.

LYMPHATIC MALFORMATIONS

Definition and Epidemiology

Lymphatic malformations are slow-flow vascular anomalies with a predilection for the head and neck. They are classified as macrocystic, microcystic, or mixed depending on the size of their fluid-filled cysts.

Etiology

The genetic basis for both syndromic and nonsyndromic LMs has recently been attributed to mutations in *PIK3CA*.[89]

Clinical Presentation

When located in the subcutaneous tissues, LMs present as soft, skin-colored nodules, whereas more superficial lesions usually appear in the skin with small pink to hemorrhagic papules. These superficial blebs and papules may bleed or drain lymphatic fluid. LMs may be complicated by spontaneous hemorrhage into the lesion, leading to pain and rapid expansion, as well as infection. Recurrent cellulitis is a

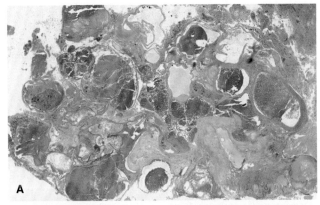

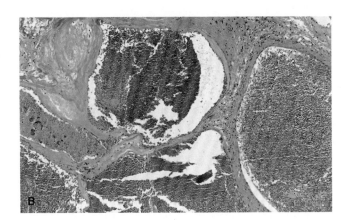

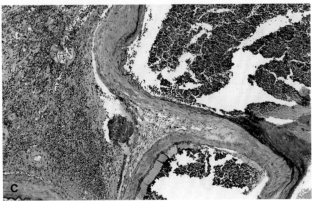

FIGURE 25-27. Arteriovenous malformation. A and B, Many malformed medium-sized vessels arranged haphazardly within the subcutis. Arteries empty directly to veins without intervening capillary beds. C, Elastic tissue stain highlights malformed elastic lamina within a muscular-walled vessel. Digital slides courtesy of Path Presenter.com.

common complication, given the stagnation of fluid within the lesion.

Histologic Findings

LM exhibits thin-walled, irregularly dilated channels that may appear empty or contain amorphous, pale eosinophilic material, often with admixed lymphocytes, histiocytes, and red blood cells (Figure 25-28). A superficial dermal component is common; pronounced hyperkeratosis and verrucous epidermal hyperplasia may overlie superficial malformed lymphatic channels. These channels may also commonly involve the reticular dermis and subcutis. Lymphoid aggregates with plasma cells, and germinal center formation may appear in the deeper aspects of these malformations. Fibrotic thickening of the reticular dermis and subcutaneous fibrous septae is common. The larger channels typical of macrocystic LM demonstrate thicker vessel walls and exhibit increased surrounding fibrous tissue, myofibroblasts, and few smooth muscle cells.[6] Immunostains for lymphatic markers, including D2-40 (podoplanin), LYVE-1, PROX1, and VEGFR-3, are helpful in differentiating LM from other malformations. D2-40 and LYVE-1 may have lower sensitivity because they stain larger channels in LM less consistently.[90] CD31 staining is variable, and CD34 is typically focal or absent.

CAPSULE SUMMARY

LYMPHATIC MALFORMATIONS

LM may be micro- or macrocystic. Anomalies previously referred to as "lymphangioma circumscriptum" are better classified as small/localized superficial LMs. Microscopic features include epidermal changes similar to those of angiokeratoma or verrucous VM (see Section "Verrucous Venous Malformation"), overlying dilated thin-walled channels in the dermis that label with D2-40 and other lymphatic immunomarkers. Stromal features include dermal and subcutaneous fibrosis, and lymphoplasmacytic inflammation.

COMBINED MALFORMATIONS

The ISSVA includes a classification for vascular malformations that are comprised by two or more vessel types. These combined malformations are extremely heterogeneous and often observed in the setting of vascular anomalies–related syndromes. For example, the large, geographic violaceous to purple stain seen in association with extremity overgrowth in Klippel-Trenaunay syndrome is

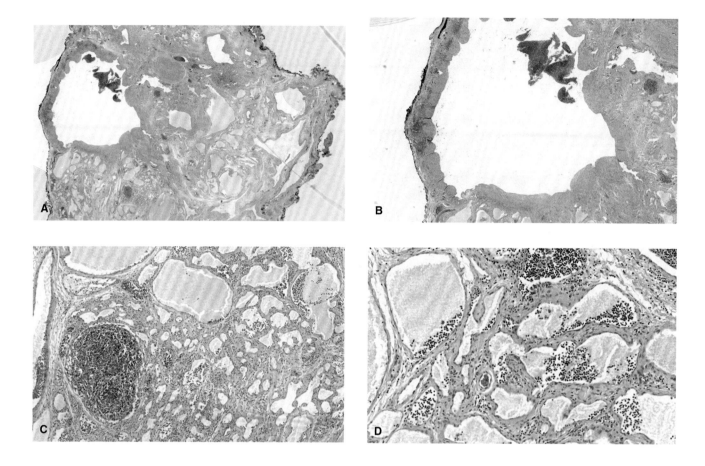

FIGURE 25-28. Lymphatic malformation (LM). A and B, Macrocystic LM. Thin-walled, dilated lymphatic channels with a predominately larger channel component. C and D, Microcystic LM. Clusters of smaller lymphatic channels with adjacent lymphoid aggregates. Digital slides courtesy of Path Presenter.com.

a capillary-lymphatic-venous malformation. Because of the heterogeneity and numerous vessel types involved, the histopathologic features of combined malformations are not well described in the literature. Histopathology typically exhibits overlapping features of the various above-described malformations. Biopsy may be most useful in confirming a malformation rather than a vascular tumor, and identifying a lymphatic component with immunostains such as PROX1 or D2-40.

OTHER VASCULAR ANOMALIES: PROVISIONALLY UNCLASSIFIED

Provisionally unclassified vascular anomalies are those that do not fit cleanly from a clinical or histopathologic standpoint into any discrete category previously outlined (Table 25-6). However, as clinical diagnoses improve and

genetic advances take place, so too will our knowledge and understanding of the biology and natural history of these uncommon vascular anomalies.

TABLE 25-6.	Provisionally unclassified vascular anomalies (ISSVA, 2014)

- Verrucous venous malformation (formerly verrucous hemangioma)
- Angiokeratoma
- MLT/CAT
- KLA
- PTEN (type) hamartoma of soft tissue/"angiomatosis" of soft tissue
- FAVA

Abbreviations: CAT, cutaneovisceral angiomatosis with thrombocytopenia; FAVA, fibroadipose vascular anomaly; KLA, kaposiform lymphangiomatosis; MLT, multifocal lymphangioendotheliomatosis with thrombocytopenia; PTEN, phosphatase and tensin homolog.

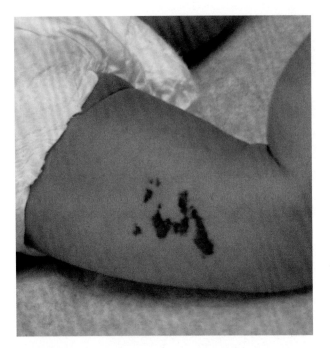

FIGURE 25-29. Verrucous venous malformation.

VERRUCOUS VENOUS MALFORMATION (FORMERLY VERRUCOUS HEMANGIOMA)

Definition and Epidemiology

Verrucous venous malformation (VVM) is an uncommon, slow-flow vascular malformation recently found to be associated with somatic mutations in *MAP3K3*.[91,92]

Clinical Presentation

VVMs most commonly occur on the lower extremity and present as well-demarcated but somewhat irregular blue to purple-colored plaques (Figure 25-29). They may become scaly and cobblestoned ("verrucous") over time and thicken. Although they are usually asymptomatic, they may become more thick and hyperkeratotic over time.

Histologic Findings

VVM demonstrates irregular papillomatous (verrucous) epidermal hyperplasia with associated hyper- and parakeratosis, above dilated, vertically oriented vessels with thin endothelial walls high in dermal papillae, and also within

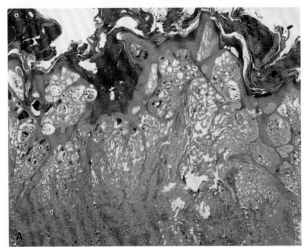

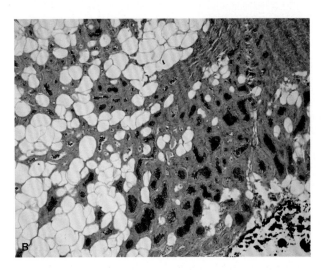

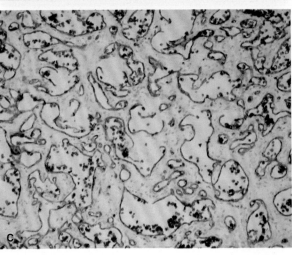

FIGURE 25-30. **Verrucous venous malformation.** A, The superficial component resembles angiokeratoma (40× magnification). B, A deeper component is also present, with small, thin-walled vessels that resemble venules in the deep dermis and superficial subcutis (100× magnification). C, Glucose transporter protein isoform-1 labels endothelial cells of lesional vessels, a helpful finding in distinguishing from angiokeratoma and other mimickers.

the deeper dermis and subcutaneous tissue (Figure 25-30). In the papillary dermis, 10 to 50 μ-diameter, thin-walled vessels are splayed between fibrotic connective tissue. The deeper component of VVM demonstrates venule-like channels with flat or hobnailed endothelium with thickened, lamellated-appearing basement membranes. The differential diagnosis includes angiokeratoma (superficially sampled VVM may be exceedingly difficult to differentiate from angiokeratoma) and other vascular malformations with hyperkeratosis and epidermal hyperplasia such as capillary-lymphatic or capillary-venous malformations.[91] Interestingly, VVM is one of the only vascular anomalies other than IH that stains positively for GLUT-1. GLUT-1 immunoreactivity within the deeper venule-like structures is an important indicator of the diagnosis of VVM.[92] D2-40 is negative in lesional vessels. Reports of Wilms tumor 1 gene staining are variable, with one report of near-complete negativity[93] and another with at least focal cytoplasmic positivity in 13 of 13 cases.[94]

CAPSULE SUMMARY

VERRUCOUS VENOUS MALFORMATION

Verrucous VM exhibits many superficial features resembling angiokeratoma, but with a deeper component with venules that notably label positively with GLUT-1, a marker otherwise largely specific to IH.

MULTIFOCAL LYMPHANGIOENDOTHELIOMATOSIS WITH THROMBOCYTOPENIA/ CUTANEOVISCERAL ANGIOMATOSIS WITH THROMBOCYTOPENIA

Definition and Epidemiology

Multifocal lymphangioendotheliomatosis with thrombocytopenia/cutaneovisceral angiomatosis with thrombocytopenia (MLT/CAT) is a very rare multifocal vascular anomaly syndrome that presents with multifocal vascular lesions and classically with associated gastrointestinal (GI) involvement. It typically presents in the neonatal period with skin lesions and severe GI bleeding and thrombocytopenia.[95,96]

Clinical Presentation

Cutaneous features include multifocal dull red to brown plaques or nodules (Figure 25-31). This is most commonly a multisystem disease, and the skin, GI tract, or other organs such as the brain may rarely be involved.

Histologic Findings

The initial report of this entity[95] described histopathologic features that included clusters of thin-walled vessels within the deep dermis and subcutis, with a notably dissecting pattern between collagen bundles in some areas. Prominent endothelial cell hobnailing was common, and intraluminal papillary projections (similar to those seen in PILA/Dabska tumor) were present (Figure 25-32). Periodic acid-Schiff stain highlighted glycogen within the papillary projections. Neither thrombi nor significant numbers of red blood cells were seen within vessels.

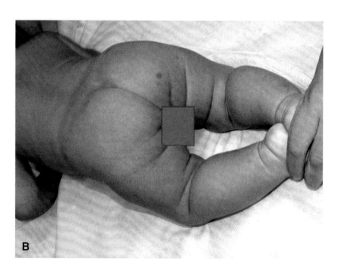

FIGURE 25-31. Multifocal lymphangioendotheliomatosis with thrombocytopenia/cutaneovisceral angiomatosis with thrombocytopenia. A, Several dark bluish papules, macules, and nodules on both shins and on the dorsum of the right foot. B, Several dark bluish papules and a nodule on the right buttock including in an area of a large Mongolian spot. Obtained with permission, Khamaysi Ziad, Bergman R. Multifocal congenital lymphangioendotheliomatosis without gastrointestinal bleeding and/or thrombocytopenia. *Am J Dermatopathol.* 2010;32(8):804-808.

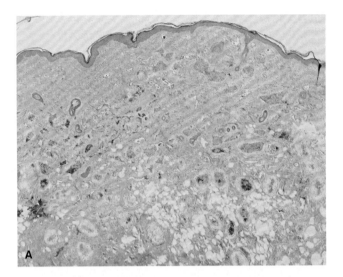

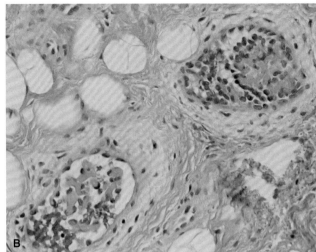

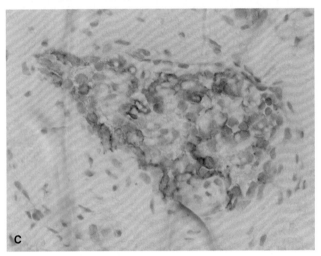

FIGURE 25-32. Multifocal lymphangioendotheliomatosis with thrombocytopenia/cutaneovisceral angiomatosis with thrombocytopenia. A, Clusters of small, thin-walled vessels within the dermis (40× magnification). B, Intraluminal papillary projections with hyaline cores, similar to those of papillary intralymphatic angioendothelioma (200× magnification). C, Endothelial cells label with LYVE-1.

Endothelial cells expressed CD31 as well as LYVE-1, but were negative for other lymphatic markers. Ki-67 labeled 10% to 15% of lesional cells.[95] Subsequent reports have described similar histologic features.[97] Essentially identical clinicopathologic findings have also been described with the term *cutaneovisceral angiomatosis with thrombocytopenia* (CAT) by authors who believe this vascular anomaly is not lymphatic in origin.[96]

CAPSULE SUMMARY

MULTIFOCAL LYMPHANGIOENDOTHELIOMATOSIS WITH THROMBOCYTOPENIA/ CUTANEOVISCERAL ANGIOMATOSIS WITH THROMBOCYTOPENIA

MLT/CAT is a rare multifocal vascular anomaly with distinctive clinical features including prominent skin and GI involvement. Microscopic findings include deeply seated, thin-walled vessels and focal features that overlap with the group of vascular tumors that exhibit intraluminal papillary projections.

KAPOSIFORM LYMPHANGIOENDOTHELIOMATOSIS

Definition and Epidemiology

Kaposiform lymphangioendotheliomatosis (KLA) is a newly described vascular anomaly with aggressive features. It shares clinical and histopathologic overlap with both KHE and generalized lymphatic anomaly.

Clinical Presentation

KLA usually presents in childhood with respiratory symptoms related to pleural effusion and hemorrhage. Cutaneous involvement is rare. Overall prognosis is poor; 50% mortality has been reported in some series.[97] KLA is difficult to classify and is thus grouped under this category because it shares some features of neoplasia (tumor) and others of a more static vascular malformation.[98] It has unique and distinctive features on histopathology.

Histologic Findings

Biopsy demonstrates "kaposiform" areas of spindled cells that are focal and may be either within lumens (intravascular) or in between (perivascular) malformed lymphatic channels. These spindle cells are clustered or sheet-like, often in parallel arrays, and may contain cytoplasmic hemosiderin granules. Cytologic atypia and mitotic figures are rare. Lymphatic immunostains such as D2-40, Lyve-1, and Prox-1 label both the spindled cells and lymphatic endothelium. The main differential diagnosis is with KHE, when the spindled component of the lesion predominates. KHE generally exhibits more frequent microthrombi, glomeruloid zones, and has more round, well-defined coalescing nodules of spindled cells. However, in most reported cases, KLA exhibits primary features of LM, with only minor spindle cell zones.[98,99]

CAPSULE SUMMARY

KAPOSIFORM LYMPHANGIOENDOTHELIOMATOSIS

KLA is a recently described entity with aggressive clinical features. Histopathology exhibits the findings of LM and KS-like spindle cell zones reminiscent of KHE.

PHOSPHATASE AND TENSIN HOMOLOG-TYPE HAMARTOMA OF SOFT TISSUE

Definition and Epidemiology

Phosphatase and tensin homolog (PTEN) hamartoma tumor syndrome (PTHTS) encompasses a group of genetic conditions because of autosomal dominant mutations in the *PTEN* gene including Cowden syndrome and Bannayan-Riley-Ruvalcaba syndrome. Individuals with PTHTS have significant phenotypical overlap including predisposition to neoplasia. Cowden syndrome is the most common presentation and is characterized by the development of multiple hamartomas as well as a high risk for the development of either benign or malignant tumors of the thyroid, breast, and endometrium.

Clinical Presentation

Clinical features include macrocephaly, trichilemmomas, and papillomas that are typically observed by the 2nd decade[100] (Figure 25-33). In addition to the development of tumors described previously, a distinctive type of vascular anomaly is associated with PTHTS. This vascular lesion has recently been described, and is a high-flow vascular malformation with the characteristic presence of adipose tissue. It is known as PTEN hamartoma of soft tissue (PHOST). It typically presents intramuscularly in the extremities of affected individuals.[101]

Histologic Findings

PHOSTs are hamartomas of abundant adipose tissue, arteries, and irregular clusters of venous channels. Arteries are

thick walled with small lumens (Figure 25-34 and 25-35). The venous channels may resemble pulmonary alveoli. Clusters of smaller vessels with prominent muscular walls are also seen, and may have prominently myxoid surrounding stroma.[101] Additional features include high-flow-type vascular zones (A-V communications), other hamartomatous elements such as bone and nerve hypertrophy, and lymphoid follicles.

CAPSULE SUMMARY

PTEN-TYPE HAMARTOMA OF SOFT TISSUE

PHOST is a vascular anomaly specific to PTEN tumor syndromes, consisting of arteries, venous channels, and smaller vessels with prominent hamartomatous soft tissue components, with the latter typically comprising greater than 50% of the bulk of the lesion.

FIBROADIPOSE VASCULAR ANOMALY (FAVA)

Definition and Epidemiology

The acronym FAVA (Fibroadipose Vascular Anomaly) has been recently given to a distinct vascular entity that is characterized by fibrofatty infiltration of muscle, unusual phlebectasia with pain, and contracture of the affected extremity. This is a distinct clinical, radiologic, and histopathologic entity that is very rarely encountered.

Clinical Presentation

Out of the isolated case reports that have been described from this entity, most patients present with painful calf masses. FAVA has a predilection for the lower extremities. Eight of the 12 cases reported showed limited ankle dorsiflexion (ie, equinus contracture). The study by Alomari et al included 18 patients with FAVA. The lesions presented from birth up to 28 years of age. Ten patients presented at birth to early childhood with mass or slight discoloration, whereas five presented in adolescence and three as adults. The anatomic locations include calf, forearm/wrist, and thigh. In three cases, the lesions were asymptomatic. Other clinical findings include phlebectasia of the affected extremity, disuse atrophy, and cutaneous lymphatic vesicles.[102-105]

Magnetic resonance imaging findings include a soft tissue lesion with a muscular epicenter. T1-weighed images show heterogeneous, high-signal intensity areas in the affected muscle. T2-weighed sequences show more intense signals. A fatty component can be present. Disruption of the intrafascial/intramuscular compartment is noted (Figure 26-36).

Histologic Findings

The most obvious findings include dense areas of fibrosis, excessive adipose tissue, a VM, and lymphoplasmacytic

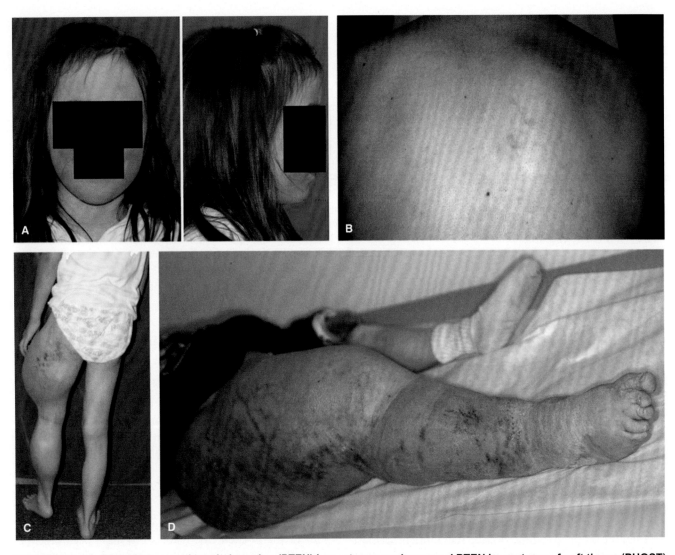

FIGURE 25-33. Phosphatase and tensin homolog (PTEN) hamartoma syndrome and PTEN hamartoma of soft tissue (PHOST). Clinical features. A, A 6-year-old girl with Bannayan-Riley-Ruvalcaba syndrome (BRRS): note macrocephaly with a square cranium and a broad, high forehead. B, An adolescent with BRRS and PHOST in the right posterior paraspinal musculature. Note the blotchy cutaneous stain. C, A boy with BRRS and large, primarily intramuscular PHOSTs of the left thigh and calf. Note the extensive cutaneous stain and the prominent veins in the thigh. D, A boy with a germline inactivation of both PTEN alleles and a massive overgrowth of the right lower extremity and pelvis. Note the cutaneous stain, prominent veins, and epidermal nevus over the first and second toes, dorsum of the foot, and the lateral aspect of the leg and thigh. Imaging features.

aggregates in the skeletal muscle. Small, irregularly muscularized venous channels are always clustered. In some cases, the vascular channels can be back-to-back, and their thin walls, that lack smooth muscle, can resemble pulmonary alveoli. In the majority of cases, large abnormal venous channels are seen, usually irregular, and sometimes with an excessive muscle layer. On a single occasion, the lesion can resemble an SCH. An abnormal lymphatic component accompanying the venous elements is seen in 25% of cases. These include clusters of small, thin-walled, channels with little to no smooth muscle, and containing lymph in the lumen.

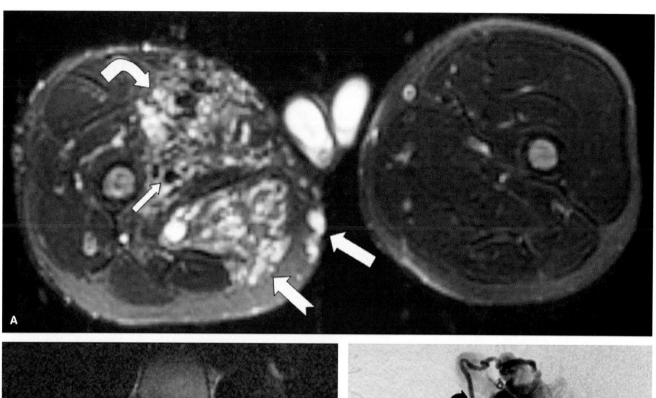

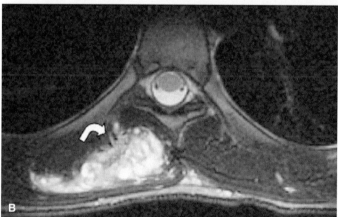

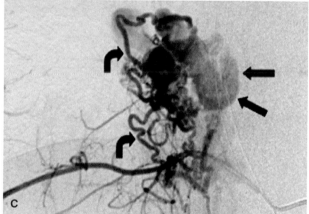

FIGURE 25-33. (*continued*) A, Extensive PHOST of the right thigh in a boy with BRRS. Infiltrative heterogenous lesion involving vastus medialis muscle (bent arrow) with increased arterial supply (small arrow). Less hypervascular lesion in semimembranosus and gracilis muscles (notched arrow). Note the venous nodules in the subcutaneous layer of the medial thigh (large arrow) (axial fat-saturated T2-weighted MR image). B, PHOST in a patient depicted in Figure 1B showing heterogenous high-signal intensity and hypervascularity evident by enlarged arterial feeders at the periphery of the lesion (arrow) (axial T2-weighted MR image with fat saturation). C, Selective right eighth intercostal arteriogram in a lesion depicted in (B) demonstrates hypervascular mass with multiple tortuous feeding arteries (bent arrows) and intratumoral shunting into dilated veins (straight arrows). MR indicates magnetic resonance. Obtained with permission, Kurek KC, Howard E, Tennant LB, et al. PTEN hamartoma of soft tissue: a distinctive lesion in PTEN syndromes. *Am J Surg Pathol.* 2012;36(5):671-687.

CAPSULE SUMMARY

The acronym FAVA has been recently given to a distinct vascular entity that is characterized by fibrofatty infiltration of muscle, unusual phlebectasia with pain, and contracture of the affected extremity. The most obvious findings include dense areas of fibrosis, excessive adipose tissue, a VM, and lymphoplasmacytic aggregates in the skeletal muscle.

Miscellaneous Vascular Entities

ECCRINE ANGIOMATOUS HAMARTOMA

Definition and Epidemiology

Eccrine angiomatous hamartoma (EAH) is a rare, benign hamartomatous proliferation comprised of eccrine glands and capillary-like structures in the skin. It is most commonly seen in children with a predilection for the extremities, but is also reported in adults.[58,59]

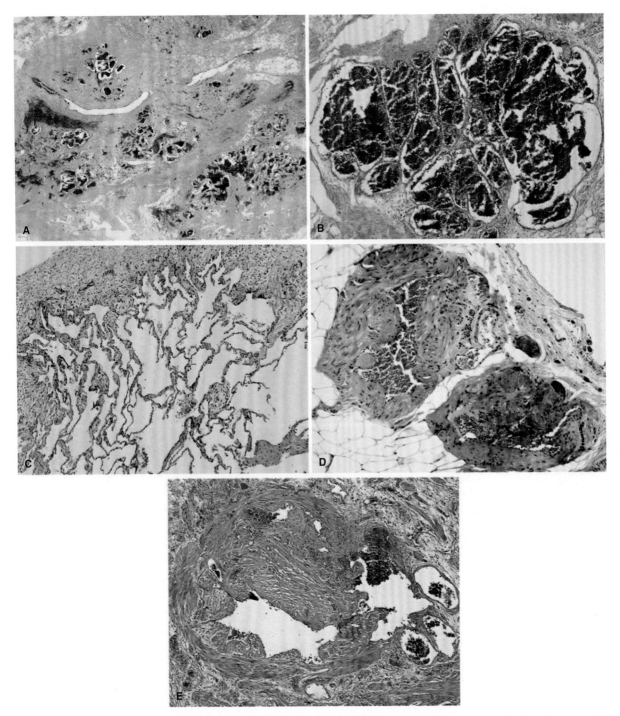

FIGURE 25-34. Phosphatase and tensin homolog hamartoma of soft tissue. Venous component. A-C, Conspicuous well-circumscribed clusters of blood-filled or empty, back-to-back, thin-walled channels. Superficial resemblance to pulmonary alveoli when empty. D and E, Some abnormal veins have uneven and striking excess of smooth muscle and highly irregular and complex lumens. Obtained with permission from Kurek KC, Howard E, Tennant LB, et al. PTEN hamartoma of soft tissue: a distinctive lesion in PTEN syndromes. *Am J Surg Pathol.* 2012;36(5):671-687.

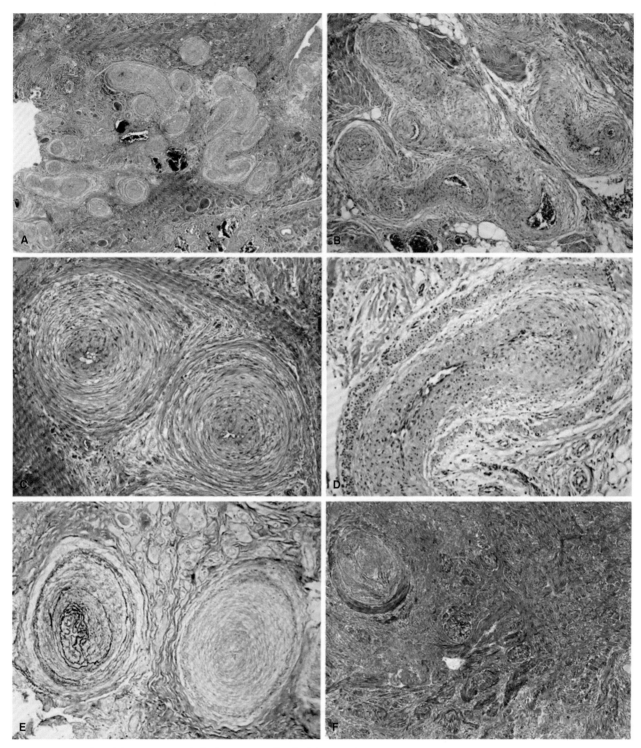

FIGURE 25-35. Arterial component. A-C, Aggregate of coiled thick-walled arteries with tiny lumens. Concentric smooth muscle hyperplasia often involving intima, media and adventitia. D, Artery with two smooth muscle layers, inner one being intimal. E, Replication and abnormal conformation of elastic laminae (Miller elastic stain). F, Smooth muscle fascicles (stained red) with no apparent vascular connection (Masson trichrome stain). Obtained with permission from Kurek KC, Howard E, Tennant LB, et al. PTEN hamartoma of soft tissue: a distinctive lesion in PTEN syndromes. *Am J Surg Pathol*. 2012;36(5):671-687.

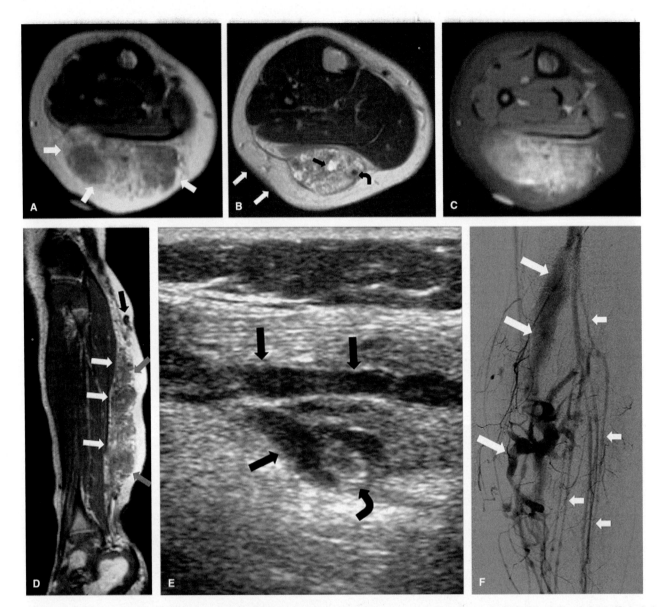

FIGURE 25-36. Magnetic resonance imaging (MRI) of a diffuse fibroadipose vascular anomaly (FAVA) of the right calf. A, Axial T1-weighted MRI. Both heads of the gastrocnemius muscle were diffusely replaced by heterogeneous soft tissue (arrows) with signal intensity higher than adjacent normal muscles. Note the transfascial fatty component of the mass. B, Axial T2-weighted MRI. The heterogeneous high-signal intensity is higher than that of the normal muscles but less intense than the fluid signal typically seen in venous malformations. Note the dilated intramuscular vein (black arrow), phlebolith (bent arrow), and thickened subcutaneous fat (white arrows). C, Axial fat-saturated T1-weighted MRI following contrast administration demonstrating moderate to strong enhancement. D, Sagittal T1-weighted MRI depicts the longitudinal distribution of the disease along the entire course of the gastrocnemius (white and gray arrows). Note subcutaneous phlebectasia (black arrow). E, Ultrasonography of a focal calf FAVA. The affected part of the gastrocnemius muscle demonstrated extensive, solid, and echogenic changes entirely replacing the normal fibrillary pattern. The dilated intramuscular veins (straight arrows) contained a clot (bent arrow) that was very tender. F, Venous phase of angiography in a diffuse calf FAVA. Note the marked phlebectasia (long arrows) of both intrafascial and extrafascial compartments. The deep veins were normal (short arrows). Obtained with permission, Alomari AI, Spencer SA, Arnold RW, et al. Fibro-adipose vascular anomaly: clinical-radiologic-pathologic features of a newly delineated disorder of the extremity. *J Pediatr Orthop.* 2014;34(1):109-117.

Clinical Presentation

The lesions are most often solitary, although multifocal presentations are reported.[106] Clinically, EAH presents as somewhat firm, rubbery nodule or plaque with erythema or hyperpigmentation (Figure 25-37). Hypertrichosis and/or hyperhidrosis may also be present.

Histologic Findings

EAH consists of a hamartomatous proliferation of eccrine glands and small vessels. Its defining feature is of hyperplastic eccrine units with closely intermingled capillary-like small vessels within the deep dermis and subcutis[107] (Figure 25-38). Additional hamartomatous elements such as increased

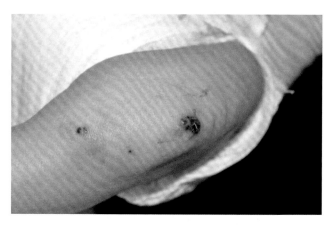

FIGURE 25-37. Eccrine angiomatous hamartoma, multifocal, on the leg of a child. Photo courtesy of Dr. Ingrid Polcari.

apocrine and follicular units, mucin, and lipomatous tissue may also be present. The overlying skin may commonly demonstrate papillomatous epidermal hyperplasia and widely dilated, thin-walled dermal vessels.[106] The differential diagnosis includes other lobulated vascular proliferations such as TA, as well as benign sweat duct tumors such as eccrine nevus. The close apposition of vessels and glands in EAH typically permits distinction from these entities.

CAPSULE SUMMARY

EAH is an uncommon hamartoma with predilection for the extremities. Microscopically, it exhibits features of a true hamartoma, with increased small vessels, eccrine glands, and often other mesenchymal elements.

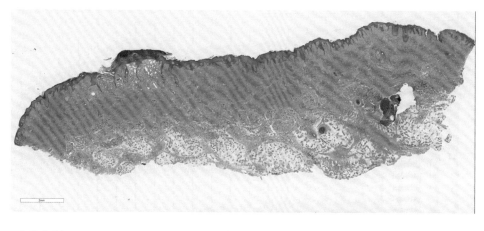

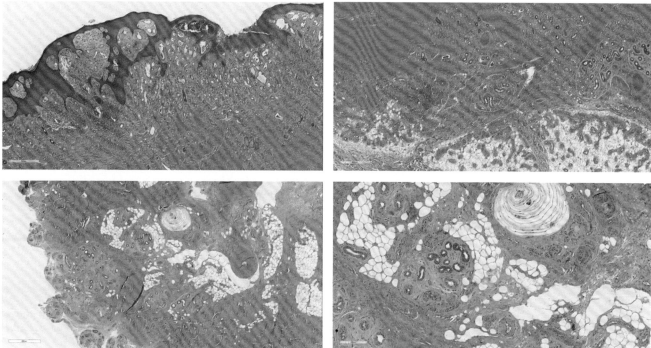

FIGURE 25-38. **Eccrine angiomatous hamartoma.** Vascular proliferation consisting mostly of clusters of capillary-like small vessels, with hamartomatous proliferation of eccrine glands. Vessel clusters are often intimately associated with eccrine gland lobules.

REFERENCES

1. Mulliken JB, Glowacki J. Classification of pediatric vascular lesions. *Plast Reconstr Surg.* 1982;70(1):120.
2. Wassef M, Blei F, Adams D, et al. Vascular anomalies classification: recommendations from the International Society for the Study of Vascular Anomalies. *Pediatrics.* 2015;136(1):e203-e214.
3. Kanada KN, Merin MR, Munden A, Friedlander SF. A prospective study of cutaneous findings in newborns in the United States: correlation with race, ethnicity, and gestational status using updated classification and nomenclature. *J Pediatr.* 2012;161(2):240-245.
4. Tollefson MM, Frieden IJ. Early growth of infantile hemangiomas: what parents' photographs tell us. *Pediatrics.* 2012;130(2):e314-e320.
5. Haggstrom AN, Drolet BA, Baselga E, et al. Prospective study of infantile hemangiomas: clinical characteristics predicting complications and treatment. *Pediatrics.* 2006;118(3):882-887.
6. Gupta A, Kozakewich H. Histopathology of vascular anomalies. *Clin Plastic Surg.* 2011;38:31–44.
7. Glowacki J, Mulliken JB. Mast cells in hemangiomas and vascular malformations. *Pediatrics.* 1982;70:48e51.
8. Olson AL, Pessin JE. Structure, function, and regulation of the mammalian facilitative glucose transporter gene family. *Annu Rev Nutr.* 1996;16:235-256.
9. Boull C, Maguiness SM. Congenital hemangiomas. *Semin Cutan Med Surg.* 2016;35(3):124-127.
10. Ayturk UM, Couto JA, Hann S, et al. Somatic activating mutations in GNAQ and GNA11 are associated with congenital hemangioma. *Am J Hum Genet.* 2016;98(4):789-795.
11. Lee PW, Frieden IJ, Streicher JL, McCalmont T, Haggstrom AN. Characteristics of noninvoluting congenital hemangioma: a retrospective review. *J Am Acad Dermatol.* 2014;70(5):899-903.
12. Berenguer B, Mulliken JB, Enjolras O, et al. Rapidly involuting congenital hemangioma: clinical and histopathologic features. *Pediatr Dev Pathol.* 2003;6:495-510.
13. Groesser L, Peterhof E, Evert M, et al. BRAF and RAS mutations in sporadic and secondary pyogenic granuloma. *J Invest Dermatol.* 2016;136(2):481-486.
14. Lim YH, Douglas SR, Ko CJ, et al. Somatic activating RAS mutations cause vascular tumors including pyogenic granuloma. *J Invest Dermatol.* 2015;135(6):1698-1700.
15. Sammut SJ, Tomson N, Corrie P. Pyogenic granuloma as a cutaneous adverse effect of vemurafenib. *N Engl J Med.* 2014;371(13):1265-1267.
16. Henning B, Stieger P, Kamarachev J, Dummer R, Goldinger SM. Pyogenic granuloma in patients treated with selective BRAF inhibitors: another manifestation of paradoxical pathway activation. *Melanoma Res.* 2016;26(3):304-307.
17. Baselga E, Wassef M, Lopez S, Hoffman W, Cordisco M, Frieden IJ. Agminated, eruptive pyogenic granuloma-like lesions developing over congenital vascular stains. *Pediatr Dermatol.* 2012;29(2):186-190.
18. Cooper PH, McAllister HA, Helwig EB. Intravenous pyogenic granuloma: a study of 18 cases. *Am J Surg Pathol.* 1979;3:221-228.
19. DiFazio F, Mogan J. Intravenous pyogenic granuloma of the hand. *J Hand Surg.* 1989;14A:310-312.
20. Hung CH, Kuo HW, Chiu YK, Huang PH. Intravascular pyogenic granuloma arising in an acquired arteriovenous malformation: report of a case and review of the literature. *Dermatol Surg.* 2004;30(7):1050-1053.
21. Weiss SW, Enzinger FM. Spindle cell hemangioendothelioma: a low-grade angiosarcoma resembling cavernous hemangioma and Kaposi's sarcoma. *Am J Surg Pathol.* 1986;10(8):521-530.
22. Requena L, Kutzner H. Hemangioendothelioma. *Semin Diagn Pathol.* 2013;30(1):29-44.
23. Kurek KC, Pansuriya TC, van Ruler MA, et al. R132C IDH1 mutations are found in spindle cell hemangiomas and not in other vascular tumors or malformations. *Am J Pathol.* 2013;182(5):1494-1500.
24. Mulliken JB, Burrows PE, Fishman SJ. *Vascular Anomalies.* 2nd ed. New York, NY: Oxford University Press; 2013.

25. Wang L, Gao T, Wang G. Expression of Prox1, D2-40, and WT1 in spindle cell hemangioma. *J Cutan Pathol.* 2014;41(5):447-450.
26. Fetsch JF, Sesterhenn IA, Miettinen M, et al. Epithelioid hemangioma of the penis: a clinicopathologic and immunohistochemical analysis of 19 cases, with special reference to exuberant examples often confused with epithelioid hemangioendothelioma and epithelioid angiosarcoma. *Am J Surg Pathol.* 2004;28:523-533.
27. Huang SC, Zhang L, Sung YS, et al. Frequent *FOS* gene rearrangements in epithelioid hemangioma: a molecular study of 58 cases with morphologic reappraisal. *Am J Surg Pathol.* 2015;39(10):1313-1321.
28. Fletcher C, Bridge JA, Hogendoorn PC, et al. *WHO Classification of Tumours of Soft Tissue and Bone.* Lyon, France: IARC; 2013.
29. Errani C, Zhang L, Sung YS, et al. A novel *WWTR1-CAMTA1* gene fusion is a consistent abnormality in epithelioid hemangioendothelioma of different anatomic sites. *Genes Chromosomes Cancer.* 2011;50:644-653.
30. Fernandez AP, Sun Y, Tubbs RR, Goldblum JR, Billings SD. FISH for MYC amplification and anti-MYC immunohistochemistry: useful diagnostic tools in the assessment of secondary angiosarcoma and atypical vascular proliferations. *J Cutan Pathol.* 2012;39(2):234-242.
31. Napekoski KM, Fernandez AP, Billings SD. Microvenular hemangioma: a clinicopathologic review of 13 cases. *J Cutan Pathol.* 2014;41(11):816-822.
32. Chang SE, Roh KH, Lee MW, et al. Microvenular hemangioma in a boy with acute myelogenous leukemia. *Pediatr Dermatol.* 2003;20(3):266-267.
33. Hudnall SD, Chen T, Brown K, et al. Human herpesvirus-8-positive microvenular hemangioma in POEMS syndrome. *Arch Pathol Lab Med.* 2003;127:1034.
34. Xu XL, Xu CR, Chen H, et al. Eruptive microvenular hemangiomas in 4 Chinese patients: clinicopathologic correlation and review of the literature. *Am J Dermatopathol.* 2010;32:837.
35. Van Vugt LJ, van der Vleuten CJM, Flucke U, Blokx WAM. The utility of GLUT1 as a diagnostic marker in cutaneous vascular anomalies: a review of literature and recommendations for daily practice. *Pathol Res Pract.* 2017;213(6):591-597.
36. Enjolras, Odile, et al. Infants with Kasabach-Merritt syndrome do not have "true" hemangiomas. *The Journal of pediatrics* 130.4 (1997): 631-640
37. Padilla RS, Orkin M, Rosai J. Acquired "tufted" angioma (progressive capillary hemangioma). A distinctive clinicopathologic entity related to lobular capillary hemangioma. *Am J Dermatopathol.* 1987;9(4):292-300.
38. Arai E, Kuramochi A, Tsuchida T, et al. Usefulness of D2-40 immunohistochemistry for differentiation between kaposiform hemangioendothelioma and tufted angioma. *J Cutan Pathol.* 2006;33(7):492-497.
39. Croteau SE, Liang MG, Kozakewich HP, et al. Kaposiform hemangioendothelioma: atypical features and risks of Kasabach-Merritt phenomenon in 107 referrals. *J Pediatr.* 2013;162(1):142-147.
40. Croteau SE, Gupta D. The clinical spectrum of kaposiform hemangioendothelioma and tufted angioma. *Semin Cutan Med Surg.* 2016;35(3):147-152.
41. Lyons LL, North PE, Lai FM-M, et al. Kaposiform hemangioendothelioma. a study of 33 cases emphasizing its pathologic, immunophenotypic, and biologic uniqueness from juvenile hemangioma. *Am J Surg Pathol.* 2004;28:559-568.
42. Debelenko LV, Perez-Atayde AR, Mulliken JB, et al. D2-40 immunohistochemical analysis of pediatric vascular tumors reveals positivity in kaposiform hemangioendothelioma. *Mod Pathol.* 2005;18:1454-1460.
43. Cheuk W, Wong KO, Wong CS, et al. Immunostaining for human herpesvirus 8 latent nuclear antigen-1 helps distinguish Kaposi sarcoma from mimickers. *Am J Clin Pathol.* 2004;121:335-342.
44. Colmenero I, Hoeger PH. Vascular tumours in infants. Part II: vascular tumours of intermediate dignity and malignant tumours. *Br J Dermatol.* 2014;171(3):474-484.
45. Dabska M. Malignant endovascular papillary angioendothelioma of the skin in childhood. Clinicopathologic study of 6 cases. *Cancer.* 1969;24(3):503-510.
46. Nayler SJ, Rubin BP, Calonje E, Chan JK, Fletcher CD. Composite hemangioendothelioma: a complex, low-grade vascular lesion mimicking angiosarcoma. *Am J Surg Pathol.* 2000;24(3):352-361.

47. McNab PM, Quigley BC, Glass LF, Jukic DM. Composite hemangioendothelioma and its classification as a low-grade malignancy. *Am J Dermatopathol.* 2013;35(4):517-522.

48. Reis-Filho JS, Paiva ME, Lopes JM. Congenital composite hemangioendothelioma: case report and reappraisal of the hemangioendothelioma spectrum. *J Cutan Pathol.* 2002;29(4):226-231.

49. Perry KD, Al-Lbraheemi A, Rubin BP, et al. Composite hemangioendothelioma with neuroendocrine marker expression: an aggressive variant. *Mod Pathol.* 2017;30(11):1589-1602.

50. Liau JY, Lee FY, Chiu CS, Chen JS, Hsiao TL. Composite hemangioendothelioma presenting as a scalp nodule with alopecia. *J Am Acad Dermatol.* 2013;69(2):e98-e99.

51. Mirra JM, Kessler S, Bhuta S, et al. The fibroma-like variant of epithelioid sarcoma: a fibrohistiocytic/myoid cell lesion often confused with benign and malignant spindle cell tumors. *Cancer.* 1992;9:1382-1395.

52. Hornick JL, Fletcher CD. Pseudomyogenic hemangioendothelioma: a distinctive, often multicentric tumor with indolent behavior. *Am J Surg Pathol.* 2011;35(2):190-201.

53. Ye C, Yu X, Zeng J, Liu H, Dai M. Pseudomyogenic hemangioendothelioma secondary to fibrous dysplasia of the left lower extremity in a 14-year-old female: a case report. *World J Surg Oncol.* 2016;14(1):198.

54. Trombetta D, Magnusson L, von Steyern FV, et al. Translocation t(7;19)(q22;q13)−a recurrent chromosome aberration in pseudomyogenic hemangioendothelioma? *Cancer Genet.* 2011;204(4):211-215.

55. Walther C, Tayebwa J, Lilljebjörn H, et al. A novel SERPINE1-FOSB fusion gene results in transcriptional up-regulation of FOSB in pseudomyogenic haemangioendothelioma. *J Pathol.* 2014;232(5):534-540.

56. Antonescu CR, Chen HW, Zhang L, et al. ZFP36-FOSB fusion defines a subset of epithelioid hemangioma with atypical features. *Genes Chromosomes Cancer.* 2014;53:951-959.

57. Hung YP, Fletcher CD, Hornick JL. FOSB is a useful diagnostic marker for pseudomyogenic hemangioendothelioma. *Am J Surg Pathol.* 2017;41(5):596-606.

58. Requena L, Santonja C, Martinez-Amo JL, Saus C, Kutzner H. Cutaneous epithelioid sarcomalike (pseudomyogenic) hemangioendothelioma: a little-known low-grade cutaneous vascular neoplasm. *JAMA Dermatol.* 2013;149(4):459-465.

59. Gantt S, Kakuru A, Wald A, Walusansa V, Corey L, Casper C, Orem J. Clinical presentation and outcome of epidemic Kaposi sarcoma in Ugandan children. *Pediatr Blood Cancer.* 2010;54(5):670-674.

60. Ziegler JL, Katongole-Mbidde E. Kaposi's sarcoma in childhood: an analysis of 100 cases from Uganda and relationship to HIV infection. *Int J Cancer.* 1996;65(2):200-203.

61. Li N, Anderson WK, Bhawan J. Further confirmation of the association of human herpesvirus 8 with Kaposi's sarcoma. *J Cutan Pathol.* 1998;25:413-419.

62. Rady PL, Hodak E, Yen A, et al. Detection of human herpesvirus-8 DNA in Kaposi's sarcomas from iatrogenically immunosuppressed patients. *J Am Acad Dermatol.* 1998;38:429-437.

63. Douglas JL, Gustin JK, Dezube B, Pantanowitz JL, Moses AV. Kaposi's sarcoma: a model of both malignancy and chronic inflammation. *Panminerva Medica.* 2007;49(3):119-138.

64. Patel RM, Goldblum JR, Hsi ED. Immunohistochemical detection of human herpes virus-8 latent nuclear antigen-1 is useful in the diagnosis of Kaposi sarcoma. *Mod Pathol.* 2004;17(4):456.

65. Weiss SW, Enzinger FM. Epithelioid hemangioendothelioma a vascular tumor often mistaken for a carcinoma. *Cancer.* 1982;50(5):970-981.

66. Antonescu CR, Le Loarer F, Mosquera JM, et al. Novel YAP1-TFE3 fusion defines a distinct subset of epithelioid hemangioendothelioma. *Genes Chromosomes Cancer.* 2013;52(8):775-784.

67. Quante M, Patel NK, Hill S, Merchant W, Courtauld E, Newman P, McKee PH. Epithelioid hemangioendothelioma presenting in the skin: a clinicopathologic study of eight cases. *Am J Dermatopathol.* 1998;20(6):541-546.

68. Mentzel T, Beham A, Calonje E, Katenkamp D, Fletcher CD. Epithelioid hemangioendothelioma of skin and soft tissues: clinicopathologic and immunohistochemical study of 30 cases. *Am J Surg Pathol.* 1997;21(4):363-374.

69. Miettinen M, Fetsch JF. Distribution of keratins in normal endothelial cells and a spectrum of vascular tumors: implications in tumor diagnosis. *Hum Pathol.* 2000;31(9):1062-1067.

70. Doyle LA, Fletcher CD, Hornick JL. Nuclear expression of CAMTA1 distinguishes epithelioid hemangioendothelioma from histologic mimics. *Am J Surg Pathol.* 2016;40(1):94-102.

71. Weedon D. Vascular Tumors. In: Weedon D, ed. *Weedon's Skin Pathology.* 3rd ed. Edinburgh, Scotland: Churchill/Livingstone/Elsevier; 2010:781-812.

72. Jeng MR, Fuh B, Blatt J, et al. Malignant transformation of infantile hemangioma to angiosarcoma: response to chemotherapy with bevacizumab. *Pediatr Blood Cancer.* 2014;61(11):2115-2117.

73. Manner J, Radlwimmer B, Hohenberger P, et al. MYC high level gene amplification is a distinctive feature of angiosarcomas after irradiation or chronic lymphedema. *Am J Pathol.* 2010;176(1):34-39.

74. Mentzel T, Schildhaus HU, Palmedo G, Büttner R, Kutzner H. Postradiation cutaneous angiosarcoma after treatment of breast carcinoma is characterized by MYC amplification in contrast to atypical vascular lesions after radiotherapy and control cases: clinicopathological, immunohistochemical and molecular analysis of 66 cases. *Mod Pathol.* 2012;25(1):75-85.

75. Shon W, Sukov WR, Jenkins SM, Folpe AL. MYC amplification and overexpression in primary cutaneous angiosarcoma: a fluorescence in-situ hybridization and immunohistochemical study. *Mod Pathol.* 2014;27(4):509-515.

76. Behjati S, Tarpey PS, Sheldon H, et al. Recurrent PTPRB and PLCG1 mutations in angiosarcoma. *Nat Genet.* 2014;46(4):376-379.

77. Piram M, Lorette G, Sirinelli D, Herbreteau D, Giraudeau B, Maruani A. Sturge-Weber syndrome in patients with facial port-wine stain. *Pediatr Dermatol.* 2012;29:32-37.

78. Shirley MD, Tang H, Gallione CJ, et al. Sturge–Weber syndrome and port-wine stains caused by somatic mutation in GNAQ. *N Engl J Med.* 2013;368(21):1971-1979.

79. Lee MS, Liang MG, Mulliken JB. Diffuse capillary malformation with overgrowth: a clinical subtype of vascular anomalies with hypertrophy. *J Am Acad Dermatol.* 2013;69(4):589-594.

80. Enjolras O. Vascular malformations. In: Bolognia JL, Jorizzo JL, Schaffer JV, eds. *Dermatology.* 3rd ed. Philadelphia, PA: WB Saunders, 2011:chap 104.

81. Greene AK, Tabler SF, Ball KL, et al. Sturge-Weber syndrome: soft-tissue and skeletal overgrowth. *J Craniofac Surg.* 2009;20(suppl 1):617-621.

82. Mills CM, Lanigan SW, Hughes J, et al. Demographic study of port wine stain patients attending a laser clinic: family history, prevalence of nevus anaemicus with results of prior treatment. *Clin Exp Dermatol.* 1997;22:166-168.

83. Sanchez-Carpintero I, Mihm MC, Mizeracki A, et al. Epithelial and mesenchymal hamartomatous changes in a mature port-wine stain: morphologic evidence for a multiple germ layer field defect. *J Am Acad Dermatol.* 2004;50:608-612.

84. Limaye N, Wouters V, Uebelhoer M, et al. Somatic mutations in an angiopoietin receptor gene TEK cause solitary and multiple sporadic venous malformations. *Nat Genet.* 2009;41(1):118.

85. Mazoyer E, Enjolras O, Bisdorff A, Perdu J, Wassef M, Drouet L. Coagulation disorders in patients with venous malformation of the limbs and trunk: a case series of 118 patients. *Arch Dermatol.* 2008;144(7):861-867.

86. Boon LM, Mulliken JB, Enjolras O, Vikkula M. Glomuvenous malformation (glomangioma) and venous malformation: distinct clinicopathologic and genetic entities. *Arch Dermatol.* 2004;140(8): 971-976.

87. Maguiness SM, Frieden IJ. Vascular birthmarks: tumors and malformations. In: Schachner LA, Hansen RC, eds. *Pediatric Dermatology.* 4th ed. Philadelphia, PA: Mosby, Elsevier; 2011.

88. Revencu N, Boon LM, Mulliken JB, et al. Parkes Weber syndrome, vein of Galen aneurysmal malformation, and other fast-flow vascular anomalies are caused by RASA1 mutations. *Hum Mut.* 2008;29(7):959-965.

89. Luks VL, Kamitaki N, Vivero MP, et al. Lymphatic and other vascular malformative/overgrowth disorders are caused by somatic mutations in PIK3CA. *J Pediatr.* 2015;166(4):1048-1054.

90. Castro EC, Galambos C. Prox-1 and VEGFR3 antibodies are superior to D2-40 in identifying endothelial cells of lymphatic malformations: a proposal of a new immunohistochemical panel to differentiate lymphatic from other vascular malformations. *Pediatr Dev Pathol.* 2009;12:187-194.

91. Tennant LB, Mulliken JB, Perez-Atayde AR, Kozakewich HP. Verrucous hemangioma revisited. *Pediatr Dermatol.* 2006;23(3):208-215.

92. Couto JA, Vivero MP, Kozakewich HP, et al. A somatic MAP3K3 mutation is associated with verrucous venous malformation. *Am J Hum Genet.* 2015;96(3):480-486.

93. Al Dhaybi R, Powell J, McCuaig C, Kokta V. Differentiation of vascular tumors from vascular malformations by expression of Wilms tumor 1 gene: evaluation of 126 cases. *J Am Acad Dermatol.* 2010;63(6):1052-1057.

94. Trindade F, Torrelo A, Requena L, et al. An immunohistochemical study of verrucous hemangiomas. *J Cutan Pathol.* 2013;40(5):472-476.

95. North PE, Kahn T, Cordisco RM, Dadra SS, Detmar M, Frieden JI. Multifocal lymphangioendotheliomatosis with thrombocytopenia: a newly recognized clinicopathological entity. *Arch Dermatol.* 2004;140:599-606

96. Prasad V, Fishman SJ, Mulliken JB, et al. Cutaneovisceral angiomatosis with thrombocytopenia. *Pediatr Dev Pathol.* 2005;8(4):407-419.

97. Piggott KD, Riedel PA, Baron HI. Multifocal lymphangioendotheliomatosis with thrombocytopenia: a rare cause of gastrointestinal bleeding in the newborn period. *Pediatrics.* 2006;117(4):e810-e813.

98. Croteau SE, Kozakewich HP, Perez-Atayde AR, et al. Kaposiform lymphangiomatosis: a distinct aggressive lymphatic anomaly. *J Pediatr.* 2014;164(2):383-388.

99. Safi F, Gupta A, Adams D, et al. Kaposiform lymphangiomatosis, a newly characterized vascular anomaly presenting with hemoptysis in an adult woman. *Ann Am Thorac Soc.* 2014;11(1):92-95.

100. Nosé V. Genodermatosis affecting the skin and mucosa of the head and neck: clinicopathologic, genetic, and molecular aspect—PTEN-Hamartoma tumor syndrome/Cowden syndrome. *Head Neck Pathol.* 2016;10(2):131-138.

101. Kurek KC, Howard E, Tenant L, et al. PTEN hamartoma of soft tissue: a distinctive lesion in PTEN syndromes. *Am J Surg Pathol.* 2012;36(5):671.

102. Alomari AI, Spencer SA, Arnold RW, et al. Fibro-adipose vascular anomaly: clinical-radiologic-pathologic features of a newly delineated disorder of the extremity. *J Pediatr Orthop.* 2014;34(1):109-117.

103. Fernandez-Pineda I, Marcilla D, Downey-Carmona FJ, Roldan S, Ortega-Laureano L, Bernabeu-Wittel J. Lower extremity fibro-adipose vascular anomaly (FAVA): a new case of a newly delineated disorder. *Ann Vasc Dis.* 2014;7(3):316-319.

104. Erickson J, McAuliffe W, Blennerhassett L, Halbert A. Fibroadipose vascular anomaly treated with sirolimus: successful outcome in two patients. *Pediatr Dermatol.* 2017;34(6):e317-e320.

105. Uller W, Fishman SJ, Alomari AI. Overgrowth syndromes with complex vascular anomalies. *Semin Pediatr Surg.* 2014;23(4):208-215.

106. Pelle MT, Pride HB, Tyler WB. Eccrine angiomatous hamartoma. *J Am Acad Dermatol.* 2002;47(3):429-435.

107. Patterson AT, Kumar MG, Bayliss SJ, Witman PM, Dehner LP, Gru AA. Eccrine angiomatous hamartoma: a clinicopathologic review of 18 cases. *Am J Dermatopathol.* 2016;38(6):413-417.

26

Histiocytic Neoplasms

Michael A. Cardis / A. Yasmine Kirkorian / Alejandro A. Gru

INTRODUCTION

A recent update in the classification of histiocytic disorders of adults and children has been proposed, which provides integration of cell of origin of these disorders, in addition to common molecular pathways that appear to be altered in this group of neoplasms. To this extent, histiocytoses can be divided into five major categories: (1) Langerhans related ("L"); (2) cutaneous and mucocutaneous ("C"); (3) malignant histiocytoses ("M"); (4) Rosai-Dorfman disease (RDD; "R"); and (5) hemophagocytic lymphohistiocytosis and macrophage activation syndrome ("H").[1] The "L" group includes Langerhans cell histiocytosis (LCH), indeterminate cell histiocytosis (ICH), Erdheim-Chester disease (ECD), mixed LCH/ECD, and the disseminated forms of juvenile xanthogranuloma (JXG). They all share clonal mutations involving genes in the MAPK pathway in >80% of cases; the "C" group incorporates the cutaneous xanthogranulomas (JXG, adult xanthogranuloma, solitary reticulohistiocytoma [SRH], benign cephalic histiocytosis [BCH], generalized eruptive histiocytosis [GEH], and progressive nodular histiocytosis [PNH]) and non–xanthogranulomatous disorders (cutaneous RDD and necrobiotic xanthogranuloma). The "R" group includes familial RDD, in addition to the sporadic extracutaneous forms (classical, extranodal, etc). The "M" group is an extraordinary rare group of disorders that include histiocytic, interdigitating dendritic cell, Langerhans cell, or indeterminate cell sarcomas. Finally, the "H" group includes the primary and secondary hemophagocytic lymphohistiocytosis. In this chapter, we will only focus on the diseases that primarily affect the skin.

GROUP "L" HISTIOCYTOSES

LANGERHANS CELL HISTIOCYTOSIS

Definition and Epidemiology

LCH (formerly histiocytosis X) represents a clonal proliferation of immature dendritic cells expressing CD1a and CD207 (langerin—surrogate marker for the presence of Birbeck granules) producing a clinical picture ranging from a focal lesion to disseminated disease affecting numerous organ tissues.[2] LCH was initially described as three different diseases, each with a unique clinical picture: eosinophilic granuloma, Hand-Schüller-Christian disease, and Letterer-Siwe disease. Although the aforementioned nomenclature has been abandoned for the use of LCH or Langerhans cell disease, they are still useful to illustrate the various clinical courses that LCH can encompass.[3,4]

Langerhans cell proliferations include reactive Langerhans cell hyperplasia, LCH, Langerhans cell sarcoma (LCS), and congenital self-healing reticulohistiocytosis (CSHR).[5,6] Debate still lingers on the nature of LCH, almost 20 years after the publication of the study with the demonstration of clonality in nonpulmonary LCH lesions.[7] Newer data now show evidence of a clonal myeloid cell origin for LCH.[8-14] Despite a rare overall incidence in the general population, LCH has a strong predilection for children and particularly an aggressive clinical course in the very young individuals, typically less than 2 years of age at diagnosis.[7,15,16] Nowadays, LCH is considered the prototypic histiocytosis from the "L" group.

LCH is most common in children and in white individuals of northern European ancestry and is usually diagnosed before age 4.[3,17] The estimated incidence of LCH in patients less than 15 years old is 4 to 5 cases per million per year.[3,18] LCH has a slight male predominance and is considered a sporadic disease, although a familial predisposition has been reported.[19]

Etiology

There has been much debate as to whether LCH represents a reactive or neoplastic illness. Evidence to support the former includes the following. LCH lesions may spontaneously resolve, there is no evidence as to the immortalization of the LCH cells in the laboratory, and proinflammatory cytokines and chemokines contribute to the pathogenesis of LCH.[3] However, in 2010, it was discovered that in a large proportion of LCH cases (greater than half of cases), there is a gain-of-function somatic mutation in lesional cells involving *BRAF (V600E)*, resulting in uncontrolled activation of the MAPK pathway (RAS/RAF/MEK/ERK).[20] It was also noted that even in wild-type *BRAF* cases of LCH, ERK remained phosphorylated, suggesting that even in those cases other mutations (such as *MAP2K1*) in the same pathway are responsible for the disease. Indeed, MAPK is active in all LCH lesions, and LCH involves a clonal proliferation of cells, thus providing strong evidence that LCH is a neoplastic disease. Berres et al found a prevalence of 64% for *BRAF* mutations in LCH and particularly a high risk of recurrence among the mutated cases.[11] Héritier et al found that the mutation showed correlation with high-risk features, increased risk of recurrence, and increased resistance to first-line therapies.[21] Whole-exome sequencing subsequently identified the presence of *MAP2K1* (*MEK1*) mutations in 7 of 21 cases of LCH with wild-type *BRAF* and in none of 20 *BRAF V600E* mutant cases. These studies implicate aberrations of the MAPK signaling pathway in the pathogenesis of LCH and strongly support a neoplastic pathogenesis.[22-25]

It has also recently been proposed that the timing and/or location at which point the disease-initiating cell acquires the mutation dictates the extent of disease, that is, mutations in premature CD34[+] progenitor cells of the hematopoietic system lead to severe disease, whereas mutations in more differentiated cell such as lesional CD207[+] cells in the skin lead to more localized disease.[2,26] The propensity for LCH to induce osteolytic lesions is thought to result from an interaction between T-lymphocytes and lesional LCH cells, causing production of cytokines that stimulate the differentiation and activation of osteoclasts that produce destructive enzymes.

Clinical Presentation

The clinical presentation of LCH is broad and ranges from a solitary osteolytic lesion (eosinophilic granuloma/unifocal LCH) to multifocal bone disease that may include the triad of osteolytic bone lesions, diabetes insipidus, and exophthalmos (Hand-Schüller-Christian disease/multifocal unisystem LCH) to an aggressive, disseminated life-threatening form of disease (Letterer-Siwe disease/disseminated multifocal multisystem LCH). Those clinical presentations were later understood to represent a spectrum of the same illness that for a while was termed histiocytosis X, a term that was later replaced by LCH.[26,27] The clinical classification of LCH is stratified into single organ system disease (SS-LCH) and multiorgan system disease (MS-LCH) in addition to unifocal versus multifocal involvement. Furthermore, MS-LCH is further classified according to whether or not there is involvement of risk organs such as the lung, liver, spleen, or bone marrow (RO-positive vs. RO-negative MS-LCH).[3] SS-LCH represents up to 70% of cases, whereas only about 10% of cases end up with RO-positive MS-LCH.[3] The most common site of involvement in SS-LCH is bone, in either a focal or multifocal pattern, followed by skin, lymph node, and lung.[17,28] The bone is involved in about 80% of LCH patients and may either be asymptomatic or produce pain. In pediatric cases, the skull is the most commonly affected site, and on plain film shows punched-out osteolytic lesions with crisp margins. Organ system involvement in MS-LCH may include a wide array of systems, but prominent ones include the bone and skin followed by the liver, spleen, and bone marrow (hematopoietic system). Almost half of all LCH cases will involve the skin to some extent during the disease course, and up to 13% of patients will have disease exclusively involving the skin at the time of diagnosis.[28] This variability in distribution and extent of involvement best explains the long list of clinical designations under the LCH umbrella.[29]

The most common presenting signs/symptoms of LCH are the following: soft tissue mass, bone pain, skin rash, fever, otorrhea, and/or lymphadenopathy.[3] Skin findings in LCH are variable and can include numerous morphologies, among which the most notorious clinical picture is that of an erythematous, scaly dermatitis in a seborrheic distribution involving the scalp, postauricular skin, axillae, and diaper area. Other morphologic findings include "blueberry muffin"–like nodules, petechia, vesicles, or red to brown papules and plaques, often with secondary changes such as erosion, crusting, bleeding, or ulceration located in the scalp, ears, flexures, or acral sites.[27,28,30] Ulcerations may occur in the axillary or inguinal folds. Isolated skin involvement by LCH is infrequent and occurs in <5% of all cases. Skin-limited LCH occurs in the form of one or multiple, often asymptomatic but occasionally erosive, papules or nodules with surrounding erythema or rarely forming masses with or without ulceration (Figure 26-1). One study documented mucosal involvement—most frequently the oral or genital mucosa—in 20% of cases with otherwise isolated skin LCH (Figure 26-2).[31] The gingiva, when involved, presents with swelling or ulceration. Bone and central nervous system (CNS) involvement can produce serious sequelae such as exophthalmos, conductive hearing loss, loss

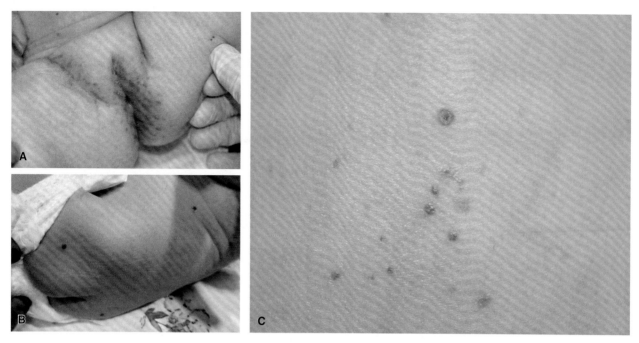

FIGURE 26-1. **Langerhans cell histiocytosis (LCH).** A, Multiple excoriated papules within the inguinal and vaginal area. B, Red-brown nodules in the back. C, The papules in LCH can have an umbilicated appearance.

of teeth, and even spinal paralysis. If the hypothalamic-pituitary axis is involved, central diabetes insipidus may ensue, as may other endocrinologic or hypothalamic symptoms. Even with treatment and cure of disease, there can be permanent complications. Prognosis is based on involvement of high-risk organ systems (liver, spleen, lung, and bone marrow), as well as response to 6 weeks of standard treatment.[2,32] Children with RO-positive MS-LCH have a mortality that ranges from 10% to 50%. Skin-limited disease portends an excellent prognosis.[3]

Systemic symptoms including fever, lymphadenopathy, hepatosplenomegaly, and cytopenias can be seen in multisystem disease, together with clinical manifestations of organ dysfunction such as diabetes insipidus in cases with pituitary involvement. Such clinical manifestations warrant the staging of LCH using bone scans and magnetic resonance imaging of the brain, in addition to blood evaluation for electrolyte imbalances.

Histologic Findings

A common unifying theme in all of these lesions/clinical entities is the histologic demonstration of Langerhans cells in aggregates despite the admixture with eosinophils, macrophages, lymphocytes, neutrophils, and non-neoplastic multinucleated giant cells.[33-36] The diagnosis of LCH can be tentatively made based on the characteristic morphologic findings of the Langerhans cells that are medium to large in size, exhibit abundant eosinophilic cytoplasm, and have a "coffee bean"–shaped grooved nuclei (Figures 26-3 and 26-4).[37] They also have fine chromatin and indistinct, small nucleoli, and scattered mitoses may be visualized. These characteristic features although best seen on cytologic preparations can also be appreciated in a well-fixed and well-prepared histologic section. Involvement of the skin may be confined to small collections of cells at the dermal-epidermal interface with variable basal vacuolar degeneration or as dense infiltrates throughout the dermis with or without the formation of eosinophilic abscesses. Marked epidermotropism

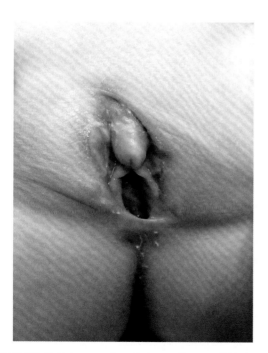

FIGURE 26-2. Vulvar erosions in Langerhans cell histiocytosis.

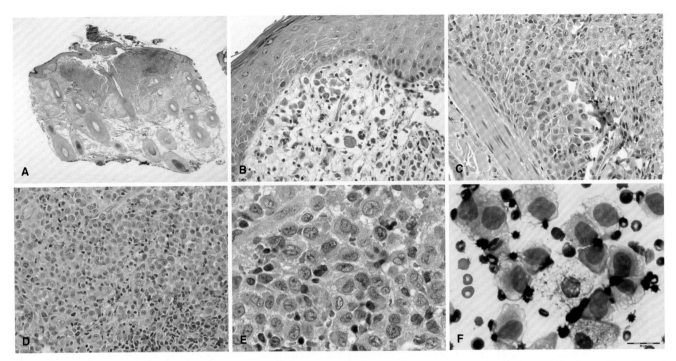

FIGURE 26-3. Langerhans cell histiocytosis (LCH)—histopathologic findings. A and B, The lesion has a folliculocentric pattern. C to E, Sheets of atypical Langerhans cells are seen with frequent nuclear grooves. F, Smear of LCH.

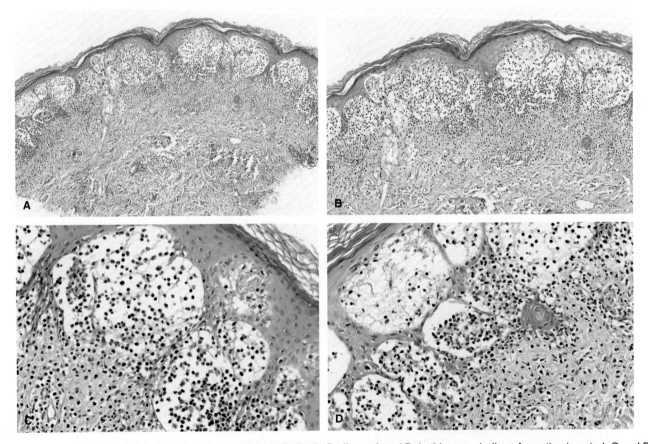

FIGURE 26-4. Langerhans cell histiocytosis—histopathologic findings. A and B, In this case, bullous formation is noted. C and D, Extensive epidermotropism is noted. Digital slides courtesy of Path Presenter.com.

is also frequently seen (Figure 26-5). Extravasated erythrocytes and a mixed inflammatory infiltrate with eosinophils, lymphocytes, neutrophils, plasma cells, and histiocytes (sometimes multinucleate giant cells, osteoclast like) are often present, and there are occasionally areas of focal necrosis.[17] The LCH cells often aggregate into granulomas. As the time course of disease progresses, macrophages tend to predominate, and xanthomatous and fibrotic change may become prominent findings.

Confirmation of the diagnosis is achieved by demonstrating Langerhans granules (Birbeck granules) on electron microscopy[38] or—more easily—by the characteristic positivity of Langerhans cells for CD1a, S-100, and langerin (Figure 26-5). The langerin immunostain is used, by many, as a surrogate marker for the presence of Birbeck granules.[39-43] Langerin (CD207), a cell surface glycoprotein receptor of the lectin family indicative of Birbeck granule formation, is highly sensitive and specific for LCH. CD207 has mostly replaced ultrastructural studies (electron microscopy) in diagnosing LCH. Langerin has similar sensitivity, but slightly less specificity for LCH when compared to CD1a.[3,33,44]

A careful distinction between reactive dermatoses with associated Langerhans cell hyperplasias and LCH is important to be made, in order to avoid overdiagnosing LCH. LCH typically fills the papillary and/or deeper dermis and sometimes can show a perifollicular and epidermal distribution. Chronic dermatoses often show increased number of perivascular and perifollicular dendritic cells that are CD1a+/langerin low to negative. Contact dermatitis shows frequent small intraepidermal clusters of Langerhans cells that lack significant cytologic atypia.[36] Immunohistochemistry for cyclin D1 and p53 has also shown an adjunct role in distinguishing reactive (negative staining) Langerhans cell hyperplasias, from neoplastic (positive staining) forms.[45,46]

Differential Diagnosis

LCH is often discernable based on its characteristic cytology and unique immunohistochemical pattern. Non-neoplastic, reactive Langerhans cell hyperplasia secondary to an exogenous inflammatory insult such as an eczematous dermatitis, bug bites, or scabies should be considered. Non-LCH disorders such as JXG and ECD may

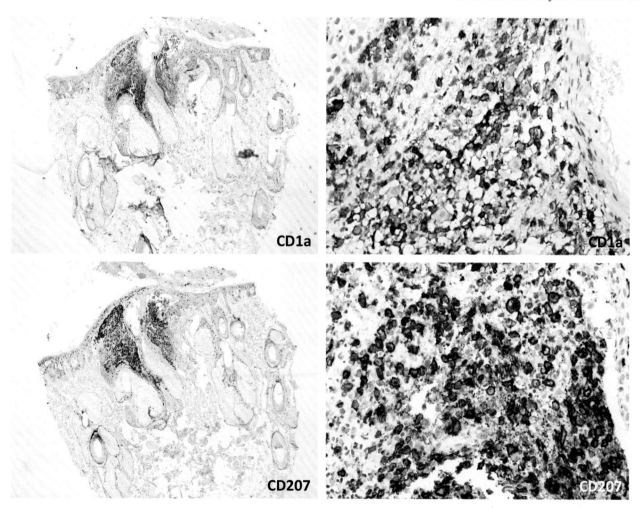

FIGURE 26-5. Langerhans cell histiocytosis—immunohistochemistry. The atypical Langerhans cells are positive for CD1a and CD207 (langerin).

mimic LCH at various time points. Other entities that may be considered include lymphoma, LCS, malignant melanoma, and cutaneous T-cell lymphoma, most of which are easily differentiated based on immunohistochemistry. Melanoma can be ruled out based on staining for melanocytic markers. Also, melanoma usually starts in the epidermis and invades deeper tissues, whereas in LCH, the infiltrate centers in the papillary dermis, is associated with a mixed cell infiltrate, and spreads up to the epidermis via epidermotropism. ECD is a multisystem histiocytosis that often involves bone, but lesions contain foamy histiocytes and a different immunoprofile than that of LCH. JXG is characterized by foamy histiocytes and Touton giant cells, although the morphology of JXG varies based on the stage of the lesion (see Section "Juvenile Xanthogranuloma").

CAPSULE SUMMARY

LANGERHANS CELL HISTIOCYTOSIS

Today LCH is considered the prototypic histiocytosis from the "L" group. LCH cells are arranged in clusters and sheets in the papillary dermis and have abundant eosinophilic cytoplasm and irregular, reniform, or folded vesicular nuclei with longitudinal grooves. Epidermotropism may be a feature. By immunohistochemistry LCH shows the following phenotypes: CD1a[+], S-100[+], CD207/langerin[+]; CD68 is variable. Birbeck granules are present on electron microscopy, but CD207 is a surrogate marker.

CONGENITAL SELF-HEALING RETICULOHISTIOCYTOSIS (HASHIMOTO-PRITZKER DISEASE)

Definition and Epidemiology

CSHR (Hashimoto-Pritzker disease), initially described by Hashimoto and Pritzker in 1973, is generally considered to be a unique, self-limited variant of LCH that presents in the neonatal period and resolves spontaneously.[47] CSHR is a disease mostly of neonates and sometimes in infants with no gender predilection.[48] It is rarely reported, but may be underestimated because of its self-limited and often short-lived clinical course.[49] The etiology is poorly understood, but it's likely related to other common forms of LCH.

Clinical Presentation

CSHR presents at birth or in the neonatal period with an eruption of red-brown papules, nodules, or vesicles in a generalized distribution and can involve the mucosa (Figure 26-6).[48] Rarely, CSHR presents as a solitary lesion. Secondary changes such as ulceration or crusting may be present. Cutaneous disease is typically self-limited, lasting weeks to months, and it rarely progresses to involve internal organs. It is difficult to predict when systemic involvement, relapse after cutaneous resolution, or a more aggressive clinical course will occur. There are no criteria for easily distinguishing CSHR from systemic LCH except for its clinical course; therefore, evaluation for systemic disease at the time of diagnosis and long-term follow-up are paramount.[49]

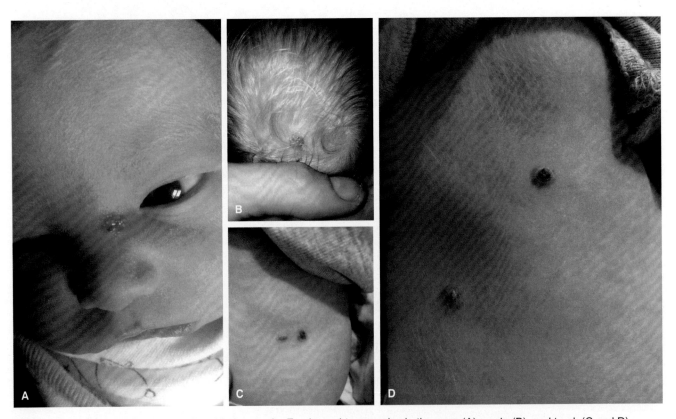

FIGURE 26-6. Congenital self-healing histiocytosis. Erosive red-tan papules in the nose (A), scalp (B), and trunk (C and D).

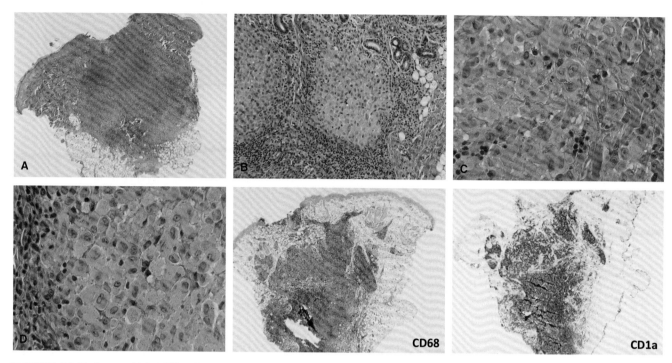

FIGURE 26-7. Congenital self-healing reticulohistiocytosis—histopathology. A, Deep dermal-based nodule with central areas of necrosis. B, The infiltrate has a nodular appearance. C and D, The infiltrate is composed of atypical Langerhans cells. The cells are positive for CD68 and CD1a.

Poor prognostic indicators are later age of onset and/or the presence of systemic involvement.[47,50,51]

Histologic Findings

The histologic picture of CSHR is similar to that of LCH, and differentiation of the two entities is primarily clinical as they likely represent polar ends of a clinical spectrum of the same disease (Figure 26-7).[47,52-54] In CSHR-LCH, lesions typically involve the deep dermis in a nodular fashion, unlike conventional LCH lesions where lesions are mainly in the upper dermis, extending to epidermis. Both clinical entities show similar staining with CD1a, S-100, and langerin. Langerhans cells of congenital self-healing LCH may show Birbeck granules similar to conventional LCH cells by electron microscopy; however, they can be separated ultrastructurally by the presence of unique cytoplasmic dense bodies containing concentrically arranged laminar structures. The differential diagnosis is similar to cases of ordinary LCH.

CAPSULE SUMMARY

CONGENITAL SELF-HEALING RETICULOHISTIOCYTOSIS (HASHIMOTO-PRITZKER DISEASE)

CSHR presents at birth or in the neonatal period with an eruption of red-brown papules, nodules, or vesicles in a generalized distribution and can involve the mucosa. Cutaneous disease is typically self-limited, lasting weeks to months, and it rarely progresses to involve internal organs. The histologic picture of CSHR is similar to that of LCH, and differentiation of the two entities is primarily clinical as they likely represent polar ends of a clinical spectrum of the same disease.

ERDHEIM-CHESTER DISEASE

Definition and Epidemiology

ECD, first reported by Erdheim and Chester as "lipid granulomatosis" in 1930, is a rare, multisystemic non-LCH that almost always affects bones, but can additionally involve almost any organ system.[55] It is characterized by a disseminated xanthogranulomatous infiltration of organs with foamy histiocytes, progressive fibrosis, and ultimately organ failure.[56] It's now included under the group "L" of histiocytosis, given the characteristic molecular profile.

ECD is rare with about 550 cases reported, and the overall prevalence is unknown. ECD is typically diagnosed in adulthood and is very uncommon in childhood,[57,58] with around 10 reported cases to date. The average age of onset is 53 years, and the male to female ratio is about 3:1.[55,57,59]

Etiology

The etiology has not been completely elucidated, but it is thought to be neoplastic in nature, representing a hematopoietic neoplasm of histiocytic origin, versus less likely a purely reactive/inflammatory process. Recently, ECD has been associated with a mutation in the *BRAF* proto-oncogene in greater than 50% of cases, establishing that the disorder is clonal in nature and supporting a neoplastic process, perhaps with a shared origin to that of LCH.[55,56,59,60] Additionally, mutations in the MAPK (such as in *NRAS*) and PIK3 pathways have been reported. Another finding in support of a Langerhans cell relationship is the fact that 20% of biopsies of ECD have coexistent LCH.[1,61] However, these data were only based on small case series and case reports.

Clinical Presentation

The disease is diagnosed most often between 40 and 60 years of age, and bone pain accompanied by fatigue is the most common presentation, with the skeletal system being involved in 95% of cases of ECD. Pathognomonic radiographic features are bilateral, symmetric, and multifocal osteosclerotic changes of the diametaphyseal regions of long bones sparing the epiphyses. This is in contrast to the lytic lesions seen in LCH, which typically affect the skull and not the long bones.[60,62] Diagnosis is based on a combination of clinical, histologic, and radiographic features. Skin involvement, which occurs in up to a third of cases, typically includes xanthoma-like papules and periorbital xanthelasma–like plaques, and less commonly red-brown papular lesions of the trunk and extremities (Figure 26-8).[57,60,63] In ECD, the periorbital plaques are often more nodular than xanthelasma and may extend into the temporal region, cheeks, or subpalpebral areas—such irregularities in addition to a normal patient lipid profile should raise the consideration that the lesions may be more than simple xanthelasma.

Clinical presentations of ECD vary broadly based on which organ systems are involved and can include: exophthalmos, papilledema, papulonodular skin lesions, endocrine dysfunction (from pituitary involvement), diabetes insipidus, lung disease, retroperitoneal fibrosis, renal failure, cardiomyopathy, and CNS disorder.[55,59] Almost all patients have extraskeletal involvement, with cardiac and neurologic involvement harboring the worst prognosis.[62] Bilateral, symmetric sclerosing bone lesions in the metaphysis of long bones, usually the distal femur and proximal tibia and fibula, are the diagnostic imaging features.[13,24,25,57,64] The 3-year mortality rate from time of diagnosis is estimated to be about 60%, and the most common causes of death include respiratory or cardiac failure.[56,65]

Histologic Findings

The histology of ECD, which is not entirely specific, shows a dense dermal infiltrate of bland, foamy histiocytes with variable amounts of intervening fibrosis, Touton giant cells, and mixed inflammatory cells such as plasma cells and lymphocytes.[66] Biopsy from involved internal sites yields comparable histologic findings (Figures 26-8 and 26-9).

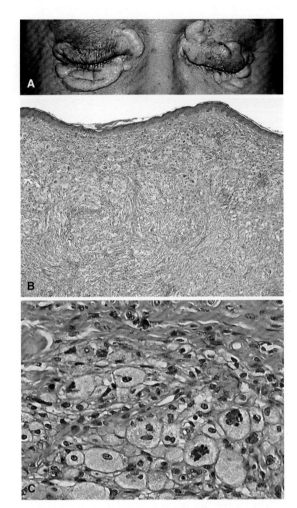

FIGURE 26-8. Erdheim-Chester disease (ECD). Xanthelasma-like tumors as cutaneous ECD manifestations. A, Large xanthelasma-like tumor around the eyes. B, Diffuse accumulation of foamy cells, fibrosis of the connective tissue (hematoxylin and eosin ×40). C, Multiple Touton giant cell and hemosiderin deposits in the dermis (hematoxylin and eosin ×400). Obtained with permission. Liersch J, Carlson JA, Schaller J. Histopathological and clinical findings in cutaneous manifestation of Erdheim–Chester disease and Langerhans cell histiocytosis overlap syndrome associated with the BRAFV600E mutation. *Am J Dermatopathol.* 2017;39(7):493-503. doi:10.1097/DAD.0000000000000793.

Cytological atypia is not a feature. ECD shares resemblance with other non-LCH such as progressed JXG, where fibrosis becomes a predominant feature. The immunohistochemical profile of the foamy macrophages is positive for CD68, CD163, CD14, and factor XIIIa and negative for S-100, CD1a, and CD207.[59] ECD-associated xanthelasma-like plaques have more multinucleate and Touton giant cells and have less fibrosis than common xanthelasma. When encountering xanthelasma-like lesions, testing for *BRAF* mutation is indicated when there is a high clinical suspicion for ECD.[63,67,68] In children, ECD can occur in association with lymphoblastic leukemias and LCH.[57,58,69,70] ECD can also have a presentation that mimics multicentric reticulohistiocytosis (MRH).[71]

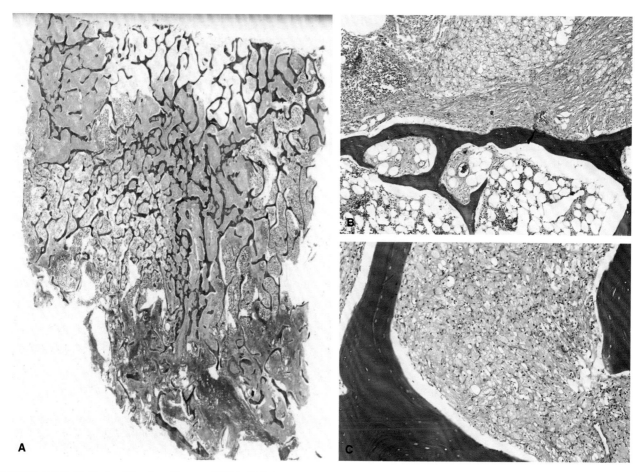

FIGURE 26-9. Erdheim-Chester disease (ECD). This bone marrow biopsy shows the classic morphologic findings of ECD involvement. A and B, There is a diffuse histiocytic infiltrate replacing most of the bone marrow space. C, The infiltrate is composed of foamy histiocytes and scattered multinucleated giant cells.

Differential Diagnosis

The clinical differential diagnosis includes other systemic diseases, such as systemic JXG, xanthoma disseminatum (XD), RDD, LCH, sarcoidosis, amyloidosis, and storage disorders. The histiocytic cells of ECD are positive for CD163 and CD68, whereas being negative for CD1a and langerin. Some cases can have partial expression of S-100. Additionally, a recent study has shown expression of the programmed cell death ligand 1 (PD-L1) protein in a subset of histiocytoses, including ECD disease, suggesting a possible role of immune checkpoint blockade in treatment. Rare cases with histologic and immunophenotypic features of ECD, but with strong ALK expression and rearrangement of the *ALK* gene, can be seen. Such cases are examples of ALK+ histiocytosis of childhood and not ECD.[72] ECD is often progressive and fatal despite aggressive therapy. The recent identification of various mutations in ECD has resulted in some success with targeted therapies, such as with vemurafenib. In a recent pangenomic analysis, all cases of ECD had at least one mutation activating the MAPK pathway.[23] In addition, in-frame fusions involving several kinases including *BRAF, ALK,* and *NTRK1* were identified in ECD without *BRAF, MAP2K1,* or *N/KRAS* point mutations.[13,24,25] ECD should

also be distinguished from JXG. As opposed to JXG, ECD more frequently harbors the *BRAF V600E* mutation. ECD also has the typical clinical and radiographic findings, not present in cases of JXG. The recently reported cases of *BRAF*-mutated JXG are now believed to be examples of ECD.[73,74]

CAPSULE SUMMARY

ERDHEIM-CHESTER DISEASE

ECD is a rare, multisystemic non-LCH that almost always affects bones, but can additionally involve almost any organ system. It is characterized by a disseminated xanthogranulomatous infiltration of organs with foamy histiocytes, progressive fibrosis, and ultimately organ failure. It is now included under the group "L" of histiocytosis, given the characteristic molecular profile. The histopathology of ECD is reminiscent of other non-LCH. There is a dense dermal infiltrate of foamy histiocytes with variable amounts of intervening fibrosis. Touton giant cells and mixed inflammatory cells are also seen. It is important to consider testing for *BRAF* mutation to help distinguish from xanthelasma if clinical suspicion exists.

INDETERMINATE DENDRITIC CELL TUMOR

Definition and Epidemiology

Indeterminate dendritic cell tumor (IDCT) is a rare histiocytic proliferative disorder that is thought to originate from dermal indeterminate histiocytes that typically share the immunophenotype of macrophages (CD68[+]) and Langerhans cells (expressing S-100 and CD1a). Indeterminate cells lack Birbeck granules—the ultrastructural pathognomonic feature of Langerhans cells—and they are nonreactive with antibodies to langerin (also known as CD207, an immunohistochemical marker that indicates the presence of Birbeck granules).[75] It was first reported by Wood et al in 1985.[76] IDCT is very rare (less than 50 reported cases), making the epidemiology and demographics difficult to assess. It can occur at any age, including childhood, but appears to be more prevalent in adults, and it has no gender predilection.[75,77-80] The updated revision of cutaneous histiocytoses includes IDCT in the "L" ("Langerhans") group.

Etiology

The cause of IDCT is unknown. Some consider the indeterminate cell to be an immature Langerhans cell that has not yet developed Birbeck granules.[76] It has been reported in association with hematologic malignancies such as B-cell lymphoma.[81] It has also been reported to be triggered by pityriasis rosea and scabies.[79] Recently, Brown et al described three cases of IDCT with an *ETV3-NCOA2* translocation.[82] That abnormality has not been identified in other histiocytic lesions, and it provides solid evidence that some IDCTs do indeed represent a neoplasm with a recurrent molecular aberration.

Clinical Presentation

IDCT is mostly a disease of the skin and usually presents as either solitary or multiple pink to red papules and nodules on the trunk, extremities, and/or head and neck, sparing the mucosa. The lesions are typically asymptomatic and may either be generalized or focal in distribution. Extracutaneous manifestations that have been reported include nodal, corneal, osseous, and genital involvement (Figure 26-10). ICH usually engenders a benign clinical course, especially when not associated with systemic illness such as hematologic malignancy, and it resolves spontaneously without treatment.[75,81]

Histologic Findings

The histologic picture of IDCT is that of a dense dermal infiltrate composed of large, monomorphous mononuclear cells with vesicular nuclei (occasionally reniform) and abundant pale cytoplasm.[83] Cases with a spindle cell morphology have been reported (Figure 26-11).[78,84] Multinucleate (Touton) and/or xanthomatized cells may be seen.[85,86] There may be scattered inflammatory cells present as well.[76] Epidermotropism is typical of ICH, but mitoses may be seen. Immunophenotype: *CD1a+, S-100+, CD68+, langerin (CD207), Birbeck granules* (Figure 26-12). An *S-100*-negative variant has been reported.[77]

Differential Diagnosis

The most important entity on the differential diagnosis is LCH, which, unlike IDCT, displays positivity for CD207 (langerin) and contains Birbeck granules. CD207 (langerin) is an immunohistochemical stain for a protein found in Birbeck granules and can be used in lieu of electron microscopy. Furthermore, in LCH, there is often epidermotropism, intercellular edema, and clinically internal involvement. Up to 50% of cases of LCH have *BRAF V600E* mutations, a feature that is much less prevalent in IDCT. Non-LCH such as JXG and generalized eruptive histiocytoma often resemble IDCT, both clinically and histologically, but the

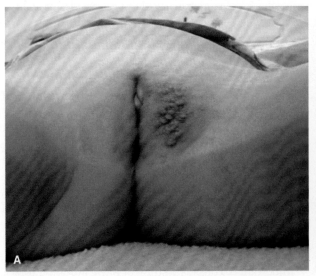
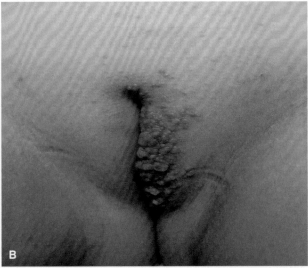

FIGURE 26-10. Indeterminate dendritic cell tumor. A and B, Multiple papules in the vulvar area.

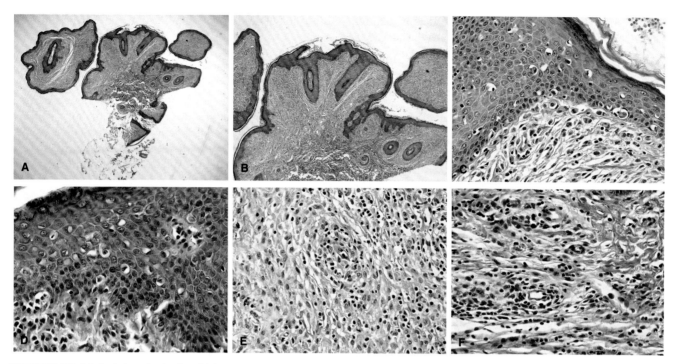

FIGURE 26-11. Indeterminate dendritic cell tumor—histopathologic findings. A and B, In this case, there is a dermal-based histiocytic proliferation accompanied by epidermal acanthosis and papillomatosis. C and D, The infiltrate shows epidermotropism. Within the dermis, the atypical histiocytes show a spindle cell appearance (E), and scattered eosinophils are seen (F).

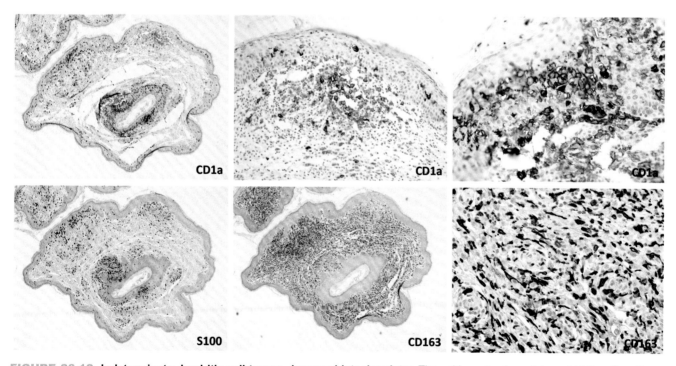

FIGURE 26-12. Indeterminate dendritic cell tumor—immunohistochemistry. The epidermotropic and dermal histiocytic cells are positive for CD1a, S-100, and CD163.

immunohistochemical profile of the disorders is distinct, with ICH demonstrating positivity for S-100 and CD1a, both of which are negative in the non-LCH disorders.

CAPSULE SUMMARY

INDETERMINATE DENDRITIC CELL TUMOR

IDCT is a rare histiocytic proliferative disorder that is thought to originate from dermal indeterminate histiocytes that typically share the immunophenotype of macrophages (CD68$^+$) and Langerhans cells (expressing S-100 and CD1a). The lesional cells are langerin negative (CD207) and show absence of Birbeck granules. The *ETV3-NCOA2* translocation has been demonstrated in a subset of cases.

GROUP "C" HISTIOCYTOSES

JUVENILE XANTHOGRANULOMA

Definition and Epidemiology

JXG (xanthogranuloma, nevoxanthoendothelioma) is a self-limited non-LCH involving proliferation of cholesterol-laden monocyte-derived macrophages that most commonly occur in the first year of life.[87] Although JXG are typically benign and confined to the skin, rarely, they may involve extracutaneous sites or be associated with other disease processes.[88] JXG is the most common form of non-LCH and is currently classified as group "C" for the cutaneous limited forms and in the "L" category for the systemic variants.[1] The exact incidence is unknown as most cases are diagnosed based upon clinical findings and without histologic confirmation. One study reported that JXG represents only 0.5% of pediatric tumors. Most cases are diagnosed in infants and young children, often in the first year or two of life.[89-91] Males are slightly affected more often than females, especially when lesions are multiple. Less commonly, JXG occurs in adolescents and young adults and in some cases may be difficult to differentiate from ECD, except for the *BRAF V600E* mutations.

Although primarily a disease of childhood, it may occur in adults as well. It is slightly more common in boys (1.5:1) and is more often reported in Caucasians. Given their transient and classically benign nature, they are likely underdiagnosed, especially by nondermatology physicians. Furthermore, JXG often presents as a small, solitary lesion that may easily be mistaken for a common benign melanocytic nevus.[92]

Etiology

The pathogenesis of JXG is poorly understood.[91] It has been postulated to represent a reactive process to an unknown stimulus or injury, but this has not been verified in studies.[92,93] There may be genetic mutations that play a role in the pathogenesis of JXG, such as that seen in several other histiocytoses like LCH and ECD, and this is currently being studied.[75,94]

JXG can be associated with neurofibromatosis type 1 (NF1) and juvenile myelomonocytic leukemia (JMML). Nearly 5% to 10% of NF1 patients and up to 30% of NF1 patients less than 2 years of age have been reported to have JXG. The presence of café au lait macules and JXG should suggest the likelihood of NF1. The association among JXG, NF1, and JMML, while well described, is poorly understood in terms of the pathogenetic relationships. JXG usually precedes JMML; however, it is unclear if JXG is a reliable marker for the subsequent development of JMML in NF1 patients. It has been suggested that mutations in the GTPase *neurofibromin*, which is present in NF1, lead to RAS dysfunction and downregulation of Fas antigen, with subsequent dysregulation of apoptosis in hematopoietic cells with the development of leukemia and JXG. Some cases of JXG follow the diagnosis of LCH.[95-102] More recently, systemic presentations of JXG with CNS involvement have shown *BRAF V600E* mutations.[73,74] The question that arises from these is: should those cases be qualified as ECD/L group lesions that haven't presented themselves with systemic findings (ie, brain only) or is there a truly separate group of JXG/*BRAF V600E*–positive tumors?

Clinical Presentation

JXG often presents very early in life. Indeed, about 10% are present at birth and up to 70% occur within the first year of life. They rarely occur in the adult population, and they are not associated with lipid abnormalities. The classic presentation of JXG is the abrupt onset of a firm, painless, and freely mobile papulonodule (Figure 26-13). JXG appears as a solitary nodule in 60% to 80% of cases, and the head and neck are the most common locations. Less common cutaneous sites include the genitalia, soles, and fingers.[64,102-104] The shape of the lesion can vary greatly, as it may be keratotic, pedunculated, linear, flat, or plaque like. The papules or nodules are usually 5 to 10 mm in diameter but can measure up to a few centimeters.[105-107] Initially, the lesion is raised and pink to erythematous in color, but over time, they become yellow-brown and may flatten as the histiocytes undergo xanthomatous transformation and regression (Figure 26-14). Regression may occur over a period of months to years with residual hyperpigmentation, atrophy, or anetoderma. Telangiectatic blood vessels or ulceration may be seen overlying the lesion, which imparts a resemblance to pyogenic granuloma. Multiple skin lesions occur infrequently, in less than 10% of cases.[89] JXG is mostly asymptomatic, but on occasion may be pruritic, painful, and/or ulcerate. The characteristic finding on dermoscopy is the "setting sun" pattern in which the center of the lesion is yellow surrounded by a circumferential orange-red rim.[108]

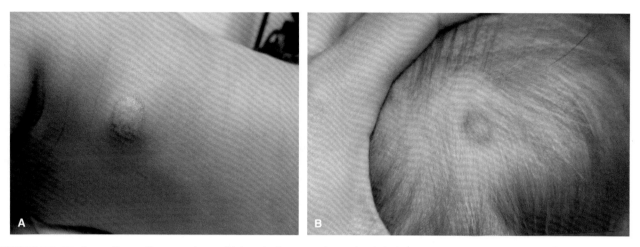

FIGURE 26-13. **Juvenile xanthogranuloma.** Mature lesions: xanthomatized plaques on the trunk (A) and scalp (B).

Although JXG is typically limited to the skin in the majority of cases, it may arise in extracutaneous sites with or without skin involvement.

JXG often resolves over the course of several years and may leave behind dyspigmentation or, more rarely, anetoderma, atrophy, or scarring.[92] Extracutaneous disease occurs in about 4% of patients, and the eye (iris followed by the eyelid) is the most common location with an overall incidence of 0.3% to 0.5%. The next most common extracutaneous sites of involvement are the lung and the liver.[75,109] Ocular involvement is usually accompanied by multiple cutaneous lesions, and complications of ocular JXG include hyphema, glaucoma, uveitis, and blindness.[91,92] CNS involvement is very rare, but is associated with poor

outcomes. The prognosis for exclusively cutaneous JXG is excellent; however, if there is systemic involvement, mortality ranges from 2% to 20%.[75]

Histologic Findings

A dense mononuclear histiocytic infiltrate in the dermis extending to the interface with the epidermis is present.[89,110,111] In smaller lesions, the infiltrate may be limited to the superficial dermis but, in larger lesions, may extend into the subcutis. There is often flattening of the epidermis with loss of the rete ridges; however, the epidermis and adnexa are spared. The infiltrate is composed of small mononuclear cells, as well as multinucleated giant cells with and

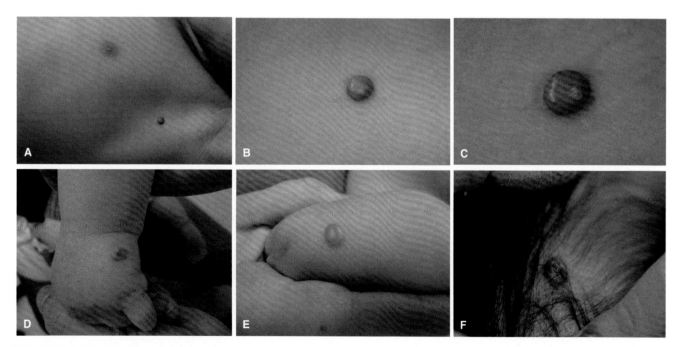

FIGURE 26-14. **Juvenile xanthogranuloma.** A to C, Early lesions show red-brown papules. D to F, Mature lesions have a yellow color, given the number of xanthomatized histiocytes.

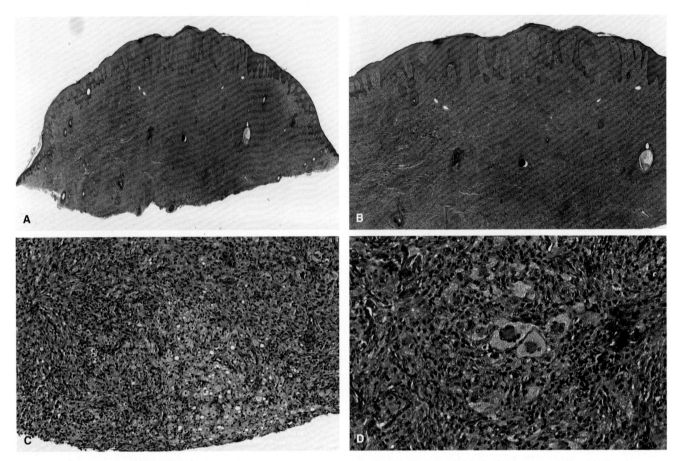

FIGURE 26-15. Juvenile xanthogranuloma—histopathologic findings. A and B, Dense dermal histiocytic infiltrate with epidermal hyperplasia. C, In this early lesion, only focal xanthomatized changes are seen. D, Scattered Touton-type giant cells are seen. Digital slides courtesy of Path Presenter.com.

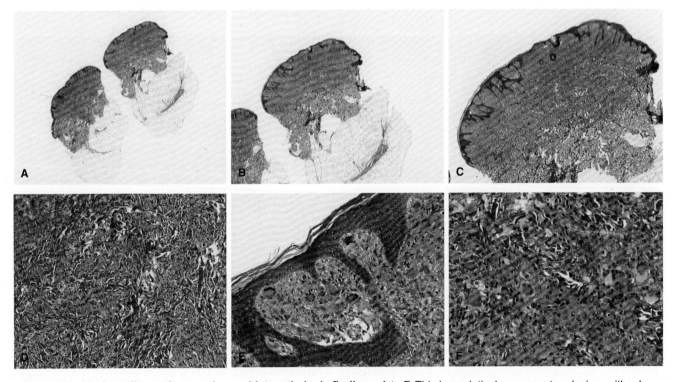

FIGURE 26-16. Juvenile xanthogranuloma—histopathologic findings. A to F, This is a relatively more mature lesion, with a larger proportion of xanthomatized histiocytes and giant cells.

without the features of Touton giant cells (Figures 26-15 and 26-16). In fact, cutaneous JXG may be devoid of giant cells, and their presence in extracutaneous lesion is often difficult to demonstrate. Lymphocytes, eosinophils, plasma cells, neutrophils, and mast cells may be scattered throughout the infiltrate or be altogether absent. The morphology of the histiocytes can vary depending on the "age" of the lesion that is often difficult to determine with any certainty. So-called early lesions are composed predominantly of mononuclear cells with abundant eosinophilic and minimally vacuolated cytoplasm. More "mature" lesions contain histiocytes with "lipidized or xanthomatized" cytoplasm with numerous fine cytoplasmic vacuoles. Touton giant cells, which are characterized by a ring or wreath of nuclei surrounded by a rim of foamy cytoplasm, are characteristic, but their presence is variable in this phase. Scalloped histiocytes with an angulated or jagged border and spindled histiocytes may also be seen. In fact, some lesions are composed predominantly of spindle cells (Figure 26-17), but the finely vacuolated interspersed mononuclear cells are the clue to the diagnosis of JXG. Not entirely surprising is the resemblance in some cases between JXG and dermatofibroma (DF). Mitotic figures may be seen, but atypical mitotic figures are absent.

The histiocytes stain positively for CD68, CD163, CD4, CD14, factor XIIIa, HLA-DR, fascin, vimentin, and lysozyme and are negative for CD1a and langerin.[89,111] The histiocytes are usually negative for S-100 but it is not unusual to encounter individual and patchy staining in some cases. Frequent admixed S-100 dendritic cells can be seen in some cases. Ultrastructural examination of "mature" lesions shows lipid vacuoles, lysosomes, cholesterol clefts, comma-shaped bodies, and myeloid bodies in the cytoplasm of the histiocytes. No Birbeck granules are present.

Differential Diagnosis

The histologic differential diagnosis of JXG varies based on the stage of the lesion, but may include reticulohistiocytoma, benign fibrous histiocytoma (DF), LCH, Spitz nevus, melanoma, and malignant fibrous histiocytoma. In early JXG in which Touton giant cells and xanthomatized histiocytes are absent, differentiating JXG from LCH may be difficult. In such cases, staining for S-100 and CD1a, both of which are positive in LCH and negative in JXG, may be used to make the diagnosis.

The lipidized variant of DF contains numerous large, foamy cells and Touton-like giant cells, reminiscent of JXG. However, areas of spindle cells in a whorled or storiform pattern may be present, and collagen trapping can be seen at the periphery of the lesion. However, the distinction between JXG and DF in an older child is a challenge, with some degree of uncertainty. DFs tend to have overlying epidermal changes, such as acanthosis, hyperpigmentation of epidermal basal cells, or folliculosebaceous induction, and often contain hemosiderin unlike JXG. Both lesions can

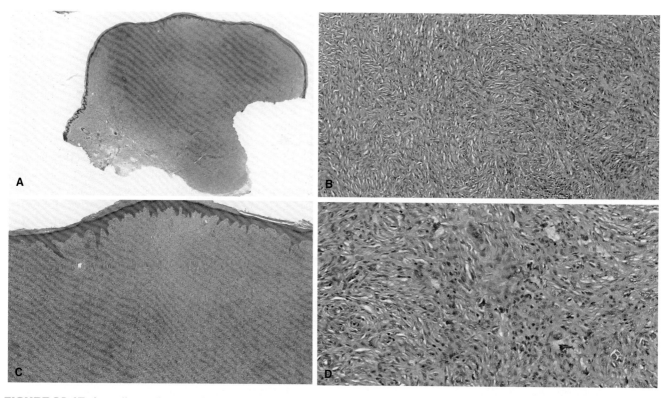

FIGURE 26-17. Juvenile xanthogranuloma—spindle cell variant. This form is a potential mimicker of dermatofibromas (DF). The lesion lacks the surface induction changes seen in DF (A and B) or the collagen "trapping" at the periphery of the lesions. The infiltrate is composed of spindle cells with admixed xanthomatized cells and Touton-type giant cells (C and D). Digital slides courtesy of Path Presenter.com.

be positive for factor XIIIa, but DFs are usually negative or only weakly positive for CD68.

Reticulohistiocytoma can also mimic JXG clinically and histologically. The histopathologic findings of reticulohistiocytoma, including the presence of densely eosinophilic "ground glass" cytoplasm, usually allow for a distinction from JXG; however, there may be immunohistochemical overlap between these lesions as the reticulohistiocytomas are also positive for CD68 and CD163, negative for CD1a, and often negative for S-100. It should be emphasized that some consider reticulohistiocytomas as histologic variants of JXG.[1,36,112] Spitz nevi can also enter the differential diagnosis; however, the melanocytic nature of the lesion can readily be demonstrated with the application of the melanocytic markers, Melan-A, HMB-45, or SOX-10. Mast cell neoplasms (mastocytomas) can also resemble JXG (when the latter are devoid of lipidized cells). Mastocytomas are characteristically positive for CD117 and tryptase and have aberrant coexpression of CD2 and CD25. α-Chloroacetate esterase (Leder stain) is positive in the mast cell granules.

Systemic JXG should also be distinguished from ALK+ histiocytosis of childhood. ALK+ histiocytosis manifests with anemia, massive hepatosplenomegaly, and thrombocytopenia. The liver shows sinusoidal infiltration by histiocytic cells with folded nuclei, fine chromatin, small nucleoli, and voluminous eosinophilic cytoplasm with occasional hemophagocytosis.[72] Therefore, when diagnosing ECD, ALK immunostain should always be performed.

CAPSULE SUMMARY

JUVENILE XANTHOGRANULOMA

JXG (xanthogranuloma, nevoxanthoendothelioma) is a self-limited non-LCH involving proliferation of cholesterol-laden monocyte-derived macrophages that most commonly occurs in the first year of life. It is the most common form of non-LCH and is currently classified as group "C" for the cutaneous limited forms and in the "L" category for the systemic variants. The infiltrate is composed of small mononuclear cells, as well as multinucleated giant cells with and without the features of Touton giant cells.

BENIGN CEPHALIC HISTIOCYTOSIS

Definition and Epidemiology

First described by Gianotti et al in 1971, BCH is an uncommon non-LCH that occurs in young children and presents as a self-healing, asymptomatic eruption of papules on the head and neck. It is benign in nature and is not associated with systemic disease or visceral involvement. BCH likely lies on a spectrum of non-LCH disorders such as Generalized eruptive histiocytosis (GEH) and JXG.[113,114] They are included under group "C."

BCH is a rare disorder that presents in infants and young children. The average age of onset is 15 months, and up to 45% of cases occur in patients less than 6 months of age. No gender predilection has been observed.[114] About 60 cases have been reported in the English literature, but the disorder may be underreported.[115,116]

Etiology

BCH is a benign proliferatory disorder of macrophage-derived histiocytes with an unknown cause that may represent a variant of JXG and GEH. It has also been postulated that BCH is an early or abortive phase of JXG or perhaps a focal clinical presentation of GEH.[117-119]

Clinical Presentation

BCH is typified by an eruption of brown to tan, flat-topped papules that range in size from about 1 to 8 mm (Figure 26-18). This condition almost always starts on the face, after which it may spread to involve the trunk and/or extremities. It does not involve mucosal or acral sites and has not been reported to affect internal organs, except in one case that was associated with infiltration of the pituitary stalk leading to diabetes insipidus.[119,120] The total number of lesions can range from as few as 5 to as many as 100. Lesions typically regress over the course of several years and can leave behind hyperpigmentation, but usually do not scar.[114,121]

Histologic Findings

The histology of BCH is characterized by a well-defined proliferation of histiocytes with oval to reniform nuclei and abundant eosinophilic cytoplasm (Figure 26-19). The infiltrate lies in the mid-upper dermis adjacent to, but sparing the epidermis, which may appear flat and atrophic. The infiltrate is often accompanied by a mixed inflammatory cell infiltrate. Xanthomatous change can occur as lesions evolve and scattered multinucleate giant cells may be present. Such findings are identical to those seen in JXG. Immunostaining of the infiltrate reveals positivity for CD68, CD163, HAM-56, and factor XIIIa and negativity for CD1a, CD 207 (langerin), and usually S-100.[117,122] Comma-shaped bodies may be seen on ultrastructural evaluation via electron microscopy, but in contrast to LCH, Birbeck granules are invariably absent.[114,118]

Differential Diagnosis

In general, the histologic differential diagnosis is the same as for JXG, and it most importantly includes LCH, which is S-100 and CD1a positive. Other non-LCH disorders such as JXG and GEH are primarily distinguished based on clinical features, as the histopathology alone is undifferentiating, especially in the early nonxanthomatous phase.[116]

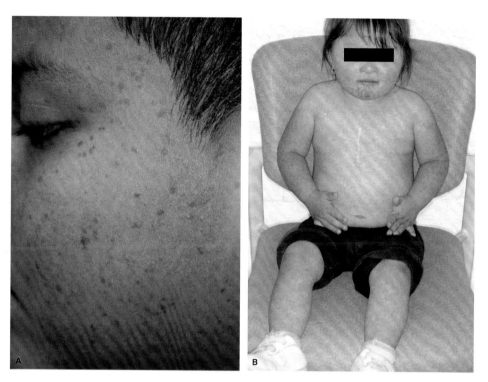

FIGURE 26-18. **Benign cephalic histiocytosis—two examples.** Small, brown-tan papules in the face (A and B).

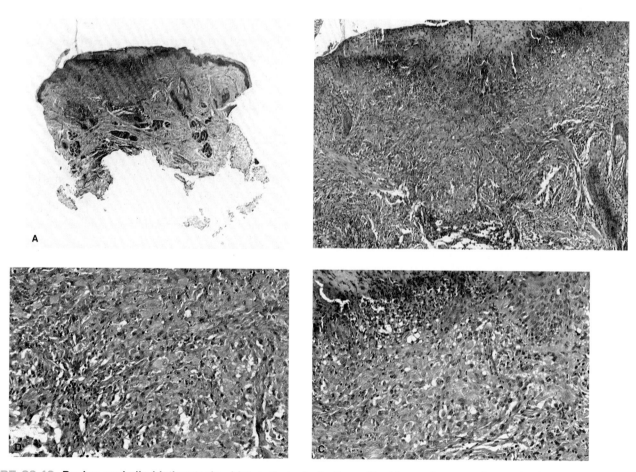

FIGURE 26-19. **Benign cephalic histiocytosis—histopathologic findings.** The biopsy shows an ulcerated epidermis (A) with a dermal-based infiltrate (B). The lesion is composed of epithelioid histiocytes and scattered multinucleated giant cells (C and D). Digital slides courtesy of Path Presenter.com.

CAPSULE SUMMARY

BENIGN CEPHALIC HISTIOCYTOSIS

Similar to JXG, BCH demonstrates a dermal CD68⁺ histiocytic infiltrate. BCH is histologically indistinguishable from other non-LCH such as JXG and GEH. The evolution of the infiltrate is marked by xanthomatization followed by fibrosis. Comma-shaped bodies can be seen on electron microscopy.

PROGRESSIVE NODULAR HISTIOCYTOSIS

Definition and Epidemiology

PNH, first described in 1978, lies on the spectrum of non-LCH most closely resembling JXG. However, unlike JXG, the skin lesions have a chronic, progressive course only rarely undergoing spontaneous resolution.[123,124] PNH is rarely reported, and there is a high degree of variance regarding the nomenclature of this disorder.

PNH is very uncommon and tends to develop in late childhood or adulthood. It is chronic in nature, distinguishing it from JXG and BCH.[124,125] It has only been reported a handful of times and the age of affected patients ranges from 9 to 62 years.

Etiology

Like the other closely related and overlapping "C" group of disorders, PNH is a proliferative disorder of dermal dendrocytes with an unknown cause. It is most similar to that of JXG, although it presents later and does not spontaneously regress over time.[123,125,126] It is possible that PNH is not a distinct entity and merely represents a distinct clinical presentation of JXG.[127]

Clinical Presentation

Clinically, PNH is characterized by the progressive appearance of asymptomatic persistent, yellow to brown superficial papules and deep nodules on the skin and rarely mucosa that enlarge over time and can lead to significant physical distortion (Figure 26-20).[125,128] The face is commonly involved and may progress to become leonine in appearance.[129] There have been various reports of PNH occurring in patients with systemic illness such as blood cancers and hypothalamic tumors, but the precise relationship between PNH and the underlying illness was unknown.[123,125,130] PNH has been reported in association with laryngeal lesions leading to respiratory failure and death.[131]

Histologic Findings

The histology of PNH closely resembles that of JXG with a dense dermal infiltrate of histiocytes with large, vacuolated cytoplasm and occasional multinucleated giant cells

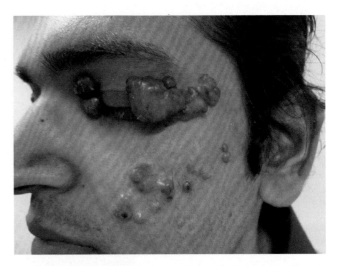

FIGURE 26-20. Progressive nodular histiocytosis. Papular and nodular lesions on the face and eyelid. Obtained with permission. Williams A, Thomas AG, Kwatra KS, Jain K. Progressive nodular histiocytosis associated with Eale's disease. *Indian J Dermatol.* 2015;60(4):388-390. doi:10.4103/0019-5154.160492.

(Figure 26-21). PNH shows a tendency toward spindled histiocytes arranged in a storiform pattern (similar to spindle cell xanthogranuloma). Scattered inflammatory cells, xanthomatized histiocytes, and variable Touton giant cells may be seen.[129,132] Similar to JXG, fibrosis becomes a prominent feature over time. The immunoprofile is identical to that of JXG, that is, positive for CD68 and HAM56, and negative for S-100 and CD1a.[123,125]

Differential Diagnosis

See the differential diagnosis for JXG. Lesions with prominent storiform architecture may also demonstrate collagen trapping at the periphery of the infiltrate reminiscent of DF; however, PNH has a different immunoprofile and does not have overlying epidermal changes similar to that of DF.[133]

CAPSULE SUMMARY

PROGRESSIVE NODULAR HISTIOCYTOSIS

The histology of PNH closely resembles JXG and shares the same immunoprofile. JXG and PNH are primarily distinguished clinically.

XANTHOMA DISSEMINATUM

Definition and Epidemiology

XD (Montgomery syndrome) is a systemic, mucocutaneous form of proliferative histiocytic disease of histiocytic origin that primarily involves the skin, respiratory tract, and mucosal sites. Unlike most forms of non-LCH, XD can cause substantial morbidity and mortality because of airway involvement

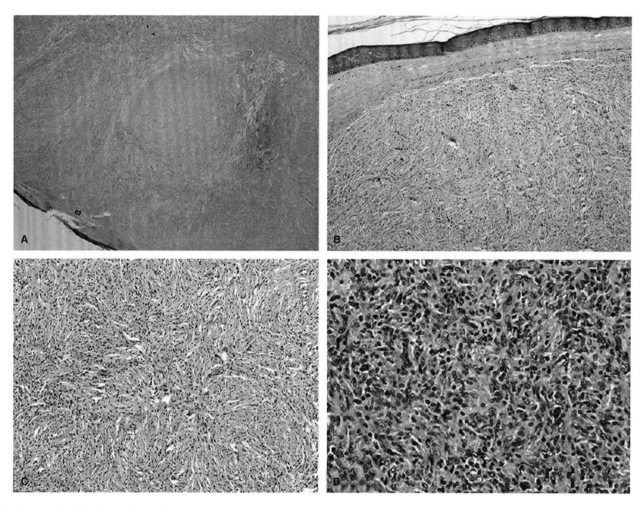

FIGURE 26-21. A, Dermal tumor with a nodular and diffuse growth pattern. Hematoxylin and eosin (H&E) ×20. B, Spindle-shaped tumor cells arranged in short fascicles. H&E ×40. C, Storiform pattern. H&E ×100. D, Histiocytes admixed with lymphocytes. H&E ×400. Obtained with permission. Williams A, Thomas AG, Kwatra KS, Jain K. Progressive nodular histiocytosis associated with Eale's disease. *Indian J Dermatol.* 2015;60(4):388-390. doi:10.4103/0019-5154.160492.

and occasional internal disease, particularly that of the bone and the CNS.[134-136] XD is very rare with around 100 reported cases. It can occur at any age, but most commonly occurs in young males, with a male to female ratio of 2.4:1.[137] Reportedly, 60% of cases occur between the ages of 5 and 25 years.[134]

Etiology

XD is a sporadic disorder and unlike most xanthomatoses, patients with XD typically are normolipidemic, with up to 20% of patients having lipid abnormalities. The cause of XD is unknown, but it is currently thought of as a reactive proliferative disorder of macrophages to an unknown antigen. Over time, the histiocytes secondarily accumulate lipid either because of increased production and increased uptake or because of decreased efflux.[135,137-139]

Clinical Presentation

Clinically, XD is characterized by a progressive eruption of numerous (often hundreds) asymptomatic yellow-brown papules, plaques, and nodules that typically first appear symmetrically in the axilla or other intertriginous sites (Figure 26-22). The eruption then spreads to the face, especially the periocular region, as well as to the trunk and extremities. XD involves the mucous membranes 40% to 60% of the time with a predilection for the respiratory tract.[134,137,140] The natural history of XD is most commonly that of persistent cutaneous disease or, less often, a progressive form with systemic involvement. The regressive type is the least common presentation and occurs in about a third of patients.[136] XD has been associated with the following systemic sequela: osteolytic bone lesions, myeloma, Waldenstrom macroglobulinemia, monoclonal gammopathy, hyper- or hypothyroidism, diabetes insipidus from infiltration of the pituitary stalk, and neurologic disorders (epilepsy, cerebellar ataxia, hydrocephalus).[137] XD with CNS involvement is rare, but when it occurs it may have a poor prognosis depending on which structures are involved.[136] The clinical findings of XD can be

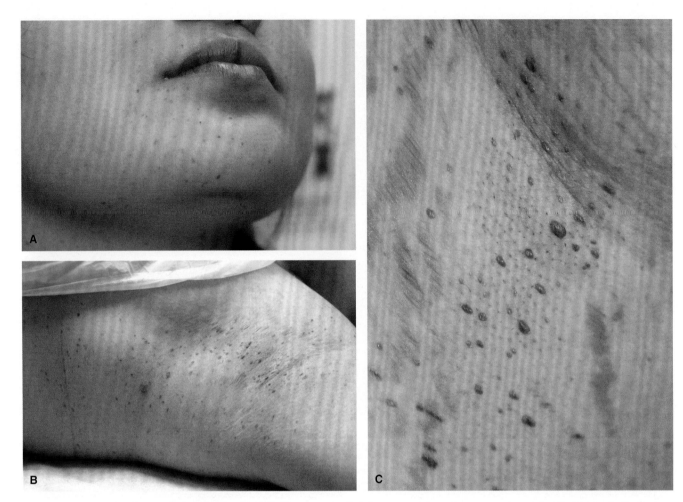

FIGURE 26-22. Xanthoma disseminatum. A to C, Numerous yellow-brown papules, plaques, and nodules that typically first appear symmetrically in the axilla or other intertriginous sites.

summarized as a triad of widespread normolipidemic xanthoma, mucous membrane involvement of the upper respiratory tract, and transient diabetes insipidus in approximately up to 40% of cases, though this triad does not occur in every patient.[114,140-142]

Histologic Findings

The histology of XD overlaps with that of the other non-LCH disorders. A diffuse dermal infiltrate of large, pleomorphic scalloped histiocytes predominates in early lesions and over time Touton and foreign body giant cells, foamy macrophages, sparse inflammatory cells, and spindled cells begin to appear. The immunoprofile of XD is as follows: CD68$^+$, factor XIIIa+, S-100$^-$, and CD1a$^-$.[134,137,143]

Differential Diagnosis

See the differential diagnosis for JXG. XD is differentiated from other non-LCH primarily on clinical grounds given the histologic overlap. Immunohistochemistry can rule out LCH.

CAPSULE SUMMARY

XANTHOMA DISSEMINATUM

XD (Montgomery syndrome) is a systemic, mucocutaneous form of proliferative histiocytic disease of histiocytic origin that primarily involves the skin, respiratory tract, and mucosal sites. Clinically, XD is characterized by a progressive eruption of numerous (often hundreds) asymptomatic yellow-brown papules, plaques, and nodules that typically first appear symmetrically in the axilla or other intertriginous sites. The histology of XD overlaps with that of the other non-LCH disorders.

SEA-BLUE HISTIOCYTE SYNDROME

Definition and Epidemiology

In 1970, sea-blue histiocyte syndrome (SBHS, OMIM 269600) was described by Silverstein as a disorder in which sea-blue histiocytes occupy various organs, especially the bone marrow, liver, and spleen.[144] The sea-blue histiocyte is a large macrophage that contains a cytoplasm filled with granules that turn blue-green in color when stained with Giemsa. It is now recognized that the disorder may either be inherited or represent a secondary phenomenon because of an underlying systemic illness. SBHS is exceptionally rare with about 60 reported cases.

Etiology

It can occur as a primary idiopathic storage disease (familial) or secondary to another disorder that leads to accumulation of lipofuscin or ceroid. Associated diseases include blood disorders (chronic myeloid leukemia, idiopathic thrombocytopenic purpura, and myelodysplastic syndromes) in which there is a high rate of intramedullary cell death via the reticuloendothelial system and inherited metabolic disorders such as Niemann-Pick disease.[37,144-154] It has also been reported in association with long-term total parenteral nutrition and with mycosis fungoides. Certain forms of SBHS may be related to mutation of the apolipoprotein E gene.[148]

Clinical Presentation

Primary SBHS usually presents with hepatosplenomegaly and hemorrhage secondary to bone marrow infiltration and subsequent thrombocytopenia. Cutaneous involvement is exceptionally rare, but it has presented as nodules and waxy plaques, eyelid swelling, and macular brown hyperpigmentation. It predominantly affects the face, but can also involve the trunk, hands, or feet. Internal involvement by SBHS can include the liver, spleen, bone marrow, lung, lymph node, retina, and nervous system. SBHS is typically a benign process when inherited (primary), but if secondary, the prognosis is related to the primary systemic disorder.[37,133,144,147]

Histologic Findings

The histology of SBHS shows a dermal infiltrate of large, monomorphic histiocytes that are arranged in a micronodular fashion and contain granules/inclusion bodies that stain blue-green with Giemsa or May-Grünwald. The cells are CD68 positive and S-100 negative. On electron microscopy, the granules appear as round dense or rod-like bodies. The granules are yellow-brown when stained with hematoxylin-eosin and turn dark blue with toluidine. They are birefringent under polarized light.

Differential Diagnosis

The main concern regarding SBHS is assessing whether the disease is primary and idiopathic or secondary to an underlying comorbidity such as hematologic or metabolic disorders.[37,133,144,147]

CAPSULE SUMMARY

SEA-BLUE HISTIOCYTE SYNDROME

This is a disorder in which sea-blue histiocytes occupy various organs, especially the bone marrow, liver, and spleen. There are dermal infiltrates of large, monomorphic histiocytes arranged in a micronodular fashion. Lesional cells contain granules/inclusion bodies that stain blue-green with Giemsa.

GENERALIZED ERUPTIVE HISTIOCYTOSIS

Definition and Epidemiology

GEH is a benign proliferative disorder of mononuclear histiocytes that is considered to lie on a spectrum among other non-LCH disorders, in particular JXG.[155] It is considered part of the group "C" category of histiocytic disorders.

GEH is extremely rare, having been reported only about 40 times in the literature since its initial description in 1963 by Winkelmann and Mullerin.[156] It usually occurs in adults, but can present in the pediatric population.[155,157]

Etiology

The etiology is unknown, largely owing to the rarity and lack of research on the condition. Furthermore, it is considered by some that GEH represents the initial presentation of several other non-LCH such as JXG, PNH, or XD. It may in fact be an early, undifferentiated form of non-LCH. More recently, the association of GEH with a translocation *LMNA-NTRK1* has been reported.[158] GEH has been previously reported in association with a variety of hematologic disorders, including chronic eosinophilic leukemia, T-cell lymphomas, and chronic and acute monocytic leukemias.[159-163]

Clinical Presentation

Clinically, GEH presents with the abrupt onset of innumerable red-brown papules and nodules that are usually several millimeters in diameter and appear on the face, trunk, and extremities (Figure 26-23). The eruption is usually asymptomatic and symmetrically distributed. The lesions may come and go in crops and can resemble molluscum contagiosum. Mucous membranes and internal organs are typically spared. Lesions can last for years prior to spontaneous resolution at which point residual hyperpigmentation may be left behind. It has occasionally been reported in association with malignancy, autoimmune disorders, and immunosuppression, but a causal relationship has not been established and the associations may be coincidental. GEH is considered to lie on a spectrum with other non-LCH, and transition from one disorder to another may occur.[155,164-166]

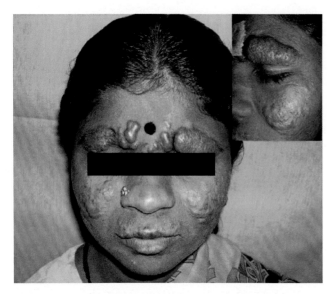

FIGURE 26-23. Generalized eruptive histiocytosis. Clinical picture of infiltrated papules, nodules, and plaques on face. Inset: Note the prominent medial eyebrow involvement and papules coalesced to form plaques on cheek. Obtained with permission. Sharath Kumar BC, Nandini AS, Niveditha SR, Gopal MG, Reeti. Generalized eruptive histiocytosis mimicking leprosy. *Indian J Dermatol Venereol Leprol.* 2011;77(4):498-502. doi:10.4103/0378-6323.82413.

Histologic Findings

GEH shows a monomorphous histiocytic infiltrate in the mid-upper dermis with sparse, scattered lymphocytes and a lack of giant cells and foamy histiocytes (Figure 26-24).

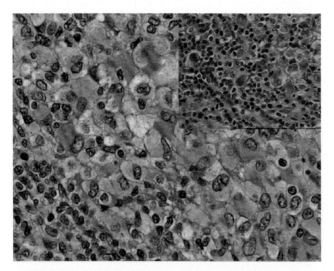

FIGURE 26-24. Generalized eruptive histiocytosis. Nodule showing large histiocytes with abundant eosinophilic to foamy cytoplasm and vesicular nucleus admixed with lymphocytes (hematoxylin and eosin, ×400). Inset: Focal granular Periodic acid–Schiff (PAS) positivity in the cytoplasm of the histiocytes (PAS, ×400) Obtained with permission. Sharath Kumar BC, Nandini AS, Niveditha SR, Gopal MG, Reeti. Generalized eruptive histiocytosis mimicking leprosy. *Indian J Dermatol Venereol Leprol.* 2011;77(4):498-502. doi:10.4103/0378-6323.82413.

It most closely resembles the histology of BCH and early JXG.[164,167] GEH shares the same phenotype as most of the other non-LCH, that is, being negative for S-100, CD1a, and CD207 and positive for CD68.

Differential Diagnosis

The differential diagnosis primarily comprises LCH and many of the forms of non-LCH, but clinically may also include sarcoidosis and urticaria pigmentosa (UP). Lack of foamy histiocytes and giant cells (including Touton giant cells) can help differentiate GEH from other non-LCH, but clinical correlation (natural history of disease, associated symptoms, etc) is the primary differentiating factor in most cases as GEH may be either an abortive or an early, undifferentiated form of another non-LCH.

CAPSULE SUMMARY

GENERALIZED ERUPTIVE HISTIOCYTOSIS

GEH is a benign proliferative disorder of mononuclear histiocytes that is considered to lie on a spectrum among other non-LCH disorders, in particular JXG. GEH has been previously reported in association with a variety of hematologic disorders, including chronic eosinophilic leukemia, T-cell lymphomas, and chronic and acute monocytic leukemias. Overlaps exists with other non-LCH in histology and immunoprofile.

PROGRESSIVE MUCINOUS HISTIOCYTOSIS

Definition and Epidemiology

Hereditary progressive mucinous histiocytosis (HPMH, OMIM 142630) is a familial, autosomal dominant form of non-LCH first described in 1988.[168] HPMH is extraordinarily rare, with less than 20 cases reported in the literature.[169-174] Unlike most forms of histiocytoses, which are sporadic, HPMH occurs in families in an autosomal dominant fashion. Sporadic cases have been reported (five total), but some authors debate whether inheritance is a required feature to make the diagnosis.[175,176] It is far more common in women, with few male patients reported to date.[168,172] No geographic preponderance has been identified.

Etiology

The cause is unknown, but given its gender predilection of females, a hormonal contribution has been suggested. No causal genetic mutation has been identified. It is thought that the involved cells in HMPH are of the mononuclear macrophage lineage.[168,175]

Clinical Presentation

At a young age, patients with HPMH begin to develop asymptomatic, skin colored to red-brown nodules on the face, extremities, and trunk that are persistent and progressive in nature. Involvement is confined to the skin sparing the mucosa. The lesions usually begin small, about 1 to 3 mm in diameter, but can increase in size up to 10 mm. Systemic involvement has not been reported and HPMH has not been associated with any comorbidities. Although HPMH is benign, unlike most forms of non-LCH, the lesions do not spontaneously regress.[168,175,177]

Histologic Findings

In the reported cases, histology is characterized by a well-circumscribed, nonencapsulated infiltrate of epithelioid, and to a lesser extent spindled, histiocytes with pale cytoplasm that are splayed between collagen bundles (reminiscent of collagen trapping) and associated with increased dermal mucin.[176] Multinucleate giant cells may be present, but xanthomatization/lipid deposition is not a feature. The circumscribed infiltrate may be separated from the epidermis by a grenz zone, and occasionally dilated vessels may be seen in association with the infiltrate.[174] The immunophenotype is not well characterized given the limited number of reports of this condition, but it is considered positive for HAM 56, vimentin, and lysozyme; variably positive for factor XIIIa and CD68; and negative for S-100 and CD1a. On electron microscopy zebra bodies are seen, similar to those encountered in lysosomal storage[168,175,178] disorders.

Differential Diagnosis

The differential diagnosis includes other forms of non-LCH, DF, Spitz nevus, acral papular mucinosis, scleromyxedema, and granuloma annulare. The hereditary nature, increase in mucin, absence of foam cells/xanthomatization, and lack of spontaneous regression help to distinguish HPMH from other non-LCH.

CAPSULE SUMMARY

PROGRESSIVE MUCINOUS HISTIOCYTOSIS

At a young age, patients with HPMH begin to develop asymptomatic, skin colored to red-brown nodules on the face, extremities, and trunk that are persistent and progressive in nature. Involvement is confined to the skin sparing the mucosa. Histologically, there is a well-circumscribed infiltrate of epithelioid and spindled histiocytes with pale cytoplasm that are splayed between collagen bundles. Increased dermal mucin and multinucleate giant cells may be seen. Zebra bodies can be present on electron microscopy.

RETICULOHISTIOCYTOMA AND RETICULOHISTIOCYTOSIS

Definition and Epidemiology

MRH is a multisystemic non-LCH that is characterized by symmetric polyarthritis, papular mucocutaneous lesions, and occasional association with underlying malignancy or systemic illness.[179] SRH (solitary epithelioid histiocytoma) primarily refers to a solitary isolated cutaneous lesion without systemic involvement. When multiple, this condition is referred to as diffuse cutaneous reticulohistiocytoma without systemic involvement.[180]

The overall incidence of MRH is unknown, but more than 300 cases of MRH have been reported in the literature.[181] MRH can develop at any age, but it is most common in the fourth decade and only rarely occurs in children. It is most common in Caucasians, and women are more likely to be affected than men by approximately a 3:1 ratio. SRH typically occurs in young adults.[179,181,182] It should be emphasized that some consider reticulohistiocytomas as histologic variants of JXG.[1,36,112]

Etiology

The pathogenesis of MRH is unknown, and it is unclear as to whether it represents an inflammatory or proliferative process. A recent theory hypothesizes that increased levels of interleukin 6 (IL-6) and TNF-α stimulate histiocytes to differentiate into osteoclasts, which leads to bone remodeling and increased resorption.[183] Up to 30% of adult cases have been associated with a wide range of hematologic and solid malignancies. MRH is not considered a paraneoplastic disorder primarily because of risk of selection bias in the literature as well as the inconsistency of associations and the lack of parallel disease course with associated malignancies.[179,182,184-186] SRH is currently regarded as a local reactive response to an unknown stimulus.[187]

Clinical Presentation

Arthritis is the most common presenting symptom of MRH and usually manifests as a symmetric polyarthritis with a predilection for the distal interphalangeal joints, wrists, elbows, shoulders, knees, hips, and feet (mimics rheumatoid arthritis). The arthritis can be very destructive in nature and can even progress to arthritis mutilans. The cutaneous eruption of MRH usually trails the arthritis by several years and presents as smooth, shiny skin colored to pink papules and nodules that range in size from several millimeters to several centimeters and favors the face, hands, and forearms. Although the cutaneous lesions tend to appear after the onset of arthritis, they may precede it or occur simultaneously. Numerous atypical cutaneous presentations of MRH have been reported, including a type that mimics dermatomyositis.[188] Involvement of the cuticle in a "coral bead" pattern is characteristic, but is not always seen. Nail dystrophy may be present as well.[184] Mucosal lesions (especially of the mouth) occur in up to half of cases and involvement of numerous other organ systems (including heart and lung leading to effusions) has been described. Systemic symptoms of fatigue, fever, and/or weight loss are common in MRH. MRH has been associated with numerous systemic illnesses including malignancy (hematologic and solid organ), tuberculosis, autoimmune disorders, and endocrine diseases. MRH is usually a self-limited disease that spontaneously remits over the course of 5 to 10 years (8 years on average); however, if malignancy associated, then the prognosis is correlated with the primary malignancy, although the natural history of the clinical manifestations does not correlate with that of the associated cancer.[179,182,188]

SRH and diffuse cutaneous RH without systemic involvement usually present as solitary or multiple asymptomatic nodular lesions on the skin respectively. They can occur anywhere on the body. SRH typically self-resolves over the course of about 6 months.[180,189]

Histologic Findings

The histologic picture of reticulohistiocytoma obtained from either cutaneous or synovial biopsy is that of a circumscribed, nodular histiocytic infiltrate composed of both plump mononuclear and multinucleate cells that have prominent nucleoli, well-defined nuclei, and an eosinophilic granular "ground glass"–appearing cytoplasm accentuated by Periodic acid–Schiff (PAS) staining (Figure 26-25).[181,189] The multinucleated giant cells may be quite large and contain anywhere from 2 to 30 nuclei, which often have crisp borders and are haphazardly arranged in the cytoplasm. Epidermal changes are variable, but can include hyperkeratosis, parakeratosis, and/or flattening of the rete ridges. The infiltrate occupies all or any part of the dermis and may extend into the subcutis on occasion. Scattered mitoses may be evident. Scattered lymphocytes usually accompany the histiocytic infiltrate, and granulocytes may or may not be present. Early lesions tend to have more inflammatory cells and less giant cells, which reverses as lesions age. Over time, lesions become more fibrotic. Reticulohistiocytoma have the following immunohistochemical profile: CD68$^+$, CD163$^+$, lysozyme+, S-100$^-$, CD1a$^-$.[186,189-191]

MRH and SRH have similar histopathologic findings; however, the infiltrate in SRH is usually more dense and circumscribed than that of MRH. Furthermore, SRH is more likely to contain xanthomatized cells and even Touton giant cells.[192]

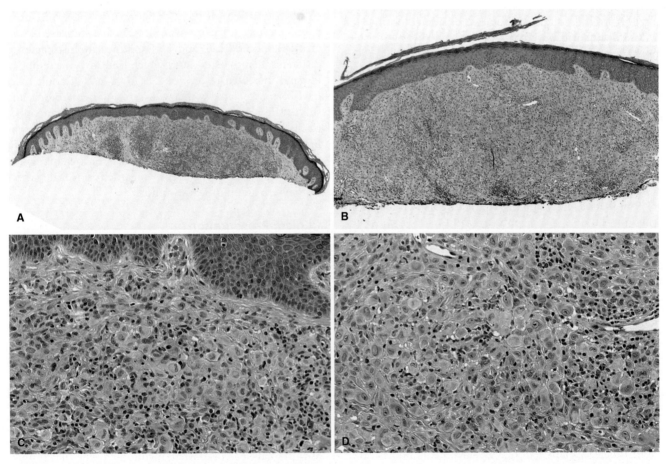

FIGURE 26-25. Reticulohistiocytoma. Nodular histiocytic infiltrate composed of both plump mononuclear and multinucleate cells that have prominent nucleoli. A dermal based histiocytic infiltrate is noted (A and B). The nodular histiocytic infiltrate composed of both plump mononuclear and multinucleate cells that have prominent nucleoli (C and D). Digital slides courtesy of Path Presenter.com.

Differential Diagnosis

The differential diagnosis of MRH/SHE includes: granuloma annulare, infectious granulomata, RDD, xanthogranuloma, epithelioid sarcoma, histiocytic sarcoma (HS), epithelioid fibrous histiocytoma (DFs), melanocytic lesions (Spitz nevus or melanoma variants), granular cell tumor, and LCH. RDD has large, atypical histiocytes that are S-100 positive and often show emperipolesis and is accompanied by a plasma cell–rich infiltrate. JXG may appear similar, but the histiocytes in MRH are epithelioid with a ground glass cytoplasm, which differs from that of JXG. Infection can be ruled out with special stains and tissue culture, and architecturally, MRH lacks nodular granulomas with or without necrosis that is often seen in an infectious granulomatous process. Epithelioid DF tends to lack giant cells, and the lesional cells are positive for factor XIIIa and negative for CD68. Melanocytic proliferations can be ruled out with melanocytic markers if needed. Epithelioid sarcoma tends to display cells with abnormal morphology arranged in nodular granulomas with central necrosis and stain with cytokeratins, and EMA and being negative for CD163 and INI-1. LCH stains with S-100, CD1a, and CD207 and contains atypical cells with reniform or folded nuclei. There is a granular cell variant of SHE that can be a mimicker of granular cell tumor; however, positivity for CD68 and negativity for S-100 of the former can help differentiate the two if needed.

CAPSULE SUMMARY

RETICULOHISTIOCYTOMA AND RETICULOHISTIOCYTOSIS

MRH is a multisystemic non-LCH that is characterized by symmetric polyarthritis, papular mucocutaneous lesions, and occasional association with underlying malignancy or systemic illness. SRH (solitary epithelioid histiocytoma) primarily refers to a solitary isolated cutaneous lesion without systemic involvement. The histopathology shows a circumscribed, nodular infiltrate composed of plump CD68+ histiocytes. Multinucleate cells with prominent nucleoli and an eosinophilic granular "ground glass" cytoplasm accentuated by PAS staining are seen. The multinucleated giant cells may be large and contain anywhere from 2 to 30 nuclei.

GROUP "R" (SYSTEMIC ROSAI–DORFMAN) AND GROUP "C" (CUTANEOUS ROSAI-DORFMAN)

ROSAI-DORFMAN DISEASE

Definition and Epidemiology

RDD (sinus histiocytosis with massive lymphadenopathy) was first described in 1969 by Rosai and Dorfman.[193] It is

a rare non-LCH characterized by abnormal proliferation of histiocytes (either nodal and/or extranodal) undergoing emperipolesis. Emperipolesis refers to active, nondestructive engulfment of lymphocytes, plasma cells, and erythrocytes by histiocytes (in contrast to phagocytosis in which engulfed entities lose their normal structure while being destroyed by lysosomal enzymes).[194,195] Two clinical forms exist, one being the classical systemic type (SRDD) and the other is an exclusively cutaneous form (CRDD) that varies in natural history and epidemiology, but shares the same histology.[196-198] SRDD with cutaneous manifestations occurs in one-third of patients,[199] whereas CRDD (disease without any other manifestations) is extremely rare.[200] Systemic disease favors young adult men and male children.[197] In contrast, CRDD favors adult white women, thus making it appear to be a distinct entity.[197,198,200] As opposed to SRDD (group "R"), CRDD is included in the group "C" of histiocytosis in the non-JXG family.

SRDD is most common in the first two decades of life (median age of onset 20.6 years), and it has a slight male predominance favoring those of African descent.[201] Its estimated prevalence is 1:200 000. The purely cutaneous form of RDD is very rare, accounting for about 3% of total RDD cases and favors older females of either Asian or Caucasian ethnicity with a median age of onset of 43.5 years.[196,202,203]

Etiology

The etiology of RDD is not completely understood, but may relate to host immune dysregulation in response to an infectious insult such as a viral infection. It has also been postulated that RDD is related to immunoglobulin G4 (IgG4)-related disease.[204-206] A recent study demonstrated that at least a subset of RDD (33% of cases in the study) are clonal in nature, demonstrating a mutation in the MAPK/ERK pathway.[195]

In two families reported to have hereditary RDD, biallelic germline mutations in *SLC29A3* have been found with phenotypic expression in the CNS, eye, inner ear, and epithelial tissues. *SLC29A3* encodes an intracellular equilibrative nucleoside transporter (hENT3).[207] RDD is mostly sporadic, but inherited cases can occur. Mutations and large deletions of greater than 50 base pairs in mitochondrial DNA have rarely been identified in tissue samples of CRDD.[208] A closely related entity, the "H syndrome," has been associated with mutations in the *SLC29A3* gene. The syndrome is characterized by numerous cutaneous findings, including: *h*yperpigmentation, *h*ypertrichosis, *h*epatosplenomegaly, *h*earing abnormalities, *h*ypogonadism, low *h*eight, *h*yperglycemia, and *h*allux valgus. The cutaneous findings in this process mimic those of RDD with a CD68+, S-100+, CD1a-, histiocytosis with emperipolesis, and abundant plasma cells.[209-211]

Clinical Presentation

SRDD is benign and self-limited, but can run a long relapsing and remitting course: it presents with fever and massive, nontender, bilateral cervical lymph node enlargement. Over 40% of patients will have extranodal involvement, the most common locations being the skin, soft tissues (including around the orbit), upper respiratory tract, salivary glands, CNS, and bone. Intrathoracic manifestations of SRDD are relatively common and present as mediastinal lymphadenopathy, airway disease, pleural effusion, cystic lung disease, and interstitial lung disease. These usually have a good prognosis.[212] Involvement of the lower respiratory tract, liver, and kidney portends a poor prognosis.[197]

Immunologic features are associated with 15% of patients with SRDD and include autoimmune hemolytic anemia and neutrophilia.[213] Such findings are a sign of poor prognosis.[197,214-216] Cutaneous lesions associated with SRDD usually present on the eyelids and malar region. These are often nonspecific and appear as multiple, focal, erythematous, brown, or xanthomatous macules, papules, pustules, nodules, or plaques (Figures 26-26 and 26-27). Some of these lesions can be as large as 4 cm in diameter. In the rare cases of pure CRDD, they present as a central plaque or nodule with satellite papules or as multiple papules and nodules that coalesce into plaques.[214,215]

The clinical course of RDD is usually protracted, but spontaneous remission usually occurs. RDD is reportedly fatal in 5% to 10% of cases, and poor outcomes usually are due to vital organ involvement or disseminated/aggressive disease.[195,201]

Histologic Findings

Histopathologically, there is an infiltrate of histiocytes with neutrophils, plasma cells, and scattered lymphocytes

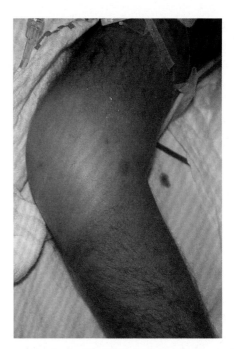

FIGURE 26-27. Cutaneous H syndrome with a presentation of Rosai-Dorfman–like changes. Hypertrichotic, hyperpigmented, edematous, and slightly indurated skin in the lower limb. Note sparing of the knee. Obtained with permission. Avitan-Hersh E, Mandel H, Indelman M, Bar-Joseph G, Zlotogorski A, Bergman R. A case of H syndrome showing immunophenotye similarities to Rosai–Dorfman disease. *Am J Dermatopathol.* 2011;33(1):47-51. doi:10.1097/DAD.0b013e3181ee547c.

densely packed in the dermis (Figure 26-28). The histiocytes are polygonal and characteristically have an abundant, foamy, lightly eosinophilic cytoplasm with feathery borders and large vesicular nuclei and small nucleoli.[197] Emperipolesis (inflammatory cells and cell fragments engulfed within histiocytes) is a very important feature that characterizes RDD. The histiocytes are characteristically positive for S-100 and negative for CD1a (Figure 26-29).[217] Multinucleated histiocytes may present as aggregates in Touton-like giant cell formation. In the cutaneous lesions, plasma cells may contain Russell bodies and present with associated xanthoma cells, fibrosis, and necrosis. CRDD differs histologically from nodal disease in that there is a greater degree of fibrosis, fewer histiocytes, and less emperipolesis. Epidermal changes are present in about half of the cases of cutaneous RDD and can include acanthosis, collarette formation, basal layer hyperpigmentation, and ulceration.[218] As a result, CRDD can be overlooked if the index of suspicion for the disease is low, perhaps contributing to its rare diagnosis.[219] The histology may also demonstrate a mixed septal and lobular panniculitis.[198] Many cases of CRDD will often elicit a "lymph node in skin" appearance. In early lesions, there may be suppurative/neutrophilic foci as well as prominent increased vascularity, whereas in older lesions emperipolesis is decreased or absent, and fibrosis

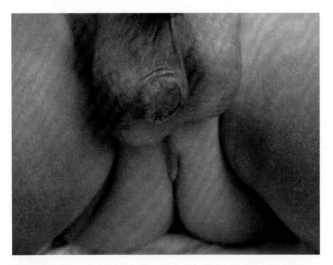

FIGURE 26-26. Cutaneous presentation of Rosai-Dorfman disease. Well-circumscribed, ulcerative lesion on right scrotum. Obtained with permission. Cole AJ, Chen C, Lorsbach RB, Honnebier BM, Gardner JM, Shalin SC. Extranodal Rosai–Dorfman disease in the scrotum of a 13-month male: a unique anatomic presentation. *Am J Dermatopathol.* 2015;37(1):88-90. doi:10.1097/DAD.0000000000000113.

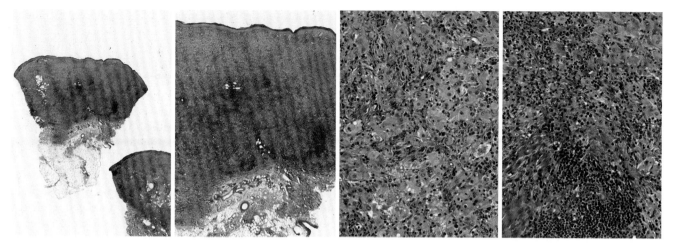

FIGURE 26-28. **Cutaneous Rosai-Dorfman disease.** A dense infiltrate of histiocytes, lymphocytes, and plasma cells is seen. The histiocytes have an epithelioid appearance. Many of them show engulfment of other inflammatory cells, "emperipolesis." Obtained with permission. Gru AA, Dehner LP. Cutaneous hematolymphoid and histiocytic proliferations in children. *Pediatr Dev Pathol.* 2018;21(2):208-251. doi:10.1177/1093526617750947.

may dominate and even overshadow the histiocytic infiltrate, making the diagnosis difficult.[202]

Histopathologic samples that are suspicious for RDD or another form of histiocytosis are stained with S-100, CD163, CD68, and CD1a. Positive staining of histiocytes with S-100 and CD68 with a negative CD1a stain suggests RDD. Positivity of all three stains suggests LCH and/or ICH. RDD can also have increased IgG4+ plasma cells.[204-206] However, the significance of this finding is not yet known. Both IgG and IgG4 stains should always be performed together, in order to properly evaluate the ratio of IgG4 to IgG+ plasma cells.

Differential Diagnosis

The differential diagnosis includes nonspecific sinus hyperplasia of the lymph node/reactive lymphoid hyperplasia, which lacks emperipolesis and is S-100 negative. Other entities to consider are leprosy, lymphoma, hemophagocytic syndromes, infection (tuberculosis, leprosy, rhinoscleroma), reticulohistiocytosis, LCH, and other non-LCH such as JXG.[137,202,203,218,220] Fortunately, the clinical and immunohistochemical features of RDD allow for easy differentiation

of most other entities. LCH has been reported to present concomitantly with RDD in a single patient, but positivity for CD1a and CD207 easily distinguishes LCH from RDD.[221] It should be noted that although characteristic, emperipolesis is not specific to RDD as it may be seen in other conditions such as B-cell lymphoma, LCH, rhinoscleroma, and cutaneous lesions of H syndrome.[196,202,222]

CAPSULE SUMMARY

ROSAI-DORFMAN DISEASE

RDD is a rare non-LCH characterized by abnormal proliferation of histiocytes (either nodal and/or extranodal) undergoing emperipolesis. The lymph node and skin pathology are similar. Characteristic RDD-associated histiocytes have a round to oval nucleus with prominent nucleoli and abundant clear to eosinophilic cytoplasm. Emperipolesis is the hallmark of RDD, but is not always visible and can be accentuated with S-100 staining. RDD has an associated predominantly lymphoplasmacytic infiltrate.

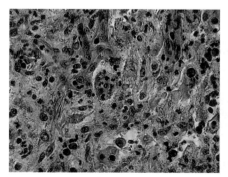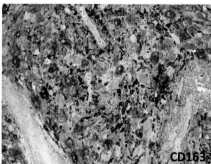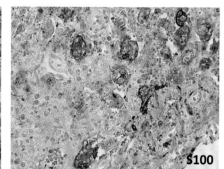

FIGURE 26-29. **Cutaneous Rosai-Dorfman disease (RDD).** High-power magnification is shown for emperipolesis. The histiocytic cells of RDD are positive for CD163 and S-100. Obtained with permission. Gru AA, Dehner LP. Cutaneous hematolymphoid and histiocytic proliferations in children. *Pediatr Dev Pathol.* 2018;21(2):208-251. doi:10.1177/1093526617750947.

GROUP "H" HISTIOCYTOSES

CYTOPHAGIC PANNICULITIS IN ASSOCIATION WITH HEMOPHAGOCYTIC LYMPHOHISTIOCYTOSIS

This process is discussed in more detail in Chapter 5.

GROUP "M" HISTIOCYTOSES

Unequivocal malignant neoplasms of monocyte/macrophage lineage are, in general, very uncommon to rare, regardless of their primary site. The skin is just one of several reported sites, and, in some cases, multifocal tumors are apparent on clinical presentation.

The past "malignant histiocytosis" was a diagnosis that today is recognized as anaplastic large cell lymphoma (ALCL) and lymphomatoid papulosis, which are CD30 T-cell proliferations with the presence of *ALK-1* translocation in subsets of ALCL. Also regarded as malignant histiocytosis in the past was histiocytic medullary reticulosis of Scott and Robb-Smith, which is recognized today as primary, or secondary hemophagocytic lymphohistiocytosis or macrophage activation syndrome.

Before a diagnosis of a malignant histiocytic lesion is made in the skin or elsewhere, it is important to keep in mind that reactive histiocytes can acquire a marked degree of atypia with nuclear enlargement, hyperchromatism, and mitotic activity.

HISTIOCYTIC SARCOMA

Definition and Epidemiology

HS is defined by the World Health Organization (WHO) as a malignancy with morphologic and immunophenotypic features that resemble those of mature tissue histiocytes.[34,223,224] HS is an aggressive neoplasm that presents across a wide range of ages, as a primary neoplasm or subsequent to a diagnosis of another hematologic malignancy. Two peaks have been reported, the first between 0 and 29 years and the second between 50 and 69 years.[224] The first peak is smaller and corresponds to the cases associated with pre-B- and T-cell leukemia/lymphoma; the second peak corresponds to those cases associated with B-cell lymphoma.[224,225] HS can present as solitary or multiple lesions involving lymph nodes or extranodal sites. The skin is the fourth most common site of extranodal involvement that can manifest as solitary or multiple lesions or as a rash. Excisional biopsy of localized lesion or a punch biopsy of a cutaneous rash usually provides adequate tissue for diagnosis with ancillary testing.

Etiology

Some cases of HS occur subsequent to or concurrent with B- or T-lymphoblastic lymphoma/leukemia or mature B-cell neoplasms such as follicular lymphoma, chronic lymphocytic leukemia, mantle cell lymphoma, extranodal marginal zone lymphoma of mucosa-associated lymphoid tissue, splenic marginal zone lymphoma, and diffuse large B-cell lymphoma. All cases associated with lymphoblastic lymphoma/leukemia are male, whereas cases associated with mature B-cell neoplasms show no sex predilection. The cases associated with lymphoblastic lymphoma/leukemia occur in children to young adults (4 years to 27 years; median age, 13 years), corresponding to the aforementioned small peak in the age distribution of HS.[225-233]

In 2008, Feldman et al provided compelling evidence that patients with follicular lymphoma and associated concurrent/subsequent HS share identical genotypic features, suggesting the possibility of transdifferentiation or dedifferentiation of the two otherwise morphologically and immunohistochemically distinctive neoplasms.[228] HS generally shares the clonal markers of the previous leukemia/lymphoma, such as *IGH* gene rearrangement, *IGK* gene rearrangement, *TCR* gamma-chain gene rearrangement, *IGH/BCL2* fusion gene (ie, a genetic hallmark of follicular lymphoma), and *CCND1-IGH* . How neoplastic B cells convert to histiocytic cells is still unknown. However, two major hypotheses have been proposed for the molecular transformation of B-cell lymphoma to HS. One is the direct transdifferentiation of neoplastic cells into malignant histiocytes. The other involves a two-step process of transformation, with first dedifferentiation of neoplastic B cells to early progenitors and subsequent redifferentiation along the histiocytic lineage. In addition, a third theoretical possibility would be the presence of a common neoplastic progenitor with differentiation along both B-cell and histiocytic/dendritic lineages.[224] Mutations in the *BRAF/HRAS* pathway have also been identified in cases of HS.[234-236]

Clinical Presentation

Lymph nodes are the most common site of presentation, although a variety of extranodal sites may be affected, particularly the gastrointestinal tract, spleen, soft tissue, and skin. Other sites of involvement include head and neck regions, salivary gland, lung, mediastinum, breast, liver, pancreas, kidney, uterus, CNS, bone, and bone marrow. Cases can be localized or disseminated. Systemic symptoms such as fever, fatigue, night sweats, weight loss, and weakness are relatively common. Lymphadenopathy is also often seen. Skin manifestations (ranging from a benign-appearing rash to solitary lesions to innumerable tumors on the trunk and extremities), intestinal obstruction, hepatosplenomegaly with associated pancytopenia and lytic bone lesions may occur.[223-225,237]

Histologic Findings

The lesion consists of a diffuse discohesive proliferation of epithelioid–spindle cells, which can have a focal whorled architecture. The nuclei are eccentric, oval, and appear convoluted or cleaved. The cytoplasm is moderate to abundant, eosinophilic to foamy, and can demonstrate evidence of phagocytosis in some areas. Nuclear pleomorphism and mitosis are often prominent (Figure 26-30). Before the era of immunostains, the above morphologic features alone were applied to arrive at a diagnosis of HS. With the advent of immunomarkers for histiocytic lineage, some of those neoplasms are now reclassified as B-cell neoplasms; one only has to recall the former appellations of "reticulum cell sarcoma" and "histiocytic lymphoma." True HSs are immunopositive for markers of macrophage lineage, CD163 and CD68 (Figure 26-31); the former is considered to be more specific.[237] S-100 can be focally positive and CD1a can be aberrantly expressed in a subset of tumors to create the diagnostic dilemma with LCS. Dendritic cell markers, CD21 and CD35, are negative as well as T- and B-cell markers.[34,237] In 2001, the WHO classification made the absence of clonal IGH (B-cell) or TCR (T-cell) gene rearrangements a requisite for diagnosis of HS, which was later retreated. Increased frequencies of these rearrangements are seen in cases with a history of lymphoma along with partial expression of T- and B-cell lineage immunohistochemical markers.[224,237]

Differential Diagnosis

The differential diagnosis includes reactive histiocytic proliferations, dendritic cell neoplasms, large cell non–Hodgkin lymphoma, especially ALCL and diffuse large cell lymphoma, malignant melanoma, epithelioid sarcoma, malignant round cell tumors, and monocytic leukemia. Reactive histiocytic proliferations can be easily distinguished on the basis of the marked degree of cellular pleomorphism seen in HS. Other dendritic cell sarcomas (interdigitating dendritic cell sarcoma) can be distinguished on the basis of a more spindle cell appearance and strong and diffuse expression of S-100. Both IDCS and HS have expression of CD68. LCH and LCS are positive for S-100, CD1a, and langerin. Some cases also have mutations of *BRAF V600E*. Malignant melanoma is very uncommon in children. The use of melanocytic markers (Melan-A, SOX-10, HMB-45, S-100) can easily distinguish between melanoma and HS. Small round cell sarcomas in children should also be considered in the differential diagnosis. Luckily, a battery of immunostains can easily distinguish them from HS. ALCLs, particularly ALK+, are common in children. The latter are strong and diffusely positive for CD30 (and ALK+). There is variable reactivity for T-cell markers, and most tumors show expression of cytotoxic markers (TIA-1, granzyme B, and perforin). Although monocytic leukemias can also enter the differential diagnosis, a diagnosis of leukemia cutis in the skin typically translates into a clinical presentation of multiple lesions. Myeloblasts and immature monocytes lack the degree of nuclear pleomorphism present in HS. The malignant cells show fine nuclear chromatin, high N/C ratio, and variable nucleoli. Expression of immature markers (CD34, CD117, and CD123) can sometimes help in the differential diagnosis.

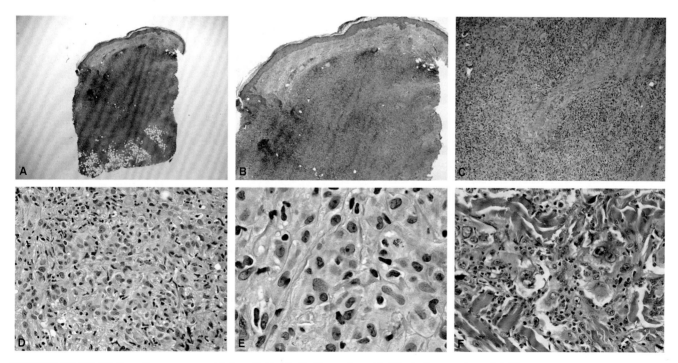

FIGURE 26-30. **Histiocytic sarcoma—histopathologic findings.** A and B, The lesion consists of a diffuse discohesive proliferation of epithelioid-spindle cells, which can have a focal whorled architecture. C, Areas of geographic necrosis mimicking epithelioid sarcoma are present. D and E, The nuclei are eccentric, oval, and appear convoluted or cleaved. F, The cytoplasm is moderate to abundant, eosinophilic to foamy, and can demonstrate evidence of phagocytosis in some areas. Nuclear pleomorphism and mitosis are often prominent.

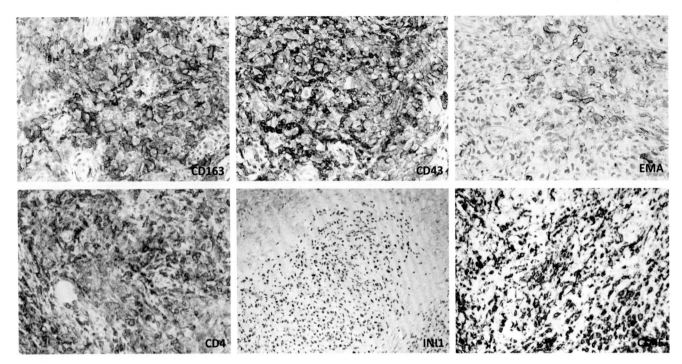

FIGURE 26-31. Histiocytic sarcoma—immunohistochemistry. The neoplastic cells are positive for CD163, CD43, focal EMA, CD4, have retained staining for INI-1 (as opposed to epithelioid sarcoma), and CD45.

CAPSULE SUMMARY

HISTIOCYTIC SARCOMA

HS is defined by the WHO as a malignancy with morphologic and immunophenotypic features that resemble those of mature tissue histiocytes. HS is an aggressive neoplasm that presents across a wide range of ages, as a primary neoplasm or subsequent to a diagnosis of another hematologic malignancy. Two peaks have been reported, the first between 0 and 29 years and the second between 50 and 69 years. HS consists of a diffuse discohesive proliferation of epithelioid-spindle cells, which can have a focal whorled architecture. The nuclei are eccentric, oval, and appear convoluted or cleaved. The cytoplasm is moderate to abundant, eosinophilic to foamy, and can demonstrate evidence of phagocytosis in some areas.

LANGERHANS CELL SARCOMA

LCS is an extremely rare high-grade malignant neoplasm with marked cytologic atypia and nuclear pleomorphism, a mitotic rate typically in excess of 50 mitoses/10 high-power field (HPF) and a morphologic appearance that resembles a dermal pleomorphic sarcoma or atypical fibroxanthoma of skin rather than LCH.[238-242] Other cytologic features that are often present include prominent nucleoli, occasional

nuclear grooves, and eccentric placement of the nucleus (Figure 26-32). In contrast to LCH, cutaneous LCS is more likely to involve the deep dermis and subcutis.[41] In a recent review, the age range of published cases of LCS was 10 to 81 years with a 1:1 male:female ratio, and 9 (29%) of 31 cases presented with cutaneous involvement. Compared to LCH, those with LCS are older and have higher stage disease and have a poorer outcome. A total of five cases have been reported in the pediatric age.

LCS is a poorly differentiated malignancy and is usually not recognized as Langerhans cell–derived neoplasm on the basis of morphology alone. This determination relies rather on the demonstration of the S-100+, CD1a+, and langerin+ immunopositivity or the finding of Birbeck granules on electron microscopy (Figure 26-33). In one study of nine cases of LCS, S-100 and CD1a were positive in all cases, but CD1a demonstrated variable staining ranging from rare positive cells to weak positivity to staining a small subset of malignant cells. In the latter study, one case was positive for Epstein-Barr virus RNA by in situ hybridization. Two of nine cases presented with skin nodules. In another report of four cases of cutaneous LCS, CD1a expression varied from weak to strong, and langerin expression ranged from absent to strong. These studies suggest that expression of the classic Langerhans cell markers may be decreased or even absent in LCS. In the setting of expression of CD1a without langerin, a diagnosis of indeterminate dendritic cell sarcoma should be considered. At least two cases have been shown to have *BRAF V600E* mutations.[242,243]

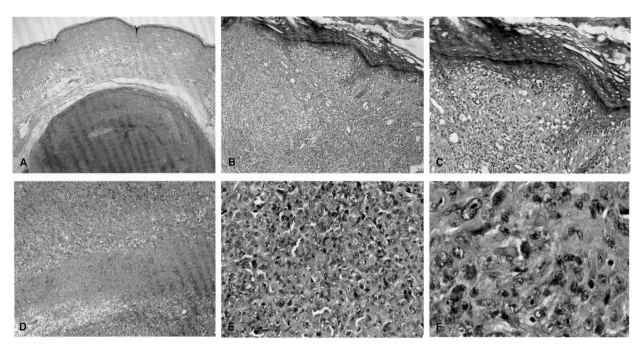

FIGURE 26-32. Langerhans cell sarcoma—histopathologic findings. A, A pleomorphic dermal tumor is present. B and C, Areas of epidermotropic markedly atypical Langerhans cells are seen. D, Necrosis is also seen. E and F, Malignant Langerhans cells show pleomorphic and vesicular nuclei with prominent nucleoli.

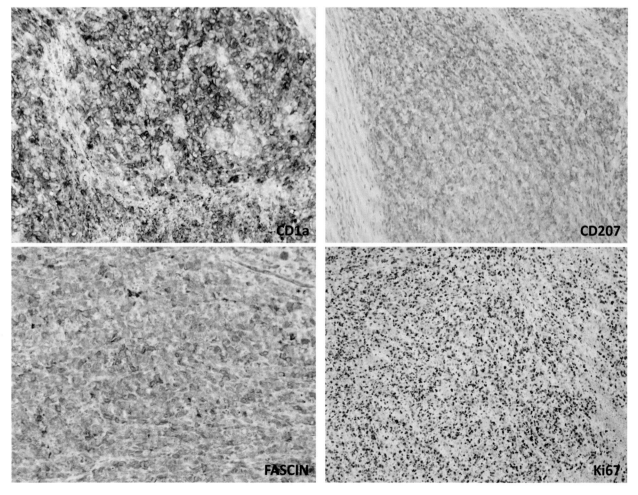

FIGURE 26-33. Langerhans cell sarcoma—immunohistochemistry. The malignant tumor is positive for CD1a, langerin (CD207), and fascin and shows a very high Ki67 proliferation index.

CAPSULE SUMMARY

LANGERHANS CELL SARCOMA

LCS is an extremely rare high-grade malignant neoplasm with marked cytologic atypia and nuclear pleomorphism, a mitotic rate typically in excess of 50 mitoses/10 HPF, and a morphologic appearance that resembles a dermal pleomorphic sarcoma or atypical fibroxanthoma of skin rather than LCH. Rare cases have been reported in children, and some of them can also harbor *BRAF* mutations.

REACTIVE HISTIOCYTOSES

INTRAVASCULAR LYMPHATIC HISTIOCYTOSIS

Definition and Epidemiology

Intravascular lymphatic histiocytosis (ILH) is a chronic, benign disorder denoted by intraluminal histiocyte hyperplasia within lymphatic vessels associated with skin pathology. It is a distinct clinical and pathologic entity from both intravascular (intracapillary) histiocytosis and reactive angioendotheliomatosis.[244]

ILH is very rare, with around 40 cases reported. It is more common in adults and slightly more prevalent in woman than in men.[245] The average age of onset is 66 years, and it is more likely to occur in patients with prior surgery, orthopedic implants, vascular disease, or rheumatoid arthritis.[244,246]

Etiology

The pathogenesis of ILH is not fully understood, but given its association with surgery as well as inflammatory and neoplastic disorders, it is hypothesized that chronic lymphatic stasis due to surgery or comorbidity may play a role in this disorder.[245,247] It has also been postulated that persistent lymphatic stasis impairs the clearance of antigens leading to a chronic inflammatory response. Finally, because ILH has been associated with a broad range of conditions, it may represent a nonspecific histologic reaction pattern.[248]

Clinical Presentation

The clinical presentation is protean and can include erythematous patches/plaques, livedo reticularis, and several other morphologies. Cutaneous lesions, which are usually painless and lack ulceration, often occur on extremities in close proximity to affected joints, be it from RA or surgery (Figure 26-34). The disease follows a chronic course and does not seem to parallel the activity of RA when associated.[244,245,247]

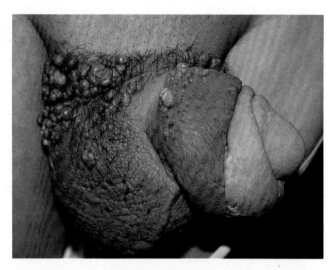

FIGURE 26-34. **Intralymphatic histiocytosis.** Scrotal and penile edema with multiple papules and vegetative lesions in a 16-year-old boy. Demirkesen C, Kran T, Leblebici C, Yücelten D, Aksu AE, Mat C. Intravascular/intralymphatic histiocytosis: a report of 3 cases. *Am J Dermatopathol.* 2015;37(10):783-789. doi:10.1097/DAD.0000000000000257.

Histologic Findings

The histology of ILH is that of dilated/ectatic reticular dermal lymphatic vessels (lymphangiectasis) with a proliferation of mononuclear, epithelioid histiocytes within their lumen. Vasculitis is not seen in ILH (Figure 26-35). The histiocytes, which may be arranged in a cluster or in more of a single-cell distribution, have an eosinophilic, vesicular cytoplasm and oval nuclei. A sparse, mixed inflammatory infiltrate may be present in the nearby dermis.[248] There is an absence of vascular proliferation and lack of thrombi, which helps differentiate ILH from reactive angioendotheliomatosis/intravascular histiocytosis.[244] The epidermis and papillary dermis are spared. D2-40, podoplanin, Prox-1, Lyve-1, CD31/34 can be used to demonstrate the association of the histiocytic proliferation within the lymphatic channels. The lesional histiocytes usually stain with CD31 and CD68, and they do not stain with S-100, CD1a, or cytokeratin markers.[249] Positive staining of histiocytes with CD31 can cause confusion as it may raise concern for a vascular tumor.

Differential Diagnosis

The histologic differential includes reactive angioendotheliomatosis/intravascular histiocytosis, intravascular lymphoma, mesothelial proliferations, glomeruloid hemangioma, metastatic carcinoma, acroangiodermatitis, and other inflammatory conditions. Immunohistochemistry can help delineate whether the affected vessels are capillary or lymphatic in nature.

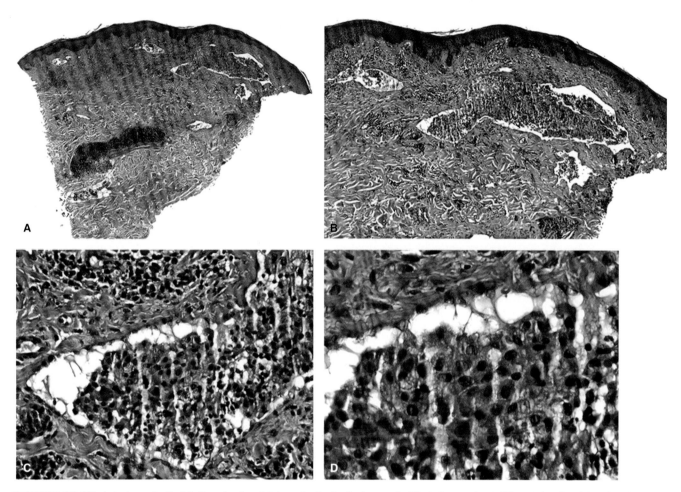

FIGURE 26-35. **Intralymphatic histiocytosis—histopathologic features.** A, Dilated vessels at different levels of the dermis. B, Intravascular collections of mononuclear epithelioid histiocytes. C, Intravascular histiocytes showed eosinophilic finely granular cytoplasm. D, Intravascular histiocytes showed vesicular oval uniform nuclei. Obtained with permission. Requena L, El-Shabrawi-Caelen L, Walsh SN, et al. Intralymphatic histiocytosis. A clinicopathologic study of 16 cases. *Am J Dermatopathol*. 2009;31(2):140-151. doi:10.1097/ DAD.0b013e3181986cc2.

CAPSULE SUMMARY

INTRAVASCULAR LYMPHATIC HISTIOCYTOSIS

ILHH is a chronic, benign disorder denoted by intraluminal histiocyte hyperplasia within lymphatic vessels associated with skin pathology. The pathogenesis of ILH is not fully understood, but given its association with surgery as well as inflammatory and neoplastic disorders, it is hypothesized that chronic lymphatic stasis due to surgery or comorbidity may play a role in this disorder. Dilated, ectatic reticular dermal lymphatic vessels (lymphangiectasis) with a luminal proliferation of mononuclear, epithelioid CD68+ histiocytes arranged in clusters or in a single-cell distribution are seen.

TUBEROUS XANTHOMAS

Definition and Epidemiology

Tuberous xanthomas (TuX) are firm, nontender, yellow subcutaneous nodules that involve trauma-prone areas of the body such as the elbows, knees, buttocks, and Achilles tendon.

TuX are rare in childhood but may occur in the setting of disorders of lipid metabolism (see Section "Etiology"). They occur in childhood because of disorders of lipid metabolism such as familial homozygous hypercholesterolemia and sitosterolemia.[250,251] Sitosterolemia may also present with intertriginous xanthomas as early as infancy.[250] In adults, there are cases of normolipemic TuX reported in association with underlying lymphoproliferative disease (especially multiple myeloma) and severe liver disease or without an underlying association.[252,253]

They present with firm, yellow-red, nontender, subcutaneous nodules that involve trauma-prone areas of the body such as the elbows, knees, buttocks, and Achilles tendon. TuX usually present as large aggregates of histiocytic cells with abundant foamy cytoplasm. Older lesions can show areas of fibrosis. Scattered multinucleated giant cells of Touton type can sometimes be seen.

CAPSULE SUMMARY

TUBEROUS XANTHOMAS

TuX are rare in childhood but may occur in the setting of disorders of lipid metabolism. TuX present with firm, yellow-red, nontender, subcutaneous nodules that involve trauma-prone areas of the body such as the elbows, knees, buttocks, and Achilles tendon.

TENDINOUS XANTHOMAS

Tendinous xanthomas (TeX) are subcutaneous tumors of lipidized histiocytes localized over tendons. TeX are rare in children but can occur in the setting of inherited or acquired disorders of lipid metabolism (see Section "Etiology"). TeX in children are seen in the setting of disorders of lipid metabolism such as cerebrotendinous xanthomatosis[254] or familial homozygous hypercholesterolemia.[251] TeX have also been reported in a child after treatment of HIV with highly active antiretroviral therapy.[255,256] TeX and TuX are a well-known side effect of ritonavir-induced hyperlipidemia in adult patients.

TeX appear as firm, skin-colored subcutaneous nodules composed of lipidized histiocytes that are located over tendons, especially the proximal finger joints, the insertion of the patellar and Achilles tendon. They do not appear yellow because the cholesterol ester is deposited deep within the tendons.[254] Over time, these TeX may fibrose, leading to interference with function, pain, and rarely spontaneous tendon rupture.[257] TeX have been reported to cause carpal tunnel syndrome and flexion contracture in a child with familial hypercholesterolemia.[258] The clinical differential diagnosis of solitary lesions would include other dermal or subcutaneous tumors such as a rheumatoid nodule, deep granuloma annulare, or a soft tissue sarcoma. Imaging with ultrasonography or clinical examination demonstrating the presence of multiple characteristic lesions should clarify the diagnosis. The histologic findings are identical to those of TuX.

CAPSULE SUMMARY

TENDINOUS XANTHOMAS

TeX are subcutaneous tumors of lipidized histiocytes localized over tendons. TeX are rare in children but can occur in the setting of inherited or acquired disorders of lipid metabolism.

VERRUCIFORM XANTHOMAS

Definition and Epidemiology

Verruciform xanthomas (VX) are rare, benign tumors of lipidized histiocytes occurring primarily on mucosal surfaces. VX in children occur primarily in the setting of genetic syndromes (see Section "Etiology").

Etiology

VX in children occur in the setting of genetic syndromes such as congenital hemidysplasia with ichthyosiform

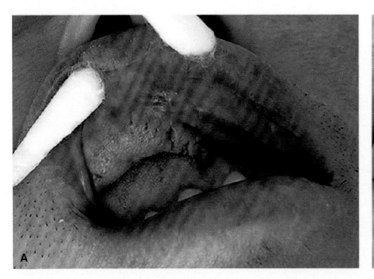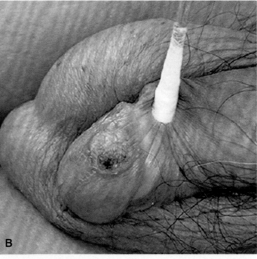

FIGURE 26-36. Verruciform xanthoma. Yellowish plaque with verrucous surface and sessile base, located on (A) upper gingival mucosa above the right incisor and canine and extending into the adjoining upper labial mucosa measuring 5 cm × 3 cm, (B) glans penis measuring 3 × 2 cm. Obtained with permission. Xue R, Su W, Pei X, Huang L, Elbendary A, Chen Z. Multiple verruciform xanthomas following bone marrow transplant. *Indian J Dermatol Venereol Leprol.* 2016;82(2):208-209.

erythroderma and limb defects (CHILD) syndrome[259,260] or primary lymphedema.[261] VX in the oral mucosa of a child have been reported in association with reactivation of Epstein-Barr virus.[262]

Clinical Presentation

VX are most commonly described as isolated, pink or yellow spongy plaques on the oral or genital mucosa (Figure 26-36). Verruciform genital-associated xanthomas are referred to as VEGAS xanthoma.[263] In children, VX have been described as verrucous papules and tumors occurring within Blaschkolinear cutaneous lesions of CHILD syndrome. In CHILD syndrome the pathogenesis of VX is thought to be related to abnormal lamellar granules and systemic lipid metabolic impairment. Nonsyndromic VX may be related to local lipid metabolic abnormality and keratinocyte degeneration

resulting from local irritation or repeated trauma.[264] In adults, most cases of VX occur as single lesions, but several concomitant oral and skin diseases have been associated with this entity, including oral lupus erythematosus, lichen planus, dystrophic epidermolysis bullosa, epidermal nevus, leukoplakia, focal acantholytic dyskeratosis, pemphigus vulgaris, chronic graft-versus-host disease, and oral squamous cell carcinoma.

Histologic Findings

Lesions typically present with papillary endothelial hyperplasia, without atypia, parakeratosis, or neutrophilic exocytosis. Sheets or large aggregates of histiocytes in the submucosa are paramount for the diagnosis (Figure 26-37). Some have classified the patterns of VX in three main forms: the most common is the verrucous form (which

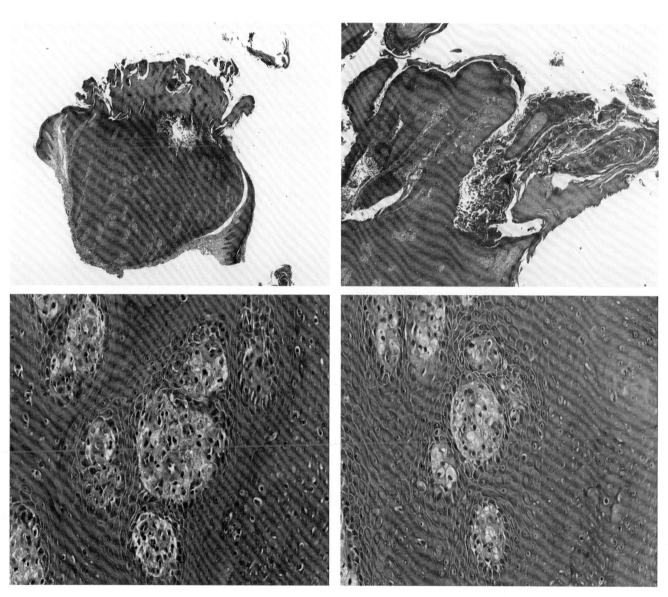

FIGURE 26-37. **Verruciform xanthoma.** There is verrucous epidermal hyperplasia with sheets of histiocytes in the dermis.

occurs in 44% of cases), followed by papillary (32%), and flat (24%). Common histiocytic markers are positive in the macrophages of the submucosa (CD68, CD163). The cells are negative for CD1a, S-100, and langerin.[265,266]

VERRUCIFORM XANTHOMAS

VX are rare, benign tumors of lipidized histiocytes occurring primarily on mucosal surfaces. VX in children occur in the setting of genetic syndromes such as CHILD syndrome or primary lymphedema. Lesions typically present with papillary endothelial hyperplasia, without atypia, parakeratosis, or neutrophilic exocytosis. Sheets or large aggregates of histiocytes in the submucosa are paramount for the diagnosis.

ERUPTIVE XANTHOMAS

Definition and Epidemiology

Eruptive xanthomas (EX) are xanthomas that appear abruptly with numerous to hundreds of lesions in the setting of hypertriglyceridemia. EX are rare in children. They typically occur in the setting of primary genetic or secondary hyperlipidemias, systemic disorders, or as a complication of certain medications (see Section "Etiology").[267-270]

Etiology

EX may occur in the setting of primary hyperlipidemia or as a secondary phenomenon in the setting of systemic illness such as poorly controlled diabetes mellitus, biliary cirrhosis, primary hypothyroidism, and nephrotic syndrome. EX may be triggered by numerous drugs such as estrogens, isotretinoin, HIV-1 protease inhibitors, and sirolimus for organ transplantation. Finally, EX may be seen in the setting of genetic syndromes including lipodystrophies and Alagille syndrome.

Clinical Presentation

EX, as the name suggests, typically present with an eruptive or explosive onset of hundreds of brown to yellow papules distributed on the hands, buttocks, and extensor surface of the extremities in the setting of extreme hypertriglyceridemia (Figure 26-38). They can occasionally be mistaken for other skin lesions, such as molluscum contagiosum.[269]

Histologic Features

The histologic findings are similar and equivalent to other forms of xanthomas.

ERUPTIVE XANTHOMAS

EX are xanthomas that appear abruptly with numerous to hundreds of lesions in the setting of hypertriglyceridemia. EX are rare in children. They typically occur in the setting of primary genetic or secondary hyperlipidemias, systemic disorders, or as a complication of certain medications.

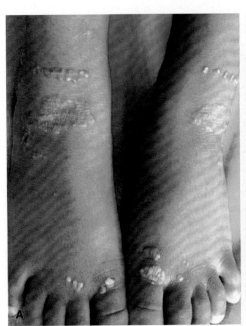
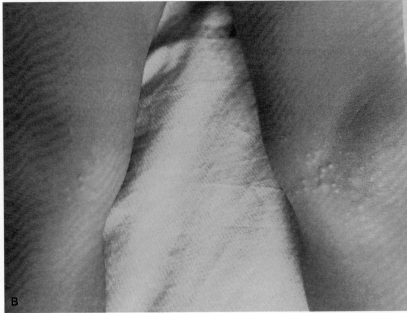

FIGURE 26-38. Eruptive xanthoma. Multiple yellow papules on the feet (A) and knees (B).

MAST CELL DISORDERS

MASTOCYTOMA

Definition and Epidemiology

Solitary mastocytoma is a form of cutaneous mastocytosis characterized by the presence of one or a few solitary cutaneous tumors comprised of clonal mast cells without systemic involvement.[271,272] Solitary mastocytomas most frequently occur in infants and children under 2 years of age, with the highest prevalence in the first month of life.[271,273] True solitary mastocytomas (isolated lesions without systemic disease) are only very rarely seen in adults and children over the age of 16, with only a handful of cases reported in the literature.[273,274] Solitary mastocytomas account for approximately 20% of cutaneous mastocytosis cases (with the remaining 80% of cases representing UP and disseminated cutaneous mastocytosis).[275,276]

Etiology

Although their etiology is not fully understood, mastocytomas often show activating mutations in the *KIT* gene.[277] KIT is a receptor tyrosine kinase and proto-oncogene that is normally expressed by mast cells.[277] Activating mutations in *KIT* are key molecular carcinogenic events in gastrointestinal stromal tumors (GISTS), as well as some melanomas and acute myeloid leukemias.[277] Contrary to the previously held notion that *KIT* mutations are generally only associated with adult mastocytosis, many recent studies have demonstrated *KIT* mutations in childhood mastocytosis.[277-280] Mastocytomas specifically have been found to have mutations in *KIT*, with one study reporting identifiable mutations in 67% of solitary mastocytomas.[277]

Clinical Presentation

Mastocytomas are typically brown or yellow-brown macules, plaques, or nodules (Figure 26-39).[281,282] The lesions are most commonly distributed on the trunk, but also occur frequently on the face and limbs.[283] Solitary mastocytomas are generally less than 1 cm in diameter..[271] The surface of the lesions may be smooth or may have a characteristic orange peel (peau d'orange) appearance.[281] Rubbing of the lesions often causes mast cell degranulation, resulting in localized swelling or wheal formation (referred to clinically as Darier's sign, Figure 26-40).[273,281] Extralesional symptoms such as flushing, pruritus, nausea, vomiting, and headaches may occur in a small subset of patients with mastocytomas and are due to release of mast cell mediators into the circulation.[281,284,285]

Patients with solitary mastocytomas have an excellent prognosis. By definition, patients do not have systemic disease.[271] The majority of mastocytomas will resolve spontaneously—in most cases within 4 to 10 years, and often by the time the patient reaches puberty.[273,283] Adult-onset

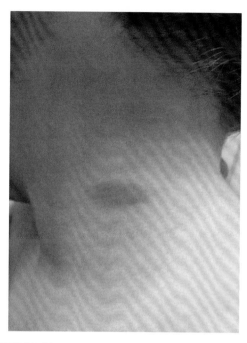

FIGURE 26-39. Solitary mastocytoma. Single brownish plaque on the neck.

mastocytomas are less likely to spontaneously involute than the typical pediatric mastocytomas.[273] However, mastocytomas that persist in any age group are often cured with complete excision.[271,286] Malignant transformation in solitary mastocytomas (primary cutaneous mast cell sarcoma) has not been described.[271]

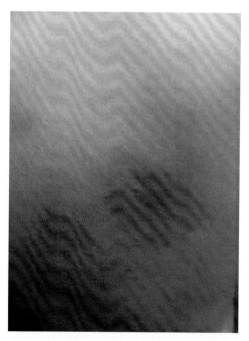

FIGURE 26-40. Darier sign. Rubbing of the lesions often causes mast cell degranulation, resulting in localized swelling or wheal formation (referred to clinically as Darier's sign).

Histologic Findings

Mastocytomas show a dense, nodular aggregate of mature mast cells in the dermis with occasional extension into the deeper levels of the dermis and subcutaneous tissues.[287] The mast cells of mastocytoma are ovoid or polygonal in shape with abundant cytoplasm and contain round to oval nuclei with inconspicuous nucleoli.[281] The cytoplasm is filled with eosinophilic to amphophilic cytoplasmic granules that contain histamine and other bioactive chemicals (Figures 26-41 and 26-42).[281]

Mastocytomas express normal mast cell markers such as CD33, CD5, CD68, CD117, tryptase, and chymase (Figure 26-43).[288,289] Mast cells also express CD45 (common leukocyte antigen).[288] Histochemical stains such as toluidine blue, Giemsa, and chloroacetate esterase (Leder stain) may also be used to highlight mast cells.[271,288] CD117 is the most sensitive marker for mast cells but is not entirely specific. Conversely, chymase is highly specific for mast cells, but less sensitive.[288] Childhood mastocytoses very rarely express aberrant immunohistochemical markers such as CD25 or CD2, with very few reported cases in the literature.[289,290] Aberrant antigen expression in solitary mastocytomas specifically is not well characterized. However, as a whole, the limited cutaneous mastocytoses (including solitary mastocytomas) express aberrant CD25 much less often than the cutaneous lesions of systemic mastocytosis.[291]

Differential Diagnosis

The differential diagnosis includes systemic mastocytosis and other forms of cutaneous mastocytosis discussed in this chapter. Cutaneous tumors with cell types that resemble

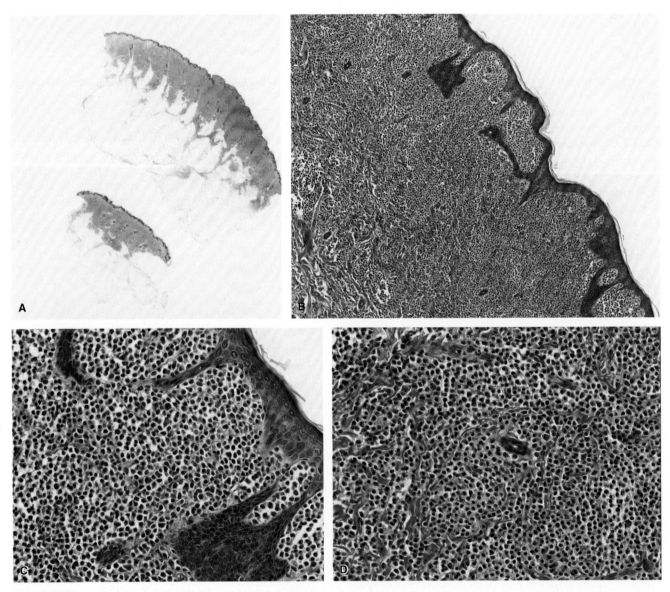

FIGURE 26-41. Solitary mastocytoma—histopathology. A and B, Localized dermal proliferation of epithelioid-appearing mast cells. C and D, The abnormal mast cells are medium in size, with abundant granular cytoplasm, and have a perivascular distribution.

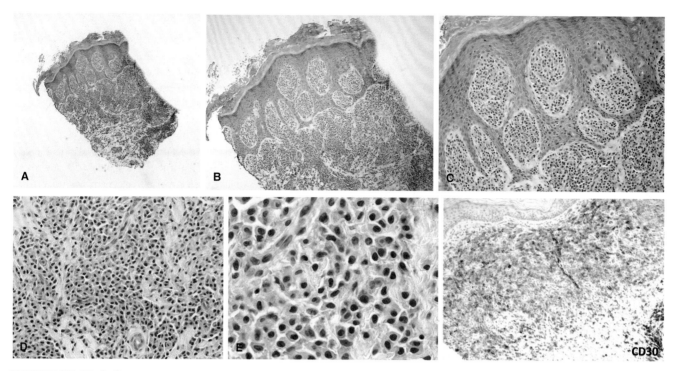

FIGURE 26-42. Solitary mastocytoma—histopathology. Another example of mastocytoma. There is a dense infiltrate in the dermis with sparing of the epidermis (A to C). The infiltrate is composed of sheets of atypical mast cells with abundant granular cytoplasm (D and E). In this particular case, there is diffuse expression of CD30.

mast cells may also be considered in the differential. Mast cells typically have a characteristic histologic appearance with amphophilic cytoplasmic granules that are uncommonly seen in other cell types.[281] Nevertheless, in certain cases mast cells may bear resemblance to melanocytes, histiocytes, and Langerhans cells.[292] LCH also frequently presents as a cutaneous tumor in infants and young children.[293] However, histologically, Langerhans cells are pale histiocytes devoid of cytoplasmic granules and demonstrate reniform or folded nuclei.[293] Langerhans cells are positive for S-100, Langerin, and CD1a whereas mast cells are negative for these markers.[290,292,293] An eosinophilic infiltrate is common in lesions of LCH,[293] but this feature has also rarely been described in cases of mastocytoma.[294,295] Histologically, mastocytomas may also bear resemblance to melanocytic nevi and even reported rarely in conjunction. Unlike junctional melanocytic nevi, mastocytomas do not typically involve the epidermis.[292] Furthermore, mastocytomas do

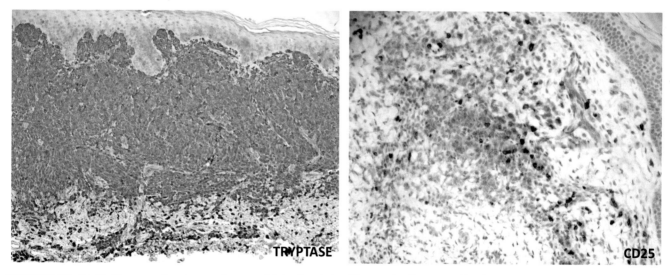

FIGURE 26-43. Solitary mastocytoma—immunohistochemistry. The mast cells are positive for tryptase and show coexpression of CD25 (a marker that is not normally expressed in mast cells).

not generally show the nesting pattern often seen in melanocytic nevi.[292] Immunohistochemical stains for S-100 protein, CD117, and melanocyte-specific markers may be used if the distinction cannot be made on histologic examination alone.

In a child or an adult with a presumed solitary cutaneous mastocytoma, systemic mastocytosis should also be considered in the differential diagnosis. Aberrant CD25 expression is more commonly seen in cases of systemic mastocytosis, and this marker may be useful for identifying patients with cutaneous mastocytosis who are more likely to have systemic disease and may require further workup.[291]

Rare cases of mastocytomas with dense eosinophilic infiltrates have been described.[294,295] The eosinophilic infiltrate may be so dense as to obscure the underlying mast cells, making the diagnosis challenging, and raising the differential consideration of LCH.[295] A histiocyte-rich pleomorphic mastocytoma has also been described. This lesion was characterized by a rich histiocytic infiltrate with enlarged, bilobed, and multinucleated mast cells.[290]

CAPSULE SUMMARY

MASTOCYTOMA

Mastoctyomas are solitary tumors comprised of clonal mast cells. Solitary mastocytomas by definition have no systemic involvement. They are most commonly seen in infants and children under the age of 2. Adult-onset solitary mastocytomas are extremely rare. Most solitary mastocytomas resolve spontaneously within a few years or by the time the child reaches puberty and do not require treatment. Solitary mastocytomas have been shown to have mutations in the *KIT* proto-oncogene.

URTICARIA PIGMENTOSA (MACULOPAPULAR CUTANEOUS MASTOCYTOSIS)

Definition and Epidemiology

UP has a clinical presentation of a cutaneous mastocytosis characterized by a rash consisting of discrete cutaneous lesions (usually macule, papules, nodules, or plaques) with abnormal mast cell infiltrates.[272,276,296] UP is the most common clinical presentation of cutaneous mastocytosis, representing 75% to 80% of all cases.[275,276] As with other forms of cutaneous mastocytosis, UP more frequently occurs in infants and children, with 80% of cases occurring in the first year of life.[272,296] In adult patients who clinically appear to have UP, further studies frequently show systemic disease, and these patients are better classified as having systemic mastocytosis with cutaneous involvement.[296,297] However, rare cases of adults with pure cutaneous UP have been described.[297] Studies have shown an equal sex predilection to slight male predominance.[276,296]

Etiology

Both childhood and adult forms of mastocytosis show mutations in the *KIT* proto-oncogene.[297] Over 80% of adults with mastocytosis show a specific *KIT* mutation: *D816V* on exon 17.[297] In contrast, only 35% of childhood mastocytosis cases (most of which are UP) have *D816V KIT* mutations.[272] Children with cutaneous mastocytosis more commonly exhibit other mutations in *KIT* involving exons 8, 9, or 11 (40% of cases) or have no *KIT* mutations whatsoever (25% of cases).[272,276] Most *KIT* mutations are sporadic, although familial forms of UP with a variety of germline mutations in *KIT* have been described.[298-303] The majority of these familial cases follow an autosomal dominant pattern of inheritance.[298-303] *KIT* activating mutations are also seen in gastrointestinal stromal tumors, as well as some melanomas and acute myeloid leukemias.[277] Some patients with germline *KIT* mutations are also prone to developing gastrointestinal stromal tumors; however, the rates of concomitant tumors in these patients are lower than would be expected, with only a few such cases described in the literature.[299,303]

Clinical Presentation

The lesions of UP are usually red or brown, oval shaped, and typically vary in size.[272] Most of the lesions are larger than 0.5 mm and may be macules, papules, nodules, or plaques (Figure 26-44).[2] The lesions can be sharply demarcated or have indistinct borders.[272] The lesions are typically symmetrically distributed on the head, neck, and extremities.[272,281] Rubbing or scratching of the rash usually results in localized swelling, wheal, or blister formation (Darier's sign) because of mast cell degranulation.[282] Itching is present in approximately half of the patients.[281] The disease only very rarely persists into adulthood.[282] Serum tryptase levels are often measured in patients with mastocytosis. Patients with isolated cutaneous mastocytosis generally have lower serum tryptase levels than those with systemic mastocytosis.[304] In children with UP, serum tryptase levels are usually within the normal range,[272,304] which is consistent with the fact that UP in children is frequently a skin-limited process. Some congenital cases can present with alopecia.

In children, UP can be subdivided into two clinically distinct variants based on the morphology of the lesions.[272] Most children with UP have a polymorphic variant, which is characterized by large lesions (usually nodules and plaques) of varying shapes and sizes.[272] Children with the polymorphic variant have the typical favorable clinical outcome of other forms of childhood cutaneous mastocytosis, and the lesions almost always resolve spontaneously by the time the patient reaches puberty.[272,304] A smaller percentage of pediatric patients with UP show lesions that are monomorphic and small (monomorphic variant).[272] Children with the monomorphic variant often have increased tryptase levels and systemic involvement. The childhood monomorphic variant of UP also frequently persists into adulthood.[282,304]

The prognosis in children is good. In most patients, the rash regresses by the time the patient reaches puberty.[282] On

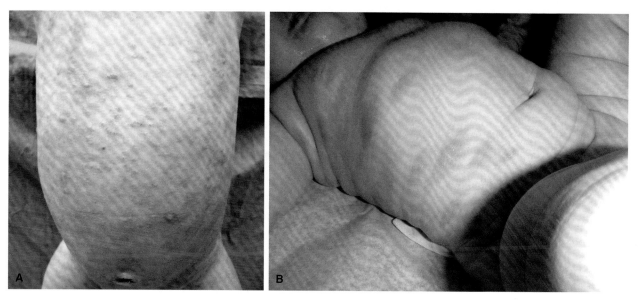

FIGURE 26-44. **Urticaria pigmentosa.** Clinical features of polymorphic variant. A, Multiple papules and nodules of varying sizes in the trunk. B, Large plaques in the chest and inguinal folds.

the other hand, adults with UP are more likely to have persistent disease and systemic involvement.[282]

Histologic Findings

Biopsies of UP lesions show an increase in dermal mast cells that is 4 to 8 times higher than that seen in normal skin and 2 to 3 times higher than that seen in inflamed skin.[2] The mast cells may be spindled or ovoid and often show characteristic amphophilic cytoplasmic granules.[282,281] The number of dermal mast cells varies from patient to patient.[282]

The infiltrate is predominantly in the upper third of the dermis, at times in proximity to the dermoepidermal junction (Figure 26-45).[305]

Mast cells express CD33, CD5, CD68, CD117, tryptase, and chymase, as well as CD45 (leukocyte common antigen).[288,306] Toluidine blue, Giemsa, and chloroacetate esterase (the Leder stain) can also be used to highlight mast cells.[270,288] CD117 is the most sensitive marker for mast cells but is not entirely specific. Conversely, chymase positivity is highly specific for mast cells, but less sensitive.[288] Tryptase has been recommended as the standard

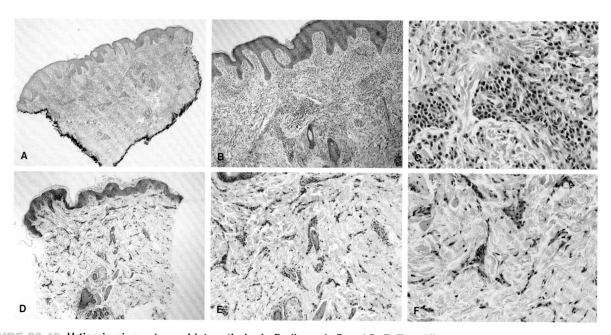

FIGURE 26-45. **Urticaria pigmentosa—histopathologic findings.** A, B and D, E, Two different examples of cases where the mast cell infiltrate is notoriously present around the vessels. C, Abundant eosinophils can be seen in the background. F, In the second case, the mast cells show a spindled appearance.

immunohistochemical marker for the identification and quantification of mast cells in mastocytosis.[270]

Differential Diagnosis

The lesions of UP may spontaneously develop edema and blistering and may be mistaken for urticaria. However, true urticaria lasts only a few hours, is migratory in nature, and is generally not hyperpigmented (UP lesions are typically red or brown in color). Many authors prefer the term *maculopapular cutaneous mastocytosis* rather than UP for this reason.[282] Bullous or blistered lesions of UP could be confused with other cutaneous bullous diseases such as bullous arthropod bites, bullous impetigo, herpes simplex virus, or linear IgA bullous diseases. Skin biopsies showing an increase in dermal mast cells help to establish the correct diagnosis.

CAPSULE SUMMARY

URTICARIA PIGMENTOSA

UP is the most common presentation of cutaneous mastocytosis in children and represents 75% to 80% of cases. Childhood cases of UP have a good prognosis. Lesions typically resolve by the time the patient reaches puberty, and patients rarely have systemic involvement. *KIT* point mutations in pediatric and adult UP appear to be different.

DIFFUSE CUTANEOUS MASTOCYTOSIS

Definition and Epidemiology

Diffuse cutaneous mastocytosis (DCM) is a rare form of cutaneous mastocytosis characterized by involvement of the entire skin by an abnormal infiltration of mast cells.[282,307] DCM is the rarest form of cutaneous mastocytosis, making up 0.6% to 8% of all cases.[307] The onset of the disease is usually in the 6 months of life and often at birth.[307] Adults rarely present with DCM.[282]

Etiology

As is the case with other forms of mastocytosis, *KIT* mutations are the suggested etiologic factor in most cases of DCM.[281] Mutations in *D816V* on exon 17 as well as mutations in exons 8 and 9 have been described.[282,281] Germline mutations in *KIT* have also been shown to cause familial forms of DCM.[308,309]

Clinical Presentation

DCM is the most severe clinical presentation of cutaneous mastocytosis and is characterized by mast cell infiltration of the entire skin.[307] Patients typically present with widespread erythema, blistering, erosions, or thickened skin (Figures 26-46 and 26-47).[307] An initial presentation with large blisters is not uncommon and may be confused for cutaneous bullous diseases.[282] The mast cell burden is higher in patients

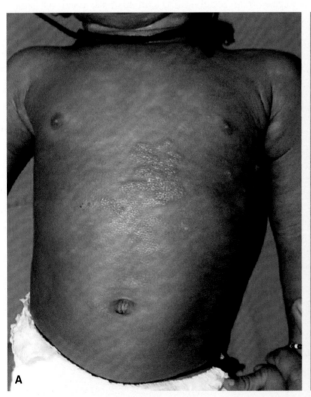
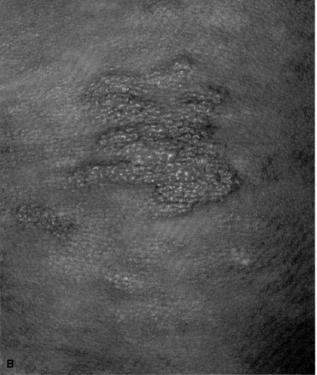

FIGURE 26-46. Diffuse cutaneous mastocytosis. A, Diffuse, erythematous, infiltrative lesions all over the trunk. B, Grouped vesicular eruptions on the epigastric region. Obtained with permission. Kumudhini S, Rao R, Salgaonkar G, Shetty S, Pai S. Granular IgM deposition at basement membrane zone in an infant with diffuse cutaneous mastocytosis. *Indian J Dermatol.* 2016;61(5):581. doi:10.4103/0019-5154.190134.

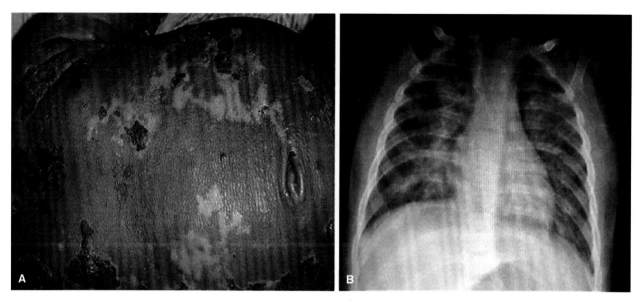

FIGURE 26-47. Diffuse cutaneous mastocytosis. A, Multiple tense bullae and erosions developed with peau d'orange–like skin on the face, scalp, and trunk. B, Bilateral pulmonary infiltration in chest x-ray. Obtained with permission. Dhar S, Maji B, Roy S, Dhar S. Diffuse cutaneous mastocytosis with bullous lesions and pulmonary involvement: a rare case. *Indian J Dermatol.* 2015;60(2):179-181. doi:10.4103/0019-5154.152522.

with DCM than in other forms of cutaneous mastocytosis, thus patients with DCM often have symptoms related to the systemic release of mast cell mediators into the circulation such as flushing, itching, gastrointestinal complaints (nausea, vomiting, diarrhea), hypotension, headaches, and, in severe cases, anaphylactic shock.[307] Rubbing or scratching of the skin in patients with DCM results in localized swelling and wheal or blister formation (Darier's sign).[307] Serum tryptase levels in DCM are often elevated and may be used to predict disease severity and prognosis.[307]

The prognosis of DCM is more guarded than that of other childhood forms of cutaneous mastocytosis.[307] This is due to the complications that may arise from an increase in circulating mast cell mediators that can cause life-threatening hypotension or anaphylaxis.[37] Because of the low incidence of DCM, the rate of this complication is not well established; however, one study demonstrated that 3 of 10 patients with DCM had an anaphylactic reaction at some point during the course of their disease.[307] The risk of developing anaphylactic reactions has been shown to be highest in the first 2 years of life and slowly declines thereafter.[307] Despite the threat of complications from mast cell mediator release, children usually achieve remission or partial remission by 3 to 5 years of age and rarely progress to systemic mastocytosis.[286,307] The disease usually resolves by adolescence.[272]

Histologic Findings

Histologic sections from biopsies of DCM show an increased number of loosely arranged mast cells throughout the dermis.[310] Normal mast cells are ovoid with round nuclei[281] and contain small, faint, amphophilic cytoplasmic granules.[281] Mast cells in DCM tend to aggregate close to vessels within the superficial dermis and within the dermal papillae.[281] The immunophenotype of DCM is similar to the other forms of cutaneous mastocytosis.

Differential Diagnosis

DCM is a rare clinical presentation of cutaneous mastocytosis that is not often encountered. The lack of macules, papules, nodules, and plaques is unusual for cutaneous mastocytosis. Because of this, the disorder is not often initially suspected.[307] Other diffuse cutaneous processes common in children are often considered, including staphylococcal scalded skin syndrome, epidermolysis bullosa acquisita, impetigo bullosa, and atopic dermatitis.[307] However, as with the other forms of cutaneous mastocytosis, DCM displays Darier's sign, and typically patients with DCM will have mediator-related symptoms.[307] Skin biopsies demonstrating an atypical mast cell infiltrate are important in confirming the diagnosis.

CAPSULE SUMMARY

DIFFUSE CUTANEOUS MASTOCYTOSIS

DCM is the most severe form of cutaneous mastocytosis and is characterized by generalized skin involvement. DCM is the rarest form of cutaneous mastocytosis and most frequently occurs in children in the first 6 months of life. Because of the high number of mast cells involved in the disease, patients often present with systemic symptoms as a result of mast cell mediator release into the circulation and can have resultant severe anaphylactic reactions.

REFERENCES

1. Emile JF, Abla O, Fraitag S, et al. Revised classification of histiocytoses and neoplasms of the macrophage-dendritic cell lineages. *Blood.* 2016;127(22):2672-2681.

2. Hutter C, Minkov M. Insights into the pathogenesis of Langerhans cell histiocytosis: the development of targeted therapies. *Immunotargets Ther.* 2016;5:81-91.

3. Morimoto A, Oh Y, Shioda Y, et al. Recent advances in Langerhans cell histiocytosis. *Pediatr Int.* 2014;56(4):451-461.

4. Gru AA, Dehner LP. Cutaneous hematolymphoid and histiocytic proliferations in children. *Pediatr Dev Pathol.* 2018;21(2):208-251.

5. Badalian-Very G, Vergilio JA, Fleming M, Rollins BJ. Pathogenesis of Langerhans cell histiocytosis. *Annu Rev Pathol.* 2013;8:1-20.

6. Stingl G, Tamaki K, Katz SI. Origin and function of epidermal Langerhans cells. *Immunol Rev.* 1980;53:149-174.

7. Willman CL, Busque L, Griffith BB, et al. Langerhans'-cell histiocytosis (histiocytosis X)—a clonal proliferative disease. *N Engl J Med.* 1994;331(3):154-160.

8. Collin M, Bigley V, McClain KL, Allen CE. Cell(s) of origin of Langerhans cell histiocytosis. *Hematol Oncol Clin North Am.* 2015;29(5):825-838.

9. Haroche J, Cohen-Aubart F, Rollins BJ. Histiocytoses: emerging neoplasia behind inflammation. *Lancet Oncol.* 2017;18(2):e113-e125.

10. Rollins BJ. Genomic alterations in Langerhans cell histiocytosis. *Hematol Oncol Clin North Am.* 2015;29(5):839-851.

11. Berres ML, Lim KP, Peters T, et al. BRAF-V600E expression in precursor versus differentiated dendritic cells defines clinically distinct LCH risk groups. *J Exp Med.* 2014;211(4):669-683.

12. Durham BH, Roos-Weil D, Baillou C, et al. Functional evidence for derivation of systemic histiocytic neoplasms from hematopoietic stem/progenitor cells. *Blood.* 2017;130(2):176-180.

13. Milne P, Bigley V, Bacon CM, et al. Hematopoietic origin of Langerhans cell histiocytosis and Erdheim-Chester disease in adults. *Blood.* 2017;130(2):167-175.

14. Milne P, Bigley V, Bacon CM, et al. Hematopoietic origin of Langerhans cell histiocytosis and Erdheim-Chester disease in adults. *Blood.* 2017;130(2):167-175.

15. Howarth DM, Gilchrist GS, Mullan BP, Wiseman GA, Edmonson JH, Schomberg PJ. Langerhans cell histiocytosis: diagnosis, natural history, management, and outcome. *Cancer.* 1999;85(10):2278-2290.

16. Salotti JA, Nanduri V, Pearce MS, Parker L, Lynn R, Windebank KP. Incidence and clinical features of Langerhans cell histiocytosis in the UK and Ireland. *Arch Dis Child.* 2009;94(5):376-380.

17. Harmon CM, Brown N. Langerhans cell histiocytosis: a clinicopathologic review and molecular pathogenetic update. *Arch Pathol Lab Med.* 2015;139(10):1211-1214.

18. Savasan S. An enigmatic disease: childhood Langerhans cell histiocytosis in 2005. *Int J Dermatol.* 2006;45(3):182-188.

19. Billings TL, Barr R, Dyson S. Langerhans cell histiocytosis mimicking malignant melanoma: a diagnostic pitfall. *Am J Dermatopathol.* 2008;30(5):497-499.

20. Zinn DJ, Grimes AB, Lin H, Eckstein O, Allen CE, McClain KL. Hydroxyurea: a new old therapy for Langerhans cell histiocytosis. *Blood.* 2016;128(20):2462-2465.

21. Héritier S, Emile JF, Barkaoui MA, et al. BRAF mutation correlates with high-risk Langerhans cell histiocytosis and increased resistance to first-line therapy. *J Clin Oncol.* 2016;34(25):3023-3030.

22. Badalian-Very G, Vergilio JA, Degar BA, et al. Recurrent BRAF mutations in Langerhans cell histiocytosis. *Blood.* 2010;116(11):1919-1923.

23. Diamond EL, Durham BH, Haroche J, et al. Diverse and targetable kinase alterations drive histiocytic neoplasms. *Cancer Discov.* 2016;6(2):154-165.

24. Emile JF, Diamond EL, Hélias-Rodzewicz Z, et al. Recurrent RAS and PIK3CA mutations in Erdheim-Chester disease. *Blood.* 2014;124(19):3016-3019.

25. Haroche J, Charlotte F, Arnaud L, et al. High prevalence of BRAF V600E mutations in Erdheim-Chester disease but not in other non-Langerhans cell histiocytoses. *Blood.* 2012;120(13):2700-2703.

26. Arico M. Langerhans cell histiocytosis in children: from the bench to bedside for an updated therapy. *Br J Haematol.* 2016;173(5):663-670.

27. Shaffer MP, Walling HW, Stone MS. Langerhans cell histiocytosis presenting as blueberry muffin baby. *J Am Acad Dermatol.* 2005;53(2 suppl 1):S143-S146.

28. Ehrhardt MJ, Humphrey SR, Kelly ME, Chiu YE, Galbraith SS. The natural history of skin-limited Langerhans cell histiocytosis: a single-institution experience. *J Pediatr Hematol Oncol.* 2014;36(8):613-616.

29. Willis B, Ablin A, Weinberg V, Zoger S, Wara WM, Matthay KK. Disease course and late sequelae of Langerhans' cell histiocytosis: 25-year experience at the University of California, San Francisco. *J Clin Oncol.* 1996;14(7):2073-2082.

30. Stein SL, Paller AS, Haut PR, Mancini AJ. Langerhans cell histiocytosis presenting in the neonatal period: a retrospective case series. *Arch Pediatr Adolesc Med.* 2001;155(7):778-783.

31. Morren MA, Vanden Broecke K, Vangeebergen L, et al. Diverse cutaneous presentations of Langerhans cell histiocytosis in children: a retrospective cohort study. *Pediatr Blood Cancer.* 2016;63(3):486-492.

32. Minkov M, Grois N, Heitger A, et al. Response to initial treatment of multisystem Langerhans cell histiocytosis: an important prognostic indicator. *Med Pediatr Oncol.* 2002;39(6):581-585.

33. Lieberman PH, Jones CR, Steinman RM, et al. Langerhans cell (eosinophilic) granulomatosis. A clinicopathologic study encompassing 50 years. *Am J Surg Pathol.* 1996;20(5):519-552.

34. Pileri SA, Grogan TM, Harris NL, et al. Tumours of histiocytes and accessory dendritic cells: an immunohistochemical approach to classification from the International Lymphoma Study Group based on 61 cases. *Histopathology.* 2002;41(1):1-29.

35. Risdall RJ, Dehner LP, Duray P, Kobrinsky N, Robison L, Nesbit ME Jr. Histiocytosis X (Langerhans' cell histiocytosis). Prognostic role of histopathology. *Arch Pathol Lab Med.* 1983;107(2):59-63.

36. Picarsic J, Jaffe R. Nosology and pathology of Langerhans cell histiocytosis. *Hematol Oncol Clin North Am.* 2015;29(5):799-823.

37. Newman B, Hu W, Nigro K, Gilliam AC. Aggressive histiocytic disorders that can involve the skin. *J Am Acad Dermatol.* 2007;56(2):302-316.

38. Motoi M, Helbron D, Kaiserling E, Lennert K. Eosinophilic granuloma of lymph nodes—a variant of histiocytosis X. *Histopathology.* 1980;4(6):585-606.

39. Valladeau J, Caux C, Lebecque S, Saeland S. Langerin: a new lectin specific for Langerhans cells induces the formation of Birbeck granules [in French]. *Pathol Biol (Paris).* 2001;49(6):454-455.

40. Valladeau J, Clair-Moninot V, Dezutter-Dambuyant C, et al. Identification of mouse langerin/CD207 in Langerhans cells and some dendritic cells of lymphoid tissues. *J Immunol.* 2002;168(2):782-792.

41. Valladeau J, Dezutter-Dambuyant C, Saeland S. Langerin/CD207 sheds light on formation of Birbeck granules and their possible function in Langerhans cells. *Immunol Res.* 2003;28(2):93-107.

42. Valladeau J, Ravel O, Dezutter-Dambuyant C, et al. Langerin, a novel C-type lectin specific to Langerhans cells, is an endocytic receptor that induces the formation of Birbeck granules. *Immunity.* 2000;12(1):71-81.

43. Chikwava K, Jaffe R. Langerin (CD207) staining in normal pediatric tissues, reactive lymph nodes, and childhood histiocytic disorders. *Pediatr Dev Pathol.* 2004;7(6):607-614.

44. Lau SK, Chu PG, Weiss LM. Immunohistochemical expression of Langerin in Langerhans cell histiocytosis and non-Langerhans cell histiocytic disorders. *Am J Surg Pathol.* 2008;32(4):615-619.

45. Grace SA, Sutton AM, Armbrecht ES, Vidal CI, Rosman IS, Hurley MY. p53 is a helpful marker in distinguishing Langerhans cell histiocytosis from Langerhans cell hyperplasia. *Am J Dermatopathol.* 2017;39(10):726-730.

46. Shanmugam V, Craig JW, Hornick JL, Morgan EA, Pinkus GS, Pozdnyakova O. Cyclin D1 is expressed in neoplastic cells of Langerhans cell histiocytosis but not reactive Langerhans cell proliferations. *Am J Surg Pathol.* 2017;41(10):1390-1396.

47. Mandel VD, Ferrari C, Cesinaro AM, Pellacani G, Del Forno C. Congenital "self-healing" Langerhans cell histiocytosis (Hashimoto-Pritzker disease): a report of two cases with the same cutaneous manifestations but different clinical course. *J Dermatol.* 2014;41(12):1098-1101.

48. Inuzuka M, Tomita K, Tokura Y, Takigawa M. Congenital self-healing reticulohistiocytosis presenting with hemorrhagic bullae. *J Am Acad Dermatol.* 2003;48(5 Suppl):S75-S77.

49. Kapur P, Erickson C, Rakheja D, Carder KR, Hoang MP. Congenital self-healing reticulohistiocytosis (Hashimoto-Pritzker disease): ten-year experience at Dallas Children's Medical Center. *J Am Acad Dermatol.* 2007;56(2):290-294.

50. Lee YH, Talekar MK, Chung CG, Bell MD, Zaenglein AL. Congenital self-healing reticulohistiocytosis. *J Clin Aesthet Dermatol.* 2014;7(2):49-53.

51. Zaenglein AL, Steele MA, Kamino H, Chang MW. Congenital self-healing reticulohistiocytosis with eye involvement. *Pediatr Dermatol.* 2001;18(2):135-137.

52. Alexis JB, Poppiti RJ, Turbat-Herrera E, Smith MD. Congenital self-healing reticulohistiocytosis. Report of a case with 7-year follow-up and a review of the literature. *Am J Dermatopathol.* 1991;13(2):189-194.

53. Oranje AP, Vuzevski VD, de Groot R, Prins ME. Congenital self-healing non-Langerhans cell histiocytosis. *Eur J Pediatr.* 1988;148(1):29-31.

54. Yurkovich M, Wong A, Lam JM. Solitary congenital self-healing Langerhans cell histiocytosis: a benign variant of Langerhans cell histiocytosis? *Dermatol Online J.* 2013;19(1):3.

55. Alotaibi S, Alhafi O, Nasr H, Eltayeb K, Elyamany G. Erdheim-Chester disease: case report with aggressive multisystem manifestations and review of the literature. *Case Rep Oncol.* 2017;10(2):501-507.

56. Estrada-Veras JI, O'Brien KJ, Boyd LC, et al. The clinical spectrum of Erdheim-Chester disease: an observational cohort study. *Blood Adv.* 2017;1(6):357-366.

57. Su HH, Wu W, Guo Y, Chen HD, Shan SJ. Pediatric Erdheim-Chester disease with aggressive skin manifestations. *Br J Dermatol.* 2018;178(1):261-264.

58. Vallonthaiel AG, Mridha AR, Gamanagatti S, et al. Unusual presentation of Erdheim-Chester disease in a child with acute lymphoblastic leukemia. *World J Radiol.* 2016;8(8):757-763.

59. Haroun F, Millado K, Tabbara I. Erdheim-Chester disease: comprehensive review of molecular profiling and therapeutic advances. *Anticancer Res.* 2017;37(6):2777-2783.

60. Neckman JP, Kim J, Mathur M, Myung P, Girardi M. Diverse cutaneous manifestations of Erdheim-Chester disease in a woman with a history of Langerhans cell histiocytosis. *JAAD Case Rep.* 2016;2(2):128-131.

61. Hervier B, Haroche J, Arnaud L, et al. Association of both Langerhans cell histiocytosis and Erdheim-Chester disease linked to the BRAFV600E mutation. *Blood.* 2014;124(7):1119-1126.

62. Nabi S, Arshad A, Jain T, Virk F, Gulati R, Awdish R. A rare case of Erdheim-Chester disease and Langerhans cell histiocytosis overlap syndrome. *Case Rep Pathol.* 2015;2015:949163.

63. Chasset F, Barete S, Charlotte F, et al. Cutaneous manifestations of Erdheim-Chester disease (ECD): Clinical, pathological, and molecular features in a monocentric series of 40 patients. *J Am Acad Dermatol.* 2016;74(3):513-520.

64. Haroche J, Abla O. Uncommon histiocytic disorders: Rosai-Dorfman, juvenile xanthogranuloma, and Erdheim-Chester disease. *Hematology Am Soc Hematol Educ Program.* 2015;2015:571-578.

65. Tsai JW, Tsou JH, Hung LY, Wu HB, Chang KC. Combined Erdheim-Chester disease and Langerhans cell histiocytosis of skin are both monoclonal: a rare case with human androgen-receptor gene analysis. *J Am Acad Dermatol.* 2010;63(2):284-291.

66. Ozkaya N, Rosenblum MK, Durham BH, et al. The histopathology of Erdheim-Chester disease: a comprehensive review of a molecularly characterized cohort. *Mod Pathol.* 2018;31(4):581-597.

67. Skinner M, Briant M, Morgan MB. Erdheim-Chester disease: a histiocytic disorder more than skin deep. *Am J Dermatopathol.* 2011;33(2):e24-e26.

68. Volpicelli ER, Doyle L, Annes JP, et al. Erdheim-Chester disease presenting with cutaneous involvement: a case report and literature review. *J Cutan Pathol.* 2011;38(3):280-285.

69. Kim S, Lee M, Shin HJ, Lee J, Suh YL. Coexistence of intracranial Langerhans cell histiocytosis and Erdheim-Chester disease in a pediatric patient: a case report. *Childs Nerv Syst.* 2016;32(5):893-896.

70. Krishna VV, James TE, Chang KT, Yen SS. Erdheim-Chester disease with rare radiological features in a 14-year old girl with pre-B acute lymphocytic leukemia and diabetes mellitus. *J Radiol Case Rep.* 2014;8(8):7-15.

71. Johnson WT, Patel P, Hernandez A, et al. Langerhans cell histiocytosis and Erdheim-Chester disease, both with cutaneous presentations, and papillary thyroid carcinoma all harboring the BRAF(V600E) mutation. *J Cutan Pathol.* 2016;43(3):270-275.

72. Chan JK, Lamant L, Algar E, et al. ALK+ histiocytosis: a novel type of systemic histiocytic proliferative disorder of early infancy. *Blood.* 2008;112(7):2965-2968.

73. Chakraborty R, Hampton OA, Abhyankar H, et al. Activating MAPK1 (ERK2) mutation in an aggressive case of disseminated juvenile xanthogranuloma. *Oncotarget.* 2017;8(28):46065-46070.

74. Techavichit P, Sosothikul D, Chaichana T, et al. BRAF V600E mutation in pediatric intracranial and cranial juvenile xanthogranuloma. *Hum Pathol.* 2017;69:118-122.

75. Li Y, Bai HX, Su C, et al. Generalized indeterminate cell histiocytosis presenting as eroded papules and crusts. *Am J Dermatopathol.* 2017;39(7):542-544.

76. Logemann N, Thomas B, Yetto T. Indeterminate cell histiocytosis successfully treated with narrowband UVB. *Dermatol Online J.* 2013;19(10):20031.

77. Bard S, Torchia D, Connelly EA, Duarte AM, Badiavas EV, Schachner LA. S100-negative indeterminate cell histiocytosis in an African American child responsive to narrowband ultraviolet B. *Pediatr Dermatol.* 2011;28(5):524-527.

78. Davick JJ, Kim J, Wick MR, Gru AA. Indeterminate dendritic cell tumor: a report of 2 new cases lacking the ETV3-NCOA2 translocation and a literature review. *Am J Dermatopathol.* 2018. doi:10.1097/DAD.0000000000001191.

79. Ghanadan A, Kamyab K, Ramezani M, et al. Indeterminate cell histiocytosis: report of a case. *Acta Med Iran.* 2014;52(10):788-790.

80. Rodríguez-Jurado R, Vidaurri-de la Cruz H, Durán-Mckinster C, Ruíz-Maldonado R. Indeterminate cell histiocytosis. Clinical and pathologic study in a pediatric patient. *Arch Pathol Lab Med.* 2003;127(6):748-751.

81. Zerbini MC, Sotto MN, de Campos FP, et al. Indeterminate cell histiocytosis successfully treated with phototherapy. *Autops Case Rep.* 2016;6(2):33-38.

82. Brown RA, Kwong BY, McCalmont TH, et al. ETV3-NCOA2 in indeterminate cell histiocytosis: clonal translocation supports sui generis. *Blood.* 2015;126(20):2344-2345.

83. Manente L, Cotellessa C, Schmitt I, et al. Indeterminate cell histiocytosis: a rare histiocytic disorder. *Am J Dermatopathol.* 1997;19(3):276-283.

84. Rosenberg AS, Morgan MB. Cutaneous indeterminate cell histiocytosis: a new spindle cell variant resembling dendritic cell sarcoma. *J Cutan Pathol.* 2001;28(10):531-537.

85. Burns MV, Ahmed A, Callahan GB, Le LQ, Cockerell C. Treatment of indeterminate cell histiocytosis with pravastatin. *J Am Acad Dermatol.* 2011;64(5):e85-e86.

86. Tóth B, Katona M, Hársing J, Szepesi A, Kárpáti S. Indeterminate cell histiocytosis in a pediatric patient: successful treatment with thalidomide. *Pathol Oncol Res.* 2012;18(2):535-538.

87. Haughton AM, Horii KA, Shao L, Daniel J, Nopper AJ. Disseminated juvenile xanthogranulomatosis in a newborn resulting in liver transplantation. *J Am Acad Dermatol.* 2008;58(2 suppl):S12-S15.

88. Fernandez-Flores A, Nicklaus I, Browne F, Colmenero I. Hemosiderotic juvenile xanthogranuloma. *Am J Dermatopathol.* 2017;39(10):773-775.

89. Dehner LP. Juvenile xanthogranulomas in the first two decades of life: a clinicopathologic study of 174 cases with cutaneous and extracutaneous manifestations. *Am J Surg Pathol.* 2003;27(5):579-593.

90. Dehner LP. Reawakening to the existence of juvenile xanthogranuloma. *Am J Surg Pathol.* 2005;29(1):119-120.

91. Janssen D, Harms D. Juvenile xanthogranuloma in childhood and adolescence: a clinicopathologic study of 129 patients from the kiel pediatric tumor registry. *Am J Surg Pathol.* 2005;29(1):21-28.

92. Hernandez-Martin A, Baselga E, Drolet BA, Esterly NB. Juvenile xanthogranuloma. *J Am Acad Dermatol.* 1997;36(3, Pt 1):355-367; quiz 368-369.

93. Pajaziti L, Hapciu SR, Pajaziti A. Juvenile xanthogranuloma: a case report and review of the literature. *BMC Res Notes.* 2014;7:174.

94. Paxton CN, O'Malley DP, Bellizzi AM, et al. Genetic evaluation of juvenile xanthogranuloma: genomic abnormalities are uncommon in solitary lesions, advanced cases may show more complexity. *Mod Pathol.* 2017;30(9):1234-1240.

95. Arachchillage DR, Carr TF, Kerr B, et al. Juvenile myelomonocytic leukemia presenting with features of neonatal hemophagocytic lymphohistiocytosis and cutaneous juvenile xanthogranulomata and successfully treated with allogeneic hemopoietic stem cell transplant. *J Pediatr Hematol Oncol.* 2010;32(2):152-155.

96. Burgdorf WH, Zelger B. JXG, NF1, and JMML: alphabet soup or a clinical issue? *Pediatr Dermatol.* 2004;21(2):174-176.

97. Fenot M, Stalder JF, Barbarot S. Juvenile xanthogranulomas are highly prevalent but transient in young children with neurofibromatosis type 1. *J Am Acad Dermatol.* 2014;71(2):389-390.

98. Ferrari F, Masurel A, Olivier-Faivre L, Vabres P. Juvenile xanthogranuloma and nevus anemicus in the diagnosis of neurofibromatosis type 1. *JAMA Dermatol.* 2014;150(1):42-46.

99. Jans SR, Schomerus E, Bygum A. Neurofibromatosis type 1 diagnosed in a child based on multiple juvenile xanthogranulomas and juvenile myelomonocytic leukemia. *Pediatr Dermatol.* 2015;32(1):e29-e32.

100. Liy-Wong C, Mohammed J, Carleton A, Pope E, Parkin P, Lara-Corrales I. The relationship between neurofibromatosis type 1, juvenile xanthogranuloma, and malignancy: A retrospective case-control study. *J Am Acad Dermatol.* 2017;76(6):1084-1087.

101. Shin HT, Harris MB, Orlow SJ. Juvenile myelomonocytic leukemia presenting with features of hemophagocytic lymphohistiocytosis in association with neurofibromatosis and juvenile xanthogranulomas. *J Pediatr Hematol Oncol.* 2004;26(9):591-595.

102. Yang CC, Chen YA, Tsai YL, Shih IH, Chen W. Neoplastic skin lesions of the scalp in children: a retrospective study of 265 cases in Taiwan. *Eur J Dermatol.* 2014;24(1):70-75.

103. Freyer DR, Kennedy R, Bostrom BC, Kohut G, Dehner LP. Juvenile xanthogranuloma: forms of systemic disease and their clinical implications. *J Pediatr.* 1996;129(2):27-37.

104. Suson K, Mathews R, Goldstein JD, Dehner LP. Juvenile xanthogranuloma presenting as a testicular mass in infancy: a clinical and pathologic study of three cases. *Pediatr Dev Pathol.* 2010;13(1):39-45.

105. Zelger B, Burgdorf WH. The cutaneous "histiocytoses". *Adv Dermatol.* 2001;17:77-114.

106. Zelger BW, Cerio R. Xanthogranuloma is the archetype of non-Langerhans cell histiocytoses. *Br J Dermatol.* 2001;145(2):369-371.

107. Zelger BW, Sidoroff A, Orchard G, Cerio R. Non-Langerhans cell histiocytoses. A new unifying concept. *Am J Dermatopathol.* 1996;18(5):490-504.

108. Song M, Kim SH, Jung DS, Ko HC, Kwon KS, Kim MB. Structural correlations between dermoscopic and histopathological features of juvenile xanthogranuloma. *J Eur Acad Dermatol Venereol.* 2011;25(3):259-263.

109. Imiela A, Carpentier O, Segard-Drouard M, Martin de Lassalle E, Piette F. Juvenile xanthogranuloma: a congenital giant form leading to a wide atrophic sequela. *Pediatr Dermatol.* 2004;21(2):121-123.

110. Marrogi AJ, Dehner LP, Coffin CM, Wick MR. Benign cutaneous histiocytic tumors in childhood and adolescence, excluding Langerhans' cell proliferations. A clinicopathologic and immunohistochemical analysis. *Am J Dermatopathol.* 1992;14(1):8-18.

111. Gru AA, Horacio Maluf MD. Contributions of Dr. Louis "Pepper" Dehner to the art of cutaneous pathology, the first pediatric dermatopathologist. *Semin Diagn Pathol.* 2016;33(6):441-449.

112. Weitzman S, Jaffe R. Uncommon histiocytic disorders: the non-Langerhans cell histiocytoses. *Pediatr Blood Cancer.* 2005;45(3):256-264.

113. Gianotti F, Caputo R, Ermacora E. Singular "infantile histiocytosis with cells with intracytoplasmic vermiform particles" [in French]. *Bull Soc Fr Dermatol Syphiligr.* 1971;78(3):232-233.

114. Jih DM, Salcedo SL, Jaworsky C. Benign cephalic histiocytosis: a case report and review. *J Am Acad Dermatol.* 2002;47(6):908-913.

115. Patsatsi A, Kyriakou A, Sotiriadis D. Benign cephalic histiocytosis: case report and review of the literature. *Pediatr Dermatol.* 2014;31(5):547-550.

116. Polat Ekinci A, Buyukbabani N, Baykal C. Novel clinical observations on benign cephalic histiocytosis in a large series. *Pediatr Dermatol.* 2017;34(4):392-397.

117. D'Auria AA, De Clerck B, Kim G. Benign cephalic histiocytosis with S-100 protein positivity. *J Cutan Pathol.* 2011;38(10):842-843.

118. Kim BC, Choi WJ, Seung NR, et al. A case of benign cephalic histiocytosis. *Ann Dermatol.* 2011;23(suppl 1):S16-S19.

119. Sidwell RU, Francis N, Slater DN, Mayou SC. Is disseminated juvenile xanthogranulomatosis benign cephalic histiocytosis? *Pediatr Dermatol.* 2005;22(1):40-43.

120. Weston WL, Travers SH, Mierau GW, Heasley D, Fitzpatrick J. Benign cephalic histiocytosis with diabetes insipidus. *Pediatr Dermatol.* 2000;17(4):296-298.

121. Koca R, Bektaş S, Altinyazar HC, Sezer T. Benign cephalic histiocytosis: a case report. *Ann Dermatol.* 2011;23(4):508-511.

122. Azulay-Abulafia L, Benez MD, Abreu Cde S, Miranda CV, Alves Mde F. Case for diagnosis. Benign cephalic histiocytosis. *An Bras Dermatol.* 2011;86(6):1222-1225.

123. Gonzalez Ruíz A, Bernal Ruíz AI, Aragoneses Fraile H, et al. Progressive nodular histiocytosis accompanied by systemic disorders. *Br J Dermatol.* 2000;143(3):628-631.

124. Taunton OD, Yeshurun D, Jarratt M. Progressive nodular histiocytoma. *Arch Dermatol.* 1978;114(10):1505-1508.

125. Glavin FL, Chhatwall H, Karimi K. Progressive nodular histiocytosis: a case report with literature review, and discussion of differential diagnosis and classification. *J Cutan Pathol.* 2009;36(12):1286-1292.

126. Kunimoto K, Uede K, Furukawa F. Progressive nodular histiocytosis. *J Dermatol.* 2010;37(12):1071-1073.

127. Guidolin L, Noguera-Morel L, Hernández-Martín A, et al. A case with juvenile xanthogranuloma and progressive nodular histiocytosis overlap. *Pediatr Dermatol.* 2017;34(2):e102-e103.

128. Torres L, Sánchez JL, Rivera A, González A. Progressive nodular histiocytosis. *J Am Acad Dermatol.* 1993;29(2, pt 1):278-280.

129. Nofal A, Assaf M, Tawfik A, et al. Progressive nodular histiocytosis: a case report and literature review. *Int J Dermatol.* 2011;50(12):1546-1551.

130. Beswick SJ, Kirk JM, Bradshaw K, Sanders DS, Moss C. Progressive nodular histiocytosis in a child with a hypothalamic tumor. *Br J Dermatol.* 2002;146(1):138-140.

131. Salunke A, Belgaumkar V, Chavan R, Dobariya R. Laryngeal involvement with fatal outcome in progressive nodular histiocytosis: a rare case report. *Indian Dermatol Online J.* 2016;7(6):516-519.

132. Chapman LW, Hsiao JL, Sarantopoulos P, Chiu MW. Reddish-brown nodules and papules in an elderly man. Progressive nodular histiocytosis. *JAMA Dermatol.* 2013;149(10):1229-1230.

133. Caputo R, Marzano AV, Passoni E, Berti E. Unusual variants of non-Langerhans cell histiocytoses. *J Am Acad Dermatol.* 2007;57(6):1031-1045.

134. Gupta P, Khandpur S, Vedi K, Singh MK, Walia R. Xanthoma disseminatum associated with inflammatory arthritis and synovitis—a rare association. *Pediatr Dermatol.* 2015;32(1):e1-e4.

135. Krishna CV, Parmar NV, Ganguly S, Kuruvila S. Xanthoma disseminatum with extensive koebnerization associated with familial hypertriglyceridemia. *JAAD Case Rep.* 2016;2(3):253-256.

136. Yang GZ, Li J, Wang LP. Disseminated intracranial xanthoma disseminatum: a rare case report and review of literature. *Diagn Pathol.* 2016;11(1):78.

137. Adışen E, Aladağ P, Özlem E, Gürer MA. Cladribine is a promising therapy for xanthoma disseminatum. *Clin Exp Dermatol.* 2017;42(6):717-719.

138. Eisendle K, Linder D, Ratzinger G, et al. Inflammation and lipid accumulation in xanthoma disseminatum: therapeutic considerations. *J Am Acad Dermatol.* 2008;58(2 suppl):S47-S49.

139. Lee EH, Kang TW, Kim SC. Successful treatment of xanthoma disseminatum with simvastatin. *J Dermatol.* 2011;38(10):1015-1017.

140. Ansarin H, Berenji Ardestani H, Tabaie SM, Shayanfar N. Xanthoma disseminatum with tumor-like lesion on face. *Case Rep Dermatol Med.* 2014;2014:621798.

141. Khezri F, Gibson LE, Tefferi A. Xanthoma disseminatum: effective therapy with 2-chlorodeoxyadenosine in a case series. *Arch Dermatol.* 2011;147(4):459-464.

142. Seaton ED, Pillai GJ, Chu AC. Treatment of xanthoma disseminatum with cyclophosphamide. *Br J Dermatol.* 2004;150(2):346-349.

143. Kim JY, Jung HD, Choe YS, et al. A case of xanthoma disseminatum accentuating over the eyelids. *Ann Dermatol.* 2010;22(3):353-357.

144. Silverstein MN. Syndrome of the sea-blue histiocyte. *Lancet.* 1970;2(7672):572.

145. Baño Aracil M, Monferrer Guardiola R, Valades Paredes MA, et al. Sea-blue histiocyte syndrome, liver cirrhosis and monoclonal gammopathy. Description of a case [in Spanish]. *An Med Interna.* 1989;6(4):199-202.

146. Bigorgne C, Le Tourneau A, Vahedi K, et al. Sea-blue histiocyte syndrome in bone marrow secondary to total parenteral nutrition. *Leuk Lymphoma.* 1998;28(5-6):523-529.

147. Candoni A, Grimaz S, Doretto P, Fanin R, Falcomer F, Bembi B. Sea-blue histiocytosis secondary to Niemann-Pick disease type B: a case report. *Ann Hematol.* 2001;80(10):620-622.

148. Faivre L, Saugier-Veber P, Pais de Barros JP, et al. Variable expressivity of the clinical and biochemical phenotype associated with the apolipoprotein E p.Leu149del mutation. *Eur J Hum Genet.* 2005;13(11):1186-1191.

149. Gahr M, Jendrossek V, Peters AM, Tegtmeyer F, Heyne K. Sea blue histiocytes in the bone marrow of variant chronic granulomatous disease with residual monocyte NADPH-oxidase activity. *Br J Haematol.* 1991;78(2):278-280.

150. Grau AJ, Weisbrod M, Hund E, Harzer K. Niemann-Pick disease type C--a neurometabolic disease through disturbed intracellular lipid transport [in German]. *Nervenarzt.* 2003;74(10):900-905.

151. Howard MR, Kesteven PJ. Sea blue histiocytosis: a common abnormality of the bone marrow in myelodysplastic syndromes. *J Clin Pathol.* 1993;46(11):1030-1032.

152. Lee RE. Histiocytic diseases of bone marrow. *Hematol Oncol Clin North Am.* 1988;2(4):657-667.

153. Papadaki HA, Michelakaki H, Bux J, Eliopoulos GD. Severe autoimmune neutropenia associated with bone marrow sea-blue histiocytosis. *Br J Haematol.* 2002;118(4):931.

154. Yamauchi K, Shimamura K. Pulmonary fibrosis and sea-blue histiocyte infiltration in a patient with primary myelofibrosis. *Eur Respir J.* 1995;8(9):1620-1623.

155. Cardoso F, Serafini NB, Reis BD, Nuñez MD, Nery JA, Lupi O. Generalized eruptive histiocytoma: a rare disease in an elderly patient. *An Bras Dermatol.* 2013;88(1):105-108.

156. Winkelmann RK, Muller SA. Generalized eruptive histiocytoma. A benign papular histiocytic reticulosis. *Arch Dermatol.* 1963;88:586-596.

157. Verma SB. Generalized eruptive histiocytomas and juvenile eruptive xanthogranulomas in a 10-year-old boy: a potpourri of exotic terms indicating the need for unification. *Int J Dermatol.* 2012;51(4):445-447.

158. Pinney SS, Jahan-Tigh RR, Chon S. Generalized eruptive histiocytosis associated with a novel fusion in LMNA-NTRK1. *Dermatol Online J.* 2016;22(8).

159. Arnold ML, Anton-Lamprecht I. Multiple eruptive cephalic histiocytomas in a case of T-cell lymphoma. A xanthomatous stage of benign cephalic histiocytosis in an adult patient? *Am J Dermatopathol.* 1993;15(6):581-586.

160. Klemke CD, Dippel E, Geilen CC, et al. Atypical generalized eruptive histiocytosis associated with acute monocytic leukemia. *J Am Acad Dermatol.* 2003;49(5 suppl):S233-S236.

161. Montero I, Gutiérrez-González E, Ginarte M, Toribio J. Generalized eruptive histiocytosis in a patient with chronic myelomonocytic leukemia. *Actas Dermosifiliogr.* 2012;103(7):643-644.

162. Shon W, Peters MS, Reed KB, Ketterling RP, Dogan A, Gibson LE. Atypical generalized eruptive histiocytosis clonally related to chronic myelomonocytic leukemia with loss of Y chromosome. *J Cutan Pathol.* 2013;40(8):725-729.

163. Ziegler B, Peitsch WK, Reiter A, Marx A, Goerdt S, Géraud C. Generalized eruptive histiocytosis associated with FIP1L1-PDGFRA-positive chronic eosinophilic leukemia. *JAMA Dermatol.* 2015;151(7):766-769.

164. Attia A, Seleit I, El Badawy N, Bakry O, Yassien H. Photoletter to the editor: Generalized eruptive histiocytoma. *J Dermatol Case Rep.* 2011;5(3):53-55.

165. Wee SH, Kim HS, Chang SN, Kim DK, Park WH. Generalized eruptive histiocytoma: a pediatric case. *Pediatr Dermatol.* 2000;17(6):453-455.

166. Wilk M, Zelger BG, Zelger B. Generalized eruptive histiocytosis with features of multinucleate cell angiohistiocytoma. *Am J Dermatopathol.* 2016;38(6):470-472.

167. Aggarwal K, Gupta S, Jain VK, Sen R, Gupta S. Generalized eruptive histiocytoma. *Indian Dermatol Online J.* 2010;1(1):27-29.

168. Requena C, Requena L, Traves V, Sanmartín O. Hereditary progressive mucinous histiocytosis: 3 different phenotypes in 3 family members. *J Cutan Pathol.* 2017;44(9):781-785.

169. Cascarino M, Caron Y, Butnaru C, Rongioletti F, Fraitag S. Sporadic progressive mucinous histiocytosis. *Ann Dermatol Venereol.* 2017;144(3):191-196.

170. Hemmati I, McLeod WA, Crawford RI. Progressive mucinous histiocytosis: importance of electron microscopy to confirm diagnosis. *J Cutan Med Surg.* 2010;14(5):245-248.

171. Narváez-Rosales V, Sáez-de-Ocariz M, Toussaint-Caire S, Ortiz-Hidalgo C, Espinosa-Rosales F. Sporadic progressive mucinous histiocytosis in a Mexican patient. *Skinmed.* 2013;11(3):175-178.

172. Schlegel C, Metzler G, Burgdorf W, Schaller M. Hereditary progressive mucinous histiocytosis: first report in a male patient. *Acta Derm Venereol.* 2010;90(1):65-67.

173. Schröder K, Hettmannsperger U, Schmuth M, Orfanos CE, Goerdt S. Hereditary progressive mucinous histiocytosis. *J Am Acad Dermatol.* 1996;35(2, Pt 2):298-303.

174. Wong D, Killingsworth M, Crosland G, Kossard S. Hereditary progressive mucinous histiocytosis. *Br J Dermatol.* 1999;141(6):1101-1105.

175. Nguyen NV, Prok L, Burgos A, Bruckner AL. Hereditary progressive mucinous histiocytosis: new insights into a rare disease. *Pediatr Dermatol.* 2015;32(6):e273-e276.

176. Young A, Olivere J, Yoo S, Martins C, Barrett T. Two sporadic cases of adult-onset progressive mucinous histiocytosis. *J Cutan Pathol.* 2006;33(2):166-170.

177. Sass U, Andre J, Song M. A sporadic case of progressive mucinous histiocytosis. *Br J Dermatol.* 2000;142(1):133-137.

178. Bork K. Hereditary progressive mucinous histiocytosis. Immunohistochemical and ultrastructural studies in an additional family. *Arch Dermatol.* 1994;130(10):1300-1304.

179. Toz B, Buyukbabani N, Inanc M. Multicentric reticulohistiocytosis: rheumatology perspective. *Best Pract Res Clin Rheumatol.* 2016;30(2):250-260.

180. Shibuya R, Tanizaki H, Kaku Y, et al. A plaque-type solitary reticulo-histiocytoma in a two-year-old boy. *Case Rep Dermatol.* 2015;7(1):7-9.

181. Tariq S, Hugenberg ST, Hirano-Ali SA, Tariq H. Multicentric reticulohistiocytosis (MRH): case report with review of literature between 1991 and 2014 with in depth analysis of various treatment regimens and outcomes. *Springerplus.* 2016;5:180.

182. Jha VK, Kumar R, Kunwar A, et al. Efficacy of vinblastine and prednisone in multicentric reticulohistiocytosis with onset in infancy. *Pediatrics.* 2016;137(6).

183. Olson J, Mann JA, White K, Cartwright VW, Bauer J, Nolt D. Multicentric reticulohistiocytosis: a case report of an atypical presentation in a 2-year-old. *Pediatr Dermatol.* 2015;32(3):e70-e73.

184. de Leon D, Chiu Y, Co D, Sokumbi O. Multicentric reticulohistiocytosis in a 5-year-old girl. *J Pediatr.* 2016;177:328-328 e1.

185. Kalajian AH, Callen JP. Multicentric reticulohistiocytosis successfully treated with infliximab: an illustrative case and evaluation of cytokine expression supporting anti-tumor necrosis factor therapy. *Arch Dermatol.* 2008;144(10):1360-1366.

186. Tan BH, Barry CI, Wick MR, et al. Multicentric reticulohistiocytosis and urologic carcinomas: a possible paraneoplastic association. *J Cutan Pathol.* 2011;38(1):43-48.

187. Caltabiano R, Magro G, Vecchio GM, Lanzafame S. Solitary cutaneous histiocytosis with granular cell changes: a morphological variant of reticulohistiocytoma? *J Cutan Pathol.* 2010;37(2):287-291.

188. Hsiung SH, Chan EF, Elenitsas R, Kolasinski SL, Schumacher HR, Werth VP. Multicentric reticulohistiocytosis presenting with clinical features of dermatomyositis. *J Am Acad Dermatol.* 2003;48(2 suppl):S11-S14.

189. Miettinen M, Fetsch JF. Reticulohistiocytoma (solitary epithelioid histiocytoma): a clinicopathologic and immunohistochemical study of 44 cases. *Am J Surg Pathol.* 2006;30(4):521-528.

190. Bogle MA, Tschen JA, Sairam S, McNearney T, Orsak G, Knox JM. Multicentric reticulohistiocytosis with pulmonary involvement. *J Am Acad Dermatol.* 2003;49(6):1125-1127.

191. West KL, Sporn T, Puri PK. Multicentric reticulohistiocytosis: a unique case with pulmonary fibrosis. *Arch Dermatol.* 2012;148(2):228-232.

192. Zelger B, Cerio R, Soyer HP, Misch K, Orchard G, Wilson-Jones E. Reticulohistiocytoma and multicentric reticulohistiocytosis. Histopathologic and immunophenotypic distinct entities. *Am J Dermatopathol.* 1994;16(6):577-584.

193. Rosai J, Dorfman RF. Sinus histiocytosis with massive lymphadenopathy. A newly recognized benign clinicopathological entity. *Arch Pathol.* 1969;87(1):63-70.

194. Al-Khateeb TH. Cutaneous Rosai-Dorfman disease of the face: a comprehensive literature review and case report. *J Oral Maxillofac Surg.* 2016;74(3):528-540.

195. Garces S, Medeiros LJ, Patel KP, et al. Mutually exclusive recurrent KRAS and MAP2K1 mutations in Rosai-Dorfman disease. *Mod Pathol.* 2017;30(10):1367-1377.

196. di Dio F, Mariotti I, Coccolini E, Bruzzi P, Predieri B, Iughetti L. Unusual presentation of Rosai-Dorfman disease in a 14-month-old Italian child: a case report and review of the literature. *BMC Pediatr.* 2016;16:62.

197. Goodman WT, Barrett TL. Disorders of Langerhans cells and macrophages. In: Bolognia JL, Jorrizzo JL, Schaffer JV, eds. *Dermatology.* Philadelphia, PA: Elsevier Saunders; 2013:1542-1544.

198. Weedon D. Cutaneous infiltrates—non-lymphoid. In: Patterson J, ed. *Weedon's Skin Pathology.* London, England: Churchill Livingstone Elsevier; 2010:959-960.

199. Chappell JA, Burkemper NM, Frater JL, Hurley MY. Cutaneous Rosai-Dorfman disease and morphea: coincidence or association? *Am J Dermatopathol.* 2009;31(5):487-489.

200. Frater JL, Maddox JS, Obadiah JM, Hurley MY. Cutaneous Rosai-Dorfman disease: comprehensive review of cases reported in the medical literature since 1990 and presentation of an illustrative case. *J Cutan Med Surg.* 2006;10(6):281-290.

201. Cai Y, Shi Z, Bai Y. Review of Rosai-Dorfman disease: new insights into the pathogenesis of this rare disorder. *Acta Haematol.* 2017;138(1):14-23.

202. Gameiro A, Gouveia M, Cardoso JC, Tellechea O. Histological variability and the importance of clinicopathological correlation in cutaneous Rosai-Dorfman disease. *An Bras Dermatol.* 2016;91(5):634-637.

203. Kutlubay Z, Bairamov O, Sevim A, Demirkesen C, Mat MC. Rosai-Dorfman disease: a case report with nodal and cutaneous involvement and review of the literature. *Am J Dermatopathol.* 2014;36(4):353-357.

204. Liu L, Perry AM, Cao W, et al. Relationship between Rosai-Dorfman disease and IgG4-related disease: study of 32 cases. Am J Clin Pathol. 2013;140(3):395-402.

205. Menon MP, Evbuomwan MO, Rosai J, Jaffe ES, Pittaluga S. A subset of Rosai-Dorfman disease cases show increased IgG4-positive plasma cells: another red herring or a true association with IgG4-related disease? *Histopathology.* 2014;64(3):455-459.

206. Wimmer DB, Ro JY, Lewis A, et al. Extranodal rosai-dorfman disease associated with increased numbers of immunoglobulin g4 plasma cells involving the colon: case report with literature review. *Arch Pathol Lab Med.* 2013;137(7):999-1004.

207. Morgan NV, Morris MR, Cangul H, et al. Mutations in SLC29A3, encoding an equilibrative nucleoside transporter ENT3, cause a familial histiocytosis syndrome (Faisalabad histiocytosis) and familial Rosai-Dorfman disease. *PLoS Genet.* 2010;6(2):e1000833.

208. Zheng M, Bi R, Li W, et al. Generalized pure cutaneous Rosai-Dorfman disease: a link between inflammation and cancer not associated with mitochondrial DNA and SLC29A3 gene mutation? *Discov Med.* 2013;16(89):193-200.

209. Molho-Pessach V, Ramot Y, Camille F, et al. H syndrome: the first 79 patients. *J Am Acad Dermatol.* 2014;70(1):80-88.

210. Tekin B1, Atay Z, Ergun T, et al. H syndrome: a multifaceted histiocytic disorder with hyperpigmentation and hypertrichosis. *Acta Derm Venereol.* 2015;95(8):1021-1023.

211. Vural S, Ertop P, Durmaz CD, et al. Skin-dominant phenotype in a patient with H syndrome: identification of a novel mutation in the SLC29A3 gene. *Cytogenet Genome Res.* 2017;151(4):186-190.

212. Cartin-Ceba R, Golbin JM, Yi ES, Prakash UB, Vassallo R. Intrathoracic manifestations of Rosai-Dorfman disease. *Respir Med.* 2010;104(9):1344-1349.

213. Grabczynska SA, Toh CT, Francis N, Costello C, Bunker CB. Rosai-Dorfman disease complicated by autoimmune haemolytic anaemia: case report and review of a multisystem disease with cutaneous infiltrates. *Br J Dermatol.* 2001;145(2):323-326.

214. Lu CI, Kuo TT, Wong WR, Hong HS. Clinical and histopathologic spectrum of cutaneous Rosai-Dorfman disease in Taiwan. *J Am Acad Dermatol.* 2004;51(6):931-939.

215. Kong YY, Lu HF, Zhu XZ, Wang J, Shi DR, Kong JC. Cutaneous Rosai-Dorfman disease [in Chinese]. *Zhonghua Bing Li Xue Za Zhi.* 2005;34(3):133-136.

216. Wang KH, Chen WY, Liu HN, Huang CC, Lee WR, Hu CH. Cutaneous Rosai-Dorfman disease: clinicopathological profiles, spectrum and evolution of 21 lesions in six patients. *Br J Dermatol.* 2006;154(2):277-286.

217. Chu P, LeBoit PE. Histologic features of cutaneous sinus histiocytosis (Rosai-Dorfman disease): study of cases both with and without systemic involvement. *J Cutan Pathol.* 1992;19(3):201-206.

218. Cole AJ, Chen C, Lorsbach RB, Honnebier BM, Gardner JM, Shalin SC. Extranodal Rosai-Dorfman disease in the scrotum of a 13-month male: a unique anatomic presentation. *Am J Dermatopathol.* 2015;37(1):88-90.

219. Kala C, Agarwal A, Kala S. Extranodal manifestation of Rosai-Dorfman disease with bilateral ocular involvement. *J Cytol.* 2011;28(3):131-133.

220. Liu G, Wang H, Yang Z, Tang T, Zhang S. Is it a metastatic disease: a case report and new understanding of Rosai-Dorfman disease? *Am J Dermatopathol.* 2016;38(6):e72-e76.

221. Litzner BR, Subtil A, Vidal CI. Combined cutaneous Rosai-Dorfman disease and localized cutaneous Langerhans cell histiocytosis within a single subcutaneous nodule. *Am J Dermatopathol.* 2015;37(12):936-939.

222. Chou TC, Tsai KB, Lee CH. Emperipolesis is not pathognomonic for Rosai-Dorfman disease: rhinoscleroma mimicking Rosai-Dorfman disease, a clinical series. *J Am Acad Dermatol.* 2013;69(6):1066-1067.

223. Dalia S, Shao H, Sagatys E, Cualing H, Sokol L. Dendritic cell and histiocytic neoplasms: biology, diagnosis, and treatment. *Cancer Control.* 2014;21(4): 290-300.

224. Takahashi E, Nakamura S. Histiocytic sarcoma: an updated literature review based on the 2008 WHO classification. *J Clin Exp Hematop.* 2013;53(1):1-8.

225. Castro EC, Blazquez C, Boyd J, et al. Clinicopathologic features of histiocytic lesions following ALL, with a review of the literature. *Pediatr Dev Pathol.* 2010;13(3):225-237.

226. Chen W, Lau SK, Fong D, et al. High frequency of clonal immunoglobulin receptor gene rearrangements in sporadic histiocytic/dendritic cell sarcomas. *Am J Surg Pathol.* 2009;33(6):863-873.

227. Dalle JH, Leblond P, Decouvelaere A, et al. Efficacy of thalidomide in a child with histiocytic sarcoma following allogeneic bone marrow transplantation for T-ALL. *Leukemia.* 2003;17(10):2056-2057.

228. Feldman AL, Minniti C, Santi M, Downing JR, Raffeld M, Jaffe ES. Histiocytic sarcoma after acute lymphoblastic leukaemia: a common clonal origin. *Lancet Oncol.* 2004;5(4):248-250.

229. Hure MC, Elco CP, Ward D, et al. Histiocytic sarcoma arising from clonally related mantle cell lymphoma. *J Clin Oncol.* 2012;30(5):e49-e53.

230. Kumar R, Khan SP, Joshi DD, Shaw GR, Ketterling RP, Feldman AL. Pediatric histiocytic sarcoma clonally related to precursor B-cell acute lymphoblastic leukemia with homozygous deletion of CDKN2A encoding p16INK4A. *Pediatr Blood Cancer.* 2011;56(2):307-310.

231. McClure R, Khoury J, Feldman A, Ketterling R. Clonal relationship between precursor B-cell acute lymphoblastic leukemia and histiocytic sarcoma: a case report and discussion in the context of similar cases. *Leuk Res.* 2010;34(2):e71-e73.

232. Shao H, Xi L, Raffeld M, et al. Clonally related histiocytic/dendritic cell sarcoma and chronic lymphocytic leukemia/small lymphocytic lymphoma: a study of seven cases. *Mod Pathol.* 2011;24(11):1421-1432.

233. Wang E, Hutchinson CB, Huang Q, et al. Histiocytic sarcoma arising in indolent small B-cell lymphoma: report of two cases with molecular/genetic evidence suggestive of a 'transdifferentiation' during the clonal evolution. *Leuk Lymphoma.* 2010;51(5):802-812.

234. Kordes M, Röring M, Heining C, et al. Cooperation of BRAF(F595L) and mutant HRAS in histiocytic sarcoma provides new insights into oncogenic BRAF signaling. *Leukemia.* 2016;30(4):937-946.

235. Liu Q, Tomaszewicz K, Hutchinson L, Hornick JL, Woda B, Yu H. Somatic mutations in histiocytic sarcoma identified by next generation sequencing. *Virchows Arch.* 2016;469(2):233-241.

236. Vaughn JL, Freitag CE, Hemminger JA, Jones JA. BRAF (V600E) expression in histiocytic sarcoma associated with splenic marginal zone lymphoma: a case report. *J Med Case Rep.* 2017;11(1):92.

237. Vos JA, Abbondanzo SL, Barekman CL, Andriko JW, Miettinen M, Aguilera NS. Histiocytic sarcoma: a study of five cases including the histiocyte marker CD163. *Mod Pathol.* 2005;18(5):693-704.

238. Black J, Coffin CM, Dehner LP. Fibrohistiocytic tumors and related neoplasms in children and adolescents. *Pediatr Dev Pathol.* 2012;15(1 suppl):181-210.

239. Chung WD, Im SA, Chung NG, Park GS. Langerhans cell sarcoma in two young children: imaging findings on initial presentation and recurrence. *Korean J Radiol.* 2013;14(3):520-524.

240. Howard JE, Dwivedi RC, Masterson L, Jani P. Langerhans cell sarcoma: a systematic review. *Cancer Treat Rev.* 2015;41(4):320-331.

241. Sagransky MJ, Deng AC, Magro CM. Primary cutaneous Langerhans cell sarcoma: a report of four cases and review of the literature. *Am J Dermatopathol.* 2013;35(2):196-204.

242. Zwerdling T, Won E, Shane L, Javahara R, Jaffe R. Langerhans cell sarcoma: case report and review of world literature. *J Pediatr Hematol Oncol.* 2014;36(6):419-425.

243. Chen W, Jaffe R, Zhang L, et al. Langerhans Cell sarcoma arising from chronic lymphocytic lymphoma/small lymphocytic leukemia: lineage analysis and BRAF V600E mutation study. *N Am J Med Sci.* 2013;5(6):386-391.

244. Mazloom SE, Stallings A, Kyei A. Differentiating intralymphatic histiocytosis, intravascular histiocytosis, and subtypes of reactive angioendotheliomatosis: review of clinical and histologic features of all cases reported to date. *Am J Dermatopathol.* 2017;39(1):33-39.

245. Demirkesen C, Kran T, Leblebici C, Yücelten D, Aksu AE, Mat C. Intravascular/intralymphatic histiocytosis: a report of 3 cases. *Am J Dermatopathol.* 2015;37(10):783-789.

246. Catalina-Fernández I, Alvárez AC, Martin FC, Fernández-Mera JJ, Sáenz-Santamaría J. Cutaneous intralymphatic histiocytosis associated with rheumatoid arthritis: report of a case and review of the literature. *Am J Dermatopathol.* 2007;29(2):165-168.

247. Grekin S, Mesfin M, Kang S, Fullen DR. Intralymphatic histiocytosis following placement of a metal implant. *J Cutan Pathol.* 2011;38(4):351-353.

248. Requena L, El-Shabrawi-Caelen L, Walsh SN, et al. Intralymphatic histiocytosis. A clinicopathologic study of 16 cases. *Am J Dermatopathol.* 2009;31(2):140-151.

249. Emanuel PO, Lewis I, Gaskin B, Rosser P, Angelo N. Periocular intralymphatic histiocytosis or localized Melkersson-Rosenthal syndrome? *J Cutan Pathol.* 2015;42(4):289-294.

250. Alam M, Garzon MC, Salen G, Starc TJ. Tuberous xanthomas in sitosterolemia. *Pediatr Dermatol.* 2000;17(6):447-449.

251. Pietroleonardo L, Ruzicka T. Skin manifestations in familial heterozygous hypercholesterolemia. *Acta Dermatovenerol Alp Pannonica Adriat.* 2009;18(4):183-187.

252. Akpinar TS, Kose M, Emet S. A rare manifestation of tuberous xanthomas. *J Gen Intern Med.* 2015;30(5):691.

253. Singh AP, Sikarwar S, Jatav OP, Saify K. Normolipemic tuberous xanthomas. *Indian J Dermatol.* 2009;54(2):176-179.

254. Degos B, Nadjar Y, Amador Mdel M, et al. Natural history of cerebrotendinous xanthomatosis: a paediatric disease diagnosed in adulthood. *Orphanet J Rare Dis.* 2016;11:41.

255. Babl FE, Regan AM, Pelton SI. Xanthomas and hyperlipidemia in a human immunodeficiency virus-infected child receiving highly active antiretroviral therapy. *Pediatr Infect Dis J.* 2002;21(3):259-260.

256. Brown CA, Lesher JL Jr, Peterson CM. Tuberous and tendinous xanthomata secondary to ritonavir-associated hyperlipidemia. *J Am Acad Dermatol.* 2005;52(5 Suppl 1):S86-S89.

257. Haacke H, Parwaresch MR. Spontaneous rupture of the Achilles tendon-a sign of hyperlipoproteinaemia (HLP) type II. *Klin Wochenschr.* 1979;57(8):397-400.

258. Yensel U, Karalezli N. Carpal tunnel syndrome and flexion contracture of the digits in a child with familial hypercholesterolaemia. *J Hand Surg Br.* 2006;31(2):154-155.

259. Kurban M, Abbas O, Ghosn S, Kibbi AG. Late evolution of giant verruciform xanthoma in the setting of CHILD syndrome. *Pediatr Dermatol.* 2010;27(5):551-553.

260. Xu XL, Huang LM, Wang Q, Sun JF. Multiple verruciform xanthomas in the setting of congenital hemidysplasia with ichthyosiform erythroderma and limb defects syndrome. *Pediatr Dermatol.* 2015;32(1):135-137.

261. Wu JJ, Wagner AM. Verruciform xanthoma in association with Milroy disease and leaky capillary syndrome. *Pediatr Dermatol.* 2003;20(1): 44-47.

262. Maldonado-Cid P, Noguera-Morel L, Beato-Merino MJ, de Lucas-Laguna R. Verruciform xanthoma associated with reactivation of Epstein-Barr virus. *Actas Dermosifiliogr.* 2013;104(5):445-446.

263. Stiff KM, Cohen PR. Vegas (verruciform genital-associated) xanthoma: a comprehensive literature review. *Dermatol Ther.* 2017;7(1):65-79.

264. Ishibashi M, Matsuda F, Oka H, Ishiko A. Abnormal lamellar granules in a case of CHILD syndrome. *J Cutan Pathol.* 2006;33(6):447-453.

265. de Andrade BA, Agostini M, Pires FR. Oral verruciform xanthoma: a clinicopathologic and immunohistochemical study of 20 cases. *J Cutan Pathol.* 2015;42(7):489-495.

266. Nowparast B, Howell FV, Rick GM. Verruciform xanthoma. A clinicopathologic review and report of fifty-four cases. *Oral Surg Oral Med Oral Pathol.* 1981;51(6):619-625.

267. Pai VV, Shukla P, Bhobe M. Combined planar and eruptive xanthoma in a patient with type IIa hyperlipoproteinemia. *Indian J Dermatol Venereol Leprol.* 2014;80(5):467-470.

268. Parihar RK, Razaq M, Saini G. Homozygous familial hypercholesterolemia. *Indian J Endocrinol Metab.* 2012;16(4):643-645.

269. Sorrell J, Salvaggio H, Garg A, Guo L, Duck SC, Paller AS. Eruptive xanthomas masquerading as molluscum contagiosum. *Pediatrics.* 2014;134(1):e257-e260.

270. Zabeen B, Khaled Z, Nahar J, et al. Hypertriglyceridemia associated with eruptive xanthomas and lipemia retinalis in newly diagnosed diabetes mellitus. *Mymensingh Med J.* 2013;22(3):591-595.

271. Valent P, Horny HP, Escribano L, et al. Diagnostic criteria and classification of mastocytosis: a consensus proposal. *Leuk Res.* 2001;25(7):603-625.

272. Hartmann K, Escribano L, Grattan C, et al. Cutaneous manifestations in patients with mastocytosis: Consensus report of the European Competence Network on Mastocytosis; the American Academy of Allergy, Asthma & Immunology; and the European Academy of Allergology and Clinical Immunology. *J Allergy Clin Immunol.* 2016;137(1):35-45.

273. Pandhi D, Singal A, Aggarwal S. Adult onset, hypopigmented solitary mastocytoma: report of two cases. *Indian J Dermatol Venereol Leprol.* 2008;74(1):41-43.

274. Khan K, Kupferman ME, Gardner JM, Ivan D. Solitary mastocytoma in an adult with an unusual clinical presentation. *J Am Acad Dermatol.* 2011;65(3):683-684.

275. Akoglu G, Erkin G, Cakir B, et al. Cutaneous mastocytosis: demographic aspects and clinical features of 55 patients. *J Eur Acad Dermatol Venereol.* 2006;20(8):969-973.

276. Meni C, Bruneau J, Georgin-Lavialle S, et al. Paediatric mastocytosis: a systematic review of 1747 cases. *Br J Dermatol.* 2015;172(3):642-651.

277. Ma D, Stence AA, Bossler AB, Hackman JR, Bellizzi AM. Identification of KIT activating mutations in paediatric solitary mastocytoma. *Histopathology.* 2014;64(2):218-225.

278. Yanagihori H, Oyama N, Nakamura K, Kaneko F. c-kit Mutations in patients with childhood-onset mastocytosis and genotype-phenotype correlation. *J Mol Diagn.* 2005;7(2):252-257.

279. Bodemer C, Hermine O, Palmerini F, et al. Pediatric mastocytosis is a clonal disease associated with D816V and other activating c-KIT mutations. *J Invest Dermatol.* 2010;130(3):804-815.

280. Lanternier F, Cohen-Akenine A, Palmerini F, et al. Phenotypic and genotypic characteristics of mastocytosis according to the age of onset. *PLoS One.* 2008;3(4):e1906.

281. Longley BJ, Henz BM. Mastocytosis. In: LeBoit PE, Burg G, Weedon D, Sarasin A, eds. *World Health Organization Classification of Tumors: Pathology and Genetics of Skin Tumors.* Lyon, France: IARC Press; 2006:226, 227-228.

282. Hartmann K, Bruns SB, Henz BM. Mastocytosis: review of clinical and experimental aspects. *J Investig Dermatol Symp Proc.* 2001;6(2):143-147.

283. Schena D, Galvan A, Tessari G, Girolomoni G. Clinical features and course of cutaneous mastocytosis in 133 children. *Br J Dermatol.* 2016;174(2):411-413.

284. Yung A. Flushing due to solitary cutaneous mastocytoma can be prevented by hydrocolloid dressings. *Pediatr Dermatol.* 2004;21(3):262-264.

285. Katoh N, Hirano S, Yasuno H. Solitary mastocytoma treated with tranilast. *J Dermatol.* 1996;23(5):335-339.

286. Heide R, Beishuizen A, De Groot H, et al. Mastocytosis in children: a protocol for management. *Pediatr Dermatol.* 2008;25(4):493-500.

287. Mihm MC, Clark WH, Reed RJ, Caruso MG. Mast cell infiltrates of the skin and the mastocytosis syndrome. *Hum Pathol.* 1973;4(2):231-239.

288. Horny HP, Valent P. Diagnosis of mastocytosis: general histopathological aspects, morphological criteria, and immunohistochemical findings. *Leuk Res.* 2001;25(7):543-551.

289. Hu S, Kuo TT, Hong HS. Mast cells with bilobed or multilobed nuclei in a nodular lesion of a patient with urticaria pigmentosa. *Am J Dermatopathol.* 2002;24(6):490-492.

290. Tran DT, Jokinen CH, Argenyi ZB. Histiocyte-rich pleomorphic mastocytoma: an uncommon variant mimicking juvenile xanthogranuloma and Langerhans cell histiocytosis. *J Cutan Pathol.* 2009;36(11):1215-1220.

291. Hollmann TJ, Brenn T, Hornick JL. CD25 expression on cutaneous mast cells from adult patients presenting with urticaria pigmentosa is predictive of systemic mastocytosis. *Am J Surg Pathol.* 2008;32(1):139-145.

292. Patterson JW. Disorders of mast cells and plasma cells. In: Patterson JW, eds. *Practical Skin Pathology: A Diagnostic Approach.* Philadelphia, PA: Elsevier Saunders; 2013:609-618.

293. Delprat C, Arico M. Blood spotlight on Langerhans cell histiocytosis. *Blood.* 2014;124(6):867-872.

294. Kuramoto Y, Tagami H. Solitary mastocytoma with massive eosinophilic infiltration. *Pediatr Dermatol.* 1994;11(3):256-257.

295. Ueng SH, Kuo TT. An unusual mastocytoma with massive eosinophilic infiltration: identification with immunohistochemistry. *Am J Dermatopathol.* 2004;26(6):475-477.

296. Brockow K. Urticaria pigmentosa. *Immunol Allergy Clin North Am.* 2004;24(2):287,316,vii.

297. Berezowska S, Flaig MJ, Rueff F, et al. Adult-onset mastocytosis in the skin is highly suggestive of systemic mastocytosis. *Mod Pathol.* 2014;27(1):19-29.

298. Pollard WL, Beachkofsky TM, Kobayashi TT. Novel R634W c-kit mutation identified in familial mastocytosis. *Pediatr Dermatol.* 2015;32(2):267-270.

299. Fett NM, Teng J, Longley BJ. Familial urticaria pigmentosa: report of a family and review of the role of KIT mutations. *Am J Dermatopathol.* 2013;35(1):113-116.

300. Zhang LY, Smith ML, Schultheis B, et al. A novel K509I mutation of KIT identified in familial mastocytosis-in vitro and in vivo responsiveness to imatinib therapy. *Leuk Res.* 2006;30(4):373-378.

301. Wohrl S, Moritz KB, Bracher A, Fischer G, Stingl G, Loewe R. A c-kit mutation in exon 18 in familial mastocytosis. *J Invest Dermatol.* 2013;133(3):839-841.

302. Wasag B, Niedoszytko M, Piskorz A, et al. Novel, activating KIT-N822I mutation in familial cutaneous mastocytosis. *Exp Hematol.* 2011;39(8):859-865.e2.

303. Beghini A, Tibiletti MG, Roversi G, et al. Germline mutation in the juxtamembrane domain of the kit gene in a family with gastrointestinal stromal tumors and urticaria pigmentosa. *Cancer.* 2001;92(3):657-662.

304. Wiechers T, Rabenhorst A, Schick T, et al. Large maculopapular cutaneous lesions are associated with favorable outcome in childhood-onset mastocytosis. *J Allergy Clin Immunol.* 2015;136(6):1581-1590.e3.

305. DiBacco RS, DeLeo VA. Mastocytosis and the mast cell. *J Am Acad Dermatol.* 1982;7(6):709-722.

306. Lange M, Niedoszytko M, Nedoszytko B, Lata J, Trzeciak M, Biernat W. Diffuse cutaneous mastocytosis: analysis of 10 cases and a brief review of the literature. *J Eur Acad Dermatol Venereol.* 2012;26(12):1565-1571.

307. Li WV, Kapadia SB, Sonmez-Alpan E, Swerdlow SH. Immunohistochemical characterization of mast cell disease in paraffin sections using tryptase, CD68, myeloperoxidase, lysozyme, and CD20 antibodies. *Mod Pathol.* 1996;9(10):982-988.

308. Wang HJ, Lin ZM, Zhang J, Yin JH, Yang Y. A new germline mutation in KIT associated with diffuse cutaneous mastocytosis in a Chinese family. *Clin Exp Dermatol.* 2014;39(2):146-149.

309. Tang X, Boxer M, Drummond A, Ogston P, Hodgins M, Burden AD. A germline mutation in KIT in familial diffuse cutaneous mastocytosis. *J Med Genet.* 2004;41(6):e88.

310. Willemze R, Ruiter DJ, Scheffer E, van Vloten WA. Diffuse cutaneous mastocytosis with multiple cutaneous mastocytomas. Report of a case with clinical, histopathological and ultrastructural aspects. *Br J Dermatol.* 1980;102(5):601-607.

27

Cutaneous Hematolymphoid Proliferations

Julia Scarisbrick / Louis P. Dehner / Alejandro A. Gru

INTRODUCTION

Primary cutaneous lymphomas are rare cutaneous neoplasms with varied clinical presentation and course. Initial examination must differentiate between primary cutaneous lymphoproliferative disorders (LPD) and secondary involvement of the skin by systemic lymphoma. In children, systemic lymphomas and leukemias are more common than primary cutaneous LPDs. Moreover, full staging investigations such as a bone marrow (BM) biopsy and imaging ensure accurate diagnosis of a primary skin lymphoma. The clinical course of primary cutaneous lymphomas differs from that of its systemic counterparts and requires a team-based approach involving hematologists, dermatologists, and other specialists. Morphologic interpretation of tumors involves the use of cytologic touch preparations, flow cytometry, fluorescence in situ hybridization (FISH), and conventional cytogenetics. The choice of molecular tools is of paramount importance as are the treatments that vary from an expectant/watchful waiting approach to aggressive chemotherapy regimens and possible allogeneic BM transplantation, depending on the histologic subtype of skin lymphoma.

Four major histologic subtypes account for most non-Hodgkin lymphomas (NHL) in the pediatric setting: Burkitt lymphoma (39%), diffuse large B-cell lymphoma (DLBCL; 16%), lymphoblastic lymphoma (28%), and anaplastic large cell lymphoma (ALCL; 10%).[1] Approximately 7% of pediatric NHL includes more unusual histologic subtypes, including cutaneous lymphomas. The epidemiologic aspects of cutaneous hematopoietic tumors in children are poorly studied, as most of them are derived from small case series that are highly biased by private consultation material from single institutions.[2] In the series by Fink-Puches et al[3](n = 69), ~35% of pediatric cutaneous lymphomas were accounted for by mycosis fungoides (MF), another ~35% by CD30+ lymphoproliferative disorders (ALCL and lymphomatoid papulosis [LyP]), and 20% included marginal zone lymphomas (MZLs) and B-lymphoblastic lymphoma. The pediatric series by Boccara et al[4] in France (n = 51) showed that nearly half of these tumors (47%) were composed by LyP, 27% by lymphoblastic lymphomas/leukemias and leukemic infiltrates by acute myeloid leukemia (AML), and approximately 10% included cases of Epstein-Barr virus (EBV)+ lymphoproliferative neoplasms and MF.

Although most cutaneous lymphomas—with MF the most common—are similar in children and adults, a disproportionate number of lesions in children have a particular clinical and immunophenotypic profile. In children, most of the hypopigmented lesions have a CD8+ phenotype and exhibit a very indolent behavior. Similarly, lymphoblastic and myeloid leukemic infiltrates are overrepresented in children, as the diseases occur with relatively greater frequency. Histiocytoses with cutaneous presentation are more frequent in children than in adults.

Mature T-Cell and NK-Cell Lymphomas

PRIMARY CUTANEOUS ALCL, ANAPLASTIC LYMPHOMA KINASE (ALK)-NEGATIVE

Definition and Epidemiology

Primary cutaneous anaplastic large cell lymphoma (PC-ALCL) is composed of large and pleomorphic cells (indistinguishable from ALK+ ALCL) with diffuse expression of CD30 in the tumor cells (greater than 75%).[5,6] The diagnosis is limited to those cases without a history of LyP or MF.[7,8] Unlike ALK+ ALCL, PC-ALCL is very rare in children compared with adults[9-14] and a diagnosis of LyP (type A or C) should first be considered. In some cases of PC-ALCL in childhood, an association with HIV infection has been documented.[9]

Clinical Presentation

Rapidly growing, asymptomatic, solitary or multiple skin nodules/tumors with a tendency to ulcerate (Figure 27-1) are the characteristic clinical presentation.[12]

Histologic Findings

Microscopically, ALCL has diffuse, cohesive sheets of large pleomorphic tumor cells, strongly CD30+, similar to ALK+ ALCL (Figures 27-2 and 27-3). Even among the conventional variants, a rich inflammatory infiltrate is present, which can lead to a misdiagnosis of an inflammatory process in the skin.[15] The neutrophilic variant (pyogenic) of PC-ALCL contains a neutrophilic-rich infiltrate (Figure 27-4). Although the conventional variant does not have a predilection for immunocompromised individuals, the pyogenic variant is

seen in those with HIV,[16] transplant recipients,[17] and hematologic malignancies, including young individuals.[10,18]

The tumors are frequently CD4+ and show expression of cytotoxic markers (TIA-1, perforin, granzyme B) (Figure 27-3). There is variable loss of T-cell antigens and, as opposed to systemic ALK+ ALCL, PC-ALCL is usually negative for epithelial membrane antigen (EMA) .[19] CD99 can also be positive.[9] The pyogenic variant can have a higher rate of CD8 and EMA (57%) expression, compared to the conventional form.[10,20] T-cell clonality has been proved in the vast majority of cases by conventional T-cell receptor (TCR) studies. ALK−ALCL have shown convergent mutations and kinase fusions that lead to constitutive activation of the JAK/STAT3 pathway, and a subset with rearrangements at the locus containing *DUSP22* and *IRF4* in chromosome 6p25 tends to be relatively monomorphic, usually lack cytotoxic granules, and have been reported to have a superior prognosis, whereas a small subset with *TP63* rearrangements are very aggressive.[21-23]

Differential Diagnosis

The clinical differential diagnosis for the pyogenic variant of PC-ALCL includes pyoderma gangrenosum, pyoderma faciale (rosacea fulminans), Sweet syndrome, leishmaniasis, deep fungal infection, or pyogenic granuloma. Bacterial cellulitis has also been described as another differential diagnostic consideration. Among neoplastic conditions, LyP is common in children (see discussion below), and tumor stage MF, which typically presents in the fifth to sixth decade, is exceedingly rare in kids; the latter two disorders are best distinguished on a clinical background. Those with transformed MF have a long-standing history of the disease and present with multiple tumors, whereas LyP has a history of self-remitting papules. ALK staining and CD30 are useful to rule out the possibility of cutaneous involvement by systemic ALK+ ALCL.[10]

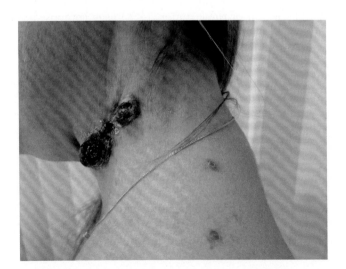

FIGURE 27-1. Cutaneous anaplastic large cell lymphoma of the neck in a girl with coexisting lymphomatoid papulosis. Large ulcerated necrotic tumors can be seen on the neck.

> **CAPSULE SUMMARY**
>
> **PRIMARY CUTANEOUS ALCL, ALK-NEGATIVE**
>
> PC-ALCL is a primary cutaneous lymphoma composed of large and pleomorphic cells (indistinguishable from ALK+ ALCL) with diffuse expression of CD30 in the tumor cells (greater than 75%). The tumor cells show variable loss of T-cell antigens, and cytotoxic marker expression. Rapidly growing, asymptomatic, solitary, or multiple skin nodules/tumors with a tendency to ulcerate are the characteristic clinical presentation.

MYCOSIS FUNGOIDES

Definition and Epidemiology

MF is the most common form of cutaneous T-cell lymphoma in both adults[24,25] and children.[4,26-29] MF in children has a characteristic clinical appearance of hypopigmented

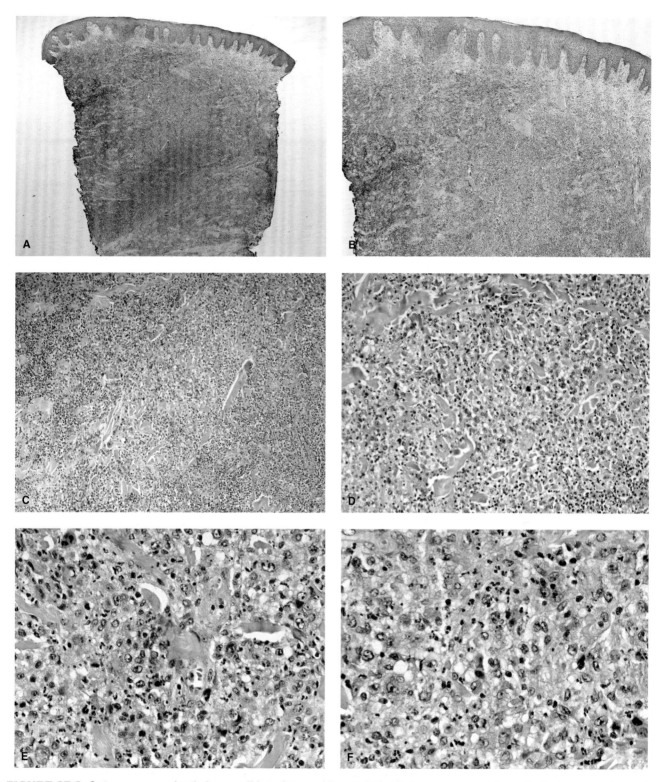

FIGURE 27-2. Cutaneous anaplastic large cell lymphoma—histopathologic findings. Diffuse dermal infiltrate sparing the surface epidermis (A and B). The malignant infiltrate dissects through the collagen bundles (C). There is a rich admixed neutrophilic inflammatory infiltrate (D). The infiltrate is composed of malignant appearing large cells with many "hallmark" cells. Eosinophils are also seen (E and F).

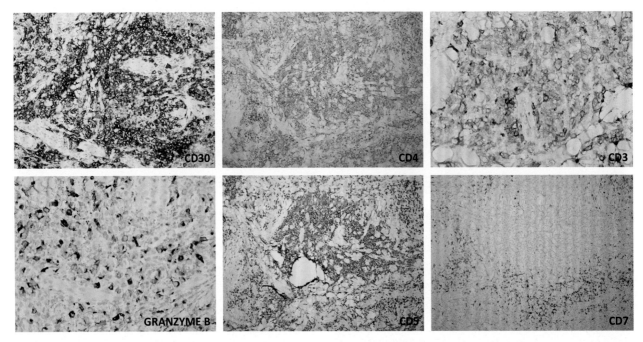

FIGURE 27-3. Cutaneous anaplastic large cell lymphoma—immunohistochemistry. The malignant cells are strong and diffusely positive for CD30 (>75%), CD4, CD3, and have patchy positivity for granzyme B. They have retained expression of CD5, whereas there is a marked loss of CD7.

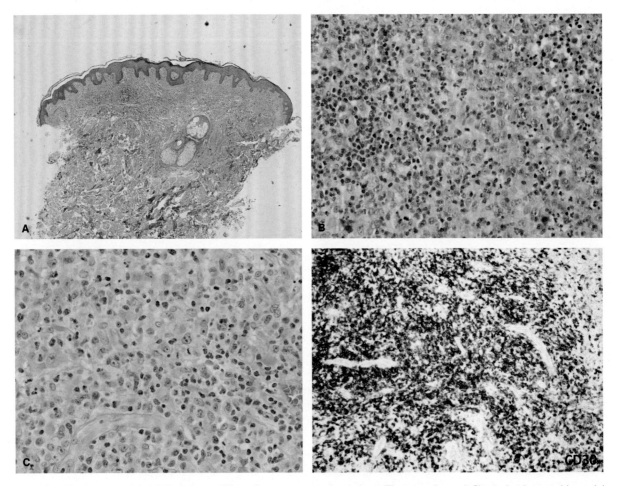

FIGURE 27-4. Cutaneous anaplastic large cell lymphoma, pyogenic variant. The very dense infiltrate is obscured by a rich acute inflammatory infiltrate with neutrophilic and numerous eosinophils (A-C). The malignant cells are unmasked by a CD30 stain.

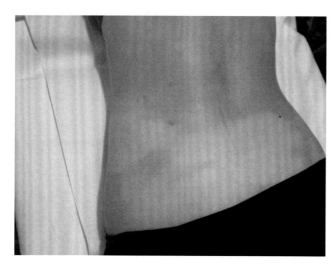

FIGURE 27-5: **Mycosis fungoides in an adolescent.** Characteristic hypopigmented patches can be seen on the lower back.

patches (Figure 27-5) and plaques that generally do not progress to the tumoral phase, and has a CD8$^+$ phenotype.[30] It has been reported in children as young as 3 years.[3,27,31-34] The male-to-female ratio is nearly equal in the pediatric setting.[27,31,34,35] Fink-Puches et al showed that MF represented almost 35% of all cutaneous lymphomas in individuals younger than 20 years.[3]

Etiology

The discovery of specific molecular rearrangements[36-40] complements advances in the mutational landscape of MF and Sézary syndrome (SS). Choi et al[36] found frequent deletions in chromatin modifying genes (*ARID1A* [62.5%], *CTCF* [12.5%], and *DNMT3A* [42.5%]). *RB1* was deleted in 25% of samples. *CARD11* and *JAK2* amplification were seen in 22.5% and 12.5% of cases, respectively. *MYC* amplification was noted in 42.5% of samples. da Silva Almeida et al[37] identified a median of 21 copy number alterations per sample (range 0-56) in SS, with characteristic recurrent gains in chromosomes 7 (5/25, 20%), 8q (13/25, 52%), and 17q (2/25, 8%), as well as recurrent deletions involving tumor-suppressor genes in 17p13.1 (*TP53*; 13/25, 52%), 13q14.2 (*RB1*; 4/25, 16%), 10q23.3 (*PTEN*, 5/25; 20%), and 12p13.1 (*CDKN1B*; 5/25, 20%). Kiel et al[38] showed numerous (n = 42) fusion genes including *TPR-MET, MYBL1-TOX, DNAJC15-ZMYM2,* and *EZH2-FOXP1,* which, albeit not recurrent, could contribute to the pathogenesis of SS. Ungewickell et al[39] found structural variation events (excluding copy number gains) in pathways related to T-cell survival and proliferation in 11% of patients with MF or SS. The structural variants were largely mutually exclusive with the TNFR2 alterations. The structural variants included *NFKB2* gene truncations in 5% (4/73) of cases with the deletion of a region whose loss generates a truncated p100 protein with predicted proteasome-independent NF-κB2

nuclear localization, as well as a deletion involving TRAF3 that increases noncanonical NF-κB signaling. A recurrent *CTLA4-CD28* fusion was also discovered.

Clinical Presentation

Clinically, pediatric and adult MF may be difficult to diagnose, partly because they can potentially mimic numerous benign inflammatory dermatoses (Figure 27-6). In fact, a diagnosis is commonly delayed and may take several years, and numerous biopsies are often required to eventually establish or consider the diagnosis before clonality studies are performed. Ackerman raised concerns about the diagnosis of MF in the pediatric setting in the past: in their review of 106 cases, it was claimed that only 23 cases had information "sufficient" for a diagnosis of hypopigmented MF.[41] Indeed, in 83 of those cases, there was no significant clinicopathologic correlation to confidently establish the diagnosis.

MF also enters into the differential diagnosis of psoriasis, tinea corporis, pityriasis lichenoides (PL), lichen aureus, atopic dermatitis, and the various hypopigmented dermatoses. Vitiligo and pityriasis alba are the two most frequent misdiagnoses in children.[42,43] In a recent case series, all children (100%, n = 69) presented at the patch stage; almost all cases had hypopigmented lesions and most of these occurred in African American children.[26] Compared with children, adults exhibit sharply demarcated, atrophic lesions with a cigarette paper appearance (Figures 27-7 and 27-8). In an earlier study by Crowley et al, of the 58 patients with MF (younger than 35 years), 17% presented with the tumor stage and approximately 4% had generalized erythroderma.[27] In another series of 46 cases, Heng et al reported that over 90% had hyperpigmented lesions.[44] The most commonly affected areas included the buttocks, trunk,

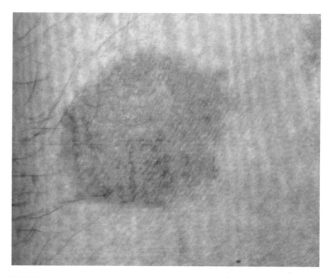

FIGURE 27-6. A patch of mycosis fungoides may be similar to other more common childhood dermatoses such as eczema or psoriasis.

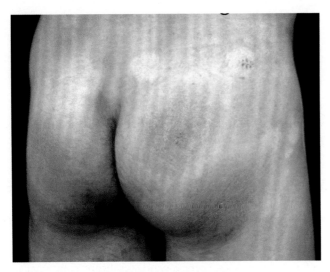

FIGURE 27-7. Distribution of patches of mycosis fungoides is more common in the "bathing suit" area.

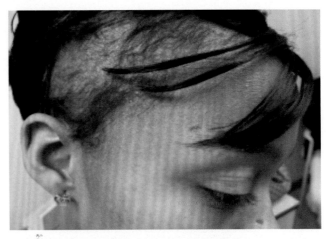

FIGURE 27-9. Mycosis fungoides, folliculotropic form. Patches of alopecia in an adolescent girl.

and extremities (sun-protected areas). About 6% of patients have solitary lesions. Rare cases of MF can present following organ transplantation.[45]

Folliculotropic MF (FMF) presents with follicular papules occasionally with an erythematous base, and follicular plugging and/or alopecia; this is the second most common clinical variant and seemingly occurs more frequently in individuals younger than 40 years (Figure 27-9) (8% of all variants).[46-50] In FMF, the lesions are usually located in the head and neck region, with the presentation of plaques

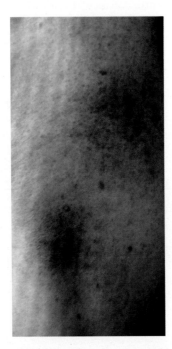

FIGURE 27-8. Patches of mycosis fungoides show poikilodermatous skin change with atrophy, telangiectasia, and dyspigmentation.

and/or tumors and intense pruritus. FMF has been associated with a worse outcome in adults and children unlike the more indolent and common patch/plaque lesions without FMF.[46] Less common clinical variants in the pediatric population include "granulomatous slack skin" or granulomatous MF,[51-55] characterized by the development of areas of pendulous, lax skin in the major skin folds (especially axillae and groins).[56] Localized pagetoid reticulosis (PR; Woringer-Kolopp disease) presents as a solitary, slowly growing erythematous and verrucous plaque on the extremities; rare cases have been reported in children.[57-59] SS is a distinctive erythrodermic cutaneous T-cell lymphoma, characterized by pruritic erythroderma, generalized lymphadenopathy, and circulating malignant cells with cerebriform nuclei. It is a disease of adults, with only rare cases in the pediatric population.[60-62] A rare clinical presentation of palmoplantar keratoderma has also been described in children.[63]

Histologic Findings

Morphologically, pediatric MF is histologically indistinguishable from that seen in adults (Figure 27-10 to 27-13). According to the series from Castano et al, the most frequent histologic findings include: lymphocytes in clusters, patchy lichenoid infiltrates, perivascular/periadnexal infiltrates, psoriasiform hyperplasia, papillary dermal fibroplasia, dermal melanophages, and Pautrier microabscesses. The infiltrate shows epidermotropism with tagging of cells along the dermal-epidermal junction.[64] The atypical lymphocytes show nuclear hyperchromasia and irregular and sometimes cerebriform nuclei. Distinctive perinuclear halos are seen surrounding the intraepidermal lesional cells. Admixed histiocytes, plasma cells, and eosinophils can be present. As the lesions progress clinically, so does the extent of the infiltrate. Large cell transformation is defined as the presence of large cells (at least 4 times the size of a small lymphocyte) comprising >25% of the infiltrate or in

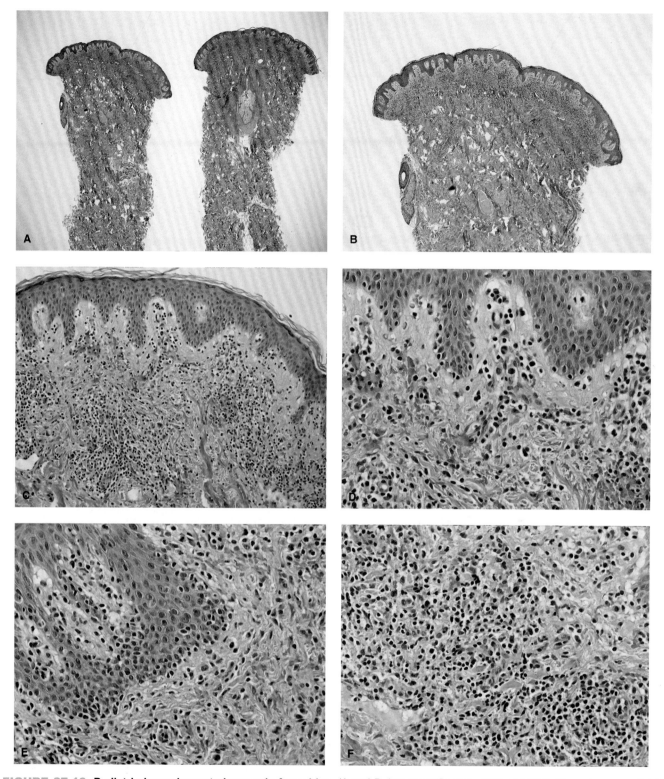

FIGURE 27-10. Pediatric hypopigmented mycosis fungoides. (A and B, low magnification—20× and 40×). There is a superficial dermal band-like infiltrate. (C and D, intermediate magnification, 100× and 200×). The infiltrate is associated with extravasation of red blood cells. There is tagging of lymphoid cells at the dermal-epidermal junction. (E and F, high magnification, 400× each). The infiltrate is composed of small- to medium-sized lymphocytes, with hyperchromasia, and irregular nuclear borders. The epidermotropic cells do not reveal definitive intraepidermal collections of lymphocytes in the form of Pautrier microabscesses. Reprinted with permission from Gru AA, Schaffer A. *Hematopathology of the skin: A clinical and pathologic approach.* 1st ed. Philadelphia, PA: Wolters Kluwer; 2017.

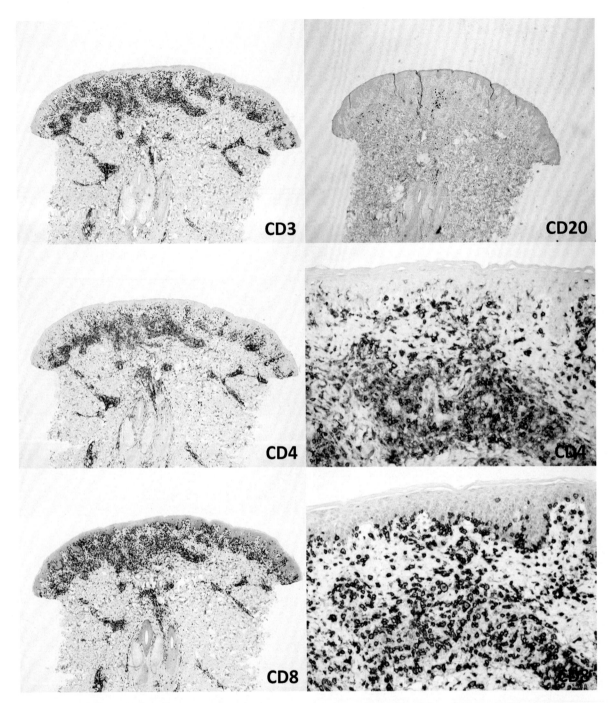

FIGURE 27-11. Pediatric hypopigmented mycosis fungoides—immunohistochemistry. CD3 is positive in the majority of the dermal and epidermal lymphocytes. CD20 is predominantly negative. CD4 shows positive staining in many of the T cells and the dermal lymphocytes. However, the vast majority of T cells in the epidermis are negative for CD4 and positive for CD8, which reveals extensive epidermotropism and tagging of cells along the dermal-epidermal junction. Reprinted with permission from Gru AA, Schaffer A. Hemato-pathology of the skin: *A clinical and pathologic approach*. 1st ed. Philadelphia, PA: Wolters Kluwer; 2017.

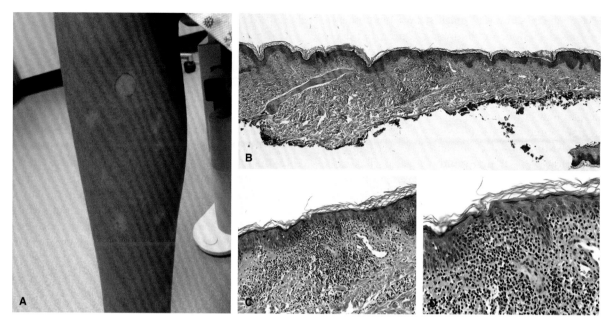

FIGURE 27-12. Pediatric mycosis fungoides, hypopigmented variant. Ill-defined hypopigmented patches are present in the leg. Histopathologically, there is an atypical infiltrate with epidermotropism. Tagging of lymphocytes along the dermal-epidermal junction is seen. The lymphocytes are small, with hyperchromasia, irregular nuclear borders, and perinuclear halos. Obtained with permission Gru A, Dehner LP. Cutaneous hematolymphoid and histiocytic proliferations in children. *Pediatr Dev Pathol.* 2018;21(2):150-207.

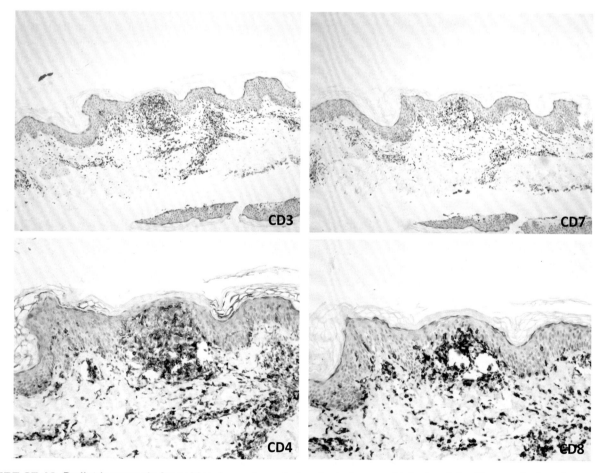

FIGURE 27-13. Pediatric mycosis fungoides, hypopigmented variant—immunohistochemistry. The neoplastic cells are positive for CD3 and CD8. The CD4:CD8 ratio is inverted. There is aberrant loss of CD7. Obtained with permission Gru A, Dehner LP. Cutaneous hematolymphoid and histiocytic proliferations in children. *Pediatr Dev Pathol.* 2018;21(2):150-207.

nodular aggregates. Only rarely has such a phenomenon been described in lesions in children.[65,66] In FMF, there is infiltration of the hair follicle epithelium with or without epidermotropism (epidermotropism is more frequently seen). The infiltrate involves the infundibulum of the hair follicle and at times deeper portions of the follicle. Follicular mucinosis may be an accompanying feature that can be better demonstrated by colloidal iron or Alcian blue stains. Additionally, FMF is often accompanied by a syringotropic infiltrate.[46] However, a Dutch study revealed that interfollicular epidermotropism is actually rare.[50] FMF is not usually accompanied by intraepidermal Pautrier microabscesses.[67] Dermal eosinophilia can be prominent, particularly during the progression of the disease, and might be a manifestation of an autoimmune response to the keratin of the hair shafts in the dermis. In granulomatous MF (GMF), dense nodular and diffuse granulomas are present in the dermis, with or without epidermotropism, and with destruction of elastic fibers and elastophagocytosis. In the PR variant of MF, prominent pagetoid epidermotropism is noted (Figure 27-14). Such cases show a very impressive clinical response to radiation treatment.

The immunophenotype of pediatric MF is different from most of the adult forms (Figures 27-11 and 27-13): hypopigmented MF is a CD8+ cytotoxic T-cell lymphoma (whereas most cases in adults are CD4+).[3,26-29,31,32,41,42,44,46,68-75] Also, CD30 expression is usually negative or reacts with only a few scattered cells (80% of cases are entirely nonreactive). Decreased expression of both CD4 and CD8 can also be seen in some cases of hypopigmented MF.[76,77] Similar to adult MF, there is usually preserved expression of CD2 and CD5 with loss of CD7. A single rare case with co-expression of CD56 has been reported with an associated indolent clinical course.[78] In FMF the infiltrate usually shows a predominance of CD4+ cells like the adult cases.[46] GMF is also a disease of CD4+ T cells. The genetics of MF and SS is less well understood in the context of the pediatric cases when compared with adult MF. T-cell gene rearrangement studies performed in pediatric MF revealed TCR clonality in approximately 64% of cases and a polyclonal result in 16% of cases. These numbers appear to be lower when compared to the adult experience of 80% clonality, which may reflect a relatively lower number of neoplastic cells in skin biopsies from children. However, sensitivity for TCR is lower in early lesions of MF (up to 60%).[79] Hodak et al revealed monoclonality in only 43% of cases.[46]

Differential Diagnosis

The differential diagnosis of MF includes a number of inflammatory dermatoses: Pityriasis alba usually presents with hypopigmented macules and patches on the face but may also affect the trunk and limbs. Histologically, there are very sparse lymphoid infiltrates, with very slight spongiosis and without the dermal fibrosis seen in MF; vitiligo consists of depigmented macules and patches in localized, segmental, or widespread distribution. The lesions are usually on the face and distal extremities. Histologically, the findings are minimal, and if present, there is a subtle perivascular infiltrate of lymphocytes with minimal epidermal involvement. As lesions evolve, there is a decrease in the number of

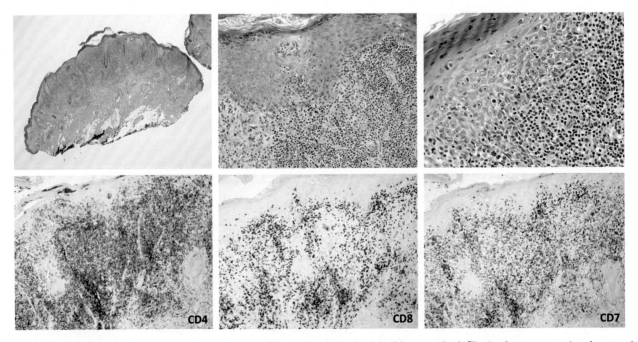

FIGURE 27-14. Pediatric mycosis fungoides, pagetoid reticulosis variant. In this case, the infiltrate shows very extensive pagetoid epidermotropism. Lymphoma cells are CD4 positive, CD8 negative, and have loss of CD7. Obtained with permission Gru A, Dehner LP. Cutaneous hematolymphoid and histiocytic proliferations in children. *Pediatr Dev Pathol.* 2018;21(2):150-207.

melanocytes at the dermal-epidermal junction, which can be proved with the use of a MART-1 immunostain. Acral pseudolymphomatous angiokeratoma of children (APACHE) can also mimic PR. A dense lymphoid infiltrate beneath the epidermis, and thick wall vessels are seen.[80] PL chronica and varioliformis acuta (PLC/PLEVA) can also share histomorphologic features. A lymphocytic vasculitis and interface changes are present in both conditions. As opposed to MF, loss of T-cell antigens (CD7) is not typical. Molecular studies (TCR rearrangement) should not be used to distinguish between both conditions, particularly if the BIOMED primers are being used, because PLC and PLEVA can have positive clonality studies in up to 25% of cases. Next generation sequencing accurately distinguishes between inflammatory dermatoses with clonal populations of cells and cutaneous T-cell lymphomas.[81] However, this technique is currently expensive and unlikely to replace TCR gene analysis in the clinical setting. Spongiotic dermatoses (eczema, contact dermatitis, etc) can also enter the differential diagnosis. The latter typically lack significant cytologic atypia of the lymphoid population or aberrant antigenic loss. If the infiltrate is positive for CD30, other CD30[+] lymphoproliferative diseases (LPDs) can enter the differential diagnosis (LyP and PC-ALCL). In children, Langerhans cell histiocytosis is also accompanied by extensive pagetoid epidermotropism of the histiocytic cells. As opposed to MF, langerhans cell histiocytosis (LCH) is positive with histiocytic markers (CD68, S100, CD1a, and Langerin), whereas it is negative for T-cell antigens. A word of caution should be made with LCH, as many cases can have clonal rearrangements of the TCR.

CAPSULE SUMMARY

MYCOSIS FUNGOIDES

MF is the most common form of cutaneous T-cell lymphoma in both adults and children. MF in children often has a characteristic clinical appearance of hypopigmented patches and plaques that generally do not progress to the tumoral phase and more frequently has a CD8[+] phenotype. More recently, folliculotropic forms have been reported with a high prevalence in this population, but without an association with a more aggressive clinical course. Loss of T-cell antigens (CD7) is common. Differential diagnosis, particularly in the hypopigmented variants, should include disorders of pigmentary alteration (pityriasis alba, vitiligo, etc).

LYMPHOMATOID PAPULOSIS

Definition and Epidemiology

Lymphomatoid papulosis (LyP) is a CD30[+] T-cell lymphoproliferative disorder characterized by recurrent crops of papulonecrotic lesions that usually prevail for 3 and 8 weeks and then resolve spontaneously.[82] The lesions are clinically "benign" appearing, but the histologic features suggest otherwise. However, the lesions may frequently heal with atrophic scarring, which may be disfiguring. LyP is the third most common type of cutaneous lymphoproliferative disorder in children.[3,83] Boys are reported to have an earlier onset of LyP compared with girls. It is estimated that between 5% and 20% of those with LyP can develop a subsequent lymphoma, usually MF, Hodgkin lymphoma, or ALCL; this proportion appears to be smaller in the pediatric setting (approximately 9%).[83-88] The frequency of LyP ranges from 16% to 47% of all skin lymphomas in children, across different case series.[2-4]

Etiology

Karai et al were the first to report a group of patients with LyP and associated rearrangements of the *IRF4-DUSP22* locus on 6p25.3.[89] The patients showed unusual histologic findings, including PR-like epidermal changes with a proliferating dermal tumor. A consistent histologic finding also included a typical periadnexal infiltrate and hallmark-like cells.

Clinical Presentation

Clinically, LyP presents with erythematous papules and nodules that become hemorrhagic and necrotic after a few days with resolution as a depigmented scar.[4,7,71,82-87,90-93] Lesions at different stages of evolution are characteristically present (Figure 27-15). In children, there is a clinical resemblance to PL, the most important disease in the differential diagnosis. The sites of predilection are the trunk and extremities, but other locations have been reported.[93] Regional LyP with crops of lesions located in a single anatomic region is seemingly more common in children.[92,93] Nearly 50% of cases in children have more than 50 lesions at one point during their clinical course.

LyP is a clinical diagnosis of self-resolving papulonecrotic lesions. Although most are CD30 positive, the histology may be varied and indistinguishable from transformed CD30-positive MF, popular MF, or PC-ALCL in some cases.

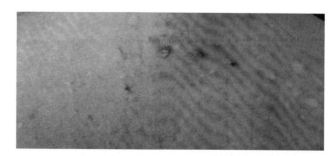

FIGURE 27-15. **Lymphomatoid papulosis (LyP).** Lesions of LyP often appear in crops; they mature from red papules and may ulcerate and tend to heal with atrophic hypopigmented scars.

Histologic Findings

Several histologic variants have been described in LyP: types A, B, C, D, E, and F (Table 27-1). None of the histologic subtypes have any prognostic significance. The importance in differentiating the various subtypes is related to the differential diagnosis that each subtype entails. Many of these lesions have substantial histopathologic overlap: Type A LyP has a wedge-shaped dermal infiltrate composed of medium to large and pleomorphic cells scattered throughout the infiltrate or are arranged in clusters (Figure 27-16). The malignant cells can show features of Hodgkin-like cells, and there is a rich background of inflammatory cells. Ulceration, edema of the dermis, and focal vasculitic changes may be present. Type B LyP is

TABLE 27-1.	Lymphomatoid Papulosis, Subtypes		
LyP Type	**Histologic Findings**	**Differential Diagnosis**	**Criteria**
Type A	• Wedge-shaped dermal infiltrate • Scattered or in small clusters arranged large CD30⁺ lymphocytes with nuclear pleomorphism and mitotes • Background infiltrate of histiocytes, eosinophils, neutrophils. • **MOST COMMON IN CHILDREN**	• Hodgkin lymphoma (primary or secondary cutaneous) • MF (transformation)	• Staging examination (in nodal HL) • Patches and plaques in MF vs self-regressing papulonodular lesions in LyP
Type B	• Epidermotropic infiltrate of small- to medium-sized lymphocytes with atypical chromatin-dense nuclei • Variable expression of CD30 (0%-77%)	• MF (patch/plaque stage) • Cutaneous γ/δ lymphoma (epidermotropic)	• Patches and plaques in MF vs self-regressing papulonodular lesions in LyP • Multiple plaques and nodules with ulceration. • IHC: Expression of TCRγ
Type C	• Nodular cohesive infiltrate of large CD30⁺ pleomorphic or anaplastic lymphocytes with abundant cytoplasm and mitotic activity. • Admixture of only few eosinophils and neutrophils.	• Anaplastic large cell lymphoma (primary cutaneous or systemic form) • MF (transformation) • Peripheral T-cell lymphoma, NOS (primary cutaneous or nodal) • Adult T-cell lymphoma/leukemia	• Clinical presentation with solitary or grouped nodules in PC-ALCL. Staging examinations in SALCL. Patches and plaques preceding tumors in MF. Lack of CD30 or expression by only a minority of tumor cells (usually <30%), Staging examinations • Integration of HTLV-1/2 in tumor cell genome.
Type D	• Epidermotropism of atypical small- to medium-sized pleomorphic lymphocytes • Deep dermal or subcutaneous perivascular infiltrates may be present. • Expression of CD8 (100%) and CD30 (90%) • **4/9 CASES IN CHILDREN**	• Pagetoid reticulosis • Primary cutaneous aggressive epidermotropic CD8⁺ cytotoxic T-cell lymphoma • Cutaneous γ/δ lymphoma	• Unilesional erythematous scaling lesion in PR (eczematous or psoriasiform clinical aspect) • Multiple rapidly evolving plaques and nodules with erosions and necrosis. • No expression of CD30! • Multiple plaques with erosions IHC: expression of TCRγ
Type E	• Angioinvasive, ie, angiocentric and angiodestructive infiltrates of mostly medium-sized pleomorphic CD30⁺ lymphocytes. • Vascular occlusion by atypical lymphocytes and/or thrombi, hemorrhage, extensive necrosis and ulceration. • Admixture of eosinophils. • Expression of CD8⁺ (70%) and CD30 (100%) • **2/16 CASES IN CHILDREN**	• Extranodal NK/T-cell lymphoma, nasal type • Cutaneous gamma/delta lymphoma • Anaplastic large cell lymphoma (primary cutaneous or systemic form) with angiocentric and angiodestructive growth)	• Association with EBV, mostly secondary cutaneous involvement (staging) • IHC: Expression of TCR gamma • Clinical presentation with solitary or grouped nodules in PC-ALCL. Staging examinations in SALCL.

Abbreviations: HL, Hodgkin lymphoma; IHC, immunohistochemistry; LyP, lymphomatoid papulosis; MF, mycosis fungoides; NOS, nodal or systemic malignant; PC-ALCL, primary cutaneous anaplastic large cell lymphoma; SALCL, systemic anaplastic large cell lymphoma.

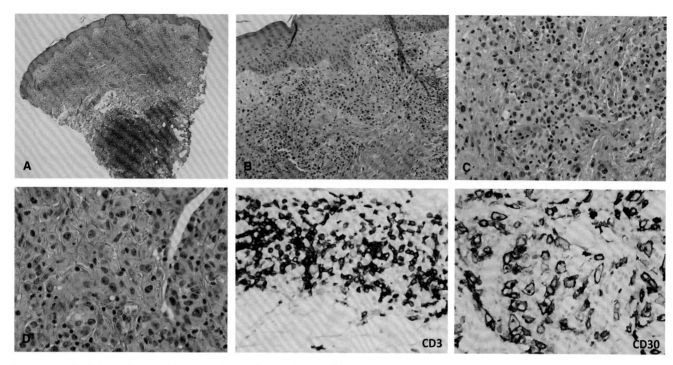

FIGURE 27-16. Lymphomatoid papulosis (LyP), type A. In LyP, there is a wedge-shaped infiltrate with only partial epidermal involvement (A and B). Malignant large and pleomorphic cells are present with a rich acute inflammatory (C and D) background. The lesional cells are positive for CD30 and have significant loss of CD3.

characterized by an epidermotropic infiltrate reminiscent of MF, whereas Type C LyP has features histologically identical to PC-ALCL. Clearly the clinical distinction is more important in a sense than the histologic findings. Cerroni et al showed that a majority of the children represented types A and C, with no examples of type B. In another pediatric series of 250 cases LyP in children, most cases belonged to type A.[88] Type D LyP mimics aggressive epidermotropic CD8+ T-cell lymphoma histologically[94]; this variant expresses other cytotoxic markers such as granzyme and TIA-1. In the latter study, 4 of the 9 patients were less than 25 years of age. Type E LyP is characterized by an angioinvasive and angiodestructive CD8+ cytotoxic T-cell infiltrate with CD30 co-expression; 2 of the 16 original patients were children.[95] Another study of 14 children with LyP revealed that 10 cases had a CD8+ cytotoxic phenotype; most cases were considered either type A or type C. Pierard et al introduced the term follicular LyP (type F) to describe a subtype with a predominant perifollicular pattern of infiltration.[96,97] A few cases of LyP (type F) have been reported in children.[98,99]

The immunophenotype of types A and C is very similar with a uniform population of CD30+ cells, with frequent CD3 and CD4 co-expression. Typically, CD8 and CD56 are negative. CD15 is usually negative but cytotoxic molecules (TIA-1 and granzyme) are positive.[100-102] Types D and E have a CD8+ phenotype. MUM1 is frequently expressed in all cases of LyP (but also in MF and PC-ALCL). Some cases of LyP can also have a *DUSP22* translocation.[89]

Differential Diagnosis

Arthropod bite reactions should be particularly considered in the differential diagnosis. Arthropod bites tend to be more itchy and do not heal with scarring. Those can also have a wedge-shaped pattern histologically of inflammation as seen in type A LyP. As opposed to LyP cases, arthropod bites never have the number of CD30+ cells, or the aberrant loss of T-cell antigens. Pseudolymphomas should also be distinguished from LyP. Although the density of the infiltrate can be similar, the number of CD30+ cells is lower in pseudolymphomas, and they also lack T-cell antigenic loss. PC-ALCL can also be seen in children, and the main distinction appears to be clinical rather than pathologic. PC-ALCL tends to be more solitary, persists for a longer period, and less frequently shows spontaneous resolution. At the molecular level, both can have the *DUSP22* translocation.

CAPSULE SUMMARY

LYMPHOMATOID PAPULOSIS

LyP is a CD30+ T-cell lymphoproliferative disorder characterized by recurrent crops of papular lesions that usually prevail for 3 and 8 weeks and then resolve spontaneously, leaving an atrophic scar. Several histologic variants have now been described in LyP: types A, B, C, D, E, and F. None of the histologic subtypes have any prognostic significance.

The first three types are CD4+, whereas types D and E are CD8+.

ANAPLASTIC LARGE CELL LYMPHOMA, ALK-POSITIVE (ALK+ ALCL)

Definition and Epidemiology

ALK+ ALCL represents approximately 10% to 30% of childhood lymphomas and is more frequent in the first three decades of life. There is a slight male predominance, and the majority of patients (70%) present with stage III or IV disease and B symptoms. The skin is the most frequent extranodal site of involvement (present in 26% of cases). Other extranodal sites include bone, soft tissues, lung, and liver.[103-106] ALK+ ALCL has a good prognosis with a 5-year survival rate of 70% to 80% in contrast to 49% and 32% 5-year survival rates for ALK-negative ALCL and peripheral T-cell lymphoma, not otherwise specified (PTCL, NOS), respectively.[107,108]

Etiology

ALK+ ALCL has rearrangements of the *ALK* gene on 2p23 with various partner genes, most typically the nucleophosmin (*NPM*) on 5q35.[109,110] Some translocations can be cryptic by conventional cytogenetic methods. Other translocation partners include nonmuscle tropomyosin (*TPM3*, 1q25 and *TPM4*, 19p13.1); amino terminus of 5-aminoimidazole-4-carboxamide ribonucleotide formyltransferase/IMP cyclohydrolase gene (*ATIC*, 2q35); TRK-fused gene (*TFG*, 3q21); clathrin heavy polypeptide gene (*CLTC*, 17q23); moesin gene (*MSN*, Xq11-12); myosin heavy chain 9 gene (*MYH9*, 22q11.2); and ALK lymphoma oligomerization partner on chromosome 17 (*ALO17*, 17q25).[105,111]

Clinical Presentation

Most cases of ALK+ ALCL present with lymphadenopathy. The most common extranodal site is the skin (26%).[112-115] Other affected sites include bone, lung, liver, and soft tissues.[105] A leukemic presentation is rare, and more frequent in the small cell variant.[116] The BM is affected in a small percentage (10%-30%) of cases.[117]

The cutaneous manifestation of ALCL, ALK+ can be precipitated by insect bites.[118,119] Lesions resemble typical arthropod bite reactions without clinical resolution. Most patients with ALCL, ALK+, or ALK− have pink papulonodular lesions.[120-122] The lesions are more frequently solitary and rarely multiple. Rare cases of isolated cutaneous ALCL, ALK+ have been reported.[123] Some uncommon clinical appearances include generalized erythroderma,[124] orbital lesions,[125] and ichthyosis.[126]

Histologic Findings

ALK+ ALCL has a variety of morphologic presentations. All cases show a malignant population of large cells with eccentric horseshoe or kidney-shaped nuclei with an eosinophilic region near the nucleus, referred to as "hallmark" cells.

In some variants, the hallmark cells can be small. Occasionally, the malignant cells can mimic Reed-Stenberg cells or their variants. There are five distinctive variants of ALK+ ALCL: common, small cell variant, Hodgkin-like pattern, lymphohistiocytic pattern, and combined forms.[111,123,127-129] Any of these patterns may present in the skin (Figures 27-17 and 27-18). The immunophenotype of ALK+ ALCL includes CD30 and ALK expression; the pattern of CD30 expression is both Golgi and cytoplasmic. Most cases are positive for EMA, TIA-1, granzyme B, and perforin, and show loss of T-cell antigens such as CD3, CD5, and CD7. Some cases can be null for all T-cell markers. CD43, CD2, and CD4 are more frequently positive.

The cellular localization of the ALK expression correlates with the pattern of translocation: the *NPM/ALK* fusion leads to both nuclear and cytoplasmic ALK staining. The ALK staining patterns in less common translocation variants include diffuse cytoplasmic (eg, *TPM3*, *ATIC*, *TFG*, *TPM4*, *MYH9*, *ALO17*), granular cytoplasmic (*CLTC*) (Figure 27-18), or membranous (*MSN*). ALCL, ALK- shows strong and diffuse expression of CD30. The pattern can be membranous, Golgi, and/or cytoplasmic. The strong and diffuse character is often a helpful clue to distinguish ALCL, ALK− from PTCL, NOS. Lack of multiple pan T-cell antigens and the expression of cytotoxic markers are characteristic. EMA and clusterin can be positive, but less frequently than in ALCL, ALK+.[108]

Lamant et al suggested a possible relationship between insect bites and the development of ALK+ ALCL[118]; this series of five patients had recent arthropod bites and developed nodal disease in the area of the skin lesions. Two of the skin biopsies revealed the presence of ALK+ cells. A complete remission was obtained after chemotherapy in all but one patient, who developed progressive disease and died. Oschlies et al[123] described a series of six children, within the context of 487 patients enrolled in the Anaplastic Large Cell Lymphoma-99 trial with disease limited to the skin; these patients had complete remissions on follow-up, and most of them were treated with surgical excision only. In all but one patient, the pattern of ALK staining was nuclear and cytoplasmic, and FISH was positive for the *ALK-NPM* translocation. Clinically, in 1 of 6 patients the lesions were solitary (maculopapules or nodules), and 1 patient had multiple lesions. Previous isolated case reports of cutaneous presentations of ALK+ ALCL have been described.[113,130,131] Despite such reports, most cases of ALK+ ALCL have associated systemic disease and require full staging.

Differential Diagnosis

From the diagnostic perspective, a diagnosis of ALK+ ALCL implies the presence of a systemic lymphoma "until proven otherwise." The rare isolated cutaneous forms are very infrequent. All patients should invariably undergo extensive

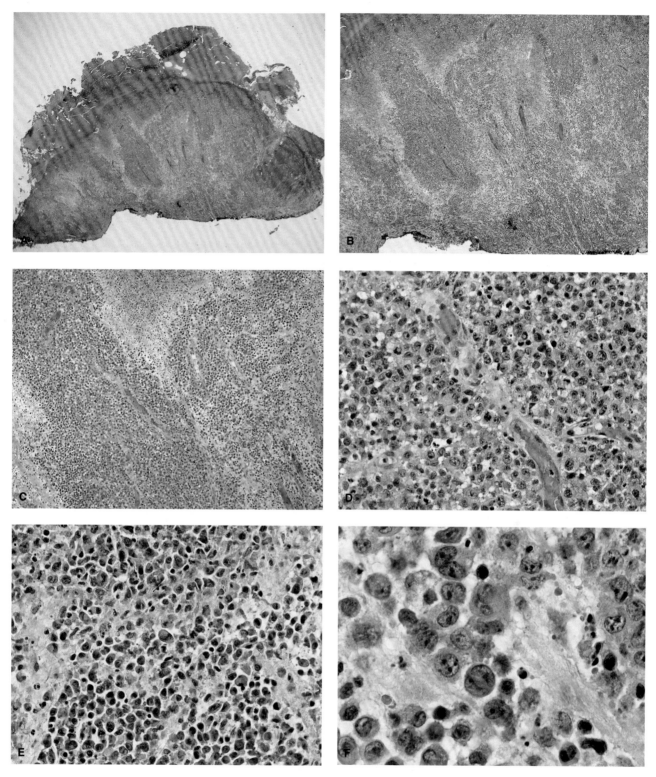

FIGURE 27-17. ALK+ Anaplastic large cell lymphoma with initial skin presentation. A dense malignant infiltrate in the dermis with surface ulceration, but sparing of the epidermis (A and B). The infiltrate shows angiotropism (C and D). It is composed of malignant large cells with frequent hallmark forms (E and F). Adapted and obtained with permission Gru AA, Voorhess PJ. A case of ALK+ anaplastic large cell lymphoma with aberrant myeloperoxidase expression and initial cutaneous presentation. *Am J Dermatopathol.* 2018;40(7):519-522.

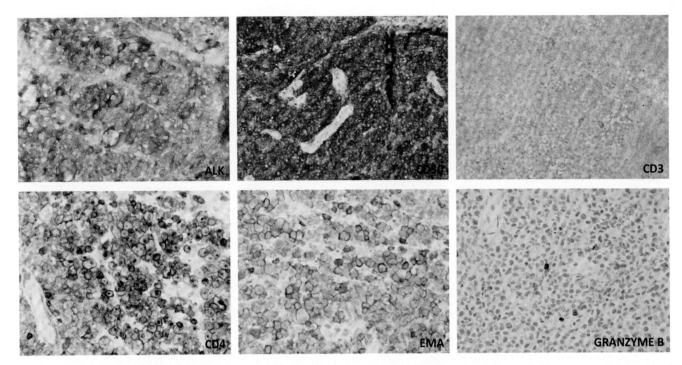

FIGURE 27-18. ALK+ Anaplastic large cell lymphoma with initial skin presentation. The large cells are positive for ALK (cytoplasmic granular staining), CD30, CD4, EMA, and weakly for granzyme B. They are negative for CD3. Adapted and obtained with permission Gru AA, Voorhess PJ. A case of ALK+ anaplastic large cell lymphoma with aberrant myeloperoxidase expression and initial cutaneous presentation. *Am J Dermatopathol.* 2018;40(7):519-522.

staging procedures. The presence of ALK+ distinguishes this process from PC-ALCL. More recently, molecular studies have proved that systemic ALK− ALCL with the presence of *DUSP22* translocations has a clinical outcome similar to cases of ALK+ ALCL. Inflammatory myofibroblastic tumors in children can also be ALK+. As opposed to ALK+ ALCL, such tumors are positive only for histiocytic markers and lack the cellular pleomorphism that is typical of ALCL cases.

CAPSULE SUMMARY

ANAPLASTIC LARGE CELL LYMPHOMA, ALK-POSITIVE

ALK+ ALCL represents approximately 10% to 30% of childhood lymphomas and is more frequent in the first three decades of life. The skin is the most frequent extranodal site of involvement (present in 26% of cases). ALK+ ALCL has a variety of morphologic presentations. All cases show a malignant population of large cells with eccentric horseshoe or kidney-shaped nuclei with an eosinophilic region near the nucleus, referred to as "hallmark" cells. The cellular localization of ALK expression correlates with the pattern of translocation: the *NPM-ALK* fusion leads to both nuclear and cytoplasmic ALK staining.

SUBCUTANEOUS PANNICULITIS-LIKE T-CELL LYMPHOMA

Definition and Epidemiology

Subcutaneous panniculitis-like T-cell lymphoma (SPTCL) is a mature T-cell lymphoma of the skin with TCR αβ expression, subcutaneous involvement, and sparing of the epidermis. It most commonly involves the extremities, occurs in different age groups (including children), and has an indolent clinical behavior.[132] SPTCLs with expression of γδ TCR have distinct clinicopathologic features and are currently classified under γδ T-cell lymphomas.[133] It is more common in women and has a predilection for younger individuals. The median age at presentation is 36 years (range 1-79). Approximately 50% of cases occurred in individuals 21-40 years old, and 19% of cases are 20-year-old or younger patients.[134] Numerous cases have been reported in children.[134-139] A subsequent study of cutaneous lymphomas in children noted that SPTCL was rare, with only 3.4% of patients in this age group.[71]

Etiology

The etiology of SPTCL remains unknown. Nearly 19% of patients with SPTCL have associated autoimmune disorders, including systemic lupus erythematosus, juvenile rheumatoid arthritis, Sjögren disease, type 1 diabetes mellitus, idiopathic thrombocytopenia, multiple sclerosis,

Raynaud disease, and Kikuchi disease.[134] Yi et al[140] showed a series of 11 cases of SPTCL initially diagnosed as autoimmune disorders; the authors divided the original diagnoses into three separate groups: (1) a group with a preceding diagnosis of erythema nodosum, pyoderma gangrenosum, lupus profundus; (2) vasculitis; (3) inflammatory myopathy-like lesions. The authors speculated that patients with inflammatory myositis and/or Behcet's represented paraneoplastic manifestations of SPTCL. Some of these patients (2/11) had elevation of antinuclear antibodies (ANA) in the serum, anti-DS DNA antibody, and one patient had an elevated antineutrophil cytoplasmic antibody. A study from the Mayo Clinic on a series of 23 patients revealed preceding diagnoses of autoimmune disorders in approximately 57% of patients, including lupus panniculitis, erythema nodosum, venous stasis, Weber-Christian disease, cellulitis, and granulomatous panniculitis of unknown etiology. The association between SPTCL and lupus erythematosus profundus (LEP) has led to the hypothesis that perhaps the two entities represent two ends of the same spectrum.[141,142] Some cases of lobular panniculitis with a CD8[+] phenotype can occur in children in association with clonal populations of T cells in the setting of congenital immune deficiency syndromes. Rare cases in association with HIV[143] and sarcoidosis have also been documented.[144] The association between certain medications and development of SPTCL has been described in patients receiving anti-TNFα therapy (etanercept),[145] and following rituximab and cyclophosphamide.[146] More unusual presentations have been reported in patients with Down syndrome,[147] cervical cancer,[148] during pregnancy,[149] and neurofibromatosis type 1.[150]

Clinical Presentation

The typical lesions consist of nodules/tumors or skin plaques, which can vary in diameter from 1 to 20 cm or more and are frequently multifocal (78%). Sometimes the nodules leave areas of lipoatrophy after resolution. Ulceration is rare (6%). The lesions present in the extremities (legs, arms) and, less frequently, on the trunk and face. Facial lesions can present with extraocular muscle palsy.[151] Rare cases in the breast have been reported.[152,153] The skin lesions often simulate other causes of panniculitis, such as EN[154] and lupus panniculitis. Other rare clinical presentations might simulate dermatomyositis,[155-156] morphea,[157] cellulitis,[158] facial edema,[159] venous stasis-like ulceration,[160] lipomembranous panniculitis,[161] eschar-like crusting,[162] erythromelalgia,[163] and alopecia.[164] The delay from the onset of symptoms to the diagnosis of SPTCL can range from 3 weeks to 10 years.[165] Systemic symptoms occur in 40% to 50% of cases, including fever, chills, night sweats, and weight loss. Cytopenias and alterations in liver enzymes often occur. Hemophagocytosis (HPS) is seen in 17% of cases[134] and is associated with high mortality (46% at 5 years). HPS is more prevalent in subcutaneous panniculitic T-cell lymphomas with γδ phenotype (45%).[166,167]

Less common clinical manifestations include lymphadenopathy, hepatosplenomegaly, pleural effusions, and BM involvement.[168,169] Systemic workup for involvement by SPTCL is usually negative for extracutaneous disease.[170,171] Transmission of the disease has been documented after allogeneic BM transplantation[145] and cardiac transplantation.[172] Some cases show spontaneous resolution.[136,173,174]

The prognosis of SPTCL in general is excellent. Approximately 60% of patients achieve complete remission, and about 12% die of the disease. Most deaths are due to hemophagocytic syndrome, which usually develops late in the disease course.[134] The 5-year overall survival is >80%.[166] The development of HPS is associated with a survival of approximately 46% at 5 years.[134,166] The largest series of SPTCL in the pediatric age group revealed a slightly higher rate of recurrences (>50%) but overall low mortality.[135] A fatal case with overlap features of lupus and HPS had been reported.[175]

Histologic Findings

A dense, nodular, interstitial, or combined lymphoid infiltrate showing adipotropism with a predilection for the subcutaneous lobule mimicking a lobular panniculitis is seen in virtually all patients (Figure 27-19).[4,71,135,136,147,176-187] Septal involvement is typically mild or absent. Extension of the infiltrate into the reticular dermis, surrounding and occasionally infiltrating sweat glands, hair follicles, and sebaceous glands can be seen.[188] Infiltration of the superficial epidermis and/or dermis is exceedingly rare and, if present, should raise the diagnostic consideration of MF with a secondary panniculitic presentation or γδ T-cell lymphoma. Rimming of neoplastic cells around adipocytes is characteristic but not pathognomonic. This pattern can also be seen in lupus panniculitis and in association with other lymphoproliferative disorders such as tumor stage MF, aggressive epidermotropic CD8[+] T-cell lymphoma, extranodal NK/T-cell lymphoma (ENKTL), γδ T-cell lymphoma, blastic plasmacytoid dendritic cell neoplasm (BPDCN), secondary DLBCL, and leukemia cutis (LC).[189] Intravascular thrombi adjacent to tissue necrosis are not uncommon, whereas angiotropism and angiodestruction are exceedingly rare. Necrosis and karyorrhexis along with nonneoplastic inflammatory infiltrates (histiocytes, small lymphocytes, and neutrophils) are often prominent and may mask the underlying neoplastic process. In such scenarios, the presence of ghost cells (necrotic malignant lymphocytes) could be useful in identifying the atypical population. Later stages might show collections of epithelioid histiocytes, granulomas, or lipomembranous changes.[161] Eosinophils and plasma cells are uncommon; however, the presence of plasma cells should raise the differential diagnosis of LEP or LEP/SPTCL overlap.[141,190-197] In cases where the presence of intralobular histiocytes with phagocytosed red blood cells or apoptotic elements are present, workup for hemophagocytic syndrome is warranted.[198] Similar to the skin findings, BM infiltration by SPTCL also shows adipocyte rimming.[168]

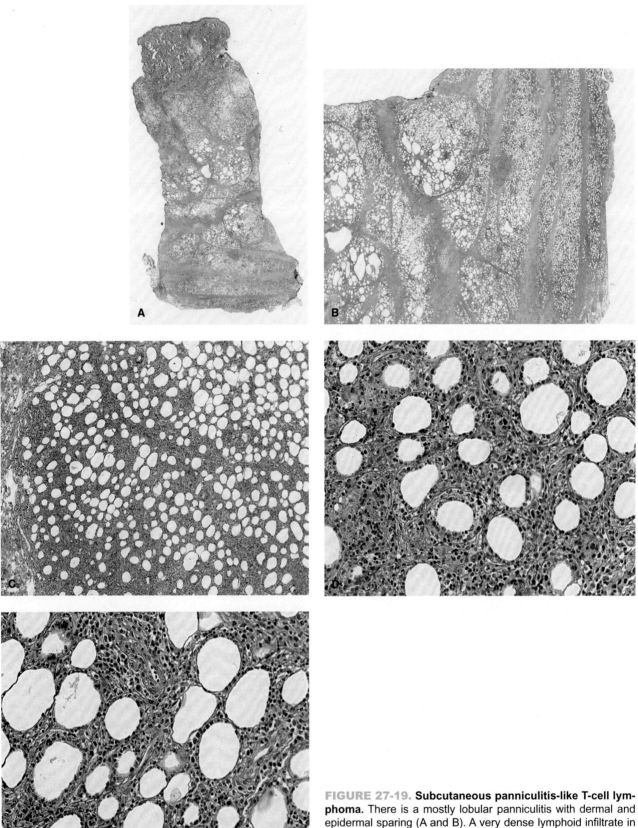

FIGURE 27-19. Subcutaneous panniculitis-like T-cell lymphoma. There is a mostly lobular panniculitis with dermal and epidermal sparing (A and B). A very dense lymphoid infiltrate in the subcutaneous lobule is seen (C). The atypical lymphocyte population shows prominent adipocyte "rimming" (D and E). Digital slides courtesy of Path Presenter.com.

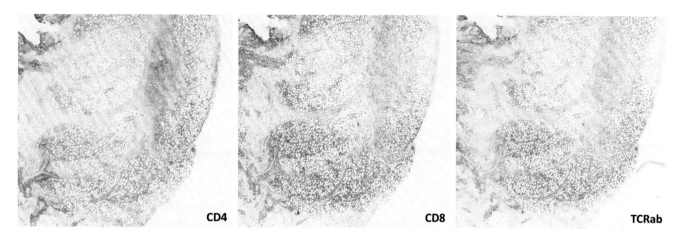

FIGURE 27-20. Subcutaneous panniculitis-like T-cell lymphoma—immunohistochemistry. The malignant infiltrate is positive for CD3 (not shown), CD8, and TCRαβ, whereas it is negative for CD4. Reprinted with permission from Gru AA, Schaffer A. *Hematopathology of the skin: A clinical and pathologic approach.* 1st ed. Philadelphia, PA: Wolters Kluwer; 2017.

The immunophenotype reveals CD3⁺, BF1⁺, CD8⁺, and cytotoxic molecules, such as TIA-1, perforin, and granzyme B. CD56 and CD30 are typically negative. Ki67 is moderately high (>50%)[199] (Figure 27-20). Loss of CD2, CD5, and/or CD7 is seen in 10%, 50%, and 44% of cases, respectively.[134] CD45RO is usually positive and CD45RA is negative. EBV has been rarely documented in patients of Asian descent.[200-204]

Differential Diagnosis

An important differential diagnosis of SPTCL is lupus panniculitis, which can present in children (Figures 27-21 and 27-22).[197] In contrast to SPTCL, lupus panniculitis presents with subcutaneous fibrosis, frequent clusters of plasmacytoid dendritic cells (CD123⁺), reactive germinal centers, and absence of the phenotype of SPTCL. Liau et al showed

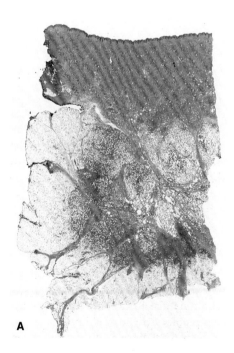

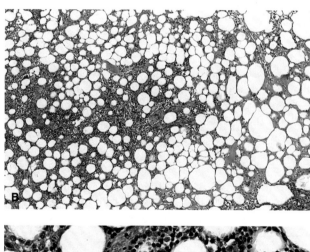

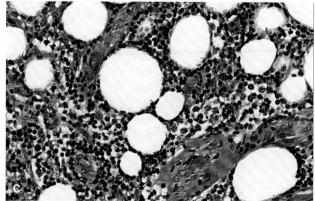

FIGURE 27-21. Lupus panniculitis. A lobular panniculitis is seen with focal lymphoid follicles (A). Areas of fibrosis are present (B). Similar to SPTCL, adipocyte rimming and cytologic atypia is evident (C). Reprinted with permission from Gru AA, Schaffer A. *Hematopathology of the skin: A clinical and pathologic approach.* 1st ed. Philadelphia, PA: Wolters Kluwer; 2017..

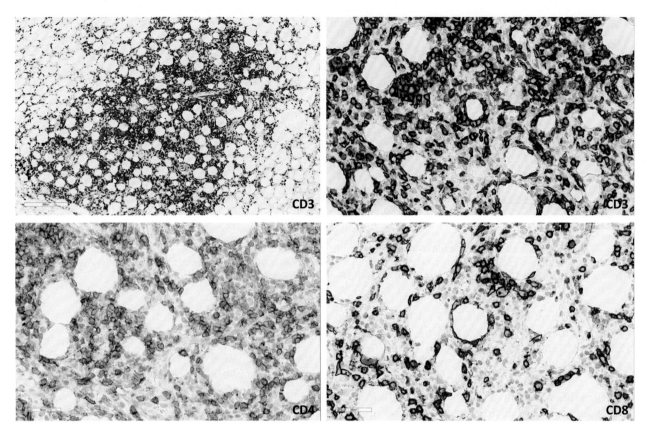

FIGURE 27-22. Lupus panniculitis—immunohistochemistry. The infiltrate is positive for CD3 and CD4, but negative for CD8. Reprinted with permission from Gru AA, Schaffer A. *Hematopathology of the skin: A clinical and pathologic approach.* 1st ed. Philadelphia, PA: Wolters Kluwer; 2017.

that the most useful criteria to distinguish LP from SPTCL include the cytologic atypia of the lymphoid cells (low in the former), presence of dermal mucin, and follicles of B cells with the formation of germinal centers. Those three features are more typical of LP and not seen in cases of SPTCL. In addition, their study showed that clusters of plasmacytoid dendritic cells (intrinsically linked to the pathogenesis of LE), as detected by CD123 immunostain, are typically seen in LP but not, or only minimally present, in SPTCL.[194] Ki67-increased proliferation is also more typical of SPTCL.[205] Pincus et al[142] have shown a series of five biopsies of patients who meet the criteria for LE and SPTCL. They proposed that some cases show histologic overlap. Those biopsies revealed the presence of dermal mucin, admixed atypical lymphocytes, interface changes, and rimming of adipocytes. Clusters of CD123+ cells were seen in the biopsies within the areas of lupus. Ki67 was elevated in all cases, and one of the cases also had a positive direct immunofluorescent study. T-cell gene rearrangement studies revealed clonal T-cell populations in all cases.

Another "reactive" panniculitis with overlap features with SPTCL and in some cases with coexistence between the two represent the so-called cytophagic histiocytic panniculitis,

a disease typically seen in children.[177,178,184,206-209] The original series of five cases[210] described patients originally believed to have Weber-Christian disease, with a chronic, intermittent course and HPS.[211] The clinical manifestations included fever, hepatosplenomegaly, ulcers, and serosal effusions. Pancytopenia, liver failure, and intravascular coagulation developed in all cases. Erythrophagocytosis or cytophagocytosis of nonerythroid cells can be seen in different organs. Marzano et al presented a series of seven cases of cytophagic panniculitis, of which four patients had SPCTL (although two of them will be categorized as γδ T-cell lymphoma by current criteria). Five of the seven patients died as a consequence of HPS. However, two of the cases had a more indolent course over several years. Although most authors will regard cytophagic panniculitis as a possible subtype of lymphoma, cases without overt clonality and aggressive course are seen, and the term should be perhaps preserved in some of these cases.[212] Cytophagic panniculitis can be associated with systemic macrophage activation syndrome and occurs isolated and in association with viral infections, connective tissue disorders, as well as malignancies.[178] Some cases occur in association with mutations of the perforin gene.[206]

SUBCUTANEOUS PANNICULITIS-LIKE T-CELL LYMPHOMA

SPTCL is a mature T-cell lymphoma of the skin with TCR αβ expression, subcutaneous involvement, and sparing of the epidermis. It most commonly involves the extremities, occurs in different age groups (including children), and has an indolent clinical behavior. The typical lesions consist of nodules/tumors or skin plaques, which can vary in diameter from 1 to 20 cm or more and are frequently multifocal. Nearly 19% of cases of SPTCL have associated autoimmune disorders. A dense, nodular, interstitial, or combined lymphoid infiltrate showing adipotropism with a predilection for the subcutaneous lobule mimicking a lobular panniculitis is seen in virtually all cases. The immunophenotype reveals CD3+, BF1+, CD8+, and cytotoxic molecules, such as TIA-1, perforin, and granzyme B.

SMALL- TO MEDIUM-SIZED CD4+ T-CELL LYMPHOPROLIFERATIVE DISORDER

Small- to medium-sized CD4+ T-cell LPD (SMPTCL) is exceedingly rare (incidence <1 per million) but has been detected in children in a minority of cases.[213] This lymphoproliferative disorder remains in a provisional category in the World Health Organization (WHO) classification.[214] The terminology in the revised classification has been modified from "lymphoma" to "LPD" to reflect this uncertain malignant potential, designating these cases as primary cutaneous CD4+ small/medium T-cell LPD. The clinical behavior is almost always indolent, with most patients presenting with localized disease. Systemic disease is rare, and conservative local management is sufficient in most patients. This may represent a limited clonal response to an unknown stimulus, not fulfilling criteria for malignancy.[23,215,216]

All cases presenting to date in children have a solitary lesion, usually a papule, nodule, or plaque in the head and neck region. The infiltrate consists of a nodular, diffuse, and interstitial infiltrate of lymphoid cells with sparing of the epidermis (Figure 27-23). There is expression of CD4, but a rich background of B cells is also encountered with the expression of germinal center markers (BCL-6, CD10, PD1, ICOS).[128,217,218] CD30 is usually negative (Figure 27-24).

AGGRESSIVE CD8-POSITIVE EPIDERMOTROPIC T-CELL LYMPHOMA (BERTI LYMPHOMA)

The original series of primary cutaneous epidermotropic CD8+ T-cell lymphoma had a single case in a child.[219] Kikuchi et al[220] subsequently described a second case in a 6-year-old girl with disseminated lesions. A multicenter study of 30 cases included 2 cases in individuals younger than 25 years. The median survival is approximately 12 months.[221] Papulonecrotic lesions in the extremities are usually present. Morphologically, these lesions typically reveal an acanthotic epidermis with prominent epidermotropism and keratinocytic necrosis. The immunophenotype includes TCRβ, TIA-1, and CD8 expression.

PRIMARY CUTANEOUS γδ T-CELL LYMPHOMA

This extraordinary rare disorder has been reported in children, but it is basically an adult condition.[4,208,222-226] Merrill et al reported the occurrence of cutaneous γδ T-cell

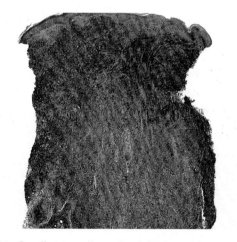
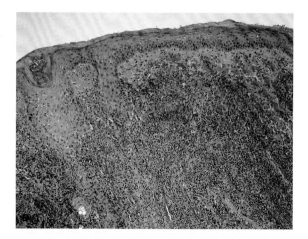

FIGURE 27-23. Small- to medium-sized CD4-positive T-cell lymphoproliferative disorder. There is a dense and vaguely nodule dermal infiltrate with sparing of the epidermis and extending very deep into the bottom of the biopsy (A and B).

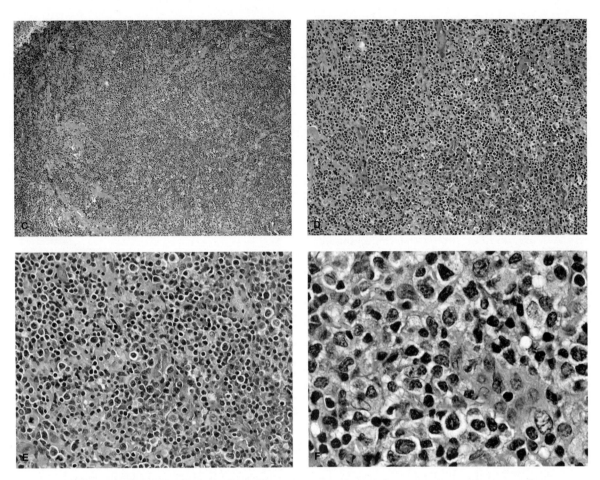

FIGURE 27-23. (*continued*) The infiltrate shows a monotonous appearance (C). Scattered larger cells are seen (D). The infiltrate is composed of a mixture of small, medium, and large pleomorphic cells (E and F). Adapted and obtained with permission Gru A, Dehner LP. Cutaneous hematolymphoid and histiocytic proliferations in children. *Pediatr Dev Pathol.* 2018;21(2):150-207.

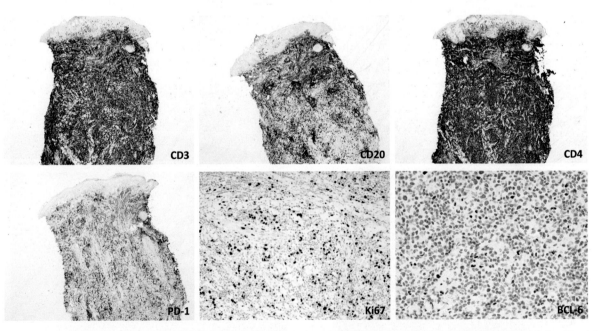

FIGURE 27-24. **Small- to medium-sized CD4-positive T-cell lymphoproliferative disorder—immunohistochemistry.** The infiltrate is diffusely positive for CD3 and CD4. CD20 shows a background very rich in B cells. PD-1 and BCL-6 are positive in a significant proportion of T cells, indicating a T$_{FH}$ phenotype. Ki67 is overall low (10%). Adapted and obtained with permission Gru A, Dehner LP. Cutaneous hematolymphoid and histiocytic proliferations in children. *Pediatr Dev Pathol.* 2018;21(2):150-207.

lymphoma (CGDTCL) in three individuals before the age of 25, including a 1-year-old child.[227] The lesions are usually found on the extremities and trunk. The malignant infiltrate is accompanied by epidermal necrosis with frequent

involvement of the subcutis. Vasculitis and ulceration can be seen, and HPS is also present. The most common immunophenotype includes CD3[+], CD4[−], CD8[−], and CD56[+/−] (Figure 27-25). The identifying feature is the presence of

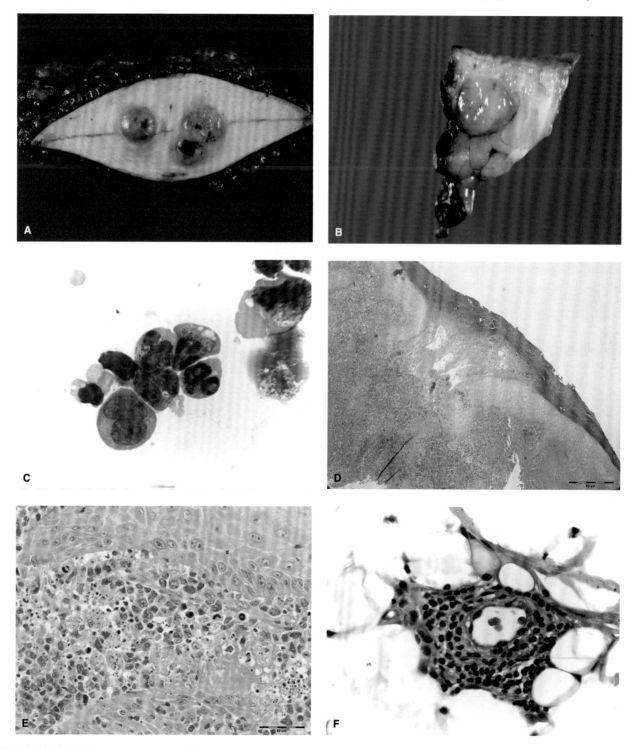

FIGURE 27-25. **Primary cutaneous γδ T-cell lymphoma.** A and B, Gross specimen from excisional biopsy. There is a dermal nodule with surface ulceration. C, Touch imprint—1000×. The malignant cells are medium to large, with pleomorphic nuclei with abnormal lobation, and numerous cytoplasmic granules. D, Low magnification—40×. The tumor is ulcerated. E and F, high magnification—400×. The infiltrate is close to the epidermis and composed of very pleomorphic cells. Focal necrosis is noted. The lymphoid infiltrate shows prominent angiotropism. Reprinted with permission from Gru AA, Schaffer A. *Hematopathology of the skin: A clinical and pathologic approach.* 1st ed. Philadelphia, PA: Wolters Kluwer; 2017.

TCRγ expression. An important differential diagnostic consideration is LyP as some cases in children can have TCRγ expression. The distinction between LyP and CGDTCL is an important one because the former is an indolent disease and the latter requires systemic chemotherapy and BM transplant. The previously reported cases of SPTCL with a γδ phenotype have now been reclassified as CGDTCL.[167]

SYSTEMIC CHRONIC ACTIVE EBV INFECTION OF T-CELL OR NK-CELL TYPE (CAEBV)

Definition and Epidemiology

This rare systemic EBV+ polyclonal, oligoclonal, or monoclonal T-cell or NK-cell lymphoproliferative disorder manifests with variable clinical severity. It was originally defined as a severe illness with a duration of more than 6 months, after a primary EBV infection with continued high titers to EBV, and evidence of major organ involvement (pneumonia, BM aplasia, uveitis, lymphadenitis, hepatitis, splenomegaly). EBV by in situ hybridization (EBER) expression has been used to document EBV in the infected tissues.[228] The updated criteria also allow for the diagnosis in the presence of symptoms that last for longer than 3 months and have high levels of EBV viremia.[23,229,230] Although the affected cells are typically T or NK cells, rare cases of B-cell derivation can occur.[231]

The disease has a strong predilection for individuals of Asian or South American descent and most notably occurs in children and adolescents.[232-235] Less frequently, chronic active EBV (CAEBV) can occur in middle age or older adults with prolonged fevers, hepatosplenomegaly, anemia, thrombocytopenia, lymphadenopathy, and cutaneous manifestations. The latter are typically in the form of mosquito bite allergy (33%), rash (26%), and hydroa vacciniforme (HV)–like manifestations. Most patients have high antibody titers (EBV VCA IgG, EBNA) as well as high EBV viremia.[229,231,234-236]

Clinical and Histologic Findings

The cutaneous findings will be discussed with the HV-like and mosquito bite allergic disorders. In other sites, such as the lymph nodes, CAEBV is characterized by paracortical hyperplasia, a polymorphous infiltrate, and a rich background of inflammatory cells that include plasma cells and granulomas at times. Some cases are accompanied by associated hemophagocytic lymphohistiocytosis (HLH), best demonstrated in BM, lymph node, and liver biopsies.[234,237] Numerous EBV+ cells are seen. When monotonous sheets of EBV+ tumor cells are noted, such cases are best classified as systemic EBV+ T-cell lymphoma of childhood (ENKTL) or aggressive NK-cell leukemia (ANKL).[238]

The prognosis of CAEBV is variable, with some patients experiencing a relatively indolent clinical course, whereas others succumb to the disease, especially in the presence of HLH. The median survival is approximately 70 to 78 months,

and adverse markers of clinical outcome include late onset (>8 years of age), thrombocytopenia, and T-cell infection (5-year survival is approximately 60% for T-cell disease and 87% for NK-cell disease).[229,231,237] T-cell clonality is sometimes associated with a more aggressive clinical course.[234]

> ### CAPSULE SUMMARY
>
> ### SYSTEMIC CHRONIC ACTIVE EBV INFECTION OF T-CELL OR NK-CELL TYPE
>
> CAEBV is defined as a severe illness with a duration of more than 3 months, after a primary EBV infection with continued high titers to EBV, and evidence of major organ involvement (pneumonia, BM aplasia, uveitis, lymphadenitis, hepatitis, splenomegaly).

SEVERE MOSQUITO BITE ALLERGY

The cutaneous manifestations of chronic active EBV infection may be precipitated by mosquito bites or vaccination.[239,240] Severe mosquito bite allergy (SMBA) is very uncommon, and most cases occur in individuals from Asia and Mexico.[241-249] This disorder is not a hypersensitive reaction in the classic sense, but is rather a cutaneous manifestation of CAEBV of NK-cell lineage, with oligoclonal or monoclonal populations of NK cells.[250]

Most patients are less than 20 years old, with a median age of 6.7.[250] Erythematous papules, macules, and plaques can subsequently evolve into bullae with ulceration and eventual scarring. Systemic symptoms are also common and include fever, lymphadenopathy, and liver dysfunction.[251,252] Recovery occurs when the systemic symptoms resolve until the next mosquito bite. Vaccinations can also sometimes elicit a similar reaction.[253] High levels of immunoglobulin-E (IgE), high EBV viremia, and NK-cell lymphocytosis (80%) are present in SMBA.[239] The skin shows epidermal necrosis with ulceration. Marked dermal edema and infiltration by neutrophils and a dense lymphoid infiltrate are noted. Vasculitis is present in the center with karyorrhectic debris and extravasated red blood cells in the dermis. The lymphoid infiltrate is composed of a mixture of CD4+, CD8+ T cells, and NK cells. EBV-positive cells represent a minority of the infiltrate (<10%).

The prognosis is variable: some patients have an indolent course with chronic protracted cutaneous manifestations, whereas others may develop fulminant HLH or progress to lymphoma, such as ANKL.[253]

HYDROA VACCINIFORME-LIKE LYMPHOPROLIFERATIVE DISEASE

Definition and Epidemiology

This chronic EBV+ LPD of childhood has a risk of progression to a systemic lymphoma.[230] Classic HV is a rare, intermittent ultraviolet light-induced vesiculopapular and scarring eruption that typically remits after adolescence.[254-256] Systemic symptoms are not usually present in HV. The estimated prevalence of HV is approximately 0.34 cases/100 000.[254] In some cases, the lesions can occur in sun-unexposed areas. Later studies have shown an association between HV and clonal proliferations of T cells; the term HV-like lymphoma (HVLL) was introduced in the WHO classification in 2008.[257] However, because of the inability to predict which patients will have an indolent course and which ones will develop overt lymphoma, the term hydroa vacciniforme-like lymphoproliferative disease (HV-LPD) has been proposed and was introduced in the new edition of the WHO monograph.[23] Other terms that have applied to describe HVLL in the past included edematous scarring vasculitic panniculitis, angiocentric cutaneous T-cell lymphoma of childhood, hydroa-like cutaneous T-cell lymphoma, and severe HV.

Most cases of HV-LPD are seen in children and adolescents from Asia, Native Americans from Central and South America (Peru, Guatemala, and Bolivia), and Mexico, and rarely occurs in adults.[255,258-266] In the Peruvian studies, approximately 50% of cases are found in the southern region of the country, correlating with a higher prevalence of early EBV infection in that area. The median age at diagnosis is 8 years. The male-to-female ratio is 2.3:1. Males with HV may have a later onset and longer duration than females. Although the disease presents in children, some patients can have persistent symptoms into adulthood.

Etiology

It has been proposed that certain populations (eg, Asian and South American) are at risk for development of lymphoma, whereas in others (North American and European), the disease has an indolent course.[254,264] Recent clinical studies suggest that HV-LPD can be successfully treated with immunomodulators (thalidomide,[267] antivirals,[268] interferon,[269] etc) rather than systemic chemotherapy, because the latter has been associated with a higher mortality among these patients.[258]

Clinical Presentation

Classical HV is characterized by a sporadic, itchy erythematous eruption in sun-exposed areas that occurs shortly (minutes to hours) after sun exposure. The eruption progresses through different stages: papules, vesicles, crusts, and, eventually, vacciniform (pox-like) scars after several weeks (Figure 27-26). Severe forms of the disease can have conjunctival and corneal ulceration and scarring. Marked facial edema is common in the more aggressive forms, associated with unilateral or bilateral eyelid compromise. Periorbital swelling can be the first manifestation of the disease.[254,255,260] The lesions can become chronic (lasting months to years) and are prone to recurrence, often characterized by temporal heterogeneity, from papules with crusts to well-formed scars in the same area.[254] When extracutaneous involvement occurs (hepatosplenomegaly, lymphadenopathy, BM infiltration), those cases are best classified as ENKTL. Fever, weight loss, and asthenia can be present.

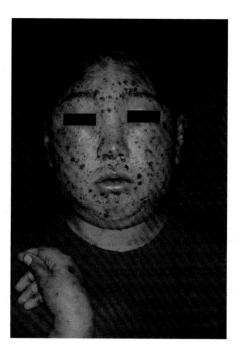
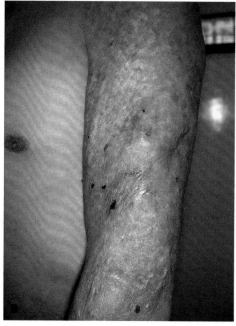

FIGURE 27-26. Hydroa vacciniforme-like lymphoproliferative disorder. Facial edema with erythematous and ulcerative crusty lesions in a child of 11 years (A). In this patient various types of injury are observed with predominantly severe scarring (B). Reprinted with permission Gru AA, Schaffer A. *Hematopathology of the Skin: A Clinical and Pathologic Approach.* Philadelphia, PA: Wolters Kluwer; 2016.

Elevations of lactate dehydrogenase (LDH) and liver enzymes are noted in one-third of patients.[258,270,271]

Histologic Findings

In HV-LPD, the lymphoid infiltrate is composed of small- to medium-sized hyperchromatic cells centered in the dermis with a perivascular/periadnexal distribution, and with associated epidermal necrosis (Figure 27-27). Spongiosis and intraepidermal vesicles are also seen. In the more aggressive forms of the disease, the cells can show significant atypia, and somewhat similar morphology to ENKTL. Mitotic figures are infrequent. Epidermotropism without Pautrier microabscesses is a common feature. Fully developed lesions are deeply infiltrative into the adipose tissue, but without significant rimming of the adipocytes as seen in SPTCL. Angiotropism with or without angionecrosis and fibrinoid changes can be seen.[258,261,263-265]

The EBV-infected cells are cytotoxic T cells (CD3+, CD8+, TIA-1+, granzyme B+, perforin+) or NK cells (CD56+).[258,261,264,265] A minority of cases can be CD4+ or CD4−/CD8−.[272-274] CD30 is occasionally positive, but LMP-1 is negative. The number of EBV+ cells is variable (Figure 27-28). The Ki-67 index is variable and is very low in some cases or as high as 50% in others. Expression of CD5, CD7, CD43, and CD25 is variable. CD57 is negative. The T cells can be positive for either TCRαβ or TCRγδ. Clonal rearrangements of the TCR can be demonstrated. Deletion of the long arm of chromosome 6 has been documented.[275]

Differential Diagnosis

The differential diagnosis includes other NK/T-cell LPD, such as ANKL and ENKTL. In the latter entities, diffuse sheets of atypical CD56+, EBER+ cells are noted. Some cases of ANKL can also show skin involvement.[276] SPTCL can have overlap in the immunophenotype, being composed of CD8+ cells. However, SPTCL is negative for CD56, lacks epidermotropism and EBV expression. Primary cutaneous γδT-cell lymphoma (PCGDL) can also be CD56+, but is more typically negative for EBV, presents in older adults, and the location is more typically truncal and in the extremities.

CAPSULE SUMMARY

HYDROA VACCINIFORME-LIKE LYMPHOPROLIFERATIVE DISEASE

Classic HV is a rare, intermittent ultraviolet light-induced vesiculopapular and scarring eruption that typically remits after adolescence. Because of the inability to predict which patients will have an indolent course and which ones will develop overt lymphoma, the term HV-LPD has been proposed and was introduced in the new edition of the WHO monograph. In HV-LPD, the lymphoid infiltrate is composed of small- to medium-sized hyperchromatic cells centered in the dermis with a perivascular/periadnexal distribution, and with associated epidermal necrosis. Spongiosis and intraepidermal vesicles are also seen.

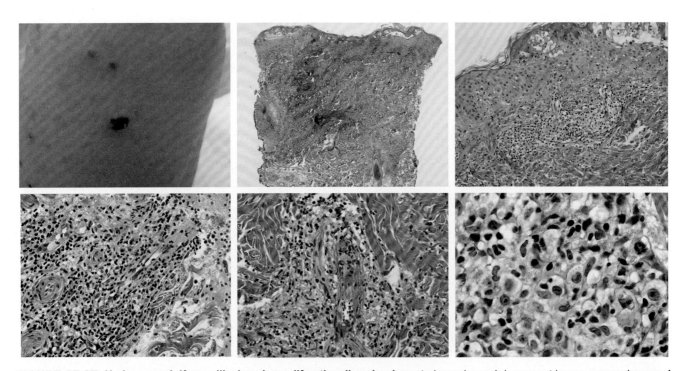

FIGURE 27-27. Hydroa vacciniforme-like lymphoproliferative disorder. A crusted papular rash is present in sun-exposed areas. A large area of epidermal necrosis is noted. There is a superficial and deep, angiotropic and perifollicular infiltrate. The infiltrate is composed of medium- to large-sized cells. Angionecrosis is proven by the presence of fibrinoid changes in the vessel walls. Obtained with permission Gru A, Dehner LP. Cutaneous hematolymphoid and histiocytic proliferations in children. *Pediatr Dev Pathol.* 2018;21(2):150-207.

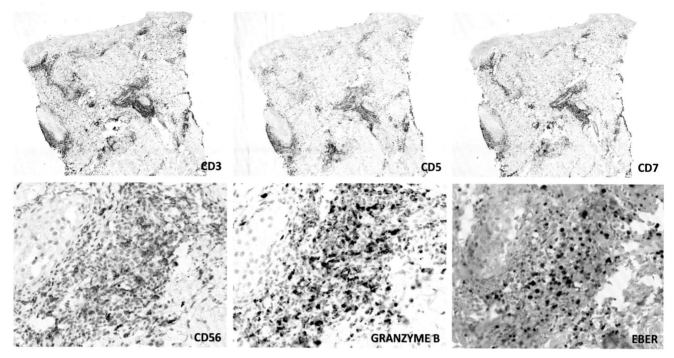

FIGURE 27-28. Hydroa vacciniforme-like lymphoproliferative disorder—immunohistochemistry. The infiltrate is positive for CD3 but shows aberrant loss of CD5. CD7 appears to be retained. Many CD56+ cells are seen. HV-LPD shows a cytotoxic phenotype that is best proved by a granzyme B immunostain. EBER is positive in the lesional cells.

EXTRANODAL NK/T-CELL LYMPHOMA

Definition and Epidemiology

ENKTL, nasal type, is a mature NHL derived by NK cells (more frequently) and sometimes T cells with extranodal (frequently upper aerodigestive) infiltration by EBV-infected cytotoxic lymphocytes with angioinvasion and necrosis.[230] In the United States, ENKTL is very rare, accounting for fewer than 1% of NHL. The disease is more prevalent in areas of Mexico, South and Central America, and Asia, where it represents nearly 6% of all NHL, and in certain areas, up to 22% to 44% of all NHL.[277,278] Overall, approximately 150 cases of ENKTL have been reported in children.[139,279,280] The median age of presentation is 13, with a male-to-female ratio of 3.25:1.

Etiology

ENKTL shows a strong association with EBV infection, irrespective of the patient's origin, which supports a direct pathogenic role of the virus in lymphomagenesis.

Clinical Presentation

The disease presents in extranodal sites, most often in the upper aerodigestive tract (70%), including the nasal cavity (by far the most frequent site), orbital soft tissue, paranasal sinuses, and palate. Some cases can present in extra nasal cavity sites, but lymph node involvement is uncommon. Most often, there are signs of local tumor infiltration: ulceration, perforation of the nasal septum (in the past, many of these cases were called midline lethal granuloma[281]), and

epistaxis are frequently seen.[230] B symptoms, such as fever, weight loss, malaise, and night sweats are also common (65% of pediatric cases) and are the second most common clinical presentation of ENKTL in children. ENKTL can also be associated with HPS, which worsens the prognosis.[282] Dissemination to the skin, gastrointestinal tract, testes, or cervical lymph nodes can also be present, whereas BM involvement is relatively uncommon. Skin involvement is present in 10% of cases of ENKTL and manifests as nodules that ulcerate and often have a necrotic center, erythematous maculopapules, cellulitis, and abscess-like swelling (Figure 27-29).

The survival rate is 30% to 40%,[283,284] but in recent years has improved with more intensive therapy including upfront radiotherapy and the steroid (dexamethasone), methotrexate, ifosfamide, L-asparaginase, and etoposide (SMILE) regimen.[285] Unfavorable prognostic factors include advanced stage (III or IV), BM or skin involvement, and high levels of EBV DNA in the serum.[283,286] Cases with extranasal presentations have a more aggressive clinical behavior, compared with the nasal ones,[287] and those with primary skin disease (and without systemic dissemination) appear to have a better prognosis.[283,284,286] Higher EBV viral load correlates with a worse outcome and disease activity.[288,289]

Histologic Findings

ENKTL has an angiocentric and angiodestructive growth pattern with coagulative necrosis, admixed apoptotic bodies, and fibrinoid change in blood vessels, even in the absence of angioinvasion (Figure 27-30).[290,291] Pseudoepitheliomatous

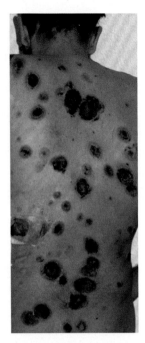

FIGURE 27-29. Extranodal NK/T-cell lymphoma. Such tumors frequently have an aggressive clinical course with numerous necrotic plaques.

changes are present in some cases. The tumor cells can exhibit a marked range in cell size. The nuclei are round or folded, have coarse or vesicular chromatin, and small inconspicuous nucleoli. Mitotic figures are frequently seen, in addition to apoptosis and karyorrhectic debris. Cytoplasmic granules are seen in some cases. Areas of geographic

necrosis can also be present. Background inflammatory cells are variable and include plasma cells, histiocytes, and neutrophils. In the skin, focal epidermotropism is seen on occasion. When the adipose tissue is affected, necrosis and rimming of the adipocytes by the malignant cells is noted, which can mimic the findings present in primary cutaneous γδ T-cell lymphoma and SPTCL. Permeation of the tumor cells into the skeletal muscle with associated myonecrosis can also be present.[230,276]

ENKTL originates from T or NK cells with a cytotoxic phenotype and[292-295] expression of cytotoxic granules (granzyme B, TIA-1, and perforin); however, most cases are derived from NK cells and are CD56+ and CD56− for surface CD3 expression yet positive for cytoplasmic CD3 subunits, including CD3ε and CD3ζ. As such, ENKTL is positive for CD3 when polyclonal anti-CD3 antibodies are applied. Most cases are positive for CD2, CD43, CD45RO, HLA-DR, CD25, CD7, and FAS (CD95), and negative for CD4, CD5, CD8, TCRγ, βF1, CD16, and CD57.[296,297] CD30 is positive in 20% to 40% of cases, particularly in cases with a rich large cell component.[279] The Ki-67 proliferation index is typically very high (>50%), even in the presence of small cell–predominant tumors. In situ hybridization studies for EBV-encoded RNA (EBER) are positive in virtually all cases.

The TCR and immunoglobulin heavy chain (*IGH*) genes are in germline configuration in ENKTL derived from NK cells. Clonal rearrangements of the TCR genes are detected in 10% to 40% of cases, particularly in those of T-cell origin.[298,299] Recent studies have demonstrated activation of the JAK-STAT signaling pathway in ENKTL.[230]

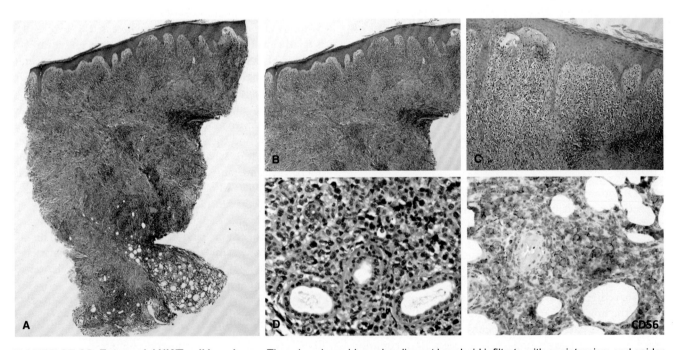

FIGURE 27-30. Extranodal NK/T-cell lymphoma. There is a dermal-based malignant lymphoid infiltrate with angiotropism and epidermal sparing (A and B). The infiltrate is composed of medium-sized cells with abundant granular cytoplasm (D). The infiltrate is diffusely positive for CD56.

Differential Diagnosis

The differential diagnosis of ENKTL in the skin includes other aggressive types of cutaneous lymphoma. PCGDL is often CD56[+], but usually lacks expression of CD5, CD4, and CD8. As opposed to ENKTL, epidermotropism is more frequently found, and the lesions show strong expression of TCRγ. Rare cases are double positive for βF1, and some cases of PCGDL are TCR silent. EBER is only rarely expressed (<5% of cases).[223] MF can rarely be CD56[+],[300,301] and, as opposed to ENKTL, shows more prominent epidermotropism and frequent formation of Pautrier microabscesses. Most cases of MF are positive for βF1, and more typically CD4 positive. Other entities included in the differential diagnosis are other EBV-associated T-cell or NK-cell lymphoproliferative disorders such as EBV+ PTCL, NOS, chronic active EBV infection, systemic EBV+ T-cell LPD of childhood, and HV-like lymphoproliferative disorder, which also occurs predominantly in children. ANKL can also be included in the differential diagnosis and shares similar immunophenotypic features to ENKTL. However, skin involvement is relatively uncommon in the ANKL disease, allowing in the clinical distinction.

The distinction of PTCL, NOS from Extranodal NK/T-cell lymphoma (ENKTL) is typically based on the EBV status, following the recommendations of the WHO classification. ENKTL are invariably EBV+, whereas PTCL, NOS in the setting of CD56 expression is EBV−. However, a recent study reported seven cases of EBV-negative ANKL, three of which had cutaneous involvement on presentation.[302] The EBV-negative cases had an aggressive clinical course similar to EBV-positive ANKL. BPDCNs also are CD56[+] and occur in children.[303,304] Morphologically, BPDCNs are composed of medium-sized cells, with fine nuclear chromatin and blastic appearance. These lesions typically lack the angiotropism and angiodestruction present in ENKTL. Immunophenotypically, BPDCN is positive for CD123, BDCA2, TCL-1, CD4 and shows variable terminal deoxynucleotidyl transferase (TdT) expression, whereas it is negative for CD3 and EBV; these markers are negative in ENKTL.

CAPSULE SUMMARY

EXTRANODAL NK/T-CELL LYMPHOMA

ENKTL, nasal type, is a mature NHL derived by NK cells (more frequently) and sometimes T cells with extranodal (frequently upper aerodigestive) infiltration by EBV infected cytotoxic lymphocytes with angioinvasion and necrosis. The lesions present clinically with midline nasal septal destruction and infiltration of the paranasal sinuses. ENKTL has an angiocentric and angiodestructive growth pattern with coagulative necrosis, admixed apoptotic bodies, and fibrinoid change in blood vessels, even in the absence of angioinvasion. The tumors are strong and diffusely CD56[+] and EBV+.

Cutaneous B-Cell Lymphomas/ Leukemias

MARGINAL ZONE LYMPHOMA

Definition and Epidemiology

MZL is a low-grade B-cell NHL composed of small, monocytoid, and lymphoplasmacytoid cells, and mature plasma cells.[305,306] Primary cutaneous MZL (PCMZL) is extraordinarily rare in children. A series from Kempf and collaborators included a total of three cases,[307] mostly in teenagers. In a study of cutaneous lymphomas in individuals younger than 20, Fink-Puches et al showed a total of seven cases of MZL. There is a slight predominance in girls, compared with boys.[308-312] More recently, Amitay-Laish et al reported a series of 11 cases of pediatric PCMZL; none of the patients had progression of the disease after a mean observation of 5.5 years.[313]

Etiology

Many cases are associated with infectious etiologies, such as *Helicobacter pylori* (in gastric mucosa-associated lymphoid tissue [MALT]), *Borrelia burgdorferi* (in cutaneous cases only in Europe) and *Chlamydia* (ocular MALT) with site specificity. More recently, IgG4 expression has been shown in cutaneous cases with prominent plasmacytic differentiation.[314] The first case of the disease reported in the United States was found in association with chronic antihistaminic use.[310] Rare cases in association with medications for attentional deficit disorders have been seen.[307] Cases in relationship to medications use usually resolve on cessation of the medication.

Clinical Presentation

The clinical findings are very similar in both adults and children, including an indolent clinical course: multiple papules, plaques, and/or nodules present on the arms, upper trunk, and face (Figure 27-31). Most recently, a 15-year-old boy with multiple lesions representing PCMZL and juxtaarticular fibrotic nodules showing a pattern of nodular sclerosis with peripheral plasma cell–rich infiltrates has been reported.[315]

Histologic Findings

Histologically, early lesions have a perivascular and periadnexal infiltrate, whereas more advanced ones may have a nodular and/or diffuse cellular infiltrate extending into the subcutaneous fat. There are small lymphocytes, lymphoplasmacytic cells, and plasma cells on routine histology (Figure 27-32). Reactive T cells may be present and can represent a significant proportion of the infiltrate. It is common to see a varying component of plasma cells, eosinophils, and histiocytes. In MZL, reactive but small and atrophic lymphoid follicles are often seen.[308,316]

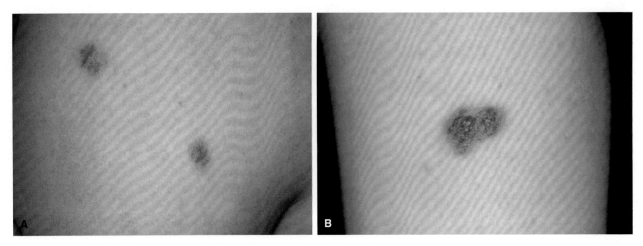

FIGURE 27-31. Primary cutaneous marginal zone lymphoma. Plaques on the left shoulder (A) and left arm (B). Obtained with permission Kempf W, Kazakov DV, Buechner SA, et al. Primary cutaneous marginal zone lymphoma in children: a report of 3 cases and review of the literature. *Am J Dermatopathol.* 2014;36(8):661-666.

By immunohistochemistry (IHC), marginal zone cells show expression of CD20, CD79a, and BCL-2, and are usually negative for CD10, CD5, and BCL-6. Co-expression of CD43 is rare in the cutaneous sites (Figure 27-33). Tumors with prominent plasma cell differentiation show expression of CD138. IgG4, although found commonly in lesions from adults, has not been seen in the pediatric group.[307,317] Clusters of PDCs, using a CD123 immunostain, can be seen. A single case in a child has been found in association with *B. burgdorferi*. In situ hybridization for kappa and lambda and/or immunohistochemical stains for surface light chains can be useful in detecting a restricted population of plasma cells. Clonality studies for *IGH* gene rearrangements are also helpful to prove a clonal population of B cells.[318] Similarly to adults, trisomy 3 can be seen using FISH, where it is the most frequent chromosomal aberration seen in this type of lymphoma in adults, with approximately 20% of studied cases displaying this anomaly, either singly or in combination with t(14;18)(q32;q21) or t(3;14)(p14.1;q32).[319-321] The t(11;18) translocation, linked to gastric and lung MALTs, has not been seen in cutaneous sites. Guitart and Gerami[322] have proposed the term atypical marginal zone hyperplasia

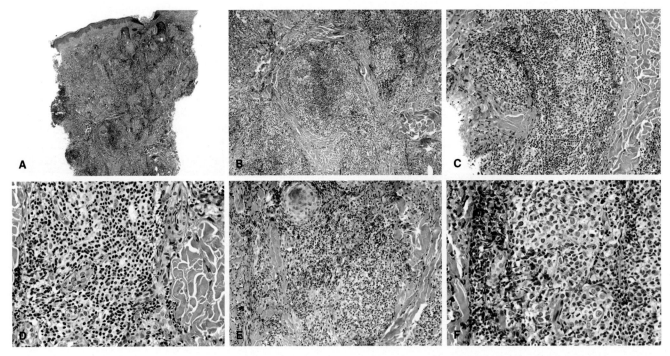

FIGURE 27-32. Cutaneous marginal zone lymphoma. There is a dermal-based infiltrate with adnexotropism and sparing of the surface epidermis (A and B). Atrophic germinal centers are seen (C and F). The infiltrate shows monocytoid cells (D and E).

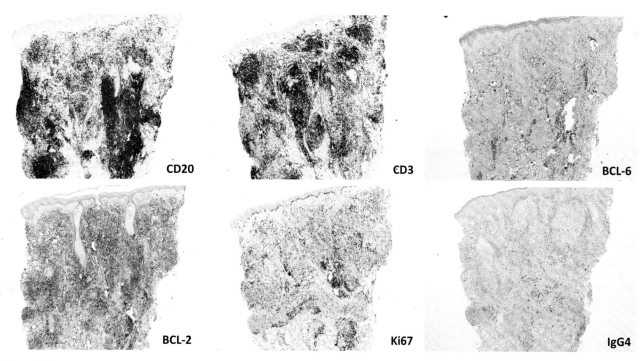

FIGURE 27-33. Cutaneous marginal zone lymphoma—immunohistochemistry. The lymphoma cells are positive for CD20. CD3 shows a rich background of T cells. The atrophic germinal centers are positive for BCL-6 but negative for BCL-2. They have a high Ki67. IgG4 is positive in abundant plasma cells.

to describe a subset of cases in young individuals with lambda restriction, and lack of BCL-2 expression. This term has been previously applied by Attygalle et al[323] to subsets of cases presenting in the tonsils of young children that are polyclonal by gene rearrangement studies and with CD43 co-expression by IHC. However, caution should be exercised, with the use of atypical marginal zone hyperplasia, as some consider those as bona fide cases of MZL.[318] Swerdlow et al have also argued that many examples of "cutaneous lymphoid hyperplasias" with the presence of germinal centers are actually examples of CMZL.[324]

Differential Diagnosis

The differential diagnosis of PCMZL in children includes Borrelia-associated lymphocytoma cutis, which mainly affects the ear lobes, nipples, and scrotum in children and presents with a solitary lesion in most patients, which contrasts with the multifocal lesions in the majority of PC-MZL.[325] The so-called tibial lymphoplasmacytic plaque occurs in the latter location.[326] Some regard this lesion within the spectrum of linear APACHE. Cutaneous plasmacytosis and plasmacytoma are now regarded as MZL. Among other B-cell lymphomas, primary cutaneous follicle center lymphoma (PC-FCL) has a germinal center phenotype (BCL-6 and with or without CD10). A prominent plasmacytic infiltrate can be seen in Melkerson-Rosenthal syndrome, usually in association with granulomas with an intralymphatic distribution.

PRIMARY CUTANEOUS FOLLICLE CENTER LYMPHOMA

Definition and Epidemiology

PC-FCL is an indolent neoplastic proliferation of B cells with a germinal center phenotype.[25] It is one of the most common forms of cutaneous B-cell lymphomas in middle age and older individuals (median 51-58 years), but extraordinarily rare in children.[327] By definition, PC-FCL is limited to the skin at the time of diagnosis, without evidence of systemic or nodal involvement, and is distinct from systemic or nodal follicular lymphoma (FL). Amitay-Laish et al reported the occurrence of a spindle cell variant of PC-FCL in a 17-year-old girl.[312] Condarco et al reported a case of PC-FCL in the scalp of an 8-year-old boy.[328] In the large series (n = 69) of pediatric cutaneous NHL from Gratz, a single case of a PC-FCL in a 20-year-old individual has been reported.[3] A case of PC-FCL in the setting of the rare congenital immunodeficiency WHIM syndrome (warts, hypogammaglobulinemia, infections, and myelokathexis) has been described.[329] Another case of PC-FCL arising in the nose and extending into the maxillary sinus and soft palate was reported in a 16-year-old boy.[330]

Clinical and Histologic Findings

It typically presents as solitary or clustered smooth, erythematous to violaceous infiltrative papules, plaques, nodules, or tumors, in the head and neck or upper trunk (Figure 27-34).[331]

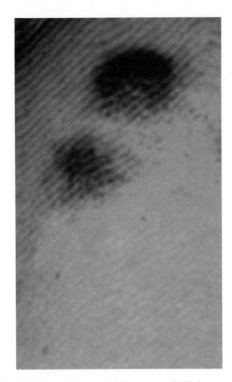

FIGURE 27-34. Primary cutaneous follicle center lymphoma. Lesions typically present as small dermal tumors and may be grouped.

Histologically, PC-FCL has a nodular, nodular and diffuse, or diffuse growth patterns in the dermis with sparing of the surface epidermis (a Grenz zone separating the infiltrate from the epidermis is invariably present)[332] (Figure 27-35). The infiltrate can extend into the adipose tissue. As opposed to systemic FL, grading has no prognostic significance as all cases of PC-FCL show an indolent course. The areas with abnormal follicles lack the tangible body macrophages present in reactive germinal centers. The neoplastic cells are composed of small cleaved centrocytes and larger centroblasts.[333-335] The lesions with a diffuse growth pattern show a predominance of centroblasts and can be potential mimickers for large B-cell lymphomas. There is a variant composed largely of spindle cells (sarcomatoid form), originally referred as "reticulohistiocytoma dorsi" or "Crosti lymphoma."[336,337] In such cases, fascicles of spindle cells admixed with areas of atypical centroblasts and centrocytes are present. One of the reported pediatric cases showed spindle cell cytology.

By IHC, PC-FCL is positive for CD19, PAX-5, CD20, CD79a, and BCL-6. CD10 is variably positive, depending on the pattern of growth (nodular growth is more typically positive, whereas diffuse growth is negative). BCL-2 is positive in approximately 50% of cases. The follicular dendritic networks can be highlighted by CD21, CD23, and D2-40 immunostains. Clonality studies can be used to demonstrate

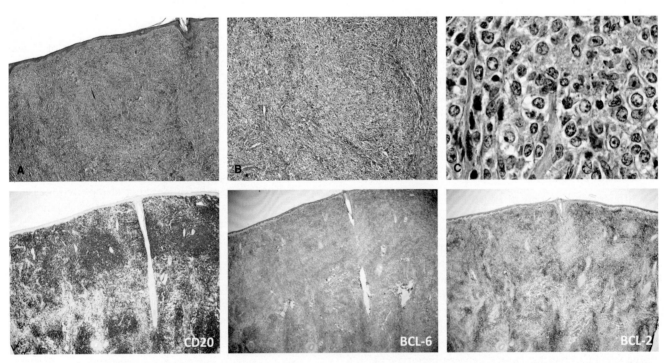

FIGURE 27-35. Primary cutaneous follicle center lymphoma: There is a dense infiltrate in the dermis with sparing of the epidermis. The infiltrate shows a nodular appearance. The poorly formed follicles lack tangible body macrophages or polarization. In this particular case, many centroblasts are present, which can potentially raise the consideration of a large B-cell lymphoma. The infiltrate is positive for CD20 and BCL-6 but negative for BCL-2. This is one of the most characteristic phenotypes of PCFCL. Obtained with permission Gru A, Dehner LP. Cutaneous hematolymphoid and histiocytic proliferations in children. *Pediatr Dev Pathol.* 2018;21(2):150-207.

rearrangement of the *IGH* gene. In situ hybridization can also show on occasion a clonal population of B cells. Translocations of the *IGH-BCL2* genes t(14;18) can be present in 18% to 41% of PC-FCL.[338,339]

Differential Diagnosis

Differential diagnostic considerations with PC-FCL include reactive lymphoid hyperplasias, PCMZL, cutaneous involvement by systemic FL, and DLBCL (particularly the so-called leg-type lymphoma). PCMZL differs in the lack of germinal center markers. Although PCMZL can show atrophic germinal centers, those typically have a very high proliferation and are rather small, in counterpart with the neoplastic follicles of PC-FCL that have a lower Ki67. In situ hybridization can help highlight a clonal population of plasma cells. Some cases of PCMZL can also show a high proportion of IgG4⁺ plasma cells. Cutaneous involvement by systemic FL has never been documented in the pediatric setting because systemic FL is a disease in older individuals and systemic pediatric FL is a more localized disease. DLBCL leg type has never been documented in the pediatric age and is a disease in older adults. Its counterpart, DLBCL-LT, presents clinically in the legs and has a nongerminal center profile (MUM1 strongly positive).

CAPSULE SUMMARY

PRIMARY CUTANEOUS FOLLICLE CENTER LYMPHOMA

PC-FCL is an indolent neoplastic proliferation of B cells with a germinal center phenotype. Although this is a disorder of middle-aged individuals, rare cases in children have been described. It typically presents as solitary or clustered smooth, erythematous to violaceous infiltrative papules, plaques, nodules, or tumors, in the head and neck or upper trunk. Histologically, PC-FCL has a nodular, nodular and diffuse, or diffuse growth patterns in the dermis with sparing of the surface epidermis. The neoplastic cells are composed of small cleaved centrocytes and larger centroblasts, the latter being more frequent in the diffuse variants. By IHC, PC-FCL is positive for CD19, PAX-5, CD20, CD79a, and BCL-6. CD10 is variably positive. BCL-2 is positive in approximately 50% of cases.

Precursor T/B-Cell Lymphoblastic Leukemias/Lymphomas

ACUTE LYMPHOBLASTIC LEUKEMIA/ LYMPHOMA

Definition and Epidemiology

Acute lymphoblastic leukemia/lymphoma (ALL) is the most common type of leukemia in childhood, representing 80% of cases.[340] In the United States, the incidence of ALL

is about 30 cases per million persons younger than 20 years of age. The peak incidence occurs between the ages of 3 and 5. There is a slightly higher incidence of ALL in boys than in girls.[341] Approximately 80% to 85% of cases are B-ALL and 10% to 15% T-ALL.[342] Although the etiology of the disease is still largely unknown, certain genetic disorders have a greater predisposition for the development of ALL, including trisomy 21 and ataxia telangiectasia. Some cases are associated with *MLL* gene rearrangements and might be secondary to chemotherapy.

Between 5% and 20% to 30% of patients develop cutaneous dissemination. Nearly 50 to 60 cases of B-ALL have been reported in children with skin involvement.[4,342-344] The frequency of cutaneous involvement in T-ALL is less well documented. However, Lee et al[345] reported an incidence of 4.3% in T-ALL and 15% in B-ALL. Approximately 33% of patients with the lymphomatous variants had cutaneous involvement, and only 1% in those with leukemic presentations.

Clinical Presentation

The lesions present as erythematous or violaceous nodules, tumors, or plaques (sometimes can be multiple). The distribution of the lesions is typically the head and neck, upper trunk, and abdomen (Figure 27-36). Kahwash and Qualman reported a series of six cases between 5 and 15 years in girls.[343] Occasional cases of aleukemic forms have been reported.[342,346-348] A single case with a congenital presentation has also been described in association with an *MLL* rearrangement.[349] Cases of T-ALL are frequently associated with a mediastinal mass (50%-65%). Many cases of ALL present in neonates with multiple blue/purple plaques or nodules on the skin, and hence the term "blueberry muffin syndrome."

Histologic Findings

The histopathologic findings for both B- and T-ALL are identical.[344,350] There is a diffuse and dense dermal infiltrate with extension into the subcutaneous tissue[4,312,342,343,347-349,351] (Figures 27-37 and 27-38). A Grenz zone is typically present with epidermal sparing. Cytologically, the infiltrate consists of small lymphoblasts with scant cytoplasm, fine nuclear chromatin, irregular nuclei, and inconspicuous nucleoli. Linear arrangements of lymphoblasts forming linear files can be noted. Infiltration of the skin adnexae is also frequently seen, as well as nerves and piloerector muscles. Mitotic activity is typically brisk.

By IHC, the blasts of B-ALL express CD19, PAX5, CD79a, and CD43. TdT and CD34 are often expressed in the malignant cells, and CD99 can be seen in >50% of cases. Expression of CD45 is dim or negative, and most cases are negative for CD20, but CD10 is present in most, but not all, cases. B-ALL with *MLL* rearrangement are typically CD15⁺ and CD10 negative. Those cases of B-ALL with the t(12;21)

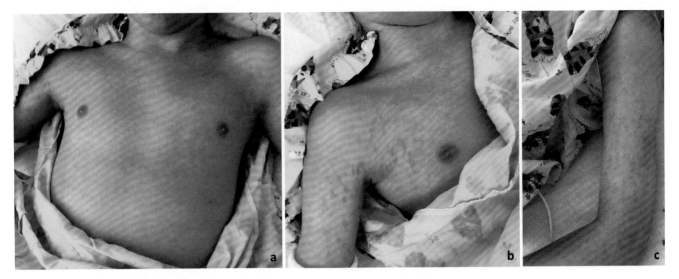

FIGURE 27-36. Acute lymphoblastic leukemia presenting as a viral exanthem (A-C).

translocation (Philadelphia chromosome) have a worse prognosis and are associated with CD10 co-expression.

The immunophenotype of cells in T-ALL usually includes positivity for TdT with variable expression of CD45, CD34, CD1a, CD10, CD2, CD3 (lineage specific), CD4, CD5, CD7, and CD8. CD4/CD8 co-expression is most frequently observed; however, co-expression is not necessarily a marker of an immature phenotype because cases of mature T-cell lymphomas have been described with dual positivity. More

reliable markers to confirm an immature phenotype include TdT, CD1a, CD99, and CD34.[352] According to the expression of specific markers, T-ALL can be subdivided into early or pro-T, pre-T, cortical-T, and medullary-T. The molecular background of T-ALL is less well understood. Cytogenetic abnormalities are frequent in T-ALL patients (50%-70%). The most common cytogenetic abnormalities involve 14q11-13, the site of TCR alpha/delta, including inv(14)(q11;q32) and deletions or translocations involving chromosomes 9, 10,

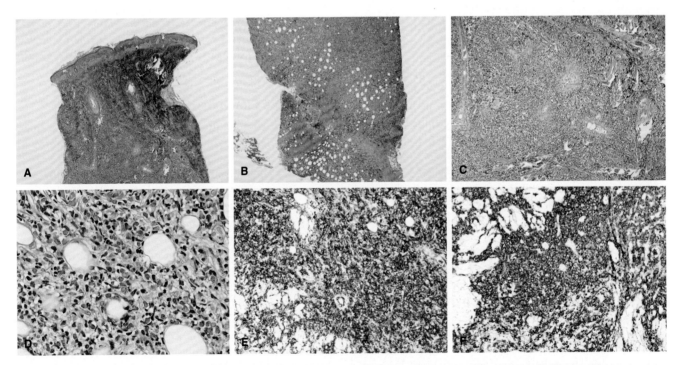

FIGURE 27-37. **Precursor B-lymphoblastic leukemia with skin involvement.** There is a diffuse dermal infiltrate with a grenz-zone (A and B). The infiltrate extends and dissect through the collagen fibers (C). It is composed of small to medium sized lymphoblasts (D) which are positive for CD34 (E) and CD10 (F).

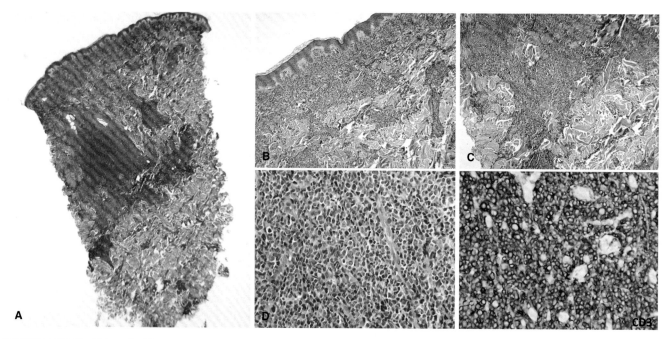

FIGURE 27-38. **T-lymphoblastic leukemia.** There is a dense infiltrate in the dermis with epidermal sparing (A and B). The infiltrate dissects through the collagen fibers (C). It is composed of immature blasts (D). The neoplastic cells are CD3-positive.

and 11 corresponding to sites of TCR α, β, and γ-subunit genes found in 47% of T-ALL. Some cases can also present in association with myeloid hyperplasia, eosinophilia, and the t(8;13)(p11;q11) aberration affecting the *FGFR1* gene. The latter has now been referred to as the 8p11 myeloproliferative disorder.[353,354] Similar to B-ALL, T-ALL are typically associated with rearrangements of the TCR.

Differential Diagnosis

The differential diagnosis can be challenging in the primary lymphomatous lesions, or its aleukemic forms. The differential diagnosis in "blueberry muffin" syndrome includes neuroblastoma, myeloid leukemia, rhabdoid tumor, and rhabdomyosarcoma. In fact, a case originally diagnosed as Ewing sarcoma (EWS) represented an example of B-ALL with CD99 co-expression.[347] However, EWS does not express B-cell antigens. Indeed, CD99, CD34, and TdT in B-ALL are useful in the differentiation from mature B-cell lymphomas in the skin, which overall are extraordinarily uncommon. In the differential diagnosis, Merkel cell carcinoma may rarely present in children[355,356] and show CD99 expression similar to B-ALL. CK20 and NSE) can help in the distinction between the two. Cutaneous involvement by neuroblastoma is also rare and might be a pitfall, but CD99 is negative in the latter.[357,358] However, CD99 expression is more typically cytoplasmic, rather than the crisp staining seen in EWS.[359] Neuroblastomas are also positive for neuroendocrine markers. Other small round cell sarcomas can be distinguished with the presence of specific markers (myogenin, desmin, etc).

CAPSULE SUMMARY

ACUTE LYMPHOBLASTIC LEUKEMIA/LYMPHOMA

ALL is the most common type of leukemia in childhood, representing 80% of cases. Approximately 80% to 85% of cases are B-ALL and 10% to 15% T-ALL. Between 5% and 20% to 30% of patients develop cutaneous dissemination: erythematous or violaceous nodules, tumors, or plaques (sometimes can be multiple). Patients with T-ALL often have a mediastinal mass. There is a diffuse and dense dermal infiltrate with extension into the subcutaneous tissue. Linear arrangement of small lymphoblasts is seen. Expression of immature markers is typical (CD34, TdT, CD99, CD1a).

Cutaneous Myeloid Neoplasms

LEUKEMIA CUTIS

Definition and Epidemiology

LC is manifested by a cutaneous infiltration of neoplastic myeloid cells, lymphoid blasts, or mature lymphoma cells. AML, particularly in those with monocytic or myelomonocytic differentiation, occur as LC.[360] However, LC is seen in association with chronic myelogenous leukemia, myelodysplastic syndrome (MDS), and ALL (T-ALL and B-ALL).[361-364]

Myeloid sarcoma, extramedullary myeloid tumor, granulocytic sarcoma, and monocytic sarcoma are often termed LC when occurring in the skin, but many now prefer the term "myeloid sarcoma" when there is a nodular infiltrate of immature blasts in the dermis.[365] In contrast, LC is the preferred term when the malignant infiltrate shows a diffuse, interstitial pattern through the dermis with the clinical appearance of a rash. LC in children may present at or soon after birth.

Rarely, cutaneous involvement by a leukemic infiltrate can occur in the absence of BM or peripheral blood involvement by acute leukemia; this then is referred to as aleukemic leukemia cutis (ALC)[346,366-374] or aleukemic myeloid sarcoma.[360,375] Byrd et al[365] proposed using aleukemic to describe those cases of extramedullary involvement in the absence of blood and BM disease for at least 1 month. The literature also includes cases described as aleukemic despite concomitant BM disease in patients who do not have circulating peripheral blasts.[376,377] An adverse prognosis has been associated with, whereas others have argued that ALC is a heterogeneous condition that can even result in spontaneous resolution without such treatment.[313,365,378-380] We have recently published a series of cases of ALC, including some with spontaneous resolution, and in two cases there was the presence of *MLL* rearrangements.[381] ALC can also be seen in association with pre-B-cell ALL[346,373,376] and in rare cases of T-cell ALL.[348,382] A monocytic phenotype and certain cytogenetic aberrations, such as t(8;21) or inv(16), are found in a disproportionate number of cases. In addition, the expression of T-cell markers and CD56 is more frequent in extramedullary myeloid blast cells.[365,383] Otsubo et al reported the development of an acute promyelocytic leukemia following ALC in association with *NPM-RARA* fusion transcript in a child.[384] Agrawal et al reported ALC in siblings at birth.[378] Interestingly, 11q23 abnormalities have been detected by FISH in some cases of congenital LC, which strongly raises the likelihood of abnormalities in the *MLL* gene.[385,386] Torrelo et al described a very aggressive clinical presentation of ALC in a newborn, clinically manifested as "blueberry muffin" skin lesions.[387] Transient abnormal myelopoiesis (TAM) is an entity characterized by the presence of blasts in the blood of children with trisomy 21, which in many cases is reversible. Cutaneous lesions with blast infiltration have been reported in children with TAM.[388-390]

Clinical Presentation

Cutaneous interstitial deposits of immature blasts present as papules, nodules, or plaques and are found in 2% to 12% of AML cases. Newborns can present with blueberry muffin appearance (Figure 27-39A and B). Although less common, LC occurs in the setting of lymphoblastic leukemias, with an estimated incidence of 1% to 3%.[391] The diagnosis of ALC is a challenging one not only because of its infrequency, but also because of the absence of concomitant blood or BM involvement. The diagnosis can also be elusive because the infiltrate can adopt a very sparse perivascular and periadnexal distribution.[392]

Histologic Findings

Morphologically, the leukemic cells are centered in the dermis and may extend into the subcutaneous tissue[393] (Figure 27-40). Epidermotropism is usually not seen. The malignant cells can disrupt the vessels and adnexal structures, and a "leukemic vasculitis" can also occur.[394] The vasculitis is thought to represent direct endothelial injury by the leukemic cells.[395] A diagnosis of LC is invariably corroborated by IHC. Because of the frequent monocytic lineage, CD34, TdT, and CD117 are often not helpful in identifying immature blasts, but Cibull et al found that CD68 and lysozyme were additionally helpful in the diagnosis.[393] The CD68 KP1 clone appears to be more specific and reliable to identify the myeloid origin of the cells.[396] In contrast, Cronin et al suggested that the combination of CD43 and CD68 was more reliable (Figure 27-41).[397] Amador-Ortiz et al., with a panel including CD117, CD33, and lysozyme, confirmed most cases of cutaneous myeloid sarcoma. The addition of CD14 and KLF-4 was also useful in achieving a greater degree of sensitivity and specificity in those lesions of monocytic lineage.[398] ERG is a more recent marker that has been used with success to help in the diagnosis of LC.[399] However, a problem with the use of immunostains is that numerous histiocytic disorders (benign and malignant) in cutaneous sites have a similar phenotype. In fact, some LCs have been masked by the presence of a prominent granulomatous reaction in the dermis, as reported by Tomasini et al[377] Ideally, correlation with the BM immunophenotypic findings of the immature blasts could be helpful. Interestingly, discrepancies in the phenotype of the immature cells in the skin and the BM have been documented, a feature that can complicate the diagnosis further.[397,398] Other molecular tools can sometimes be helpful in establishing a diagnosis, such as *MLL* rearrangements (Figure 27-42) by FISH or *NPM1* and *FLT3-ITD* mutations by PCR analysis.

Differential Diagnosis

In the setting of a clinical context and history of AML, the findings of an immature infiltrate in the dermis are strongly suggestive of a diagnosis of LC. However, one should be aware of the possibility that patients with AML or MDS can develop Sweet syndrome, particularly the histiocytoid variant. The latter can be associated with a somewhat immature infiltrate in the dermis, lacks expression of immature markers (CD34, CD123, CD117), and has myeloperoxidase positivity. Many have argued that a diagnosis of histiocytoid Sweet syndrome reflects an "immature myeloid infiltrate" in the skin. Other diagnostic

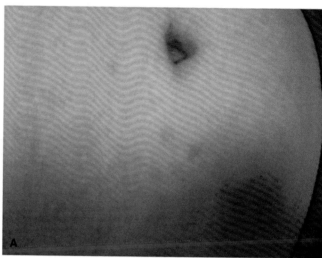

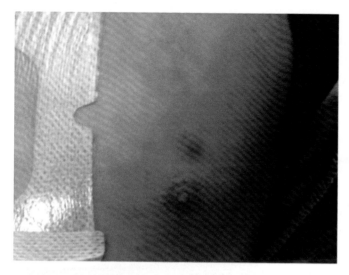

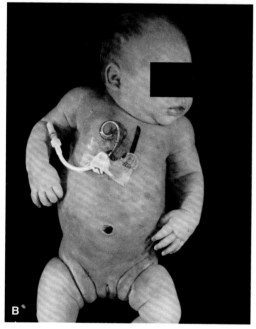

FIGURE 27-39. A, Small red papules and nodules on the upper chest and lower abdomen in a case of aleukemic leukemia cutis. Obtained with permission. Gru AA et al. Pediatric aleukemic leukemia cutis: report of 3 cases and review of the literature. *Am J Dermatopathol.* 2015 Jun;37(6):477-84. B, Clinical postmortem photograph of a patient with congenital leukemia with a cutaneous presentation resulting in a "blueberry muffin" appearance. Reprinted with permission Gru AA, Schaffer A. *Hematopathology of the Skin: A Clinical and Pathologic Approach.* Philadelphia, PA: Wolters Kluwer; 2016.

considerations that can mimic LC, particularly in newborns and small infants, are cutaneous deposits of extramedullary hematopoiesis (EMH). As opposed to LC, most EMH deposits have a predominance of erythroid precursors. Rare megakaryocytes can be seen. On many occasions, an etiologic cause for EMH (viral infection—CMV, HSV, etc) can be encountered in children.

CAPSULE SUMMARY

LEUKEMIA CUTIS

LC is manifested by a cutaneous infiltration of neoplastic myeloid cells, lymphoid blasts, or mature lymphoma cells. AML, particularly those with monocytic or

myelomonocytic differentiation, may present as LC. Myeloid sarcoma, extramedullary myeloid tumor, granulocytic sarcoma, and monocytic sarcoma are often termed LC when occurring in the skin, but many now prefer the term "myeloid sarcoma" when there is a nodular infiltrate of immature blasts in the dermis. Aleukemic LC occurs in the absence of BM involvement by leukemia. Cutaneous interstitial deposits of immature blasts present as papules, nodules, or plaques, and are found in 2% to 12% of AML cases. Morphologically, the leukemic cells are centered in the dermis and may extend into the subcutaneous tissue. Because of the frequent monocytic differentiation of the malignant cells, often the immature markers (CD34, CD117, and TdT) are negative in the cells.

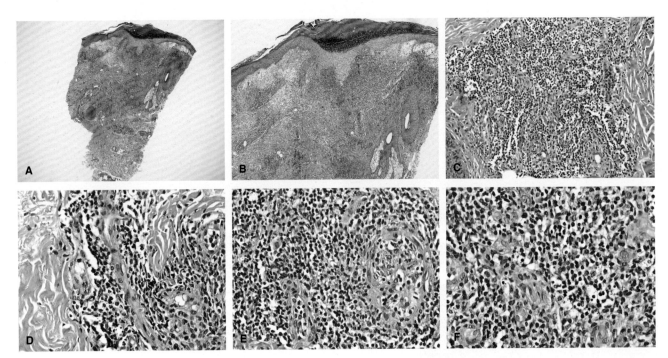

FIGURE 27-40. **A leukemic infiltrate is present in the dermis with a focus of acute folliculitis (A and B).** The infiltrate shows an interstitial and perivascular distribution (C and D). It is composed of medium-sized cells, with fine chromatin and variable nucleoli (E and F).

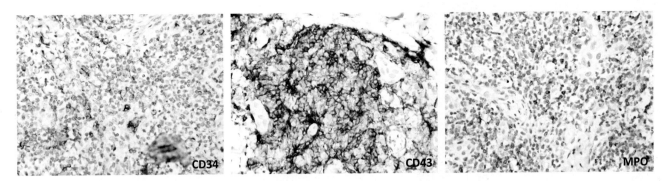

FIGURE 27-41. **Leukemia cutis—immunohistochemistry.** The infiltrate is weakly positive for CD34 but more diffusely positive for MPO and CD43.

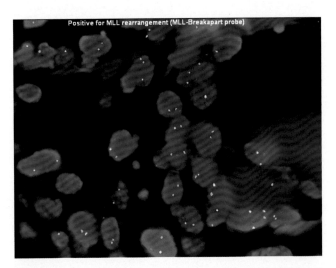

FIGURE 27-42. *MLL* **rearrangement in a case of aleukemic leukemia cutis arising in a myeloid neoplasm after treatment for osteosarcoma.** A break-apart probe was used.

BLASTIC PLASMACYTOID DENDRITIC CELL NEOPLASM

Definition and Epidemiology

BPDCN is an extremely rare subtype of acute leukemia and was formerly known as blastic natural killer (NK)–cell lymphoma or CD4⁺/CD56⁺ hematodermic neoplasm.[400-403] Once postulated to originate from NK-lineage precursors, accumulating phenotypic, functional, and genetic evidence has pointed to its derivation from hematopoietic precursors with commitment to the plasmacytoid dendritic cell lineage, cells which are positive for CD123.[402,404-408] BPDCN is rare in children,[303,400,409-412] and the largest series from BPDCN in the pediatric setting was reported by Jegalian et al.[304]

Clinical Presentation

Clinically, most adults have cutaneous lesions at diagnosis (85%), but the opposite has been found in children: Seven of the 29 cases (24%) lacked cutaneous disease at presentation, with disease confined to the BM, peripheral blood, lymph nodes, spleen, and/or liver.[304] Skin lesions can be multiple (>60% of the time) or single. The lesions range from tumors and nodules to plaques and patches that are brown, erythematous, or violaceous (Figure 27-43). A characteristic clinical finding is that the lesions are bruise-like or hemorrhagic in appearance. They may be found anywhere on the body, especially the scalp, face, trunk, and extremities. Those without cutaneous disease at presentation had 100% survival at 60 months follow-up. Most adults relapsed within the first year of diagnosis with BM and central nervous system involvement (approximately 33% of cases). The disease has an overall survival of approximately 74% in children.[304]

Histologic Findings

Morphologically, BPDCN in children tends to have smaller sized cells and a lymphoblast-like appearance of the blasts. In adults, BPDCN has a more pleomorphic appearance (Figure 27-44). Cutaneous lesions of BPDCN are characterized by a dermal infiltrate composed of sheets of neoplastic cells. The infiltrate is typically diffuse but can often show an accentuated periadnexal or perivascular distribution. The epidermis is characteristically spared with an underlying Grenz zone. The cells are typically intermediate to large with round nuclei and finely dispersed "blastic" chromatin. Nuclear contours are irregular and may be notched, folded, or occasionally show moderate pleomorphism. Nucleoli are usually inconspicuous, but one to several prominent nucleoli can be present. With hematoxylin and eosin staining, the cytoplasm is pale to eosinophilic, agranular, and usually scant, but can be moderate to abundant in some cases.

CD123, CD4, and CD56 positivity, the most common BPDCN immunophenotypic profile, is not specific as these markers are also expressed in both AML and ALL (Figures 27-44 and 27-45).[411] However, cases without cutaneous involvement also expressed other BPDCN markers, including BDCA-4, CD303/BDCA-2, CD2AP, and TCL1. CD68 (KP1) is generally negative, but focal punctate staining is seen in a minority of cases. Strong staining for CD68 should raise suspicion of acute or chronic myeloid leukemia with monocytic differentiation.[304] Myeloid cell nuclear differentiation antigen (MNDA) can be used effectively to distinguish between LC and BPDCN, as only LC is positive.[413] Additionally, S100 expression is seen in approximately 75% of pediatric cases, compared with only 25% of cases in the adult population.[414] The genetics of this disease is poorly understood, but a recent case was reported with *EWSR* gene rearrangement, an important diagnostic consideration in the pediatric population.[415] *TET2* is the most common mutated gene (36% to 80%)[416]; other recurrent somatic mutations include *IKZF3* and *ZEB2* (12% to 16%),[416] *ASXL1* (32%), *NPM1* (10%), and *RAS* (9% to 27%).[417] Gene expression profiling has demonstrated a unique signature, distinct from AML and ALL.[418] Compared with normal PDCs, BPDCN has shown increased expression of genes involved in Notch signaling and NFKB activation.

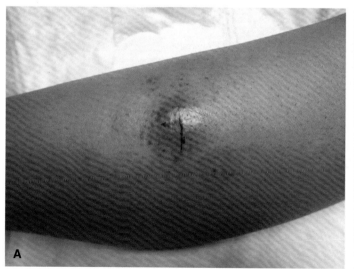
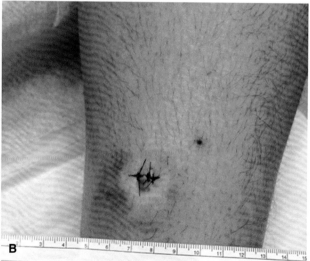

FIGURE 27-43. Blastic plasmacytoid dendritic cell neoplasm. Solitary 2.1 cm indurated red-brown nodule with smaller violaceous macules at the periphery (A). Single bruise-like subcutaneous nodule (B). Adapted and obtained with permission from Nguyen CM, Stuart L, Skupsky H, Lee YS, Tsuchiya A, Cassarino DS. Blastic plasmacytoid dendritic cell neoplasm in the pediatric population: a case series and review of the literature. *Am J Dermatopathol.* 2015;37(12):924-928.

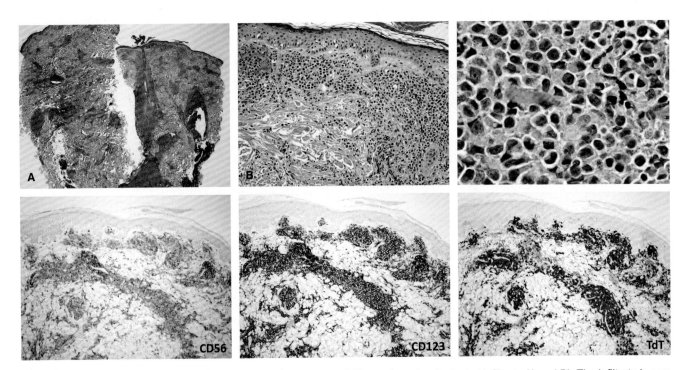

FIGURE 27-44. Blastic plasmacytoid dendritic cell neoplasm. Diffuse adnexotropic dermal infiltrate (A and B). The infiltrate is composed of blastic cells with variable pleomorphism (C). The infiltrate is positive for CD56, CD123, and TdT.

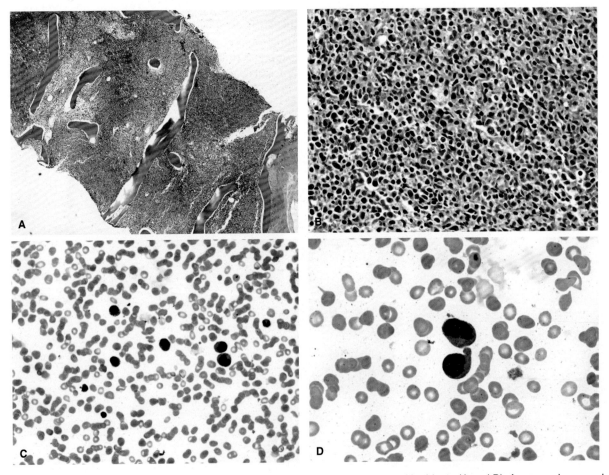

FIGURE 27-45. Bone marrow dissemination. The marrow space is diffusely replaced by blasts (A and B). A smear shows a plasmacytoid appearance of the malignant cells (C and D).

Differential Diagnosis

The most closely related lesions that mimic BPDCN are the clonal, tumoral proliferations of PDCs that can occur in the skin, lymph nodes, BM, and spleen secondary to a variety of myeloid neoplasms with monocytic differentiation. Tumoral PDC proliferations can most reliably be distinguished from BPDCN by a Ki-67 index (usually <10% in PDC proliferations and >30% in BPDCN). When positive, TdT is also helpful in excluding a tumoral PDC proliferation, because these are uniformly negative.

Acute monocytic leukemias, myelomonocytic leukemia, and juvenile myelomonocytic leukemia frequently have significant cutaneous localization. These are also often positive for CD4, CD56, and CD123, making their distinction from BPDCN even more difficult. Thorough cytochemical analysis and immunophenotyping is necessary for definitive classification. If available, Wright-Giemsa–stained cytologic preparations will often show cytoplasmic granules. When granules are present, myeloperoxidase and/or lysozyme will usually be positive, excluding BPDCN from the differential diagnosis. Less mature myeloid neoplasms may lack cytoplasmic granules but will be positive for CD13, CD34, and/ or CD117, excluding BPDCN. CD68 is positive in both BPDCN and other myeloid neoplasms but shows distinctive dot-like cytoplasmic positivity in BPDCN as opposed to the diffuse cytoplasmic staining seen in other lesions.

The expression of CD4, other T-cell antigens, TdT, and cutaneous infiltration raises the possibility of a cutaneous T-cell leukemia/lymphoma. Absence of CD3, CD5, and CD8, and the absence of a *TCR* gene rearrangement support BPDCN. NK-cell leukemia also needs to be included in the differential diagnosis of BPDCN. Both entities express CD56, but NK-cell leukemia often shows distinctive areas of angiodestruction and necrosis. NK-cell leukemia will also be positive for EBV studies and will express cytoplasmic CD3 and granzyme B by IHC, both of which are absent in BPDCN.

CAPSULE SUMMARY

BLASTIC PLASMACYTOID DENDRITIC CELL NEOPLASM

BPDCN is a rare, distinct form of myeloid precursor neoplasm differentiated toward PDCs. It is characterized by early, often isolated skin lesions that almost inevitably progresses to systemic and BM involvement with a poor prognosis. The skin lesions have a characteristic bruise-like or hemorrhagic appearance. The diagnosis requires thorough immunophenotyping to exclude a number of other pathologies with similar clinical and histomorphologic features.

EXTRAMEDULLARY HEMATOPOIESIS

Definition and Epidemiology

EMH is defined as nonneoplastic extramedullary erythropoiesis that is typically seen secondary to intrauterine infections and hemoglobinopathies. The most common sites for EMH are spleen, and liver, but almost any organ can be involved. Skin involvement is an extremely rare manifestation.[419]

Etiology

The original TORCH syndrome complex includes intrauterine infections by *Toxoplasma gondii*, rubella virus, cytomegalovirus, and herpes simplex virus, types 1 and 2. Dermal erythropoiesis is mostly associated with toxoplasma, CMV, and rubella infections.[420] The commonest hematologic etiologies causing reactive erythropoiesis include erythroblastosis fetalis, hereditary spherocytosis, and twin-twin transfusion syndrome.[421]

Clinical Presentation

The clinical presentation of EMH is similar to those of other cutaneous metastases, such as the presence of pink or red-violaceous macules, papules, and nodules, typically on the trunk. Bulla formation, hemorrhage, and ulcerations have been also observed.[422,423] The clinical features of blueberry muffin baby include nonblanching, violaceous macules or firm, dome-shaped papules (<1 cm). The lesions are mostly generalized with preference to the trunk, head, and neck. The lesions typically resolve by 3 to 6 weeks after birth and often leave light brown macular discoloration.

Histologic Findings

Histopathologically, there are clusters of normoblastic erythropoiesis with nucleated red blood cell precursors in the dermis (Figure 27-46). Myeloid and megakaryocytic elements as well as dermal fibrosis are not typically present. CD61, factor VIIIra, and CD31 can be used to demonstrate the megakaryocytes, glycophorin A, or hemoglobin for erythroid precursors, and CD34, CD117, and TdT for blasts. Megakaryocytes can be small and hypolobulated and might be missed without CD61 staining.

Differential Diagnosis

The differential diagnosis of blueberry muffin appearance includes congenital LC, Langerhans cells histiocytosis, congenital vascular malformations such as multifocal hemangiomas and lymphangioendotheliomatosis, glomangiomas, and blue rubber bleb nevus syndrome.

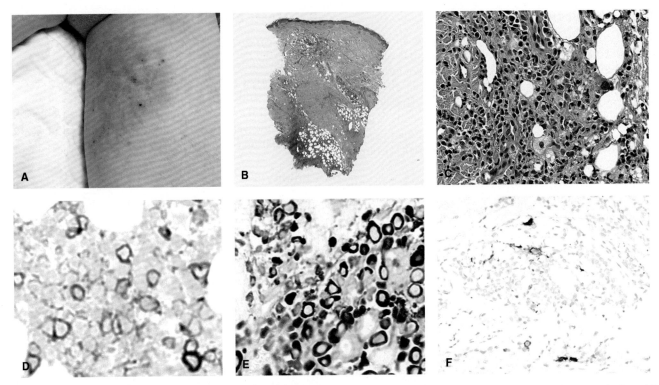

FIGURE 27-46. Extramedullary hematopoiesis. A, Extramedullary hematopoiesis presenting as pink, erythematous patch. B and C, Dermal perivascular infiltrates stained with hematoxylin and eosin show scattered blasts, immature myeloid forms, eosinophils, erythroid elements, and dysmorphic hypolobulated megakaryocytes. D, Megakaryocytes are decorated by CD61. E, Scattered blasts express C-Kit. F, Immature myeloid cells are highlighted by myeloperoxidase. A, Photo courtesy of Urvi Patel, MD, Washington University School of Medicine in St. Louis; reprinted with permission Gru AA, Schaffer A. *Hematopathology of the Skin: A Clinical and Pathologic Approach.* Philadelphia, PA: Wolters Kluwer; 2016.

CAPSULE SUMMARY

EXTRAMEDULLARY HEMATOPOIESIS

EMH is defined as nonneoplastic extramedullary erythropoiesis that is typically seen secondary to intrauterine infections and hemoglobinopathies. Skin involvement is an extremely rare manifestation. The clinical presentation of EMH is similar to those of other cutaneous metastases, such as the presence of pink or red-violaceous macules, papules, and nodules, typically on the trunk, or as "blueberry muffin." Histopathologically, there are clusters of normoblastic erythropoiesis with nucleated red blood cell precursors in the dermis.

REFERENCES

1. O'Suoji C, Welch JJ, Perkins SL, et al. Rare pediatric non-Hodgkin lymphomas: a report from Children's Oncology Group Study ANHL 04B1. *Pediatr Blood Cancer.* 2016;63(5):794-800.
2. Kempf W, Kazakov DV, Belousova IE, Mitteldorf C, Kerl K. Paediatric cutaneous lymphomas: a review and comparison with adult counterparts. *J Eur Acad Dermatol Venereol.* 2015;29(9):1696-1709.
3. Fink-Puches R, Chott A, Ardigo M, et al. The spectrum of cutaneous lymphomas in patients less than 20 years of age. *Pediatr Dermatol.* 2004;21(5):525-533.
4. Boccara O, Blanche S, de Prost Y, Brousse N, Bodemer C, Fraitag S. Cutaneous hematologic disorders in children. *Pediatr Blood Cancer.* 2012;58(2):226-232.
5. Beljaards RC, Kaudewitz P, Berti E, et al. Primary cutaneous CD30-positive large cell lymphoma: definition of a new type of cutaneous lymphoma with a favorable prognosis. A European Multicenter Study of 47 patients. *Cancer.* 1993;71(6):2097-2104.
6. Ralfkiaer E, Willemze R, Paulli M, Kadin ME. *CD30-positive T-cell lymphoproliferative disorders.* 4th ed. Lyon, France: International Agency for Research on Cancer; 2008.
7. Willemze R, Beljaards RC. Spectrum of primary cutaneous CD30 (Ki-1)-positive lymphoproliferative disorders. A proposal for classification and guidelines for management and treatment. *J Am Acad Dermatol.* 1993;28(6):973-980.
8. Kempf W. CD30+ lymphoproliferative disorders: histopathology, differential diagnosis, new variants, and simulators. *J Cutan Pathol.* 2006;33 suppl 1:58-70.
9. Kumar S, Pittaluga S, Raffeld M, Guerrera M, Seibel NL, Jaffe ES. Primary cutaneous CD30-positive anaplastic large cell lymphoma in childhood: report of 4 cases and review of the literature. *Pediatr Dev Pathol.* 2005;8(1):52-60.
10. Papalas JA, Van Mater D, Wang E. Pyogenic variant of primary cutaneous anaplastic large-cell lymphoma: a lymphoproliferative disorder with a predilection for the immunocompromized and the young. *Am J Dermatopathol.* 2010;32(8):821-827.
11. Sciallis AP, Law ME, Inwards DJ, et al. Mucosal CD30-positive T-cell lymphoproliferations of the head and neck show a clinicopathologic spectrum similar to cutaneous CD30-positive T-cell lymphoproliferative disorders. *Mod Pathol.* 2012;25(7):983-992.

12. Tomaszewski MM, Moad JC, Lupton GP. Primary cutaneous Ki-1(CD30) positive anaplastic large cell lymphoma in childhood. *J Am Acad Dermatol.* 1999;40(5, pt 2):857-861.

13. Vaid R, Cohen B. Primary cutaneous CD30 positive anaplastic large cell lymphoma in an adolescent. *Pediatr Dermatol.* 2009;26(6):721-724.

14. Mahajan VK, Jindal R. Primary cutaneous anaplastic large cell lymphoma in a child simulating primary cutaneous Hodgkin's disease. *Indian J Dermatol Venereol Leprol.* 2016;82(1):98-101.

15. Camisa C, Helm TN, Sexton C, Tuthill R. Ki-1-positive anaplastic large-cell lymphoma can mimic benign dermatoses. *J Am Acad Dermatol.* 1993;29(5, pt 1):696-700.

16. Jhala DN, Medeiros LJ, Lopez-Terrada D, Jhala NC, Krishnan B, Shahab I. Neutrophil-rich anaplastic large cell lymphoma of T-cell lineage. A report of two cases arising in HIV-positive patients. *Am J Clin Pathol.* 2000;114(3):478-482.

17. Salama S. Primary "cutaneous" T-cell anaplastic large cell lymphoma, CD30+, neutrophil-rich variant with subcutaneous panniculitic lesions, in a post-renal transplant patient: report of unusual case and literature review. *Am J Dermatopathol.* 2005;27(3):217-223.

18. Kong YY, Dai B, Kong JC, Lu HF, Shi DR. Neutrophil/eosinophil-rich type of primary cutaneous anaplastic large cell lymphoma: a clinico-pathological, immunophenotypic and molecular study of nine cases. *Histopathology.* 2009;55(2):189-196.

19. de Bruin PC, Beljaards RC, van Heerde P, et al. Differences in clinical behaviour and immunophenotype between primary cutaneous and primary nodal anaplastic large cell lymphoma of T-cell or null cell phenotype. *Histopathology.* 1993;23(2):127-135.

20. Plaza JA, Feldman AL, Magro C. Cutaneous CD30-positive lymphoproliferative disorders with CD8 expression: a clinicopathologic study of 21 cases. *J Cutan Pathol.* 2013;40(2):236-247.

21. Wang X, Boddicker RL, Dasari S, et al. Expression of p63 protein in anaplastic large cell lymphoma: implications for genetic subtyping. *Hum Pathol.* 2017;64:19-27.

22. Onaindia A, Montes-Moreno S, Rodriguez-Pinilla SM, et al. Primary cutaneous anaplastic large cell lymphomas with 6p25.3 rearrangement exhibit particular histological features. *Histopathology.* 2015;66(6):846-855.

23. Swerdlow SH, Campo E, Pileri SA, et al. The 2016 revision of the World Health Organization classification of lymphoid neoplasms. *Blood.* 2016;127(20):2375-2390.

24. Burg G, Kempf W, Cozzio A, et al. WHO/EORTC classification of cutaneous lymphomas 2005: histological and molecular aspects. *J Cutan Pathol.* 2005;32(10):647-674.

25. Willemze R, Jaffe ES, Burg G, et al. WHO-EORTC classification for cutaneous lymphomas. *Blood.* 2005;105(10):3768-3785.

26. Castano E, Glick S, Wolgast L, et al. Hypopigmented mycosis fungoides in childhood and adolescence: a long-term retrospective study. *J Cutan Pathol.* 2013;40(11):924-934.

27. Crowley JJ, Nikko A, Varghese A, Hoppe RT, Kim YH. Mycosis fungoides in young patients: clinical characteristics and outcome. *J Am Acad Dermatol.* 1998;38(5, pt 1):696-701.

28. El-Shabrawi-Caelen L, Cerroni L, Medeiros LJ, McCalmont TH. Hypopigmented mycosis fungoides: frequent expression of a CD8+ T-cell phenotype. *Am J Surg Pathol.* 2002;26(4):450-457.

29. Pope E, Weitzman S, Ngan B, et al. Mycosis fungoides in the pediatric population: report from an International Childhood Registry of Cutaneous Lymphoma. *J Cutan Med Surg.* 2010;14(1):1-6.

30. Cervini AB, Torres-Huamani AN, Sanchez-La-Rosa C, et al. Mycosis fungoides: experience in a pediatric hospital [in English, Spanish]. *Actas Dermosifiliogr.* 2017;108(6):564-570.

31. Koch SE, Zackheim HS, Williams ML, Fletcher V, LeBoit PE. Mycosis fungoides beginning in childhood and adolescence. *J Am Acad Dermatol.* 1987;17(4):563-570.

32. Peters MS, Thibodeau SN, White JW Jr, Winkelmann RK. Mycosis fungoides in children and adolescents. *J Am Acad Dermatol.* 1990;22(6, pt 1):1011-1018.

33. Wain EM, Orchard GE, Whittaker SJ, Spittle MF, Russell-Jones R. Outcome in 34 patients with juvenile-onset mycosis fungoides: a clinical, immunophenotypic, and molecular study. *Cancer.* 2003;98(10):2282-2290.

34. Zackheim HS, McCalmont TH, Deanovic FW, Odom RB. Mycosis fungoides with onset before 20 years of age. *J Am Acad Dermatol.* 1997;36(4):557-562.

35. Tan E, Tay YK, Giam YC. Profile and outcome of childhood mycosis fungoides in Singapore. *Pediatr Dermatol.* 2000;17(5):352-356.

36. Choi J, Goh G, Walradt T, et al. Genomic landscape of cutaneous T cell lymphoma. *Nat Genet.* 2015;47(9):1011-1019.

37. da Silva Almeida AC, Abate F, Khiabanian H, et al. The mutational landscape of cutaneous T cell lymphoma and Sezary syndrome. *Nat Genet.* 2015.

38. Kiel MJ, Sahasrabuddhe AA, Rolland DC, et al. Genomic analyses reveal recurrent mutations in epigenetic modifiers and the JAK-STAT pathway in Sezary syndrome. *Nat Commun.* 2015;6:8470.

39. Ungewickell A, Bhaduri A, Rios E, et al. Genomic analysis of mycosis fungoides and Sezary syndrome identifies recurrent alterations in TNFR2. *Nat Genet.* 2015;47(9):1056-1060.

40. Wang L, Ni X, Covington KR, et al. Genomic profiling of Sezary syndrome identifies alterations of key T cell signaling and differentiation genes. *Nat Genet.* 2015;47(12):1426-1434.

41. Werner B, Brown S, Ackerman AB. "Hypopigmented mycosis fungoides" is not always mycosis fungoides! *Am J Dermatopathol.* 2005;27(1):56-67.

42. Ngo JT, Trotter MJ, Haber RM. Juvenile-onset hypopigmented mycosis fungoides mimicking vitiligo. *J Cutan Med Surg.* 2009;13(4):230-233.

43. Zackheim HS, McCalmont TH. Mycosis fungoides: the great imitator. *J Am Acad Dermatol.* 2002;47(6):914-918.

44. Heng YK, Koh MJ, Giam YC, Tang MB, Chong WS, Tan SH. Pediatric mycosis fungoides in Singapore: a series of 46 children. *Pediatr Dermatol.* 2014;31(4):477-482.

45. Amin A, Burkhart C, Groben P, Morrell DS. Primary cutaneous T-cell lymphoma following organ transplantation in a 16-year-old boy. *Pediatr Dermatol.* 2009;26(1):112-113.

46. Hodak E, Amitay-Laish I, Feinmesser M, et al. Juvenile mycosis fungoides: cutaneous T-cell lymphoma with frequent follicular involvement. *J Am Acad Dermatol.* 2014;70(6):993-1001.

47. Alikhan A, Griffin J, Nguyen N, Davis DM, Gibson LE. Pediatric follicular mucinosis: presentation, histopathology, molecular genetics, treatment, and outcomes over an 11-year period at the Mayo Clinic. *Pediatr Dermatol.* 2013;30(2):192-198.

48. Hess Schmid M, Dummer R, Kempf W, Hilty N, Burg G. Mycosis fungoides with mucinosis follicularis in childhood. *Dermatology.* 1999;198(3):284-287.

49. Santos-Briz A, Canueto J, Garcia-Dorado J, Alonso MT, Balanzategui A, Gonzalez-Diaz M. Pediatric primary follicular mucinosis: further evidence of its relationship with mycosis fungoides. *Pediatr Dermatol.* 2013;30(6):e218-e220.

50. van Doorn R, Scheffer E, Willemze R. Follicular mycosis fungoides, a distinct disease entity with or without associated follicular mucinosis: a clinicopathologic and follow-up study of 51 patients. *Arch Dermatol.* 2002;138(2):191-198.

51. Convit J, Kerdel F, Goihman M, Rondon AJ, Soto JM. Progressive, atrophying, chronic granulomatous dermohypodermitis. Autoimmune disease? *Arch Dermatol.* 1973;107(2):271-274.

52. Helm KF, Cerio R, Winkelmann RK. Granulomatous slack skin: a clinicopathological and immunohistochemical study of three cases. *Br J Dermatol.* 1992;126(2):142-147.

53. LeBoit PE, Beckstead JH, Bond B, Epstein WL, Frieden IJ, Parslow TG. Granulomatous slack skin: clonal rearrangement of the T-cell receptor beta gene is evidence for the lymphoproliferative nature of a cutaneous elastolytic disorder. *J Invest Dermatol.* 1987;89(2):183-186.

54. Noto G, Pravata G, Miceli S, Arico M. Granulomatous slack skin: report of a case associated with Hodgkin's disease and a review of the literature. *Br J Dermatol.* 1994;131(2):275-279.

55. Wieser I, Wohlmuth C, Duvic M. Granulomatous mycosis fungoides in an adolescent-A rare encounter and review of the literature. *Pediatr Dermatol.* 2016;33(5):e296-e298.

56. Camacho FM, Burg G, Moreno JC, Campora RG, Villar JL. Granulomatous slack skin in childhood. *Pediatr Dermatol.* 1997;14(3):204-208.

57. Matsuzaki Y, Kimura K, Nakano H, Hanada K, Sawamura D. Localized pagetoid reticulosis (Woringer-Kolopp disease) in early childhood. *J Am Acad Dermatol.* 2009;61(1):120-123.

58. Mendese GW, Beckford A, Krejci N, Mahalingam M, Goldberg L, Gilchrest BA. Pagetoid reticulosis in a prepubescent boy successfully treated with photodynamic therapy. *Clin Exp Dermatol.* 2012;37(7):759-761.

59. Miedler JD, Kristjansson AK, Gould J, Tamburro J, Gilliam AC. Pagetoid reticulosis in a 5-year-old boy. *J Am Acad Dermatol.* 2008;58(4):679-681.

60. Ai WZ, Keegan TH, Press DJ, et al. Outcomes after diagnosis of mycosis fungoides and Sezary syndrome before 30 years of age: a population-based study. *JAMA Dermatol.* 2014;150(7):709-715.

61. LeBoit PE, Abel EA, Cleary ML, et al. Clonal rearrangement of the T cell receptor beta gene in the circulating lymphocytes of erythrodermic follicular mucinosis. *Blood.* 1988;71(5):1329-1333.

62. Meister L, Duarte AM, Davis J, Perez JL, Schachner LA. Sezary syndrome in an 11-year-old girl. *J Am Acad Dermatol.* 1993;28(1):93-95.

63. Magro CM, Nguyen GH. Keratoderma-like T cell dyscrasia: a report of 13 cases and its distinction from mycosis fungoides palmaris et plantaris. *Indian J Dermatol Venereol Leprol.* 2016;82(4):395-403.

64. Smoller BR, Santucci M, Wood GS, Whittaker SJ. Histopathology and genetics of cutaneous T-cell lymphoma. *Hematol Oncol Clin North Am.* 2003;17(6):1277-1311.

65. Romero M, Haney M, Desantis E, Zlotoff B. Mycosis fungoides with focal CD 30 transformation in an adolescent. *Pediatr Dermatol.* 2008;25(5):565-568.

66. Carrie E, Buzyn A, Fraitag S, Hermine O, Bodemer C. Transformed juvenile-onset mycosis fungoides: treatment by bone marrow transplantation with graft-versus-lymphoma effect [in French]. *Ann Dermatol Venereol.* 2007;134(5, pt 1):471-476.

67. Gerami P, Guitart J. The spectrum of histopathologic and immunohistochemical findings in folliculotropic mycosis fungoides. *Am J Surg Pathol.* 2007;31(9):1430-1438.

68. Ben-Amitai D, Michael D, Feinmesser M, Hodak E. Juvenile mycosis fungoides diagnosed before 18 years of age. *Acta Derm Venereol.* 2003;83(6):451-456.

69. Hanna S, Walsh N, D'Intino Y, Langley RG. Mycosis fungoides presenting as pigmented purpuric dermatitis. *Pediatr Dermatol.* 2006;23(4):350-354.

70. Lu D, Patel KA, Duvic M, Jones D. Clinical and pathological spectrum of CD8-positive cutaneous T-cell lymphomas. *J Cutan Pathol.* 2002;29(8):465-472.

71. Moon HR, Lee WJ, Won CH, et al. Paediatric cutaneous lymphoma in Korea: a retrospective study at a single institution. *J Eur Acad Dermatol Venereol.* 2014;28(12):1798-1804..

72. Neuhaus IM, Ramos-Caro FA, Hassanein AM. Hypopigmented mycosis fungoides in childhood and adolescence. *Pediatr Dermatol.* 2000;17(5):403-406.

73. Quaglino P, Zaccagna A, Verrone A, Dardano F, Bernengo MG. Mycosis fungoides in patients under 20 years of age: report of 7 cases, review of the literature and study of the clinical course. *Dermatology.* 1999;199(1):8-14.

74. Wang T, Liu YH, Zheng HY, et al. Hypopigmented mycosis fungoides in children: a clinicopathological study of 6 cases [in Chinese]. *Zhonghua Yi Xue Za Zhi.* 2010;90(46):3287-3290.

75. Whittam LR, Calonje E, Orchard G, Fraser-Andrews EA, Woolford A, Russell-Jones R. CD8-positive juvenile onset mycosis fungoides: an immunohistochemical and genotypic analysis of six cases. *Br J Dermatol.* 2000;143(6):1199-1204.

76. Singh ZN, Tretiakova MS, Shea CR, Petronic-Rosic VM. Decreased CD117 expression in hypopigmented mycosis fungoides correlates with hypomelanosis: lessons learned from vitiligo. *Mod Pathol.* 2006;19(9):1255-1260.

77. Hodak E, David M, Maron L, Aviram A, Kaganovsky E, Feinmesser M. CD4/CD8 double-negative epidermotropic cutaneous T-cell lymphoma: an immunohistochemical variant of mycosis fungoides. *J Am Acad Dermatol.* 2006;55(2):276-284.

78. Wain EM, Orchard GE, Mayou S, Atherton DJ, Misch KJ, Russell-Jones R. Mycosis fungoides with a CD56+ immunophenotype. *J Am Acad Dermatol.* 2005;53(1):158-163.

79. Pimpinelli N, Olsen EA, Santucci M, et al. Defining early mycosis fungoides. *J Am Acad Dermatol.* 2005;53(6):1053-1063.

80. Ramsay B, Dahl MC, Malcolm AJ, Wilson-Jones E. Acral pseudolymphomatous angiokeratoma of children. *Arch Dermatol.* 1990;126(11):1524-1525.

81. Kirsch IR, Watanabe R, O'Malley JT, et al. TCR sequencing facilitates diagnosis and identifies mature T cells as the cell of origin in CTCL. *Sci Transl Med.* 2015;7(308):308ra158.

82. Macaulay WL. Lymphomatoid papulosis. A continuing self-healing eruption, clinically benign--histologically malignant. *Arch Dermatol.* 1968;97(1):23-30.

83. Nijsten T, Curiel-Lewandrowski C, Kadin ME. Lymphomatoid papulosis in children: a retrospective cohort study of 35 cases. *Arch Dermatol.* 2004;140(3):306-312.

84. Kunishige JH, McDonald H, Alvarez G, Johnson M, Prieto V, Duvic M. Lymphomatoid papulosis and associated lymphomas: a retrospective case series of 84 patients. *Clin Exp Dermatol.* 2009;34(5):576-581.

85. Zackheim HS, Jones C, Leboit PE, Kashani-Sabet M, McCalmont TH, Zehnder J. Lymphomatoid papulosis associated with mycosis fungoides: a study of 21 patients including analyses for clonality. *J Am Acad Dermatol.* 2003;49(4):620-623.

86. Miquel J, Fraitag S, Hamel-Teillac D, et al. Lymphomatoid papulosis in children: a series of 25 cases. *Br J Dermatol.* 2014;171(5):1138-1146.

87. Martorell-Calatayud A, Hernandez-Martin A, Colmenero I, et al. Lymphomatoid papulosis in children: report of 9 cases and review of the literature [in Spanish]. *Actas Dermosifiliogr.* 2010;101(8):693-701.

88. Wieser I, Wohlmuth C, Nunez CA, Duvic M. Lymphomatoid papulosis in children and adolescents: a systematic review. *Am J Clin Dermatol.* 2016;17(4):319-327.

89. Karai LJ, Kadin ME, Hsi ED, et al. Chromosomal rearrangements of 6p25.3 define a new subtype of lymphomatoid papulosis. *Am J Surg Pathol.* 2013;37(8):1173-1181.

90. Bekkenk MW, Geelen FA, van Voorst Vader PC, et al. Primary and secondary cutaneous CD30(+) lymphoproliferative disorders: a report from the Dutch Cutaneous Lymphoma Group on the long-term follow-up data of 219 patients and guidelines for diagnosis and treatment. *Blood.* 2000;95(12):3653-3661.

91. de Souza A, Camilleri MJ, Wada DA, Appert DL, Gibson LE, el-Azhary RA. Clinical, histopathologic, and immunophenotypic features of lymphomatoid papulosis with CD8 predominance in 14 pediatric patients. *J Am Acad Dermatol.* 2009;61(6):993-1000.

92. Scarisbrick JJ, Evans AV, Woolford AJ, Black MM, Russell-Jones R. Regional lymphomatoid papulosis: a report of four cases. *Br J Dermatol.* 1999;141(6):1125-1128.

93. Thomas GJ, Conejo-Mir JS, Ruiz AP, Linares Barrios M, Navarrete M. Lymphomatoid papulosis in childhood with exclusive acral involvement. *Pediatr Dermatol.* 1998;15(2):146-147.

94. Saggini A, Gulia A, Argenyi Z, et al. A variant of lymphomatoid papulosis simulating primary cutaneous aggressive epidermotropic CD8+ cytotoxic T-cell lymphoma. Description of 9 cases. *Am J Surg Pathol.* 2010;34(8):1168-1175.

95. Kempf W, Kazakov DV, Scharer L, et al. Angioinvasive lymphomatoid papulosis: a new variant simulating aggressive lymphomas. *Am J Surg Pathol.* 2013;37(1):1-13.

96. Pierard GE. A reappraisal of lymphomatoid papulosis and of its follicular variant. *Am J Dermatopathol.* 1981;3(2):179-181.

97. Pierard GE, Ackerman AB, Lapiere CM. Follicular lymphomatoid papulosis. *Am J Dermatopathol.* 1980;2(2):173-180.

98. Kempf W, Kazakov DV, Baumgartner HP, Kutzner H. Follicular lymphomatoid papulosis revisited: a study of 11 cases, with new histopathological findings. *J Am Acad Dermatol.* 2013;68(5):809-816.

99. Ross NA, Truong H, Keller MS, Mulholland JK, Lee JB, Sahu J. Follicular lymphomatoid papulosis: an eosinophilic-rich follicular subtype masquerading as folliculitis clinically and histologically. *Am J Dermatopathol.* 2016;38(1):e1-e10.

100. Kummer JA, Vermeer MH, Dukers D, Meijer CJ, Willemze R. Most primary cutaneous CD30-positive lymphoproliferative disorders have a CD4-positive cytotoxic T-cell phenotype. *J Invest Dermatol.* 1997;109(5):636-640.

101. Kadin ME. Common activated helper-T-cell origin for lymphomatoid papulosis, mycosis fungoides, and some types of Hodgkin's disease. *Lancet.* 1985;2(8460):864-865.

102. Kaudewitz P, Burg G, Stein H, Klepzig K, Mason DY, Braun-Falco O. Monoclonal antibody patterns in lymphomatoid papulosis. *Dermatol Clin.* 1985;3(4):749-757.

103. Benharroch D, Meguerian-Bedoyan Z, Lamant L, et al. ALK-positive lymphoma: a single disease with a broad spectrum of morphology. *Blood.* 1998;91(6):2076-2084.

104. Criscione VD, Weinstock MA. Incidence of cutaneous T-cell lymphoma in the United States, 1973-2002. *Arch Dermatol.* 2007;143(7):854-859.

105. Delsol G, Falini B, Muller-Hermelink HK, et al. *Anaplastic Large Cell Lymphoma (ALCL), ALK-Positive.* 4th ed. Lyon, France: International Agency for Research on Cancer; 2008.

106. Falini B, Pileri S, Zinzani PL, et al. ALK+ lymphoma: clinico-pathological findings and outcome. *Blood.* 1999;93(8):2697-2706.

107. Bajor-Dattilo EB, Pittaluga S, Jaffe ES. Pathobiology of T-cell and NK-cell lymphomas. *Best Prac Res Clin Haematol.* 2013;26(1):75-87.

108. Savage KJ, Harris NL, Vose JM, et al. ALK- anaplastic large-cell lymphoma is clinically and immunophenotypically different from both ALK+ ALCL and peripheral T-cell lymphoma, not otherwise specified: report from the International Peripheral T-Cell Lymphoma Project. *Blood.* 2008;111(12):5496-5504.

109. de Leval L. Molecular classification of ganglionic T cell lymphomas. pathological and diagnostic implications [in French]. *Bull Mem Acad R Med Belg.* 2010;165(1-2):99.

110. de Leval L, Bisig B, Thielen C, Boniver J, Gaulard P. Molecular classification of T-cell lymphomas. *Crit Rev Oncol/Hematol.* 2009;72(2):125-143.

111. Kinney MC, Higgins RA, Medina EA. Anaplastic large cell lymphoma: twenty-five years of discovery. *Arch Pathol Lab Med.* 2011;135(1):19-43.

112. Ando K, Tamada Y, Shimizu K, et al. ALK-positive primary systemic anaplastic large cell lymphoma with extensive cutaneous manifestation. *Acta Derm Venereol.* 2010;90(2):198-200.

113. Chan DV, Summers P, Tuttle M, et al. Anaplastic lymphoma kinase expression in a recurrent primary cutaneous anaplastic large cell lymphoma with eventual systemic involvement. *J Am Acad Dermatol.* 2011;65(3):671-673.

114. Hosoi M, Ichikawa M, Imai Y, Kurokawa M. A case of anaplastic large cell lymphoma, ALK positive, primary presented in the skin and relapsed with systemic involvement and leukocytosis after years of follow-up period. *Int J Hematol.* 2010;92(4):667-668.

115. Ogunrinade O, Lin O, Steinhertz P, Pulitzer M. ALK-positive (2p23 rearranged) anaplastic large cell lymphoma with localization to the skin in a pediatric patient. *J Cutan Pathol.* 2015;42(3):182-187.

116. Bayle C, Charpentier A, Duchayne E, et al. Leukaemic presentation of small cell variant anaplastic large cell lymphoma: report of four cases. *Br J Haematol.* 1999;104(4):680-688.

117. Fraga M, Brousset P, Schlaifer D, et al. Bone marrow involvement in anaplastic large cell lymphoma. Immunohistochemical detection

of minimal disease and its prognostic significance. *Am J Clin Pathol.* 1995;103(1):82-89.

118. Lamant L, Pileri S, Sabattini E, Brugieres L, Jaffe ES, Delsol G. Cutaneous presentation of ALK-positive anaplastic large cell lymphoma following insect bites: evidence for an association in five cases. *Haematologica.* 2010;95(3):449-455.

119. Piccaluga PP, Ascani S, Fraternali Orcioni G, et al. Anaplastic lymphoma kinase expression as a marker of malignancy. Application to a case of anaplastic large cell lymphoma with huge granulomatous reaction. *Haematologica.* 2000;85(9):978-981.

120. Hoshina D, Arita K, Mizuno O, et al. Skin involvement in ALK-negative systemic anaplastic large-cell lymphoma. *J Am Acad Dermatol.* 2012;67(4):e159-e160.

121. Marschalko M, Eros N, Hollo P, et al. Secondary ALK negative anaplastic large cell lymphoma in a patient with lymphomatoid papulosis of 40 years duration. *Am J Dermatopathol.* 2010;32(7):708-712.

122. Querfeld C, Khan I, Mahon B, Nelson BP, Rosen ST, Evens AM. Primary cutaneous and systemic anaplastic large cell lymphoma: clinicopathologic aspects and therapeutic options. *Oncology.* 2010;24(7):574-587.

123. Oschlies I, Lisfeld J, Lamant L, et al. ALK-positive anaplastic large cell lymphoma limited to the skin: clinical, histopathological and molecular analysis of 6 pediatric cases. A report from the ALCL99 study. *Haematologica.* 2013;98(1):50-56.

124. Hanafusa T, Igawa K, Takagawa S, et al. Erythroderma as a paraneoplastic cutaneous disorder in systemic anaplastic large cell lymphoma. *J Eur Acad Dermatol Venereol.* 2012;26(6):710-713.

125. Mencia-Gutierrez E, Gutierrez-Diaz E, Salamanca J, Martinez-Gonzalez MA. Cutaneous presentation on the eyelid of primary, systemic, CD30+, anaplastic lymphoma kinase (ALK)-negative, anaplastic large-cell lymphoma (ALCL). *Int J Dermatol.* 2006;45(6):766-769.

126. Rodis DG, Liatsos GD, Moulakakis A, Pirounaki M, Tasidou A. Paraneoplastic cerebellar degeneration: initial presentation in a patient with anaplastic T-cell lymphoma, associated with ichthyosiform cutaneous lesions. *Leuk Lymphoma.* 2009;50(8):1369-1371.

127. Ferreri AJ, Govi S, Pileri SA, Savage KJ. Anaplastic large cell lymphoma, ALK-positive. *Crit Rev Oncol Hematol.* 2012;83(2):293-302.

128. Jaffe ES, Nicolae A, Pittaluga S. Peripheral T-cell and NK-cell lymphomas in the WHO classification: pearls and pitfalls. *Mod Pathol.* 2013;26 suppl 1:S71-87.

129. Vassallo J, Lamant L, Brugieres L, et al. ALK-positive anaplastic large cell lymphoma mimicking nodular sclerosis Hodgkin's lymphoma: report of 10 cases. *Am J Surg Pathol.* 2006;30(2):223-229.

130. Beylot-Barry M, Groppi A, Vergier B, Pulford K, Merlio JP. Characterization of t(2;5) reciprocal transcripts and genomic breakpoints in CD30+ cutaneous lymphoproliferations. *Blood.* 1998;91(12):4668-4676.

131. Kadin ME, Pinkus JL, Pinkus GS, et al. Primary cutaneous ALCL with phosphorylated/activated cytoplasmic ALK and novel phenotype: EMA/MUC1+, cutaneous lymphocyte antigen negative. *Am J Surg Pathol.* 2008;32(9):1421-1426.

132. Jaffe ES, Gaulard P, Ralfiaer E. *Subcutaneous Panniculitis-Like T-cell Lymphoma.* 4th ed. Lyon, France: International Agency for Research on Cancer; 2008.

133. Slater DN. The new World Health Organization-European Organization for Research and Treatment of Cancer classification for cutaneous lymphomas: a practical marriage of two giants. *Br J Dermatol.* 2005;153(5):874-880.

134. Willemze R, Jansen PM, Cerroni L, et al. Subcutaneous panniculitis-like T-cell lymphoma: definition, classification, and prognostic factors: an EORTC Cutaneous Lymphoma Group Study of 83 cases. *Blood.* 2008;111(2):838-845.

135. Huppmann AR, Xi L, Raffeld M, Pittaluga S, Jaffe ES. Subcutaneous panniculitis-like T-cell lymphoma in the pediatric age group:

a lymphoma of low malignant potential. *Pediatr Blood Cancer.* 2013;60(7):1165-1170.

136. Kawachi Y, Furuta J, Fujisawa Y, Nakamura Y, Ishii Y, Otsuka F. Indolent subcutaneous panniculitis-like T cell lymphoma in a 1-year-old child. *Pediatr Dermatol.* 2012;29(3):374-377.

137. Gupta V, Arava S, Bakhshi S, Vashisht KR, Reddy R, Gupta S. Subcutaneous panniculitis-like T-cell lymphoma with hemophagocytic syndrome in a child. *Pediatr Dermatol.* 2016;33(2):e72-e76.

138. Johnston EE, LeBlanc RE, Kim J, et al. Subcutaneous panniculitis-like T-cell lymphoma: Pediatric case series demonstrating heterogeneous presentation and option for watchful waiting. *Pediatr Blood Cancer.* 2015;62(11):2025-2028.

139. Mellgren K, Attarbaschi A, Abla O, et al. Non-anaplastic peripheral T cell lymphoma in children and adolescents-an international review of 143 cases. *Ann Hematol.* 2016;95(8):1295-1305.

140. Yi L, Qun S, Wenjie Z, et al. The presenting manifestations of subcutaneous panniculitis-like T-cell lymphoma and T-cell lymphoma and cutaneous gammadelta T-cell lymphoma may mimic those of rheumatic diseases: a report of 11 cases. *Clin Rheumatol.* 2013;32(8):1169-1175.

141. Bosisio F, Boi S, Caputo V, et al. Lobular panniculitic infiltrates with overlapping histopathologic features of lupus panniculitis (lupus profundus) and subcutaneous T-cell lymphoma: a conceptual and practical dilemma. *Am J Surg Pathol.* 2014;39(2):206-211.

142. Pincus LB, LeBoit PE, McCalmont TH, et al. Subcutaneous panniculitis-like T-cell lymphoma with overlapping clinicopathologic features of lupus erythematosus: coexistence of 2 entities? *Am J Dermatopathol.* 2009;31(6):520-526.

143. Joseph LD, Panicker VK, Prathiba D, Damodharan J. Subcutaneous panniculitis-like T cell lymphoma in a HIV positive patient. *J Assoc Physicians India.* 2005;53:314-316.

144. Iqbal K, Bott J, Greenblatt D, et al. Subcutaneous panniculitis-like T-cell lymphoma in association with sarcoidosis. *Clin Exp Dermatol.* 2011;36(6):677-679.

145. Michot C, Costes V, Gerard-Dran D, Guillot B, Combes B, Dereure O. Subcutaneous panniculitis-like T-cell lymphoma in a patient receiving etanercept for rheumatoid arthritis. *Br J Dermatol.* 2009;160(4):889-890.

146. Schmutz JL, Trechot P. Subcutaneous panniculitis-like T-cell lymphoma following treatment with rituximab and cyclophosphamide [in French]. *Ann Dermatol Venereol.* 2013;140(3):246-247.

147. Mixon B, Drach L, Monforte H, Barbosa J. Subcutaneous panniculitis-like T-cell lymphoma in a child with trisomy 21. *Fetal Pediatr Pathol.* 2010;29(6):380-384.

148. Swain M, Swarnalata G, Bhandari T. Subcutaneous panniculitis-like T-cell lymphoma in a case of carcinoma cervix. *Indian J Med Paediatr Oncol.* 2013;34(2):104-106.

149. Reimer P, Rudiger T, Muller J, Rose C, Wilhelm M, Weissinger F. Subcutaneous panniculitis-like T-cell lymphoma during pregnancy with successful autologous stem cell transplantation. *Ann Hematol.* 2003;82(5):305-309.

150. Reich A, Butrym A, Mazur G, et al. Subcutaneous panniculitis-like T-cell lymphoma in type 1 neurofibromatosis: a case report. *Acta Dermatovenerol Croat.* 2014;22(2):145-149.

151. Leonard GD, Hegde U, Butman J, Jaffe ES, Wilson WH. Extraoular muscle palsies in subcutaneous panniculitis-like T-cell lymphoma. *J Clin Oncol.* 2003;21(15):2993-2995.

152. Gualco G, Chioato L, Harrington WJ Jr, Weiss LM, Bacchi CE. Primary and secondary T-cell lymphomas of the breast: clinico-pathologic features of 11 cases. *Appl Immunohistochem Mol Morphol.* 2009;17(4):301-306.

153. Jeong SI, Lim HS, Choi YR, et al. Subcutaneous panniculitis-like T-cell lymphoma of the breast. *Korean J Radiol.* 2013;14(3):391-394.

154. Risulo M, Rubegni P, Sbano P, et al. Subcutaneous panniculitis lymphoma: erythema nodosum-like. *Clin Lymphoma Myeloma.* 2006;7(3):239-241.

155. Chiu HY, He GY, Chen JS, Hsiao PF, Hsiao CH, Tsai TF. Subcutaneous panniculitis-like T-cell lymphoma presenting with clinicopathologic features of dermatomyositis. *J Am Acad Dermatol.* 2011;64(6):e121-e123.

156. Kaieda S, Idemoto A, Yoshida N, Ida H. A subcutaneous panniculitis-like T-cell lymphoma mimicking dermatomyositis. *Intern Med.* 2014;53(13):1455.

157. Troskot N, Lugovic L, Situm M, Vucic M. From circumscribed scleroderma (morphea) to subcutaneous panniculitis-like T-cell lymphoma: case report. *Acta Dermatovenerol Croat.* 2004;12(4):289-293.

158. Tzeng HE, Teng CL, Yang Y, Young JH, Chou G. Occult subcutaneous panniculitis-like T-cell lymphoma with initial presentations of cellulitis-like skin lesion and fulminant hemophagocytosis. *J Formos Med Assoc.* 2007;106(2 suppl):S55-S59.

159. Velez NF, Ishizawar RC, Dellaripa PF, et al. Full facial edema: a novel presentation of subcutaneous panniculitis-like T-cell lymphoma. *J Clin Oncol.* 2012;30(25):e233-e236.

160. Weenig RH, Daniel Su WP. Subcutaneous panniculitis-like T-cell lymphoma presenting as venous stasis ulceration. *Int J Dermatol.* 2006;45(9):1083-1085.

161. Weenig RH, Ng CS, Perniciaro C. Subcutaneous panniculitis-like T-cell lymphoma: an elusive case presenting as lipomembranous panniculitis and a review of 72 cases in the literature. *Am J Dermatopathol.* 2001;23(3):206-215.

162. Ghosh SK, Roy D, Mondal P, Bhunia D, Dutta DP. Subcutaneous panniculitis-like T-cell lymphoma with unusual eschar-like crusting. *Dermatol Online J.* 2014;20(2).

163. Thomas J, Maramattom BV, Kuruvilla PM, Varghese J. Subcutaneous panniculitis like T cell lymphoma associated with erythromelalgia. *J Postgrad Med.* 2014;60(3):335-337.

164. Torok L, Gurbity TP, Kirschner A, Krenacs L. Panniculitis-like T-cell lymphoma clinically manifested as alopecia. *Br J Dermatol.* 2002;147(4):785-788.

165. Hahtola S, Burghart E, Jeskanen L, et al. Clinicopathological characterization and genomic aberrations in subcutaneous panniculitis-like T-cell lymphoma. *J Invest Dermatol.* 2008;128(9):2304-2309.

166. Koh MJ, Sadarangani SP, Chan YC, et al. Aggressive subcutaneous panniculitis-like T-cell lymphoma with hemophagocytosis in two children (subcutaneous panniculitis-like T-cell lymphoma). *J Am Acad Dermatol.* 2009;61(5):875-881.

167. Parveen Z, Thompson K. Subcutaneous panniculitis-like T-cell lymphoma: redefinition of diagnostic criteria in the recent World Health Organization-European Organization for Research and Treatment of Cancer classification for cutaneous lymphomas. *Arch Pathol Lab Med.* 2009;133(2):303-308.

168. Gao J, Gauerke SJ, Martinez-Escala ME, et al. Bone marrow involvement by subcutaneous panniculitis-like T-cell lymphoma: a report of three cases. *Mod Pathol.* 2014;27(6):800-807.

169. Ghobrial IM, Weenig RH, Pittlekow MR, et al. Clinical outcome of patients with subcutaneous panniculitis-like T-cell lymphoma. *Leuk Lymphoma.* 2005;46(5):703-708.

170. Babb A, Zerizer I, Naresh KN, Macdonald D. Subcutaneous panniculitis-like T-cell lymphoma with extracutaneous dissemination demonstrated on FDG PET/CT. *Am J Hematol.* 2011;86(4):375-376.

171. Huang CT, Yang WC, Lin SF. Positron-emission tomography findings indicating the involvement of the whole body skin in subcutaneous panniculitis-like T cell lymphoma. *Ann Hematol.* 2011;90(7):853-854.

172. Berg KD, Brinster NK, Huhn KM, et al. Transmission of a T-cell lymphoma by allogeneic bone marrow transplantation. *N Engl J Med.* 2001;345(20):1458-1463.

173. Hathaway T, Subtil A, Kuo P, Foss F. Efficacy of denileukin diftitox in subcutaneous panniculitis-like T-cell lymphoma. *Clin Lymphoma Myeloma.* 2007;7(8):541-545.

174. Messeguer F, Gimeno E, Agusti-Mejias A, San Juan J. Primary cutaneous CD4+ small- to medium-sized pleomorphic T-cell lymphoma:

report of a case with spontaneous resolution [in Spanish]. *Actas Dermosifiliogr.* 2011;102(8):636-638.

175. Ma L, Bandarchi B, Glusac EJ. Fatal subcutaneous panniculitis-like T-cell lymphoma with interface change and dermal mucin, a dead ringer for lupus erythematosus. *J Cutan Pathol.* 2005;32(5):360-365.

176. Acree SC, Tovar JP, Pattengale PK, et al. Subcutaneous panniculitis-like T-cell lymphoma in two pediatric patients: an HIV-positive adolescent and a 4-month-old infant. *Fetal Pediatr Pathol.* 2013;32(3):175-183.

177. Ali SK, Othman NM, Tagoe AB, Tulba AA. Subcutaneous panniculitic T cell lymphoma mimicking histiocytic cytophagic panniculitis in a child. *Saudi Med J.* 2000;21(11):1074-1077.

178. Bader-Meunier B, Fraitag S, Janssen C, et al. Clonal cytophagic histiocytic panniculitis in children may be cured by cyclosporine A. *Pediatrics.* 2013;132(2):e545-e549.

179. Bittencourt AL, Vieira M, Carvalho EG, Cunha C, Araujo I. Subcutaneous panniculitis-like T-cell lymphoma (SPTL) in a child with spontaneous resolution. *Case Rep Oncol Med.* 2011;2011:639240.

180. Grassi S, Borroni RG, Brazzelli V. Panniculitis in children. *G Ital Dermatol Venereol.* 2013;148(4):371-385.

181. Kobayashi R, Yamato K, Tanaka F, et al. Retrospective analysis of non-anaplastic peripheral T-cell lymphoma in pediatric patients in Japan. *Pediatr Blood Cancer.* 2010;54(2):212-215.

182. Lim GY, Hahn ST, Chung NG, Kim HK. Subcutaneous panniculitis-like T-cell lymphoma in a child: whole-body MRI in the initial and follow-up evaluations. *Pediatr Radiol.* 2009;39(1):57-61.

183. Merritt BY, Curry JL, Duvic M, Vega F, Sheehan AM, Curry CV. Pediatric subcutaneous panniculitis-like T-cell lymphoma with features of hemophagocytic syndrome. *Pediatr Blood Cancer.* 2013;60(11):1916-1917.

184. Moraes AJ, Soares PM, Zapata AL, Lotito AP, Sallum AM, Silva CA. Panniculitis in childhood and adolescence. *Pediatr Int.* 2006;48(1):48-53.

185. Nagai K, Nakano N, Iwai T, et al. Pediatric subcutaneous panniculitis-like T-cell lymphoma with favorable result by immunosuppressive therapy: a report of two cases. *Pediatr Hematol Oncol.* 2014;31(6):528-533.

186. Rajic L, Bilic E, Femenic R, et al. Subcutaneous panniculitis-like T-cell lymphoma in a 19 month-old boy: a case report. *Coll Antropol.* 2010;34(2):679-682.

187. Yim JH, Kim MY, Kim HO, Cho B, Chung NG, Park YM. Subcutaneous panniculitis-like T-cell lymphoma in a 26-month-old child with a review of the literature. *Pediatr Dermatol.* 2006;23(6):537-540.

188. Hoque SR, Child FJ, Whittaker SJ, et al. Subcutaneous panniculitis-like T-cell lymphoma: a clinicopathological, immunophenotypic and molecular analysis of six patients. *Br J Dermatol.* 2003;148(3):516-525.

189. Lozzi GP, Massone C, Citarella L, Kerl H, Cerroni L. Rimming of adipocytes by neoplastic lymphocytes: a histopathologic feature not restricted to subcutaneous T-cell lymphoma. *Am J Dermatopathol.* 2006;28(1):9-12.

190. Cassis TB, Fearneyhough PK, Callen JP. Subcutaneous panniculitis-like T-cell lymphoma with vacuolar interface dermatitis resembling lupus erythematosus panniculitis. *J Am Acad Dermatol.* 2004;50(3):465-469.

191. Fraga J, Garcia-Diez A. Lupus erythematosus panniculitis. *Dermatol Clin.* 2008;26(4):453-463, vi.

192. Gonzalez EG, Selvi E, Lorenzini S, et al. Subcutaneous panniculitis-like T-cell lymphoma misdiagnosed as lupus erythematosus panniculitis. *Clin Rheumatol.* 2007;26(2):244-246.

193. Li JY, Liu HJ, Wang L. Subcutaneous panniculitis-like T-cell lymphoma accompanied with discoid lupus erythematosus. *Chin Med J.* 2013;126(18):3590.

194. Liau JY, Chuang SS, Chu CY, Ku WH, Tsai JH, Shih TF. The presence of clusters of plasmacytoid dendritic cells is a helpful feature for differentiating lupus panniculitis from subcutaneous panniculitis-like T-cell lymphoma. *Histopathology.* 2013;62(7):1057-1066.

195. Massone C, Kodama K, Salmhofer W, et al. Lupus erythematosus panniculitis (lupus profundus): clinical, histopathological, and molecular analysis of nine cases. *J Cutan Pathol.* 2005;32(6):396-404.

196. Rose C, Leverkus M, Fleischer M, Shimanovich I. Histopathology of panniculitis—aspects of biopsy techniques and difficulties in diagnosis. *J Dtsch Dermatol Ges.* 2012;10(6):421-425.

197. Weingartner JS, Zedek DC, Burkhart CN, Morrell DS. Lupus erythematosus panniculitis in children: report of three cases and review of previously reported cases. *Pediatr Dermatol.* 2012;29(2):169-176.

198. Ikeda E, Endo M, Uchigasaki S, et al. Phagocytized apoptotic cells in subcutaneous panniculitis-like T-cell lymphoma. *J Eur Acad Dermatol Venereol.* 2001;15(2):159-162.

199. Sen F, Rassidakis GZ, Jones D, Medeiros LJ. Apoptosis and proliferation in subcutaneous panniculitis-like T-cell lymphoma. *Mod Pathol.* 2002;15(6):625-631.

200. Go RS, Wester SM. Immunophenotypic and molecular features, clinical outcomes, treatments, and prognostic factors associated with subcutaneous panniculitis-like T-cell lymphoma: a systematic analysis of 156 patients reported in the literature. *Cancer.* 2004;101(6):1404-1413.

201. Kong YY, Dai B, Kong JC, et al. Subcutaneous panniculitis-like T-cell lymphoma: a clinicopathologic, immunophenotypic, and molecular study of 22 Asian cases according to WHO-EORTC classification. *Am J Surg Pathol.* 2008;32(10):1495-1502.

202. Nemoto Y, Taniguchi A, Kamioka M, et al. Epstein-Barr virus-infected subcutaneous panniculitis-like T-cell lymphoma associated with methotrexate treatment. *Int J Hematol.* 2010;92(2):364-368.

203. Soylu S, Gul U, Kilic A, Heper AO, Kuzu I, Minareci BG. A case with an indolent course of subcutaneous panniculitis-like T-cell lymphoma demonstrating Epstein-Barr virus positivity and simulating dermatitis artefacta. *Am J Clin Dermatol.* 2010;11(2):147-150.

204. Wang L, Yang Y, Liu W, et al. Subcutaneous panniculitis-like T-cell lymphoma: expression of cytotoxic-granule-associated protein TIA-1 and its relation with Epstein-Barr virus infection [in Chinese]. *Zhonghua Bing Li Xue Za Zhi.* 2000;29(2):103-106.

205. LeBlanc RE, Tavallaee M, Kim YH, Kim J. Useful parameters for distinguishing subcutaneous panniculitis-like T-cell lymphoma from lupus erythematosus panniculitis. *Am J Surg Pathol.* 2016;40(6):745-754.

206. Chen RL, Hsu YH, Ueda I, et al. Cytophagic histiocytic panniculitis with fatal haemophagocytic lymphohistiocytosis in a paediatric patient with perforin gene mutation. *J Clin Pathol.* 2007;60(10):1168-1169.

207. Li MT, Zeng XF, Zhang FC, Tang FL. Cytophagic histiocytic panniculitis: a report of 6 cases with literature review [in Chinese]. *Zhonghua Nei Ke Za Zhi.* 2004;43(8):576-579.

208. Marzano AV, Berti E, Paulli M, Caputo R. Cytophagic histiocytic panniculitis and subcutaneous panniculitis-like T-cell lymphoma: report of 7 cases. *Arch Dermatol.* 2000;136(7):889-896.

209. Pasqualini C, Jorini M, Carloni I, et al. Cytophagic histiocytic panniculitis, hemophagocytic lymphohistiocytosis and undetermined autoimmune disorder: reconciling the puzzle. *Ital J Pediatr.* 2014;40(1):17.

210. Crotty CP, Winkelmann RK. Cytophagic histiocytic panniculitis with fever, cytopenia, liver failure, and terminal hemorrhagic diathesis. *J Am Acad Dermatol.* 1981;4(2):181-194.

211. Raciborska A, Gadomski A, Wypych A, Maldyk J, Gutowska-Grzegorczyk G. [5-year old boy with Weber-Christian Syndrome or histiocytic cytophagic panniculitis? Diagnostic difficulties. Case presentation]. *Med Wieku Rozwoj.* 2004;8(2, pt 1):201-208.

212. Fardet L, Galicier L, Vignon-Pennamen MD, et al. Frequency, clinical features and prognosis of cutaneous manifestations in adult patients with reactive haemophagocytic syndrome. *Br J Dermatol.* 2010;162(3):547-553.

213. Alberti-Violetti S, Torres-Cabala CA, Talpur R, et al. Clinicopathological and molecular study of primary cutaneous CD4+ small/medium-sized pleomorphic T-cell lymphoma. *J Cutan Pathol.* 2016;43(12):1121-1130.

214. Baum CL, Link BK, Neppalli VT, Swick BL, Liu V. Reappraisal of the provisional entity primary cutaneous CD4+ small/medium pleomorphic T-cell lymphoma: a series of 10 adult and pediatric patients and review of the literature. *J Am Acad Dermatol.* 2011;65(4):739-748.

215. Garcia-Herrera A, Colomo L, Camos M, et al. Primary cutaneous small/medium CD4+ T-cell lymphomas: a heterogeneous group of tumors with different clinicopathologic features and outcome. *J Clin Oncol.* 2008;26(20):3364-3371.

216. Grogg KL, Jung S, Erickson LA, McClure RF, Dogan A. Primary cutaneous CD4-positive small/medium-sized pleomorphic T-cell lymphoma: a clonal T-cell lymphoproliferative disorder with indolent behavior. *Mod Pathol.* 2008;21(6):708-715.

217. Beltraminelli H, Leinweber B, Kerl H, Cerroni L. Primary cutaneous CD4+ small-/medium-sized pleomorphic T-cell lymphoma: a cutaneous nodular proliferation of pleomorphic T lymphocytes of undetermined significance? A study of 136 cases. *Am J Dermatopathol.* 2009;31(4):317-322.

218. Volks N, Oschlies I, Cario G, Weichenthal M, Folster-Holst R. Primary cutaneous CD4+ small to medium-size pleomorphic T-cell lymphoma in a 12-year-old girl. *Pediatr Dermatol.* 2013;30(5):595-599.

219. Berti E, Tomasini D, Vermeer MH, Meijer CJ, Alessi E, Willemze R. Primary cutaneous CD8-positive epidermotropic cytotoxic T cell lymphomas. A distinct clinicopathological entity with an aggressive clinical behavior. *Am J Pathol.* 1999;155(2):483-492.

220. Kikuchi Y, Kashii Y, Gunji Y, et al. Six-year-old girl with primary cutaneous aggressive epidermotropic CD8+ T-cell lymphoma. *Pediatr Int.* 2011;53(3):393-396.

221. Guitart J, Martinez-Escala ME, Subtil A, et al. Primary cutaneous aggressive epidermotropic cytotoxic T-cell lymphomas: reappraisal of a provisional entity in the 2016 WHO classification of cutaneous lymphomas. *Mod Pathol.* 2017;30(5):761-772.

222. Garcia-Herrera A, Song JY, Chuang SS, et al. Nonhepatosplenic gammadelta T-cell lymphomas represent a spectrum of aggressive cytotoxic T-cell lymphomas with a mainly extranodal presentation. *Am J Surg Pathol.* 2011;35(8):1214-1225.

223. Guitart J, Weisenburger DD, Subtil A, et al. Cutaneous gammadelta T-cell lymphomas: a spectrum of presentations with overlap with other cytotoxic lymphomas. *Am J Surg Pathol.* 2012;36(11):1656-1665.

224. Magro CM, Wang X. Indolent primary cutaneous gamma/delta T-cell lymphoma localized to the subcutaneous panniculus and its association with atypical lymphocytic lobular panniculitis. *Am J Clin Pathol.* 2012;138(1):50-56.

225. Tripodo C, Iannitto E, Florena AM, et al. Gamma-delta T-cell lymphomas. *Nat Rev Clin Oncol.* 2009;6(12):707-717.

226. Kerbout M, Mekouar F, Bahadi N, et al. A rare pediatric case of cutaneous gamma/delta T-cell lymphoma. *Ann Biol Clin (Paris).* 2014;72(4):483-485.

227. Merrill ED, Agbay R, Miranda RN, et al. Primary cutaneous T-cell lymphomas showing gamma-delta (gammadelta) phenotype and predominantly epidermotropic pattern are clinicopathologically distinct from classic primary cutaneous gammadelta T-cell lymphomas. *Am J Surg Pathol.* 2017;41(2):204-215.

228. Straus SE. The chronic mononucleosis syndrome. *J Infect Dis.* 1988;157(3):405-412.

229. Kimura H, Morishima T, Kanegane H, et al. Prognostic factors for chronic active Epstein-Barr virus infection. *J Infect Dis.* 2003;187(4):527-533.

230. Ko YH, Chan JKC, Quintanilla-Martinez L. Virally associated T-cell and NK-cell neoplasms. In: Jaffe ES, Arber DA, Campo E, Harris NL, Quintanilla-Martinez L, eds. *Hematopathology.* 2nd ed. Philadelphia, PA: Elsevier; 2016.

231. Kimura H, Hoshino Y, Kanegane H, et al. Clinical and virologic characteristics of chronic active Epstein-Barr virus infection. *Blood.* 2001;98(2):280-286.

232. Cho EY, Kim KH, Kim WS, Yoo KH, Koo HH, Ko YH. The spectrum of Epstein-Barr virus-associated lymphoproliferative disease in Korea: incidence of disease entities by age groups. *J Korean Med Sci.* 2008;23(2):185-192.

233. Hong M, Ko YH, Yoo KH, et al. EBV-positive T/NK-cell lymphoproliferative disease of childhood. *Korean J Pathol.* 2013;47(2):137-147.

234. Ohshima K, Kimura H, Yoshino T, et al. Proposed categorization of pathological states of EBV-associated T/natural killer-cell lymphoproliferative disorder (LPD) in children and young adults: overlap with chronic active EBV infection and infantile fulminant EBV T-LPD. *Pathol Int.* 2008;58(4):209-217.

235. Okano M, Matsumoto S, Osato T, Sakiyama Y, Thiele GM, Purtilo DT. Severe chronic active Epstein-Barr virus infection syndrome. *Clin Microbiol Rev.* 1991;4(1):129-135.

236. Cohen JI, Kimura H, Nakamura S, Ko YH, Jaffe ES. Epstein-Barr virus-associated lymphoproliferative disease in non-immunocompromised hosts: a status report and summary of an international meeting, 8-9 September 2008. *Ann Oncol.* 2009;20(9):1472-1482.

237. Kimura H, Hoshino Y, Hara S, et al. Differences between T cell-type and natural killer cell-type chronic active Epstein-Barr virus infection. *J Infect Dis.* 2005;191(4):531-539.

238. Gru AA, Jaffe ES. Cutaneous EBV-related lymphoproliferative disorders. *Semin Diagn Pathol.* 2017;34(1):60-75.

239. Ishihara S, Ohshima K, Tokura Y, et al. Hypersensitivity to mosquito bites conceals clonal lymphoproliferation of Epstein-Barr viral DNA-positive natural killer cells. *Jpn J Cancer Res.* 1997;88(1):82-87.

240. Kawa K, Okamura T, Yagi K, Takeuchi M, Nakayama M, Inoue M. Mosquito allergy and Epstein-Barr virus-associated T/natural killer-cell lymphoproliferative disease. *Blood.* 2001;98(10):3173-3174.

241. Cho JH, Kim HS, Ko YH, Park CS. Epstein-Barr virus infected natural killer cell lymphoma in a patient with hypersensitivity to mosquito bite. *J Infect.* 2006;52(6):e173-e176.

242. Chung JS, Shin HJ, Lee EY, Cho GJ. Hypersensitivity to mosquito bites associated with natural killer cell-derived large granular lymphocyte lymphocytosis: a case report in Korea. *Korean J Intern Med.* 2003;18(1):50-52.

243. Fan PC, Chang HN. Hypersensitivity to mosquito bite: a case report. *Gaoxiong Yi Xue Ke Xue Za Zhi.* 1995;11(7):420-424.

244. Hidano A, Kawakami M, Yago A. Hypersensitivity to mosquito bite and malignant histiocytosis. *Jpn J Exp Med.* 1982;52(6):303-306.

245. Ishihara S, Okada S, Wakiguchi H, Kurashige T, Hirai K, Kawa-Ha K. Clonal lymphoproliferation following chronic active Epstein-Barr virus infection and hypersensitivity to mosquito bites. *Am J Hematol.* 1997;54(4):276-281.

246. Ishihara S, Okada S, Wakiguchi H, Kurashige T, Morishima T, Kawa-Ha K. Chronic active Epstein-Barr virus infection in children in Japan. *Acta Paediatr.* 1995;84(11):1271-1275.

247. Ohsawa T, Morimura T, Hagari Y, et al. A case of exaggerated mosquito-bite hypersensitivity with Epstein-Barr virus-positive inflammatory cells in the bite lesion. *Acta Derm Venereol.* 2001;81(5):360-363.

248. Tokura Y, Tamura Y, Takigawa M, et al. Severe hypersensitivity to mosquito bites associated with natural killer cell lymphocytosis. *Arch Dermatol.* 1990;126(3):362-368.

249. Tsai WC, Luo SF, Liaw SJ, Kuo TT. Mosquito bite allergies terminating as hemophagocytic histiocytosis: report of a case [in Chinese]. *Taiwan Yi Xue Hui Za Zhi.* 1989;88(6):639-642, 629.

250. Ishihara S, Yabuta R, Tokura Y, Ohshima K, Tagawa S. Hypersensitivity to mosquito bites is not an allergic disease, but an Epstein-Barr virus-associated lymphoproliferative disease. *Int J Hematol.* 2000;72(2):223-228.

251. Asada H, Saito-Katsuragi M, Niizeki H, et al. Mosquito salivary gland extracts induce EBV-infected NK cell oncogenesis via CD4 T cells in patients with hypersensitivity to mosquito bites. *J Invest Dermatol.* 2005;125(5):956-961.

252. Tokura Y, Matsuoka H, Koga C, et al. Enhanced T-cell response to mosquito extracts by NK cells in hypersensitivity to mosquito bites associated with EBV infection and NK cell lymphocytosis. *Cancer Sci.* 2005;96(8):519-526.

253. Tokura Y, Ishihara S, Tagawa S, Seo N, Ohshima K, Takigawa M. Hypersensitivity to mosquito bites as the primary clinical manifestation of a juvenile type of Epstein-Barr virus-associated natural killer cell leukemia/lymphoma. *J Am Acad Dermatol.* 2001;45(4):569-578.

254. Gupta G, Man I, Kemmett D. Hydroa vacciniforme: a clinical and follow-up study of 17 cases. *J Am Acad Dermatol.* 2000;42(2, pt 1):208-213.

255. Iwatsuki K, Satoh M, Yamamoto T, et al. Pathogenic link between hydroa vacciniforme and Epstein-Barr virus-associated hematologic disorders. *Arch Dermatol.* 2006;142(5):587-595.

256. Iwatsuki K, Yamamoto T, Tsuji K. Hypersensitivity to mosquito bites and hydroa vacciniforme [in Japanese]. *Nihon Rinsho.* 2006;64 Suppl 3:657-661.

257. Quintanilla-Martinez L, Kimura H, Jaffe ES. *EBV+ T-cell Lymphoproliferative Disorders of Childhood.* 4th ed. Lyon, France: International Agency for Research on Cancer; 2008.

258. Barrionuevo C, Anderson VM, Zevallos-Giampietri E, et al. Hydroa-like cutaneous T-cell lymphoma: a clinicopathologic and molecular genetic study of 16 pediatric cases from Peru. *Appl Immunohistochem Mol Morphol.* 2002;10(1):7-14.

259. Boddu D, George R, Nair S, Bindra M, L GM. Hydroa vacciniforme-like lymphoma: a case report from India. *J Pediatr Hematol Oncol.* 2015;37(4):e223-e226.

260. Iwatsuki K, Ohtsuka M, Akiba H, Kaneko F. Atypical hydroa vacciniforme in childhood: from a smoldering stage to Epstein-Barr virus-associated lymphoid malignancy. *J Am Acad Dermatol.* 1999;40(2, pt 1):283-284.

261. Magana M, Sanguéza P, Gil-Beristain J, et al. Angiocentric cutaneous T-cell lymphoma of childhood (hydroa-like lymphoma): a distinctive type of cutaneous T-cell lymphoma. *J Am Acad Dermatol.* 1998;38(4):574-579.

262. Oono T, Arata J, Masuda T, Ohtsuki Y. Coexistence of hydroa vacciniforme and malignant lymphoma. *Arch Dermatol.* 1986;122(11):1306-1309.

263. Plaza JA, Sanguéza M. Hydroa vacciniforme-like lymphoma with primarily periorbital swelling: 7 cases of an atypical clinical manifestation of this rare cutaneous T-cell lymphoma. *Am J Dermatopathol.* 2015;37(1):20-25.

264. Quintanilla-Martinez L, Ridaura C, Nagl F, et al. Hydroa vacciniforme-like lymphoma: a chronic EBV+ lymphoproliferative disorder with risk to develop a systemic lymphoma. *Blood.* 2013;122(18):3101-3110.

265. Rodriguez-Pinilla SM, Barrionuevo C, Garcia J, et al. EBV-associated cutaneous NK/T-cell lymphoma: review of a series of 14 cases from Peru in children and young adults. *Am J Surg Pathol.* 2010;34(12):1773-1782.

266. Sanguéza M, Plaza JA. Hydroa vacciniforme-like cutaneous T-cell lymphoma: clinicopathologic and immunohistochemical study of 12 cases. *J Am Acad Dermatol.* 2013;69(1):112-119.

267. Beltran BE, Maza I, Moises-Alfaro CB, et al. Thalidomide for the treatment of hydroa vacciniforme-like lymphoma: report of four pediatric cases from Peru. *Am J Hematol.* 2014;89(12):1160-1161.

268. Lysell J, Wiegleb Edstrom D, Linde A, et al. Antiviral therapy in children with hydroa vacciniforme. *Acta Derm Venereol.* 2009;89(4):393-397.

269. Gambichler T, Al-Muhammadi R, Boms S. Immunologically mediated photodermatoses: diagnosis and treatment. *Am J Clin Dermatol.* 2009;10(3):169-180.

270. Chen HH, Hsiao CH, Chiu HC. Hydroa vacciniforme-like primary cutaneous CD8-positive T-cell lymphoma. *Br J Dermatol.* 2002;147(3):587-591.

271. Wu YH, Chen HC, Hsiao PF, Tu MI, Lin YC, Wang TY. Hydroa vacciniforme-like Epstein-Barr virus-associated monoclonal T-lymphoproliferative disorder in a child. *Int J Dermatol.* 2007;46(10):1081-1086.

272. Cho KH, Lee SH, Kim CW, et al. Epstein-Barr virus-associated lymphoproliferative lesions presenting as a hydroa vacciniforme-like eruption: an analysis of six cases. *Br J Dermatol.* 2004;151(2):372-380.

273. Demachi A, Nagata H, Morio T, et al. Characterization of Epstein-Barr virus (EBV)-positive NK cells isolated from hydroa vacciniforme-like eruptions. *Microbiol Immunol.* 2003;47(7):543-552.

274. Morizane S, Suzuki D, Tsuji K, Oono T, Iwatsuki K. The role of CD4 and CD8 cytotoxic T lymphocytes in the formation of viral vesicles. *Br J Dermatol.* 2005;153(5):981-986.

275. Zhang Y, Nagata H, Ikeuchi T, et al. Common cytological and cytogenetic features of Epstein-Barr virus (EBV)-positive natural killer (NK) cells and cell lines derived from patients with nasal T/NK-cell lymphomas, chronic active EBV infection and hydroa vacciniforme-like eruptions. *Br J Haematol.* 2003;121(5):805-814.

276. Chan JK, Quintanilla-Martinez L, Ferry JA, Peh SC. *Extranodal NK/T-Cell Lymphoma, Nasal Type.* 4th ed. Lyon, France: International Agency for Research on Cancer; 2008.

277. Greer JP, Mosse CA. Natural killer-cell neoplasms. *Curr Hematol Malig Rep.* 2009;4(4):245-252.

278. Lima M. Aggressive mature natural killer cell neoplasms: from epidemiology to diagnosis. *Orphanet J Rare Dis.* 2013;8:95.

279. Termuhlen AM. Natural killer/T-cell lymphomas in pediatric and adolescent patients. *Clin Adv Hematol Oncol.* 2017;15(3):200-209.

280. Huang Y, Xie J, Ding Y, Zhou X. Extranodal Natural Killer/T-Cell Lymphoma in Children and Adolescents: A Report of 17 Cases in China. *Am J Clin Pathol.* 2016;145(1):46-54.

281. Dickson RJ. Radiotherapy of lethal mid-line granuloma. *J Chronic Dis.* 1960;12:417-427.

282. Chan JK, Sin VC, Wong KF, et al. Nonnasal lymphoma expressing the natural killer cell marker CD56: a clinicopathologic study of 49 cases of an uncommon aggressive neoplasm. *Blood.* 1997;89(12):4501-4513.

283. Chim CS, Ma SY, Au WY, et al. Primary nasal natural killer cell lymphoma: long-term treatment outcome and relationship with the International Prognostic Index. *Blood.* 2004;103(1):216-221.

284. Barrionuevo C, Zaharia M, Martinez MT, et al. Extranodal NK/T-cell lymphoma, nasal type: study of clinicopathologic and prognosis factors in a series of 78 cases from Peru. *Appl Immunohistochem Mol Morphol.* 2007;15(1):38-44.

285. Yamaguchi M, Suzuki R, Kwong YL, et al. Phase I study of dexamethasone, methotrexate, ifosfamide, L-asparaginase, and etoposide (SMILE) chemotherapy for advanced-stage, relapsed or refractory extranodal natural killer (NK)/T-cell lymphoma and leukemia. *Cancer Sci.* 2008;99(5):1016-1020.

286. Huang WT, Chang KC, Huang GC, et al. Bone marrow that is positive for Epstein-Barr virus encoded RNA-1 by in situ hybridization is related with a poor prognosis in patients with extranodal natural killer/T-cell lymphoma, nasal type. *Haematologica.* 2005;90(8):1063-1069.

287. Au WY, Weisenburger DD, Intragumtornchai T, et al. Clinical differences between nasal and extranasal natural killer/T-cell lymphoma: a study of 136 cases from the International Peripheral T-Cell Lymphoma Project. *Blood.* 2009;113(17):3931-3937.

288. Wang XM, Xu CG. Diagnostic value of serum levels of BamHI-W, LMP-1 and BZLF1 in NK/T-cell lymphoma [in Chinese]. *Zhonghua Xue Ye Xue Za Zhi.* 2013;34(1):36-40.

289. Wang ZY, Liu QF, Wang H, et al. Clinical implications of plasma Epstein-Barr virus DNA in early-stage extranodal nasal-type NK/T-cell lymphoma patients receiving primary radiotherapy. *Blood.* 2012;120(10):2003-2010.

290. Chan JK. Natural killer cell neoplasms. *Anat Pathol.* 1998;3:77-145.

291. Liang X, Graham DK. Natural killer cell neoplasms. *Cancer.* 2008;112(7):1425-1436.

292. Ohshima K, Suzumiya J, Shimazaki K, et al. Nasal T/NK cell lymphomas commonly express perforin and Fas ligand: important mediators of tissue damage. *Histopathology.* 1997;31(5):444-450.

293. Nagata H, Konno A, Kimura N, et al. Characterization of novel natural killer (NK)-cell and gammadelta T-cell lines established from primary lesions of nasal T/NK-cell lymphomas associated with the Epstein-Barr virus. *Blood.* 2001;97(3):708-713.

294. Kanavaros P, Lescs MC, Briere J, et al. Nasal T-cell lymphoma: a clinicopathologic entity associated with peculiar phenotype and with Epstein-Barr virus. *Blood.* 1993;81(10):2688-2695.

295. Cuadra-Garcia I, Proulx GM, Wu CL, et al. Sinonasal lymphoma: a clinicopathologic analysis of 58 cases from the Massachusetts General Hospital. *Am J Surg Pathol.* 1999;23(11):1356-1369.

296. Hasserjian RP, Harris NL. NK-cell lymphomas and leukemias: a spectrum of tumors with variable manifestations and immunophenotype. *Am J Clin Pathol.* 2007;127(6):860-868.

297. Kuo TT, Shih LY, Tsang NM. Nasal NK/T cell lymphoma in Taiwan: a clinicopathologic study of 22 cases, with analysis of histologic subtypes, Epstein-Barr virus LMP-1 gene association, and treatment modalities. *Int J Surg Pathol.* 2004;12(4):375-387.

298. Swerdlow SH, Jaffe ES, Brousset P, et al. Cytotoxic T-cell and NK-cell lymphomas: current questions and controversies. *Am J Surg Pathol.* 2014;38(10):e60-e71.

299. Jhuang JY, Chang ST, Weng SF, et al. Extranodal natural killer/T-cell lymphoma, nasal type in Taiwan: a relatively higher frequency of T-cell lineage and poor survival for extranasal tumors. *Hum Pathol.* 2015;46(2):313-321.

300. Kempf W, Kazakov DV, Broekaert SM, Metze D. Pediatric CD8(+) CD56(+) non-poikilodermatous mycosis fungoides: case report and review of the literature. *Am J Dermatopathol.* 2014;36(7):598-602.

301. Poppe H, Kerstan A, Bockers M, et al. Childhood mycosis fungoides with a CD8+ CD56+ cytotoxic immunophenotype. *J Cutan Pathol.* 2015;42(4):258-264.

302. Nicolae A, Ganapathi KA, Pham TH, et al. EBV-negative aggressive NK-cell leukemia/lymphoma: clinical, pathologic, and genetic features. *Am J Surg Pathol.* 2017;41(1):67-74.

303. Ferrandiz-Pulido C, Lopez-Lerma I, Sabado C, Ferrer B, Pisa S, Garcia-Patos V. Blastic plasmacytoid dendritic cell neoplasm in a child. *J Am Acad Dermatol.* 2012;66(6):e238-e240.

304. Jegalian AG, Buxbaum NP, Facchetti F, et al. Blastic plasmacytoid dendritic cell neoplasm in children: diagnostic features and clinical implications. *Haematologica.* 2010;95(11):1873-1879.

305. Isaacson PG, Chott A, Nakamura S, et al. *Extranodal Marginal Zone Lymphoma of Mucosa-Associated Lymphoid Tissue (MALT lymphoma).* 4th ed. Lyon, France: International Agency for Research on Cancer; 2008.

306. Taddesse-Heath L, Pittaluga S, Sorbara L, Bussey M, Raffeld M, Jaffe ES. Marginal zone B-cell lymphoma in children and young adults. *Am J Surg Pathol.* 2003;27(4):522-531.

307. Kempf W, Kazakov DV, Buechner SA, et al. Primary cutaneous marginal zone lymphoma in children: a report of 3 cases and review of the literature. *Am J Dermatopathol.* 2014;36(8):661-666.

308. Sharon V, Mecca PS, Steinherz PG, Trippett TM, Myskowski PL. Two pediatric cases of primary cutaneous B-cell lymphoma and review of the literature. *Pediatr Dermatol.* 2009;26(1):34-39.

309. Park MY, Jung HJ, Park JE, Kim YC. Pediatric primary cutaneous marginal zone B-cell lymphoma treated with intralesional rituximab. *Eur J Dermatol.* 2010;20(4):533-534.

310. Sroa N, Magro CM. Pediatric primary cutaneous marginal zone lymphoma: in association with chronic antihistamine use. *J Cutan Pathol.* 2006;33 suppl 2:1-5.

311. Zambrano E, Mejia-Mejia O, Bifulco C, Shin J, Reyes-Mugica M. Extranodal marginal zone B-cell lymphoma/maltoma of the lip in a child: case report and review of cutaneous lymphoid proliferations in childhood. *Int J Surg Pathol.* 2006;14(2):163-169.

312. Amitay-Laish I, Feinmesser M, Ben-Amitai D, et al. Juvenile onset of primary low-grade cutaneous B-cell lymphoma. *Br J Dermatol.* 2009;161(1):140-147.

313. Amitay-Laish I, Tavallaee M, Kim J, et al. Paediatric primary cutaneous marginal zone B-cell lymphoma: does it differ from its adult counterpart? *Br J Dermatol.* 2017;176(4):1010-1020.

314. Brenner I, Roth S, Puppe B, Wobser M, Rosenwald A, Geissinger E. Primary cutaneous marginal zone lymphomas with plasmacytic differentiation show frequent IgG4 expression. *Mod Pathol.* 2013;26(12):1568-1576.

315. Ghatalia P, Porter J, Wroblewski D, Carlson JA. Primary cutaneous marginal zone lymphoma associated with juxta-articular fibrotic nodules in a teenager. *J Cutan Pathol.* 2013;40(5):477-484.

316. Salama S. Primary cutaneous B-cell lymphoma and lymphoproliferative disorders of skin: current status of pathology and classification. *Am J Clin Pathol.* 2000;114 suppl:S104-S128.

317. De Souza A, Ferry JA, Burghart DR, et al. IgG4 expression in primary cutaneous marginal zone lymphoma: a multicenter study. *Appl Immunohistochem Mol Morphol.* 2018;26(7):462-467.

318. Swerdlow SH. Cutaneous marginal zone lymphomas. *Semin Diagn Pathol.* 2017;34(1):76-84.

319. Streubel B, Lamprecht A, Dierlamm J, et al. T(14;18)(q32;q21) involving IGH and MALT1 is a frequent chromosomal aberration in MALT lymphoma. *Blood.* 2003;101(6):2335-2339.

320. Streubel B, Simonitsch-Klupp I, Mullauer L, et al. Variable frequencies of MALT lymphoma-associated genetic aberrations in MALT lymphomas of different sites. *Leukemia.* 2004;18(10):1722-1726.

321. Streubel B, Vinatzer U, Lamprecht A, Raderer M, Chott A. T(3;14)(p14.1;q32) involving IGH and FOXP1 is a novel recurrent chromosomal aberration in MALT lymphoma. *Leukemia.* 2005;19(4):652-658.

322. Guitart J, Gerami P. Is there a cutaneous variant of marginal zone hyperplasia? *Am J Dermatopathol.* 2008;30(5):494-496.

323. Attygalle AD, Liu H, Shirali S, et al. Atypical marginal zone hyperplasia of mucosa-associated lymphoid tissue: a reactive condition of childhood showing immunoglobulin lambda light-chain restriction. *Blood.* 2004;104(10):3343-3348.

324. Swerdlow SH, Quintanilla-Martinez L, Willemze R, Kinney MC. Cutaneous B-cell lymphoproliferative disorders: report of the 2011 Society for Hematopathology/European Association for Haematopathology workshop. *Am J Clin Pathol.* 2013;139(4):515-535.

325. Boudova L, Kazakov DV, Sima R, et al. Cutaneous lymphoid hyperplasia and other lymphoid infiltrates of the breast nipple: a retrospective clinicopathologic study of fifty-six patients. *Am J Dermatopathol.* 2005;27(5):375-386.

326. Moulonguet I, Hadj-Rabia S, Gounod N, Bodemer C, Fraitag S. Tibial lymphoplasmacytic plaque: a new, illustrative case of a recently and poorly recognized benign lesion in children. *Dermatology.* 2012;225(1):27-30.

327. Senff NJ, Hoefnagel JJ, Jansen PM, et al. Reclassification of 300 primary cutaneous B-Cell lymphomas according to the new WHO-EORTC classification for cutaneous lymphomas: comparison with previous classifications and identification of prognostic markers. *J Clin Oncol.* 2007;25(12):1581-1587.

328. Condarco T, Sagatys E, Prakash AV, Rezania D, Cualing H. Primary cutaneous B-cell lymphoma in a child. *Fetal Pediatr Pathol.* 2008;27(4-5):206-214.

329. Yoshii Y, Kato T, Ono K, et al. Primary cutaneous follicle center lymphoma in a patient with WHIM syndrome. *J Eur Acad Dermatol Venereol.* 2016;30(3):529-530.

330. Ghislanzoni M, Gambini D, Perrone T, Alessi E, Berti E. Primary cutaneous follicular center cell lymphoma of the nose with maxillary sinus involvement in a pediatric patient. *J Am Acad Dermatol.* 2005;52(5 suppl 1):S73-S75.

331. Senff NJ, Noordijk EM, Kim YH, et al. European Organization for Research and Treatment of Cancer and International Society for Cutaneous Lymphoma consensus recommendations for the management of cutaneous B-cell lymphomas. *Blood.* 2008;112(5):1600-1609.

332. Bergman R, Kurtin PJ, Gibson LE, Hull PR, Kimlinger TK, Schroeter AL. Clinicopathologic, immunophenotypic, and molecular characterization of primary cutaneous follicular B-cell lymphoma. *Arch Dermatol.* 2001;137(4):432-439.

333. Cerroni L, Arzberger E, Putz B, et al. Primary cutaneous follicle center cell lymphoma with follicular growth pattern. *Blood.* 2000;95(12):3922-3928.

334. Cerroni L, Kerl H. Primary cutaneous follicle center cell lymphoma. *Leuk Lymphoma.* 2001;42(5):891-900.

335. Cerroni L, Kerl H. Cutaneous follicle center cell lymphoma, follicular type. *Am J Dermatopathol.* 2001;23(4):370-373.

336. Berti E, Alessi E, Caputo R. Reticulohistiocytoma of the dorsum (Crosti's disease) and other B-cell lymphomas. *Semin Diagn Pathol.* 1991;8(2):82-90.

337. Berti E, Alessi E, Caputo R, Gianotti R, Delia D, Vezzoni P. Reticulohistiocytoma of the dorsum. *J Am Acad Dermatol.* 1988;19(2, pt 1):259-272.

338. Abdul-Wahab A, Tang SY, Robson A, et al. Chromosomal anomalies in primary cutaneous follicle center cell lymphoma do not portend a poor prognosis. *J Am Acad Dermatol.* 2014;70(6):1010-1020.

339. Streubel B, Scheucher B, Valencak J, et al. Molecular cytogenetic evidence of t(14;18)(IGH;BCL2) in a substantial proportion of primary cutaneous follicle center cell lymphomas. *Am J Surg Pathol.* 2006;30(4):529-536.

340. Borowitz M, Chan CH. *B Lymphoblastic Leukaemia/Lymphoma, not Otherwise Specified.* 4th ed. Lyon, France: International Agency for Research on Cancer; 2008.

341. Hunger SP, Mullighan CG. Acute lymphoblastic leukemia in children. *N Engl J Med.* 2015;373(16):1541-1552.

342. Sander CA, Medeiros LJ, Abruzzo LV, Horak ID, Jaffe ES. Lymphoblastic lymphoma presenting in cutaneous sites. A clinicopathologic analysis of six cases. *J Am Acad Dermatol.* 1991;25(6, pt 1):1023-1031.

343. Kahwash SB, Qualman SJ. Cutaneous lymphoblastic lymphoma in children: report of six cases with precursor B-cell lineage. *Pediatr Dev Pathol.* 2002;5(1):45-53.

344. Boccara O, Laloum-Grynberg E, Jeudy G, et al. Cutaneous B-cell lymphoblastic lymphoma in children: a rare diagnosis. *J Am Acad Dermatol.* 2012;66(1):51-57.

345. Lee WJ, Moon HR, Won CH, et al. Precursor B- or T-lymphoblastic lymphoma presenting with cutaneous involvement: a series of 13 cases including 7 cases of cutaneous T-lymphoblastic lymphoma. *J Am Acad Dermatol.* 2014;70(2):318-325.

346. Ansell LH, Mehta J, Cotliar J. Recurrent aleukemic leukemia cutis in a patient with pre-B-cell acute lymphoblastic leukemia. *J Clin Oncol.* 2013;31(20):e353-e355.

347. Hsiao CH, Su IJ. Primary cutaneous pre-B lymphoblastic lymphoma immunohistologically mimics Ewing's sarcoma/primitive neuroectodermal tumor. *J Formos Med Assoc.* 2003;102(3):193-197.

348. Taniguchi S, Hamada T, Kutsuna H, Ishii M. Lymphocytic aleukemic leukemia cutis. *J Am Acad Dermatol.* 1996;35(5, pt 2):849-850.

349. Frontanes A, Montalvo F, Valcarcel M. Congenital leukemia with leukemia cutis: a case report. *Bol Asoc Med P R.* 2012;104(1):52-54.

350. Muljono A, Graf NS, Arbuckle S. Primary cutaneous lymphoblastic lymphoma in children: series of eight cases with review of the literature. *Pathology.* 2009;41(3):223-228.

351. Yang CC, Chen YA, Tsai YL, Shih IH, Chen W. Neoplastic skin lesions of the scalp in children: a retrospective study of 265 cases in Taiwan. *Eur J Dermatol.* 2014;24(1):70-75.

352. Savage NM, Johnson RC, Natkunam Y. The spectrum of lymphoblastic, nodal and extranodal T-cell lymphomas: characteristic features and diagnostic dilemmas. *Hum Pathol.* 2013;44(4):451-471.

353. Inhorn RC, Aster JC, Roach SA, et al. A syndrome of lymphoblastic lymphoma, eosinophilia, and myeloid hyperplasia/malignancy associated with t(8;13)(p11;q11): description of a distinctive clinicopathologic entity. *Blood.* 1995;85(7):1881-1887.

354. Cortelazzo S, Ponzoni M, Ferreri AJ, Hoelzer D. Lymphoblastic lymphoma. *Crit Rev Oncol Hematol.* 2011;79(3):330-343.

355. Koksal Y, Toy H, Talim B, Unal E, Akcoren Z, Cengiz M. Merkel cell carcinoma in a child. *J Pediatr Hematol Oncol.* 2009;31(5):359-361.

356. Marzban S, Geramizadeh B, Farzaneh MR. Merkel cell carcinoma in a 17-year-old boy, report of a highly aggressive fatal case and review of the literature. *Rare Tumors.* 2011;3(3):e34.

357. Isaacs H Jr. Cutaneous metastases in neonates: a review. *Pediatr Dermatol.* 2011;28(2):85-93.

358. Vanchinathan V, Marinelli EC, Kartha RV, Uzieblo A, Ranchod M, Sundram UN. A malignant cutaneous neuroendocrine tumor with features of Merkel cell carcinoma and differentiating neuroblastoma. *Am J Dermatopathol.* 2009;31(2):193-196.

359. Magro G, Longo FR, Angelico G, Spadola S, Amore FF, Salvatorelli L. Immunohistochemistry as potential diagnostic pitfall in the most common solid tumors of children and adolescents. *Acta Histochem.* 2015;117(4-5):397-414.

360. Aboutalebi A, Korman JB, Sohani AR, et al. Aleukemic cutaneous myeloid sarcoma. *J Cutan Pathol.* 2013;40(12):996-1005.

361. Desch JK, Smoller BR. The spectrum of cutaneous disease in leukemias. *J Cutan Pathol.* 1993;20(5):407-410.

362. Kaiserling E, Horny HP, Geerts ML, Schmid U. Skin involvement in myelogenous leukemia: morphologic and immunophenotypic heterogeneity of skin infiltrates. *Mod Pathol.* 1994;7(7):771-779.

363. Cho-Vega JH, Medeiros LJ, Prieto VG, Vega F. Leukemia cutis. *Am J Clin Pathol.* 2008;129(1):130-142.

364. Su WP, Buechner SA, Li CY. Clinicopathologic correlations in leukemia cutis. *J Am Acad Dermatol.* 1984;11(1):121-128.

365. Byrd JC, Edenfield WJ, Shields DJ, Dawson NA. Extramedullary myeloid cell tumors in acute nonlymphocytic leukemia: a clinical review. *J Clin Oncol.* 1995;13(7):1800-1816.

366. Bachmeyer C, Turc Y, Fraitag S, Delmer A, Aractingi S. Aleukemic monoblastic leukemia cutis [in French]. *Ann Dermatol Venereol.* 2003;130(8-9, pt 1):773-775.

367. Barzilai A, Lyakhovitsky A, Goldberg I, Meytes D, Trau H. Aleukemic monocytic leukemia cutis [in French]. *Cutis.* 2002;69(4):301-304.

368. Daoud MS, Snow JL, Gibson LE, Daoud S. Aleukemic monocytic leukemia cutis. *Mayo Clinic Proc.* 1996;71(2):166-168.

369. Gil-Mateo MP, Miquel FJ, Piris MA, Sanchez M, Martin-Aragones G. Aleukemic "leukemia cutis" of monocytic lineage. *J Am Acad Dermatol.* 1997;36(5, pt 2):837-840.

370. Hejmadi RK, Thompson D, Shah F, Naresh KN. Cutaneous presentation of aleukemic monoblastic leukemia cutis—a case report and review of literature with focus on immunohistochemistry. *J Cutan Pathol.* 2008;35 suppl 1:46-49.

371. Heskel NS, White CR, Fryberger S, Neerhout RC, Spraker M, Hanifin JM. Aleukemic leukemia cutis: juvenile chronic granulocytic leukemia presenting with figurate cutaneous lesions. *J Am Acad Dermatol.* 1983;9(3):423-427.

372. Imanaka K, Fujiwara K, Satoh K, et al. A case of aleukemic monocytic leukemia cutis treated with total body electron therapy. *Radiat Med.* 1988;6(5):229-231.

373. Kishimoto H, Furui Y, Nishioka K. Guess what. B-cell acute lymphoblastic leukemia with aleukemic leukemia cutis. *Eur J Dermatol.* 2001;11(2):151-152.

374. Iliadis A, Koletsa T, Georgiou E, Patsatsi A, Sotiriadis D, Kostopoulos I. Bilateral aleukemic myeloid sarcoma of the eyelids with indolent course. *Am J Dermatopathol.* 2016;38(4):312-314.

375. Jung HD, Kim HS, Park YM, Kim HO, Lee JY. Multiple granulocytic sarcomas in a patient with longstanding complete remission of acute myelogenous leukemia. *Ann Dermatol.* 2011;23(suppl 2):S270-S273.

376. Zengin N, Kars A, Ozisik Y, Canpinar H, Turker A, Ruacan S. Aleukemic leukemia cutis in a patient with acute lymphoblastic leukemia. *J Am Acad Dermatol.* 1998;38(4):620-621.

377. Tomasini C, Quaglino P, Novelli M, Fierro MT. "Aleukemic" granulomatous leukemia cutis. *Am J Dermatopathol.* 1998;20(4):417-421.

378. Agrawal AK, Guo H, Golden C. Siblings presenting with progressive congenital aleukemic leukemia cutis. *Pediatr Blood Cancer.* 2011;57(2):338-340.

379. Kanegane H, Nomura K, Abe A, et al. Spontaneous regression of aleukemic leukemia cutis harboring a NPM/RARA fusion gene in an infant with cutaneous mastocytosis. *Int J Hematol.* 2009;89(1):86-90.

380. Landers MC, Malempati S, Tilford D, Gatter K, White C, Schroeder TL. Spontaneous regression of aleukemia congenital leukemia cutis. *Pediatr Dermatol.* 2005;22(1):26-30.

381. Gru AA, Coughlin CC, Schapiro ML, et al. Pediatric aleukemic leukemia cutis: report of 3 cases and review of the literature. *Am J Dermatopathol.* 2015;37(6):477-484.

382. Najem N, Zadeh VB, Badawi M, Kumar R, Al-Otaibi S, Al-Abdulraz-zaq A. Aleukemic leukemia cutis in a child preceding T-cell acute lymphoblastic leukemia. *Pediatr Dermatol.* 2011;28(5):535-537.

383. Zebisch A, Cerroni L, Beham-Schmid C, Sill H. Therapy-related leukemia cutis: case study of an aggressive disorder. *Ann Hematol.* 2003;82(11):705-707.

384. Otsubo K, Horie S, Nomura K, Miyawaki T, Abe A, Kanegane H. Acute promyelocytic leukemia following aleukemic leukemia cutis harboring NPM/RARA fusion gene. *Pediatr Blood Cancer.* 2012;59(5):959-960.

385. Monpoux F, Lacour JP, Hatchuel Y, et al. Congenital leukemia cutis preceding monoblastic leukemia by 3 months. *Pediatr Dermatol.* 1996;13(6):472-476.

386. Monpoux F, Sirvent N, Sudaka I, Mariani R. Acute congenital monoblastic leukemia and 9;11 translocation: a case [in French]. *Pediatrie.* 1992;47(10):691-694.

387. Torrelo A, Madero L, Mediero IG, Bano A, Zambrano A. Aleukemic congenital leukemia cutis. *Pediatr Dermatol.* 2004;21(4):458-461.

388. Bidet A, Dulucq S, Aladjidi N. Transient abnormal myelopoiesis (TAM) in a neonate without Down syndrome. *Br J Haematol.* 2015;168(1):2.

389. Krawczyk J, McDermott M, Irvine AD, O'Marcaigh A, Storey L, Smith O. Skin involvement in Down syndrome transient abnormal myelopoiesis. *Br J Haematol.* 2012;157(3):280.

390. Winckworth LC, Chonat S, Uthaya S. Cutaneous lesions in transient abnormal myelopoiesis. *J Paediatr Child Health.* 2012;48(2):184-185.

391. Boggs DR, Wintrobe MM, Cartwright GE. The acute leukemias. Analysis of 322 cases and review of the literature. *Medicine (Baltimore).* 1962;41:163-225.

392. Martinez-Escaname M, Zuriel D, Tee SI, Fried I, Massone C, Cerroni L. Cutaneous infiltrates of acute myelogenous leukemia simulating inflammatory dermatoses. *Am J Dermatopathol.* 2013;35(4):419-424.

393. Cibull TL, Thomas AB, O'Malley DP, Billings SD. Myeloid leukemia cutis: a histologic and immunohistochemical review. *J Cutan Pathol.* 2008;35(2):180-185.

394. Jones D, Dorfman DM, Barnhill RL, Granter SR. Leukemic vasculitis: a feature of leukemia cutis in some patients. *Am J Clin Pathol.* 1997;107(6):637-642.

395. Seckin D, Senol A, Gurbuz O, Demirkesen C. Leukemic vasculitis: an unusual manifestation of leukemia cutis. *J Am Acad Dermatol.* 2009;61(3):519-521.

396. Harris NL, Demirjian Z. Plasmacytoid T-zone cell proliferation in a patient with chronic myelomonocytic leukemia. Histologic and immunohistologic characterization. *Am J Surg Pathol.* 1991;15(1):87-95.

397. Cronin DM, George TI, Sundram UN. An updated approach to the diagnosis of myeloid leukemia cutis. *Am J Clin Pathol.* 2009;132(1):101-110.

398. Amador-Ortiz C, Hurley MY, Ghahramani GK, et al. Use of classic and novel immunohistochemical markers in the diagnosis of cutaneous myeloid sarcoma. *J Cutan Pathol.* 2011;38(12):945-953.

399. Xu B, Naughton D, Busam K, Pulitzer M. ERG Is a Useful immunohistochemical marker to distinguish leukemia cutis from nonneoplastic leukocytic infiltrates in the skin. *Am J Dermatopathol.* 2016;38(9):672-677.

400. Feuillard J, Jacob MC, Valensi F, et al. Clinical and biologic features of CD4(+)CD56(+) malignancies. *Blood.* 2002;99(5):1556-1563.

401. Meyer N, Petrella T, Poszepczynska-Guigne E, et al. CD4+ CD56+ blastic tumor cells express CD101 molecules. *J Invest Dermatol.* 2005;124(3):668-669.

402. Petrella T, Bagot M, Willemze R, et al. Blastic NK-cell lymphomas (agranular CD4+CD56+ hematodermic neoplasms): a review. *Am J Clin Pathol.* 2005;123(5):662-675.

403. Facchetti F, Jones D, Petrella T. *Blastic Plasmacytoid Dendritic Cell Neoplasm.* 4th ed. Lyon, France: International Agency for Research on Cancer; 2008.

404. Chaperot L, Bendriss N, Manches O, et al. Identification of a leukemic counterpart of the plasmacytoid dendritic cells. *Blood.* 2001;97(10):3210-3217.

405. Chaperot L, Perrot I, Jacob MC, et al. Leukemic plasmacytoid dendritic cells share phenotypic and functional features with their normal counterparts. *Eur J Immunol.* 2004;34(2):418-426.

406. Dijkman R, van Doorn R, Szuhai K, Willemze R, Vermeer MH, Tensen CP. Gene-expression profiling and array-based CGH classify CD4+CD56+ hematodermic neoplasm and cutaneous myelomonocytic leukemia as distinct disease entities. *Blood.* 2007;109(4):1720-1727.

407. Marafioti T, Paterson JC, Ballabio E, et al. Novel markers of normal and neoplastic human plasmacytoid dendritic cells. *Blood.* 2008;111(7):3778-3792.

408. Petrella T, Comeau MR, Maynadie M, et al. "Agranular CD4+ CD56+ hematodermic neoplasm" (blastic NK-cell lymphoma) originates from a population of CD56+ precursor cells related to plasmacytoid monocytes. *Am J Surg Pathol.* 2002;26(7):852-862.

409. Chang SE, Choi HJ, Huh J, et al. A case of primary cutaneous CD56+, TdT+, CD4+, blastic NK-cell lymphoma in a 19-year-old woman. *Am J Dermatopathol.* 2002;24(1):72-75.

410. Eguaras AV, Lo RW, Veloso JD, Tan VG, Enriquez ML, Del Rosario ML. CD4+/CD56+ hematodermic neoplasm: blastic NK cell lymphoma in a 6-year-old child: report of a case and review of literature. *J Pediatr Hematol Oncol.* 2007;29(11):766-769.

411. Julia F, Dalle S, Duru G, et al. Blastic plasmacytoid dendritic cell neoplasms: clinico-immunohistochemical correlations in a series of 91 patients. *Am J Surg Pathol.* 2014;38(5):673-680.

412. Rossi JG, Felice MS, Bernasconi AR, et al. Acute leukemia of dendritic cell lineage in childhood: incidence, biological characteristics and outcome. *Leuk Lymphoma.* 2006;47(4):715-725.

413. Johnson RC, Kim J, Natkunam Y, et al. Myeloid cell nuclear differentiation antigen (MNDA) expression distinguishes extramedullary presentations of myeloid leukemia from blastic plasmacytoid dendritic cell neoplasm. *Am J Surg Pathol.* 2016;40(4):502-509.

414. Jegalian AG, Facchetti F, Jaffe ES. Plasmacytoid dendritic cells: physiologic roles and pathologic states. *Adv Anat Pathol.* 2009;16(6):392-404.

415. Cao Q, Liu F, Niu G, Xue L, Han A. Blastic plasmacytoid dendritic cell neoplasm with EWSR1 gene rearrangement. *J Clin Pathol.* 2014;67(1):90-92.

416. Menezes J, Acquadro F, Wiseman M, et al. Exome sequencing reveals novel and recurrent mutations with clinical impact in blastic plasmacytoid dendritic cell neoplasm. *Leukemia.* 2014;28(4):823-829.

417. Stenzinger A, Endris V, Pfarr N, et al. Targeted ultra-deep sequencing reveals recurrent and mutually exclusive mutations of cancer genes in blastic plasmacytoid dendritic cell neoplasm. *Oncotarget.* 2014;5(15):6404-6413.

418. Sapienza MR, Fuligni F, Agostinelli C, et al. Molecular profiling of blastic plasmacytoid dendritic cell neoplasm reveals a unique pattern and suggests selective sensitivity to NF-kB pathway inhibition. *Leukemia.* 2014;28(8):1606-1616.

419. Fraga GR, Caughron SK. Cutaneous myelofibrosis with JAK2 V617F mutation: metastasis, not merely extramedullary hematopoiesis! *Am J Dermatopathol.* 2010;32(7):727-730.

420. Epps RE, Pittelkow MR, Su WP. TORCH syndrome. *Semin Dermatol.* 1995;14(2):179-186.

421. Hoss DM, McNutt NS. Cutaneous myelofibrosis. *J Cutan Pathol.* 1992;19(3):221-225.

422. Kuo T. Cutaneous extramedullary hematopoiesis presenting as leg ulcers. *J Am Acad Dermatol.* 1981;4(5):592-596.

423. Mizoguchi M, Kawa Y, Minami T, Nakayama H, Mizoguchi H. Cutaneous extramedullary hematopoiesis in myelofibrosis. *J Am Acad Dermatol.* 1990;22(2, pt 2):351-355.

28

Medication-Induced Hypersensitivity Reactions

Grace L. Lee / Barbara Reichert / Alejandro A. Gru / Benjamin H. Kaffenberger

Medication-induced hypersensitivity reactions are an important cause of morbidity, and even mortality within the pediatric population. Fortunately, they tend to be less frequent than those seen in adults, likely related to fewer medications concurrently used.[1] Dermatopathology plays an important role in distinguishing low-risk idiosyncratic drug eruptions from high-risk immunologic reactions. In addition to the risks of severe toxicity, if the diagnosis is not properly made, medical and economic costs can be substantial with misdiagnoses.[2] The causative drug often will not be apparent by histopathology and clinicians should be directed to validate criteria to assess the etiology such as the Naranjo or Alden scores.[3,4] This chapter distinguishes three general drug eruption presentations: the classic idiosyncratic drug reactions, chemotherapy and targeted oncologic associated eruptions, and severe cutaneous adverse reactions.

Classic Idiosyncratic Drug Reactions

Classic idiosyncratic eruptions in this chapter will focus on immediate-type reactions (or urticarial), serum sickness–like reactions, morbilliform eruptions, fixed drug eruptions, and acneiform eruptions. Epidemiologically, these five form the majority of typical drug eruptions, particularly in the hospital setting where the morbilliform eruption will be, by far, the most common.[5-8] Children produce a unique challenge in that these eruptions can often mimic viral hypersensitivity reactions that are far more frequent

compared to adults. Fortunately, children tend to be on fewer medications than adults, which allows easier evaluation of drug causality.

IMMEDIATE-TYPE URTICARIAL HYPERSENSITIVITY REACTION

Definition and Epidemiology

Immediate-type or type 1 hypersensitivity reactions are the classic urticarial reaction that occurs within minutes to a few hours after drug administration.[9] These reactions occur as 5% to 20% of all drug eruptions.[6,8,10]

Etiology

Immediate-type hypersensitivity reactions occur because of preformed immunoglobulin E autoantibodies recognizing the drug, excipient, or metabolite. Any medicine can be a potential cause, although antibiotics tend to have the highest risk.

Clinical Presentation

Classically, this will present as near-immediate urticarial plaques developing across the body, often times with arcuate, annular, or figurate appearances (Figure 28-1). Pruritus is common, although scale should not be seen. Patients can also have associated angioedema, including periocular, hand, and perioral edema, and may be accompanied by oral swelling, wheezing, and anaphylaxis. In the absence of angioedema, the eruptions will often clear within hours to a few days of stopping the offending medication.

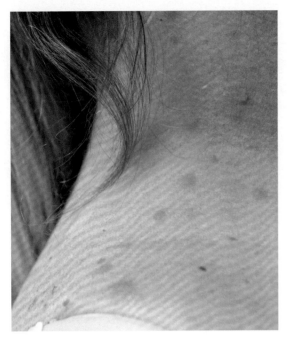

FIGURE 28-1. Urticaria: scattered erythematous, edematous papules, and plaques over the upper body.

Histologic Findings

Microscopically, the stratum corneum and epidermis will not demonstrate any irregularity and only minimal spongiosis. Dermal edema can be prominent, with a sparse perivascular infiltrate of lymphocytes with or without mast cells and eosinophils.[11] Upon close examination of the vessels, marginating neutrophils may be seen.

Differential Diagnosis

Urticaria can be challenging and be confused with normal skin when there is minimal edema. However, the lack of interface dermatitis and minimal perivascular lymphocyte extravasation should differentiate urticaria from a morbilliform drug eruption. Urticarial vasculitis is another consideration, but should show typical features of fibrinous necrosis of the vessel walls and more extensive red blood cell extravasation.

CAPSULE SUMMARY

IMMEDIATE-TYPE URTICARIAL HYPERSENSITIVITY REACTION

Urticaria is one of the most common types of drug reactions, but often will be obvious to the clinician on the basis of appearance and time course. Pathologically, it will be characterized by a lack of injury to the epidermis, with dermal edema, and marginating neutrophils within the superficial blood vessels.

SERUM SICKNESS–LIKE REACTION

Definition and Epidemiology

Serum sickness itself is a rare condition typically associated with infusion of foreign proteins such as horse antithymocyte globulin. It is the classic type 3 hypersensitivity reaction involving immune complex development and tissue deposition resulting in hypocomplementemia, urticaria, vasculitis, fever, arthralgia, and often kidney damage. Serum sickness–like reactions are characterized by urticaria, arthritis, and fever, but do not have life-threatening risks that true serum sickness does.

Serum sickness is very rare. Serum sickness–like reactions are reported at less than 1% of all drug eruptions and primarily in children under 5.[12]

Etiology

In clinical practice, cefaclor is the most common medication associated with this reaction pattern. Other rarely reported etiologies include other cephalosporins, penicillins, minocycline, infliximab, and insulin.[13] Interestingly, unlike true serum sickness, serum sickness–like reactions tend to be triggered most often by small molecules and not proteins.

Clinical Presentation

Patients present with urticarial eruption, arthritis, and fevers,[14] which resolve upon drug withdrawal, without long-term complications. The eruption tends to occur 1 to 3 weeks after starting the therapy, in contrast to immediate-type hypersensitivity eruptions.

Histologic Findings

The histology is generally indistinguishable from common urticaria and thus it is imperative for the clinician to recognize that the fevers and arthralgias are not typical for a simple urticarial eruption.

Differential Diagnosis

Urticaria must be distinguished clinically. Urticarial vasculitis should be distinguished by the fibrinoid vessel wall necrosis, and may be concerning for true serum sickness if the patient has been treated with foreign proteins. Systemic lupus erythematosus and juvenile idiopathic arthritis are considerations in a young patient presenting with arthralgias, fevers, and rashes, but the pathology should distinguish these cases, without interface pattern changes. Viral hypersensitivity reactions would also be in the differential, particularly parvovirus and Epstein-Barr virus, but generally the clinician should recognize the eruption as fixed and thus not urticarial, in these cases. Pathologically, more interface dermatitis and superficial lymphocyte infiltration should be seen instead of urticarial features.

SERUM SICKNESS–LIKE REACTION

Serum sickness–like reactions are rare eruptions that should be distinguished from true serum sickness. They are most often seen in children associated with antibiotics, such as cefaclor, and consist of the triad of urticarial eruption, arthralgias, and fevers.

MORBILLIFORM DRUG ERUPTION (MACULOPAPULAR/EXANTHEMATOUS)

Definition and Epidemiology

The classic drug exanthem, is a delayed-type hypersensitivity reaction, presenting with diffuse macules, papules, and patches of erythema of the trunk and extremities. This form of drug eruption typically accounts for 30% to 90% of total drug eruptions.[1,6,10,15]

Etiology

Morbilliform drug eruptions present after metabolite or other drug-antigen internalization, and presentation to the lymphocytes resulting in a specific delayed-type reaction. Many medications can cause this eruption, but antibiotics, particularly penicillins, cephalosporins, sulfa antibiotics, and aromatic antiepileptics most commonly are associated.

Clinical Presentation

The eruption typically begins on the trunk as scattered, small erythematous blanching papules (Figure 28-2). Over the next several days, these papules progress in a centrifugal pattern. Centrally, the papules fade to macules and coalesce into patches. This eruption generally does not affect the face, palms/soles, cause lymphadenopathy, nor is it associated with an enanthem. These features would be suspicious for severe cutaneous adverse reactions or a viral etiology.[16,17]

Histologic Findings

The histology of these eruptions is not specific, but typically the inflammation is perivascular and is confined to superficial dermis, containing lymphocytes with or without eosinophils and neutrophils (Figure 28-3).[18] A total of 50% of cases may have associated interface changes, and similarly, only 50% of cases have eosinophils present in the inflammatory infiltrate.[15]

Differential Diagnosis

The differential diagnosis contains other causes of drug eruptions, viral hypersensitivity reactions, severe cutaneous

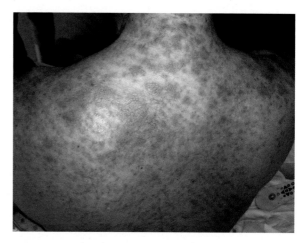

FIGURE 28-2. Morbilliform eruption: coalescing macules and papules over the trunk and spreading to the extremities. The etiology in this case was a cephalosporin antibiotic.

adverse drug reactions, and graft-versus-host disease. Unfortunately, quantitating eosinophils in the inflammatory infiltrates has not been associated with differentiation of these hypersensitivity reactions or in distinguishing graft-versus-host disease;[19,20] thus it is imperative for clinicopathologic correlation for the final diagnosis.

MORBILLIFORM DRUG ERUPTION

Morbilliform eruptions are the most commonly diagnosed form of drug eruptions. Pathologically, they are characterized by superficial perivascular inflammation potentially with interface dermatitis, but at present, drug, viral, or graft-versus-host disease cannot be differentiated reliably without clinicopathologic correlation.

FIXED DRUG ERUPTION

Definition and Epidemiology

Fixed drug eruption is a recurrent, perfectly annular, eruption that will reoccur in the exactly same location with repeated ingestion of the offending medication.

The fixed drug eruption has a variable frequency and generally occurs as 5% to 30% of all drug eruptions.[1,6]

Etiology

This is another form of a delayed-type hypersensitivity reaction, but one where cytotoxic T cells are the primary effector cell.[21] The most common causes for fixed drug eruptions are terbinafine,-azole antifungals, trimethoprim-sulfamethoxazole and sulfa drugs, penicillin and cephalosporin antibiotics, tetracycline antibiotics, nonsteroidal anti-inflammatory drugs, and over-the-counter decongestants.[22]

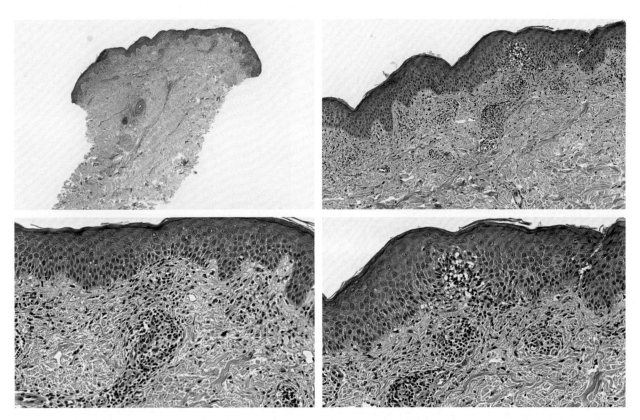

FIGURE 28-3. Morbilliform reaction—histopathologic findings. A mild degree of spongiosis and acanthosis is noted. The more prominent manifestations are in the dermis, where a superficial and perivascular inflammatory infiltrate is noted, with numerous dermal eosinophils. Focal interface changes are present (bottom right panel). Digital slides courtesy of Path Presenter.com.

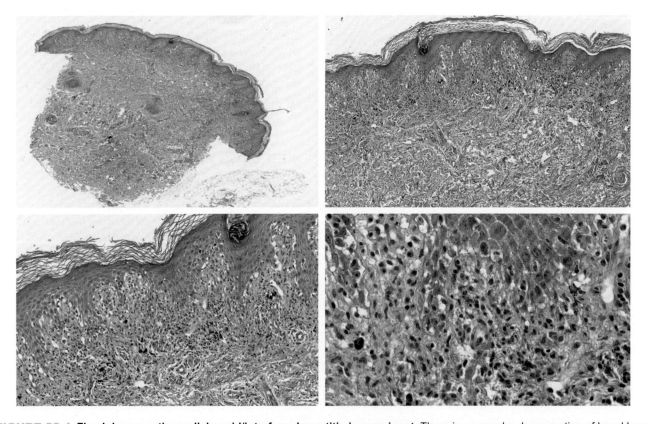

FIGURE 28-4. Fixed drug reaction; a lichenoid/interface dermatitis is prominent. There is a vacuolar degeneration of basal keratinocytes and frequent dyskeratotic cells. Pigment incontinence in the dermis is noted. The dermal inflammatory infiltrate also shows the presence of eosinophils. Digital slides courtesy of Path Presenter.com.

Clinical Presentation

Fixed drug eruptions almost always present as a single or multiple, clustered, perfectly annular, sharply demarcated, dusky, erythematous patches. Patients will generally describe burning as opposed to itching.[21] The most common locations are the perioral skin, dorsal hands and feet, and glans penis. Occasionally, the eruption can generalize, but typically can still be distinguished from Stevens-Johnson syndrome by the lack of significant mucosal involvement.

Histologic Findings

Pathologically, this eruption will look very similar to that of Stevens-Johnson syndrome with an interface dermatitis and keratinocyte necrosis that can be full thickness. In contrast to Stevens-Johnson syndrome, eosinophils may be more abundant, and often pigment dropout and melanophages will be visible from a previous reaction (Figure 28-4).

Differential Diagnosis

The consistent locations and rapid onset after drug use should be highly supportive of the diagnosis. However, erythema multiforme (EM) may also present similarly clinically. Histologically, it may not be distinguishable if the pigment dropout is not present. Stevens-Johnson syndrome and EM should be ruled out with clinicopathologic correlation by the locations of involvement, targetoid versus homogeneous patches, microorganism etiology (EM), and by substantial mucosal involvement.

CAPSULE SUMMARY

FIXED DRUG ERUPTION

Fixed drug eruptions are another common idiosyncratic eruption. Pathologically, they look very similar to those of EM or Stevens-Johnson syndrome, but they may be distinguished by tissue eosinophils and melanophages.

ACNEIFORM ERUPTION

Definition and Epidemiology

Acneiform eruption is a follicle-based pustular eruption over the upper body, head, and neck triggered by a drug. This eruption is generally considered rare or is not lumped with other causes of drug eruptions, except in the case of epidermal growth factor inhibitors, where the incidence of papulopustular eruptions can be as high as 90% of patients.[23-26]

Etiology

Acneiform eruptions may occur from many different etiologies, especially corticosteroids, lithium, and hormone supplements.[27] The similar papulopustular eruption of epidermal growth factor inhibitors, and mammalian target of rapamycin inhibitors is common and is addressed in the section on cancer.

Clinical Presentation

Papules and pustules over the upper chest and back, and most dense over the face and neck. Typically, comedones are not seen.

Histologic Findings

A follicular-based pustule or multiple pustules, folliculitis, and ruptured follicular structures are the typical features seen in acneiform drug reactions. (Figure 28-5). Usually, the follicles will not have significant bacterial or yeast colonization, although demodex may be present.

Differential Diagnosis

Acute generalized exanthematous pustulosis and diseases of subcorneal pustules need to be distinguished from the follicular pustules in this type of drug eruption. Demodex and malassezia folliculitis could also be considered if there is a high density of organisms in the follicles. Lastly, normal adolescent acne could be a mimicker, but typically children will notice the flare with one of the common etiologies of this eruption.

CAPSULE SUMMARY

ACNEIFORM ERUPTION

Acneiform eruption is a papular and pustular drug eruption that does not coalesce like the other drug eruptions. Typically, the eruption does not contain comedones, and the extent of the follicular inflammation should distinguish this eruption from acute generalized exanthematous pustulosis (AGEP) and other subcorneal pustular diseases.

CUTANEOUS ADVERSE EVENTS ASSOCIATED WITH TUMOR NECROSIS FACTOR INHIBITION

Definition and Epidemiology

A spectrum of toxicities, including paradoxical skin inflammation, psoriasis, palmoplantar eczema, cutaneous lupus, as well as infusion reactions can be seen with tumor necrosis factor inhibitors. Overall, these reactions are not infrequent. Paradoxical skin disease of psoriasis, eczematous, or other inflammatory skin diseases occurs in 5% to 10% of patients undergoing treatment with tumor necrosis factor (TNF) inhibitors for inflammatory bowel disease, whereas the rate is only 0.1% among patients treated for rheumatoid arthritis.[28] Including events such as infusion and injection site reactions, dermatologic toxicities can occur in 25% of patients.[29]

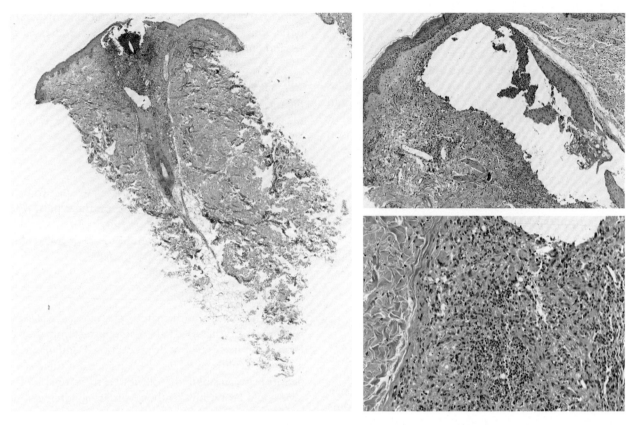

FIGURE 28-5. Acneiform eruption in association with epidermal growth factor receptor inhibitors. A pustular folliculitis and peri-folliculitis is present. At the edges of the inflamed follicle, focal granulomatous changes are present.

Etiology

Injection site reactions and infusion reactions relate to the immunogenicity of the antibody; however, the paradoxical skin inflammation is suspected to be caused by a signal loop downstream from the TNF inhibitor or increased interferon signaling.[28,29]

Clinical Presentation

The presentations are highly variable. Most commonly, psoriasis, generally of the palmoplantar subtype, dermatitis, or drug-induced lupus are reported. Less common presentations include vasculitis with palpable purpura or cutaneous lymphoma.[30] These diseases generally mimic classic forms of disease, with a preponderance of palmoplantar involvement. TNF-associated lupus may or may not affect the skin.[31] Infusion reactions occur only in patients receiving infusions, such as infliximab, and present cutaneously with an urticarial eruption or angioedema. Injection site reactions are highly variable on the basis of the therapy but tend to present with injection site pain and short-lived erythema.

Histologic Findings

Similarly, the histopathology of these diverse eruptions will mimic their classic forms of skin disease (Figure 28-6): psoriasiform forms are typical with regular elongation of the rete, intracorneal collections of neutrophils, superficial papillary dermal vessel dilatation, and a decreased granular cell layer. Other drug reactions can show features of pustular psoriasis or AGEP. As opposed to the classic forms of psoriasis, dermal eosinophils are frequently seen.

Differential Diagnosis

The differential diagnosis includes the same skin diseases developing in a de novo fashion; however, the recent initiation of a TNF inhibitor should trigger the consideration of a paradoxical immune effect.

CAPSULE SUMMARY

CUTANEOUS ADVERSE EVENTS ASSOCIATED WITH TUMOR NECROSIS FACTOR INHIBITION

There are many paradoxical skin diseases associated with the TNF inhibitors. With the frequency of use in children with inflammatory bowel disease and arthropathies, dermatologists should be aware of the various immune-mediated events. Whether the TNF inhibitor is changed, stopped, or continued, children who have developed psoriasis tend to partially or completely clear primarily with topical corticosteroids.[32]

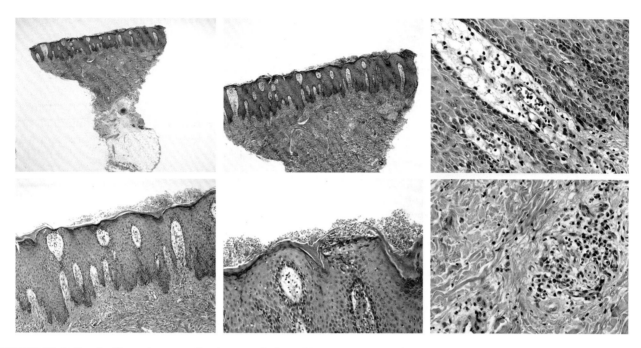

FIGURE 28-6. Psoriasiform drug reaction in association with tumor necrosis factor blockers. Psoriasiform epidermal acanthosis with regular elongation of the rete is seen. Dilatation of the superficial papillary dermal vessels is also present. Within the stratum corneum and superficial epidermis, collections of neutrophils are seen. Within the dermis, scattered eosinophils are seen, more numerous in number to what could be seen in cases of psoriasis.

Cutaneous Toxicity Reactions From Chemotherapeutic Agents in Children

Cancer remains the second leading cause of death in children aged 5 to 14 years, with accidents being the leading cause.[33] The top five most common cancers in children are acute lymphoblastic leukemia, brain and central nervous system tumors, neuroblastoma, non-Hodgkin lymphoma (particularly anaplastic lymphoma kinase + anaplastic large cell lymphoma), and Wilms tumor.[33] Chemotherapeutic agents can be effective, but may cause cutaneous adverse reactions; the most common are addressed in the following section.

TOXIC ERYTHEMA OF CHEMOTHERAPY

Definition and Epidemiology

Chemotherapy can cause direct cytotoxic cutaneous toxicity. Toxic erythema of chemotherapy is a clinical term that encompasses a spectrum of reactions, including acral erythema, eccrine squamous syringometaplasia, malignant intertrigo,[34] and neutrophilic eccrine hidradenitis (chemotherapy-induced) among others.[35] These reactions favor acral sites, intertriginous areas (particularly the scrotum), and also elbows and knees.[35]

The incidence of toxic erythema is unclear, but is thought to be rare in children. A few cases of acral erythema caused by oral methotrexate and cytarabine (AraC) have been reported in children.[36-38] As these eruptions are caused by traditional cytotoxic therapies, they may be underreported because they are no longer novel.

Etiology

The most common chemotherapeutic agents associated with toxic erythema of chemotherapy include AraC, anthracyclines, 5-fluorouracil (5-FU), capecitabine, taxanes, and methotrexate.

Clinical Presentation

The clinical characteristics of toxic erythema of chemotherapy include well-demarcated erythematous or edematous patches or plaques on the hands and feet, intertriginous zones, elbows, knees, and ears, usually appearing 2 days to 3 weeks following the administration of the chemotherapeutic agent (Figure 28-7). There is associated pain, burning, and pruritus. Some lesions may have a dusky hue and/or bullae within the area of erythema. These symptoms should subside spontaneously and may have associated desquamation. This reaction may recur with repeat chemotherapy administration.[35] Acral erythema is characterized by painful erythema of bilateral palms and soles with symmetrically well-demarcated borders, progressing into bullous formation.

Histologic Findings

Pathology will often distinguish the forms of toxic erythema of chemotherapy from competing diagnoses like drug eruptions and leukemia cutis. It is typically characterized by

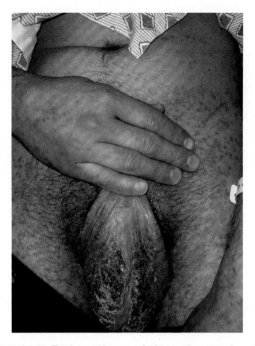

FIGURE 28-7. Toxic erythema of chemotherapy. A malignant intertrigo-like presentation in a young man undergoing therapy for Hodgkin lymphoma. Note that the duskiness is similar to that of Stevens-Johnson syndrome; however, this is typically associated with cytotoxic chemotherapy and occurs in intertriginous locations.

epidermal dysmaturation, syringosquamous metaplasia, and neutrophils within the sweat gland apparatus (Figure 28-8).

Differential Diagnosis

This must be distinguished from Sweet syndrome, leukemia cutis, and conventional morbilliform drug eruptions. These conditions can be differentiated with minimal neutrophilic infiltrate, without edema or vasculitis, and without leukemic cell infiltration. The conventional morbilliform eruption can be distinguished by the degree of epidermal dysmaturation, necrosis, and sweat gland metaplasia, but they may coexist, so it is important to collaborate with the clinician on the final diagnosis.

CAPSULE SUMMARY

TOXIC ERYTHEMA OF CHEMOTHERAPY

Toxic erythema of chemotherapy is a broadly encompassing term that brings together a shared pathophysiology of many previously individually described forms of epidermal dysmaturation and disruption secondary to cytotoxic chemotherapy. It is typified by epidermal dysmaturation, keratinocyte necrosis, syringosquamous metaplasia, and neutrophilic infiltrates in the sweat glands.

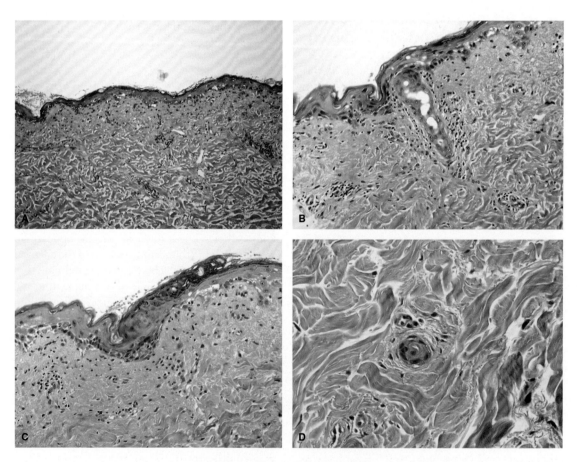

FIGURE 28-8. Toxic erythema of chemotherapy—histopathologic findings. Epidermal atrophy, dysmaturation ("actinic keratosis-like"), and interface changes are seen. Squamous metaplasia of the eccrine ducts is present.

MUCOSITIS

Definition and Epidemiology

Mucositis is characterized by inflammation, erosions, and/or ulceration of oral mucosa typically caused by radiation or chemotherapy. The prevalence of mucositis is high, with reports from ranging from 45% to 58% in children who undergo chemotherapy.[39]

Etiology

The exact mechanism is unclear but is thought to be caused by (1) direct drug-induced cytotoxic effects on the oral epithelial cells resulting in cell apoptosis and (2) indirect effects of secondary superimposed infections including Candida, herpes simplex virus, neutropenia. Several classes of chemotherapy agents can cause mucositis, with mTOR inhibitors being the most frequent.[40]

Clinical Presentation

Patients may develop erythema with associated edema and erythema 5 to 8 days after chemotherapy treatment. The nonkeratinized mucosal surfaces, including the buccal and labial mucosa, ventral and lateral surfaces of the tongue, floor of the mouth, and soft palate, are affected more.[41]

Histologic Findings

Pathologically, the findings are very similar to those of toxic erythema of chemotherapy because of the pathogenesis, and if biopsies are performed, they tend to demonstrate extensive necrosis throughout the mucosa, with neutrophilic infiltration of the submucosa (Figure 28-9).

Differential Diagnosis

Thrush and herpes simplex reactivation needs to be ruled out in this setting. Pseudohyphae on the biopsy should confirm oral thrush, whereas herpes simplex should be considered with any multinucleate cells with the typical steel gray coloration and can be confirmed using immunohistochemistry.

CAPSULE SUMMARY

MUCOSITIS

Mucositis is a common event after cytotoxic chemotherapy, and excluding secondary infections is important.

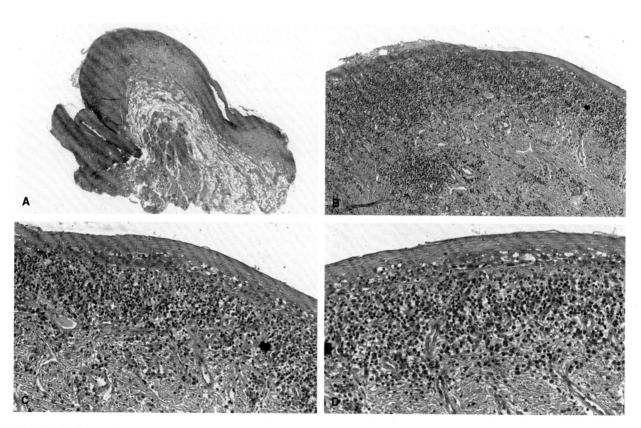

FIGURE 28-9. Lichenoid mucositis in association with chemotherapy. Mucosal necrosis is present, in association with a very dense lichenoid lymphoplasmacytic infiltrate. Keratinocyte necrosis is also seen. Digital slides courtesy of Path Presenter.com.

PAPULOPUSTULAR ERUPTION

Definition and Epidemiology

This type of reaction is associated with epidermal growth factor receptor (EGFR) inhibitor therapy in a dose-dependent fashion and is characterized by the development of papules and pustules typically in a seborrheic distribution.[24] There are limited studies done in pediatric patients, but this reaction is well documented in the adult population, and may occur in up to 90% of patients with some EGFR inhibitors.[42-45]

Etiology

EGFR has been shown to play a role in controlling IL-1 and TNF-induced inflammation at the hair-follicle level. Thus by inhibiting this receptor, the end result is excessive pustular inflammation.[46] The most common etiologies are the EGFR inhibitors, but the protooncogene BRAF and MAPK/ERK Kinase (MEK) inhibitors also have a high rate of papulopustular eruptions.[47-50]

Clinical Presentation

The rash often develops 1 to 2 weeks after starting targeted inhibitor therapy in a dose-dependent fashion. The eruption has predilection for a seborrheic distribution on the central face, nose, cheeks, forehead, chin, scalp, neck and retroauricular area, upper shoulders, and upper trunk (Figure 28-10). The pustules should be sterile but may be secondarily infected with *Staphylococcus aureus*.[51]

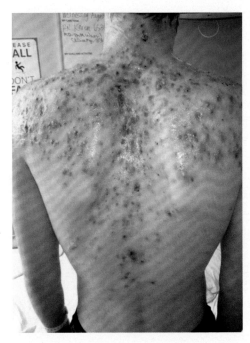

FIGURE 28-10. Papulopustular eruption: Numerous inflammatory papules and pustules without comedones over the upper body.

Histologic Findings

The eruption is very similar to that of acne with the exception of comedones (Figure 28-5). Typically, follicular and perifollicular neutrophilic and lymphocytic inflammation is seen with a potential for follicular rupture.[18]

Differential Diagnosis

Acne and rosacea are histopathologically indistinguishable. Excluding subcorneal pustular dermatoses like AGEP is critical.

CAPSULE SUMMARY

PAPULOPUSTULAR ERUPTION

The papulopustular eruption, typically from EGFR, BRAF, or MEK inhibitors in cancer therapeutics, is an exceedingly common eruption in susceptible patients. Because it is well described, it is unlikely that many pediatric patients will receive a biopsy, but confirming the follicular nature should ensure that this is not a more severe form of a drug eruption.

PERSISTENT SERPENTINE SUPRAVENOUS HYPERPIGMENTATION

Definition and Epidemiology

First described by Hrushesky in 1980, persistent serpentine supravenous hyperpigmentation is a rare reaction characterized by linear hyperpigmentation of the skin overlying veins from intravenous chemotherapy treatment infused into a peripheral vein.

Although rare, the typical cases are associated with 5-FU, actinomycin, cyclophosphamide, cisplatin, docetaxel, taxanes, fotemustine, nitrogen mustard, nitrourea, and pemetrexed.

Etiology

The etiology is unclear, but is believed to be a possible cytotoxic effect on the vascular epithelium.[52]

Clinical Presentation

It presents as a symptomatic serpentine erythema overlying veins on the upper extremities at sites of intravenous infusion several hours after the infusion. There is residual hyperpigmentation a few weeks after the initial onset of symptoms. Treatment is supportive, and the pigment may last anywhere from a few months to more than a year after completion of treatment.[53]

Histologic Findings

Biopsies in the acute phase will typically demonstrate interface dermatitis, with keratinocyte necrosis, potentially epidermal dysmaturation, dermal edema, and superficial perivascular infiltrates. In the chronic phase, melanophages and pigment incontinence will be more obvious.

Differential Diagnosis

The peculiar nature along the vein after an infusion is very indicative. Superficial venous thrombophlebitis should be excluded, in which case a biopsy would demonstrate papillary dermal edema without other histopathologic changes. Because of the depth of the pathology, the final corroboration would require a venous duplex for confirmation.

CAPSULE SUMMARY

PERSISTENT SERPENTINE SUPRAVENOUS HYPERPIGMENTATION

This is a rare pigmented eruption that occurs along the superficial veins, causing acute necrosis of the epidermis and secondary pigment incontinence.

FLAGELLATE HYPERPIGMENTATION

Definition and Epidemiology

Flagellate hyperpigmentation appears as multiple curvilinear streaks on the skin and may be caused by a variety of medications, but especially bleomycin.[54] This reaction is uncommon but may be underreported,[55,56] and is most often reported from bleomycin, part of the regimen for Hodgkin lymphoma and some testicular cancers.

Etiology

Bleomycin is an antibiotic, isolated from *Streptomyces verticillus*, with antineoplastic properties.[57] The exact mechanism by which bleomycin causes hyperpigmentation is unclear, but some hypotheses include excess itching in the acute phase, causing localized increased in melanogenesis, similar to postinflammatory hyperpigmentation.[57]

Clinical Presentation

The rash is characterized by pruritic linear erythema that can thicken over time, leaving residual hyperpigmentation.[56] The onset of flagellate erythema is variable, from a few hours to 9 weeks, and the streaks may be present up to 6 months.[54] The reaction is independent of the route of bleomycin administration or the types of cancer treated, but has been associated with cumulative dose ranging between 90 and 285 mg.[56]

Histologic Findings

The pathology is generally nonspecific with slight spongiosis, superficial lymphocytic infiltration, dermal edema, and melanophages and pigment incontinence in the papillary dermis.

Differential Diagnosis

Clinically, the findings are unique, particularly in the cancer patient on bleomycin, although it has also been reported with Shiitake mushroom farmers. Pathologically, these findings can be similar to those of other pigment anomalies after chemotherapy and require clinicopathologic correlation to arrive at the diagnosis of flagellate hyperpigmentation.

CAPSULE SUMMARY

FLAGELLATE HYPERPIGMENTATION

This is a clinically unique phenomenon, typically related to bleomycin that shows features of mild inflammation with pigment incontinence and melanophages pathologically.

PIGMENTARY CHANGES

Definition and Epidemiology

Patients may develop localized or generalized hypo-or hyperpigmentation following traditional chemotherapy but also with tyrosine kinase inhibitors (TKI). The severity of clinical presentation appears to be dose dependent.[58]

Forty-one percent of 118 patients and thirty-three percent of 24 patients taking imatinib developed depigmentation.[59,60] This rate is higher than that typical for traditional cytotoxic chemotherapies.

Etiology

Imatinib, dasatinib, and nilotinib are a group of tyrosine kinase inhibitors—targeting *bcr-abl*, c-kit, and platelet-derived growth factor receptors—that are used to treat chronic myelogenous leukemia and B-lymphoblastic leukemia.[24] The variable presentation of cutaneous eruption appears to be related to the inhibition of c-kit. C-kit is important in melanocyte biology, and by inhibiting the tyrosine kinase pathway, patients on tyrosine kinase inhibitors can develop depigmentation as well as paradoxical hyperpigmentation.[58]

Clinical Presentation

Patients, especially those with darker skin, may develop vitiligo-like depigmentation in patchy or generalized fashion after the initiation of tyrosine kinase inhibitors.[24] The onset of symptoms may range from 4 weeks to several months.[58]

Histologic Findings

Increased basal melanin pigmentation, in addition to a mild superficial perivascular lymphohistiocytic inflammation, melanin pigment incontinence, and melanophages are typical in cases of hyperpigmentation, whereas hypopigmentation will look like normal skin with decreased melanin staining and potentially perifollicular fibrosis (Figure 28-11).

Differential Diagnosis

Flagellate hyperpigmentation, melasma, vitiligo, and other drug pigmentation are in the differential, but these require clinicopathologic correlation to differentiate.

CAPSULE SUMMARY

PIGMENTARY CHANGES

Tyrosine kinase inhibitors, through effects on the c-kit pathway, can result in generalized hypo-or hyperpigmentation of the skin, which pathologically is similar to other diseases of hypo-and hyperpigmentation, thus requiring clinicopathologic correlation. Some cytotoxic chemotherapies can have similar effects.

Severe Cutaneous Adverse Reactions

Severe cutaneous adverse drug reactions (SCARs) are rare and potentially life-threatening. These include AGEP, drug reaction with eosinophilia and systemic symptoms (DRESS), Stevens-Johnson syndrome, and toxic epidermal necrolysis. Approximately one-third of adverse drug reactions in children are cutaneous, but most are mild. Only 2% to 6.7% of all cutaneous reactions are life-threatening, and the incidence is likely lower in children.[61] The histologic features of SCARs in children are not fully characterized, particularly in DRESS, where the diagnosis is often made clinically. As a whole, the histologic findings of SCARs in children resemble those seen in adults.

ACUTE GENERALIZED EXANTHEMATOUS PUSTULOSIS

Definition and Epidemiology

AGEP is an uncommon SCAR most commonly caused by a medication. It is characterized by the eruption of nonfollicular sterile pinpoint pustules with an erythematous base.[62]

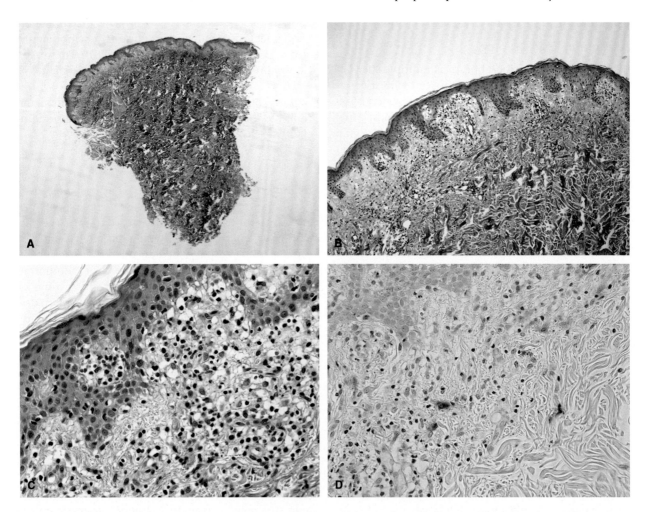

FIGURE 28-11. Pigmented purpuric-like eruption in association with a tyrosine kinase inhibitor. A dense perivascular lymphocytic infiltrate is present, in addition to interface changes (vacuolar alteration of basal keratinocytes). Hemosiderin deposits are noted by an iron stain (bottom right panel).

The incidence of AGEP is low at 1 to 5 cases per million patients per year, and the mean age of patients is 56 years.[63] Although the exact incidence is not known in pediatric patients, it is thought to be less common in children than in adults. Several cases of AGEP have been described in children in the literature. Mortality is lower than in other SCARs, with an average overall rate of less than 5%.[62]

Etiology

AGEP is thought to be a T-cell-mediated disease with a predominant Th1 cytokine profile. Accordingly, patch testing can often be helpful in diagnosis.[62] Medications are almost exclusively the cause of AGEP in adults, whereas in children, AGEP has been documented in the absence of any medication exposure. Viral infections or vaccinations are suspected culprits in these cases.[64] Medications most often associated with AGEP include antibiotics (65%), particularly macrolides and beta-lactams. Several other medications have been implicated, such as calcium channel blockers and nonsteroidal anti-inflammatory drugs.[64] Microbes, including parvovirus B19, Chlamydia pneumonia, and cytomegalovirus, have been reported as well.[62]

Clinical Presentation

AGEP is unique among the SCAR group of reactions in its relatively rapid onset and resolution after discontinuation of the culprit medication. Onset typically occurs only 1 to 2 days after drug initiation, and the condition resolves with 2 weeks of drug discontinuation.[62] Patients typically present with high fever and a cutaneous eruption of nonfollicular sterile pinpoint pustules atop an erythematous, edematous background on the face and intertriginous areas (Figure 28-12). This eruption generalizes within a matter of hours. Mucous membrane involvement is uncommon, helping to distinguish this from Stevens-Johnson syndrome or toxic epidermal necrolysis. Lab work demonstrates leukocytosis with neutrophilia, hypocalcemia, and sometimes eosinophilia.

Histologic Findings

Pediatric cases of AGEP have shown histologic features similar to those of adults. AGEP is characterized histologically by intra-and subcorneal pustules with papillary dermal edema.[65] Pustules contain eosinophils and neutrophils (Figure 28-13). Spongiosis can be seen, as well as exocytosis of neutrophils and necrotic keratinocytes.[66]

Differential Diagnosis

AGEP must be distinguished histologically from pustular psoriasis. Eosinophils in the inflammatory infiltrate are more indicative of AGEP and are not generally seen in pustular psoriasis. Histologic features of psoriasis, including parakeratosis, mitotic figures, and dilated blood vessels, are generally

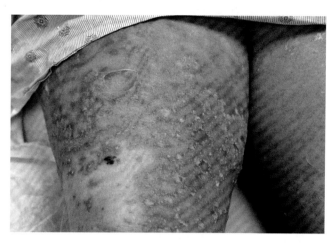

FIGURE 28-12. Acute generalized exanthematous pustulosis: superficial pustules coalescing into lakes of pus. This reaction was secondary to vancomycin.

absent in AGEP. In a study of 102 cases of adult AGEP, the histologic findings did not differ between patients with or without history of psoriasis.[66]

CAPSULE SUMMARY

ACUTE GENERALIZED EXANTHEMATOUS PUSTULOSIS

Histologic features of AGEP are similar to those cases seen in adults. It is characterized by intra-and subcorneal pustules containing eosinophils and neutrophils overlying papillary dermal edema. Differentiating this disease from pustular psoriasis requires clinicopathologic correlation.

DRUG REACTION WITH EOSINOPHILIA AND SYSTEMIC SYMPTOMS (DRESS)

Definition and Epidemiology

DRESS, also known as drug-induced hypersensitivity syndrome and drug-induced delayed multiorgan hypersensitivity syndrome, is a severe life-threatening systemic hypersensitivity reaction to a medication. It is characterized by fever, widespread cutaneous eruption, facial edema, peripheral eosinophilia, and internal organ involvement.[67,68]

The incidence of DRESS is 1 per 1000 to 10 000 drug exposures. Mortality ranges from 10% to 40%. DRESS is infrequently reported in children and is likely underdiagnosed in this population.[67]

Etiology

DRESS is thought to be a type IV hypersensitivity reaction and is associated with enzymatic defects in the metabolism of certain drugs. Drugs most commonly implicated in DRESS include aromatic anticonvulsants such as

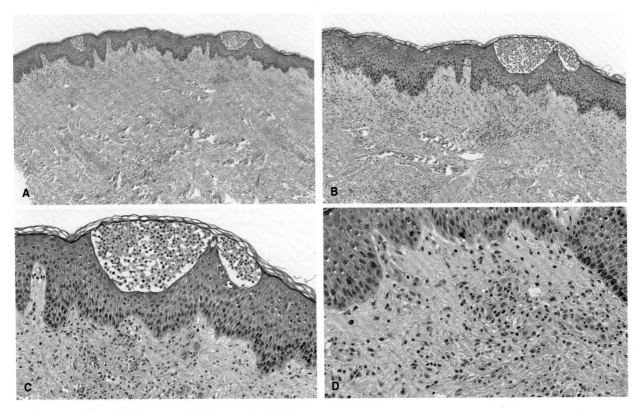

FIGURE 28-13. Acute generalized exanthematous pustulosis. Intracorneal pustules containing abundant neutrophils are present. Within the dermis, a mostly neutrophilic perivascular infiltrate is present, with sparse eosinophils. Digital slides courtesy of Path Presenter.com.

phenytoin, carbamazepine, and phenobarbital, as well as sulfonamides. In a multicenter study by Misirlioglu et al, antibiotics were the most common offending agent in children with DRESS.[61,67] Viral infections, particularly the herpes virus family, have also been implicated, in particular herpes virus 6 reactivation, herpes virus 7, Epstein-Barr virus, and cytomegalovirus.[69]

Clinical Presentation

DRESS is characterized by fever, widespread cutaneous eruption, facial edema, peripheral eosinophilia, and internal organ involvement, typically presenting within 6 weeks of exposure to the offending drug.[67,68] Cutaneous findings are present in 75% of patients with DRESS. Although there is not a single cutaneous morphology that characterizes DRESS, the eruption often begins with facial edema, particularly periorbitally, followed by erythema and pruritus. A more widespread eruption usually begins on the face and upper trunk, which can be urticarial, exanthematous, morbilliform, EM-like, or nonspecific.[70] Internal organ involvement is a hallmark of DRESS. The liver is the most frequently affected organ in children and adults,[61] with renal involvement also common, although any organ can be affected. Mucous membrane involvement is rare.[71] Lab work reveals peripheral eosinophilia, atypical lymphocytosis, as

well as hepatic and renal abnormalities when these organs are involved.

Histologic Findings

Much like the cutaneous findings in DRESS, this reaction can vary histologically. Most research on the histopathologic findings of DRESS have been performed in adults, whereas many cases of DRESS in children are diagnosed without cutaneous biopsy. In adults, focal interface dermatitis, a superficial perivascular lymphocytic infiltrate, and erythrocyte extravasation are often seen in DRESS (Figure 28-14). These are relatively nonspecific findings that can be seen in generic drug–induced dermatitis. Although peripheral eosinophilia is a hallmark of this disease, eosinophils are not typically seen in cutaneous biopsy specimens.[70] Although helpful as an aid to diagnosis, laboratory testing and clinicopathologic correlation are required to make a definitive diagnosis of DRESS.

Differential Diagnosis

The histopathologic differential diagnosis of DRESS includes primarily other drug eruptions. Eczematous, interface, AGEP-like, and erythema-multiforme-like histologic patterns have all been observed in cases of DRESS. The presence of two or three of these patterns in a single biopsy

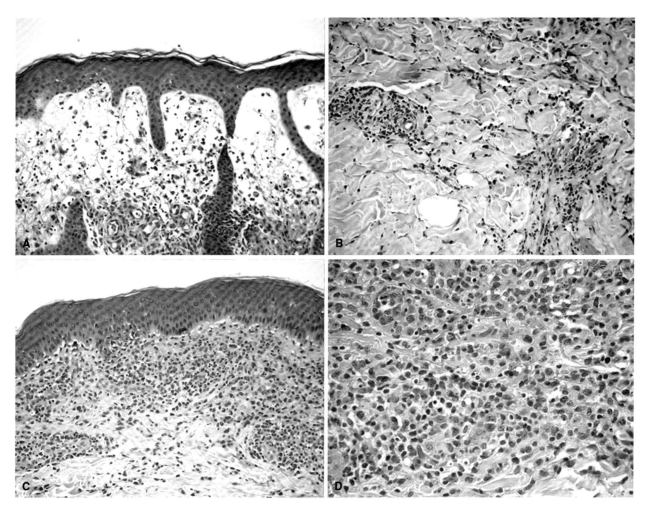

FIGURE 28-14. **The histopathologic findings of drug reaction with eosinophilia and systemic symptoms (DRESS).** Histopathology of DRESS mainly with dermal edema with scarce epidermal involvement (A) and a perivascular and interstitial infiltrate of lymphocytes and eosinophils with extravasated erythrocytes but no vasculitis (B); a pseudolymphomatous reaction with a dense dermal infiltrate of large and atypical lymphocytes, with some mitotic figures, associated with vacuolization of the basal layer (C and D). Reprinted with permission from Margarida G, Cardoso JC, Gouveia MP, et al. Histopathology of the Exanthema in DRESS Is Not Specific but May Indicate Severity of Systemic Involvement. *Am J Dermatopathol.* 2016;38(6):423-433.

is more common in DRESS than in nondrug-induced dermatoses and may be helpful in differentiating DRESS from these other eruptions.[72]

CAPSULE SUMMARY

DRUG REACTION WITH EOSINOPHILIA AND SYSTEMIC SYMPTOMS

The histopathologic findings of DRESS in pediatric patients are not well studied. DRESS shows various histologic patterns, usually characterized by focal interface dermatitis, a superficial perivascular lymphocytic infiltrate, and erythrocyte extravasation. The presence of multiple reaction patterns in a single biopsy can be a histologic clue in the diagnosis of DRESS.

STEVENS-JOHNSON SYNDROME AND TOXIC EPIDERMAL NECROLYSIS

Definition and Epidemiology

Stevens-Johnson syndrome (SJS) and toxic epidermal necrolysis (TEN) are rare, life-threatening diseases characterized by necrosis and detachment of the epidermis, skin sloughing, and mucous membrane erosion. The two diseases exist on a spectrum, with SJS being characterized by a detachment of less than 10% of the body surface area (BSA) and TEN being characterized by a detachment of more than 30% of the BSA. Those with an involvement of 10% to 30% BSA are considered to have SJS–TEN overlap.[73]

The incidences of SJS and TEN are reported to be 1 to 7 and 1 to 2 cases per million, respectively;[74] however, little is known about the incidence of pediatric SJS and TEN, as

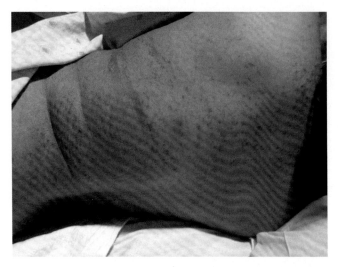

FIGURE 28-15. Stevens-Johnson syndrome: coalescent patches of cutaneous necrosis and dusky bullae with atypical targetoid figures. This is in the early phase of disease and prior to erosions.

most studies include limited numbers of cases. Gerull et al report an incidence of SJS and TEN combined, in pediatric patients, of 0.5 cases per million person-years.[75] The mortality of pediatric SJS, SJS–TEN overlap, and TEN are reported to be 0%, 4.0%, and 16.0%, respectively.[74]

Etiology

The cause of SJS and TEN is not fully understood, but it is thought to be an autoimmune reaction incited by a medication or virus. Fas ligand overexpression leads to dermoepidermal junction separation and resultant skin sloughing. SJS and TEN are most commonly caused by drugs, including sulfonamides, hydantoins, nonsteroidal anti-inflammatory drugs, and penicillins.[76]

Clinical Presentation

TEN and SJS typically begin 1 to 2 weeks after a culprit medication is introduced. There is often a prodrome of fever, malaise, and respiratory symptoms or sore throat. The earliest cutaneous findings are painful atypical macular targets or dusky macules found on the trunk that then spread to the face and extremities (Figure 28-15). These lesion coalesce into large bullae and the skin easily sloughs off. Tangential pressure can cause detachment of the epidermis from the dermis, known as a positive Nikolsky sign. Severe mucous membrane involvement is characteristic of this disease, including the eyes, mouth, lungs, anogenital region, and any mucosal surface.[77] Children are able to maintain hemodynamic stability until a later stage of the disease, up until a point of rapid decompensation. Children are at particular risk for airway compromise early in the disease.

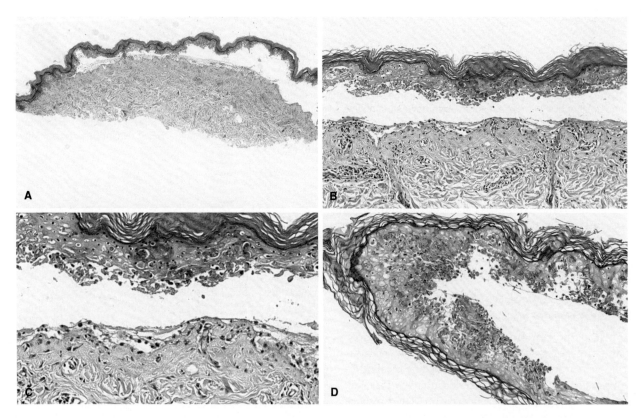

FIGURE 28-16. Stevens-Johnson syndrome/toxic epidermal necrolysis—histopathologic findings. A subepidermal blister is present, produced by the marked interface changes. Areas of transepidermal necrosis are prominent. Digital slides courtesy of Path Presenter.com.

Edema of the anatomically small airways of children can quickly reduce the size of the airway and impede airflow.[76] Predictors of mortality from these diseases in the pediatric population include renal failure, malignancy, septicemia, bacterial infection, and epilepsy.[74]

Histologic Findings

The histologic findings of pediatric SJS and TEN are similar to those of adults with these diseases. SJS and TEN are histologically identical. They are characterized histologically by confluent full-thickness epidermal necrosis and minimal to no superficial perivascular inflammatory infiltrate made up primarily of CD8[+] cytotoxic T cells and NK cells (Figure 28-16). The stratum corneum is typically a normal basket-weave pattern, indicating an acute process. Immunofluorescence is negative. Basal layer vacuolization can also be seen.[73]

Differential Diagnosis

SJS and TEN must be distinguished histologically from EM. EM demonstrates individual necrotic keratinocytes at all levels of the epidermis; however, this necrosis is typically not confluent, as it is in SJS and TEN. Inflammation is more prominent in EM than in SJS and TEN. Vacuolar interface dermatitis, as well as superficial and perivascular inflammation, is seen, consisting primarily of lymphocytes. Similar to SJS and TEN, the stratum corneum maintains its normal basket-weave orthokeratosis. Spongiosis with intraepidermal and/or subepidermal bullae can be seen.[73]

CAPSULE SUMMARY

STEVENS-JOHNSON SYNDROME AND TOXIC EPIDERMAL NECROLYSIS

The histologic findings of pediatric SJS and TEN are similar to those of adults. These diseases are characterized histologically by full-thickness epidermal necrosis with separation of the epidermis from the dermis, with minimal underlying inflammation in the dermis.

REFERENCES

1. Apaydin R, Bilen N, Dökmeci S, Bayramgürler D, Yildirim G. Drug eruptions: a study including all inpatients and outpatients at a dermatology clinic of a university hospital. *J Eur Acad Dermatol Venereol.* 2000;14:518-520.
2. Sastre J, Manso L, Sanchez-García S, Fernández-Nieto M. Medical and economic impact of misdiagnosis of drug hypersensitivity in hospitalized patients. *J Allergy Clin Immunol.* 2012;129(2):566-567. doi:10.1016/j.jaci.2011.09.028.
3. Sassolas B, Haddad C, Mockenhaupt M, et al. ALDEN, an algorithm for assessment of drug causality in Stevens–Johnson syndrome and toxic epidermal necrolysis: comparison with case–control analysis. *Clin Pharmacol Ther.* 2010;88(1):60-68. doi:10.1038/clpt.2009.252.
4. Naranjo C, Busto U, Sellers E, et al. A method for estimating the probability of adverse drug reactions. *Clin Pharmacol Titer.* 1981;30(2):239-245.
5. Nigen S, Knowles SR, Shear NH. Drug eruptions: approaching the diagnosis of drug-induced skin diseases. *J Drugs Dermatol.* 2003;2(3):278-299.
6. Saha A, Das NK, Hazra A, Gharami RC, Chowdhury SN, Datta PK. Cutaneous adverse drug reaction profile in a tertiary care out patient setting in Eastern India. *Indian J Pharmacol.* 2012;44(6):792-797. doi:10.4103/0253-7613.103304.
7. Puavilai S, Noppakun N, Sitakalin C, et al. Drug eruptions at five institutes in Bangkok. *J Med Assoc Thail.* 2005;88(11):1642-1650.
8. Puavilai S, Choonhakarn C. Drug eruptions in Bangkok: A 1-year study at Ramathibodi Hospital. *Int J Dermatol.* 1998;37(10):747-751. doi:10.1046/j.1365-4362.1998.00378.x.
9. Bircher AJ, Scherer Hofmeier K. Drug hypersensitivity reactions: Inconsistency in the use of the classification of immediate and nonimmediate reactions. *J Allergy Clin Immunol.* 2012;129(1):263-264. doi:10.1016/j.jaci.2011.08.042.
10. Jhaj R, Uppal R, Malhotra S, Bhargava VK. Cutaneous adverse reactions in in-patients in a tertiary care hospital. *Indian J Dermatol Venereol Leprol.* 65(1):14-17.
11. Barzilai A, Sagi L, Baum S, et al. The Histopathology of Urticaria Revisited-Clinical Pathological Study. *Am J Dermatopathol.* 2017;39(10):753-759. doi:10.1097/DAD.0000000000000786.
12. Knowles SR, Uetrecht J, Shear NH. Idiosyncratic drug reactions: the reactive metabolite syndromes. *Lancet.* 2000;356(9241):1587-1591. doi:10.1016/S0140-6736(00)03137-8.
13. Dodiuk-Gad R, Laws P, Shear N. Epidemiology of severe drug hypersensitivity. *Semin Cutan Med Surg.* 2014;33(1):2-9. doi:10.12788/j.sder.0057.
14. Hebert AA, Sigman ES, Levy ML. Serum sickness-like reactions from cefaclor in children. *J Am Acad Dermatol.* 1991;25(5, pt 1):805-808.
15. Gerson D, Sriganeshan V, Alexis JB. Cutaneous drug eruptions: a 5-year experience. *J Am Acad Dermatol.* 2008;59(6):995-999. doi:10.1016/j.jaad.2008.09.015.
16. Drago F, Rampini P, Rampini E, Rebora A. Atypical exanthems: morphology and laboratory investigations may lead to an aetiological diagnosis in about 70% of cases. *Br J Dermatol.* 2002;147:255-260.
17. Drago F, Paolino S, Rebora A, et al. The challenge of diagnosing atypical exanthems: a clinico-laboratory study. *J Am Acad Dermatol.* 2012;67(6):1282-1288.doi:10.1016/j.jaad.2012.04.014.
18. Lee JJ, Kroshinsky D, Hoang MP. Cutaneous reactions to targeted therapy. *Am J Dermatopathol.* 2017;39(2):67-82. doi:10.1097/DAD.0000000000000504.
19. Seitz CS, Rose C, Kerstan A, Trautmann A. Drug-induced exanthems: correlation of allergy testing with histologic diagnosis. *J Am Acad Dermatol.* 2013;69(5):721-728. doi:10.1016/j.jaad.2013.06.022.
20. Marra DE, McKee PH, Nghiem P. Tissue eosinophils and the perils of using skin biopsy specimens to distinguish between drug hypersensitivity and cutaneous graft-versus-host disease. *J Am Acad Dermatol.* 2004;51(4):543-546. doi:10.1016/j.jaad.2004.02.019.
21. Özkaya E. Fixed drug eruption: state of the art. *JDDG.* 2008;6(3):181-188. doi:10.1111/j.1610-0387.2007.06491.x.
22. Sehgal VN, Srivastava G. Fixed drug eruption (FDE): changing scenario of incriminating drugs. *Int J Dermatol.* 2006;45(8):897-908. doi:10.1111/j.1365-4632.2006.02853.x.
23. Ra HS, Shin SJ, Kim JH, Lim H, Cho BC, Roh MR. The impact of dermatological toxicities of anti-cancer therapy on the dermatological quality of life of cancer patients. *J Eur Acad Dermatol Venereol.* 2013;27(1):53-59. doi:10.1111/j.1468-3083.2012.04466.x.
24. Reyes-Habito CM, Roh EK. Cutaneous reactions to chemotherapeutic drugs and targeted therapy for cancer: Part II. Targeted therapy. *J Am Acad Dermatol.* 2014;71(2):217.e1-217.e11. doi:10.1016/j.jaad.2014.04.013.
25. Thatcher N, Nicolson M, Groves RW, et al. Expert consensus on the management of erlotinib-associated cutaneous toxicity in the U.K. *Oncologist.* 2009;14(8):840-847. doi:10.1634/theoncologist.2009-0055.

26. Bergman H, Walton T, Del Bel R, et al. Managing skin toxicities related to panitumumab. *J Am Acad Dermatol.* 2014;71(4):1-6. doi:10.1016/j.jaad.2014.06.011.

27. Zeichner JA. *Acneiform Eruptions in Dermatology: A Differential Diagnosis.* New York, NY: Springer; 2014:1-478.

28. Fiorino G, Danese S, Pariente B, Allez M. Paradoxical immune-mediated inflammation in inflammatory bowel disease patients receiving anti-TNF-α agents. *Autoimmun Rev.* 2014;13(1):15-19. doi:10.1016/j.autrev.2013.06.005.

29. Mocci G, Marzo M, Papa A, Armuzzi A, Guidi L. Dermatological adverse reactions during anti-TNF treatments: focus on inflammatory bowel disease. *J Crohn's Colitis.* 2013;7(10):769-779. doi:10.1016/j.crohns.2013.01.009.

30. Moustou AE, Matekovits A, Dessinioti C, Antoniou C, Sfikakis PP, Stratigos AJ. Cutaneous side effects of anti-tumor necrosis factor biologic therapy: a clinical review. *J Am Acad Dermatol.* 2009;61(3):486-504. doi:10.1016/j.jaad.2008.10.060.

31. Lowe GC, Henderson CL, Grau RH, Hansen CB, Sontheimer RD. A systematic review of drug-induced subacute cutaneous lupus erythematosus. *Br J Dermatol.* 2011;164(3):465-472. doi:10.1111/j.1365-2133.2010.10110.x.

32. Romiti R, Araujo KM, Steinwurz F, Denadai R. Anti-tumor necrosis factor α-related psoriatic lesions in children with inflammatory bowel disease: case report and systematic literature review. *Pediatr Dermatol.* 2016;33(2):e174-e178. doi:10.1111/pde.12820.

33. Ward E, Desantis C, Robbins A, Kohler B, Jemal A. Childhood and adolescent cancer statistics, 2014. *CA Cancer J Clin.* 2014;64(2):83-103. doi:10.3322/caac.21219.

34. Smith SM, Milam PB, Fabbro SK, Gru AA, Kaffenberger BH. Malignant intertrigo: a subset of toxic erythema of chemotherapy requiring recognition. *JAAD Case Reports.* 2016;2(6):476-481. doi:10.1016/j.jdcr.2016.08.016.

35. Bolognia JL, Cooper DL, Glusac EJ, Haven N. Toxic erythema of chemotherapy: a useful clinical term. *J Am Acad Dermatol.* 2008;59(3):524-529. doi:10.1016/j.jaad.2008.05.018.

36. Ozmen S, Dogru M, Bozkurt C, Kocaoglu AC. Probable cytarabine-induced acral erythema: report of 2 pediatric cases. *J Pediatr Hematol Oncol.* 2013;35(1):e11-e13. doi:10.1097/MPH.0b013e3182580ba0.

37. Werchniak AE, Chaffee S, Dinulos JGH. Methotrexate-induced bullous acral erythema in a child. *J Am Acad Dermatol.* 2005;52(5 suppl 1):S93-S95. doi:10.1016/j.jaad.2004.11.065.

38. Varela CR, McNamara J, Antaya RJ. Acral erythema with oral methotrexate in a child. *Pediatr Dermatol.* 2007;24(5):541-546. doi:10.1111/j.1525-1470.2007.00513.x.

39. Gandhi K, Datta G, Ahuja S, Saxena T, Datta AG. Prevalence of oral complications occurring in a population of pediatric cancer patients receiving chemotherapy. *Int J Clin Pediatr Dent.* 2017;10(2):166-171.

40. Belum VR, Washington C, Pratilas CA, Sibaud V, Boralevi F, Lacouture ME. Dermatologic adverse events in pediatric patients receiving targeted anticancer therapies: a pooled analysis. *Pediatr Blood Cancer.* 2015;62(5):798-806. doi:10.1002/pbc.25429.

41. Rodríguez-Caballero A, Torres-Lagares D, Robles-García M, Pachón-Ibáñez J, González-Padilla D, Gutiérrez-Pérez JL. Cancer treatment-induced oral mucositis: a critical review. *Int J Oral Maxillofac Surg.* 2012;41(2):225-238. doi:10.1016/j.ijom.2011.10.011.

42. Friedman MD, Lacouture M, Dang C. Dermatologic adverse events associated with use of adjuvant lapatinib in combination with paclitaxel and trastuzumab for HER2-positive breast cancer: a case series analysis. *Clin Breast Cancer.* 2016;16(3):e69-e74. doi:10.1016/j.clbc.2015.11.001.

43. Lacouture ME. Mechanisms of cutaneous toxicities to EGFR inhibitors. *Nat Rev Cancer.* 2006;6(10):803-812. doi:10.1038/nrc1970.

44. Drucker AM, Wu S, Dang CT, Lacouture ME. Risk of rash with the anti-HER2 dimerization antibody pertuzumab: a meta-analysis. *Breast Cancer Res Treat.* 2012;135(2):347-354. doi:10.1007/s10549-012-2157-7.

45. Lacouture ME, Mitchell EP, Piperdi B, et al. Skin toxicity evaluation protocol with panitumumab (STEPP), a Phase II, open-label, randomized trial evaluating the impact of a pre-emptive skin treatment regimen on skin toxicities and quality of life in patients with metastatic colorectal cancer. *J Clin Oncol.* 2010;28(8):1351-1357. doi:10.1200/JCO.2008.21.7828.

46. Rodeck U. Skin toxicity caused by EGFR antagonists-an autoinflammatory condition triggered by deregulated IL-1 signaling? *J Cell Physiol.* 2009;218(1):32-34. doi:10.1002/jcp.21585.

47. Belum VR, Fischer A, Choi JN, Lacouture ME. Dermatological adverse events from BRAF inhibitors: a growing problem. *Curr Oncol Rep.* 2013;15(3):249-259. doi:10.1007/s11912-013-0308-6.

48. Anforth RM, Blumetti TCMP, Kefford RF, et al. Cutaneous manifestations of dabrafenib (GSK2118436): a selective inhibitor of mutant BRAF in patients with metastatic melanoma. *Br J Dermatol.* 2012;167(5):1153-1160. doi:10.1111/j.1365-2133.2012.11155.x.

49. Lacroix J-P, Wang B. Prospective case series of cutaneous adverse effects associated with dabrafenib and trametinib. *J Cutan Med Surg.* 2016;21(1):54-59. doi:10.1177/1203475416670368.

50. Long GV, Stroyakovskiy D, Gogas H, et al. Dabrafenib and trametinib versus dabrafenib and placebo for Val600 BRAF-mutant melanoma: a multicentre, double-blind, phase 3 randomised controlled trial. *Lancet.* 2015;386(9992):444-451. doi:10.1016/S0140-6736(15)60898-4.

51. Segaert S, Chiritescu G, Lemmens L, Dumon K, Van Cutsem E, Tejpar S. Skin toxicities of targeted therapies. *Eur J Cancer.* 2009;45(suppl 1):295-308. doi:10.1016/S0959-8049(09)70044-9.

52. Jain V, Bhandary S, Prasad GN, Shenoi SD. Serpentine supravenous streaks induced by 5-fluorouracil. *J Am Acad Dermatol.* 2005;53(3):529-530. doi:10.1016/j.jaad.2005.01.128.

53. Marcoux D, Anex R, Russo P. Persistent serpentine supravenous hyperpigmented eruption as an adverse reaction to chemotherapy combining actinomycin and vincristine. *J Am Acad Dermatol.* 2000;43(3):540-546. doi:10.1067/mjd.2000.106239.

54. Lee HY, Lim KH, Ryu Y, Song SY. Bleomycin-induced flagellate erythema: a case report and review of the literature. *Oncol Lett.* 2014;8(2):933-935. doi:10.3892/ol.2014.2179.

55. Yaris N, Çakir M, Kalyoncu M, Aysenur O. Bleomycin induced hyperpigmentation with yolk sac tumor. *Indian J Pediatr.* 2007;74(5):505-506. doi:10.1007/s12098-007-0089-8.

56. Silveira JCG, Da Cunha BM, Estrella RR. Bleomycin-induced flagellate dermatitis. *An Bras Dermatol.* 2006;81(1):83-85. doi:10.1055/s-2004-814507.

57. Khmamouche MR, Debbagh A, Mahfoud T, et al. Flagellate erythema secondary to bleomycin: a new case report and review of the literature. *J Drugs Dermatol.* 2014;13(8):983-984.

58. Brazzelli V, Grasso V, Borroni G. Imatinib, dasatinib and nilotinib: a review of adverse cutaneous reactions with emphasis on our clinical experience. *J Eur Acad Dermatol Venereol.* 2013;27(12):1471-1480. doi:10.1111/jdv.12172.

59. Arora B, Kumar L, Sharma A, Wadhwa J, Kochupillai V. Pigmentary changes in chronic myeloid leukemia patients treated with imatinib mesylate. *Ann Oncol.* 2004;15(2):358-359. doi:10.1093/annonc/mdh068.

60. Aleem A. Hypopigmentation of the skin due to imatinib mesylate in patients with chronic myeloid leukemia. *Hematol Oncol Stem Cell Ther.* 2009;2(2):358-361. doi:10.1016/S1658-3876(09)50026-X.

61. Dibek Misirlioglu E, Guvenir H, Bahceci S, et al. Severe cutaneous adverse drug reactions in pediatric patients: a multicenter study. *J Allergy Clin Immunol Pract.* 2017;5(3):757-763. doi:10.1016/j.jaip.2017.02.013.

62. Szatkowski J, Schwartz RA. Acute generalized exanthematous pustulosis (AGEP): a review and update. *J Am Acad Dermatol.* 2015;73(5):843-848. doi:10.1016/j.jaad.2015.07.017.

63. de Sousa AS, Lara OA, Papaiordanou F, Marchioro GS, Tebcherani AJ. Acute generalized exanthematous pustulosis x Von Zumbusch's pustular psoriasis: a diagnostic challenge in a psoriatic patient. *An Bras Dermatol.* 2015;90(4):557-560. doi:10.1590/abd1806-4841.20153256.

64. Ersoy S, Paller AS, Mancini AJ. Acute generalized exanthematous pustulosis in children. *Arch Dermatol*. 2004;140:1172-1173.

65. Poeschl MD, Hurley MY, Goyal SD, Vidal CI. Targetoid eruptions: answer. *Am J Dermatopathol*. 2014;36(10):838. doi:10.1097/DAD.0000000000000168.

66. Halevy S, Kardaun SH, Davidovici B, Wechsler J. The spectrum of histopathological features in acute generalized exanthematous pustulosis: a study of 102 cases. *Br J Dermatol*. 2010;163(6):1245-1252. doi:10.1111/j.1365-2133.2010.09967.x.

67. Vignesh P, Kishore J, Kumar A, et al. A young child with Eosinophilia, Rash, and multisystem illness: drug rash, eosinophilia, and systemic symptoms syndrome after receipt of fluoxetine. *Pediatr Dermatol*. 2017;34(3):e120-e125. doi:10.1111/pde.13131.

68. Newell BD, Moinfar M, Mancini AJ, Nopper AJ. Retrospective analysis of 32 pediatric patients with anticonvulsant hypersensitivity syndrome (ACHSS). *Pediatr Dermatol*. 2009;26(5):536-546. doi:10.1111/j.1525-1470.2009.00870.x.

69. Silva-Feistner M, Ortiz E, Rojas-Lechuga MJ, Muñoz D. Síndrome de sensibilidad a fármacos con eosinofilia y síntomas sistémicos en pediatría. Caso clínico. *Rev Chil Pediatr*. 2017;88(1):164-168. doi:10.1016/j.rchipe.2016.05.010.

70. Borroni G, Torti S, Pezzini C, et al. Histopathologic spectrum of Drug Reaction with Eosinophilia and Systemic Symptoms (DRESS): a diagnosis that needs clinico-pathological correlation. *G Ital Dermatol Venereol*. 2014;149(3):291-300.

71. Segal AR, Doherty KM, Leggott J, Zlotoff B. Cutaneous reactions to drugs in children. *Pediatrics*. 2007;120(4):e1082-e1096. doi:10.1542/peds.2005-2321.

72. Ortonne N, Valeyrie-Allanore L, Bastuji-Garin S, et al. Histopathology of drug rash with eosinophilia and systemic symptoms syndrome: a morphological and phenotypical study. *Br J Dermatol*. 2015;173(1):50-58. doi:10.1111/bjd.13683.

73. Schwartz RA, McDonough PH, Lee BW. Toxic epidermal necrolysis: Part II. Prognosis, sequelae, diagnosis, differential diagnosis, prevention, and treatment. *J Am Acad Dermatol*. 2013;69(2):187.e1-187.e16. doi:10.1016/j.jaad.2013.05.002.

74. Hsu DY, Brieva J, Silverberg NB, Paller AS, Silverberg JI. Pediatric Stevens-Johnson syndrome and toxic epidermal necrolysis in the United States. *J Am Acad Dermatol*. 2017;76(5):811-817.e4. doi:10.1016/j.jaad.2016.12.024.

75. Gerull R, Nelle M, Schaible T. Toxic epidermal necrolysis and Stevens-Johnson syndrome: A review. *Crit Care Med*. 2011;39(6):1521-1532. doi:10.1097/CCM.0b013e31821201ed.

76. Rizzo JA, Johnson R, Cartie RJ. Pediatric toxic epidermal necrolysis: experience of a tertiary burn center. *Pediatr Dermatol*. 2015;32(5):704-709. doi:10.1111/pde.12657.

77. Harris V, Jackson C, Cooper A. Review of toxic epidermal necrolysis. *Int J Mol Sci*. 2016;17(12):1-11. doi:10.3390/ijms17122135.

Index

Note: Page numbers followed by *f* and *t* indicates figures and tables respectively.

ss